The
CODER'S
HANDBOOK

2007

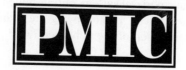

ISBN 1-57066-416-1

Practice Management Information Corporation
4727 Wilshire Boulevard
Los Angeles, California 90010
http://www.pmiconline.com

Printed in the United States of America

OTHER PMIC TITLES OF INTEREST

RISK MANAGEMENT TITLES
Malpractice Depositions
Medical Risk Management
Preparing for Your Deposition
Preventing Emergency Malpractice
Testifying in Court

FINANCIAL MANAGEMENT TITLES
A Physician's Guide to Financial Independence
Business Ventures for Physicians
Financial Valuation of Your Practice
Personal Money Management for Physicians
Personal Pension Plan Strategies for Physicians
Securing Your Assets

DICTIONARIES AND OTHER REFERENCE TITLES
Drugs of Abuse
Health and Medicine on the Internet
Medical Acronyms and Abbreviations
Medical Phrase Index
Medical Word Building
Medico Mnemonica
Medico-Legal Glossary
Spanish/English Handbook for Medical Professionals

MEDICAL REFERENCE AND CLINICAL TITLES
Advance Medical Directives
Clinical Research Opportunities
Gastroenterology: Problems in Primary Care
Manual of IV Therapy
Medical Care of the Adolescent Athlete
Medical Procedures for Referral
Neurology: Problems in Primary Care
Orthopaedics: Problems in Primary Care
Patient Care Emergency Handbook
Patient Care Flowchart Manual
Patient Care Procedures for Your Practice
Physician's Office Laboratory
Pulmonary Medicine: Problems in Primary Care
Questions and Answers on AIDS

OTHER PMIC TITLES OF INTEREST

CODING AND REIMBURSEMENT TITLES

Collections Made Easy!
CPT Coders Choice®, Thumb Indexed
CPT & HCPCS Coding Made Easy!
CPT Easy Links
CPT Plus!
DRG Plus!
E/M Coding Made Easy!
Getting Paid for What You Do
HCPCS Coders Choice®, Color Coded, Thumb Indexed
Health Insurance Carrier Directory
HIPAA Compliance Manual
ICD-9-CM, Coders Choice®, Thumb Indexed
ICD-9-CM Coding for Physicians' Offices
ICD-9-CM Coding Made Easy!
ICD-9-CM, Home Health Edition
Medical Fees in the United States
Medicare Compliance Manual
Medicare Rules & Regulations
Physicians Fee Guide
Reimbursement Manual for the Medical Office

PRACTICE MANAGEMENT TITLES

Accounts Receivable Management for the Medical Practice
Achieving Profitability With a Medical Office System
Encyclopedia of Practice and Financial Management
Managed Care Organizations
Managing Medical Office Personnel
Marketing Strategies for Physicians
Medical Marketing Handbook
Medical Office Policy Manual
Medical Practice Forms
Medical Practice Handbook
Medical Staff Privileges
Negotiating Managed Care Contracts
Patient Satisfaction
Performance Standards for the Laboratory
Professional and Practice Development
Promoting Your Medical Practice
Starting in Medical Practice
Working With Insurance and Managed Care Plans

**AVAILABLE FROM YOUR LOCAL MEDICAL
BOOK STORE OR CALL 1-800-MED-SHOP**

FOREWORD

The Coder's Handbook is a comprehensive coding, compliance and terminology reference designed for medical office, hospital, and health insurance company personnel involved in the coding and reimbursement process.

As experienced coders know, and beginning coders quickly learn, the CPT™, HCPCS and ICD-9-CM coding books by themselves do not have all the information needed to select and report CPT, HCPCS and ICD-9-CM codes for medical services and procedures. As a result, coders frequently have to research terminology, coding, and compliance questions and issues before selecting codes and completing health insurance claim forms...typically consulting several resources in the process.

The Coder's Handbook provides answers to the most common coding, compliance, coverage, reimbursement and terminology questions encountered by medical coding personnel. The reference begins with a list of over 8,000 medical abbreviations, acronyms and eponyms, includes sections covering CPT, HCPCS, and ICD-9-CM coding, beautiful anatomical illustrations, and completion of the CMS-1500 health insurance claim form, and ends with a listing of over 4,000 CPT codes with critical coverage and compliance information.

James B. Davis, Publisher

DISCLAIMER

This publication is designed to offer basic information regarding medical terminology, coding and billing of medical services, supplies and procedures using the CPT™, HCPCS, and ICD-9-CM coding systems, and selected information regarding Medicare coverage and compliance issues. The information presented is based on a thorough analysis of the CPT, HCPCS and ICD-9-CM coding systems, information obtained from official U.S. government resources, and the experience and interpretations of the author. Though all of the information has been carefully researched and checked for accuracy and completeness, neither the author nor the publisher accept any responsibility or liability with regard to errors, omissions, misuse or misinterpretation.

CONTENTS

INTRODUCTION

Coding and medical terminology is the *language* of medical billing and reimbursement. Fluency in this language is required for all medical personnel involved in the processes of billing for medical services, chart abstracting, coding, medical transcription, and reimbursement management.

If the medical practice insurance billing staff is not fluent in this language, the practice will not receive the reimbursement it deserves and audit liability will increase. If hospital coders and patient accounting personnel are not fluent in this language, the hospital will not be paid properly and likewise may find itself with higher audit liability. If health insurance company claims processing personnel are not fluent in this language, claims processing errors may be made which result in improper denial or low payment of claims, or improper payment or overpayment of claims.

To a beginning coder, the coding and reimbursement process may appear at first to be simple and easy. Just find out what the doctor did for the patient, take a CPT book, look up the procedure and get the CPT code. Then find out what the doctor's diagnosis is, take an ICD-9-CM book, look up the diagnosis and get the ICD-9-CM code. Type everything on the HCFA1500 health insurance claim form . . . mail it in . . .and get paid. What could be easier than that?

Experienced coders know that the process of selecting the correct CPT, HCPCS and ICD-9-CM codes to report medical services and procedures is actually very complicated and complex. Not only do you have to select the correct CPT and ICD-9-CM codes, you have to know: 1) how to interpret, decipher, and transfer medical acronyms, eponyms and abbreviations, 2) when to use HCPCS procedure codes instead of CPT procedure codes, 3) how to sequence multiple procedure codes properly, 4) when to use CPT or HCPCS modifiers, 5) how to sequence multiple ICD-9-CM diagnosis codes, 5) when a medical report is required to support your procedures, 6) if a procedure is covered by Medicare, 7) if there are special billing rules or payment policies for Medicare, and a variety of other rules, regulations, policies and procedures.

The Coder's Handbook is designed to answer the most common coding, compliance, coverage, reimbursement and terminology questions encountered by medical coding personnel involved in the coding and reimbursement process. The book is divided into four comprehensive sections.

MEDICAL ACRONYMS, EPONYMS AND ABBREVIATIONS

This section includes over 8,000 medical acronyms, abbreviations and eponyms with definitions. The language or nomenclature of medicine, with its heavy emphasis on Latin and Greek etymology, is further complicated by the proliferation of medical acronyms, eponyms and abbreviations. These were originally designed to 1) reduce the amount of writing by doctors when writing orders or making medical record entries, 2) facilitate the abstracting of medical records, particularly for tests and medications, and 3) to simplify and standardize the communication process among medical personnel.

Medical nomenclature is an evolving language. New words, phrases, acronyms, eponyms, and abbreviations appear frequently as diseases and illnesses are discovered or understood more clearly, new diagnostic and operative procedures are developed, and new technology is implemented. While the fundamentals of the nomenclature are easy after the basics have been mastered, the constant additions requires regular review and updates of medical terminology resources.

CPT AND HCPCS CODING

Selection of the proper CPT and/or HCPCS procedure codes has a tremendous impact on reimbursement for the medical practice. In addition, proper reporting of CPT and/or HCPCS codes helps to protect your medical practice in the event of an audit by Medicare or other health insurance carriers.

The CPT coding system provides a uniform coding language that accurately describes medical, surgical and diagnostic procedures and services, and to provide an effective means for reliable communication among physicians, hospitals, and health insurance companies. Likewise, the HCPCS Level II coding system provides a uniform coding language for reporting durable medical equipment, orthotics, prosthetics, supplies, materials and injections to the Medicare program. HCPCS Level II also includes codes for procedures and services which are not included in the CPT coding system. Codes from either system may be reported independently or together, depending upon the status of the patient.

This section includes a comprehensive tutorial covering CPT and HCPCS procedure coding. The section covers CPT and HCPCS procedure coding basics, common coding and billing issues, coding of evaluation and management services, and coding of surgery, radiology, laboratory and medicine services. In addition, the section includes 24 large size, full-color anatomical illustrations with CPT cross-references.

ICD-9-CM CODING

Selection of the proper ICD-9-CM diagnosis codes also has a tremendous impact on reimbursement for the medical practice. Likewise, the proper reporting of ICD-9-CM codes helps to protect your medical practice in the event of an audit by Medicare or other health insurance carriers.

This section includes a comprehensive tutorial covering ICD-9-CM diagnosis coding. The section covers ICD-9-CM diagnosis coding basics, special Medicare requirements for diagnosis coding, diagnosis coding and billing issues, combination coding, coding suspected conditions, specialty coding, coding manifestations, and the use of V-codes and E-codes. In addition, the section includes 24 large size, full-color anatomical illustrations with ICD-9-CM cross-references.

COVERAGE AND COMPLIANCE

Knowing and understanding the various policies, procedures, rules, restrictions, limitations, and opportunities involved in reporting CPT codes for medical services and procedures can have a significant impact on your reimbursement and your audit liability. However, with over 7,000 CPT codes and over 2,000 HCPCS Level II codes, it is virtually impossible for anyone to know all the rules for each and every code. In addition, the rules for Medicare may be different than for other health insurance plans, and the rules change frequently.

This section includes over 4,000 CPT codes with guidelines designed to help you answer important coding and compliance questions about specific CPT codes. The CPT codes listed in this section include short and simple descriptions plus annotations regarding follow-up periods, assistant surgery, billing supply charges, and add-on procedures.

TERMINOLOGY

Understanding the coding and compliance process requires a fundamental working knowledge of the words and acronyms used by medical professionals, government agencies and health insurance carriers to describe services, benefits and reimbursement policies. While many publications place the terminology section in an appendix at the back of the book, we feel that you should have an opportunity to review and learn the terminology before you encounter it within the text itself. Following is a comprehensive list of billing, coding, compliance, HIPAA and reimbursement words, terms and acronyms, including some that may not appear in the text of the book.

AAPCC: Average adjusted per capita cost

ABA: American Bar Association

Ability to add attributes: One possible capability of a digital signature technology, for example, the ability to add a time stamp as part of a digital signature.

Abstract: The collection of information from the medical record via hard copy or electronic instrument.

Abuse: A range of the following improper behaviors or billing practices including, but not limited to: billing for a non-covered service; misusing codes on the claim (i.e., the way the service is coded on the claim does not comply with national or local coding guidelines or is not billed as rendered); or inappropriately allocating costs on a cost report.

Access: The ability to obtain needed medical care.

Access: The ability or the means necessary to read, write, modify, or communicate data/information or otherwise make use of any system resource (HIPAA).

Access authorization: Information-use policies/procedures that establish the rules for granting and/or restricting access to a user, terminal, transaction, program, or process.

Access control: A method of restricting access to resources, allowing only privileged entities access. (PGP, Inc.) Types of access control include, among others, mandatory access control, discretionary access control, time-of-day, classification, and subject-object separation.

Access controls: The protection of sensitive communications transmissions over open or private networks so that it cannot be easily intercepted and interpreted by parties other than the intended recipient.

Access establishment: The security policies, and the rules established therein, that determine an entity's initial right of access to a terminal, transaction, program, or process.

Access level: A level associated with an individual who may be accessing information (for example, a clearance level) or with the information which may be accessed (for example, a classification level).

Access modification: The security policies, and the rules established therein, that determine types of, and reasons for, modification to an entity's established right of access to a terminal, transaction, program, or process.

Accident and health insurance: Health insurance under which benefits are payable in case of disease, accidental injury or accidental death.

Accountability: The property that ensures that the actions of an entity can be traced uniquely to that entity.

Accreditation: An evaluative process in which a healthcare organization undergoes an examination of its policies, procedures, and performance by an external organization ("accrediting body") to ensure that it is meeting predetermined criteria. It usually involves both on- and off-site surveys.

Accreditation cycle for M+C deeming: The duration of CMS's recognition of the validity of an accrediting organization's determination that a Medicare+Choice Organization (M+C organization) is "fully accredited."

Accreditation for deeming: Some states use the findings of private accreditation organizations, in part or in whole, to supplement or substitute for state oversight of some quality related standards. This is referred to as "deemed compliance" with a standard. Accreditation for Participation state requirement that plans must be accredited to participate in the Medicaid managed care program.

Act: The Social Security Act. Titles referred to are titles of that Act.

Actual charge: One of the factors determining a physician's payment for a service under Medicare; equivalent to the billed or submitted charge. See Customary, Prevailing and Reasonable.

Actuarial balance: The difference between the summarized income rate and the summarized cost rate over a given valuation period.

Actuarial deficit: A negative actuarial balance.

Actuarial rates: One half of the expected monthly cost of the SMI program for each aged enrollee (for the aged actuarial rate) and one half of the expected monthly cost for each disabled enrollee (for the disabled actuarial rate) for the duration the rate is in effect.

Actuarial soundness: A measure of the adequacy of Hospital Insurance (HI) and Supplementary Medical Insurance (SMI) financing as determined by the difference between trust fund assets and liabilities for specified periods.

Actuarial status: A measure of the adequacy of the financing as determined by the difference between assets and liabilities at the end of the periods for which financing was established.

Acute: Refers to the condition that is the primary reason for the current encounter.

ADA: American Dental Association

Addenda: Official updates to ICD-9-CM published continuously since 1986 that become effective on October 1st of each year.

Adjusted average per capita cost (AAPCC): An estimate of the average per capita cost incurred by Medicare per beneficiary in the fee-for-service system, adjusted by county for age, sex, and program entitlement.

Adjusted historical payment basis (AHPB): The average historical payment in a specific locality for a specific service.

Administrative agent: See Carrier.

Administrative costs: A general term that refers to Medicare and Medicaid administrative costs, as well as CMS administrative costs.

Administrative data: Information that is collected, processed, and stored in automated information systems. Administrative data include enrollment or eligibility information, claims information, and managed care encounters. The claims and encounters may be for hospital and other facility services, professional services, prescription drug services, laboratory services, or other services.

Administrative expenses: Expenses incurred by the Department of Health and Human Services and the Department of the Treasury in administering the SMI program and the provisions of the Internal Revenue Code relating to the collection of contributions.

Administrative procedures to guard data integrity, confidentiality and availability: Documented, formal practices to manage (1) the selection and execution of security measures to protect data, and (2) the conduct of personnel in relation to the protection of data.

Administrator: The Administrator of the Center for Medicare and Medicaid Services (CMS).

Admission date: The date the patient was admitted for inpatient care, outpatient service, or start of care. For an admission notice for hospice care, enter the effective date of election of hospice benefits.

Admitting diagnosis code: Code indicating patient's diagnosis at admission.

Adult living care facility: To be used when billing services rendered at a residential care facility that houses beneficiaries who cannot live alone but who do not need around-the-clock skilled medical services. The facility services do not include a medical component.

Adverse: Any response to a drug that is noxious and unintended and occurs with proper dosage.

Adverse selection: A health plan with a disproportionate percentage of enrollees who are more likely to file claims and use services because of existing health risk conditions.

Advisory Council on Social Security: Prior to the enactment of the Social Security Independence and Program Improvements Act of 1994 (Public Law 103-296) on August 15, 1994, the Social Security Act required the appointment of an Advisory Council every 4 years to study and review the financial status of the OASDI and Medicare programs.

AFDC: Aid to Families with Dependent Children

Aftercare: An encounter for something planned in advance, for example, cast removal.

Age/Sex rating: A method of structuring capitation payments based on enrollee/membership age and sex.

Aged enrollee: An individual aged 65 or over, who is enrolled in the SMI program.

AHFS: American Hospital Formulary Service.

AHPB: Adjusted Historical Payment Basis

Algorithm: A rule or procedure containing conditional logic for solving a problem or accomplishing a task.

Alliance: A regional health insurance purchasing entity specified in the Clinton administration's health system reform proposal that would enroll individuals, collect premiums, purchase enrollee's health insurance from participating health plans, and enforce the rules that manage health plan competition.

Allowed charge (approved charge): Payment for a physician service under the customary, prevailing and reasonable system; includes the payment from Medicare and the beneficiary's coinsurance, but not any balance bill. See Balance Bill; Coinsurance; Customary, Prevailing and Reasonable.

Alphabetic index: The portion of ICD-9-CM that lists definitions and code sets in alphabetic order. Also referred to as Volume 2.

Alternative Delivery System (ADS): A system of delivering healthcare benefits that is different from traditional indemnity systems. An HMO is an example of an ADS.

Ambulance (air or water): An air or water vehicle specifically designed, equipped, and staffed for life saving and transporting the sick or injured.

Ambulance (land): A land vehicle specifically designed, equipped, and staffed for life saving and transporting the sick or injured.

Ambulatory Surgical Center (ASC): A freestanding facility, other than a physician's office, where surgical and diagnostic services are provided on an ambulatory basis.

Amortization: Process of the gradual retirement of an outstanding debt by making periodic payments to the trust fund.

Anniversary: The beginning of a benefit year for a subscriber group.

Annual deductible: See Deductible.

ANSI: American National Standards Institute

Appeal: A process whereby the provider and/or beneficiary (or representative) exercises the right to request a review of a contractor determination to deny Medicare coverage or payment for a service in full or in part.

Approved charge: See Allowed Charge or Reasonable Charge.

Assets: Treasury notes and bonds guaranteed by the federal government, and cash held by the trust funds for investment purposes.

Assignment [Medicare]: The term used to refer to a physician's decision to accept Medicare's allowed charge as payment in full; a guarantee not to balance bill. See Balance Bill/Extra Bill, Nonparticipating Physician, Participating Physician and Supplier Program.

Assignment of benefits: A procedure whereby the subscriber authorizes the carrier to make payment of allowable benefits directly to the provider.

Assistant-at-surgery: An individual who actively assists in performing a surgery.

Attachment(s): Information, hard copy or electronic, related to a particular claim. Attachments may be structured (such as Certificates of Medical Necessity) or non-structured (such as an Operative Report). Though attachments may be submitted separately, it is common to say the attachment was "submitted with the claim."

Attending physician: Number of the licensed physician who would normally be expected to certify and recertify the medical necessity of the number of services rendered and/or who has primary responsibility for the patient's medical care and treatment.

Audit controls: The mechanisms employed to record and examine system activity.

Authoritative approval: Method or type of approval that requires a determination that the service is likely to have a diagnostic or therapeutic benefit for the patient for whom it is intended.

Authorization control: The mechanism for obtaining consent for the use and disclosure of health information.

Automated claim review: Claim review and determination made using system logic (edits). Automated claim reviews never require the intervention of a human to make a claim determination.

Automatic logoff: After a pre-determined time of inactivity (for example, 15 minutes), an electronic session is terminated.

Availability: The property of being accessible and usable upon demand by an authorized entity.

Average market yield: A computation that is made on all marketable interest-bearing obligations of the United States. It is computed on the basis of market quotations as of the end of the calendar month immediately preceding the date of such issue.

Balance bill/extra bill: Physician's charges exceeding the Medicare allowed charge.

Balance billing: Billing the beneficiary for any fee in excess of that allowed by the health insurance carrier.

Basic Health Services: Benefits defined under Subpart A, Section 100.102 of the Federal HMO Regulations that must be offered by all federally qualified HMOs.

Beneficiary: A person eligible to receive benefits under a health care plan. Under Part B of Medicare, Americans over 65, many disabled individuals, and certain individuals with end-stage renal disease can become beneficiaries by paying a monthly premium.

Beneficiary survey: A 1988 survey of a national sample of beneficiaries regarding assignment, participation, balance billing, and understanding of the Medicare program. The survey was sponsored by PPRC and conducted by Mathematical Policy Research.

Benefit package: Services covered by a health insurance plan and the financial terms of such coverage, including cost sharing and limitations on amounts of services.

Benefit payments: The amounts disbursed for covered services to beneficiaries after the deductible and coinsurance amounts have been deducted.

Benefit period: An alternate name for "spell of illness."

Blue Cross: Nonprofit, community service organizations, providing in-hospital health care services to their subscribers. Some Blue Cross plans have converted to for-profit status recently.

Blue Shield: Nonprofit voluntary organization which provides subscribers with coverage for expenses (other than hospital costs). May also serve as the carrier for programs like Medicare.

BMAD: Part B Medicare Annual Data Files

Bonus: Means a payment a physician or entity receives beyond any salary, fee-for-service payments, capitation or returned withhold. Bonuses and other compensation that are not based on referral or utilization levels (such as bonuses based solely on quality of care, patient satisfaction or physician participation on a committee) are not considered in the calculation of substantial financial risk.

Bonus payment: An additional amount paid by Medicare for services provided by physicians in Health Professional Shortage Areas (HPSAs).

Budget Neutrality: For the Medicare program, adjustment of payment rates when policies change so that total spending under the new rules is expected to be the same as it would have been under the previous payment rules.

Bundling: The use of a single payment for a group of related procedures or services.

Capitation: A set dollar payment per patient per unit of time (usually per month) that is paid to cover a specified set of services and administrative costs without regard to the actual number of services provided. The services covered may include a physician's own services, referral services or all medical services. The set dollar payment may be a percent of the premium that the managed care organization collects for a beneficiary; the capitation received from CMS would be considered a premium for this purpose.

Carrier: The health insurance company which writes and administers the health insurance policy.

Carrier (Medicare): A private contractor who administers claims for Part B Medicare services.

Case management: Monitoring and coordinating the delivery of health services for individual patients to enhance care and manage costs. Often used for patients with specific diagnoses or who require high-cost or extensive health care services.

Case mix: Is the distribution of patients into categories reflecting differences in severity of illness or resource consumption.

Case mix index: The average DRG relative weight for all Medicare admissions.

Cash basis: The costs of the service when payment was made rather than when the service was performed.

Cash indemnity benefits: Payments to subscribers for covered services that require submission of an health insurance claim. Subscribers may assign such payments directly to providers.

Category: Refers to diagnoses codes listed within a specific three-digit category, for example category 250, Diabetes Mellitus.

Cause: That which brings about any condition or produces an effect.

CBS: Current Beneficiary Survey

Center for Medicare and Medicaid Services: Formerly known as HCFA (Health Care Financing Administration), this branch of the Department of Health and Human Services oversees the Medicare and Medicaid programs.

Certification: The technical evaluation performed as part of, and in support of, the accreditation process that establishes the extent to which a particular computer system or network design and implementation meet a pre-specified set of security requirements. This evaluation may be performed internally or by an external accrediting agency.

CF: Conversion Factor

Chain of trust partner agreement: Contract entered into by two business partners in which it is agreed to exchange data and that the first party will transmit information to the second party, where the data transmitted is agreed to be protected between the partners. The sender and receiver depend upon each other to maintain the integrity and confidentiality of the transmitted information. Multiple such two-party contracts may be involved in moving information from the originator to the ultimate recipient.

CHAMPUS [Civilian Health and Medical Program of the Uniformed Services]: A federally funded comprehensive health benefits program designed to provide eligible beneficiaries a supplement to medical care in military and Public Health Service facilities.

Charge reduction (Medicare): The percentage difference between a provider's billed charge and the Medicare allowed charge.

Chronic: An illness or condition continuing over a long period of time or recurring frequently.

Claim: A demand to the carrier, by the insured person, for payment of benefits under a policy.

Claim form: A form used to present claim information in an organized manner to the carrier. See CMS1500.

Claims examiner: The carrier's employee who is responsible for handling claims as they are received from patients and medical offices.

Classification: Protection of data from unauthorized access by the designation of multiple levels of access authorization clearances to be required for access, dependent upon the sensitivity of the information.

Clearing house: A public or private entity that processes or facilitates the processing of nonstandard data elements of health information into standard data elements.

Clinic-without-walls: A practice setting designed to preserve physician autonomy/independence while taking advantage of the benefits inherent in a large group practice. Results when several independent practices combine into one corporate entity.

Clinical Performance Measure (CPM): This is a method or instrument to estimate or monitor the extent to which the actions of a health care practitioner or provider conform to practice guidelines, medical review criteria, or standards of quality.

CMP: Competitive Medical Plan

CMS: Center for Medicare and Medicaid Services

CMS1500: (Formerly referred to as HCFA1500) A universal health insurance claim form that is mandated for Medicare billing and generally accepted by all health insurance carriers.

CMS agent: Any individual or organization, public or private, with whom CMS has a contractual arrangement to contribute to or participate in the Medicare survey and certification process.

CMS directed improvement process: A CMS directed improvement project is any project where CMS specifies the subject, size, pace, data source, analytic techniques, educational intervention techniques, or impact measurement model. These projects may be developed by CMS in consultation with Networks, the health care community, and other interested people.

COB: See Coordination of benefits

COBRA: Consolidated Omnibus Budget Reconciliation Act of 1985. P.L. 99-272, enacted April 1986

Code set: Code Set means any set of codes used for encoding data elements, such as tables of terms, medical concepts, medical diagnostic codes, or medical procedure codes.

Coding: A mechanism for identifying and defining medical services, procedures, illnesses, injuries, signs, symptoms, ill-defined conditions, drugs and supplies.

Coinsurance: A provision of a plan by which the beneficiary shares in the cost of certain covered expenses on a percentage basis. Also known as copayment.

Combination: An ICD-9-CM code that combines a diagnosis with an associated secondary process or combination.

Commercial MCO: A Commercial MCO is a health maintenance organization, an eligible organization with a contract under 11876 or a Medicare-Choice organization; a provider sponsored organization, or any other private or public organization, which meets the requirements of 11902(w). These MCOs provide comprehensive services to commercial and/or Medicare enrollees, as well as Medicaid enrollees.

Common working file (CWF): A new CMS data reporting system which will combine Part A and Part B claims in a common file.

Community Mental Health Center (CMHC): A facility that provides the following services: Outpatient services, including specialized outpatient services for children, the elderly, individuals who are chronically ill, and residents of the CMHC's mental health services area who have been discharged from inpatient treatment at a mental health facility.

Community Rating: A method for establishing health insurance premiums whereby an insurer's premium is the same for all individuals in a premium class with a specific geographic area.

Community Rating Area (CRA): Under community rating, a defined geographic area for which each insurer must establish a single set of health insurance premiums.

Competitive medical plan (CMP): A health plan that is eligible under TEFRA 1982 to enter into a Medicare risk contract in return for a capitation payment, but which does not satisfy the requirements to be a federally qualified HMO. See Capitation, Federally Qualified HMO.

Complaint (of fraud or abuse): A statement, oral or written, alleging that a provider or beneficiary received a Medicare benefit of monetary value, directly or indirectly, overtly or covertly, in cash or in kind, to which he or she is not entitled under current Medicare law, regulations, or policy. Included are allegations of misrepresentation and violations of Medicare requirements applicable to persons or entities that bill for covered items and services.

Complication: The occurrence of two or more diseases in the same patient at the same time.

Comprehensive inpatient rehabilitation facility: A facility that provides comprehensive rehabilitation services under the supervision of a physician to inpatients with physical disabilities. Services include physical therapy, occupational therapy, speech pathology, social or psychological services, and orthotics and prosthetics services.

Comprehensive MCO (Comp-MCO): A MCO is a health maintenance organization, an eligible organization with a contract under 11876 or a Medicare-Choice organization; a provider sponsored organization or any other private or public organization, which meets the requirements of 11902(w). These MCOs provides comprehensive services to both commercial and/or Medicare, as well as Medicaid enrollees.

Comprehensive medical insurance: A policy designed to give the protection offered by both a basic and a major medical health insurance policy.

Comprehensive Outpatient Rehabilitation Facility (CORF): A facility that provides comprehensive rehabilitation services under the supervision of a physician to outpatients with physical disabilities. Services include physical therapy, occupational therapy, and speech pathology services.

Concurrent: When a patient is being treated by more than one provider for different care conditions at the same time.

Confidentiality: The property that information is not made available or disclosed to unauthorized individuals, entities or processes.

Consent and Authorization (Basic Rule): A covered entity may use or disclose PHI only: with the consent of the individual for treatment, payment, or health care operations with the authorization of the individual for all other uses or disclosures as permitted under this rule for certain public policy purposes.

Consumer Price Index (CPI): A measure of the average change in prices over time in a fixed group of goods and services.

Consumer self-report data: Data collected through survey or focus group. Surveys may include Medicaid beneficiaries currently or previously enrolled in a MCO or PHP. The survey may be conducted by the state or a contractor to the state.

Consumer survey data: Data collected through a survey of those Medicaid beneficiaries who are enrolled in the program and have used the services. The survey may be conducted by the state or by the managed care entity (if the managed care entity reports the results to the state).

Context-based access: An access control based on the context of a transaction (as opposed to being based on attributes of the initiator or target). The "external" factors might include time of day, location of the user, strength of user authentication, etc.

Contingency: Funds included in the trust fund to serve as a cushion in case actual expenditures are higher than those projected at the time financing was established. Since the financing is set prospectively, actual experience may be different from the estimates used in setting the financing.

Contingency margin: An amount included in the actuarial rates to provide for changes in the contingency level in the trust fund. Positive margins increase the contingency level, and negative margins decrease it.

Contingency plan: A plan for responding to a system emergency. The plan includes performing backups, preparing critical facilities that can be used to facilitate continuity of operations in the event of an emergency, and recovering from a disaster.

Continuity of signature capability: The public verification of a signature shall not compromise the ability of the signer to apply additional secure signatures at a later date.

Continuous Ambulatory Peritoneal Dialysis (CAPD): A type of dialysis where the patient's peritoneal membrane is used as the dialyzer. The patient dialyzes at home, using special supplies, but without the need for a machine. See peritoneal dialysis.

Continuous Cycling Peritoneal Dialysis (CCPD): A type of dialysis where the patient generally dialyzes at home and utilizes an automated peritoneal cycler for delivering dialysis exchanges. See peritoneal dialysis.

Continuous Quality Improvement (CQI): A process, which continually monitors program performance. When a quality problem is identified, CQI develops a revised approach to that problem and monitors implementation and success of the revised approach. The process includes involvement at all stages by all organizations, which are affected by the problem and/or involved in implementing the revised approach.

Contractor policy: Policy developed by CMS contractors (PSC, AC, FI, or carrier) and used to make coverage and coding determinations. It is developed when there is an absence of national coverage policy for a service or all of the uses of a service, there is a need to interpret national coverage policy, or local coding rules are needed.

Conventions: Refers to the use of certain abbreviations, punctuation, symbols, type faces, and other instructions that must be clearly understood in order to use ICD-9-CM.

Conversion factor (CF): A dollar value, specific to the four general categories of service: medical, surgical, lab and radiology, that is used with a relative value scale to calculate fees for services and procedures.

Conversion factor update: Annual percentage change in each Medicare Fee Schedule conversion factor, established by the Congress or the default formula under Volume Performance Standards.

Conversion privilege: The right of an individual insured under a group plan to convert to an individual plan if the individual leaves the group.

Coordinated care plan: A plan that includes a CMS-approved network of providers that are under contract or arrangement with the M+C organization to deliver the benefit package approved by CMS. Coordinated care plans include plans offered by health maintenance organizations (HMOs), provider-sponsored organizations (PSOs), preferred provider organizations (PPOs), as well as other types of network plans (except network MSA plans).

Coordination of benefits: A program that determines which plan or insurance policy will pay first if two health plans or insurance policies cover the same benefits. If one of the plans is a Medicare health plan, Federal law may decide who pays first.

Copayment: See Coinsurance.

Cost-Based Health Maintenance Organization (HMO/Competitive Medical Plan, CMP): A type of managed care organization that will pay for all of the enrollees/members' medical care costs in return for a monthly premium, plus any applicable deductible or co-payment.

Cost of practice index (Medicare): A measurement of the differences across geographic areas of the cost of operating a medical practice.

Cost rate: The ratio of the cost (or outgo, expenditures, or disbursements) of the program on an incurred basis during a given year to the taxable payroll for the year. In this context, the outgo is defined to exclude benefit payments and administrative costs for those uninsured persons for whom payments are reimbursed from the general fund of the Treasury, and for voluntary enrollees who pay a premium to be enrolled.

Cost report: The report required from providers on an annual basis in order to make a proper determination of amounts payable under the Medicare program.

Cost sharing: The portion of payment for health expenses that the beneficiary must pay, including the deductibles, copayments, coinsurance, and extra bill.

Cost shifting: A situation wherein a healthcare provider compensates for the effect of lower revenue from one payer by increasing charges to another payer.

Counter signatures: It shall be possible to prove the order of application of signatures. This is analogous to the normal business practice of countersignatures, where some party signs a document which has already been signed by another party.

Coverage decision: A decision by a health plan or insurer whether to pay for or provide a medical service or technology for particular clinical indications.

Covered earnings: Earnings in employment covered by the HI program.

Covered employment: All employment and self-employment creditable for Social Security purposes. Almost every kind of employment and self-employment is covered under the program.

Covered services: Services for which SMI pays, as defined and limited by statute. Covered services include most physician services, care in outpatient departments of hospitals, diagnostic tests, DME, ambulance services, and other health services that are not covered by the HI program.

Covered worker: A person who has earnings creditable for Social Security purposes on the basis of services for wages in covered employment and/or on the basis of income from covered self-employment. The number of HI covered workers is slightly larger than the number of OASDI covered workers because of different coverage status for federal employment.

CPR: Customary, Prevailing and Reasonable

CPRI: Computer-based Patient Record Institute

CPT [Current procedural terminology]: A system of procedure codes and descriptions published annually by the American Medical Association. This procedure coding system is accepted by virtually all commercial health insurance carriers and is required by Medicare and Medicaid.

Credentialing: The process by which a managed care organization deems a physician competent to provide medical services to plan members.

Criteria: The expected levels of achievement or specifications against which performance can be assessed.

Cross-over patient: A patient who has both Medicare and Medicaid coverage.

Current procedural terminology: See CPT.

Custodial care facility: A facility, which provides room, board, and other personal assistance services, generally on a long-term basis and which does not include a medical component.

Customary charge: The provider's standard charge for a given service. Typically calculated by health insurance carriers as the provider's median charge for the service over a prior 12 month period.

Customary, prevailing and reasonable (Medicare): Current method of payment for physician services by Medicare. Payment for service is limited to the lowest of 1) the billed charge, 2) the customary charge, or 3) the prevailing charge in the community.

CWF: Common Working File

Data: A sequence of symbols to which meaning may be assigned.

Data authentication: The corroboration that data has not been altered or destroyed in an unauthorized manner. Examples of how data corroboration may be assured include the use of a check sum, double keying, a message authentication code, or digital signature.

Data backup: A retrievable, exact copy of information.

Data backup plan: A documented and routinely updated plan to create and maintain, for a specific period of time, retrievable exact copies of information.

Data integrity: The property that data has not been altered or destroyed in an unauthorized manner.

Data storage: The retention of health care information pertaining to an individual in an electronic format.

Date of filing and date of submission: The day of the mailing (as evidenced by the postmark) or hand-delivery of materials, unless otherwise defined.

Date of receipt: The date on the return receipt of "return receipt requested" mail, unless otherwise defined.

DEA: Data Encryption Algorithm

Deductible: A stipulated amount which the covered person must pay toward the cost of medical treatment before the benefits of the program go into effect.

Deductible carryover: A feature whereby covered charges in the last three months of the year may be carried over to be counted toward the next year's deductible.

Deemed status: Designation that an M+C organization has been reviewed and determined "fully accredited" by a CMS-approved accrediting organization for those standards within the deeming categories that the accrediting organization has the authority to deem.

Deemed wage credit: See Non-contributory or deemed wage credits.

Deeming authority: The authority granted by CMS to accrediting organizations to determine, on CMS's behalf, whether a M+C organization evaluated by the accrediting organization is in compliance with corresponding Medicare regulations.

DEFRA: Deficit Reduction Act of 1984. P.L. 98-369, enacted July 1984.

Demographic assumptions: See Assumptions.

Demographic data: Data that describe the characteristics of enrollee populations within a managed care entity. Demographic data include but are not limited to age, sex, race/ethnicity, and primary language.

Demonstrations: Projects and contracts that CMS has signed with various health care organizations. These contracts allow CMS to test various or specific attributes such as payment methodologies, preventive care, social care, etc., and to determine if such projects/pilots should be continued or expanded to meet the health care needs of the Nation. Demonstrations are used to evaluate the effects and impact of various health care initiatives and the cost implications to the public.

Department of Health and Human Services (DHHS): DHHS administers many of the "social" programs at the Federal level dealing with the health and welfare of the citizens of the United States. (It is the "parent" of CMS.)

Department, The: The Department of Health and Human Services.

Dependents: The spouse and children of the insured as defined in the health insurance contract.

Determination: A decision made to either pay in full, pay in part, or deny a claim. See also Initial Claim Determination.

Diagnosis: A written description of the reason(s) for the procedure, service, supply or encounter.

Diagnosis code: The first of these codes is the ICD-9-CM diagnosis code describing the principal diagnosis (for example, the condition established after study to be chiefly responsible for causing this hospitalization). The remaining codes are the ICD-9-CM diagnosis codes corresponding to additional conditions that coexisted at the time of admission, or developed subsequently, and which had an effect on the treatment received or the length of stay.

Diagnosis-related groups (DRGs): A classification system that groups patients according to diagnosis, type of treatment, age, and other relevant criteria. Under the prospective payment system, hospitals are paid a set fee for treating patients in a single DRG category, regardless of the actual cost of care for the individual.

Dialysate: Dialysate or the dialysate fluid is the solution used in dialysis to remove excess fluids and waste products from the blood.

Dialysis: A process by which dissolved substances are removed from a patient's body by diffusion from one fluid compartment to another across a semi-permeable membrane. The two types of dialysis that are currently commonly in use are hemodialysis and peritoneal dialysis.

Dialysis center (renal): A hospital unit that is approved to furnish the full spectrum of diagnostic, therapeutic, and rehabilitative services required for the care of the ESRD dialysis patients (including inpatient dialysis) furnished directly or under arrangement.

Dialysis facility (renal): A unit (hospital based or freestanding) which is approved to furnish dialysis services directly to ESRD patients.

Dialysis station: A portion of the dialysis patient treatment area, which accommodates the equipment necessary to provide a hemodialysis or peritoneal dialysis treatment. This station must have sufficient area to house a chair or bed, the dialysis equipment, and emergency equipment if needed. Provision for privacy is ordinarily supplied by drapes or screens.

Digital signature: An electronic signature based upon cryptographic methods of originator authentication, computed by using a set of rules and a set of parameters such that the identity of the signer and the integrity of the data can be verified.

Direct costs: The labor, supply and equipment costs directly attributable to the provision of a specific service.

Disability: For Social Security purposes, the inability to engage in substantial gainful activity by reason of any medically determinable physical or mental impairment that can be expected to result in death or to last for a continuous period of not less than 12 months. Special rules apply for workers aged 55 or older whose disability is based on blindness. The law generally requires that a person be disabled continuously for 5 months before he or she can qualify for a disabled worker cash benefit. An additional 24 months is necessary to qualify under Medicare.

Disability income insurance: A form of health insurance that provides periodic payments to replace income when the insured is unable to work as a result of illness, injury or disease.

Disabled enrollee: An individual under age 65 who has been entitled to disability benefits under Title II of the Social Security Act or the Railroad Retirement system for at least 2 years and who is enrolled in the SMI program.

Disaster recovery: The process whereby an enterprise would restore any loss of data in the event of fire, vandalism, natural disaster, or system failure.

Disaster recovery plan: Part of an overall contingency plan. The plan for a process whereby an enterprise would restore any loss of data in the event of fire, vandalism, natural disaster, or system failure.

Discretionary access control: Discretionary Access Control (DAC) is used to control access by restricting a subject's access to an object. It is generally used to limit a user's access to a file. In this type of access control it is the owner of the file who controls other users' accesses to the file.

Discretionary spending: Outlays of funds subject to the Federal appropriations process.

Disposal: The final disposition of electronic data, and/or the hardware on which electronic data is stored.

Disproportionate Share Hospital (DSH): A hospital with a disproportionately large share of low-income patients. Under Medicaid, states augment payment to these hospitals. Medicare inpatient hospital payments are also adjusted for this added burden.

DMERC: Four contracted regional carriers which process Medicare claims for DME, orthotics, prosthetics and supplies. Providers are required to obtain supplier numbers and disclose ownership prior to submitting claims.

Documentation: Written security plans, rules, procedures, and instructions concerning all components of an entity's security.

Down coding: A process used by health insurance carriers to reduce the value of billed procedures by changing the codes submitted to ones of lower value. Procedure code and procedure description mismatch, and diagnosis code not supporting the level of care are the two most common opportunities for health insurance carrier down-coding.

DRG: Diagnosis Related Groups

DRG Coding: The DRG categories used by hospitals on discharge billing. See also Diagnosis-related groups (DRGs).

Dual choice: A health benefit offered by an employer which permits eligible employees a choice of health plans.

Dual eligibles: Medicare beneficiaries who also receive the full range of Medicaid benefits offered in their state.

Durable Medical Equipment (DME): Purchased or rented items such as hospital beds, iron lungs, oxygen equipment, seat lift equipment, wheelchairs, and other medically necessary equipment prescribed by a health care provider to be used in a patient's home which are covered by Medicare.

Durable Medical Equipment Regional Carrier: See DMERC

E codes: Specific ICD-9-CM codes used to identify the cause of injury, poisoning or other adverse effects.

EDI: Electronic Data Interchange

Edit: Logic within the Standard Claims Processing System (or PSC Supplemental Edit Software) that selects certain claims, evaluates or compares information on the selected claims or other accessible source, and depending on the evaluation, takes action on the claims, such as pay in full, pay in part, or suspend for manual review.

Effectiveness: The net health benefits provided by a medical service or technology for typical patients in community practice settings.

Efficacy: The net health benefits provided by a medical service or technology under ideal conditions, usually in controlled, expert settings with carefully selected patients.

Efficient: Activities performed effectively with minimum of waste or unnecessary effort, or producing a high ratio of results to resources.

EHNAC: Electronic Healthcare Network Accreditation Commission

Electronic claim: A claim form which is processed and delivered from one computer to another via some form of magnetic media (magnetic tape, diskette) or via telecommunications (telephone link).

Electronic Data Interchange (EDI): Refers to the exchange of routine business transactions from one computer to another in a standard format, using standard communications protocols.

Electronic media questionnaire: A process that large employers can use to complete their requirements for supplying IRS/SSA/CMS Data Match information electronically.

Electronic signature: The attribute that is affixed to an electronic document to bind it to a particular entity. An electronic signature process secures the user authentication (proof of claimed identity, such as by biometrics—fingerprints, retinal scans, hand written signature verification—tokens or passwords) at the time the signature is generated; creates the logical manifestation of signature (including the possibility for multiple parties to sign a document and have the order of application recognized and proven) and supplies additional information such as time stamp and signature purpose specific to that user; and ensures the integrity of the signed document to enable transportability, interoperability, independent verifiability, and continuity of signature capability. Verifying a signature on a document verifies the integrity of the document and associated attributes and verifies the identity of the signer. There are several technologies available for user authentication, including passwords, cryptography, and biometrics.

Eligibility: Refers to the process whereby an individual is determined to be eligible for health care coverage through the Medicaid program. Eligibility is determined by the state. Eligibility data are collected and managed by the state or by its Fiscal Agent. In some managed care waiver programs, eligibility records are updated by an enrollment broker, who assists the individual in choosing a managed care plan to enroll in.

E/M: Evaluation and management services

EMC: Electronic Media Claim

Emergency mode operation: Access controls in place that enable an enterprise to continue to operate in the event of fire, vandalism, natural disaster, or system failure.

Emergency mode operation plan: Part of an overall contingency plan. The plan for a process whereby an enterprise would be able to continue to operate in the event of fire, vandalism, natural disaster, or system failure.

Emergency room (Hospital): A portion of the hospital where emergency diagnosis and treatment of illness or injury is provided.

Employee: For purposes of the Medicare Secondary Payer (MSP) provisions, an employee is an individual who works for an employer, whether on a full- or part-time basis, and receives payment for his/her work.

Employer: Individuals and organizations engaged in a trade or business, plus entities exempt from income tax such as religious, charitable, and educational institutions, the governments of the United States, Puerto Rico, the Virgin Islands, Guam, American Samoa, the Northern Marianna Islands, and the

District of Columbia, and the agencies, instrumentalities, and political subdivisions of these governments.

Employer bulletin board service: An electronic bulletin board service offered by the COB Contractor. Employers that have to report on less than 500 workers can fulfill their requirements under the Internal Revenue Service/Social Security Administration/Health Care Financing Administration (IRS/SSA/CMS) Data Match law by downloading from the internet a questionnaire entry application from the bulletin board. The information will be processed through several logic and consistency edits. Once the employer has completed the information, he or she will return the completed file through the bulletin board.

Encounter data: Detailed data about individual services provided by a capitated managed care entity. The level of detail about each service reported is similar to that of a standard claim form. Encounter data are also sometimes referred to as "shadow claims."

Encryption: Transforming confidential plain text into cipher text to protect it. Also called encipherment. An encryption algorithm combines plain text with other values called keys, or ciphers, so the data becomes unintelligible. Once encrypted, data can be stored or transmitted over unsecured lines. Decrypting data reverses the encryption algorithm process and makes the plain text available for further processing.

End-Stage Renal Disease (ESRD): Permanent kidney failure. That stage of renal impairment that appears irreversible and permanent, and requires a regular course of dialysis or kidney transplantation to maintain life.

End-stage renal disease treatment facility: A facility, other than a hospital, which provides dialysis treatment, maintenance, and/or training to patients or caregivers on an ambulatory or home-care basis.

Enrollee hotlines: Toll-free telephone lines, usually staffed by the state or enrollment broker that beneficiaries may call when they encounter a problem with their MCO/PHP. The people who staff hotlines are knowledgeable about program policies and may play an "intake and triage" role or may assist in resolving the problem.

Enrollment: The process by which a person eligible for Medicaid becomes a member of a managed care plan. Enrollment data refer to the managed care plan's information on Medicaid eligible individuals who are plan members. The managed care plan gets its enrollment data from the Medicaid program's eligibility system.

Enterprise liability: The assumption of liability by a health care organization for all negligent injuries to patients under its care, thereby relieving individual practitioners of all personal liability for such injuries.

Entity assets: Assets which the reporting entity has authority to use in its operations (for example, management has the authority to decide how funds are used or management is legally obligated to use funds to meet entity obligations).

Entity authentication: (1) The corroboration that an entity is the one claimed. (ISO 7498-2, as cited in the HISB draft Glossary of Terms Related to Information Security In Health Care Information Systems. (2) A communications/network mechanism to irrefutably identify authorized users, programs, and processes, and to deny access to unauthorized users, programs and processes.

EOB: Explanation of benefits. A form included with a check from the health insurance carrier which explains the benefits that were paid and/or charges that were rejected.

EOMB: Explanation of Medicare Benefits

Eponyms: Medical procedures or conditions named after a person or a place.

EQRO: External Quality Review Organization

Equipment control (into and out of site): Documented security procedures for bringing hardware and software into and out of a facility and for maintaining a record of that equipment. This includes, but is not limited to, the marking, handling, and disposal of hardware and storage media.

Equivalency review: The process CMS employs to compare an accreditation organization's standards, processes and enforcement activities to the comparable CMS requirements, processes and enforcement activities.

ESRD eligibility requirements: To qualify for Medicare under the renal provision, a person must have ESRD and either be entitled to a monthly insurance benefit under Title II of the Act (or an annuity under the Railroad Retirement Act), be fully or currently insured under Social Security (railroad work may count), or be the spouse or dependent child of a person who meets at least one of the two last requirements. There is no minimum age for eligibility under the renal disease provision. An Application for Health Insurance Benefits Under Medicare for Individuals with Chronic Renal Disease, Form CMS-43 (effective October 1, 1978) must be filed.

ESRD facility: A facility, which is approved to furnish at least one specific, ESRD service. These services may be performed in a renal transplantation center, a renal dialysis facility, self-dialysis unit, or special purpose renal dialysis facility.

ESRD network: All Medicare approved ESRD facilities in a designated geographic area specified by CMS.

ESRD network organization: The administrative governing body of the ESRD Network and liaison to the Federal Government.

ESRD patient: A person with irreversible and permanent kidney failure who requires a regular course of dialysis or kidney transplantation to maintain life.

ESRD services: The type of care or service furnished to an ESRD patient. Such types of care are transplantation, dialysis, outpatient dialysis, staff assisted dialysis, home dialysis, and self-dialysis and home dialysis training.

Essential community providers: Providers such as community health centers that have traditionally served low-income populations. The Clinton administration's health reform proposal includes special payment rules to these organizations for five years.

Etiology: The cause(s) or origin of a disease.

Evaluation and management services: Nontechnical services provided by most physicians for the purpose of diagnosing and treating diseases and counseling and evaluating patients.

Exclusions: Specific services or conditions which the policy will not cover or which are covered at a limited rate.

Exclusive Provider Organization (EPO): A provider network similar to a PPO wherein a patient must pay the entire cost of any care obtained outside the EPO network of providers. EPO providers typically are paid for services rendered instead of by capitation.

Expenditure: The issuance of checks, disbursement of cash, or electronic transfer of funds made to liquidate an expense regardless of the fiscal year the service was provided or the expense was incurred. When used in the discussion of the Medicaid program, expenditures refer to funds spent as reported by the states. The same as an Outlay.

Expenditure limit: A maximum level of spending for the health sector as a whole or for particular categories of services; usually set by the government to be achieved through rate setting or premium limits.

Expense: Funds actually spent or incurred providing goods, rendering services, or carrying out other mission related activities during a period. Expenses are computed using accrual accounting techniques which recognize costs when incurred and revenues when earned and include the effect of accounts receivables and accounts payable on determining annual income.

Experience rating: A system used by insurers to set premium levels based on the insured's past loss history. For example, rating may be based on service utilization for health insurance or on liability experience for professional liability insurance.

Explanation of benefits: See EOB.

Extended care services: In the context of this report, an alternate name for "skilled nursing facility services."

External Quality Review Organization (EQRO): The organization with which the state contracts to evaluate the care provided to Medicaid managed eligibles. Typically the EQRO is a peer review organization. It may conduct focused medical record reviews (for example, reviews targeted at a particular clinical condition) or broader analyses on quality. While most EQRO contractors rely on medical records as the primary source of information, they may also use eligibility data and claims/encounter data to conduct specific analyses.

Facility security plan: A plan to safeguard the premises and building(s) (exterior and interior) from unauthorized physical access, and to safeguard the equipment therein from unauthorized physical access, tampering, and theft.

False negatives: Occur when the medical record contains evidence of a service that does not exist in the encounter data. This is the most common problem in partially or fully capitated plans because the provider does not need to submit an encounter in order to receive payment for the service, and therefore may have a weaker incentive to conform to data collection standards.

False positives: Occurs when the encounter data contain evidence of a service that is not documented in the patient's medical record. If the medical record contains complete information on the patient's medical history, a false positive may be considered a fraudulent service. In a fully capitated environment, however, the provider would receive no additional reimbursement for the submission of a false positive encounter.

Federal general revenues: Federal tax revenues (principally individual and business income taxes) not earmarked for a particular use.

Federally qualified health center: A facility located in a medically underserved area that provides Medicare beneficiaries preventive primary medical care under the general supervision of a physician.

Federally qualified HMO: An HMO that has satisfied certain federal qualifications pertaining to organizational structure, provider contracts, health service delivery information, utilization review/quality assurance, grievance procedures, financial status, and marketing information.

Fee for service (FFS): Refers to paying medical providers for individual services rendered. UCR, CPR and Fee Schedules are examples of fee for service systems.

Fee schedule: A list of predetermined payments for medical services.

Fee schedule payment areas: Geographic areas within which payment under the fee schedule will be equal. Analogous to localities under current payment policies. See Geographic Adjustment Factor.

Fee-screen year: A specified period of time in which SMI-recognized fees pertain. The fee-screen year period has changed over the history of the program.

FEHB: Federal Employees Health Benefits.

FFS: Fee-for-Service

FICA: Federal Insurance Contribution Act Payroll Tax. Medicare's share of FICA is used to fund the HI trust fund.

Financial data: Data regarding the financial the status of managed care entities (e.g. the medical loss ratio).

Financial interchange: Provisions of the Railroad Retirement Act providing for transfers between the trust funds and the Social Security Equivalent Benefit Account of the Railroad Retirement program in order to place each trust fund in the same position as if railroad employment had always been covered under Social Security.

Fiscal Intermediary (FI): An entity with whom CMS contracts under section 1816 of the Act to process claims and make payments for Medicare Part A and Part B services.

Fiscal year: The accounting year of the U.S. Government. Since 1976, each fiscal year has begun October 1 of the prior calendar year and ended the following September 30th. For example, fiscal year 2001 began October 1, 2000 and ended September 30, 2001.

Fixed capital assets: The net worth of facilities and other resources.

FMAP (Federal Medical Assistance Percentage): The portion of the Medicaid program which is paid by the Federal government.

FMFIA (Federal Managers' Financial Integrity Act): A program to identify management inefficiencies and areas vulnerable to fraud and abuse and to correct such weaknesses with improved internal controls.

Focused studies: State required studies that examine a specific aspect of health care (such as prenatal care) for a defined point in time. These projects are usually based on information extracted from medical records or MCO/PHP administrative data such as enrollment files and encounter/claims data. State staff, EQRO staff, MCO/PHP staff or more than one of these entities may perform such studies at the discretion of the state.

Formal mechanism for processing records: Documented policies and procedures for the routine, and non-routine, receipt, manipulation, storage, dissemination, transmission, and/or disposal of health information.

Fraud: The intentional deception or misrepresentation that an individual knows, or should know, to be false, or does not believe to be true, and makes, knowing the deception could result in some unauthorized benefit to himself or some other person(s).

Frequency distribution: An exhaustive list of possible outcomes for a variable, and the associated probability of each outcome. The sum of the probabilities of all possible outcomes from a frequency distribution is 100 percent.

Full capitation (FUL): The plan or Primary Care Case Manager is paid for providing services to enrollees through a combination of capitation and fee-for-service reimbursements.

Full Program Safeguard Contractor (PSC): For the purposes of this umbrella SOW, a full PSC is one that performs all of the fundamental activities contained in Section 3, General Requirements, under a Task Order.

Fully accredited: Designation that all the elements within all the accreditation standards for which the accreditation organization has been approved by CMS have been surveyed and fully met or have otherwise been determined to be acceptable without significant adverse findings, recommendations, required actions or corrective actions.

Fully capitated (FUL): A stipulated dollar amount established to cover the cost of all health care services delivered for a person.

GAF: Geographic Adjustment Factor

Gaming: Gaining advantage by using improper means to evade the letter or intent of a rule or system.

Gatekeeper: A primary care physician in an HMO who reviews and evaluates patients for referral to specialists. The gatekeeper's mission is to reduce unnecessary services and costs.

Geographic adjustment factor (GAF): The adjustment made to a service's fee in the Medicare Fee Schedule to determine the correct payment in each fee schedule payment area. As defined in OBRA89, the geographic adjustment factor is created by combining three separate adjustment factors, one for each component of the Medicare Fee Schedule: physician work, practice expense, and malpractice expense. The adjustment factors for physician work, practice expense, and malpractice are based on the same measures that underlie the GPCI. See Fee Schedule Payment Areas, Geographic Cost of Practice Index.

Geographic practice cost index (GPCI): An index summarizing the prices of inputs to physician services in an area relative to national average prices. The GPCI is based on three components, reflecting the opportunity cost of physician work, the costs of goods and services that comprise practice expenses, and malpractice expenses.

Global service: A group of clinically related services that are treated as a single unit for the purpose of coding, billing and payment.

Global surgery policy: The payment policy in the Medicare Fee Schedule that specifies the surgical procedure and the related services and visits that are included in a global surgical fee.

GPCI: Geographic Practice Cost Index

Grievances and complaints: Information about grievances and complaints submitted to the health plan.

Group contract: A contract between an HMO and a subscribing group of beneficiaries which specifies rates, performance, relationships, schedule of benefits, and other conditions, usually for a 12 month period.

Group Health Plan (GHP): A health plan that provides health coverage to employees, former employees, and their families, and is supported by an employer or employee organization.

Group model HMO: An HMO that pays a medical group a negotiated, per capita rate, which the group distributes among its physicians, often under a salaried arrangement.

Guaranteed issue: The requirement that each insurer and health plan accept everyone who applies for coverage and guarantees the renewal of that coverage as long as the applicant pays the premium.

Guidelines: Guidelines are systematically developed by appropriate groups to assist practitioner and patient decisions about appropriate health care for specific clinical circumstances.

Harvard relative value study: A study completed at Harvard University to develop a resource-based relative value scale.

HCPCS: Heath care Common Procedure Coding System. A two-level coding system, consisting of CPT, and National or Level II codes used to report and bill services provided to Medicare patients. See Coding, Current Procedural Terminology.

Health Care Prepayment Plan (HCPP): A type of managed care organization. In return for a monthly premium, plus any applicable deductible or co-payment, all or most of an individual's physician services will be provided by the HCPP. The HCPP will pay for all services it has arranged for (and any emergency services) whether provided by its own physicians or its contracted network of physicians. If a member enrolled in an HCPP chooses to receive services that have not been arranged for by the HCPP, he/she is liable for any applicable Medicare deductible and/or coinsurance amounts, and any balance would be paid by the regional Medicare carrier.

Health Care Quality Improvement Program (HCQIP): A program which supports the mission of CMS to assure health care security for beneficiaries. The mission of HCQIP is to promote the quality, effectiveness, and efficiency of services to Medicare beneficiaries by strengthening the community of those committed to improving quality, by monitoring and improving quality of care; by communicating with beneficiaries and health care providers, practitioners; and by plans to promote informed health choices, to protect beneficiaries from poor care, and to strengthen the infrastructure.

Health information: "Health information," as defined in section 1171 of the Act, means any information, whether oral or recorded in any form or medium, that 1) is created or received by a health care provider, health plan, public health authority, employer, life insurer, school or university, or health care clearinghouse; and 2) relates to the past, present, or future physical or mental health or condition of an individual; the provision of health care to an individual; or the past, present, or future payment for the provision of health care to an individual.

Health Insurance Claims Number (HICN): The number assigned by the Social Security Administration to an individual identifying him/her as a Medicare beneficiary. This number is shown on the beneficiary's insurance card and is used in processing Medicare claims for that beneficiary.

Health Insuring Organization (HIO): An entity that provides for or arranges for the provision of care and contracts on a prepaid capitated risk basis to provide a comprehensive set of services.

Health Maintenance Organization (HMO): Competitive medical plans, including Medicare + Choice, that have contracts with CMS on a prospective capitation payment basis for providing health care to Medicare beneficiaries.

Health Maintenance Organization/Federally Qualified (HMO/FQ): A public or private organization that contracts on a prepaid capitated risk basis to provide a comprehensive set of services and is federally qualified.

Health Maintenance Organization/State Plan Defined (HMO/SPD): A public or private organization that contracts on a prepaid capitated risk basis to provide a comprehensive set of services and is state plan defined.

Health plan: An organization that acts as an insurer for an enrolled population. May be structured as a fee-for-service or managed care plan.

Health Plan Purchasing Cooperative (HPPC): A health insurance purchasing entity advanced by some health system reform proposals to enroll individuals, collect premiums, purchase enrollee's health insurance from participating health plans, and enforce the rules that manage health plan competition. Also known as an Alliance.

Health Professional Shortage Areas [HPSAs]: Replaces Health Manpower Shortage Areas [HMSAs]. A Health Professional Shortage Area means any of the following which the Secretary of the Department of Health and Human Services determines has a shortage of health manpower: (1) an urban or rural area (which need not conform to the geographic boundaries of a political subdivision and which is a rational area for the delivery of health services); (2) a population group; (3) a public nonprofit private medical facility. Designated HPSAs can apply for National Health Services Corps (NHSC) personnel, or be eligible for the NHSC scholarship program or health profession student loan program.

Hearing: A procedure that gives a dissatisfied claimant an opportunity to present reasons for the dissatisfaction and to receive a new determination based on the record developed at the hearing. Hearings are provided for in 11842(b)(3)(C) of the Act.

HHS: Department of Health and Human Services (also referred to as DHHS).

Hierarchy: A system that ranks items one above another.

High risk area: A potential flaw in management controls requiring management attention and possible corrective action.

HISB: Health Care Informatics Standards Board

HMO: An organization that provides comprehensive health services to its members in return for a fixed prepaid fee. There are four types of HMOs: group, staff, independent practice association, and network.

HMO Act: Health Maintenance Organization Act of 1973, P.L. 93-222, enacted December 1973.

HMO regulatory agency: A state agency with the authority to grant or deny an HMO the right to do business in a state.

Home: Location, other than a hospital or other facility, where the patient receives care in a private residence.

Home Health Agency (HHA): A public agency or private organization that is primarily engaged in providing the following services in the home: skilled nursing services, other therapeutic services (such as physical, occupational, or speech therapy), and home health aide services.

Home patients: Medically-able individuals, who have their own dialysis equipment at home and after proper training, perform their own dialysis treatment alone or with the assistance of a helper.

Hospice: A provider of care for the terminally ill. Delivered services generally include home health care, nursing care, physician services, medical supplies, and short-term inpatient hospital care. A facility, other than a patient's home, in which palliative and supportive care for terminally ill patients and their families are provided.

Hospital assumptions: These include differentials between hospital labor and non-labor indices compared with general economy labor and non-labor indices; rates of admission incidence; the trend toward treating less complicated cases in outpatient settings; and continued improvement in DRG coding.

Hospital coinsurance: For the 61st through 90th day of hospitalization in a benefit period, a daily amount for which the beneficiary is responsible, equal to one-fourth of the inpatient hospital deductible; for lifetime reserve days, a daily amount for which the beneficiary is responsible, equal to one-half of the inpatient hospital deductible. See Lifetime reserve days.

Hospital input price index: An alternate name for "hospital market basket."

Hospital Insurance (HI): The Medicare program that covers specified inpatient hospital services, posthospital skilled nursing care, home health services, and hospice care for aged and disabled individuals who meet the eligibility requirements. Also known as Medicare Part A.

Hospital market basket: The cost of the mix of goods and services (including personnel costs but excluding nonoperating costs) comprising routine, ancillary, and special care unit inpatient hospital services.

HPSA: Health Professional Shortage Area

HSQB: Health Standards and Quality Bureau, CMS

ICD-9-CM: International Classification of Diseases, 9th Revision, Clinical Modification. A standardized system of describing diagnoses by code numbers developed and maintained by the World Health Organization.

ICD-10: International Classification of Diseases, 10th Revision.

Improvement plan: A plan for measurable process or outcome improvement. The plan is usually developed cooperatively by a provider and the Network. The plan must address how and when its results will be measured.

Inappropriate utilization: Utilization of services that are in excess of a beneficiary's medical needs and condition (overutilization) or receiving a capitated Medicare payment and failing to provide services to meet a beneficiary's medical needs and condition (underutilization).

Incidence: The frequency of new occurrences of a condition within a defined time interval. The incidence rate is the number of new cases of specific disease divided by the number of people in a population over a specified period of time, usually one year.

Income rate: The ratio of income from tax revenues on an incurred basis (payroll tax contributions and income from the taxation of OASDI benefits) to the HI taxable payroll for the year.

Incurred basis: The costs based on when the service was performed rather than when the payment was made.

Indemnity schedule: See Schedule of Allowances.

Independent laboratory: A freestanding clinical laboratory meeting conditions for participation in the Medicare program and billing through a carrier. A laboratory certified to perform diagnostic and/or clinical tests independent of an institution or a physician's office.

Independent Practice Association [IPA]: An HMO that contracts with individual physicians to provide services to HMO members in a negotiated per capita or fee-for-service rate. Physicians maintain their own offices and can contract with other HMO's and see other fee-for-service patients.

Independent verifiability: The capability to verify the signature without the cooperation of the signer. Technically, it is accomplished using the public key of the signatory, and it is a property of all digital signatures performed with asymmetric key encryption.

Indicator: A key clinical value or quality characteristic used to measure, over time, the performance, processes, and outcomes of an organization or some component of health care delivery.

Information: Data to which meaning is assigned, according to context and assumed conventions.

Information access control: Formal, documented policies and procedures for granting different levels of access to health care information.

Initial (claim) determination: The first adjudication made by a carrier or fiscal intermediary (for example, the affiliated contractor) following a request for Medicare payment or the first determination made by a PRO either in a prepayment or postpayment context.

Initial Enrollment Questionnaire (IEQ): A questionnaire sent to a patient to find out if that patient has other insurance that should pay his medical bills before Medicare. See Medicare Secondary Payer.

Inpatient hospital: A facility, other than psychiatric, which primarily provides diagnostic, therapeutic (both surgical and nonsurgical) and rehabilitation services by or under the supervision of physicians to patients admitted for a variety of medical conditions.

Inpatient hospital deductible: An amount of money that is deducted from the amount payable by Medicare Part A for inpatient hospital services furnished to a beneficiary during a spell of illness.

Inpatient hospital services: These services include bed and board, nursing services, diagnostic or therapeutic services, and medical or surgical services.

Inpatient psychiatric facility: A facility that provides inpatient psychiatric services for the diagnosis and treatment of mental illness on a 24-hour basis, by or under the supervision of a physician.

Insurance clerk: One of the health care professional's employees who has been assigned the very important job of managing health insurance claims in the medical office.

Insured: The person who represents the family unit in relation to the health insurance program. Usually the employee whose employment makes this coverage possible.

Insurer: An insurer of a group health plan is an entity that, in exchange for payment of a premium, agrees to pay for GHP-covered services received by eligible individuals. See Carrier.

Integrity controls: Security mechanism employed to ensure the validity of the information being electronically transmitted or stored.

Interest: A payment for the use of money during a specified period.

Interfund borrowing: The borrowing of assets by a trust fund (OASI, DI, HI, or SMI) from another of the trust funds when one of the funds is in danger of exhaustion. Interfund borrowing was authorized only during 1982-1987.

Intermediary: A private or public organization that is under contract to CMS to determine costs of, and make payments to, providers for HI and certain SMI services.

Intermediary hearing: That hearing provided for in 42 CFR 1405.1809.

Intermediary/program safeguard contractor determination: A determination as defined in 42 CFR 1405.1801 under the definition for Intermediary Determination.

Intermediate assumptions: See Assumptions.

Intermediate care facility/mentally retarded: A facility which primarily provides health-related care and services above the level of custodial care to mentally retarded individuals but does not provide the level of care available in a hospital or skilled nursing facility.

Intermediate entities: Entities which contract between an MCO or one of its subcontractors, and a physician or physician group, other than physician groups themselves. An Independent Practice Association is considered to be an intermediate entity if it contracts with one or more physician groups in addition to contracting with individual physicians.

Internal audit: The in-house review of the records of system activity (for example, logins, file accesses, security incidents) maintained by an organization.

Internal controls: Management systems and policies for reasonably documenting, monitoring, and correcting operational processes to prevent and detect waste and to ensure proper payment.

Internal Revenue Service/Social Security Administration/Health Care Financing Administration Data Match (IRS/SSA/CMS Data Match): A process by which information on employers and employees is provided by the IRS and SSA and is analyzed by CMS for use in contacting employers concerning possible periods of MSP. This information is used to update the CWF-Medicare Common Working File.

Interoperability: The applications used on either side of a communication, between trading partners and/or between internal components of an entity, being able to read and correctly interpret the information communicated from one to the other.

Intermediary: An health insurance carrier, or data processing company, designed to receive and process Medicare or Medicaid claims on behalf of the government.

International classification of diseases: See ICD-9-CM.

Intragovernmental assets, liabilities: Assets or liabilities that arise from transactions among federal entities.

Inventory: Formal, documented identification of hardware and software assets.

IPA: See Independent Practice Association

ISO: International Organization for Standardization

Key: An input that controls the transformation of data by an encryption algorithm.

Late effect: A residual effect (condition produced) after the acute phase of an illness or injury has ended.

LCL: Lowest Charge Level Limit

Level II codes: See HCPCS

Liability determination: Determination based on 11879 or 11870 or 11842(L) of the Act, of whether the beneficiary and the provider did not and could not have been reasonably expected to know that payment would not be made for services.

Licensed by the state as a risk-bearing entity: An entity that is licensed or otherwise authorized by the state to assume risk for offering health insurance or health benefits coverage. The entity is authorized to accept prepaid capitation for providing, arranging, or paying for comprehensive health services under an M+C contract. Designation that an M+C organization has been reviewed and determined "fully accredited" by a CMS-approved accrediting organization for those standards within the deeming categories that the accrediting organization has the authority to deem.

Lifetime reserve days: Under HI, each beneficiary has 60 lifetime reserve days that he or she may opt to use when regular inpatient hospital benefits are exhausted. The beneficiary pays one-half of the inpatient hospital deductible for each lifetime reserve day used.

Limited License Practitioner (LLP): A professional licensed to perform certain health services in independent practice; for example, podiatrists, dentists, optometrists and chiropractors.

Limiting charge: The maximum amount that a nonparticipating physician is permitted to charge a Medicare beneficiary for a service.

Line item: Service or item specific detail of claim.

Living donor kidney transplant: The surgical procedure of excising a kidney from a living donor and implanting it into a suitable recipient.

LLP: Limited License Practitioner

Local codes: See HCPCS

Locality [Medicare]: A geographic area for which a carrier calculates prevailing charges. Localities can be states, aggregations of counties, parts of counties, metropolitan zip code areas, or townships.

Long range: The next 75 years.

Long-term disability income insurance: A provision to pay benefits to a covered disabled person as long as he or she remains disabled, up to a specified period.

M+C organization (Medicare+Choice): A public or private entity organized and licensed by a state as a risk-bearing entity (with the exception of provider sponsored organization receiving waivers) that is certified by CMS as meeting the M+C contract requirements. See 42 C.F.R. 1 422.2.

M+C plan: Health benefits coverage offered under a policy or contract offered by a Medicare+Choice Organization under which a specific set of health benefits are offered at a uniform premium and uniform level of cost-sharing to all Medicare beneficiaries residing in the service area of the M+C plan. See 42

C.F.R. 1 422.2. An M+C plan may be a coordinated care plan (with or without point of service options), a combination of an M+C medical savings account (MSA) plan and a contribution into an M+C MSA established in accordance with 42 CFR part 422.262, or an M+C private fee-for-service plan. See 42 C.F.R. 1 422.4(a).

MAAC: Maximum Allowable Actual Charge. A limitation on billed charges for Medicare services provided by non-participating physicians. For physicians with charges exceeding 115 percent of the prevailing charge for nonparticipating physicians, MAACs limit increases in actual charges to 1 percent a year. For physicians whose charges are less than 115 percent of the prevailing, MAACs limit actual charge increases so they may not exceed 115 percent. See Actual Charge, Nonparticipating Physician.

MAC: Mandatory Access Control

MAF: Medical Assistance Facility

Main term: Refers to listings the Alphabetic Index of ICD-9-CM appearing in **boldface** type.

Maintenance of record of access authorizations: Ongoing documentation and review of the levels of access granted to a user, program, or procedure accessing health information.

Maintenance records: Documentation of repairs and modifications to the physical components of a facility (for example, hardware, software, walls, doors, locks).

Major medical insurance: Health insurance to finance the expense of major illnesses and injuries. Major medical policies usually include a substantial deductible clause. Above the initial deductible, major medical insurance is characterized by large benefit maximums.

Managed care: Any system of health service payment or delivery arrangements where the health plan attempts to control or coordinate use of health services by its enrolled members in order to contain health expenditures, improve quality, or both. Arrangements often involve a defined delivery system of providers with some form of contractual arrangement with the plan.

Managed Care Organization (MCO): Managed Care Organizations are entities that serve Medicare or Medicaid beneficiaries on a risk basis through a network of employed or affiliated providers. The term generally includes HMOs, PPOs, and Point of Service plans. In the Medicaid arena, other organizations may set up managed care programs to respond to Medicaid managed care. These organizations include Federally Qualified Health Centers, integrated delivery systems, and public health clinics. It is a health maintenance organization, an eligible organization with a contract under 11876 or a Medicare-Choice organization, a provider-sponsored organization, or any other private or public organization, which meets the requirements of 11902 (w) to provide comprehensive services.

Managed care payment suspension: See Suspension of payments. Includes Health Maintenance Organizations (HMO), Competitive Medical Plans (CMP), and other plans that provide health services on a prepayment basis, based either on cost or risk, depending on the type of contract they have with Medicare. See also Medicare+Choice.

Managed care system: Integrates the financing and delivery of appropriate health care services to covered individuals by means of arrangements with selected providers to furnish a comprehensive set of health care services to members, explicit criteria for the selection of health care provides, and significant financial incentives for members to use providers and procedures associated with the plan. Managed care plans typically are labeled as HMOs (staff, group, IPA, and mixed models), PPOs, or Point of Service plans. Managed care services are reimbursed via a variety of methods including capitation, fee-for-service, and a combination of the two.

Managed competition: An approach to health system reform in which health plans compete to provide health insurance coverage for enrollees. Typically, enrollees would sign up with a health plan purchasing entity and would be offered a choice of health plans during an open enrollment season.

Management Service Organization (MSO): An entity which provides practice management and other support services, such as marketing, billing, financial management, nursing pools, staff recruitment, etc. to medical groups.

Mandatory Access Control (MAC): A means of restricting access to objects that are based on fixed security attributes assigned to users and to files and other objects. The controls are mandatory in the sense that they cannot be modified by users or their programs.

Mandatory spending: Outlays for entitlement programs (Medicare and Medicaid) that are not subject to the Federal appropriations process.

Manifestation: Characteristic signs or symptoms of an illness.

Manual claim review: Review, pre- or postpayment, that requires the intervention of PSC personnel.

Market baskets: See Hospital market basket.

Mass immunization center: A location where providers administer pneumococcal pneumonia and influenza virus vaccination and submit these services as electronic media claims, paper claims, or using the roster billing method. This generally takes place in a mass immunization setting, such as a public health center, pharmacy, or mall but may include a physician's office setting (4408.8, Part 3 of MCM).

Material weakness: A serious flaw in management controls requiring high-priority corrective action.

Maximum fee schedule: A compensation arrangement in which a participating physician agrees to accept the Schedule of Allowances as his total fee for covered services.

Maximum tax base: Annual dollar amount above which earnings in employment covered under the HI program are not taxable. Beginning in 1994, the maximum tax base is eliminated under HI.

Maximum taxable amount of annual earnings: See Maximum tax base.

Maximums: The top limit of the amount a carrier will pay for a specific benefit or policy during a specified time period.

MCCA: Medicare Catastrophic Coverage Act of 1988, P.L. 100-360, enacted July 1, 1988 and repealed December 13, 1989.

MCO: Managed Care Organization

MCO/PHP standards: These are standards that states set for plan structure, operations, and the internal quality improvement/assurance system that each MCO/PHP must have in order to participate in the Medicaid program.

Measurement: The systematic process of data collection, repeated over time or at a single point in time.

Media controls: Formal, documented policies and procedures that govern the receipt and removal of hardware/software (for example, diskettes, tapes) into and out of a facility.

Medicaid: A state/federal government sponsored medical assistance program to enable eligible recipients to obtain essential medical care and services.

Medicaid Management Information System (MMIS): A CMS approved system that supports the operation of the Medicaid program. The MMIS includes the following types of sub-systems or files: recipient eligibility, Medicaid provider, claims processing, pricing, SURS, MARS, and potential encounter processing.

Medicaid MCO: A Medicaid MCO provides comprehensive services to Medicaid beneficiaries, but not commercial or Medicare enrollees.

Medicaid-only MCO (MCAID-MCO): A Medicaid-only MCO is an MCO that provides comprehensive services to Medicaid beneficiaries, but not commercial or Medicare enrollees.

Medicare: A nationwide, federally administered health insurance program authorized in 1965 to cover the cost of hospitalization, medical care, and some related services for most people over age 65. In 1972, coverage was extended to people receiving Social Security Disability Insurance payments for 2 years, and people with ESRD. Medicare consists of two separate but coordinated programs: Part A (HI, hospital insurance) and Part B (SMI, supplementary medical insurance). Almost all persons who are aged 65 or over or disabled and who are entitled to HI are eligible to enroll in the SMI program on a voluntary basis by paying a monthly premium. Health insurance protection is available to Medicare beneficiaries without regard to income. The health insurance program for the aged and disabled under Title XVIII of the Act.

Medicare Catastrophic Coverage Act of 1988: P.L. 100-330, enacted and repealed in 1989. Established ICD-9-CM coding requirements for all Medicare claims.

Medicare contractor: A collective term for carriers and intermediaries.

Medicare Economic Index (MEI): An index often used in the calculation of the increases in the prevailing charge levels that help to determine allowed charges for physician services. In 1992 and later, this index is considered in connection with the update factor for the physician fee schedule.

Medicare Fee Schedule [MFS]: The resource based fee schedule currently used by Medicare to pay for physicians' services. This method replaced the customary, prevailing and reasonable (CPR) payment method in the first quarter of 1992. This fee schedule is based on resource costs, and composed of factors representing physician work and practice costs.

Medicare handbook: The Medicare Handbook provides information on such things as how to file a claim and what type of care is covered under the Medicare program. This handbook is given to all beneficiaries when first enrolled in the program.

Medicare Payment Advisory Commission (MedPAC): A commission established by Congress in the Balanced Budget Act of 1997 to replace the Prospective Payment Assessment Commission and the Physician Payment Review Commission. MedPAC is directed to provide the Congress with advice and recommendations on policies affecting the Medicare program.

Medicare risk contract: A contract between Medicare and an HMO or competitive medical plan under which the plan provides Medicare covered services for enrollees and receives monthly capitated payments from Medicare, thereby assuming health insurance risk for its enrollees.

Medicare Secondary Payer (MSP): Any situation when another insurance policy, plan, or program pays your medical bills before Medicare.

Medicare trust funds: Treasury accounts established by the Social Security Act for the receipt of revenues, maintenance of reserves, and disbursement of payments for the HI and SMI programs.

Medicare+Choice: An expanded set of options, established by the Balanced Budget Act of 1997, for the delivery of health care under Medicare. Most Medicare beneficiaries can choose to receive benefits through the original fee-for-service program or through one of the following Medicare+Choice plans: (1) coordinated care plans (such as health maintenance organizations, provider sponsored organizations, and preferred provider organizations); (2) Medical Savings Account (MSA)/High Deductible plans (through a demonstration available to up to 390,000 beneficiaries); or (3) private fee-for-service plans.

Medigap insurance: Private health insurance policies designed to supplement Medicare coverage. Benefits may include payment of Medicare deductibles, coinsurance, and balance bills, and payment for services not covered by Medicare.

MEI: Medicare Economic Index

Message: A digital representation of information.

Message authentication: Ensuring, typically with a message authentication code, that a message received (usually via a network) matches the message sent.

Message authentication code: Data associated with an authenticated message that allows a receiver to verify the integrity of the message.

Message integrity: The assurance of unaltered transmission and receipt of a message from the sender to the intended recipient.

MFS: Medicare Fee Schedule

Military service wage credits: Credits recognizing that military personnel receive other cash payments and wages in kind (such as food and shelter) in addition to their basic pay. Noncontributory wage credits of $160 are provided for each month of active military service from September 16, 1940 through December 31, 1956. For years after 1956, the basic pay of military personnel is covered under the Social Security program on a contributory basis. In addition to contributory credits for basic pay, noncontributory wage credits of $300 are granted for each calendar quarter in which a person receives pay for military service from January 1957 through December 1977. Deemed wage credits of $100 are granted for each $300 of military wages in years after 1977. (The maximum credits allowed in any calendar year are $1,200.) See also Quinquennial military service determinations and adjustments.

Military Treatment Facility (MTF): A medical facility operated by one or more of the Uniformed Services. An MTF also refers to certain former U.S. Public Health Services (USPHS) facilities now designated as Uniformed Service Treatment Facilities (USTF).

Modality: Methods of treatment for kidney failure/ESRD. Modality types include transplant, hemodialysis, and peritoneal dialysis.

Model fee schedule: The sample fee schedule developed by CMS in 1990 from Phase I of the Hsaio study.

Modified average-cost method: Under this system of calculating summary measures, the actuarial balance is defined as the difference between the arithmetic means of the annual cost rates and the annual income rates, with an adjustment included to account for the offsets to cost that are due to (1) the starting trust fund balance and (2) interest earned on the trust fund.

Modifiers: Codes used supplementally with CPT or HCPCS codes to indicate that the service has been changed in some way.

Monitoring: A planned, systematic, and ongoing process to gather and organize data, and aggregate results in order to evaluate performance.

Monitoring of MCO/PHP Standards: Activities related to the monitoring of standards that have been set for plan structure, operations, and quality improvement/assurance to determine that standards have been established, implemented, and adhered to.

Morbidity: A diseased state, often used in the context of a "morbidity rate"—the rate of disease or proportion of diseased people in a population. In common clinical usage, any disease state, including diagnosis and complications is referred to as morbidity.

Morbidity rate: The rate of illness in a population. The number of people ill during a time period divided by the number of people in the total population.

Mortality rate: The death rate often made explicit for a particular characteristic (e.g. gender, sex, or specific cause of death). Mortality rate contains three essential elements: the number of people in a population exposed to the risk of death (denominator), a time factor, and the number of deaths occurring in the exposed population during a certain time period (the numerator).

MR/UR (Medical Review/Utilization Review): Contractor reviews of Medicare claims to ensure that the service was necessary and appropriate.

MSA: Metropolitan Statistical Area

MSP: Medicare Secondary Payor

MUA: Medically Underserved Area

Multi-employer group health plan: A group health plan that is sponsored jointly by two or more employers or by employers and employee organizations.

Multiple coding: Refers to the need to use more than one ICD-9-CM code to fully identify coding for a condition.

Multiple employer plan: A health plan sponsored by two or more employers. These are generally plans that are offered through membership in an association or a trade group.

Multiple signatures: It will be possible for multiple parties to sign a document. Multiple signatures are conceptually and simply appended to the document.

National coverage policy: A policy developed by CMS that indicates whether and under what circumstances certain services are covered under the Medicare program. It is published in CMS regulations, published in the Federal Register as a final notice, contained in a CMS ruling, or issued as a program instruction.

National Improvement Projects: Health care quality improvement projects developed by a group consisting of representatives of some or all of the following groups: CMS, Public Health Service, Networks, renal provider, and consumer communities. The object is to use statistical analysis to identify better patterns of care and outcomes, and to feed the results of the analysis back into the provider community to improve the quality of care provided to renal Medicare beneficiaries. Each project has a particular clinical focus.

National standard per visit rates: National rates for each six home health disciplines based on historical claims data. Used in payment of LUPAs and calculation of outliers.

NCQA: National Council for Quality Assurance

NCSC: National Computer Security Center

NCVHS: National Committee on Vital and Health Statistics

Need-to-know procedures for personnel access: A security principle stating that a user should have access only to the data he or she needs to perform a particular function.

NIST: National Institutes of Standards and Technology

No-fault insurance: Automobile insurance that provides coverage against injury or loss without the need to determine responsibility for an accident.

Noncontributory or deemed wage credits: Wages and wages-in-kind that were not subject to the HI tax but are deemed as having been. Deemed wage credits exist for the purposes of (1) determining HI program eligibility for individuals who might not be eligible for HI coverage without payment of a premium were it not for the deemed wage credits; and (2) calculating reimbursement due the HI trust fund from the general fund of the Treasury. The first purpose applies in the case of providing coverage to persons during the transitional periods when the HI program began and when it was expanded to cover federal employees; both purposes apply in the cases of military service wage credits and deemed wage credits granted for the internment of persons of Japanese ancestry during World War II.

Non-covered service: A service that does not meet the requirements of a Medicare benefit category, that is statutorily excluded from coverage on grounds other than 1862(a)(1), or is not reasonable and necessary under 1862(a)(1).

Non-entity assets: Assets that are held by an entity but are not available to the entity. These are also amounts that, when collected, cannot be spent by the reporting entity.

Nonparticipating physician (Medicare): A physician who does not sign a Medicare participation agreement, and therefore is not obligated to accept assignment on all claims. Frequently defined as NonPar. See Participating Physician.

Nonrepudiation: Strong and substantial evidence of message integrity and of the identity of the signer, sufficient to prevent a party from successfully denying the origin, submission or delivery of the message and the integrity of its contents.

NUBC: National Uniform Billing Committee

NUCC: National Uniform Claim Committee

Nursing Facility: A facility which primarily provides skilled nursing care and relate to residents. It also provides services for the rehabilitation of injured, disabled, or sick persons on a regular basis. It is health related care services above the level of custodial care to other than mentally retarded individuals.

Obligation: Budgeted funds committed to be spent.

Office: Location, other than a hospital, skilled nursing facility (SNF), military treatment facility, community health center, state or local public health clinic, or intermediate care facility (ICF), where the health professional routinely provides health examinations, diagnosis, and treatment of illness or injury on an ambulatory basis.

Offset: The recovery by Medicare of a non-Medicare debt by reducing present or future Medicare payments and applying the amount withheld to the indebtedness. (Examples are Public Health Service debts or Medicaid debts recovered by CMS). See also Recoupment and Suspension of Payments.

OHMO: Office of Health Maintenance Organizations. A department of DHHS which has the responsibility for directing the federal HMO program.

OIG: Office of the Inspector General

Old-Age, Survivors, and Disability Insurance (OASDI): The Social Security programs that pay for (1) monthly cash benefits to retired-worker (old-age) beneficiaries, their spouses and children, and survivors of deceased insured workers; and (2) monthly cash benefits to disabled-worker beneficiaries and their spouses and children, and for providing rehabilitation services to the disabled.

Ombudsman: An ombudsman is an individual who assists enrollees in resolving problems they may have with their MCO/PHP. An ombudsman is a neutral party who works with the enrollee, the MCO/PHP, and the provider (as appropriate) to resolve individual enrollee problems.

On-site reviews: Reviews performed on-site at the MCO/PHP health care delivery system sites to assess the physical resources and operational practices in place to deliver health care.

OPM: Office of Personnel Management. The federal agency that administers and directs the Federal Employees Health Benefits (FEHP) plans.

Organ: Refers to a human kidney, liver, heart, or pancreas.

Organ procurement: The process of acquiring donor kidneys in the ESRD program.

Organ Procurement Organization (OPO): An organization that performs or coordinates the retrieval, preservation, and transportation of organs and maintains a system of locating prospective recipients for available organs.

Other managed care arrangement: Used if the plan is not considered either a PCCM, PHP, Comprehensive MCO, Medicaid-only MCO, or HIO.

Other unlisted facility: Other service facilities not previously identified.

Outcome: The result of performance (or nonperformance) of a function or process. The consequences of a medical intervention on a group of patients.

Outcome data: Data that measure the health status of people enrolled in managed care resulting from specific medical and health interventions (for example, the incident of measles among plan enrollees during the calendar year).

Outcome indicator: An indicator that assesses what happens or does not happen to a patient following a process; agreed upon desired patient characteristics to be achieved; undesired patient conditions to be avoided.

Outlay: The issuance of checks, disbursement of cash, or electronic transfer of funds made to liquidate an expense regardless of the fiscal year the service was provided or the expense was incurred. When used in the discussion of the Medicaid program, outlays refer to amounts advanced to the states for Medicaid benefits.

Outlier: Additions to a full episode payment in cases where costs of services delivered are estimated to exceed a fixed loss threshold. Outliers are computed as part of Medicare claims payment by pricer software.

Outpatient hospital: A portion of a hospital which provides diagnostic, therapeutic (both surgical and nonsurgical), and rehabilitation services to sick or injured persons who do not require hospitalization or institutionalization. Part of a hospital providing services covered by SMI, including services in an emergency room or outpatient clinic, ambulatory surgical procedures, medical supplies such as splints, or laboratory tests billed by the hospital.

Overpayment assessment: A decision that an incorrect amount of money has been paid for Medicare services and a determination of what that amount is.

Overvalued procedure: A procedure considered to be overpriced based on its relative value.

Panel size: Means the number of patients served by a physician or physician group. If the panel size is greater than 25,000 patients, then the physician group is not considered to be at substantial financial risk because the risk is spread over the large number of patients. Stop loss and beneficiary surveys would not be required.

PAR: Participating Physician and Supplier Program

Part A: The Medicare Hospital Insurance program which covers hospital and related post-hospital services. As an entitlement program, it is available without payment of a premium. Beneficiaries are responsible for an initial deductible per spell of illness and coinsurance for some services.

Part A premium: A monthly premium paid by or on behalf of individuals who wish for and are entitled to voluntary enrollment in the Medicare Hospital Insurance (HI) program. These individuals are those who are aged 65 and older, are uninsured for social security or railroad retirement, and do not otherwise meet the requirements for entitlement to Part A. Disabled individuals who have exhausted other entitlement are also qualified. These individuals are those not now entitled but who have been entitled under section 226(b) of the Act, who continue to have the disabling impairment upon which their entitlement was based, and whose entitlement ended solely because the individuals had earnings that exceeded the substantial gainful activity amount (as defined in section 223(d)(4) of the Act).

Part B: The Medicare Supplementary Medical Insurance program (SMI), which covers the costs of physician services, outpatient lab, x-ray, DME and certain other services. As a voluntary program, Part B requires payment of a monthly premium. Beneficiaries are responsible for a deductible and coinsurance payment for most covered services.

Part B of Medicare: Medicare Supplementary Medical Insurance also referred to as "SMI." Medicare insurance that pays for inpatient hospital stay, care in a skilled nursing facility, home health care, and hospice care. Part B is the supplementary or "physicians" insurance portion of Medicare. It was established in Title XVIII of the Social Security Act of 1965 as amended, and covers services of physicians/other suppliers, outpatient care, medical equipment and supplies, and other medical services not covered by the hospital insurance part of Medicare.

Partial Capitation (PAR): A plan is paid for providing services to enrollees through a combination of capitation and fee-for-service reimbursements.

Partially Capitated (PAR): A stipulated dollar amount established for certain health care services while other services are reimbursed on a cost or fee-for-service basis.

Participating hospitals: Those hospitals that participate in the Medicare program.

Participating physician: A physician who signs a participation agreement, agreeing to accept assignment on all Medicare claims for a period of one year. Frequently referred to as PAR.

Participating physician and supplier program (PAR): a program which provides financial and administrative incentives for physicians and suppliers to agree in advance to accept assignment on all Medicare claims for a period of one year.

Password: Confidential authentication information composed of a string of characters.

Pattern analysis: The clinical and statistical analysis of data sets. Frequently used ESRD data sets include the PMMIS, USRDS, the core indicators, Network files, or CMS analytic files.

Pay-as-you-go financing: A financing scheme in which taxes are scheduled to produce just as much income as required to pay current benefits, with trust fund assets built up only to the extent needed to prevent exhaustion of the fund by random fluctuations.

Payment rate: The total amount paid for each unit of service rendered by a healthcare provider, including both the amount covered by the insurer and the consumer's cost sharing.

Payment safeguards: Activities to prevent and recover inappropriate Medicare benefit payments including MSP, MR/UR, provider audits, and fraud and abuse detection.

Payment suspension: Suspension of Payments.

Payroll taxes: Taxes levied on the gross wages of workers.

PCF: Patient Compensation Fund

Peer review: Evaluation of a physician's performance by other physicians, usually within the same geographic area and medical specialty.

Peer Review Organization (PRO): An organization that reviews the medical necessity and the quality of care provided to Medicare beneficiaries to ensure that health care services are medically necessary, appropriate, provided in a proper setting, and are of acceptable quality.

Percentile: A number that corresponds to one of the equal divisions of the range of a variable in a given sample and that characterizes a value of the variable as not exceeded by a specified percentage of all the values in the sample. For example, a score higher that 97 percent of those attained is said to be in the 97th percentile.

Performance: The way in which an individual, group, or organization carries out or accomplishes its important functions or processes.

Performance assessment: Involves the analysis and interpretation of performance measurement data to transform it into useful information for purposes of continuous performance improvement.

Performance improvement projects: Projects that examine and seek to achieve improvement in major areas of clinical and non-clinical services. These projects are usually based on information such as enrollee characteristics, standardized measures, utilization, diagnosis and outcome information, data from surveys, and grievance and appeals processes. They measure performance at two periods of time to ascertain if improvement has occurred. These projects are required by the state and can be of the MCO/PHPs choosing or prescribed by the state.

Performance measures: A gauge used to assess the performance of a process or function of any organization. Quantitative or qualitative measures of the care and services delivered to enrollees (process) or the end result of that care and services (outcomes). Performance measures can be used to assess other aspects of an individual or organization's performance such as access and availability of care, utilization of care, health plan stability, beneficiary characteristics, and other structural and operational aspects of health care services. Performance measures included here may include measures calculated by the state (from encounter data or another data source) or measures submitted by the MCO/PHP.

Peritoneal dialysis: A procedure that introduces dialysate into the abdominal cavity to remove waste products through the peritoneum (a membrane which surrounds the intestines and other organs in the abdominal cavity). It functions in a manner similar to that of the artificial semi-permeable membrane in the hemodialysis machine. Three forms of peritoneal dialysis are continuous ambulatory peritoneal dialysis, continuous cycling peritoneal dialysis, and intermittent peritoneal dialysis.

Personnel clearance procedure: A protective measure applied to determine that an individual's access to sensitive unclassified automated information is admissible. The need for and extent of a screening process is normally based on an assessment of risk, cost, benefit, and feasibility as well as other protective measures in place. Effective screening processes are applied in such a way as to allow a range of implementation, from minimal procedures to more stringent procedures commensurate with the sensitivity of the data to be accessed and the magnitude of harm or loss that could be caused by the individual.

Personnel security: The procedures established to ensure that all personnel who have access to sensitive information have the required authority as well as appropriate clearances.

Personnel security policy/procedure: Formal, documentation of policies and procedures established to ensure that all personnel who have access to sensitive information have the required authority as well as appropriate clearances.

Physical access controls (limited access): Those formal, documented policies and procedures to be followed to limit physical access to an entity while ensuring that properly authorized access is allowed.

Physical safeguards: Protection of physical computer systems and related buildings and equipment from fire and other natural and environmental hazards, as well as from intrusion. Also covers the use of locks, keys, and administrative measures used to control access to computer systems and facilities.

Physician group: A partnership, association, corporation, individual practice association (IPA), or other group that distributes income from the practice among members. An IPA is considered to be a physician group only if it is composed of individual physicians and has no subcontracts with other physician groups.

Physician Hospital Organization (PHO): A separate legal entity owned by a hospital and participating physicians which can contract with health insurance companies, HMOs or self-insured employers for the provision of medical services.

Physician Incentive Plan (PIP): Any compensation arrangement at any contracting level between an MCO and a physician or physician group that may directly or indirectly have the effect of reducing or limiting services furnished to Medicare or Medicaid enrollees in the MCO. MCOs must disclose physician incentive plans between the MCO itself and individual physicians and groups and, also, between groups or intermediate entities (for example, certain IPAs or Physician-Hospital Organizations) and individual physicians and groups. *See* 42 C.F.R. 1 422.208(a).

Physicians Practice Cost and Income Survey (PPCIS): A survey sponsored by CMS of a national sample of physicians regarding practice characteristics, costs and reimbursement, conducted by the National Opinion Research Center in 1984 with a follow-up in 1987.

PIN: Personal Identification Number. A code used to report performing physicians and group numbers. PIN stands for Provider Identification Number and is commonly known as the provider number.

PLI: Professional Liability Insurance

Point-of-service plan: A managed care plan that combines features of both prepaid and fee-for-service health insurance. Health plan enrollees decide whether to use network or non-network providers at the time care is needed and usually are charged sizable copayments for selecting the latter.

Policy/guidelines on work station use: Documented instructions and procedures delineating the proper functions to be performed at an employees workstation, the manner in which those functions are to be performed, and the physical attributes of the surroundings, of a specific computer terminal site or type of site, dependant upon the sensitivity of the information accessed from that site.

Policy holder: See Insured.

Postpayment review: The review of a claim after a determination and payment has been made to the provider or beneficiary.

Potential fraud case: A case developed after the PSC has substantiated an allegation of fraud.

Potential payments: The maximum anticipated total payments (based on the most recent year's utilization and experience and any current or anticipated factors that may affect payment amounts) that could be received if use or costs of referral services were low enough. These payments include amounts paid for services furnished or referred by the physician/group, plus amounts paid for administrative costs. The only payments not included in potential payments are bonuses or other compensation not based on referrals (for example, bonuses based on patient satisfaction or other quality of care factors).

PPO: Preferred Provider Organization

PPRC: Physician Payment Review Commission

PPS: Prospective Payment System

Practice expense: The cost of nonphysician resources incurred by the physician to provide physician services. Examples are salaries and the cost of fringe benefits received by nurses, physician assistants and receptionists who are employed by the physician, and the expenses associated with purchase and use of medical equipment and supplies in the physician's office.

Practice guidelines: Clinical recommendations for patient care, based on knowledge of effectiveness of medical practices and procedures.

Preauthorization: See Precertification.

Precertification: The process of obtaining permission to perform a service from the health insurance carrier before the service is performed. Sometimes referred to as preauthorization.

Predetermination: The process of obtaining an estimate of what an health insurance carrier will pay for service(s) before the service(s) is/are performed.

Preferred Provider Organization (PPO): A managed care health plan that contracts with networks or panels of providers to furnish services and be paid on a negotiated fee schedule. Enrollees are offered a financial incentive to use providers on the preferred list, but may use non-network providers as well. See Social Security Act Section 1852(e)(2)(D), 42 U.S.C. 1139w-22(e)(2)(D).

Premium: An amount paid periodically to purchase medical health insurance benefits.

Prepaid Health Plan (PHP): A prepaid managed care entity that provides less than comprehensive services on an at-risk basis or one that provides any benefit package on a non-risk basis.

Prepayment review: The review of claims prior to determination and payment.

Present value: The lump-sum amount of a future stream of payments that, if invested today, together with interest earnings would be just enough to meet each of the payments as it fell due. At the time of the last payment, the invested fund would be exactly zero.

Prevailing charge: One of the factors determining a physician's payment for service under Medicare. Currently set at the 75th percentile of customary charges for all physicians in a locality.

Prevalence: The number of existing cases of a disease or condition in a given population at a specific time.

Pricer: Software modules in Medicare claims processing systems, specific to certain benefits, used in pricing claims, most often under prospective payment systems.

Primary Care Case Management (PCCM): A program where the state contracts directly with primary care providers who agree to be responsible for the provision and/or coordination of medical services to Medicaid recipients under their care. Currently, most PCCM programs pay the primary care physician a monthly case management fee in addition to reimbursing services on a fee-for-service basis.

Primary Care Case Management Provider: A provider (usually a physician, physician group practice, or an entity employing or having other arrangements with such physicians, but sometimes also including nurse practitioners, nurse midwives, or physician assistants) who contracts to locate, coordinate, and monitor covered primary care (and sometimes additional services).

Primary carrier: The health insurance carrier which has first responsibility under Coordination of Benefits.

Primary code: The ICD-9-CM code that defines the main reason for the current encounter.

PRO: See Peer Review Organization

Procedure for emergency access: Documented instructions for obtaining necessary information during a crisis.

Procedures for verifying access authorizations prior to physical access: Formal, documented policies and instructions for validating the access privileges of an entity prior to granting those privileges.

Process: The goal-directed, interrelated series of actions, events, mechanisms, or steps.

Process improvement: A methodology utilized to make improvements to a process through the use of continuous quality improvement methods.

Process indicator: A gauge that measures a goal-directed interrelated series of actions, events, mechanisms, or steps.

Productivity investments: Spending aimed at increasing contractor operational efficiency and productivity through improved work methods, or application of technology.

Professional component: The part of the relative value or fee for a procedure that represents physician work.

Professional Liability Insurance (PLI): The health insurance physicians must purchase to help protect themselves from the financial risks associated with malpractice claims and awards.

Profiles: Data segregated by specific time period (quarterly, annually) and target area (facility, state) for the purpose of identifying patterns.

Profiling: Expressing a pattern of practice as a rate (costs or services) or outcome (morbidity, mortality) collected over time for a defined population of patients to compare with other practice patterns.

Program management: CMS operational account. Program management supplies the agency with the resources to administer Medicare, the Federal portion of Medicaid, and other Agency responsibilities. The components of program management are Medicare contractors, survey and certification, research, and administrative costs.

Program Management and Medical Information System (PMMIS): An automated system of records that contains records primarily of current Medicare-eligible ESRD patients, but also maintains historical information on people no longer classified as ESRD patients because of death or successful transplantation or recovery of renal function. The PMMIS contains medical information on patients and the services that they received during the course of their therapy. In addition, it contains information on ESRD facilities and facility payment. Beginning January 1, 1995, the PMMIS collects information on all dialysis and kidney transplant patients.

Projection error: Degree of variation between estimated and actual amounts.

Proof of eligibility: Evidence of eligibility for health insurance benefits.

ProPAC: Prospective Payment Assessment Committee

Prospective Payment System (PPS): A method of reimbursement in which Medicare payment is made based on a predetermined, fixed amount. The payment amount for a particular service is derived based on the classification system of that service (for example, DRGs for inpatient hospital services).

Protected Health Information (PIH): Individually identifiable health information transmitted or maintained in any form or medium, which is held by a covered entity or its business associate. Identifies the individual or offers a reasonable basis for identification. Is created or received by a covered entity or an employer. Relates to a past, present, or future physical or mental condition, provision of health care or payment for health care.

Provider: Any Medicare provider (for example, hospital, skilled nursing facility, home health agency, outpatient physical therapy, comprehensive outpatient rehabilitation facility, end-stage renal disease facility, hospice, physician, non-physician provider, laboratory, supplier) providing medical services covered under Medicare Part B. Any organization, institution, or individual that provides health care services to Medicare beneficiaries. Physicians, ambulatory surgical centers, and outpatient clinics are some of the providers of services covered under Medicare Part B.

Provider survey data: Data collected through a survey or focus group of providers who participate in the Medicaid program and have provided services to enrolled Medicaid beneficiaries. The state or a contractor of the state may conduct the survey.

Proxy: An index of known values that likely approximates an index for which values are unavailable. The proxy is used as a "stand-in" for the unavailable index.

Psychiatric facility (partial hospitalization): A facility for the diagnosis and treatment of mental illness on a 24-hour basis by, or under, the supervision of a physician.

Psychiatric residential treatment center: A facility or distinct part of a facility for psychiatric care that provides a total 24-hour therapeutically planned and professionally staffed group living and learning environment.

Public key: One of the two keys used in an asymmetric encryption system. The public key is made public, to be used in conjunction with a corresponding private key.

QA: Quality Assurance

QMB: Qualified Medicare Beneficiary

Quality: Defined by the Institute of Medicine as the degree to which health services for individuals and populations increase the likelihood of desired outcomes and are consistent with current professional knowledge.

Railroad retirement: A federal insurance program similar to Social Security designed for workers in the railroad industry. The provisions of the Railroad Retirement Act provide for a system of coordination and financial interchange between the Railroad Retirement program and the Social Security program.

Random sample: A random sample is a group selected for study, which is drawn at random from the universe of cases by a statistically valid method.

Rate setting: An approach to cost containment where the government establishes payment rates for all payers for various categories of health services.

RBRVS: Resource Based Relative Value Scale. A government mandated relative value system, based on a study conducted at Harvard University, that is to be used for calculating national fee schedules for services provided to Medicare patients.

Real-wage differential: The difference between the percentage increases before rounding in (1) the average annual wage in covered employment, and (2) the average annual CPI.

Reasonable charge: The amount Medicare will pay for a covered service. This is usually the lowest of the actual, customary and prevailing charges.

Reasonable cost: FIs and carriers use CMS guidelines to determine reasonable costs incurred by individual providers in furnishing covered services to enrollees. Reasonable cost is based on the actual cost of providing such services, including direct and indirect cost of providers and excluding any costs that are unnecessary in the efficient delivery of services covered by the program.

Reasonable-cost basis: The calculation to determine the reasonable cost incurred by individual providers when furnishing covered services to beneficiaries. The reasonable cost is based on the actual cost of providing such services, including direct and indirect costs of providers, and excluding any costs that are unnecessary in the efficient delivery of services covered by a health insurance program.

Recipient: An individual covered by the Medicaid program. Now referred to as a beneficiary.

Recoupment: The recovery by Medicare of any Medicare debt by reducing present or future Medicare payments and applying the amount withheld to the indebtedness.

Referral services: Means any specialty, inpatient, outpatient, or laboratory services that are ordered or arranged, but not furnished directly. Certain situations may exist that should be considered referral services for purposes of determining if a physician/group is at substantial financial risk. For example, an MCO may require a physician group/physician to authorize "retroactive" referrals for emergency care received outside the MCO's network. If the physician group/physician's payment from the MCO can be affected by the utilization of emergency care, such as a bonus if emergency referrals are low, then these emergency services are considered referral services and need to be included in the calculation of substantial financial risk. Also, if a physician group contracts with an individual physician or another group to provide services that the initial group cannot provide itself, any services referred to the contracted physician group/physician should be considered referral services.

Regional Office (RO): CMS has ten ROs that work closely together with Medicare contractors in their assigned geographical areas on a day-to-day basis. Four of these ROs monitor network contractor performance, negotiate contractor budgets, distribute administrative monies to contractors, work with contractors when corrective actions are needed, and provide a variety of other liaison services to the contractors in their respective regions.

Rehabilitation: A restorative process through which an individual with ESRD develops and maintains self-sufficient functioning consistent with his/her capability.

Reject status: The encounter data did not pass the "front-end" edit process. M+C organization needs to correct the data and resubmit.

Relative Value (RV): A value that reflects a comparison with an arbitrary standard.

Relative value scale: An index that assigns specific numeric values to medical services. Multiplying the relative value by a conversion factor results in a fee.

Release of information: The patient's signature indicating consent to the release of information necessary for settlement of his or her health insurance claim.

Removal from access lists: The physical eradication of an entity's access privileges.

Removal of user account(s): The termination or deletion of an individual's access privileges to the information, services, and resources for which they currently have clearance, authorization, and need-to-know when such clearance, authorization and need-to-know no longer exists.

Renal transplant center: A hospital unit that is approved to furnish transplantation and other medical and surgical specialty services directly for the care of ESRD transplant patients, including inpatient dialysis furnished directly or under arrangement.

Reopening: An action taken, after all appeal rights are exhausted, to re-examine or question the correctness of a determination, a decision, or cost report otherwise final.

Report procedures: The documented formal mechanism employed to document security incidents.

Residential substance abuse treatment facility: A facility which provides treatment for substance (alcohol and drug) abuse to live-in residents who do not require acute medical care. Services include individual and group therapy and counseling, family counseling, laboratory tests, drugs and supplies, psychological testing, and room and board.

Residual: The long-term condition(s) resulting from a previous acute illness or injury.

Residual factors: Factors other than price, including volume of services, intensity of services, and age/sex changes.

Resource-Based Relative Value Scale (RBRVS) : A scale of national uniform relative values for all physicians' services. The relative value of each service must be the sum of relative value units representing physicians' work, practice expenses net of malpractice expenses, and the cost of professional liability insurance.

Resource costs: The costs of the inputs used by an efficient physician to provide a service or procedure, including both the costs of the physician's own time and effort and the costs of nonphysician inputs. The apparently redundant use of "resource" with "costs" is a convention used to indicate the average costs of an efficient physician, as distinguished from cost-based reimbursement such as that used for hospitals prior to the prospective payment system.

Response procedures: The documented formal rules/instructions for actions to be taken as a result of the receipt of a security incident report.

Revenue: The recognition of income earned and the use of appropriated capital from the rendering of services in the current period.

Revenue code: Payment codes for services or items in FL 42 of the UB-92 found in Medicare and/or NUBC (National Uniform Billing Committee) manuals (42X, 43X, etc.).

Review of claims: Using information on a claim or other information requested to support the services billed, to make a determination.

Rights of individuals: Rights provided to individuals under HIPAA legislation include the right to: receive notice of information practices, see and copy own records, request corrections, obtain accounting of disclosures, request restrictions and confidential communications, and file complaints.

Risk analysis: A process whereby cost-effective security/control measures may be selected by balancing the costs of various security/control measures against the losses that would be expected if these measures were not in place.

Risk-based Health Maintenance Organization (HMO)/Competitive Medical Plan (CMP): A type of managed care organization. After any applicable deductible or co-payment, all of an enrollee/member's medical care costs are paid for in return for a monthly premium. However, due to the "lock-in" provision, all of the enrollee/member's services (except for out-of-area emergency services) must be arranged for by the risk-HMO. Should the Medicare enrollee/member choose to obtain service not arranged for by the plan, he/she will be liable for the costs. Neither the HMO nor the Medicare program will pay for services from providers that are not part of the HMO's health care system/network.

Risk management: Risk is the possibility of something adverse happening. Risk management is the process of assessing risk, taking steps to reduce risk to an acceptable level and maintaining that level of risk.

Role-Based Access Control (RBAC): An alternative to traditional access control models (discretionary or non-discretionary access control policies) that permits the specification and enforcement of enterprise-specific security policies in a way that maps more naturally to an organization's structure and business activities. With RBAC, rather than attempting to map an organization's security policy to a relatively low-level set of technical controls (typically, access control lists), each user is assigned to one or more predefined roles, each of which has been assigned the various privileges needed to perform that role.

Rule out: Refers to a method used to indicate that a condition is probable, suspected or questionable but unconfirmed.

Rural Health Clinic (RHC): An outpatient facility that is primarily engaged in furnishing physicians' and other medical and health services and that meets other requirements designated to ensure the health and safety of individuals served by the clinic. The clinic must be located in a medically under-served area that is not urbanized as defined by the U.S. Bureau of Census.

RVS: Relative Value Scale

RVU: Relative Value Unit

Sanction policy: Organizations must have policies and procedures regarding disciplinary actions which are communicated to all employees, agents and contractors. For example, verbal warnings, notice of disciplinary action placed in personnel files, removal of system privileges, termination of employment, or contract penalties (ASTM E 1869). In addition to enterprise sanctions, employees, agents, and contractors must be advised of civil or criminal penalties for misuse or misappropriation of health information. Employees, agents and contractors, must be made aware that violations may result in notification to law enforcement officials and regulatory, accreditation and licensure organizations.

Sanctions: Administrative remedies and actions (exclusion or civil monetary penalties) available to the Office of the Inspector General (OIG) to deal with questionable, improper, or abusive behaviors of providers under the Medicare, Medicaid, or any state health programs.

Schedule of allowances: A list of specific amounts which the carrier will pay toward the cost of medical services provided.

SDO: Standards Development Organization

Secondary carrier: The health insurance carrier which is second in responsibility under Coordination of Benefits.

Secondary code: ICD-9-CM code(s) listed after the primary code that further indicate the cause(s) for the current encounter or define the need for higher levels of care.

Secretary: The Secretary of Health and Human Services.

Secure work station location: Physical safeguards to eliminate or minimize the possibility of unauthorized access to information. For example, locating a terminal used to access sensitive information in a locked room and restricting access to that room to authorized personnel or by not placing a terminal used to access patient information in any area of a doctor's office where the screen contents can be viewed from the reception area.

Security: Security encompasses all of the safeguards in an information system, including hardware, software, personnel policies, information practice policies, disaster preparedness, and the oversight of all these areas. The purpose of security is to protect both the system and the information it contains from unauthorized access from without and from misuse from within. Through various security measures, a health information system can shield confidential information from unauthorized access, disclosure and misuse, thus protecting privacy of the individuals who are the subjects of the stored data.

Security awareness training: All employees, agents, and contractors must participate in information security awareness training programs. Based on job responsibilities, individuals may be required to attend customized education programs that focus on issues regarding use of health information and responsibilities regarding confidentiality and security.

Security configuration management: Measures, practices and procedures for the security of information systems should be coordinated and integrated with each other and other measures, practices and procedures of the organization so as to create a coherent system of security. (OECD Guidelines, as cited in NIST Pub 800-14).

Security incident procedures: Formal, documented instructions for reporting security breaches.

Security management process: A process that encompasses the creation, administration and oversight of policies to ensure the prevention, detection, containment, and correction of security breaches. It involves risk analysis and risk management, including the establishment of accountability, management controls (policies and education), electronic controls, physical security, and penalties for the abuse and misuse of its assets, both physical and electronic.

Security policy: The framework within which an organization establishes needed levels of information security to achieve the desired confidentiality goals. A policy is a statement of information values, protection responsibilities, and organization commitment for a system (OTA, 1993). The American Health Information Management Association recommends that security policies apply to all employees, medical staff members, volunteers, students, faculty, independent contractors, and agents.

Security testing: A process used to determine that the security features of a system are implemented as designed and that they are adequate for a proposed applications environment. This process includes hands-on functional testing, penetration testing, and verification.

Self-dialysis: Dialysis performed with little or no professional assistance (except in emergency situations) by an ESRD patient who has completed an appropriate course of training, in a dialysis facility or at home.

Self-employment: Operation of a trade or business by an individual or by a partnership in which an individual is a member.

Self-Employment Contribution Act (SECA) Payroll Tax: Medicare's share of SECA is used to fund the HI trust fund.

Sequencing: The process of listing procedure and/or diagnosis codes in the proper order on the health insurance claim form.

Sequester: The reduction of funds to be used for benefits or administrative costs from a federal account based on the requirements specified in the Gramm-Rudman-Hollings Act.

Service: Medical care and items such as medical diagnosis and treatment, drugs and biologicals, supplies, appliances, equipment, medical social services, and use of hospital or SNF facilities (42 CFR 400.202).

Severity modifier: An adjustment that reflects the effect of patient factors, such as severity of illness, comorbidity, or risk of complications, on the relative work required to deliver a service.

Short range: The next 10 years.

Site-of-service differential: The difference in the amount paid when the same service is performed in different practice settings, for example, an outpatient visit in a physician's office or a hospital clinic.

Skilled Nursing Facility (SNF): A facility (which meets specific regulatory certification requirements) which primarily provides inpatient skilled nursing care and related services to patients who require medical, nursing, or rehabilitative services but does not provide the level of care or treatment available in a hospital.

SMI: Supplementary Medical Insurance. Medicare Part B which helps pay for services other than hospital (Part A) services.

SMI premium: Monthly premium paid by those individuals who have enrolled in the voluntary SMI program.

SMS: Socioeconomic Monitoring System

SNF coinsurance: For the 21st through 100th day of extended care services in a benefit period, a daily amount for which the beneficiary is responsible, equal to one-eighth of the inpatient hospital deductible.

Social Security Act: Public Law 74-271, enacted on August 14, 1935, with subsequent amendments. The Social Security Act consists of 20 titles, four of which have been repealed. The HI and SMI programs are authorized by Title XVIII of the Social Security Act.

Social Security Administration (SSA): The Federal agency that, among other things, determines initial entitlement to and eligibility for Medicare benefits.

Socioeconomic Monitoring System (SMS): A system of annual and supplemental surveys of physicians directed by the American Medical Association Center for Health Policy Research. The SMS provides information on a range of characteristics including physician's earnings, expense, work patterns, and fees.

Special public-debt obligation: Securities the U.S. Government issued exclusively to the OASI, DI, HI, and SMI trust funds and other federal trust funds. Section 1841(a) of the Social Security Act provides that the public-debt obligations issued for purchase by the SMI trust fund shall have maturities fixed with due regard for the needs of the funds. The usual practice in the past has been to spread the holdings of special issues, as of every June 30, so that the amounts maturing in each of the next 15 years are approximately equal. Special public-debt obligations are redeemable at par at any time.

Specialty contractor: A Medicare contractor that performs a limited Medicare function, such as coordination of benefits, and statistical analysis.

Specialty differential: A difference in the amount paid for the same service when performed by physicians in different specialties. Eliminated from the Medicare program in 1992.

Specificity: Refers to the requirement to code to the highest number of digits possible when selecting ICD-9-CM codes.

Spell of illness: A period of consecutive days, beginning with the first day on which a beneficiary is furnished inpatient hospital or extended care services, and ending with the close of the first period of 60 consecutive days thereafter in which the beneficiary is in neither a hospital nor a skilled nursing facility.

SSI: Supplemental Security Income

Staff assisted dialysis: Dialysis performed by the staff of the renal dialysis center or facility.

Staff model HMO: An HMO in which physicians practice solely as employees of the HMO and usually are paid a salary.

Standard claims processing system: Certain computer systems currently used by carriers and Fiscal Intermediaries to process Medicare claims. For physician and lab claims, the system is Electronic Data Systems (EDS); for facility and other Part A provider claims the system is the Fiscal Intermediary Standard System (FISS), formerly known as the Florida Shared System (FSS); and for supplier claims the system is the Viable Information Processing System (VIPS).

State certification: Inspections of Medicare provider facilities to ensure compliance with Federal health, safety, and program standards.

State licensure agency: A state agency that has the authority to terminate, sanction, or prosecute fraudulent providers under state law.

State or local public health clinic: A facility maintained by either state or local health departments that provides ambulatory primary medical care under the general direction of a physician.

State survey: Under 11864 of the Act, CMS has entered into agreements with agencies of state governments, typically the agency that licenses health facilities within the state Health Departments, to conduct surveys of Medicare participating providers and suppliers for purposes of determining compliance with Medicare requirements for participation in the Medicare program.

Status location: An indicator on a claim record describing the queue where the claim is currently situated and the action that needs to be performed on the claim.

Stochastic model: An analysis involving a random variable. For example, a stochastic model may include a frequency distribution for one assumption. From the frequency distribution, possible outcomes for the assumption are selected randomly for use in an illustration.

Subject/object separation: Access to a subject does not guarantee access to the objects associated with that subject. Subject is defined as an active entity, generally in the form of a person, process, or device that causes information to flow among objects or changes the system state. Technically, a process/domain pair. (Glossary of INFOSEC and INFOSEC Related Terms—Idaho state University) Object is defined as a passive entity that contains or receives information. Access to an object potentially implies access to the information it contains. Examples of objects are: records blocks, pages, segments, files, directories, directory trees, and programs, as well as bits, bytes, words, fields, processors, video displays, keyboards, clocks, printers, network nodes, etc. A type of access control.

Subscriber: See Insured.

Substantial financial risk: Means an incentive arrangement that places the physician or physician group at risk for amounts beyond the risk threshold, if the risk is based on the use or costs of referral services. The risk threshold is 25%. However, if the patient panel is greater than 25,000 patients, then the physician group is not considered to be at substantial financial risk because the risk is spread over the large number of patients. Stop loss and beneficiary surveys would not be required.

Summarized cost rate: The ratio of the present value of expenditures to the present value of the taxable payroll for the years in a given period. In this context, the expenditures are on an incurred basis and exclude costs for those uninsured persons for whom payments are reimbursed from the general fund of the Treasury, and for voluntary enrollees, who pay a premium in order to be enrolled. The summarized cost rate includes the cost of reaching and maintaining a "target" trust fund level, known as a contingency fund ratio. Because a trust fund level of about 1 year's expenditures is considered to be an adequate reserve for unforeseen contingencies, the targeted contingency fund ratio used in determining summarized cost rates is 100 percent of annual expenditures. Accordingly, the summarized cost rate is equal to the ratio of (1) the sum of the present value of the outgo during the period, plus the present value of the targeted ending trust fund level, plus the beginning trust fund level, to (2) the present value of the taxable payroll during the period.

Summarized income rate: The ratio of (1) the present value of the tax revenues incurred during a given period (from both payroll taxes and taxation of OASDI benefits), to (2) the present value of the taxable payroll for the years in the period.

Superbill: A multi-part form which provides sufficient information so that patients may file their own health insurance claim forms.

Supplemental edit software: A system, outside the Standard Claims Processing System, which allows further automation of claim reviews. It may be designed using the logic, or expertise of a medical professional.

Supplemental health services: Benefits offered by an HMO that exceed their basic health service requirements.

Supplementary Medical Insurance (SMI): The Medicare program that pays for a portion of the costs of physicians' services, outpatient hospital services, and other related medical and health services for voluntarily insured aged and disabled individuals. Also known as Part B.

Supplier: Providers, other than practitioners, of health care services. Under Medicare, these include independent labs, durable medical equipment suppliers, ambulance services, orthotists, prosthetists, and portable X-ray providers.

Survey and certification process: The activity conducted by state survey agencies or other CMS agents under the direction of CMS and within the scope of applicable regulations and operating instructions and under the provisions of 11864 of the Act whereby surveyors determine compliance or noncompliance of Medicare providers and suppliers with applicable Medicare requirements for participation. The survey and certification process for each provider and supplier is outlined in detail in the state Operations and Regional Office Manuals published by CMS.

Suspension of payments: The withholding of payment by an Fiscal Intermediary or carrier from a provider or supplier of an approved Medicare payment amount before a determination of the amount of the overpayment exists.

Sustainable growth rate: A system for establishing goals for the rate of growth in expenditures for physicians' services.

Systematic: Pursuing a defined objective(s) in a planned, step by step manner.

Table of allowances: See Schedule of allowances.

Tabular list: The portion of ICD-9-CM that lists codes and definitions in numeric order. Also known as Volume 1.

Tax and donations: State programs under which funds collected by the state through certain health care related taxes and provider-related donations were used to effectively increase the amount of Federal Medicaid reimbursement without a comparable increase in state Medicaid funding or provider reimbursement levels.

Tax rate: The percentage of taxable earnings, up to the maximum tax base, that is paid for the HI tax.

Taxable earnings: Taxable wages and/or self-employment income under the prevailing annual maximum taxable limit.

Taxable payroll: A weighted average of taxable wages and taxable self-employment income. When multiplied by the combined employee-employer tax rate, it yields the total amount of taxes incurred by employees, employers, and the self-employed for work during the period.

Taxable self-employment income: Net earnings from self-employment—generally above $400 and below the annual maximum taxable amount for a calendar or other taxable year—less any taxable wages in the same taxable year.

Taxable wages: Wages paid for services rendered in covered employment up to the annual maximum taxable amount.

Taxation of benefits: Beginning in 1994, up to 85 percent of an individual's or a couple's OASDI benefits is potentially subject to federal income taxation under certain circumstances. The revenue derived from taxation of benefits in excess of 50 percent, up to 85 percent, is allocated to the HI trust fund.

Taxes: See Payroll taxes.

Technical component: The part of the relative value or fee for a procedure that represents the costs of doing the procedure excluding physician work.

Technical security mechanisms: The processes that are put in place to guard against unauthorized access to data that is transmitted over a communications network.

Technical security services: The processes that are put in place (1) to protect information and (2) to control and monitor individual access to information.

TEFRA: Tax Equity and Fiscal Responsibility Act of 1982. P.L. 97-248, enacted September 1982.

Telephone callback: A method of authenticating the identity of the receiver and sender of information through a series of "questions" and "answers" sent back and forth establishing the identity of each. For example, when the communicating systems exchange a series of identification codes as part of the initiation of a session to exchange information, or when a host computer disconnects the initial session before the authentication is complete, and the host calls the user back to establish a session at a predetermined telephone number.

Term insurance: A type of insurance that is in force for a specified period of time.

Termination procedures: Formal, documented instructions, which include appropriate security measures, for the ending of an employee's employment, or an internal/external user's access.

Testing and revision: (1) Testing and revision of contingency plans refers to the documented process of periodic testing to discover weaknesses in such plans and the subsequent process of revising the documentation if necessary. (2) Testing and revision of programs should be restricted to formally authorized personnel.

Third party administrator (TPA): An administrative organization other than the health insurance company or healthcare provider that collects health insurance premiums, pays claims and provides administrative services.

Token: A physical item used to provide identity. Typically an electronic device that can be inserted in a door or a computer system to obtain access.

Tort reform: Changes in the legal rules governing medical malpractice lawsuits.

Training: Education concerning the vulnerabilities of the health information in an entity's possession and ways to ensure the protection of that information.

Transient patients: Patients who receive treatments on an episodic basis and are not part of a facilities regular caseload (for example, patients who have not been permanently transferred to a facility for ongoing treatments).

Transplant: The surgical procedure that involves removing a functional organ from either a deceased or living donor and implanting it in a patient needing a functional organ to replace their nonfunctional organ.

Transportability: A signed document can be transported (over an insecure network) to another system, while maintaining the integrity of the document.

Trauma Code Development (TCD): An MSP investigation process triggered by receipt of a Medicare claim with a diagnosis indicating traumatic injury.

True negatives: These are eligibles who have not received any services through the managed care plan, as evidenced by the absence of a medical record and any encounter data. True negatives signify potential access problems and should be investigated by the managed care plan.

Trust fund: Separate accounts in the U.S. Treasury, mandated by Congress, whose assets may be used only for a specified purpose. For the SMI trust fund, monies not withdrawn for current benefit payments and administrative expenses are invested in interest-bearing federal securities, as required by law; the interest earned is also deposited in the trust fund.

Trust fund ratio: A short-range measure of the adequacy of the trust fund level. Defined as the assets at the beginning of the year expressed as a percentage of the outgo during the year.

TW: Total Work

UCR [Usual, customary and reasonable]: A method of determining benefits by comparing the physician's charges to those of his or her peers in the same community and specialty.

UI: Urban Institute

Unbundling: The process of coding, billing and requesting payment for services that are generally included in a global charge.

Underwriter: See Carrier.

Unique user identification: The combination name/number assigned and maintained in security procedures for identifying and tracking individual user identity.

Unit input intensity allowance: The amount added to, or subtracted from, the hospital input price index to yield the prospective payment system (PPS) update factor.

Upcoding: The process of selecting a code for a service that is more intense, extensive, or has a higher charge, than the service actually provided.

UPIN [Unique physician identification number]: A unique code number used to identify referring and ordering physicians.

URVG: Uniform Relative Value Guide

Usual, customary, and reasonable: See UCR

User authentication: The provision of assurance of the claimed identity of an entity.

User-based access: A security mechanism used to grant users of a system access based upon the identity of the user.

Utilization management: A process that measures the use of resource such as staff, facilities and services to determine medical necessity, cost effectiveness, and conformity to criteria for best use.

Utilization review: The process of reviewing services provided to determine if those services were medically necessary and appropriate.

Utilization summary data: Data that is aggregated by the capitated managed care entity (for example, the number of primary care visits provided by the plan during the calendar year).

V codes: Specific ICD-9-CM codes used to identify encounters for reasons other than illness or injury, for example, immunization.

Valuation period: A period of years that is considered as a unit for purposes of calculating the status of a trust fund.

Virus checking: A computer program that identifies and disables: 1) A "virus" computer program, typically hidden, that attaches itself to other programs and has the ability to replicate. (Unchecked virus programs result in undesired side effects generally unanticipated by the user.) 2) A type of programmed threat. A code fragment (not an independent program) that reproduces by attaching to another program. It may damage data directly, or it may degrade system performance by taking over system resources which are then not available to authorized users. 3) Code embedded within a program that causes a copy of itself to be inserted in one or more other programs. In addition to propagation, the virus usually performs some unwanted function.

Vocational Rehabilitation (VR): The process of facilitating an individual in the choice of or return to a suitable vocation. When necessary, assisting the patient to obtain training for such a vocation. Vocational rehabilitation can also mean preparing an individual—regardless of age, status (whether U.S. citizen or immigrant) or physical condition (disability other than ESRD)—to cope emotionally, psychologically, and physically with changing circumstances in life, including remaining at school or returning to school, work, or work equivalent (homemaker).

Volume (behavioral) offset: The change in the volume of services that occurs in reaction to a change in fees. A 50 percent volume offset means that half of the savings from fee reductions will be offset by increase volume of services.

Volume performance standard (VPS): A mechanism included in OBRA89 to adjust fee updates based on how annual increases in actual expenditures compare to previously determined performance standard rates of increase.

Voluntary agreement: Agreements between CMS and various insurers and employers to exchange Medicare information and group health plan eligibility information for the purpose of coordinating health benefit payments.

Voluntary enrollee: Certain individuals aged 65 or older or disabled, who are not otherwise entitled to Medicare and who opt to obtain coverage under Part A by paying a monthly premium.

WEDI: Workgroup for Electronic Data Interchange

Withhold: Means a percentage of payment or set dollar amounts that are deducted from the payment to the physician group/physician that may or may not be returned depending on specific predetermined factors.

Workers' compensation: State laws which provide coverage of medical expenses for employees who are injured during performance of their work.

Year of exhaustion: The first year in which a trust fund is unable to pay benefits when due because the assets of the fund are exhausted.

ACRONYMS AND ABBREVIATIONS

To the lay person, medical documents are intimidating, and for good reason. Not only are they filled with lots of Latin terms and phrases, but they also contain an endless assortment of abbreviations. Supposedly these stand for something important, but what?

This chapter is designed to help you answer that question. It translates those seemingly meaningless letters into something meaningful.

Nearly all medical personnel who enter information on a patient's chart write in cryptic symbols. Even medical journals and textbooks rely extensively on such conventions. Deciphering this jargon is vitally important, whether you are a patient taking control of your own healthcare, or a health science student taking a test.

Take for example **A.K.A.**, which many people would read as "also known as." Its predominant medical meaning is "above the knee amputation."

And many abbreviations have more than one meaning. For example, **B.S.** can mean Bachelor of Science, or barium swallow (an x-ray), or blood sugar, or bowel sounds, or Blue Shield. Without a comprehensive list of the possible definitions, as you will find in this book, an inappropriate connotation might be assigned to a term.

Acronyms are words that are formed from the initial letter or letters of words in a phrase. You might already know from television that **MASH** stands for **M**obile **A**rmy **S**urgical **H**ospital. From this book, you will also learn that a **BRAT** is a diet of **b**ananas, **r**ice cereal, **a**pples and **t**oast; that **MOM** is **m**ilk **o**f **m**agnesia; and that **PET** means **p**ositron **e**mission **t**omography.

Eponyms use the name of a person to describe a disease or other phenomenon. It is certainly an honor for the named person, but less descriptive for the medical reader. **Hansen disease** just doesn't have the same impact as leprosy, and **VonWillebrand disease** doesn't carry the connotation of hemophilia. The book translates these and other eponyms into their more descriptive medical terms.

Who should use this book? Anyone who needs to accurately decode and interpret medical records and information.

Of course this includes health care workers, medical transcriptionists, and students. This book can even be used by fiction writers who want to add realism to their stories of hospital intrigue and physician romance.

But in today's changing health environment, it is increasingly important for patients to know exactly what their doctors are diagnosing; to know what treatments are being prescribed; and to know what their medical insurance is being billed.

The most difficult part in compiling entries for this book was in stopping. New acronyms, eponyms and abbreviations are created every day. Hopefully this will answer the vast majority of information needs you have.

A

a	accommodation • acid, acidity • alpha • ampere • anode • anterior • area • artery, arterial • asymmetric • at • axial • before (*ante*) • water (*aqua*)
ā	before (*ante*)
A	abnormal • absorbence • adenine • adenosine • adult • age • allergy • alpha • alternate • alveolar • ampere • Angstrom unit • anterior • area • atropine • axial • axillary (temperature) • symbol for mass number • water (*aqua*) • year (*annus*)
A₂	aortic second sound
A-II	angiotensin II
āā	of each (*ana*)
A-a	alveolar-arterial (gradient)
AA	achievement age • Alcoholics Anonymous • amino acid • anticipatory avoidance • aplastic anemia • arteries • Associate in Arts (degree) • atomic absorption (spectrophotometer) • author's alteration • automobile accident
aaa	amalgam
AAA	abdominal aortic aneurysm • acquired aplastic anemia • acute anxiety attack • addiction, autoimmune disease and aging • American Academy of Allergy • American Academy of Anatomists • American Allergy Association • androgenic anabolic agent • aromatic amino acids
AAAAA	aphasia, agnosia, apraxia, agraphia, alexia
AAAHC	American Association for Ambulatory Health Care
AAAI	American Academy of Allergy and Immunology
AAAS	American Association for the Advancement of Science
AABA	American Anorexia and Bulemia Association
AABB	American Association of Blood Banks
AAC	antibiotic-associated colitis

AACCN	American Association of Critical Care Nurses
AACHP	American Association for Comprehensive Health Planning
AACIA	American Association for Clinical Immunology and Allergy
AACN	American Association of Critical-Care Nurses • American Association of Colleges of Nursing
AAD	American Academy of Dermatology • antibiotic-associated diarrhea
AADP	American Academy of Denture Prosthetics
AADR	American Academy of Dental Radiology
AADS	American Academy of Dental Schools
A-aDO$_2$	alveolar-arterial oxygen difference (gradient)
AAE	active assistive exercise • acute allergic encephalitis • Affirmative Action Employer • American Association of Endodontists
AAF	acetic-alcohol formalin (fixing fluid) • acetylaminofluorene • ascorbic acid factor
AAFA	Asthma and Allergy Foundation of America
AAFP	American Academy of Family Physicians • American Academy of Family Practice
AAGP	American Academy of General Practice
AAHA	American Association for Homes for the Aging
AAHP	American Association of Health Plans
AAHPERD	American Alliance for Health, Physical Education, Recreation and Dance
AAI	American Association of Immunologists
AAID	American Academy of Implant Dentistry
AAIN	American Association of Industrial Nurses
AAKP	American Association of Kidney Patients
AAL	anterior axillary line
AAMA	American Association of Medical Assistants
AAMC	American Association of Medical Colleges

AAMD	American Association on Mental Deficiency
AAME	acetylargenine methyl ester
AAMRL	American Association of Medical Records Librarians
AAMS	acute aseptic meningitis syndrome
AAMSI	American Association for Medical Systems and Informatics
AAMT	American Association for Medical Transcription
AAN	American Academy of Neurology • American Academy of Nursing • amino acid nitrogen
AANA	American Anorexia Nervosa Association • American Association of Nurse-Anesthetists
AANN	American Association of Neuroscience Nurses
AANS	American Academy of Neurological Surgery • American Association of Neurological Surgeons
AAO	American Academy of Ophthalmology • American Academy of Otolaryngolgy • American Association of Orthodontists • American Association of Osteopathy
AAOG	American Association of Obstetricians and Gynecologists
AAOHN	American Association of Occupational Health Nurses
AAOO	American Academy of Ophthalmology and Otolaryngology
AAOP	American Academy of Oral Pathology
AAOS	American Academy of Orthopaedic Surgeons
AAP	air at atmospheric pressure • American Academy of Pediatrics • American Association of Pathologists • American Academy of Pedodontics • American Academy of Periodontology
AAPA	American Academy of Physician Assistants
AAPB	American Association of Pathologists and Bacteriologists
AAPC	annual average per capita
AAPCC	average annual per capita cost
A-a pCO_2	alveolar-arterial pCO2 (gradient)
AAPMR	American Academy of Physical Medicine and Rehabilitation

AAPS	American Association of Physicians and Surgeons
AAR	Australian antigen radioimmunoassay
AARC	American Association for Respiratory Care
AAROM	active assist range of motion
AARP	American Association of Retired Persons
AAS	acute abdominal series • anthrax antiserum • aortic arch syndrome • atomic absorption spectrophotometry
AASEC	American Association of Sex Educators and Counselors
AAT	acute abdominal tympany • alpha-1 antitrypsin
AAU	acute anterior uveitis
AAV	adeno-associated virus
ab	abortion, abort • about
Ab	abortion • antibody, antibodies
AB	abortion • Aid to the Blind • alcian blue • antibiotic • apex beat • asthmatic bronchitis • axiobuccal • Bachelor of Arts (*Artium Baccalaureus*)
A/B	acid-based ratio
A&B	apnea and bradycardia
ABA	abscisic acid • American Board of Anesthesiology
ABAI	American Board of Allergy and Immunology
AbAP	antibody-against-panel
ABBS	American Brittle Bone Society
ABC	airway, breathing, circulation • antigen-binding capacity • apnea, bradycardia, cyanosis • applesauce, bananas, cereal (diet) • aspiration, biopsy, cytology • atomic, biological, chemical • axiobuccocervical
ABC&C&C	airway, breathing, circulation, cervical spine, consciousness level
ABCRS	American Board of Colon and Rectal Surgery
abd	abdomen, abdominal • abduction, abductor
ABD	American Board of Dermatology

ABDA	American Board of Disability Analysts
abdom	abdomen, abdominal
ABE	acute bacterial endocarditis • trivalent antitoxin for types A, B, and E botulism
ABEM	American Board of Emergency Medicine
ABFP	American Board of Family Practices
ABG	arterial blood gases • axiobuccogingival
ABIM	American Board of Internal Medicine
ABL	a-beta-lipoproteinemia • antigen-binding lymphocytes • axiobuccolingual
ABLB	alternate binaural loudness balance (test)
ABMS	American Board of Medical Specialties
abn	abnormal
ABNM	American Board of Nuclear Medicine
abnorm	abnormal
ABNS	American Board of Neurological Surgery
ABO	absent bed occupant • American Board of Ophthalmology • American Board of Otolaryngology • major blood group system
ABOG	American Board of Obstetrics and Gynecology
ABOS	American Board of Orthopaedic Surgery
ABP	Adriamycin, bleomycin, prednisone • androgen-binding protein • arterial blood pressure
ABPA	acute bronchopulmonary asthma
ABPM	American Board of Preventive Medicine
ABPMR	American Board of Physical Medicine and Rehabilitation
ABPN	American Board of Psychiatry and Neurology
ABPS	American Board of Plastic Surgery
ABR	absolute bed rest • American Board of Radiology • auditory brain-stem response

abras	abrasion
abs	absent, absence • absolute • absorbence
ABS	acute brain syndrome • American Board of Surgery
absc	abscissa
abs feb	in the absence of fever (*absente febre*)
absorb	absorption
abstr	abstract
ABT	autologous bone marrow transplantation
ABTS	American Board of Thoracic Surgery
ABU	American Board of Urology
ABVD	Adriamycin, bleomycin, vinblastine, dacarbazine
ABVE	American Board of Vocational Evaluators
abx	antibiotics
ABY	acid bismuth yeast agar
ac	acetyl • acute • alternating current • before meals (*ante cibum*) • assisted control
Ac	actinium
AC	acetylcholine • acetylcysteine • acid • acromioclavicular • acute • adherent cell • admission certification • adrenal cortex • Adriamycin, cyclophosphamide • air conduction • alternating current • anodal closure • anterior chamber • anticoagulant • anti-inflammatory corticoid • aortic closure • atriocarotid • auriculucarotid • axiocervical
A/C	albumin-coagulin ratio
ACA	adenocarcinoma • American College of Anesthesiologists • aminocaproic acid • anterior cerebral artery • Automatic Clinical Analyzer
acad	academy
ACAT	acyl CoA: cholesterol acyltransferase
ACB	American Council of the Blind • aortocoronary (saphenous vein) bypass • arterialized capillary blood

acc	acceleration • accident • accommodation • according
ACC	adenoid cystic carcinoma • alveolar-cell carcinoma • ambulatory care center • American College of Cardiology • American College of Cryosurgery • anodal closure contraction • aplasia cutis congentia
A-CCC	Advanced Certification Continuity of Care
accel	acceleration
AcCh	acetylcholine
ACCl	anodal closure clonus
accid	accident
AcCoA	acetylcoenzyme A
accom	accommodation
ACCP	American College of Chest Physicians
accum	accumulation
ACD	absolute cardiac dullness • acid-citrate-dextrose (solution) • anterior chest diameter • area of cardiac disease
ACDF	anterior cervical discectomy and fusion
ACE	acute care of the elderly • adrenal cortical (adrenocortical) extract • aerobic chair exercises • angiotensin-converting enzyme
ACEP	American College of Emergency Physicians
ACF	accessory clinical findings
ac-G	accelerator globulin
ACG	American College of Gastroenterology • angiocardiogram, angiocardiography • apexcardiogram, apexcardiography
ACGME	Accreditation Council for Graduate Medical Education
ACh	acetylcholine
ACH	adrenal cortical (adreocortical) hormone • arm, chest height
ACHA	American College of Hospital Administrators
AChE	acetylcholinesterase
AChR	acetylcholine receptor

ACI	after-care instructions • anticlonus index
ACIDS	acquired cellular immunodeficient syndrome
ACIP	Advisory Committee on Immunization Practices
ACL	anterior cruciate ligament
ACLA	American Clinical Laboratory Association
ACLS	advance cardiac life support
ACN	acute conditioned necrosis
ACNM	American College of Nurse-Midwives
ACNP	American College of Neuropsychopharmacology
ACOEM	American College of Occupational and Environmental Medicine
ACOG	American College of Obstetricians and Gynecologists
ACOMS	American College of Oral and Maxillofacial Surgeons
ACOS	American College of Osteopathic Surgeons
ACP	acyl-carrier protein • American College of Pathologists • American College of Physicians • aspirin, caffeine, phenacetin • Association of Clinical Pathologists
ac phos	acid phosphate
ACMP	American College of Preventive Medicine
ACPP	adrenocorticopolypeptide
ACPPD	average cost per patient day
ACPS	acrocephalopolysyndactyly
ACR	American College of Radiology • anticonstipation regimen • adjusted community rate • American College of Rheumatology
ACS	acute confusional state • ambulatory care services • American Cancer Society • American Celiac Society • American College of Surgeons • anodal closing sound • antireticular cytotoxic serum • aperture current setting • abdominal compartment syndrome
ACSM	American College of Sports Medicine
ACSW	Academy of Certified Social Workers

act	active, activity
ACT	achievement through counseling and treatment • activated clotting time • activated coagulation time • anticoagulant therapy • asthma care training
ACTD	actinomycin D
ACTe	anodal closure tetanus
ACTH	adrenocorticotropic hormone
activ	activity
ACTN	adrenocorticotropin
ACTP	adrenocorticotropic polypeptide
ACU	acute care unit • ambulatory care unit
ACV	assist control ventilation
ACVD	acute cardiovascular disease
AC/W	acetone in water
ad	let there be added (*adde*) • to, toward, up to (*ad*)
AD	achievement drive • addicted to drugs • admitting diagnosis • advanced directive • after discharge • alcohol dehydrogenase • Alzheimer's disease • adenoidal degeneration • anodal duration • autosomal dominant • average deviation • right atrium (*atrium dextrum*) • right ear (*auris dextra*) • axiodistal
ADA	American Dental Association • American Diabetes Association • American Dietetic Association • Americans with Disabilities Act • adenosine deaminase
ADAA	American Dental Assistants Association • Anxiety Disorders Association of America
ADAMHA	Alcohol, Drug Abuse and Mental Health Administration
ADAS	Alzheimer's Disease Assessment Scale
AdC	adrenal cortex
ADC	Aid to Dependent Children • albumin, dextrose, catalase • anodal duration contraction • average daily census • axiodistalcervical
ADCC	antibody-dependent cellular cytotoxicity

add	adduction, adductor • let there be added (*adde*)
ADD	attention deficit disorder
ad def an	to the point of fainting (*ad defectionem animi*)
ADE	acute disseminated encephalitis
ADEA	Age Discrimination in Employment Act
ADEM	acute disseminated encephalomyelitis
adeq	adequate
ADG	axiodistogingival
ADH	adhesions • alcohol dehydrogenase • antidiuretic hormone • Adult Day Health
ADHA	American Dental Hygienists Association
ADHD	attention-deficit/hyperactivity disorder
adhib	to be administered (*adhibendus*)
ADI	acceptable daily intake • axiodistoincisal
adj	adjunct • claims adjustor
ADL	activities of daily life, activities of daily living
ad lib	freely, as desired (*ad libitum*)
adm	administrator, administration • admit, admission
AdM	adrenal medulla
ADM	administrative medicine • adriamycin
ADME	absorption, distribution, metabolism, excretion
admov	apply, let be applied (*admove, admoveatur*)
ADN	Associate Degree in Nursing
ADO	axiodisto-occlusal
ADP	adenosine diphosphate • area diastolic pressure • automated data processing
ADPKD	autosomal dominant polycystic kidney disease
ADPL	average daily patient load

ADR	Acceptable Dental Remedies • actual death rate • adverse drug reaction
ADRN	Associate Degree Registered Nurse
ADS	antibody deficient syndrome • antidiuretic substance
adst feb	while fever is present (*adstante febre*)
ADT	adenosine triphosphate • admission, discharge, transfer • algar-gel diffusion test • alternate day treatment • automated dithionite test • placebo ("Any Desired Thing")
ADTe	anodal duration tetanus
adv	against (*adversum*)
A-DV	arterial-deep venous difference
advert	advertisement
ADX	adrenalectomized
AE	above elbow • acrodermatitis enteropthica • activation energy • airplane ear
A/E	above elbow
AEA	alcohol, ether, acetone
AEC	at earliest convenience • Atomic Energy Commission
AED	automatic external defibrillator • Academy for Eating Disorders • anti-epileptic drugs
aeg	the patient (*aeger, aegra*)
AEG	air encephalogram
AEL	acute erythroleukemia
AEM	analytical electron microscope
AEP	admission evaluation protocol • auditory evoked potential • average evoked potential
aer	aerosol
AER	acoustic evoked response • albumin excretion rate • aldosterone excretion rate • auditory evoked response • average evoked response
AES	antieosinophilic sera

aet	at the age of, aged (*aetas*)
aetat	of age (*aetatis*)
AEV	avian erythroblastosis virus
AEVS	automated eligibility verification system
af	audiofrequency
AF	acid-fast • albumin free (tuberculin) • amniotic fluid • aortic flow • aortofemoral • Arthritis Foundation • atrial fibrillation • atrial flutter • audio frequency • auricular fibrillation
AFA	alcohol-formalin-acetic acid (solution)
AFB	acid-fast bacillus • American Foundation for the Blind
AFB1	aflatoxin B1
AFCR	American Federation for Clinical Research
AFDC	Aid to Families with Dependent Children
aff	afferent
AFH	adenfibromatous hyperplasia • anterior facial height
AFI	amaurotic familial idiocy
AFib	atrial fibrillation
AFIP	Armed Forces Institute of Pathology
AFMS	Affective Family Member Syndrome
AFO	ankle-foot orthosis (splint)
AFP	alpha-fetoprotein
AFR	ascorbic free radical
AFRD	acute febrile respiratory disease
AFRI	acute febrile respiratory illness
AFS	American Fertility Society
AFTC	apparent free testosterone concentration
AFX	atypical fibroxanthoma
ag	atrial gallop

Ag	antigen • silver (*argentum*)
AG	aminoglutethimide • anitglobulin • antigravity • atrial gallop • axiogingival
A/G	albumin-globulin ratio
AGA	accelerated growth area • American Gastroenterological Association • American Geriatrics Association • appropriate for gestational age
AgCI	silver chloride
AGD	agar gel diffusion
AGE	acute gastroenteritis • angle of greatest extension
AGEPC	acetyl glyceryl ether phosphoryl choline
AGF	angle of greatest flexion
agg	agglutinate, agglutination
AGG	agammaglobulinemia
aggl	agglutinate, agglutination
aggreg	aggregation
AGGS	anti-gas gangrene serum
agit	shake (*agita*)
agit bene	shake well (*agita bene*)
agit vas	the vial being shaken (*agitato vase*)
AGL	acute granulocytic leukemia
AGMK	African green monkey kidney
AGN	acute glomerulonephritis • agnosia
AgNO$_3$	silver nitrate
AGOS	American Gynecological and Obstetrical Society
AGPA	American Group Practice Association
AGS	adrenogenital syndrome • American Geriatrics Society
agt	agent
AGT	antiglobulin test • adrenoglomerulotrophin

AGTH	adrenoglomerulotropin
AGTT	abnormal glucose tolerance test
AGV	aniline gentian violet
AH	abdominal hysterectomy • amenorrhea and hirsutism • antihyaluronidase • arterial hypertension • hypermetropic astigmatism
A&H	accident and health insurance
AHA	acquired hemolytic anemia • American Heart Association • American Hospital Association • autoimmune hemolytic anemia • alpha hydroxy acids
AHC	acute hemorrhagic conjunctivitis • acute hemorrhagic cystitis
AHCPR	Agency for Health Care Policy and Research (of the Dept. of Health and Human Services)
AHD	antihypertensive drug • arteriosclerotic heart disease • atherosclerotic heart disease • autoimmune hemolytic disease
AHE	acute hemorrhagic encephalomyelitis
AHEC	area health-education center
AHF	antihemolytic factor • antihemophilic factor
AHFS	American Hospital Formulary Service
AHFS-DI	American Hospital Formulary Service-Drug Information
AHG	antihemophilic globulin • anithuman globulin
AHGS	acute herpetic gingival stomatitis
AHH	arylhydrocarbon hydroxylase
AHIMA	American Health Information Management Association
AHIP	assisted health insurance plan
AHN	Assistant Head Nurse
AHNA	American Holistic Nurses Association
AHP	acute hemorrhagic pancreatitis • allied health professionals
AHR	autonomic hyperreflexia
AHRQ	Agency for Healthcare Research and Quality

AHTG	anithuman thymocytic globulin
AHTP	antihuman thymocytic plasma
AI	accidentally incurred • aortic insufficiency • apical impulse • artificial insemination • artificial intelligence • atherogenic index • atrial insufficiency • axioincisal • first auditory area • anaphylatoxin inhibitor
AIB	aminoisobutyric acid
AIBA	aminoisobutyric acid
AIBS	American Institute of Biological Sciences
AICAR	aminoimidazole caboxamide ribonucleotide
AICD	Automatic Implantable Cardioverter Defibrillator
AICF	autoimmune complement fixation
AID	acute infectious disease • Agency for International Development • artificial insemination donor
AIDS	acquired immune deficiency syndrome
AIE	acute infective endocarditis
AIF	aortic-iliac-femoral
AIG	anti-immunoglobulin
AIH	artificial insemination, homologous
AIHA	autoimmune hemolytic anemia
AIHD	acquired immune hemolytic disease
AII	second auditory area
AIL	angioimmunoblastic lymphadenopathy
AILC	adult independent living center
AILD	angioimmunoblastic lymphadenopathy with dysproteinemia
AIM	artificial intelligence in medicine
AIMS	abnormal involuntary movement scale
AIP	acute idiopathic pericarditis • acute inflammatory polyneuropathy • acute intermittent porphyria • annual implementation plan • average intravascular pressure

AIS	androgen insensitivity syndrome
AIT	administrator-in-training
AIU	absolute iodine uptake
AIUM	American Institute of Ultrasound in Medicine
AIVR	accelerated idioventricular rhythm
AJ	ankle jerk
AJAO	American Juvenile Arthritis Organization
AJC	American Joint Commission (Study for Cancer Staging and End Results Reporting)
AJN	American Journal of Nursing
AK	above knee
AKA	above-knee amputation • also known as
AK amp	above-knee amputation
AKBR	arterial ketone body ratio
AKV	acrokeratosis verruciformis
Al	aluminum
AL	adaptation level • alignment mark • arterial line • axiolingual
Ala	alanine
ALa	axiolabial
ALA	American Lung Association • aminolevulinic acid dehydrase
ALaG	axiolabiogingival
alb	albumin • white (*albus*)
alc	alcohol, alcoholism
ALC	alternative level of care • avian leukosis complex • axiolinguocervical
Alc R	alcohol rub
ALD	adrenoleukodystrophy • alcoholic liver disease • aldolase
ALE	allowable limits of error

alg	algebraic
ALG	antilymphocytic globulin • axiolinguogingival
ALH	anterior lobe hormone • anterior lobe of hypophysis
A-line	arterial line
ALJ	administrative law judge
alk	alkaline
alk agents	alkylating agents
alk phos	alkaline phosphate
alk p'tase	alkaline phosphatase
all	allergy
ALL	acute lymphatic leukemia • acute lymphoblastic leukemia • acute lymphocytic leukemia
ALLO	atypical legionnaires-like organism
ALMI	anterolateral myocardial infarction
ALMV	anterior leaflet of mitral valve
ALN	anterior lymph node
ALO	axiolunguo-occlusal
ALOH	average length of hospitalization
ALOS	average length of stay
ALP	acute lupus pericarditis • alkaline phosphatase • anterior lobe of pituitary
ALROS	American Laryngological, Rhinological and Otological Society
ALS	advanced life support • amyotropic lateral sclerosis • antilymphocytic serum
alt	alternate • altitude
ALT	alanine (amino) transaminase
ALT/AST	ratio of serum alanine aminotransferase to serum asparate aminotransferase
ALTB	acute laryngotracheobronchitis

alt dieb	every other day (*alternis diebus*)
alt hor	every other hour (*alternis horis*)
alt noc	every other night (*alternis noctus*)
alv	alveolar
ALW	arch-loop-whorl (system)
am	ametropia • amyl • before noon (*ante meridien*) • meter-angle • myopic astigmatism
Am	americium
AM	actomyosin • ambulatory • amethopterin • ampere meter • amplitude modulation • anovular menstruation • arousal mechanism • aviation medicine • axiomesial • before noon (*ante meridien*) • myopic astigmatism
AMA	against medical advice • American Medical Association • antimitochondrial antibody
AMA-DE	American Medical Association-Drug Evaluations
amb	ambient • ambiguous • ambulance • ambulatory
AMC	academic medical center • arthrogryposis multiplex congenita • axiomesiocervical
AMCHA	aminomethylcyclohexanecarboxylic acid
AMD	age-related macular degeneration
AME	Agreed Medical Examiner
AMEEGA	American Medical Electroencephalographic Assocation
AMEL	Aero-Medical Equipment Laboratory
Amer	American
AMEND	Aiding Mothers Experiencing Neonatal Death
AMESLAN	American Sign Language
AMG	axiomesiogingival
AMH	Accreditation Manual for Hospitals • automated medical history • mixed astigmatism with myopia predominating
AMHT	automated multiphasic health testing

AMI	acute myocardial infarction • amitriptyline • anterior myocardial infarction • axiomesioincisal
AML	acanthiomeatal line • acute myeloblastic leukemia • acute myeogenous leukemia • acute myeloid leukemia • acute myelomonocytic leukemia • automated Medicare log
Am Lev	aminolevulinic acid
AMM	agnogenic myeloid metaplasia
ammon	ammonia
AMol	acute monoblastic leukemia • acute monocytic leukemia
AMO	axiomesio-occlusal
AMOL	acute monocytic leukemia
amor	amorphous
amp	ampere • amplification • ampule • amputate, amputation
AMP	accelerated mental process • adenosine monophosphate (adenylate, adenylic acid) • amphetamine • ampicillin • average mean pressure
AMPAC	American Medical Political Action Committee
amp-hr	ampere-hour
AMPS	acid mucopolysaccharide
AMPT	alpha-methylparatyrosine
AMR	alternate motion rate
AMRS	automated Medical-record system
AMS	altered mental status • auditory memory span • automated multiphasic screening
amt	amount
AMT	American Medical Technologists
amu	atomic mass unit
AMV	avian myeloblastosis virus
AMVI	acute mesenteric vascular insufficiency
AMVL	anterior mitral valve leaflet

AMWA	American Medical Women's Association • American Medical Writer's Association
An	actinon • anisometropia • anode, anodal • antigen
A_n	normal atmosphere
AN	acne neonatorum • anesthesia services • anorexia nervosa • anterior • avascular necrosis
ana	each (*ana*)
ANA	American Neurological Association • American Nurses' Association • antinuclear antibody
ANAD	anorexia nervosa and associated disorders • National Association of Anorexia Nervosa and Associated Disorders
anal	analgesic • analysis, analyst, analytic, analyze
ANAP	agglutination negative, absorption positive
anat	anatomy, anatomical
ANC	acid-neutralizing capacity • Army Nurse Corps
AnCC	anodal closure contraction
ANCC	anodal closure contraction • American Nurse Credentialing Center
AND	administratively necessary days • anterior nasal discharge
ANDA	Abbreviated New Drug Application
ANDTe	anodal duration tetanus
anes	anesthesia, anesthesiology
anesth	anesthesia, anesthesiology
an ex	anode excitation
ANF	American Nurses' Federation • American Nurses' Foundation • antinuclear factor
ang	angle
ANG	angiogram, angiography
angio	angiogram
anh	anhydrous

ANLL	acute nonlymphocytic leukemia
annot	annotation
ANoA	anodal opening contraction
ANOVA	analysis of variance
ANP	adult nurse practitioner • advanced nurse practitioner
ANRL	antihypertensive neural renomedullary lipids
ANS	anterior nasal spine • arterionephrosclerosis • autonomic nervous system
ANSI	American National Standards Index • American National Standards Institute
ant	antenna • anterior
ANT	aminonitrothiazol • anterior
antag	antagonist
ante	before *(ante)*
anti-coag	anticoagulant
anti-HAV	antibody to hepatitis A virus
anti-HBc	antibody to hepatitis B core antigen
anti-HBe	antibody to hepatitis Be antigen
anti-HBs	antibody to hepatitis B surface antigen
anti-log	antilogarithm
ant pit	anterior pituitary
ant sup spine	anterior superior spine
ANTU	alpha-naphthylthiourea
ANUG	acute necrotizing ulcerative gingivitis
Ao	aorta
AO	achievement orientation • anodal opening • aortic opening
A + O x 4	alert and oriented to person, place, time and date
AOA	American Osteopathic Association
AOB	alcohol on breath

AOC	abridged ocular chart • anodal opening contraction
AOCl	anodal opening clonus
AOD	arterial occlusive disease
AODM	adult-onset diabetes mellitus
AOE	arising out of (the) employment
AOL	acro-osteolysis
AOM	acute otitis media
AOMA	American Occupational Medical Association
AONE	American Organization of Nurse Executives
AOO	anodal opening odor
AOP	anodal opening picture
AORN	Association of Operating Room Nurses
aor regurg	aortic regurgitation
aort sten	aortic stenosis
AOS	anodal opening sound
AOTA	American Occupational Therapy Association
AOTe	anodal opening tetanus
AOTF	American Occupational Therapy Foundation
AoV	aortic valve
ap	apothecary • before dinner (*ante prandium*)
AP	acid phosphatase • action potential • alkaline phosphatase • alum-precipitated • angina pectoris • anterior pituitary • antero-posterior • antipyrine • aortic pressure • apical pulse • appendectomy, appendix • arterial pressure • artificial pneumo-thorax • attending physician • axiopulpal • Alzheimer's Program • abruptio placenta
A/P	ascites-plasma ratio
A&P	anatomy and physiology • anterior and posterior • auscultation and palpation • auscultation and percussion
$A_2=P_2$	second aortic sound equals second pulmonic sound

$A_2 > P_2$	second aortic sound greater than second pulmonic sound
$A_2 < P_2$	second aortic sound less than second pulmonic sound
APA	Administrative Procedures Act • aldosterone-producing adenoma • American Pharmaceutical Association • American Physiotherapy Association • American Podiatry Association • American Psychiatric Association • antipernicious anemia (factor)
APACHE	acute physiology and chronic health evaluation system
AP/AHC	Accreditation Program/Ambulatory Health Care
APB	atrial premature beat
APC	acute pharyngoconjunctival fever • adenoidal-pharyngeal-congunctival (virus) • aspirin, phenacetin, caffeine • atrial premature contraction • adenomatous polyposis coli
APC-C	aspirin, phenacetin and caffeine with codeine
APD	action potential duration • anteroposterior diameter • atrial premature depolarization
APE	anterior pituitary extract
APF	animal protein factor
APG	ambulatory patient group • ambulatory patient groups
A.P.G.A.R.	adaptability, partnership, growth, affection, resolve (family screening - not the same as Apgar scoring systems for newborns)
APH	antepartum hemorrhage • anterior pituitary hormone
APhA	American Pharamaceutical Association
APHA	American Public Health Association
AP/HC	Accreditation Program/Home Health Care
API	ankle-arm pressure index
APIC	Association for Practitioners in Infection Control
APK	antiparkinsonian
APL	accelerated painless labor • acute promyelocytic leukemia • anterior pituitary-like substance • A Programming Language
AP&L	anteroposterior and lateral

AP&Lat	anteroposterior and lateral
AP/LTC	Accreditation Program/Long Term Care
APN	advanced practice nurse
APO	adverse patient occurrences
APORF	acute postoperative renal failure
app	appendix • applied • approximate
APP	appendix
appar	apparatus • apparent
AP/PF	Accreditation Program/ Psychiatric Facilities
appl	appliance • applicable • application • applied
applan	flattened (*applanatus*)
appoint	appointment
approx	approximate
appt	appointment
APPT	Adolescent-Pediatric Pain Tool
appy	appendectomy
APR	abdominoperineal resection • accelerator-produced radiopharmaceuticals • anterior pituitary reaction • Acute Physical Rehab
aprax	apraxia
APS	acute physiology score • adenosine phosphisulfate • Adult Protective Services
APSAC	anisoylated plasminogen streptokinase activator complex
APT	alum-precipitated toxoid
APTA	American Physical Therapy Association
APTC	ambulatory psoriasis treatment center
APTD	Aid to the Permanently and Totally Disabled
aPTT	activated partial thromboplastin time
APTT	activated partial thrombosplastin time

APUD	amine precursor uptake and decarboxylation cells
APVD	anomalous pulmonary venous drainage
aq	aqueous • water (*aqua*)
AQ	accomplishment quotient • achievement quotient • anxiety quotient
aq bull	boiling water (*aqua bulliens*)
aq com	common water (*aqua communis*)
aq dest	distilled water (*aqua destillata*)
aq ferv	hot water (*aqua fervens*)
aq frig	cold water (*aqua frigida*)
aq mar	sea water (*aqua marina*)
aq pur	pure water (*aqua pura*)
aq tep	tepid water (*aqua tepida*)
aqu	aqueous
Ar	argon
AR	abnormal record • achievement ration • active resistance exercises • alarm reaction • analytic reagent • aortic regurgitation • artificial respiration • autosomal recessive
A/R	accounts receivable • apical-radial
Ara	arabinose
ARA	American Rheumatism Association
Ara-A	adenine arabinoside
Ara-C	cytosine arabinoside
ARBOR	arthropod-borne (virus)
ARBOW	artificial rupture of bag of waters
ARC	AIDS-related complex • alcohol rehabilitation center • American Red Cross • American Refugee Committee • anomalous retinal correspondence
Arch	archives

ARD	acute respiratory disease • anorectal dressing • antimicrobial removal device
ARDS	acute respiratory distress syndrome • adult respiratory distress syndrome
ARF	acute renal failure • acute respiratory failure • acute rheumatic fever
ARFC	autorosette-forming cells
arg	silver (*argentum*)
Arg	arginine
ARI	acute respiratory infection
ARM	artificial rupture of membranes
ARMD	age-related macular degeneration
ARN	Association of Rehabilitation Nurses
AROA	autosomal recessive ocular albinism
AROM	artificial rupture of membranes
ARP	absolute refractory period
ARRD	Asthma, Rhinitis, & other Respiratory Diseases
ARRT	American Registry of Radiologic Technologies
ARS	antirabies serum
ARS-A	arylsulfatase A
art	artery, arterial • artificial
ART	accelerated recovery technique • Accredited Record Technician • automated reagin test • arthritis
artif	artificial
ARV	AIDS-related virus • antiretroviral
As	arsenic
AS	acute salpingitis • androsterone sulfate • ankylosing spondylitis • antiserum • anxiety state • aortic stenosis • aqueous suspension • arteriosclerosis • astigmatism • arterial stenosis • left ear (*auris sinistra*) • sickle cell trait (hemoglobin, genotype)

A-S	Adams-Stokes (disease, syndrome)
A/S	sickle cell trait (hemoglobin, genotype)
ASA	acetylsalicylic acid (aspirin) • American Society of Anesthesiologists • American Standards Association • argininosuccinic acid
ASAP	as soon as possible
ASAPS	American Society for Aesthetic Plastic Surgery
ASAS	American Society of Abdominal Surgery • argininosuccinate synthetase
ASAT	aspartate aminotransferase
ASC	altered state of consciousness • ambulatory surgical center
Asc-A	ascending aorta
ASCH	American Society for Clinical Hypnosis
ASCLT	American Society of Clinical Laboratory Technicians
ASCP	American Society of Clinical Pathologists
ASCRS	American Society of Cataract and Refractive Surgery
ASCVD	arteriosclerotic cardiovascular disease
ASD	aldosterone secretion defect • anterior sagittal diameter • atrial septal defect
ASDC	Association of Sleep Disorders Centers
ASE	axilla, shoulder, elbow
ASET	American Society of Electroencepholographic Technologists
ASF	aniline, sulfur, formaldehyde
AsH	hypermetropic astigmatism
ASH	antistreptococcal hyalurodinase • asymmetric septal hypertrophy
ASHD	arteriosclerotic heart disease
ASHRM	American Society of Hospital Risk Managers
ASIA	American Spinal Injury Association
ASIS	anterior superior iliac spine

ASL	American Sign Language • antistreptolysin • assisted living
ASLC	acute self-limited colitis
ASL-O	antistreptolysin-O
AsM	myopic astigmatism
ASMI	anteroseptal myocardial infarction
Asn	asparagine
ASO	antistreptolysin-O • arteriosclerosis obliterans • administrative services only
ASOA	American Society of Ophthalmic Administrators
ASOT	antistreptolysin-O titer
Asp	asparagine • asparate
ASP	area systolic pressure
ASPAN	American Society of Plastic and Reconstructive Surgeons
ASPVD	arteriosclerotic peripheral vascular disease
ASQ	Abbreviated Symptom Questionnaire
ASR	aldosterone secretion rate
ASRT	American Society of Radiologic Technologists
ASS	anterior superior spine
assby	assembly
AS-SCORE	assessing severity: Age of patient, Systems involved, Stage of disease, COmplications, REsponse to therapy
assn	association
assoc	associate, association
asst	assistant
Ast	astigmatism
AST	antistreptolysin titer • Aphasia Screening Test • aspartate aminotransferase
ASTM	American Society for Testing Materials
ASTO	antistreptolysin-O

As tol	as tolerated
ASTR	American Society of Therapeutic Radiologists
ASV	antisiphon valve • anti-snake venom
A-SV	arterial-superficial venous disease
ASVD	arteriosclerotic vascular disease
Asx	asymptomatic
at	airtight • atom
At	astatine
AT	abdominal tympany • achievement test • adjunctive therapy • antithrombin • atraumatic • Aquatic Therapy • atrial tachycardia
A-T	ataxia-telangiectasia
AT-III	antithrombin-III
AT_{10}	dihydrotachysterol
ATA	alimentary toxic aleukia • atmosphere absolute (pressure at sea level)
ATB	antibiotics • atrial tachycardia with block
ATC	around the clock
ATCC	American Type Culture Collection
ATD	admission, transfer, discharge • antithyroid drugs
ATDN	AIDS Treatment Data Network
at fib	atrial fibrillation
ATG	antithrombocyte globulin
ATH	acute toxic hepatitis
ATL	Achilles tendon lengthening • adult T-cell leukemia • atypical lymphocytes
ATLL	adult T-cell leukemia/lymphoma
ATLS	advanced trauma life support
atm	atmosphere, atmospheric
ATM	acute transverse myelitis

ATN	acute tubular necrosis
AT/NC	atraumatic/normocephalic
at no	atomic number
ATNR	asymmetrical tonic neck reflex
ATP	adenosine triphosphate
ATPase	adenosine triphosphatase
ATPD	ambient temperature and pressure, dry
ATPS	ambient temperature and pressure, saturated
atr	atrophy
ATR	Achilles tendon reflex
ATR FIB	atrial fibrillation
ATS	antitetanic serum • antithymocyte serum • anxiety tension state • atherosclerosis
at wt	atomic weight
Au	gold (*aurum*)
^{198}Au	colloidal gold
AU	Angstrom Unit • antitoxin unit • Australia antigen • both ears (*aures unitas*), each ear (*auris uterque*)
AUA	American Urological Association
AUC	area under concentration • blood concentration curve (area under the curve)
AUD	auditory
AUL	acute undifferentiated leukemia
aus	auscultation
ausc	auscultation
auscul	auscultation
aux	auxiliary
av	average • avoirdupois

AV	aortic valve • arteriovenous • atrioventricular • avoirdupois
AVA	arteriovenous anastomosis
$AvCDO_2$	arteriovenous oxygen content difference
AVD	apparent volume of distribution
avdp	avoirdupois
AVE	active voluntary euthanasia • agreed vocation evaluator
AVF	augmented voltage unipolar left foot lead (ECG)
AVH	acute viral hepatitis
AVI	air velocity index
AVL	augmented voltage unipolar left arm lead (ECG)
AVM	arteriovenous malformation
AVN	arterioventricular node
$A-VO^2$	arteriovenous oxygen difference
AVP	antiviral protein
AVR	aortic valve replacement • augmented voltage unipolar right arm lead (ECG)
AVRT	atrioventricular reciprocating tachycardia
AVS	arteriovenous shunt • aortic valve stenosis
AVT	Allen vision test
AW	anterior wall
A&W	alive and well
AWF	adrenal weight factor
AWHONN	Association for Women's Health, Obstetric and Neonatal Nurses
AWI	anterior wall infarction • area wage index
AWMI	anterior wall myocardial infarction
AWOL	absent without leave
AWS	alcohol withdrawal syndrome

ax	axilla, axillary • axis, axial
Ax	axilla, axillary
ax grad	axial gradient
Az	nitrogen (*azote*)
AZ	Aschheim-Zondek test
AZOOR	acute zonal occult outer retinopathy
AZQ	diaziquone
AZT	Aschheim-Zondek test • zidovudine
AzUR	6-azauridine

B

b	twice (*bis*)
B	bacillus • balnium • barometric • base • bath • Baume scale • behavior • Benoist scale • bicuspid • bilateral • black • blood • blue • body • born • boron • both • brother • buccal • gauss (unit of magnetic induction)
Ba	barium
BA	Bachelor of Arts • bile acid • blood alcohol • boric acid • brachial artery • bronchial asthma • buccoaxial • *Bacillus anthracis*
B/A	backache
BAA	benzoyl arginine amide
BAC	bacterial antigen complex • blood alcohol concentration
BACOP	bleomycin, Adriamycin, cyclophosphamide, oncovin, prednisone
bact	bacteriology • bacterium, bacteria, bacterial
BaEn	barium enema
BAEP	brain-stem auditory evoked potential
BAER	brain-stem auditory evoked response
BAG	buccoaxiogingival
BAIB	beta-aminobutyric acid

bal	balance
BAL	British anti-Lewisite (dimercaprol) • bronchoalveolar lavage
bals	balsam
BaM	barium meal
BAO	basal acid output
BAO/MAO	ratio of basal acid output to maximal acid output
BAP	blood agar plate • brachial artery pressure
bar	barometer, barometric
barbs	barbiturates
BASH	body acceleration synchronous with heartbeat
BASIC	Beginner's All-Purpose Symbolic Instruction Code
baso	basophil
BAT	basic assurance test • best available technology • brown adipose tissue
batt	battery
BB	bath blanket • bed bath • blood bank • both bones • break- through bleeding • breast biopsy • buffer base
BBA	Bachelor of Business Administration • born before arrival • Balanced Budget Act of 1997
BBB	blood-brain barrier • bundle branch block
BBBB	bilateral bundle branch block
BBC	brombenzylcyanide
BBMG	bedside blood glucose management
BBS	bilateral breath sounds
BBT	basal body temperature
BC	birth control • blood culture • Blue Cross • board-certified • bone conduction • Bowman's capsule • buccocervical
B&C	board and care
BCAA	branched chain amino acid(s)

BC/BS	Blue Cross/Blue Shield
BCC	basal-cell carcinoma • birth control clinic
BCDDP	Breast Cancer Detection Demonstration Program
BCDF	B cell differentiation factors
BCE	basal-cell epithelioma
BCF	basophil chemotactic factor
BCG	bacillus Calmette-Guerin • ballistocardiogram • bicolor guaiac • bromocresol green
BCGF	B cell growth factors
BCH	basal-cell hyperplasia
BCI	Basic and Clinical Immunology
BCLS	basic cardiac life support
BCM	body cell mass
BCNU	bischloroethylnitrosourea
BCP	birth control pill • bromocresol purple
BCS	battered child syndrome • Budd-Chiari Syndrome
BCVA	best corrected visual acuity
bd	twice daily (*bis die*)
BD	base of prism down • basophilic degeneration • bed • benzodiazepine • bile duct • birth defect • board • borderline dull • brain dead • bucco distal
BD/1000	bed days per thousand
BDC	burn-dressing change
BDE	bile duct exploration
BDMS	Bureau of Data Management and Strategy
BDS	Bachelor of Dental Surgery
BDP	Brain Injury Day Program
BDSc	Bachelor of Dental Science
Be	Baume scale • beryllium

BE	*Bacillen Emulsion* • bacterial endocarditis • barium enema • base excess • below elbow • board-eligible • Barrett's esophagus
BEAM	Brain Electrical Activity Mapping
BEE	basal energy expenditure
beg	began, begin, beginning
beh	behavior, behavioral
BEI	butanol-extractable iodine
bepti	bionomics, environment, *Plasmodium*, treatment, immunity (malaria epidemiology)
BES	balanced electrolyte solution
bet	between
bev	billion electron-volts
BF	bentonite flocculation • blood flow • body fat • bone fragment • boy friend • buffered
B/F	bound-free ratio
BFM	bendroflumethiazide
BFP	biologic false-positive
BFR	blood filtration rate • blood flow rate • bone formation rate
BFR sol	buffered Ringer's solution
BFT	bentonite flocculation test
BFU-E	burst-forming units-erythroid
BG	bicolor guaiac test • blood glucose • Bordet-Gengou (agar, bacillus phenomenon) • buccogingival
BGG	bovine gamma globulin
BH	bill of health • bundle of His
BHA	butylated hydroxyanisole
BHC	benzene hexachloride
BHCDA	Bureau of Health Care Delivery & Assistance
BHI	bone healing index

BHIB	beef heart infusion broth
BHL	biologic half-life
BHP	Bureau of Health Professionals
BHRD	Bureau of Health Resources Development
BHS	beta-hemolytic streptococci
BHT	butylated hydroxytoluene
BH/VH	body hematocrit-venous hematocrit ratio
Bi	bismuth
BI	base of prism in • bifocal • bone injury • Braille Institute
bib	drink (*bibe*)
BIB	brought in by
Bicarb	bicarbonate
bid	twice daily (*bis in die*)
BID	brought in dead
bif	bifocal
BIH	benign intracranial hypertension
bihor	during two hours (*bihorium*)
Bi. Isch.	between ischial tuberosities
bil	bilateral • bilirubin
bilat	bilateral
bili	bilirubin
bin	twice a night (*bis in nocte*)
BIO	biofeedback
biol	biologic, biology
BIP	background interference procedure • bacterial intravenous protein • biparietal • bismuth iodoform paraffin
BIPP	back injury prevention program • bismuth iodoform paraffin paste
BIR	basic incidence rate

bis	twice (*bis*)
Bi sp	bispinous
bi wk	twice a week
BJ	biceps jerk
B-J	Bence-Jones protein
Bk	berkelium
BK	below knee
BKA	below-knee amputation
BKTT	below knee to toe
BKV	BK virus
BKWC	below knee walking cast
bl	bleeding • blood
BL	blood loss • body lean • buccolingual • Burkitt's lymphoma
BLB	Boothby, Lovelace, Bulbulian (mask)
bl cult	blood culture
bld	blood
BLE	both lower extremities
Bleo	bleomycin
BLESS	bath, laxative, enema, shampoo, shower
BLFG	bilateral firm (hand) grips
BLG	Beta-lactoglobin
BLIP	beta-lactamase inhibitory protein
BLLS	bilateral leg strength
BLM	bleomycin
BLN	bronchial lymph nodes
BlP	blood pressure
BLS	basic life support • blood sugar

BM	Bachelor of Medicine • basal metabolism • basement membrane • bone marrow • bowel movement • buccomesial • behavior management
BMA	British Medical Association
BMB	bone marrow biopsy
BMC	bone marrow depression • Bureau of Medical Devices
BMD	bone mineral density
BMI	body mass index
BMK	birthmark
BMMP	benign mucous membrane pemphigus
BMN	bone marrow necrosis
BMPAN	basic metabolic panel
BPD	borderline personality disorder
BMQA	Board of Medical Quality Assurance
BMR	basal metabolic rate
BMS	Bachelor of Medical Science
BMT	bone marrow transplant
BMZ	basement membrane zone
BNA	*Basle Nomina Anatomica* (nomenclature)
BNDD	Bureau of Narcotics and Dangerous Drugs
BNO	bladder neck obstruction
BO	base of prism out • body odor • bowel • bowels open • bucco- occlusal
B/O	because of
B&O	belladonna and opium
BOA	born out of asepsis
BOB	Bureau of Biologics
BOD	biochemical oxygen demand
BOEA	ethyl biscoumacetate

bol	pill (*bolus*)
BOM	bilateral otitis media
BOR	bowels open regularly
bot	bottle
BOW	bag of waters (amniotic sac)
BP	barometric pressure • bathroom privileges • bedpan • biparietal • birthplace • blood pressure • body part • boiling point • British Pharmacopeia • brinchopleural • buccopulpal • bypass
BPB	bromphenol blue
BPD	biparietal diameter • blood pressure decreased • bronchopulmonary dysplasia • biliopancreatic diversion
BPF	bronchopleural fistual
BPH	benign prostatic hypertrophy
BPI	blood pressure increased
BPIG	bacterial polysaccharide immune globulin
BPL	beta-propiolactone
BPM	beats per minute
BPPV	benign paroxysmal positional vertigo
BPRS	Brief Psychiatric Rating Scale
BPV	benign paroxysmal vertigo • benign positional vertigo • bovine papilloma virus
Bq	becquerel
BQA	Board of Quality Assurance • Bureau of Quality Assurance
br	branch • breath • brother
bR	bacteriorhodopsin
Br	bromine • bronchitis • brown
BR	bathroom • bedrest • *Brucella* • Blindness Rehabilitation
BRAT	bananas, rice cereal, applesauce and toast (diet)
BRB	bright red blood

BRBPR	bright red blood per rectum
BRH	Bureau of Radiological Health
BRM	biological response modifier
bronch	bronchoscope, bronchoscopy
BRP	bathroom privileges • bilirubin production
BS	Bachelor of Science • Bachelor of Surgery • barium swallow • blood sugar • bispecific • Blue Shield • bowel sounds • breath sounds
B&S	Bartholin's and Skene's glands
BSA	beef serum albumin • body surface area • bovine serum albumin
BSB	body surface burned • breath sounds bilateral
BSC	bedside commode
BSD	bedside drainage
BSE	breast self-examination
BSER	brain-stem evoked response
BSF	basal skull fracture
BSL	blood sugar level
BSN	Bachelor of Science in Nursing • bowel sounds normal
BSNA	bowel sounds normal and active
BSO	bilateral salpingo-oophorectomy
BSOM	bilateral serous otitis media
BSp	bronchospasm
BSP	bromosulfophthalein
BSPA	bowel sounds present and active
BSPIS	Body Substance Precautions and Isolation Systems
BSR	blood sedimentation rate
BSS	balanced salt solution • black silk suture • buffered saline solution

BST	blood serologic test • brief-stimulus therapy
BSU	British Standard Unit
BSV	Batten-Spielmyer-Vogt (syndrome)
BSW	Bachelor of Social Work
BT	bedtime • bitemporal • bladder tumor • bleeding time • body temperature • brain tumor • bulbotruncal
BTB	breakthrough bleeding • bromthymol blue
BTFS	breast tumor frozen section
BTM	bilateral tympanic membranes
BTPS	body temperature, pressure, saturated
BTS	bioptic telescopic spectacle
BTU	British thermal unit
Bu	bilirubin • butyl
BU	base of prism up • below the umbilicus • Bodansky unit • Burn Unit • buccal
BUDR	5-bromodeoxyuridine
BUE	both upper extremities
BUN	blood urea nitrogen
BUS	Bartholin's, urethral, and Skene's glands
BV	basilic vein • biological value • blood vessel • blood volume • bulboventricular
B/V	binging and vomiting
B&V	binging and vomiting
BVAD	biventricular assistive device
BVE	biventricular enlargement
BVI	Better Vision Institute
BVRT	Benton Visual Retention Test
BW	below waist • biologic warfare • birth weight • blood Wasserman • body water • body weight

B&W	black and white (cascara and milk of magnesia)
BWC	Bureau of Workers' Compensation
BWS	battered woman syndrome
Bx	biopsy
BX	biopsy • Blue Cross
BX/BS	Blue Cross/Blue Shield
Bz-Ty-PABA	benzoyl-tyrosyl-para-aminobenzoic acid (test)

C

c	calorie (small calorie, gram calorie) • capacity • capillary • contact • cubic • curie • cycle • hundred (*centum*)
$\bar{c}$	with (*cum*)
C	calorie (large calorie, kilocalorie) • canine tooth • carbohydrate • carbon • cathode • Caucasian • Celsius • centigrade • cerebrospinal fluid • certified • cervical (nerve, vertebra) • cesarean (section) • chest • cholesterol • clearance • clonus • closure • coarse • cocaine • coeffecient • color sense • complement • compound • concentration • content • contraction • cortex • coulomb (electrical unit) • cylinder • cytosine • gallon (*congius*) • hundred (*centum*) • rib (*costa*)
C'	complement
c^2	square centimeter
c^{14}	radioactive carbon
C'-3	component of complement in serum
C1-C7	cervical vertebrae 1 through 7
C1-C9	complement C1 through C9
C-I to C-V	controlled substances-Schedules I thru V
ca	about, approximately (*circa*)
Ca	calcium • cancer • *Candida* • carcinoma • cathode

CA	cancer • carcinoma • cardiac arrest • cholic acid • chronological age • Cocaine Anonymous • cold agglutinin • common antigen • compressed air • conditioned abstinence • coronary artery • cortisone acetate • croup-associated (virus) • cytosine arabinoside
c/a	Clinitest/Acetest
CAAT	computer assisted axial tomography
CAB	coronary artery bypass • combined androgen blockade
CABG	coronary artery bypass graft
CaBP	calcium-binding protein
CAC	cardiac accelerator center • circulating anticoagulant
CaC_2	calcium carbide
CaCC	cathodal closure contraction
$CaCl_2$	calcium chloride
$CaCO_3$	calcium carbonate
CaC_2O_4	calcium oxalate
CACX	cancer of the cervix
CAD	computer-assisted dialogue • coronary artery disease
CaDTe	cathodal duration tetanus
CaEdTA	edathamil calcium disodium
CAF	contract administration fees • cyclophosphamide, Adriamycin, fluorouracil
CAG	chronic atrophic gastritis
CAH	chronic active hepatitis • chronic aggressive hepatitis • congenital adrenal hyperplasia
CAI	computer-assisted instruction • confused artificial insemination
cal	caliber • calorie (small or gram calorie)
Cal	calorie (large calorie, kilocalorie)
Calb	albumin clearance
calc	calculate, calculated

CALD	chronic active liver disease
calef	warmed (*calefactus*)
CALLA	common acute lymphocytic leukemia antigen
Cam	amylase clearance
CAM	chorioallantoic membrane • complimentary alternative medicine • cell adhesion molecules
cAMP	cyclic adenosine monophosphate
c amplum	heaping spoonful, tablespoonful (*cochleare amplum*)
CAN	*Candida* • cord (umbilical) around the neck • chronic anovulatory disorder
canc	canceled
CaO	calcium oxide (quick lime)
CAO	chronic airway obstruction
CaO_2	arterial oxygen content
CaOC	cathodal opening contraction
$Ca(OH)_2$	calcium hydroxide
ca ox	calcium oxalate
cap	capacity • capillary • capsule • community action program • let him take (*capiat*)
CAP	choramphenicol • College of American Pathologists • Computerized Automated Psychophysiological (device)
CAPD	continuous ambulatory peritoneal dialysis
cardiol	cardiology
CAS	cerebral arteriosclerosis • Chemistry Abstract Service • chronic anovulation syndrome
$CaSO_4$	calcium sulfate
CASS	Coronary Artery Surgery Study
CAT	cataract • Children's Apperception Test • chronic abdominal tympany • computerized axial tomography
cath	cathartic • catheter, catheterize, catheterization • cathode

cauc	Caucasian
cav	cavity
CAV	congenital absence of vagina • congenital adrenal virilism • croup-associated virus
CAVB	complete atrioventricular block
CAVH	continuous arteriovenous hemodialysis
Cb	columbium
CB	Bachelor of Surgery (*Chirurgiae Baccalaureus*) • ceased breathing • chronic bronchitis
C-B	chest-back
CBA	chronic bronchitis with asthma
CBBB	complete bundle branch block
CBC	complete blood count
CBCME	computer-based continuing medical education
CBD	closed bladder drainage • common bile duct
CBE	clinical breast exam
CBF	capillary blood flow • cerebral blood flow
CBG	corticosteroid-binding globulin • cortisol-binding globulin
Cbl	cobalamin
CBO	Congressional Budget Office
CBOC	completion of bed occupancy care
CBR	carotid bodies resected • chemical, bacteriologic and radiologic • complete bed rest • crude birth rate
CBS	chronic brain syndrome
CBV	circulating blood volume
CBW	chemical and biological warfare
CBZ	carbamazepine epoxide
cc	cubic centimeter

CC	cell culture • cellular compartment • chief (current) complaint • circulatory collapse • coeffecient of correlation certified • complications and co-morbidities • compound cathartic • concave • cord compression • coronary collateral • corpus callosum • costochondral • critical condition • current complaint
C&C	confirmed and compatible
CCA	chick-cell agglutination • chimpanzee coryza agent • cholangiocarcinoma • circumflex coronary artery • common carotid artery • congenital contractual arachnodactyly
CCAT	conglutinating complement absorption test
CCB	calcium channel blockers
CCBV	central circulating blood volume
CCC	cathodal closure contraction • central counteradaptive changes • chronic calculous cholecystitis • California Compensation Cases
CCCR	closed chest cardiac resuscitation
CCD	calibration curve data • charge-coupled device
CCF	cephalin-cholesterol flocculation (test) • congestive cardiac failure • crystal-induced chemotactic factor
CCHF	Congo-Crimean hemorrhagic fever
CCI	chronic coronary insufficiency
CCK	cholecystokinin
CCK-GB	cholecystokinin-gallbladder (cholecystogram)
CCK-PZ	cholecystokinin-pancreozymin
CCM	Certified Case Manager
CCMA	Certified Case Manager Administration
CCMC	Commission for Case Manager Certification
CCME	Coordinating Council for Medical Education
CCMS	clean-catch midstream urinalysis
CCNS	cell-cycle nonspecific (agent)

CCNSC	Cancer Chemotherapy National Service Center
CCNU	chloroethylcyclohexylnitrosourea (lomustine)
CCP	Crippled Children's Program • Code of Civil Procedure
CCPD	continuous cycled peritoneal dialysis
C_{cr}	creatinine clearance
CCRC	continuing care retirement community
CCRN	Certified Critical Care Registered Nurse
CCS	casualty clearing station • cell-cycle specific (agent) • Critical Care Services
cct	circuit
CCT	carotid compression tomography • chocolate-coated tablet • closed cerebral trauma • coated compressed tablet • controlled cord traction
CCTe	cathodal closure tetanus
CCU	cardiac care unit • coronary care unit • critical care unit
CCW	counterclockwise
cd	caudal • candela
Cd	cadmium • coccygeal
CD	cardiovascular deconditioning • cardiovascular disease • caudal • cesarean-delivered • cesarean delivery • chemical dependency • civil defense • common duct • communicable disease • constant drainage • contagious disease • convulsive disorder • Crohn's disease • curative dose • current diagnosis • cystic duct • diagonal conjugate diameter of pelvic inlet (*conjugata diagonalis*) • cluster designation (for antigens)
C&D	cystoscopy and dilatation
CD_{50}	median curative dose
CDA	congenital dyserythropoietic anemia
CDAA	chlorodiallylacetamide
C&DB	cough and deep breathe

CDC	calculated day of confinement • Center for Disease Control & Prevention
CDCA	chenodeoxycholic acid
CDE	canine distemper encephalitis • Certified Diabetes Educator • common duct exploration
CDEC	Commission on Disability Examiner Certification
cdf	cumulative distribution function
CDH	congenital dislocation of hip • congenital diaphragmatic hernia
CDMS	Certified Disability Management Specialist • Commission on Disability Management Specialists
CDMSC	Certification of Disability Management Specialists Committee
CDNA	complementary deoxyribonucleic acid • copy deoxyribonucleic acid
CDP	comprehensive discharge planning • constant distending pressure • cytidine diphosphate • cytidine diphosphocholine • complete decongestive physiotherapy
CDS	cul-de-sac
CDT	carbon dioxide therapy
Cdyn	dynamic compliance
Ce	cerium
CE	California encephalitis • cardiac enlargement • cardiac enzyme • cerebral embolus • chloroform-ether • cholesterol esters • clinical emphysema • conjugated estrogens • constant error • continuing education • stroke • capsule endoscopy • claims examiner
CEA	carcinoembryonic antigen • crystalline egg albumin
CEAC	Certification in Environmental Access for Consultants and Contractors
CED	chronic enthusiasm disorder • chronic erythema disorder • cultural/ethnic diversity • chole-enteral diversion
CEEV	Central European encephalitis virus
CEF	chick embryo fibroblast (vaccine)

Cel	Celsius
CELO	chick embryo lethal orphan (virus)
CEM	conventional-transmission electron microscope
cemf	counter-electromotive force
CEN	Certified Emergency Nurse
cent	centigrade • central
CEO	congenital erythropoietic porphyria • counter-electrophoresis • counterimmunoelectrophoresis
Ceph-floc	cephalin flocculation (test)
CEQ	Council on Environmental Quality
CER	capital expenditure review • conditioned emotional response
cert	certificate • certified
cerv	cervical
CES	central excitatory state
CESD	cholesterol ester storage disease
CESI	cervical epidural steroid injection
CEU	continuing education unit
ct	compare (*confer*)
Cf	californium • carrier
CF	carbolfuchsin • cardiac failure • chest and left leg • Christmas factor • citrovorum factor • complement fixation • contractile force • count fingers (visual acuity test) • cystic fibrosis
C'F	complement fixing
C/F	count fingers (visual acuity test)
CFA	complement-fixing antibody • complete Freund adjuvant
CFC	colony-forming cell • continuous-flow centrifugation
CFF	critical fusion frequency (test) • Cystic Fibrosis Foundation
CFFA	cystic fibrosis factor activity

Cf-Fe	carrier-bound iron (*ferrum*)
CFI	chemotactic factor inactivator • complement fixation inhibition test
CFO	chief financial officer
CFR	Code of Federal Regulations
CFS	cancer family syndrome
CFT	complement fixation test
CFU	colony-forming unit
CFU-C	colony-forming unit-culture
CFU-E	colony-forming unit-erythroid
CFU-S	colony-forming unit-spleen
CFW	cancer-free white (mouse)
cg	centigram
CG	center of gravity • cholecystogram, cholecystography • chorionic gonadotropin • chronic glomerulonephritis • colloidal gold • control group • phosgene ("choking gas")
CGC	Certified Gastrointestinal Clinician
CGD	chromosomal gonadal dysgenesis • chronic granulomatous disease
CGH	chorionic gonadotropic hormone
CGL	chronic granulocytic anemia • chronic granulocytic leukemia
cgm	centigram
CGM	central gray matter
cGMP	cyclic guanosine monophosphate
CGN	chronic glomerulonephritis • Convalescent Growing Nursery
CGP	chorionic growth-hormone prolactin
cgs	centimeter-gram-second (system)
CGS	catgut suture • centimeter-gram-second (system)
CGTT	cortisone-glucose tolerance test

ch	chest • chief • child • chronic
CH	cholesterol • convalescent hospital • crown-heel length
C&H	cocaine and heroin
CHA	congenital hypoplastic anemia
ChAc	choline acetyltransferase
CHAMPUS	Civilian Health and Medical Program of the Uniformed Services
CHAMPVA	Civilian Health and Medical Program of the Veterans Administration
CHAP	Child Health Assessment Program
chart	a paper (*charta*)
ChB	Bachelor of Surgery (*Chirurgiae Baccalaureus*)
CHB	complete heart block
CHC	Community Health Center
ChD	Doctor of Surgery (*Chirurgiae Doctor*)
CHD	congenital heart disease • coronary heart disease
ChE	cholinesterase
chem	chemical, chemistry
CHEOPS	Children's Hospital of Eastern Ontario Pain Scale
CHF	congestive heart failure
chg	change
CHI	creatinine height index
CHIP	Comprehensive Health Insurance Plan • Children's Health Insurance Program – Title 21
chl	chloroform
CHL	chloramphenicol
ChM	Master of Surgery (*Chirurgiae Magister*)
CHN	Certified Hemodialysis Nurse • community health network • community health nurse
CHO	carbohydrate • Chinese hamster ovary (cell)

CH_2O	carbohydrate
Chol	cholesterol
CHP	child psychiatry • comprehensive health plan
ch px	chicken pox
chr	chronic
chron	chronic
CHS	Chediak-Higashi syndrome
CHSS	Cooperative Health Statistics System
Ci	curie
CI	cardiac index • cardiac insufficiency • cerebral infarction • chain-initiating • chemotherapeutic index • coeffecient of intelligence • colloidal iron • Colour Index • crystalline insulin • cumulative injury
cib	food (*cibus*)
CIBD	chronic inflammatory bowel disease
CIB HA	congenital inclusion-body hemolytic anemia
CIC	cardiac inhibitor center • Certified Infection Control • circulating immune complex (titer)
CICU	cardiac (coronary) intensive care unit
CID	Central Institute for the Deaf • chick infective dose • cytomegalic inclusion disease
CIDS	cellular immunodeficiency syndrome
CIE	counterimmunoelectrophoresis
CIF	claims inquiry forms • cloning inhibiting factor
CIH	carbohydrate-induced hyperglycemia
Ci-hr	curie – hour
CIL	Center for Independent Living • Central Identification Laboratory
CILHI	Central Identification Laboratory - Hawaii
CIM	cortically induced movement

C_{in}	insulin clearance
C In	insulin clearance
CIN	cerebriform intradermal nevus • cervical intraepithelial neoplasia • Computers in Nursing
CIR	Comprehensive Inpatient Rehabilitation
CIRB	California Worker's Compensation Inspection Rating Bureau
circ	circular • circumcision • circumference
Circ	circulating, circulation, circulatory
CIRR	cirrhosis
CIS	carcinoma in situ • central inhibitory state • clinical information systems
cit	citrate
CIT	combined intermittent therapy
CIV	continuous intravenous (infusion)
CJD	Creutzfeldt-Jakob disease
ck	check
CK	creatine kinase
CK-BB	isoenzyme of creatine kinase with brain subunits
CKD	chronic kidney disease
CK-MB	isoenzyme of creatine kinase with muscle and brain subunits
CK-MM	isoenzyme of creatine kinase with muscle subunits
cl	centiliter • clavicle • clinic • closure • corpus luteum
Cl	chloride • chlorine
CL	capacity of the lung • chest and left arm • *Clostridium* • corpus luteum • critical list • current liabilities • cycle length
CL	compliance of the lungs
CLA	cervicolinguoaxial
CLAS	career ladder advancement system • culturally and linguistically appropriate service

CLBBB	complete left bundle branch block
CLCP	Certified Life Care Planner
CL/CP	cleft lip, cleft palate
CLD	chronic liver disease
CLH	chronic lobular hepatitis
clin	clinic, clinical
CLIP	cerebral lipidosis without visceral involvement and with onset of disease past infancy • corticotrophin-like intermediate lobe peptide
CLL	cholesterol-lowering lipid • chronic lymphatic leukemia • chronic lymphocytic leukemia
CLMA	Clinical Laboratory Management Association
CLML	Current List of Medical Literature
CLN	computer liaison nurse
CLO	cod liver oil
CIP	Clinical Pathology
Cl pal	cleft palate
CLS	clinical laboratory scientist
CLSP	clinical laboratory specialist
CLT	clinical laboratory technician • clinical laboratory technologist • clot lysis time
clysis	hypodermoclysis
cm	centimeter • complications • costal margin • tomorrow morning (*cras mane*)
Cm	curium
C_m	maximum clearance
CM	case manager • chloroquine and mepacrine • chondromalacia • circular muscle • competing message • congenital malformation • contrast media • costal margin • Master of Surgery
C&M	cocaine and morphine

cm^3	cubic centimeter
CMA	Canadian Medical Association • certified medical assistant
CMAC	Case Management Administrator Certified
c magnum	tablespoon, tablespoonful (*cochleare magnum*)
CMAP	compound muscle action potential
CMB	carbolic methylene blue
CMC	carboxymethylcellulose • carpometacarpal • Chloromycetin • Case Manager, Certified
CMCN	Certified Manager Care Nurse
CMD	cerebromacular degeneration
CME	cervical mediastinal exploration • continuing medical education • cystoid macular edema
CMF	cyclophosphamide, methotrexate, fluorouracil
CMFP	cyclophosphamide, methotrexate, fluorouracil, prednisone
CMFVP	cyclophosphamide, methotrexate, fluorouracil, vincristine, prednisone
CMG	cystometrogram
CMGN	chronic membranous glomerulonephritis
CMHC	Community Mental Health Center
CMI	carbohydrate metabolism index • cell-mediated immunity • Cornell Medical Index
CMID	cytomegalic inclusion disease
c/min	cycles per minute
CMIR	cell-mediated immune response
CMIS	Case Management Information Systems
CMIT	Current Medical Information and Terminology
CML	cell-mediated lympholysis • chronic myelocytic leukemia • chronic myelogenous leukemia
cmm	cubic millimeter
cm/m^2	centimeters per square meter

CMM	cutaneous malignant melanoma
CMS	Center for Medicare and Medicaid Services
CMN	cystic medial necrosis
cMo	centimorgan
CMO	cardiac minute output
C-MOPP	cyclophosphamide, mechlorethamine, Oncovin, procarbazine, prednisone
CMP	competitive medical plans • cytidine monophosphate
CMR	cerebral metabolic rate • cystic medical necrosis
CMRG	cerebral metabolic rate of glucose
CMRNG	chromosomally mediated resistant *Neisseria gonorrhoeae*
CMRO	cerebral metabolic rate of oxygen
cms	to be taken tomorrow morning (*cras mane sumendus*)
CMSA	Case Management Society of America
CMSC	Certified Medical Staff Coordinator
cm/sec	centimeters per second
CMSS	Council of Medical Specialty Societies
CMSUA	clean, midstream urinalysis
CMT	catechol-O-methyltransferase • Charcot-Marie-Tooth • Current Medical Technology
CMV	cytomegalovirus
cn	tomorrow night (*cras nocte*)
CN	caudate nucleus • Charge Nurse • clinical nursing • congenital nystagmus • cranial nerve • cyanogen
CNA	Canadian Nurses Association • certified nurse assistant • chart not available
Cn-Cbl	cyanocobalamin
CNE	chronic nervous exhaustion
CNH	community nursing home
CML	community nursing liaison

CNM	certified nurse-midwife • clinical nurse manager
CNOR	Certified Nurse, Operating Room
CNP	constant negative pressure
CNRN	Certified Neuroscience Registered Nurse
cns	to be taken tomorrow night (*cras nocte sumendus*)
CNS	central nervous system • clinical nurse-specialist • computerized notation system
CNSD	chronic nonspecific diarrhea • Certified Nutrition Support Dietitian
CNSN	Certified Nutrition Support Nurse
CNV	contingent negative variation
co	cutoff
Co	cobalt • coenzyme
^{60}Co	radioactive cobalt
CO	carbon monoxide • cardiac output • castor oil • co-insurance • compound • cross-over • central office
C/O	complains of
CO_2	carbon dioxide
Co I	coenzyme I (diphosphopyridine nucleotide, nicotinamide adenine dinucleotide)
Co II	coenzyme II (triphosphopyridine nucleotide, nicotinamide adenine dinucleotide phosphate)
CoA	coenzyme A
COAD	chronic obstructive airway disease
coag	coagulation
COAP	cyclophosphamide, Oncovin, cytosine arabinoside, prednisone
COB	coordination of benefits
COBOL	Common Business Oriented Language
COBRA	Consolidated Omnibus Budget Reconciliation Act (1985)
COBS	Cesarean-obtained barrier-sustained

COBT	chronic obstruction of biliary tract
coc	coccygeal • coccyx
COC	cathodal opening contraction • combination of oral contraceptive • calcifying odontogenic cyst
cochl	spoonful (*cochleare*)
cochl amp	heaping spoonful (*cochleare amplum*)
cochl mag	tablespoon (*cochleare magnum*)
cochl parv	teaspoon (*cochleare parvum*)
COCL	cathodal opening clonus
coct	boiling (*coctio*)
cod	codeine
COD	cause of death • chemical oxygen demand • condition on discharge
CODA	Cadaveric Organ Donor Act • Co-Dependents Anonymous
COE	course of the employment
coef	coefficient
coeff	coefficient
COEPS	cortically originating extrapyramidal system
C of A	coarctation of aorta
COGTT	cortisone-primed oral glucose tolerance test
COH	carbohydrate
COHb	carboxyhemoglobin
COHgb	carboxyhemoglobin
COHN	Certified Occupational Health Nurse
COHN-CM	Certified Occupational Health Nurse – Case Manager
COHN–S	Certified Occupational Health Nurse – Specialist
COHN-S/CM	Certified Occupational Health Nurse – Specialist/Case Manager
col	colony • color • strain (cola)

COL	cost of living
colat	strained (*colatus*)
COLD	chronic obstructive lung disease
cold agg	cold agglutinin
coll	collect, collection • college • colloidal • eyewash (*collyrium*)
collut	mouthwash (*collutorium*)
collyr	eyewash (*collyrium*)
COM	cyclophosphamide, Oncovin, methotrexate
COMA	cyclophosphamide, Oncovin, methotrexate, cytosine arabinoside
comb	combination
ComC	Committee Chairperson
COMLA	cyclophosphamide, Oncovin, methotrexate, leucovorin, cytosine arabinoside
comm	committee, commission, commissioner
commun dis	communicable disease
comp	compare, comparative, comparable • composition • compound • compression
compd	compound
compet	competition
compl	complete, completed • complication
complic	complicating, complication
COMT	catechol-O-methyltransferase
CON	certificate of need
ConA	concunavalin A
conc	concentrated, concentration
concis	cut (*concisus*)
cond	condense, condensed • condition
cond ref	conditioned reflex

cond resp	conditioned response
conf	conference
cong	congenital • congress • gallon (*conglius*)
congen	congenital
congr	congruent
conjug	conjugated, conjugation
cons	keep (*conserva*)
const	constant
cont	containing • contents • continue, continued
cont rem	let the medicine be continued (*continuatur remedium*)
contrx	contraction
conv	convalescent, convalescence
coord	coordination
COP	capillary osmotic pressure • colloid osmotic pressure
COPD	chronic obstructive pulmonary disease
COPE	chronic obstructive pulmonary emphysema
COPP	cyclophosphamide, Oncovin, procarbazine, prednisone
coq	boil (*coque*)
CoQ	coenzyme Q
coq in s a	boil in sufficient water (*coque in sufficiente aqua*)
cos s a	boil properly (*coque secundum artem*)
cor	corrected • heart (*cor*)
CoR	Congo red
COR	Comprehensive Outpatient Rehabilitation Facility • coronary • heart (*cor*) • Conditioned Orientation Response
CORF	comprehensive outpatient rehabilitation facilities
corr	correct, corrected • correlate
cort	cortex, cortical

CORT	Certified Operating Room Technician
cos	change of shift • cosine
CO_2T	total carbon dioxide content
COTA	Certified Occupational Therapy Assistant
COTe	cathodal opening tetanus
COTH	Council of Teaching Hospitals
COTRANS	Coordinated Transfer Application System
COTS	commercial off-the-shelf software
coul	coulomb (electrical unit)
cp	chemically pure • centipoise
CP	candle power • capillary pressure • cerebellopontile • cerebellopontine • cerebral palsy • chemically pure • chloropurine • chloroquine and primaquine • chronic pyelonephritis • cleft palate • clinical pathways • constant pressure • coproporphyrin • cor pulmonale • creatine phosphate • critical pathways • cyclophosphamide • capital payments
C&P	cystoscopy and pyelogram
CPA	Canadian Physiotherapy Association • cardiopulmonary arrest • carotid phonoangiography • costophrenic angle • cyproterone acetate
CPAC	competitive pricing advisory committee
CPAN	Certified Post-Anesthesia Nurse
C_{pah}	Para-aminohippurate clearance
CPA/OBG	carotid phonoangiography/oculoplethysmography
CPAP	continuous (constant) positive airway pressure
c parvum	teaspoonful (*cochleare parvum*)
CPB	cardiopulmonary bypass • competitive protein binding
CPBA	competitive protein-binding analysis • competitive protein-binding assay
CPBS	cardiopulmonary bypass surgery

CPC	chronic passive congestion • clinical pathologic correlation • clinicopathologic conference • community psychiatric center
CPCRA	Community Programs for Clinical Research on AIDS
cpd	compare • compound
CPD	cephalopelvic disproportion • citrate phosphate dextrose solution • continuous peritoneal dialysis
CPD-A	citrate phosphate dextrose-adenine solution
CPDD	calcium pyrophosphate deposition disease
CPDM	Certified Professional in Disability Management
CPE	chronic pulmonary emphysema • cytopathic effect • cytopathogenic effect
CPEHS	Consumer Protection and Environmental Health Service
CPF	clot-promoting factor
CPGM	capillary blood glucose monitoring
CPGN	chronic progressive glomerulonephritis
CPH	Certificate in Public Health • chronic persistent hepatitis
CPHA	Committee on Professional and Hospital Activities • community public health agency
CPHQ	Certified Professional in Healthcare Quality
CPI	constitutional psychopathic inferiority • consumer price index • coronary prognostic index • cost-patient index • competitive price index
CPIB	chlorophenoxyisobutyrate
CPID	chronic pelvic inflammatory disease
CPK	creatine phosphokinase
CPK-BB (CPK$_1$)	a CPK isoenzyme (CPK$_1$)
CPK-MB (CPK$_2$)	a CPK isoenzyme (CPK$_2$)
CPK-MM (CPK$_3$)	a CPK isoemzyme (CPK$_3$)
cpm	counts per minute
CPM	continuous passive motion • counts per minute

CPMG	Carr-Purcell-Meiboom-Gill (spin-echo technique)
CPN	chronic polyneuropathy • chronic pyelonephritis
CPNP	Certified Pediatric Nurse Practitioner
CPP	cerebral perfusion pressure • cyclopentanophenanthrene • chronic pelvic pain
CPPB	continuous (constant) positive-pressure breathing
CPPD	calcium pyrophosphate dihydrate
CP&PD	chest percussion and postural drainage
CPPV	continuous (constant) positive-pressure ventilation
CPQA	Certified Professional in Quality Assurance
CPR	cardiac and pulmonary rehabilitation • cardiopulmonary resuscitation • computer-based patient records • cortisol production rate
cps	counts per second • cycles per second
CPS	Child Protective Services • chloroquine, pyrimethamine, sulfisoxazole
CPSC	Consumer Product Safety Commission
CPSII	carbamoyl phosphate synthetase II
CPT	chest physiotherapy • combining power test • Current Procedural Terminology
CPT-4	Current Procedural Terminology
CPU	central processing unit (computer)
CPUR	Certified Professional Utilization Review
CPX	complete physical examination
CPZ	chlorpromazine • Compazine
CQ	chloroquine and quinine
CQI	continuous quality improvement
Cr	chromium • creatinine • crisis

CR	cardiorespiratory • central ray • chest and right arm • closed reduction • clot retraction • coefficient of fat retention • colon resection • complete remission • complete response • conditioned reflex, response • controlled release • cranial • creatinine • cresol red • critical ratio • crown-rump (length) • cyanosis retinae • cardiac rehabilitation
C & R	compromise and release
CRA	central retinal artery
CRAB	Central Registry at Bethesda
CRBBB	complete right bundle branch block
CRC	colorectal carcinoma • Certified Rehabilitation Counselor • Commission on Rehabilitation Counseling
CRD	chronic renal disease • chronic respiratory disease • completely randomized design • complete reaction of degeneration
CRE	cumulative radiation effect
creat	creatinine
CREG	cross-reactive group (of HLA antigens)
CREST	calcinosis cutis, Raynaud's phenomenon, esophageal dysfunctional hypermotility, scelodactyly, telangiectasia (syndrome)
CRF	chronic renal failure • citrovorum rescue factor • corticotropin-releasing factor
CRH	corticotropin-releasing hormone
crit	criteria • critical
Crit	hematocrit
CRL	crown-rump length
CRM	certified raw milk • cross-reacting material
CRNA	Certified Registered Nurse-Anesthetist
CRO	cathode-ray oscilloscope
CROS	contralateral routing of signal
CrP	creatinine phosphate

CRP	community resource professional • C-reactive protein • cysticretinal pigmentation
CRPA	C-reactive protein antiserum
CRPS	complex regional pain syndrome
CRRN	Certified Rehabilitation Registered Nurse
CRRN-A	Certified Rehabilitation Registered Nurse – Advanced
CRS	Chinese restaurant syndrome • colon-rectal surgery • congenital rubella syndrome
CRST	calcinosis cutis, Raynaud's phenomenon, sclerodactyly, telangiectasia (syndrome)
CRT	cathode-ray tube • certified • complex reaction time • community resource trainee
CRTT	certified respiratory therapy technician
CRV	central retinal vein
CRVO	central retinal vein occlusion
crys	crystal, crystalline, crystallized
cryst	crystal, crystalline, crystallized
cs	case • conscious • consciousness
Cs	cesium
^{137}Cs	radioactive cesium
CS	cat scratch • central supply • cesarean section • chronic schizophrenia • clinical stage • completed stroke • conditioned stimulus • conjuctival secretions • coronary sinus • corpus striatum • corticosteroid • current strength • cycloserine
C&S	conjunctiva and sclera • culture and sensitivity • culture and susceptibility
CSB	chemical stimulation of the brain
CSBO	complete small bowel obstruction
CSCT	comprehensive support care team
CSD	cat scratch disease • celiac sprue disease
C-section	Cesarean section

CSF	cerebrospinal fluid • colony-stimulating factor
CSFP	cerebrospinal fluid pressure
CSF-WR	cerebrospinal fluid - Wasserman reaction
CSI	cholesterol saturation index
CSLU	chronic stasis leg ulcer
CSM	cerebrospinal meningitis • circulation, sensation, mobility • Consolidated Standards Manual
CSN	carotid sinus nerve • Certified School Nurse
CSNR	carotid sinus nerve resection
CSNS	carotid sinus nerve stimulation • carotid sinus nerve stimulator
CSOM	chronic serous otitis media
C-spine	cervical spine
CSR	central supply room • Cheyne-Stokes respiration • corrected sedimentation rate • cortisol secretion rate
CSS	chewing, sucking, swallowing
Cst	static compliance
CST	contraction stress test • convulsive shock therapy
CSU	catheter specimen of urine
CSUF	continuous slow ultrafiltration
CT	calcitonin • cardiothoracic • chemotherapy • circulation time • clotting time • coated tablet • compressed tablet • computerized tomography • connective tissue • Coombs' test • corneal transplant • coronary thrombosis • corrective therapy • crutch training • cytotechnologist • continuing trauma
CTA	clear to auscultation • clinical teaching associate • cytoplasmic tubular aggregates • cytotoxic assay
CTAB	cetyltrimethylammonium bromide
CTB	ceased to breathe • chronic tuberculosis
CTBA	cetrimonium bromide
CTBM	cetyltrimethylammonium bromide

CTC	chlortetracycline
CTCL	cutaneous T-cell lymphoma
CTD	carpal tunnel decompression • cumulative trauma disorder
CTF	Colorado tick fever
C/TG	cholesterol-triglyceride ratio
CTICU	cardiothoracic intensive care unit
CTL	cytotoxic lymphocytes
CTP	cytidine triphosphate
ctr	center • control
CTR	cardiothoracic ratio • carpal tunnel release
CTS	carpal tunnel syndrome • composite treatment score • computerized tomographic scanner
CTU	cardiothoracic unit • centigrade thermal unit
CTUWSD	chest tube under water seal drainage
CTX	Cytoxan • cervical traction
CTZ	chemoreceptor trigger zone • chlorothiazide
cu	cubic • curie
CU_μ	cubic micron
Cu	copper (*cuprum*)
C_u	urea clearance
CU	cause unknown • clinical unit • control unit • convalescent unit • curie
CUC	chronic ulcerative colitis
cu cm	cubic centimeter
CUD	congenital urinary (tract) deformities
cu ft	cubic foot
CUG	cystourethrogram
cu in	cubic inch
cuj	of which (*cujus*)

cuj lib	of any you desire (*cujus libet*)
cult	culture
cu m	cubic meter
cum	cumulative report
cu mm	cubic millimeter
cur	curative • current
CUR	cystourethrocele
CURN	Certified Urological Registered Nurse
cu yd	cubic yard
cv	tomorrow evening (*cras vespere*)
CV	cardiovascular • cell volume • central venous • cerebrovascular • closing volume • coefficient of variation • concentrated volume • conduction velocity • conjugate diameter of pelvic inlet • constant volume • corpuscular volume • cresyl violet • critical value • curriculum vitae
CVA	cardiovascular accident • cerebrovascular accident • costovertebral angle
CVC	central venous catheter • crying vital capacity
CVD	cardiovascular disease • cerebrovascular disease • color-vision deviant
CVE	Certified Vocational Evaluation
CVI	cerebrovascular insufficiency
CVN	central venous nutrient
CVO	obstetric conjugate diameter of pelvic inlet (*conjugata vera obstetrica*)
C_VO_2	mixed venous oxygen content
CVP	cardiac valve procedure • central venous pressure • cyclophosphamide, vincristine, prednisone
CVP lab	cardiovascular-pulmonary laboratory
CVPP	cyclophosphamide, vincristine, prednisone, procarbazine
CVPR	central venous pressure report

CVR	cardiovascular-renal • cardiovascular-respiratory • cerebrovascular resistance
CVS	cardiovascular surgery • cardiovascular system • chorionic villi sampling • clean-voided specimen
cw	cell wall • common wart • continuous-wave
CW	Case Worker • chemical warfare • chest wall • Children's Ward • clockwise • continuous-wave • crutch walking
CWBTS	capillary whole-blood true sugar
CWCI	California Worker's Compensation Institute
cwop	childbirth without pain
CWP	childbirth without pain • coal workers' pneumoconiosis
CWS	cold water soluble
cwt	hundredweight
Cx	cervix • convex
CX	circumflex artery
CXR	chest x-ray
CY	calendar year • cyanogen
c/y	Children and Youth Project of Maternal and Child Health Program
CYCLO	cyclophosphamide • cyclopropane
Cyd	cytidine
cyl	cylinder, cylindrical
CYL	casein yeast lactate
Cys	cysteine • cystoscopy
Cysto	cystoscopy
Cyt	Cytosine
cytol	cytologic, cytology
CZI	crystalline zinc insulin

D

d	date • day • deceased, dead, died • degree • density • deuterium • dextro- (right, clockwise) • dose • give (*da*)
/d	daily, per day
D	date • daughter • day • dead space • deciduous • decreased • density • dermatologist, dermatology • deuterium • deviation • dextrorotatory • dextrose • diameter • died • diffusion coefficient • diopter • disease • distal • diverticulum • divorced • dorsal • dorsal vertebra • dose • duration • right (*dexter*) • vitamin D unit
DA	degenerative arthritis • delayed action • developmental age • direct admission • direct agglutination • disability assistance • dispense as directed • dopamine • ductus arteriosus
D/A	date of admission
DAA	double aortic arch
DAB	diaminobutyric acid • dimethylaminoazobenzene
DAD	delayed after depolarization
DADDS	diacetyldiaminodiphenyl sulfone
DAF	decay-activating factor
DAFT	Draw-a-Family Test
DAGT	direct antiglobulin test
DAH	disordered action of the heart
DAI	diffuse axonal injury
dal	decaliter
DALA	delta-aminolevulinic acid
DAM	degraded amyloid • diacetylmonoxime
dAMP	deoxyadenosine monophosphate (deoxyadenylate)
DAO	diamine oxidase
DAP	Department of Applied Physiology • dihydroxyacetone phosphate • Draw-A-Person test

DAPT	direct agglutination pregnancy test • Draw-A-Person Test
DAR	daily affective rhythm
DARP	drug abuse rehabilitation program
DASD	direct access storage device
DASP	double antibody solid phase
DAT	delayed action tablet • diet as tolerated • differential agglutination titer • differential aptitude test • diptheria antitoxin • direct anti-globulin test
dau	daughter
DAUNO	daunorubicin
DAW	dispense as written
db	decibel
dB	decibel
DB	date of birth • dextran blue • distobuccal • diabetes
D/B	date of birth
DBA	dibenzanthracene
DBCL	dilute blood clot lysis (method)
DBE	synthetic estrogen
DBF	disturbed bowel function
DBH	dopamine beta-hydroxylase
DBI	development at birth index • phenformin
DBI-TD	phenformin hydrochloride
dbl	double
DBM	diabetic management
DBMS	data-base management system
DBO	distobucco-occlusal
DBP	diastolic blood pressure • dibutylphthalate • distobuccopupal
DBT	dialectical behavior therapy

dc	discontinue
DC	Dental Corps • diagnostic center • diagonal conjugate • dihydrocodeine • dephenylarsine cyanide • direct Coombs' (test) • direct current • Direction Circular • discharge(d) • discontinue • distocervical • Doctor of Chiropractic • donor cells
D/C	diarrhea/constipation • discontinue
D&C	dilatation and curettage
DCA	deoxycholate-citrate agar • desoxycorticosterone acetate
DCB	dilutional cardiopulmonary bypass
DC&B	dilatation, curettage and biopsy
DCc	double concave
DCC	day care center • deletion colon carcinoma
DCCN	Dimensions of Critical-Care Nursing
DCCT	Diabetes Control and Complications Trial
DCE-MRI	dynamic contrast-enhanced magnetic resonance imaging
DCF	day care facility • direct centrifugal flotation method
DCG	desoxycorticosterone glucoside • disodium cromoglycate
DCH	delayed cutaneous hypersensitivity
DCI	dichloroisoproterenol
dCMP	deoxycytidine monophosphate
DCN	delayed conditioned necrolysis
DCP	dicalcium phosphate • discharge plan, discharge planner
DCR	direct cortical response • direct critical response
DCS	dorsal column stimulator
DCT	direct Coombs' test • distal convoluted tubule
DCTMA	desoxycorticosterone triphenylacetate
dCTP	deoxycytidine triphosphate
DCU	Diabetes Care Unit

DCx	double coverage
DCX	double convex
DD	dependent drainage • developmental disability • diaper dermatitis • disability determination • disc diameter • differential diagnosis • DiGuglielmo disease • double dose • dry dressing • development delays
DDA	DDT metabolite excreted in urine
DDAVP	desamino-D-arginine vasopressin
DDB	donor directed blood
DDC	diethyldithiocarbamic acid
DDD	degenerative disc disease • dense-deposit disease • dichloro-diphenyl-dichloroethane
DDE	DDT metabolite that accumulates in fatty tissue • direct data entry
DDGB	double-dose gallbladder (choloecystogram)
DDR	discharged during referral
DDS	diaminodiphenylsulfone • Doctor of Dental Surgery • dystrophy-dystonia syndrome
DDSc	Doctor of Dental Science
DDST	Denver Developmental Screening Test
DDT	dichloro-diphenyl-trichloroethane (chlorophenothane)
DDVP	dichlorovinyl-dimethyl-phosphate (dichlorvos)
DDx	differential diagnosis
DE	digestive energy • dose equivalent
D&E	dilatation and evacuation
DEA	dehydroepiandrosterone • Drug Enforcement Agency
DEAE	diethylaminothanol • diethylaminoethyl
DEAE-D	diethylaminoethyl dextran
DEB	diethylbutanediol • dystrophic epidermolysis bullosa • Disability Evaluation Bureau
DEBA	diethylbarbaturic acid

debil	debility
dec	deceased • decompose, decomposed • decreased • pour off (*decanta*)
deca-	ten
dec'd	deceased
decel	deceleration
deci-	one-tenth
decoct	decoction
decomp	decompose, decomposed, decomposition
decr	decrease, decreased
decub	lying down (*decbitus*)
de d in d	from day to day (*de die in diem*)
def	defecate, defecation • deficient, deficiency • definite • definition
DEF	decayed, extracted or filled (teeth)
defic	deficiency
defib	defibrillate
deform	deformity
deg	degeneration • degree
degen	degeneration
degult	let it be swallowed (*deglutiatur*)
DEHS	Division of Emergency Health Services
del	delivery • delusion
Dem	Demerol (meperidine)
DEM	Department of Emergency Medicine
denom	denominator
dent	dental • let it be given (*dentur*)
dep	dependent
DEP	diethylpropanediol

depr	depressed, depression
dept	department
De R	reaction of degeneration
deriv	derive, derivation, derivative
derm	dermatology, dermatologist
DES	diethylstilbestrol
desat	desaturation
desc	descent, descending
DESI	Drug Efficacy Study Implementation
dest	distilled (*destillata*)
det	determine • let it be given (*detur*)
DET	diethyltryptamine
detn	detention
dets	let it be given and labeled (*detur et signatur*)
DEU	Disability Evaluation Unit
dev	develop, development • deviate, deviation
DEV	duck embryo vaccine
devel	develop, development
DEXA	dual energy X-ray absorptiometry
DF	decayed and filled (teeth) • degrees of freedom (a statistical parameter) • dorisflexion • dry gas phase fractional concentration
DFA	diet for age • direct fluorescent antibody (technique)
DFDD	difluorodiphenyldichloroethane
DFDT	difluorophenyltrichloroethane
DFMC	daily fetal movement count
DFO	deferoxamine (desferrioxamine)
DFP	disopropylfluorophosphate
DFR	dialysate filtration rate

DFS	disease-free survival • dead fetus syndrome
DFT_4	dialyzable free thyroxine 4
DFU	dead fetus in utero
dg	decigram
DG	deoxyglucose • diagnose, diagnosis, diagnostic • diglyceride
dGDP	deoxyguanosine diphosphate
DGI	disseminated gonococcal infection
dgm	decigram
dGMP	deoxyguanosine monophosphate (deoxyguanylate)
dGTP	deoxyguanosine triphosphate
DGVB	dextrose, gelatin, Veronal buffer
DH	delayed hypersensitivity • dermatitis herpetiformis • diffuse and histiocytic
DHA	dehydroepiandrosterone • dihydroxyacetone
DHE	dihydroergotamine
DHEA	dehydropiandrosterone
DHEAS	dehydroepiandrosterone sulfate
DHEW	Department of Health, Education and Welfare
DHF	dengue hemorrhagic fever
DHFR	dihydrofolate reductase
DHHS	Department of Health and Human Services
DHL	diffuse histiocytic lymphoma
DHMO	Dental Health Maintenance Organization
DHO	deiterium hydrogen oxide
DHPR	dihydropteridine reductase
DHS	Department of Health Services • direct health service • duration of hospital stay
DHSM	dihydrostreptomycin

DHSQ	Division of Health Standards and Quality
DHT	dihydrotachysterol • dihydrotestosterone
DHy	Doctor of Hygiene
Di	Diego blood group
DI	deterioration index • diabetes insipidus • disability insurance • distoincisal • double indemnity
D/I	Date of Injury
dia	diameter • diatherm
DIA	Division of Industrial Accidents
diab	diabetes, diabetic
diag	diagnosis, diagnostic • diagonal • diagram
diam	diameter
diath	diathermy
DIB	disability insurance benefit
DIC	diffuse intravascular coagulation • drug information center
DIDMOAD	diabetes insipidus, diabetes mellitus, optic atrophy, deafness
dieb alt	on alternate days (*diebus alternis*)
dieb tert	every third day (*diebus tertiis*)
dif	differential blood count • differential leukocyte count
DIF	diffuse interstitial fibrosis • direct immunofluorescence
Diff	difference, different • differential • differential blood count • differential leukocyte count
diff diag	differential diagnosis
DIFP	diisopropyl fluorophosphonate
dig	digitalis
Dig	digitalis
dil	dilute, diluted, dilution
dilat	dilate, dilated, dilation, dilatation
DILD	diffuse infiltrative lung disease

dilut	dilute, diluted, dilution
dim	dimension • diminish • diminutive
DIM	one-half (*dimidius*)
dIMP	deoxyinosine monophosphate (deoxyinosinate)
d in p aeq	divide into equal parts (*divide in partes aequales*)
diopt	diopter
DIP	desquamative interstitial pneumonia • distal interphalangeal
DIPC	diffuse interstitial pulmonary calcification
DIPF	diisopropylphosphofluoridate
diph	diphtheria
DIPJ	distal interphalangeal joint
dir	direct
dis	disabled • disease • distance
disc	discontinue
disch	discharge, discharged
DISH	diffuse idiopathic skeletal hyperostosis
disloc	dislocate, dislocation
disp	dispense, dispensary
dissd	dissolved
dissem	disseminate, disseminated, dissemination
dist	distal • distill, distilled • distribute, distribution • disturbance
distill	distillation
DIT	diiodotyrosine
div	divergence • divide, division • divorced
DJD	degenerative joint disease
DKA	diabetic ketoacidosis
dkg	dekagram

dkl	dekaliter
dkm	dekameter
DKS	deoxyketosteroids
dl	deciliter
DL	danger list • diffusing capacity of the lung • direct laryngoscopy • distolingual • Donath-Landsteiner (test)
DLa	distolabial
DlaI	distolabioincisal
DLaP	distolabiopulpal
DLB	diffuse and lymphoblastic
DLCO	diffusing capacity of the lung
DLCO-SB	single-breath diffusing capacity of the lung for carbon monoxide
DLE	discoid lupus erythematosus • disseminated lupus erythematosus
DLI	distolinguoincisal
dm	decimeter
DM	diabetes mellitus • diastolic murmur • disease management • dopamine • double minute • membrane-diffusing capacity
DMA	dimethyladenosine • directed memory access • District Medical Advisor
DMABA	dimethylaminobenzaldehyde
DMAPN	dimethylaminopropionitrile
DMARD	disease-modifying antirheumatic drug
DMAT	disaster medical assistance team
DMCT	dimethylchlortetracycline
DMD	Doctor of Dental Medicine (*Dentariae Medicinae Doctor*)
DME	direct medical education • Director of Medical Education • durable medical equipment
DMEC	Disability Management Employer Coalition, Inc.

DMERC	durable medical equipment regional carriers
DMF	decayed, missing or filled (teeth)
DMFO	eflorinthine
DMFS	decayed, missing or filled surfaces
DMHS	Department of Mental Health Services
DMI	diaphragmatic myocardial infarction • Documentation of Medical Import
DMM	dimethylmyleran
DMN	dimethylnitrosamine
DMNA	dimethylnitrosamine
DMO	dimethyloxazolidinedione
DMOC	diabetes mellitus out of control
DMOOC	diabetes mellitus out of control
DMP	dimethylphosphate • dimethylphthalate
DMPA	depomedroxyprogesterone acetate
DMPE	3, 4 – dimethoxyphenylethylamine
DMS	delayed muscle soreness • dermatomyositis • Director of Medical Services • Disease Management Society
DMSA	dimercaptosuccinic acid
DMSO	dimethylsulfoxide
DMT	dimethyltryptamine (hallucinogenic drug)
DN	dicrotic notch • dibucaine number
D/N	dextrose-nitrogen ratio
DNA	deoxyribonucleic acid
DNase	deoxyribonuclease
DNB	dinitrobenzene
DNCB	dinitrochlorobenzene
DNE	Director of Nursing Education
DNFB	dinitrofluorbenzene

DNI	do not intubate
DNOC	dinotro-o-cresol
DNP	deoxyribonucleoprotein • dinitrophenyl
DNPH	dinitrophenylhydrazine
DNPM	dinitrophenylmorphine
DNR	daunorubicin • do not report • do not resuscitate
DNS	deviated nasal septum • Director of Nursing Service • dysplastic nevus system
D5/NS	5% dextrose in normal saline
DO	diamine oxidase • dissolved oxygen • disto-occlusal • Doctor of Osteopathy • doctor's orders
D & O	Decision and Order (of the Rehabilitation Unit)
DOA	date of admission • dead on arrival
DOAC	data operations and analysis center
DOB	date of birth • doctor's order book
doc	diabetes out of control • document, documentation
DOC	deoxycholate • deoxycorticosterone • diabetes out of control • drug of choice
DOCA	deoxycorticosterone acetate
DOC-SR	deoxycorticosterone secretion rate
DOD	Department of Defense
DOE	desoxyephedrine • dyspnea on exertion
DOES	disorders of excessive somnolence
DOI	Date of Injury
dom	dominant
DOM	dimethoxymethylamphetamine
DON	Director of Nurses
DOOC	diabetes out of control
DOOR	deafness, onchyo-osteodystrophy and mental retardation

DOPA	dihydroxyphenylalamine
DOPAC	dihydroxyphenylacetic acid
DOPS	diffuse obstructive pulmonary syndrome
dos	dose, dosage
DOS	day of surgery
DOT	Dictionary of Occupational Titles • died on (operating) table • directly observant therapy
DOU	Definitive Observation Unit
doz	dozen
DP	data processing • deep pulse • dementia praecox • diastolic pressure • diffusion pressure • digestible protein • diphosgene • disopyramide phosphate • displaced person • distal pancreatectomy • distopulpal • Doctor of Pharmacy • Doctor of Podiatry • donor's plasma • dorsalis pedis • dyspnea
DPA	diphenylamine
DPAHC	Durable Power of Attorney for Health Care
DPD	diffuse pulmonary disease
DPDA	phosphorodiamidic anhydride
DPDL	diffuse poorly differentiated lymphocytic
DPDT	double-pole, double-throw (switch)
DPG	diphosphoglycerate • displacement placentogram
DPH	Department of Public Health • diphenylhydantoin • Diploma in Public Health • Doctor of Public Health
DPL	diagnostic peritoneal lavage
dpm	disintegrations per minute
DPM	Doctor of Podiatric Medicine
DPN	diphosphopyridine nucleotide
DPNH	diphosphopyridine nucleotide, reduced form
DPO	designated provider organization
DPP	documented poor prognosis

dps	disintegrations per second
DPST	double-pole, single-throw (switch)
DPT	diphtheria, pertussis and tetanus toxoid • diphtheria toxoid-pertussis vaccine-tetanus toxoid immunization • Demerol, Phenergan and Thorazine
DPTI	diastolic pressure-time index
DQ	deterioration quotient • development quotient
dr	dram • dressing
Dr	doctor
DR	degeneration reaction • delivery room • diabetic retinopathy • diagnostic radiology • diurnal rhythm • dorsal root
DRA	despite resuscitation attempts
DRE	direct rectal exam • digital rectal exam
DRF	daily replacement factor
DRG	Diagnosis Related Group
$D(Rh_0)$	blood antigen
drng	drainage
DRQ	discomfort relief quotient
DRS	data retrieval system
drsg	dressing
DRTC	Diabetes Research and Training Center
DS	dead (air) space • dehydroepiandrosterone sulfate • depolarizing shift • density standard • desynchronized sleep • dextran sulfate • dextrose in saline • dilute strength • dioptic strength • Doctor of Science • donor's serum • double-stranded • double-strength • Down Syndrome • duration of systole
D-S	Doerfler-Stewart (test)
DSA	digital subtraction angiography
DSAP	disseminated superficial actinic porokeratosis
DSB	drug-seeking behavior

DSC	Doctor of Surgical Chiropody
DSCG	disodium cromoglycate
DSCM	Disease State Case Management
DSD	dry sterile dressing
dsg	dressing
DSH	deliberate self-harm • disproportionate share hospital
DSI	drug-seeking index
DSM	Diagnostic and Statistical Manual of Mental Disorders • disease state management
DSM-III-R	Diagnostic and Statistical Manual of Mental Disorders – Third Edition, Revised
DSS	dengue shock syndrome • decision support system
DST	desensitization test • dexamethasone suppression test
D-stix	dextrostix
DSVP	downstream venous pressure
Dt	duration of tetany
DT	delirium tremens • Dietetic Services • diphtheria and tetanus toxoids • distance test • doubling time (of tumor size) • duration of tetany • dietician
DtaP	diphtheria and tetanus toxoide and acellular pertussis vaccine
DTBC	d-tubocurarine
dtd	give of such a dose (*datur talis dosis*)
DTH	delayed-type hypersensitivity
DTIC	dacarbazine
DTM	dermatophyte test medium
DTN	diphtheria toxin, normal
DTNB	dithiobisnitrobenzoic acid
DTP	diphtheria toxoid-tetanus toxoid-pertussis vaccine immunization • distal tingling on percussion
DTPA	diethylenetriamine penta-acetic acid

DTR	deep tendon reflex
DTS	discrete time sample
DTX	detoxification
DU	deoxyuridine • diagnosis undetermined • diffuse and undifferentiated • dog unit • duodenal ulcer
DUB	dysfunctional uterine bleeding
DUG	drug use guidelines
DUI	driving under the influence
DUL	diffuse undifferentiated lymphoma
dUMP	deoxyuridine monophosphate (deoxyuridylate)
DUR	Drug Usage Review
dur dolor	while the pain lasts (*durante dolore*)
DUS	Doppler Ultrasound Stethescope
dUTP	deoxyuridine triphosphate
dv	double vision
DV	dependent variable • dilute volume • direct vision • distance vision • double vibration
D&V	diarrhea and vomiting
DVA	duration of voluntary apnea (test)
DVI	Digital Vascular Imaging
DVM	Doctor of Veterinary Medicine
DVMS	Doctor of Veterinary Medicine and Surgery
DVS	Doctor of Veterinary Science • Doctor of Veterinary Surgery
DVT	deep venous thrombus
DVVC	direct visualization of vocal chords
DW	distilled water • dry weight
D/W	dextrose in water
D_5W	5% dextrose in water
DWC	Department of Worker's Compensation

DWC-100	Employee Claim Form
DWDL	diffuse, well-differentiated, lymphocytic
DWI	driving while intoxicated
Dx	diagnosis
DX	dextran
DXM	dexamethasone
DXR	deep x-ray
DXRT	deep x-ray therapy
DXT	deep x-ray therapy
Dy	dysprosium
DYS	dysphasia
DZ	dizygotic, dizygous

E

e	base of natural-logarithm system (approximately 2.71828) • electronic charge • electron • from (*ex*)
E	electrode potential • electromotive force • emmetropia • enema • energy • enzyme • epidural • epinephrine • erythrocyte • *Escherichia* • experimenter • expired (gas) • extinction coefficient • eye
E_1	estrone
E_2	estradiol
E_3	estriol
ea	each
EA	early antigen • educational age • electroanesthesia • environmental assessment • erythrocyte antibody • employing agency
E&A	evaluate and advise
EAA	essential amino acid
EAB	extra-anatomic bypass
EAC	erythrocyte antibody complement • external auditory canal

EACA	epsilon-aminocaproic acid
EACD	eczematous allergic contact dermatitis
EACH	essential access community hospital
ead	the same (*eadem*)
EAD	early after-depolarization
EAE	experimental allergic encephalomyelitis
EAHF	eczema, asthma, hay fever
EAI	electronically assisted instruction
EAL	electronic artificial larynx
EAM	external acoustic meatus
EAMG	experimental allergic myasthenia gravis
EAN	experimental allergic rhinitis
EANG	epidemic acute nonbacterial gastroenteritis
EAP	employee assistance program • epiallopregnanolone
EaR	reaction of degeneration (*Entartungs Reaktion*)
EAT	equine-assistance therapy
EB	elementary body • Epstein-Barr virus
EBAA	Eye Bank Association of America
EBBS	equal bilateral breath sounds
EBCDIC	extended binary-coded decimal interchange code
EBD	enrollee bad debt
EBF	erythroblastosis fetalis
EBI	emetine bismuth iodine
EBL	estimated blood loss
EBM	expressed breast milk
EBNA	Epstein-Barr virus nuclear antigen
EBP	epidural blood patch • estradiol-binding protein
EBS	electric brain stimulator

EBV	Epstein-Barr virus
EC	electron capture • emergency center • enteric-coated • entrance complaint • Enzyme Commission • expiratory center • extra-cellular compartment
E-C	ether-chloroform
E/C	estriol-creatinine ratio
ECA	electrocardioanalyzer • epidemiological catchment area
ECBO	enteric cytopathogenic bovine orphan (virus)
ECC	emergency cardiac care • external cardiac compression • extracorporeal circulation
ECCE	extracapsular cataract extraction
ECD	electron-capture detector
ECF	extended-care facility • extracellular fluid • eosinophil chemotactic factor • Employee Claim (or Benefits) Form
ECF-A	eosinophilic chemotactic factor of anaphylaxis
ECFMG	Educational Council for Foreign Medical Graduates
ECG	electrocardiogram, electrocardiography
echo	echoencephalogram, echoencephalography
Echo	echocardiogram
ECHO	electronic computing health oriented • enteric cytopathogenic human orphan (virus)
ECI	extracorporeal irradiation • electrocerebral inactivity
ECL	extension of cost limits
eclec	eclectic
ECM	egg crate mattress • erythema chronicum migrans • extracellular matrix
ECMO	enteric cytopathogenic monkey orphan (virus) • extracorporeal membrane oxygenation
ECOG	Eastern Cooperative Oncology Group
E coli	*Escherichia coli*
econ	economic

ECP	electronic claims processing • external counter-pulsation • Extended Care Pathway
ECPO	enteric cytopathogenic porcine orphan (virus)
ECPOG	electrochemical potential gradient
ECS	electrocerebral silence • electroconvulsive shock • electronic claims submission
ECSO	enteric cytopathogenic swine orphan (virus)
ECT	electroconvulsive therapy • enteric-coated tablet
ECU	extensorcarpularis
ECV	extracellular volume
ECW	extracellular water
ed	editor
ED	effective dose • emergency department • epidural • erythema dose • erectile dysfunction
ED_{50}	median effective dose
EDAP	Eating Disorders Awareness and Prevention
EDB	early dry breakfast • ethylene dibromide
EDC	effective dynamic compliance • estimated date of confinement
ED&C	electrodesiccation and curettage
Ed.D.	Doctor of Education
EDD	end-diastolic dimension • estimated discharge date • expected date of delivery
edent	edentulous
edit	editorial
EDN	electrodesiccation
EDP	electronic data processing • emergency department physician • end diastolic pressure
EDR	effective direct radiation • electrodermal response • expected death rate

EDRF	endothelium-derived relaxing factor • endothelial-derived relaxant factor
EDS	Ehlers-Danlos syndrome • extended date stream
EDTA	edetate disodium • edetic acid • ethylene-diaminetetra-acetic acid
educ	education
EDV	end-diastolic volume
EDx	electrodiagnosis
EE	embryo extract • equine encephalitis • eye and ear • employee
EEC	enteropathogenic *E. coli*
EEE	eastern equine encephalomyelitis
EEG	electroencephalogram, electroencephalography
EENT	eye, ear, nose and throat
EEOC	Equal Employment Opportunity Commission
EEP	end-expiratory pressure
EERP	extended endocardial resection procedure
EES	erythromycin ethylsuccinate
EF	ejection fraction • elongation factor • equivalent focus • erythroblastosis fetalis • erythrocytic fragmentation • exophthalmic factor • extended-field (radiotherapy) • extrinisic factor
EFA	Epilepsy Foundation of America • essential fatty acids
EFAD	essential fatty acid deficiency
EFE	endocardial fibroelastosis
eff	effect(s), effective • efferent • efficient
EFM	electronic fetal monitoring
EFP	effective filtration pressure
EFR	effective filtration rate • Employers First Report of Occupational Injury
eg	for example (*exempli gratia*)

EGA	estimated gestational age
EGC	epithelioid A globoid cells
EGD	esophagogastroduodenoscopy
EGF	epidermal growth factor
EGFR	epidermal growth factor receptor
EGG	electrogastrogram
EGHP	employer group health plan
EGOT	erythrocyte gluathione reductase
EGTA	esophageal gastric tube airway • egtazic acid
eH	oxidation-reduction potential
E_h	oxidation-reduction potential
EH	enlarged heart • essential hypertension • endometrial hyperplasia
E&H	environment and heredity
EHBF	estimated hepatic blood flow • extrahepatic blood flow
EHBFF	extrahepatic blood flow factor
EHC	exterohepatic circulation • enterhepatic clearance
EHDP	disodium etidronate • ethane hydroxydiphosphate
EHF	exophthalmos-hyperthyroid factor
EHH	esophageal hiatal hernia
EHIP	employee health insurance plan
EHL	effective half-life
EHPT	Eddy hot plate test
EHSDS	experimental health services delivery system
EIA	enzyme immunoassay • exercise-induced asthma
EIS	Epidemic Intelligence Service
EIT	erythrocyte iron turnover
EJ	elbow jerk

ejusd	of the same (*ejusdem*)
EKC	epidemic keratoconjunctivitis
EKG	electrocardiogram
EKY	electrokymogram
EL	effective-level • exercise limit
E-L	Eaton-Lambert syndrome
elb	elbow
ELB	early light breakfast
elect	electric, electricity
ELF	elective low forceps (delivery)
ELG	eligible
ELISA	enzyme-linked immunosorbent assay
elix	elixir
ELM	Early Language Milestone Scale
ELT	euglobulin lysis time
elytes	electrolytes
em	electromagnetic
EM	effective masking • electron microscope • emergency medicine • emmetropia
E-M	Embden-Meyerhof (glycolytic pathway)
E&M	endocrine and metabolic
EMA	emergency medical attendant
Emb	embryo, embryology
EMB	eosin methylene blue • ethambutol
EMC	encephalomyocarditis
EMCRO	Experimental Medical Care Review Organization
EMD	electromagnetic dissociation
emer	emergency

emf	electromotive force
EMF	electromotive force • endomycardial fibrosis • erythrocyte maturation factor
EMG	electromyogram, electromyography • exophthalmos, macroglossia, and gigantism
EMGN	extra-membranous glomerulonephritis
EMI	electromagnetic interference
EMIC	emergency maternity and infant care
EMIT	enzyme-multiplied immunoassay technique
emot	emotion, emotional
emp	as directed (*ex modo praescripto*) • plaster (*emplastrum*)
EMPEP	erythrocyte membrane protein electrophoretic pattern
EMR	electromagnetic radiation
EMS	early morning specimen • Emergency Medical Service • Emergency Medical System
EMT	emergency medical technician • emergency medical treatment
emu	electromagnetic unit
emul	emulsion
en	enema
EN	enteral nutrition • erythema nodosum
ENA	extractable nuclear antigen
enem	enema
ENG	electronystagmography
enl	enlarged
ENL	erythema nodosum leprosum
ENNS	Early Neonatal Neurobehavior Scale
eNO	exhaled nitric acid
ENS	enteric nervous system
ENT	ear, nose and throat

environ	environment, environmental
enz	enzyme
EO	ethylene oxide
EOA	Equal Opportunity Act • esophageal obturator airway • examination, opinion and advice
EOB	explanation of benefits
EOC	episode of care
eod	every other day
EOD	environmental and occupational disorders
EOE	Equal Opportunity Employer
EOF	end of field • end of title
EOG	electro-oculogram, electro-oculography • electro-olfactogram
EOI	evidence of insurability
EOL	end-of-life
EOM	extraocular movement • extraocular muscles
EOMB	explanation of medical benefits • Explanation of Medicare Benefits
EOP	endogenous opioid peptides
eos	eosinophil
EOS	eligibility on-site
EP	extopic pregnancy • electrophoresis • emergency physician • endogenous pyrogen • erythrocyte protoporphyrin • esophoria • evoked potential
EPA	Environmental Protection Agency • erect posteroanterior
EPC	epilepsia partialis continua
EPCG	endoscopic pancreatocholangiography
EPD	equilibrium peritoneal dialysis
EPEA	expense per equivalent admission
EPEC	enteripathogenic *E. coli*

EPF	exophthalmos-producing factor
EPI	epinephrine
EPIC	European Prospective Investigation of Cancer and Nutrition
epil	epilepsy
epis	episiotomy
EPITH	epithelium, epithelial
EPO	exclusive provider organization
EPP	equal pressure point • erythropoietic protoporphyria
EPPS	Edwards Personal Preference Schedule
EPR	electron paramagnetic resonance • electrophrenic respiration
EPS	elastosis perforans serpiginosa • exophthalmos-producing substance • expressed prostrate secretions • extrapyramidal symptoms • extrapyramidal syndrome
EPSDT	early and periodic screening, diagnosis and treatment
EPSE	extrapyramidal side effects
EPSP	excitatory postsynaptic potential
EPTS	existed prior to service
eq	equal • equation • equilibrium • equivalent
EQ	educational quotient
EQA	external quality assessment
equilib	equilibrium
equip	equipment
equiv	equivalent
Er	erbium
ER	emergency room • endoplasmic reticulum • equivalent roentgen • estradiol receptor • estrogen receptor • evoked response • extended release • external resistance • external rotation • employer
ERA	electric response audiometry • evoked response audiometry
ERBF	effective renal blood flow

ERC	endoscopic retrograde cholangiography
ERCP	endoscopic retrograde cannulization of pancreas • endoscopic retrograde cholangio-pancreatography
ERD	evoked response detector
erf	error function
ERF	Education and Research Foundation (AMA)
erg	energy unit
ERG	electrolyte replacement with glucose • electroretinogram, electroretinography
ERIA	electroradio-immuno assay
ERISA	Employee Retirement Income Security Act
ERO	external review organization
ERP	early receptor potential • effective refractory period • emergency room physician • endoscopic retrograde pancreatography • estrogen receptor protein • endocardial resection procedure
ERPF	effective renal plasma flow
ERT	estrogen replacement therapy
ERV	expiratory reserve volume
Ery	*Erysipelothrix*
Es	einsteinium • electrical stimulation • estriol
ES	Emergency Service • end stage • end-to-side • (graded compression) elastic stockings
ESB	electrical stimulation of the brain
Esch	*Escherichia*
ESD	end-systolic dimension • esophagus, stomach and duodenum
ESE	electrostatic unit (*electrostatische Einheit*)
ESF	erythropoietic-stimulating factor
ESFI	epidural steroid facet injection
ESG	electrospinogram • estrogen

ESH	elastic support hose
ESN	educationally subnormal
ESO	esophagus
esp	especially
ESP	Economic Stabilization Program • electrosensitive point • end systolic pressure • extrasensory perception
ESR	electron spin resonance • erythrocyte sedimentation rate
ESRD	end-stage renal disease
ess	essential, essentially
ESS	empty sella syndrome
est	estimated
EST	electroshock therapy
esu	electrostatic unit
ESU	electrostatic unit • electrosurgical unit
ESV	end-systolic volume
ESWL	extracorporeal shock wave lithotripsy
et	and (*et*) • etiology
Et	ethyl
ET	educational therapy • endotracheal • endotracheal tube • entero-stomal therapy, therapist • esotropia, esotropic • eustachian tube • exercise treadmill
ETA	endotracheal aspirates • ethionamide
et al	and others (*et alii*)
E_TCO_2	end-tidal carbon dioxide concentration
ETD	estimated time of death
ETEC	enterotoxigenic *Escherichia coli*
ETF	electron-transferring flavoprotein
eth	ether
ETI	ejective time index

etiol	etiology
ET-NANB	enterically transmitted non-A, non-B hepatitis
EtO	ethylene oxide
Et_2O	ether
ETO	estimated time of ovulation
ETOH	ethyl alcohol
ETP	elective termination of pregnancy
ETR	effective thyroxine ratio
ETT	endotracheal tube • exercise tolerance test • exercise treadmill test
Eu	europium
EUA	examination under anesthesia
EUC	end user computing
EUCD	emotionally unstable character disorder
ev	electron-volt • eversion
eV	electron-volt
EV	extravascular
evac	evacuated, evacuation
eval	evaluate, evaluation
evap	evaporate, evaporation
EVR	evoked visual response
EW	emergency ward
EWL	evaporative water loss
Ex	examination • exercise • former
exam	examination, examiner
exc	except • excision
exec	executive
exhib	let it be given (*exhibeatur*)

exist	existing
exp	expected • expired • exponent
exper	experimental
expir	expiration, expiratory
expn	expression
exptl	experimental
ext	extensor • exterior • external • extract, extraction • extremity, extremities • spread (extend)
Ext FHR	external fetal heart rate (monitoring)
ext fl	fluid extract
extrap	extrapolate, extrapolation
EY	ophthalmologic disease

F

f	frequency
F	brother (*frater*) • facies • Fahrenheit • failure • family • farad, farady • father • fecal • fellow • female • fetal • field (visual) • fluorine • flutter wave • foot • force • formula, formulary • fractional concentration • French (catheter size) • function • fusion beat • make (*fac*) • son (*filus*)
FA	Family Anonymous • Fanconi's anemia • fatty acid • femoral artery • fertilization antigen • field ambulance • filterable agent • filtered air • first aid • fluorescent antibody • folic acid • forearm • fortified aqueous (solution) • fusaric acid
F & A	findings and award
FAAN	Fellow of the American Academy of Nursing
FAB	French-American-British (Cooperative Group, classification) • functional arm brace
FAC	fluorouracil, Adriamycin, cyclophosphamide • free-standing ambulatory care
FACA	Fellow of the American College of Anesthesiologists • Federal Advisory Committee Act

FACD	Fellow of the American College of Dentists
FACHA	Fellow of the American College of Hospital Administrators
FACNM	Fellow of the American College of Nuclear Medicine
FACOG	Fellow of the American College of Obstetrics and Gynecology
FACP	Fellow of the American College of Physicians
FACS	fluorescense-activated cell sorter
FACSM	Fellow of the American College of Sports Medicine
FAD	flavin adenine dinucleotide
$FADH_2$	flavin adenine dinucleotide, reduced form
FAHM	Fellow of the Academy for Healthcare Management
FAI	functional aerobic impairment
fam	family
FAMA	Fellow of the American Medical Association • fluorescent antibody membrane antigen (test)
fam doc	family doctor
FAMILIES	Financial Support, Advocacy, Medical Management, Love, Information, Education and Structural Support
FANA	fluorescent antinuclear antibody
FAOTA	Fellow of the American Occupational Therapy Association
FAP	familial adenomatous polyposis
FAPHA	Fellow of the American Public Health Association
far	farad, faradic
FAR	flight aptitude rating
F^{AR}	immediate good function followed by accelerated rejection
FASA	Freestanding Ambulatory Surgery Association
fasc	bundle (*fasciculus*)
FASC	freestanding ambulatory surgery center
FAT	fluorescent antibody test
FB	fingerbreadth • foreign body

FBCOD	foreign body cornea left eye
FBCOS	foreign body cornea right eye
FBG	fasting blood glucose
FBI	flossing, brushing, irrigation
FBM	fetal breathing movements
FBP	fibrin breakdown products • fructose biphosphate
FBS	fasting blood sugar • feedback signal • feedback system • fetal bovine serum
FBU	fingers below umbilicus
Fc	foot-candle
FC	finger count • fluorocytosine • Foley catheter • functional class
F/C	fever and chills
FCC	follicular center cell • fracture-compound, comminuted
FCE	functional capacity evaluation
FCP	final common pathway
FCSA	Federal Controlled Substances Act
FD	family doctor • fatal dose • fibrinogen derivative • fixed and dilated • focal distance • forceps delivery • freeze-dried • feeding disorders
FD_{50}	median fatal dose
F/D	fracture dislocation
FDA	Food and Drug Administration
DD&C Act	Food and Drug Cosmetic Act
FDF	fast death factor
fdg	feeding
FDG	fluoro-18-deoxyglucose
FDIU	fetal death in utero
FDNB	fluorodinitrobenzene

FDO	formula-driven overpayment
FDP	fibrin degradation products
FDRA	food and drug reactions and anaphylaxis
Fe	iron (*ferrum*)
FE	fatty ester • fetal erythroblastosis
FEAR	false expectations about reality
feb dur	while the fever lasts (*febre durante*)
FEC	freestanding emergency center
FECG	fetal electrocardiogram
$FeCl_3$	ferric chloride
FeCN	ferricyanide
FECT	fibro-elastic connective tissue
FEEG	fetal electroencephalogram
FEF	forced expiratory flow
FEHB	Federal Employees Health Benefits Program
FEHBP	Federal Employees Health Benefits Program
FEKG	fetal electrocardiogram
FEL	familial erythrophagocytic lymphohistiocytosis
FELA	Federal Employers' Liability Act
FELV	feline leukemia virus
fem	female • thigh (*femoris*)
FEP	free erythrocyte protoporphyrin
ferv	boiling (*fervens*)
FES	functional electrical stimulation
FETI	fluorescence energy transfer immunoassay
Fe/TIBC	iron saturation of serum transferrin
FEV	forced expiratory volume
FEV_1	one-second forced expiratory volume

FEV$_1$/FVC	ratio of one-second forced expiratory volume to forced vital capacity
ff	following • forced fluids
FF	fat-free • filtration fraction • fixing fluid • flat feet • force fluids • foster father • fresh frozen • fundus firm
FFA	female-female adaptor • free fatty acid
FFC	free from chlorine
FFD	focus-to-film distance (x-ray)
FFDW	fat-free dry weight
FFF	fair, fat and forty
FFI	Family Functioning Index • free from infection
FFP	Federal Financial Participation • fresh frozen plasma
FFS	fat-free supper • fee-for-service • flexible fiberoptic sigmoidoscopy
FFT	flicker fusion threshold
FFWW	fat-free wet weight
fg	femtogram
FGF	fibroblast growth factors
FGT	female genital tract
FH$_4$	folacin
FH	family history • fetal heart • Frankfort horizontal (plane of the skull)
FHC	family health center
FHMI	family history of mental illness
FHNH	fetal heart not heard
FHR	fetal heart rate
FHS	fetal heart sounds
FHT	fetal heart tones
FHVP	free hepatic venous pressure
FHx	family history

FI	fiscal intermediary
FIA	fluorescence immunoassay • Freedom of Information Act
fib	fibrillation
FICA	Federal Insurance Contribution Act
FICD	Fellow of the International College of Dentists
FICS	Fellow of the International College of Surgeons
FID	flame-ionization detector • fraud investigation database
FIF	formaldehyde-induced fluorescence
fig	figure
FIGLU	formiminoglutamic acid
FIGO	International Federation of Obstetricians and Gynecologists
FIH	fat-induced hyperglycemia
filt	filter
FIN	fine intestinal needle
FiO_2	fractional inspiratory oxygen
FIO_2	forced inspiratory oxygen
fist	fistula
FIT	Food Intolerance Testing
FITC	fluorescein isothyiocyanate, conjugated
5-FU	5-fluorouracil
FJRM	full joint range of motion
fl	flexion • fluid
FL	focal length
fla	let it be done according to the rule (*fiat lege artis*)
fld	field • fluid
fl dr	fluid dram
flex	flexion
FLEX	Federation Licensing Examination

flor	flowers
fl oz	fluid ounce
Fluo	fluothane
fluores	fluorescence, fluorescent
fm	make a mixture (*fiat mistura*)
Fm	fermium
FM	fetal movements • flavin mononucleotide • frequency modulation
F/M	future medical (denoting future medical treatment or benefits)
FMAP	federal medical assistance percentage
FMC	Foundation for Medical Care
FMD	fibromuscular dysplasia • foot and mouth disease
FME	full-mouth extraction • Formal Medical Evaluation
fMet	formylmethionine
FMF	familial Mediterranean fever
FMG	foreign medical graduate
FMH	fat-mobilizing hormone • fetal-maternal hemorrhage
FML	fluorometholone
FMLA	Family and Medical Leave Act
FMN	flavin mononucleotide
$FMNH_2$	flavin mononucleotide, reduced form
FMP	first menstrual period
FMR	Friend-Moloney-Rauscher (virus)
FMS	false memory syndrome • fat-mobilizing substance • full mouth series
FMTC	familial medullary thyroid carcinoma
FMX	full-mouth x-rays
fn	function

FN	false-negative • finger to nose (coordination test) • Field Nurse
FNA(C)	fine needle aspiration (cytology)
FNH	focal nodular hyperplasia
fn p	fusion point
FNP	Family Nurse Practitioner
FNTC	fine needle transhepatic cholangiography
FO	focus out • foramen ovale • fronto-occipital
FOB	fecal occult blood • fiberoptic bronchoscopy • foot of bed
FOBT	fecal occult blood test
FOC	functional ovarian cyst
FOIA	Freedom of Information Act
FOM	figure of merit (measure of diagnostic value per radionuclide radiation dose)
for	foreign
FOR	forensic
fort	strong (*fortis*)
FORTRAN	Formula Translation
found	foundation
fp	freezing point
FP	false-positive • family physician • family planning • flat plate • family practice, family practitioner • Federation Proceedings • flavin phosphate • fluid pressure • frozen plasma • fluticosone propionate
FPC	family practice center • fish protein concentrate • frozen packed cells
FPG	fasting plasma glucose
FPHx	family psychiatric history
FPIA	fluorescence polarization immunoassay
fpm	feet per minute

FPM	filter paper microscopic (test)
FPMP	Federal Preventive Medicine Program
FPP	Faculty Practice Plan
fps	feet per second • foot-pound-second (system)
FPS	foot-pound-second (system)
FQHC	federally qualified health centers
fr	from
Fr	francium
FR	flocculation reaction • French (catheter size)
F&R	force and rhythm
FRA	fluorescent rabies antibody (test) • right frontoanterior
frac	fracture
fract dos	in divided doses (*fracta dosi*)
frag	fragile • fragment
FRC	frozen red cells • functional residual capacity
FRCP	Fellow of the Royal College of Physicians
FRCS	Fellow of the Royal College of Surgeons
freq	frequency
FRF	follicle-stimulating hormone-releasing factor
FRH	follicle-stimulating hormone-releasing hormone
Fried	Friedman's test
frig	refrigerator
FRJM	full-range joint movement
FROM	full range of motion
FRS	Fellow of the Royal Society • first rank symptoms (Schneider's)
FRT	full recovery time
FRV	functional residual volume

FS	factor of safety • fracture - simple • forearm supinated • frozen section • full soft • full strength
FSB	fetal scalp blood
FSBG	finger-stick blood gas
FSC	fracture - simple, comminuted
FSD	focus-to-skin distance (x-ray)
FSF	fibrin-stabilizing factor
FSGS	focal segmental glomerulosclerosis
FSH	follicle-stimulating hormone
FSH/LH-RH	follicle-stimulating hormone and luteinizing hormone releasing hormone
FSH-RF	follicle-stimulating hormone-releasing factor
FSI	foam stability index
FSP	fibrin split products
FSS	fetal skin sampling
ft	foot • let it be made (*fiat*)
ft^2	square foot
ft^3	cubic foot
Ft	ferritin
FT	full-term
FT_3	free triiodothyronine
FT_4	free thyroxine
FTA	fluorescent treponemal antibody
FTA-ABS	fluorescent treponemal antibody absorption (test)
F-TAG	fast-binding target-attaching globulin
FTBD	full-term born dead
ft c	foot-candle
FTC	Federal Trade Commission
FTE	full-time employee • full-time equivalent

FTF	fingertips to floor
FTFD	full-time, full duty
FTI	free thyroxine index
ft lb	foot-pound
FTND	full-term normal delivery
FTP	failure to progress
FTSG	full-thickness skin graft
FTT	failure to thrive
FU	fat unit • fecal urobilinogen • Finsen unit • fluorouracil • follow-up • fractional analysis
FU-I, FU-II	first, second set of follow-up data
FUB	functional uterine bleeding
FUDR	fluorodeoxyuridine
func	function, functional
FUO	fever of undetermined origin • fever of unknown origin
fu p	fusion point
FUT	fibrinogen uptake test
FV	femoral vein
FVC	false vocal chord • forced vital capacity • functional vital capacity
FWB	full-weight-bearing
FWHM	full width at half maximum
FWR	Felix-Weil reaction
FWW	front-wheel walker
Fx	fracture • friction
FY	fiscal year
FYI	for your information
FZ	focal zone • frozen section

G

g	gas • grain • gram
G	gastrin • gauge • gauss • gender • giga- • gingival • glucose • good • gram • gravid, gravida • gravity • Greek • guanine • guanosine • Newtonian constant of gravitation
Ga	gallium
GA	gastric analysis • general anesthesia • general assistance • gingivoaxial
GABA	gamma-aminobutyric acid
GAD	glutamic acid decarboxylase
GAF	global assessment of functioning
GAG	glycosaminoglycan
gal	galactose • gallon
GAL	guardian ad litem
gal/min	gallons per minute
GALT	gut-associated lymphoid tissue
galv	galvanic
gang	ganglion, ganglionic
GAO	Government Accounting Office
GAPD	glyceraldenyde-3-phosphate dehydrogenase
garg	gargle
GAS	general adaptation syndrome • generalized arteriosclerosis • Global Assessment Scale • Group A streptococcus
Gas Anal F&T	gas analysis, free and total
GASCVD	generalized arteriosclerotic cardiovascular disease
GASP	Group Against Smokers' Pollution
gastroc	gastrocnemius
GATB	General Aptitude Test Battery
GAW	airway conductance

GB	gall-bladder • Guillain-Barré (syndrome)
GBA	gingivobuccoaxial
GBBS	group B beta-hermolytic streptococcus
GBG	glycerine-rich gamma glycoprotein
GBGase	glycine-rich gamma glycoproteinase
GBM	glomerular basement membrane
GBS	gallbladder series • group B streptococcus • Guillain-Barré Syndrome
GC	gas chromatography • gastrointestinal catastrophe • glucocorticoid • gonococcus, gonococcal • guanine-cytosine
GCA	giant-cell arteritis
g-cal	gram calorie (small calorie)
GCFT	gonorrhea complement fixation test
GCI	gestational carbohydrate intolerance
g-cm	gram-centimeter
GCS	general clinical service • Glasgow coma scale
G-CSF	granulocyte colony-stimulating factor
Gd	gadolinium
GD	given dose • Graves' disease
GDM	gestational diabetes mellitus
GDP	guanosine diphosphate
GDTP	goal-directed therapy program
Ge	germanium
GE	gastroenterology
GEF	gonadotrophin enhancing factor
gen	general • genus
geom	geometric
GEP	gastroenteropancreatic (endocrine system)

GER	gastroesophageal reflux
GERD	gastroesophageal reflux disease
GET	gastric emptying time
GF	gastric fistula • germ-free • girlfriend • globule fibril • glomerular filtration • grandfather • growth fraction
GFAP	glial fibrillory acidic protein
GFR	glomerular filtration rate
GG	Gamma globulin • glyceryl guaiacolate
GGE	generalized glandular enlargement
GGT	gamma-glutamyltransferase • gamma-glutamyltranspeptidase
GGTP	gamma-glutamyltranspeptidase
GH	general hospital • growth hormone
GHA	Group Health Association
GHAA	Group Health Association of America
GHb	glycosylated hemoglobin
GHB	glycosylated hemoglobin
GHBP	growth hormone-binding protein
GHPP	Genetically Handicapped Persons Program
GHQ	general health questionnaire
GHRF	growth hormone-releasing factor
GHRH	growth hormone-releasing hormone
GHRIF	growth hormone releasing-inhibiting factor
GI	gastrointestinal • Gingival Index • globin insulin • glomerular index • growth-inhibiting
GIBF	gastrointestinal bacterial flora
GIFT	gamete intra-Fallopian transfer
GIGO	garbage in, garbage out (computer data)
GIK	glucose-insulin-potassium

GII	gastrointestinal infection
GIP	gastric inhibitory peptide • gastric inhibitory polypeptide
GIS	gastrointestinal series
GIT	gastrointestinal tract
GITT	glucose-insulin tolerance test
GIV	gastrointestinal virus
GIX	an insecticidal compound
GK	galactokinase
GKR	gamma knife radiosurgery
gl	gland, glands
GL	greatest length
GLA	gingivolinguaxial
glc	glaucoma
GLC	gas-liquid chromatography
GLI	glucagon-like immunoreactivity
Gln	glutamine
Glob	globular • globulin
glu	glucose
Glu	glutamate
Gluc	glucose
glucur	glucuronide
glu ox	glucose oxidase
glut max	gluteus maximus
glut med	gluteus medius
GLV	Gross leukemia virus
Gly	glycine
glyc	glycerin
gm	gram

Gm	gram
GM	grand mal (epilepsy) • grandmother
GMC	General Medical Council
gm cal	gram calorie (small calorie)
GM-CSF	granulocyte-macrophage colony-stimulating factor
GME	graduate medical education
GMENAC	Graduate Medical Education National Advisory Committee
GMK	green monkey kidney
GML	glabellomeatal line
gm-m	gram-meter
GMP	guanosine monophosphate (guanylate, guanylic acid)
GM&S	general medical and surgical
GMT	geometric mean titer
GMW	gram molecular weight
GN	glomerulonephritis • gonococcus • graduate nurse • gram-negative
G/N	glucose-nitrogen ratio
GNB	Gram negative bacillus
GNC	General Nursing Council • Gram negative cocci
gnd	ground
GND	Gram negative diplococci
GNP	gerontological nurse-practitioner
GNR	Gram negative rods
GnRH	gonadotropin-releasing hormone
GNS	gerontological nurse-specialist
GNTP	graduate nurse transition program
GO	glucose oxidase
GOE	gas, oxygen, ether • Guide for Occupational Exploration

GOG	gynecological oncology group
GOK	God only knows
GOR	general operating room
GOT	glutamic-oxaloacetic transaminase
govt	government
GP	general paralysis • general paresis • general practice, general practitioner • gram-positive • group • guinea pig
GPB	glossopharyngeal breathing
GPC	gastric parietal cells • Gram positive cocci
G-6-PD	glucose-6-phosphate dehydrogenase
GPEP	General Professional Education of the Physician
GPI	general paralysis of the insane • Gingival-Periodontal Index
GPM	general preventive medicine
GPN	graduate practical nurse
GPO	group purchasing organization
GPP	general payment provisions
GPPP	group practice prepayment plan
GPR	Gram positive rods
GPT	glutamic-pyruvic transaminase
GpTh	group therapy
gr	grain • gravity
Gr	Greek
GR	gamma ray • gastric resection • general relief
GRA	Gombarts reducing agent
grad	by degrees • gradient • gradually • graduate
GRAE	generally recognized as effective
GRAN	Gombarts reducing agent - negative
GRAS	generally recognized as safe

grav	gravid, gravida • gravity
GRAY	Gombarts reducing agent - positive
GRE	Graduate Record Examination
GR-FeSV	Gardner-Rasheed feline sarcoma virus
GRH	growth hormone-releasing hormone
GRID	Ga-Related Immune Deficiency
GRN	geriatric resource nurse
GRS	gross
GRS & MIC	gross and microscopic
GRT	graduate respiratory therapist
GS	gallstone • general surgeon, general surgery • glomerular sclerosis • glucosamine sulfate
GSA	Gerontological Society of America
GSC	gas-solid chromatography
GSE	gluten-sensitive enteropathy • grips strong and equal
GSH	glutathione, reduced form
GSR	galvanic skin response • generalized Schwartzman reaction
GSSG	glutathione, oxidized form
GSW	gunshot wound
gt	drop (*gutta*)
GT	gait training • gastrostomy tube • glucose tolerance
GTF	glucose tolerance factor
GTH	gonadotropic hormone
GTN	glomerulotubulonephritis
GTP	guanosine triphosphate
GTR	granulocyte turnover rate
gtt	drops (*guttae*)
GTT	gelatin-tellurite-taurocholate (agar) • glucose tolerance test

GU	gastric ulcer • genitourinary • gonococcal urethritis
guid	guidance
GUS	genitourinary system
GV	gentian violet
GVA	general visceral afferent
GVE	general visceral efferent
GVH	graft-versus-host
GVHD	graft-versus-host disease
GVHR	graft-versus-host reaction
GW	gigawatt
G/W	glucose in water
GXT	graded exercise test
Gy	gray
GY	gynecological disease
Gyn	gynecologic, gynecology, gynecologist

H

h	height • high • horizontal • hour • hypermetropia • hyperopia, hyperopic • hypodermic • Planck's constant
H	height • henry (unit of electrical inductance) • heroin • histamine • history • Holzknecht unit • husband • hydrogen
^{2}H	deuterium
^{3}H	tritium
H_1	histamine receptor type 1
H_2	histamine receptor type 2
H^{+}	hydrogen ion
Ha	hahnium
HA	headache • heated aerosol • hemadsorbent • hemagglutination • hepatic adenoma • hepatitis A • hyaluronic acid • hyperalimentation

HA^1	hemadsorption virus, type 1
HA^2	hemadsorption virus, type 2
HAA	hepatitis A antibody • hepatitis-associated antigen
HAAb	hepatitis A antibody
HAAg	hepatitis A antigen
HAART	highly aggressive antiretroviral therapy
HABA	hydroxyazobenzenebenzoic acid
HAD	hospital administration
HAE	hereditary angioneurotic edema
HAGG	hyperimmune antivariola gamma globulin
HAI	hemagglutination inhibition
halluc	hallucination
HAMA	human anti-mouse antibody
HaMSV	Harvey murine sarcoma virus
HANE	hereditary angioneurotic edema
harm	harmonic
HAP	home antibiotic program • Hospital Accreditation Program
HARPPS	Heat, Absence of use, Redness, Pain, Pus, Swelling (symptoms of infection)
HAS	hypertensive arteriosclerosis
HASHD	hypertensive arteriosclerotic heart disease
HASP	Hospital Admission and Surveillance Program
HAT	hospital arrival time • hypoxanthine-aminopterin-thymidine (medium)
HATG	horse anti-human thymocyte globulin
HATT	hemagglutination treponemal test
HAV	hepatitis A virus
Hb	hemoglobin

HB	heart block • hemoglobin • hepatitis B • His bundle • hospital based
H-B	Hill-Burton Act (funds)
HbA	normal adult hemoglobin
HBAb	hepatitis B antibody
HBAg	hepatitis B antigen
HbAS	hemoglobin A and hemoglobin S (sickle-cell trait)
HBcAB	antibody to hepatitis B core antigen
HbCO	carboxyhemoglobin
HBD	has been drinking • hydroxybutyrate dehydrogenase
HBDH	hydroxybutyrate dehydrogenase
HBeAg	hepatitis B e antigen
HbF	fetal hemoglobin
HBGM	home blood glucose monitoring
HBI	hepatobiliary imaging
HBIG	hepatitis B immune globulin
HbO_2	oxyhemoglobin
HBO	hospital benefits organization • hyperbaric oxygen
HBP	high blood pressure • hospital based physician
HbS	sickle-cell hemoglobin • sulfhemoglobin
HBsAB	antibody to hepatitis B surface antigen
HBsAg	hepatitis B surface antigen
HBV	hepatitis B vaccine • hepatitis B virus
HC	head compression • health care • Hickmann catheter • high-calorie • home care • hospital corps • hospital course • house call • hydranencephaly • hydrocodone • hydrocortisone • hypertrophic cardiomyopathy
HCA	health care assistant • hypothalmic chronic anovulation • heterocyclic antidepressant
HCC	health-care corporation • hepatocellular carcinoma

HCD	health care delivery • heavy-chain disease
HCEC	Hospital Care Evaluation Committee
HCFA	Health Care Financing Administration
hCG	human chorionic gonadotropin
HCG	human chorionic gonadotropin
HCHO	formaldehyde
HCI	hydrochloric acid
HCL	hairy-cell leukemia
HCM	hypertrophic cardiomyopathy
HCN	hydrocyanic acid
HCO	health care organization
HCO_3	bicarbonate
HCP	hereditary coproporphyria • hexacholorophene
HCPCS	Health Care Procedure Coding System
HCPOTP	health care practitioner other than physician
HCPP	health care prepayment plan
HCQIP	Health Care Quality Improvement Program
HCRIS	Hospital Cost Report Information System
hCS	human chorionic somatomammotropin
HCS	human chorionic somatomammotropin
hCT	human calcitonin • human chorionic thyrotropin
Hct	hematocrit
HCT	hematocrit • human calcitonin • human chorionic thyrotropin
HCTZ	hydrochlorothiazide
HCV	Hepatitis C virus
HCVD	hypersensitive cardiovascular disease
HCW	health care worker

hd	at bedtime (*hora decubitus*)
HD	Hansen's disease • hearing distance • heart disease • hemodialysis • herniated disc • high density • hip disarticulation • Hodgkin's disease
HDC	histidine decarboxylase • human diploid cell • high-dose chemotherapy • HCFA Data Center
HDCS	human diploid-cell strain
HDCV	human diploid-cell vaccine
HDF	host defensive factor
HDI	high-definition imaging
HDL	high density lipoprotein
HDL-C	high-density lipoprotein cholesterol
HDLP	high-density lipoprotein
HDLW	distance at which a watch is heard by the left ear
HDN	hemolytic disease of the newborn
HDRW	distance at which a watch is heard by the right ear
HDS	health delivery system
HDU	hemodialysis unit
HDV	hepatitis-D virus
He	helium
HE	hemoglobin electrophoresis • hereditary elliptocytosis
H&E	hematoxylin and eosin (stain) • hereditary and environment
HEAT	human erythrocyte agglutination test
HEC	hospital ethics committee
HED	unit of roentgen-ray dosage (*Haut-Einheits-Dosis*) • hypohidrotic ectodermal dysplasia
HEDIS	Health plan Employer Data and Information Set
HEENT	Head, Eyes, Ears, Nose and Throat
HEK	human embryonic kidney

HEL	human embryonic lung
HeLa cells	cultured strain of carcinoma cells used for study
HELLP	Hemolysis, Elevated Liver enzymes, Low Platelets syndrome
Hem	hemolysis, hemolytic • hemorrhage • hemorrhoids
hemi	hemiplegia
HEMPAS	hereditary erythroblastic multinuclearity with positive acidified serum
HEP	Home Exercise Program
HEPA	high-efficiency particulate air
HES	hydroxyethyl starch • hypereosinophilic syndrome
HeSCA	Health Sciences Communications Association
HETP	hexaethyltetraphosphate
HEV	hepatitis-E virus • human enteric virus
HEW	Health, Education, and Welfare
HEX	Handicapped Educational Exchange
Hf	hafnium • half
HF	Hageman factor • hard-filled (capsules) • heart failure • hemorrhagic factor • high-frequency
HFAK	hollow-fiber artificial kidney
HFC	hard-filled capsules
HFJV	high-frequency jet ventilation
HFOV	high-frequency oscillatory ventilation
HFPPV	high-frequency positive-pressure ventilation
Hfr	high frequency
HFRS	hemorrhagic fever with renal syndrome
HFUPR	hourly fetal urine production rate
HFV	high-frequency ventilation
Hg	hemoglobin • mercury
HG	human gonadotropin • hyperemesis gravidarum

Hgb	hemoglobin
HgbF	fetal hemoglobin
HGF	human growth factor • hyperglycemic- glygogenolytic factor (glucagon)
hGG	human gamma globulin
HGG	human gamma globulin
HGH	human growth hormone
HGO	hepatic glucose output
HGP	hypogastric plexus
HG-PRT	hypoxanthine-guanine phospho-ribosyl-transferase
HH	hard of hearing • home hyperalimentation
H/H	hemoglobin/hematocrit
HHA	home health agency • home health aide
HHb	reduced hemoglobin
HHC	home health care • hereditary hemochromatosis
HHCC	home health cost containment
HHD	hypertensive heart disease
HHFM	high-humidity face mask
HHN	hand-held nebulizer • home health nurse
HHNKS	hyperglycemic, hyperosmolar nonketotic syndrome
HHO	home health organization
HHS	Health and Human Services (Department) • home health services
HHT	hereditary hemorrhagic telangiectasia
HHV6	human herpes virus 6
HI	health insurance • hemagglutination inhibition • hepatic insufficiency • head injury • hospital insurance
HIA	HCFA Information Architecture
HIAA	hydroxyindoleacetic acid

HIC	health information center • health insurance claims • health insurance company
H-ICD-A	Hospital (version)-International Classification of Diseases-Adapted
HICN	cyanmethemoglobin
HID	headache, insomnia, depression • herniated intervertebral disk
HIFC	hog intrinsic factor concentrate
HiHb	hemiglobin
H inf	hypodermoclysis infusion
HINN	Hospital Issued Notice of Non-Coverage
HIOMT	hydroxyindole-O-methyl transferase
HIP	health insurance plan
HIPP	Health Insurance Premium Program
HiPro	high protein
His	histidine
HIS	Hospital Information Service
Hist	histidinemia • history
HIV	human immunodeficiency virus
HIVD	herniated intervertebral disc
HJ	Howell-Jolly bodies
HJR	hepatojugular reflux
HK	human kidney (cells)
H-K	hand-to-knee (coordination)
HKAFO	hip-knee-ankle-foot orthosis
HKO	hip-knee orthosis (splint)
hl	hectoliter
Hl	hypermetropia, latent • hyperopia, latent
HL	half-life • hearing level • hearing loss • hectoliter • hyperlipidemia

H/L	heparin lock • latent hyperopia • low risk heart disease
H&L	heart and lung
HL7	Health Level Seven
HLA	histocompatibility leukocyte antigen • histocompatibility locus antigen • homologous leukocytic antibodies • human leukocyte antigen • human lymphocyte antigen
HLA-A,B,C,D	varieties of human leukocyte antigen
HLA-DR	human histocompatibility leukocyte antigen
hLH	human luteinizing hormone
HLI	hemolysis inhibition
HLP	hyperlipoproteinemia
HLR	heart-lung resuscitation
HLHS	hypoplastic left heart syndrome
HLTK	Holmium YAG laser thermokeratoplasty
hm	hectometer
HM	severe chronic heart disease
Hm	manifest hypermetropia • manifest hyperopia
HMC	heroin, morphine, cocaine
HMD	hyaline membrane disease
HME	heat, massage, exercise • home medical equipment
HMEIA	Health Manpower Education Initiative Award
hMG	human menopausal gonadotropin
HMG	human menopausal gonadotropin • Healthcare Management Guidelines
HMG-CoA	3-hydroxy 3-methylglutaryl coenzyme-A reductase
HMI	healed myocardial infarction
HMM	hexamethylmelamine
HMO	health maintenance organization • heart minute output
HMP	hexose monophosphate

HMPG	hydroxymethoxyphenylglycol
HMSA	Health Manpower Shortage Area
HMSN	hereditary motor and sensory neuropathy
HMW	high-molecular-weight
HMW-NCF	high-molecular-weight neurophil chemotactic factor
HMX	heat, massage, exercise
hn	tonight (*hoc nocte*)
HN	head nurse
H&N	head and neck
HN_2	mechlorethamine (nitrogen mustard)
HNP	herniated nucleus pulposus
HNPCC	hereditary nonpolyposis colorectal cancer
hnRNA	heterogeneous nuclear ribonucleic acid
HNV	has not voided
Ho	holmium
HO	house officer
h/o	history of
HO-1/HO-2	first-year house officer, second year house officer
H_2O	water
H_2O_2	hydrogen peroxide
HOB	head of bed
HOCM	hypertrophic obstructive cardiomyopathy
hoc vesp	tonight (*hoc vespere*)
HOD	hyperbaric oxygen drenching
Hoff	Hoffman (reflex)
HOH	hard of hearing
HOL	HCFA on-line

HOME	Home Observation for the Management of the Environment • home-oriented maternity experience
homolat	homolateral
HOP	high oxygen pressure
HOPA	hospital-based organ procurement agency
HOPD	hospital out-patient department
HOPE	healthcare options plan entitlement
hor	horizontal
hor decub	at bedtime (*hora decubitus*)
hor interm	at the intermediate hours (*horis intermediis*)
horiz	horizontal
hor som	at bedtime (*hora somni*)
hor un spatio	at the end of an hour (*horae unius spatio*)
hosp	hospital, hospitalization
HOT	human old tuberculin
hp	horsepower
Hp	haptoglobin
HP	health plan • health professional • hemiparesis • hemiplegia • highly purified • high potency • high power • high pressure • hot pack • hot pad • house physician • hydrostatic pressure • hyperphoria • hypoparathyroidism
H&P	history and physical
HPA	hypothalamic-pituitary-adrenal (axis)
HPD	hemtoporphyrin derivative
H&PE	history and physical examination
hpf	high power field
HPF	high power field
HPFH	hereditary persistence of fetal hemoglobin
hPG	human pituitary gonadotropin

HPG	human pituitary gonadotropin
HPGe	high-purity germanium
HPI	history of present illness
hPL	human placental lactogen
HPL	human placental lactogen
HPLC	high-performance liquid chromatography • high-pressure liquid chromatography
HPM	Harding-Passey melanoma
hpn	hypertension
HPN	hypertension • home parenteral nutrition
HPO	high-pressure oxygen (hyperbaric oxygen)
HPP	hereditary pyropoikikocytosis
HPPH	hydroxyphenylphenylthydantoin
HPR	hospital peer review
HPRT	hypoxanthine-guanine phosphoribosyl transferase
HPS	Hanta-virus pulmonary syndrome
HPT	hyperparathyroidism
HPTH	hyperparathyroidism
HPV	human papillomavirus
HPVD	hypertensive pulmonary vascular disease
HPX	high-peroxide-containing (cells)
HQCB	Healthcare Quality Certification Board
hr	hour
HR	heart rate • hemorrhagic retinopathy • human resources
HRA	Health Resources Administration • high right atrial (ECG recording)
HRCT	high resolution computer tomography
HRF	histamine releasing factor
HRG	Health Research Group

HRIG	human rabies immune globulin
HRL	head rotated left
HRLA	human retrovirus-like agent
HRQL	health-related quality of life
HRR	Hardy-Rand-Rittler (color vision test kit) • head rotated right
HRS	hepatorenal syndrome
HRSA	Health Resources and Services Administration
HRT	hormone replacement therapy
hs	at bedtime (*hora somni*) • half-strength
HS	half-strength • heart sounds • heme synthetase • hereditary spherocytosis • herpes simplex • house surgeon • severe acute heart disease
HSA	Hazardous Substances Act • Health Services Administration • health services area • human serum albumin • hypersomnia-sleep apnea (syndrome)
HSAN	hereditary sensory and autonomic neuropathy
HSC	Hand-Schüller-Christian
HSCD	Hand-Schüller-Christian disease
HSD	hypoactive sexual desire disorder
HSDI	Health Self Determination Index
HSE	herpes simplex encephalitis
HSES	hemorrhagic shock and encephalopathy syndrome
HSF	hydrozine-sensitive factor
HSG	herpes simplex genitalis • hysterosalpingogram
HSIM	Health Status Improvement and Management
HSL	herpes simplex labialis
HSM	hepatosplenomegaly • holosystolic murmur
HSN	Hanson-Street nail • herpes simplex neonatorium
HSP	Health Systems Plan • Henoch-Schönlein purpura • Hospital Specific Payment • hospice care

HSQ	home screening questionnaire
HSQB	Health Standards and Quality Bureau
HSR	homogeneously staining regions
HSS	Hallervorden-Spatz syndrome
HSTS	human-specific thyroid stimulator
HSV	herpes simplex virus • highly selective vagotomy
ht	height
Ht	hypermetropia, total • hyperopia, total
HT	Hashimoto's thyroiditis • histologic technician • home treatment • Hubbard tank • hydrotherapy • hydroxytryptamine • hypertropia • hypodermic tablet
5-HT	5-hydroxytryptamine
HTACS	human thyroid ademylate cyclose stimulators
HTB	hot tub bath
HTC	homozygous typing cells
HTL	histologic technologist
HTLV	human T-cell leukemia virus • human T-cell lymphotropic virus
HTN	hypertension
HTP	House-Tree-Person (test) • hydroxytryptophan
hTS	human thyroid stimulator
HTS	hemangioma-thrombocytopenia syndrome
HU	heat unit • hydroxyurea • hyperemia unit
HuIFN	human interferon
HUIS	high-dose urea in invert sugar
HUM	heat, ultrasound, massage
HUAM	Home Uterine Activity Monitoring
HUP	Hospital Utilization Project
HURT	hospital utilization review team

HUS	hemolytic-uremic syndrome
HV	Hanta virus • high-voltage • hospital visit • hyperventilation
HVA	homovanillic acid
HVD	hypertensive vascular disease
HVE	hepatic vascular exclusion • high-voltage electrophoresis
HVH	herpesvirus hominis
HVHMA	herpesvirus hominis membrane antigen
HVL	half-value layer
HVT	half-value thickness
HWB	hot water bottle
HWS	hot-water soluble
Hx	history • hypoxanthine
HXM	hexamethylmelamine
hy	hysteria
Hy	hydraulics • hydrostatics • hypermetropia • hyperopia
hyd	hydration
hydro	hydrotherapy
hyg	hygiene
hyp	hydroxyproline • hyperresonance • hypertrophy
hyperten	hypertension
hypn	hypertension
hypno	hypnosis
hypo	hypodermic injection
hys	hysteria, hysterical
hyst	hysterectomy
Hz	hertz
HZ	herpes zoster

HZFO	hamster zona-free ovum (test)
HZO	herpes zoster oticus
HZV	herpes zoster virus

I

i	incisor (deciduous)
I	inactive • incisor (permanent) • increased • index • induction • insoluble • inspiration, inspired (gas) • intake • intensity (electrical, luminous, magnetic, radioactive) • internal medicine • internist • iodine
I_2	iodine
$^{125}I, {}^{131}I$	radioactive isotopes of iodine commonly used in medicine
^{127}I	stable iodine
IA	immunobiologic activity • impedance angle • incurred accidentally • infantile apnea • intra-amniotic • intra-aortic • intra-arterial • intra-articular
I & A	information and assistance office (officer)
IAA	indoleacetic acid
IAB	intra-aortic balloon • intermittent androgen blockade
IABC	intra-aortic balloon counterpulsation
IABP	intra-aortic balloon pump
IABPA	intra-aortic balloon pumping assistance
I-Ac	imideazoleacetic acid
IAC	internal auditory canal • interposed abdominal compression
IADH	inappropriate antidiuretic hormone
IADL	Instrument Activities of Daily Living (scale)
IAEA	International Atomic Energy Agency
IAET	International Association for Enterostomal Therapy
IAFI	infantile amaurotic familial idiocy
IAHA	immune-adherence hemagglutination
i-amniot	intra-amniotic

IANC	International Anatomical Nomenclature Committee
IAP	intermittent acute porphyria
IARC	International Agency for Research on Cancer
i-arter	intra-arterial
IAS	intra-amniotic saline (infusion)
IASD	interatrial septal defect
IAT	indirect antiglobulin test • iodine-azide test
IAV	intermittent assisted ventilation
IB	immune body • inclusion body • index of body build • infectious bronchitis
IBC	iron-binding capacity
IBD	infectious bowel disease • inflammatory bowel disease • irritable bowel disease
IBF	immunoglobulin-binding factor
IBI	intermittent bladder irrigation
ibid	the same, in the same place (*ibidem*)
IBNR	incurred but not reported
IBP	iron-binding protein
IBR	infectious bovine rhinotracheitis
IBS	irritable bowel syndrome
IBU	international benzoate unit
IBV	infectious bronchitis virus
IBW	ideal body weight
ic	between meals (*inter cibos*)
IC	infection control • information content • inhibitory concentration • inspiratory capacity • inspiratory center • intensive care • intercarpal • intercostal • intermediate care • interstitial cell • intracarotid • intracellular • intracerebral • intracranial • intracutaneous • intraductal carcinoma • irritable colon
IC_{50}	median inhibitory concentration

iCA	ionized calcium
ICA	intercountry adoption • internal carotid artery
ICAM-1	intercellular adhesion molecule 1
ICAM-2	intercellular adhesion molecule 2
i-card	intracardial
ICC	intensive coronary care • intermittent clean catheterization
ICCE	intracapsular cataract extraction
ICCU	intensive coronary care unit
ICD	implantable cardioverter defibrillator • International Classification of Diseases • isocitric dehydrogenase • intrauterine contraceptive device
ICD-A	International Classification of Diseases - Adapted
ICD-9	International Classification of Diseases - Ninth Revision
ICD-9-CM	International Classification of Diseases - Ninth Revision - Clinical Modification
ICDH	isocitric dehydrogenase
ICE	ifosfamide, carboplatin, etoposide
ICES	ice, compression, elevation, support
ICF	intermediate-care facility • intracellular fluid
ICF/MR	intermediate-care facility for the mentally retarded
ICG	indocyanine green
ICM	intercostal margin
ICN	intensive care nursery • International Council of Nurses
i-coch	intracochlear
ICP	infection control practitioner • intracranial pressure
ICPMM	incisors, canines, premolars, molars
ICR	distance between iliac crests • intrastromal corneal ring
ICRC	infant care review committee
ICRP	International Commission on Radiological Protection

IRCU	International Commission on Radiological Units and Measurements
ICS	intercostal space • International College of Surgeons • injury compensation specialist
ICSH	interstitial cell-stimulating hormone (luteinizing hormone)
ict	icterus
iCT	immunoreactive calcitonin
ICT	inflammation of connective tissue • insulin-coma therapy • intensive conventional therapy
ict ind	icterus index
ICU	infant care unit • intermediate care unit • intensive care unit
i-cut	intracutaneous
ICW	intensive care ward • intracellular water
id	the same (*idem*)
ID	identification • immunodiffusion • immunoglobulin deficiency • inclusion disease • infectious disease • infective dose • inhibitory dose • inside diameter • intradermal
I&D	incision and drainage
ID_{50}	median effective dose
IDA	iminodiacetic acid • iron-deficiency anemia
IDAT	indirect antiglobulin test
IDD	insulin-dependent diabetes • intraspinal drug delivery
IDDF	investigational drug data form
IDDM	insulin-dependent diabetes mellitus
IDDS	investigational drug data sheet
IDE	investigational drug exemption
IDEA	Individuals with Disabilities Education Act
i-derm	intradermal
IDET	intradiscal electrothermal therapy • intradiscal electrothermy

IDFN	integrated delivery and financing network
IDFS	integrated delivery and financing system
IDL	intermediate-density lipoprotein
IDM	infant of diabetic mother
IDP	inosine diphosphate
IDS	integrated delivery system(s)
IDT	intradermal test
IDU	idoxuridine
IDUR	idoxuridine
IDV	intermittent demand ventilation
ie	that is (*id est*)
IE	immunoelectrophoresis • infective endocarditis
I/E	inspiratory/expiratory
IEA	intravascular erythrocyte aggregation • Insurance Education Association
IEC	intra-epithelia carcinoma
IED	intermittent explosive disorder
IEE	inner enamel epithelium
IEF	isoelectric focusing
IEM	inborn error of metabolism
IEOP	immunoelectric-osmophoresis
IEP	immunoelectrophoresis • isoelectric point
IF	immunofluorescence • inhibiting factor • initiation factor • interferon • intermediate frequency • interstitial fluid • intrinsic factor • involved-field (radiotherapy)
IFA	immunofluorescent assay • indirect fluorescent antibody
IFE	immunofixation electrophoresis
IFN	interferon
iG	immunoreactive gastrin

Ig	immunoglobulin
IG	immune globulin • immunoglobulin • Inspector General
IgA	immunoglobulin A
IgD	immunoglobulin D
IgE	immunoglobulin E
IGF	insulin-like growth factor(s)
IGFBP	IGF-binding proteins
IgG	immunoglobulin G
IGIV	immune globulin intravenous
IgM	immunoglobulin M
IgQ	immunoglobulin quantitation
IGR	intrauterine growth retardation
IGT	impaired glucose tolerance
IH	indirect hemagglutination • infectious hepatitis • inhibiting hormone • inpatient hospital
IHA	immune hemolytic anemia • indirect hemagglutination
IHD	ischemic heart disease
IHO	idiopathic hypertrophic osteoarthropathy • Institute of Human Origins
IHP	idiopathic hypopituitarism
IHS	Indian Health Service
IHSA	iodinated human serum albumin
^{131}IHSA	radioiodinated (radioactive iodine-labeled) human serum albumin
IHSS	idiopathic hypertrophic subaortic stenosis • In-Home Support Services
II	icterus index • image intensifier • insurance index
IICP	increased intracranial pressure
IICU	infant intensive care unit
IID	insulin-independent diabetes

IIE	idiopathic ineffective erythropoiesis
IIF	indirect immunofluorescence
IIIVC	infrahepatic interruption of the inferior vena cava
IIS	intermittent infusion sets
I-J	ileojejunal
IL	incisolingual • independent laboratory • insensible weight loss • interleukin intermediary letter
ILA	insulin-like activity
I-Lac	imidazolelactic acid
ILBBB	incomplete left bundle branch block
Ilc	isoleucine
Ile	isoleucine
i-lesion	intralesional
IM	Index Medicus • infectious mononucleosis • internal medicine • intramedullary • intramuscular
IMA	Industrial Medicine Association
IMC	immediate care • Industrial Medical Council
IMCU	intermediate care unit
IMD	Institution for Mental Disease
ImD_{50}	median immunizing dose
IME	indirect medical education • independent medical examination • independent medical examiner
IMF	intermaxillary fixation
IMI	immunologically measurable insulin
immat	immature
immed	immediate
immob	immobilize
ImmU	immunizing unit
immunol	immunology, immunological

IMN	internal mammary nodes
imp	important • impression • improved
IMP	incomplete male pseudohermaphroditism • inosine monophosphate
IMPA	incisal mandibular plane angle
impair	impaired, impairment
Impx.	impaction
IMR	infectious mononucleosis receptors
IMS	Indian Medical Services
IMSC	internal mammary supraclavicular
ImU	international milliunit
IMV	intermittent mandatory ventilation
IMViC	indole, methyl red, Voges-Proskauer, citrate
in	inch
In	indium
IN	icterus neonatorum • internist • intranasal
INAH	isoniazid (isonicotinic acid hydrazide)
inc	incomplete • inconclusive • incontinent • increase
Inc AB	incomplete abortion
incl	including • inclusive
IncO$_2$	incubator oxygen
incompat	incompatible
incompl	incomplete
incr	increase, increased, increasing • increment
inc(R)	increase (relative)
incur	incurable
in d	daily (*in dies*)
ind	independent

IND	Investigational New Drug
indic	indicative, indication
INDM	infant of nondiabetic mother
indust	industry, industrial
inf	infant, infancy, infantile • infect, infected, infection, infectious • inferior • infirmary • infusion • pour in (*infunde*)
infarct	infarction
inf dis	infectious disease
infect	infection, infectious
infl	influence
inflam	inflamed, inflammation, inflammatory
info	information
infx	infection
ing	inguinal
ingest	ingestion
inh	inhalation
INH	isoniazid (isonicotinic acid hydrazide)
inhal	inhalation
inhib	inhibit, inhibition, inhibitor
INI	intranasal insulin • intranuclear inclusion (agent)
inj	inject, injection • injury, injurious
inject	injection
inj enem	let an enema be given (*injiciatur enema*)
in-lb	inch-pound
INN	International Nonproprietary Names
innerv	innervation, innerved
Ino	inosine
inoc	inoculate, inoculated, inoculation

inop	inoperable
inorg	inorganic
Inorg phos	inorganic phosphorus
INPRONS	information processing in the central nervous system
IN PRO PER	not represented by a lawyer (*in propia persona*)
INR	International Normalized Ratio
INS	insert • insurance
insol	insoluable
insp	inspiration
inst	institute • instrument
instil	instilled, instillation
instr	instructor
insuff	insufficiency, insufficient
int	integral • intermittent • internal • internist • intestinal
int cib	between meals (*inter cibos*)
intest	intestine, intestinal
Int FHR	internal fetal heart rate
INTH	intrathecal
Int Med	internal medicine
intox	intoxication
int rot	internal rotation
in utero	within the uterus
inv	inverse • inversion • involuntary
Io	ionium
IO	inferior oblique • intestinal obstruction • intraocular
I&O	intake and output
IOC	intern on call
IOFB	intraocular foreign body

IOL	intraocular lens
IOML	infraorbitomeatal line
IOP	intraocular pressure
IOPA	independent organ procurement agency
IORT	intraoperative radiotherapy
IOTA	information overload testing aid
IOV	initial office visit
IP	incisoproximal • incubation period • infection prevention • initial pressure • inpatient • International Pharmacopeia • interphalangeal • intraperitoneal • isoelectric point
IPA	independent practice association • individual practice association • isopropyl alcohol
IPC	intermittent pneumatic compression
IPD	immediate pigment darkening • intermittent peritoneal dialysis
IPE	interstitial pulmonary emphysema
i-periton	intraperitoneal
IPF	infection-potentiating factor
IPG	impedance plethysmography
IPH	idiopathic pulmonary hemosiderosis • interphalangeal
IPJ	interphalangeal joint
IPL	interpupillary line
i-pleur	intrapleural
IPN	interim progress note
IPP	inpatient pharmacy • intermittent positive pressure
IPPA	inspection, palpatation, percussion, auscultation
IPPB	intermittent positive-pressure breathing
IPPBA	intermittent positive-pressure breathing apparatus
IPPF	International Planned Parenthood Foundation

IPPR	intermittent positive-pressure respiration
IPPV	intermittent positive-pressure ventilation
IPR	independent professional review
IPRA	Independent Professional Review Agents
IPS	(Medicare) Interim Payment System
IPSP	inhibitory postsynaptic potential
IPTG	isopropylthiogalactoside
IPTH	immunoreactive parathyroid hormone
IPV	inactivated poliovirus vaccine
IQ	intelligence quotient
Ir	immune response (genes) • iridium
IR	immunoreactive • inferior rectus • infrared • internal resistance • internal rotation • inversion-recovery • irritant reaction
IRB	Institutional Review Board • intern/resident to bed ratio
IRBBB	incomplete right bundle branch block
IRC	inspiratory reserve capacity • International Red Cross • internal revenue code • Internet relay chat
IRD	immune renal disease
IRDS	idiopathic respiratory distress syndrome • infant respiratory distress syndrome
IRGI	immunoreactive glucagon
IRHGH	immunoreactive human growth hormone
IRHS	inpatient rehabilitation hospital services
IRI	immunoreactive insulin
irid	iridescent
IRI/G	ratio of immunoreactive insulin to glucose
IRM	innate releasing mechanism • Institute of Rehabilitation Medicine • information resources management
IRMA	immunoradiometric assay

IRO	International Refugee Organization
IRP	immunoreactive proinsulin • International Reference Preparation
IRR	intrarenal reflux
irrig	irrigated, irrigation
IRV	inspiratory reserve volume
IS	immune serum • incentive spirometer • induced sputum • intensity of services • intercostal space • interspace • interventricular septum • intraspinal • inventory of systems • island
ISA	International Symbol of Access • intrinsic sympathomimetic activity
ISC	International Statistical Classification • interstitial cell • irreversibly sickled cell
ISD	initial sleep disturbance • isosorbide dinitrate
ISDN	integrated services digital network
ISE	ion-selective electrode
ISF	interstitial fluid
ISG	immune serum globulin
ISO	International Standards Organization
isoenz	isoenzymes
isol	isolation
isom	isometric
ISP	distance between iliac spines • intraspinal
ISR	Institute of Surgical Research
IST	insulin shock therapy
ISW	interstitial water
ISY	intrasynovial
IT	information technologies • inhalation therapy • intertrochanteric • intertuberous • intimal thickening • intrathecal • intrathoracic

ITFF	intertrochanteric femoral fracture
ITFS	incomplete testicular feminization syndrome
IT Fx	intertrochanteric fracture
i-thec	intrathecal
ITP	idiopathic thrombocytopenic purpura • inosine triphosphate
ITPA	Illinois Test of Psycholinguistic Abilities
ITQ	Infant Temperament Questionnaire
ITR	intratracheal
i-trach	intratracheal
ITT	insulin tolerance test • intent to treat • iron tolerance test
i-tumor	intratumoral
ITX	intertriginous xanthoma
IU	immunizing unit • international unit • intrauterine
IUCD	intrauterine contraceptive device
IUD	intrauterine death • intrauterine device
IUDR	idoxuridine
IUFB	intrauterine foreign body
IUFD	intrauterine fetal distress
IUGR	intrauterine growth rate • intrauterine growth retardation
IUP	intrauterine pregnancy
IUPAC	International Union of Pure and Applied Chemistry
IUPC	intrauterine pressure catheter
IV	interventricular • intervertebral • intravascular • intravenous • intraventricular
IVAC	intravenous automated controller
IVC	inferior vena cava • inspired vital capacity • intravenous cholangiogram, intravenous cholangiography
IVCD	intraventricular conduction defect • intraventricular conduction delay

IVD	intervertebral disk
IVE	independent vocational evaluator
IVF	intravascular fluid • intravenous fluid
IVGTT	intravenous glucose tolerance test
IVH	intravenous hyperalimentation • intraventricular hemorrhage
IVIG	intravenous immunoglobulin
IVJC	intervertebral joint complex
IVLBW	infant of very low birth weight
IVOX	intravascular oxygenator
IVP	intravenous pyelogram • intraventricular pressure • intravenous push
IVPB	intravenous piggyback
IVPF	isovolume pressure flow (curve)
IVRT	isovolumic relaxation time
IVS	interventricular septum
IVSD	interventricular septal defect
IVSS	intravenous Solu-Set
IVT	intravenous transfusion • isovolumic time
IVU	intravenous urography
IW	injured worker
IWI	inferior wall infarction
IWL	insensible water loss
IWMI	inferior wall myocardial infarction
IZS	insulin zinc suspension

J

J	joint • joule • Joule's equivalent • journal • juice
JA	job analysis
JAI	juvenile amaurotic idiocy

JAMA	Journal of the American Medical Association
JAN	Job Accommodation Network
jaund	jaundice
JCAH	Joint Commission on Accreditation of Hospitals
JCAHO	Joint Commission on Accreditation of Healthcare Organizations
jct	junction
JEE	Japanese equine encephalitis
jej.	jejunum
JFS	Jewish Family Services
JG	juxtaglomerular
JGA	juxtaglomerular apparatus
JI	jejunoileal
JIB	jejunoileal bypass
JJ	jaw jerk
JL	joint line
JMD	juvenile macular degeneration
JND	just noticeable difference
jnt	joint
JOB	Job Opportunities for the Blind
JOC	joint operating committees
JODM	juvenile-onset diabetes mellitus
jour	journal
J-P	Jackson-Pratt drain
JPC	junctional premature contracture
JRA	juvenile rheumatoid arthritis
jt	joint
JUA	Joint Underwriting Association

junct	junction
juv	juvenile
JVD	jugular venous distention

K

k	rate or velocity constant
K	absolute zero (Kelvin) • cathode • dissociation constant • electrostatic capacity • equilibrium constant • Kelvin • keratometer • kilo- • permeability coeffecient • potassium (*kallium*) • thousand (kilo)
^{0}K	degrees Kelvin (absolute temperature)
K$^+$	potassium ion
Ka	cathode • kallikrein
KA	ketoacidosis • King-Armstrong (unit)
KAF	conglutinogen activity factor
KAFO	knee-ankle-foot orthosis
KAP	knowledge, aptitude, practices
kb	kilobase
KB	ketone bodies • knowledge base
K-B	Kleihauer-Betke (stain)
KBr	potassium bromide
kc	kilocycle
KC	kathodal closure • keratoconjunctivitis • kilocycle
K-C	knee-chest
kcal	kilocalorie (large calorie)
KCC	kathodal closure contraction
KCF	key clinical findings
kCi	kilocurie
KCl	potassium chloride
kcps	kilocycles per second

KCS	keratoconjunctivitis sicca
kc/sec	kilocycles per second
KCT	kathodal closure tetanus
KD	kathodal duration • knitted Dacron
KD	dissociation constant
K/D	Keto-Diastix
kdal	kilodalton
KDC	Kidney Disease Treatment Center
K/DOQI	Kidney Disease Outcomes Quality Initiative
KDT	kathodal duration tetanus
KDTC	Kidney Disease Treatment Center
KE	kinetic energy
KED	Kendrick Extrication Device
kev	kiloelectron-volt
keV	kiloelectron-volt
KFD	kinetic family drawings
kg	kilogram
kg-cal	kilogram-calorie (large calorie)
kg-m	kilogram-meter
KGS	ketogenic steroid
KHb	potassium hemoglobinate
KHN	Knoop hardness number
kHz	kilohertz
K_i	inhibition constant
KI	Krönig's isthmus • potassium iodide
KID	keratitis, ichthyosis, and deafness
kilo	kilogram
KiMSV	Kirsten murine sarcoma virus

kJ	kilojoule
KJ	knee jerk
KJL	knee joint line
KK	knee kick
kl	kiloliter
KL bac	Klebs-Löffler bacillus
KLH	keyhole-limpet hemocyanin
KLS	kidney, liver, spleen
km	kilometer
Km	Michaelis constant
KM	kanamycin • Kussmaul (respirations)
kMc	kilomegacycle
kMcps	kilomegacycles per second
KMIS	keratomileusis-in-situ
$KMnO_4$	postassium permanganate
KO	keep open • knock out
KOC	kathodal opening contraction
KOH	potassium hydroxide
KP	keratitic precipitates • keratitis punctata
kPa	kilopascal (unit of pressure)
KPE	Kilman phacoemulsification
Kr	kiloroentgen • krypton
KRP	Kolmer test with Reiter protein
KS	Kaposi's sarcoma • ketosteroid • Kochleffel syndrome • hyphoscoliosis
KTP	potassium titanyl phosphate
KU	Kimbel unit
KUB	kidneys, ureters, bladder

kv	kilovolt
kV	kilovolt
kVA	kilovolt-ampere
KVO	keep vein open
kvp	kilovolts peak
kw	kilowatt
kW	kilowatt
KW	Keith-Wagener scale of retinopathy • Kirschner wire
kw-hr	kilowatt-hour
K-wire	Kirschner wire

L

l	levo- (left, counterclockwise) • liter
L	coefficient of induction • *Lactobacillus* • lateral • lambert (unit of brightness) • Latin • left (counterclockwise) • length • lethal • levorotatory • Lewisite • licensed • ligament • light • light sense • liter • low, lower, lowest • lumbar • lumen • pound (*libra*)
L1-L5	lumbar vertebrae 1 through 5
La	lanthanum
LA	lactic acid • Latin American • left angle • left arm • left atrial (pressure) • left atrium • left auricle • leucine aminopeptidase • linoleic acid • local anesthetic • long-acting
L&A	light and accommodation
LAA	left atrial abnormality • leukocyte ascorbic acid
lab	laboratory
lab proc	laboratory procedure
lac	laceration
LAC	long arm cast
lact	lactate, lactating

LAD	lactic acid dehydrogenase • left anterior descending • left axis deviation • linoleic acid depression
LADCA	left anterior descending coronary artery
LAE	left atrial enlargement
LAF	laminar air flow
LAFB	left anterior fascicular block
LAH	left anterior hemiblock • left atrial hypertrophy
LAHB	left anterior hemiblock
LAI	left atrial involvement
LAIT	latex agglutination inhibition test
LAK	lymphokine-activated killer cells
LaL	labiolingual
Lam	laminectomy
LAN	local area network
L Ant	left anterior
LAO	left anterior oblique
lap	laparotomy
LAP	left atrial pressure • leucine aminopeptidase • leukocyte alkaline phosphatase • lyophilized anterior pituitary • leukocyte adhesion protein
LAPMS	long arm posterior molded splint
LAR	left arm recumbent
LARC	leukocyte automatic recognition computer
LAS	linear alkylate sulfonate • local adaptation syndrome
LASER	light amplification by stimulated emission of radiation
LASIK	laser-assisted in situ keratomileusis
L-Asp	L-asparaginase
LASS	labile aggregation-stimulating substance
LAST	Leukocyte-Antigen Sensitivity Testing

lat	lateral • latitude
lat dol	to the painful side (*lateri dolenti*)
LATR	Laser Assisted Turbinate Resection
LATS	long-acting thyroid stimulator
LATSP	long-acting thyroid stimulator protector
LAV	lymphadenopathy-associated virus
LAVH	laparoscopy-assisted vaginal hysterectomy
lb	pound (*libra*)
LB	laser bullectomy • live birth • low back
L-B	Liebermann-Burchard (reaction)
L&B	left and below
LBB	left breast biopsy • left bundle branch
LBBB	left bundle branch block
LBBsB	left bundle branch system block
LBBX	left breast biopsy examination
LBCD	left border of cardiac dullness
LBD	left border dullness
lb-ft	pound-feet, pound-foot
LBH	length, breadth, height
LBM	last bowel movement • lean body mass
LBNP	lower-body negative pressure
LBP	low back pain • low blood pressure
LBRF	louse-borne relapsing fever
LBT	lupus band test
LBVP	luminal balloon valvuloplasty
LBW	low birth weight

LC	laparoscopic cholecystectomy • lactation consultant • left ear, cold stimulus • leisure counseling • lethal concentration • linguocervical • liquid capsule • living children • low-calorie • Labor Code
LCA	left coronary artery
LCAH	life care at home
LCAT	lecithin-cholesterol-acyltransferase (deficiency)
LCCA	left common carotid artery
LCCS	low cervical cesarean section
LCD	liquid-crystal display
LCFA	long-chain fatty acid
LCGME	Liaison Committee on Graduate Medical Education
LCh	Licentiate in Surgery (*Chirurgia*)
LCIS	lobular carcinoma in situ
LCL	Levinthal-Coles-Lille (bodies) • lower control limits • lateral collateral ligament
LCM	left costal margin • lymphocytic choriomeningitis
LCME	Liaison Committee on Medical Education
LCP	Legg-Calve-Perthes' disease • life care plan , life care planning, life care planner
LCSW	licensed clinical social worker
LCT	lymphocytotoxicity test
LCU	life change units
LD	lactic dehydrogenase • learning disability • left deltoid • lethal dose • light difference (perception) • linguodistal • living donor • low dosage • Lyme disease
LD_{50}	median lethal dose
LDA	left dorsoanterior
LDB	legionnaires' disease bacterium
LDC	leukocyte differential count
LDD	lumbar disc disease

LDGF	leukocyte-derived growth factors
LDH	lactic dehydrogenase
LDL	low-density lipoprotein
LDL-C	low-density lipoprotein cholesterol
LDLP	low-density lipoprotein
LDP	left dorsoposterior
LDR	labor, delivery, recovery
LDRP	labor, delivery, recovery, post-partum
LDS	Licentiate in Dental Surgery
LDUH	low-dose unfractionated heparin
Le	Leonard (cathode ray unit)
LE	left eye • lower extremity • lupus erythematosus
LED	light-emitting diode • lupus erythematosus disseminatus
LEP	limited English proficiency
LES	local excitatory state • lower esophageal sphincter
LET	linear energy transfer
Leu	leucine
lev	levator muscle
Lf	limit of flocculation (unit)
LF	low forceps (delivery) • low frequency
LFA	left femoral artery • left forearm • left frontoanterior
LFA-1	leukocyte function-associated antigen 1
LFA-2	leukocyte function-associated antigen 2
LFA-3	leukocyte function-associated antigen 3
LFD	least fatal dose • low fat diet • low forceps delivery
LFH	left femoral hernia
LFL	left frontolateral
LFP	left frontoposterior

LFPS	Licentiate of the Faculty of Physicians and Surgeons
LFT	latex flocculation test • left frontotransverse • liver function test
lg	large
LG	laryngectomy • left gluteal, left gluteus • linguogingival
LGA	large for gestational age
LGB	Landry-Guillain-Barré (syndrome)
LGH	lactogenic hormone
LGL	Lown-Ganong-Levine (syndrome)
LGN	lateral geniculate nucleus
LGV	lymphogranuloma venereum
LH	left hand • luteinizing hormone • lues hereditaria
L & H	United States Longshore and Harbor Workers' Act
LHH	left homonymous hemianopsia
LHP	left hemiparesis • left hemiplegia
LHRF	luteinizing hormone-releasing factor
LHRH	luteinizing hormone-releasing hormone
LHS	left heart strain
LHV	left hepatic vein
Li	lithium
LIA	leukemia-associated inhibitory activity • lysine-iron agar
LIBC	latent iron-binding capacity
LIC	left iliac crest • left internal carotid • leisure-interest class
LICA	left internal carotid artery
LICM	left intercostal margin
LICS	left intercostal space
LIF	left iliac fossa • leukocyte inhibitory factor
LIFE	Longitudinal Interval Follow-up Evaluation

lig	ligament
LIH	left inguinal hernia
LIMA	left internal mammary artery
lin	linear
linim	liniment
LIP	lymphoid interstitial pneumonia
liq	liquid • liquor
LIRBM	liver, iron, red bone marrow
LIS	lobular in situ • low intermittent suction
LISS	low-ionic-strength saline solution
lith	lithotomy
LK	lamellar keratectomy • left kidney
LKS	liver, kidneys, spleen
LL	left lateral • left leg • left lung • lepromatous leprosy • lower lid
LLat	left lateral
L LAT	left lateral
LLB	long-leg brace
LLBCD	left lower border of cardiac dullness
LLC	long-leg cast • lower level of care
LLD	*Lactobacillus lactis*, Dorner factor (vitamin B12) • left lateral decubitus (position)
LLE	left lower extremity
LLL	left lower lobe
LLLI	La Leche League International
LLM	localized leukocyte mobilization
LLO	*Legionella*-like organisms
LLPMS	long leg posterior molded splint
LLQ	left lower quadrant

LLR	left lateral rectus
LLSB	left lower sternal border
LLT	left lateral thigh
lm	lumen
LM	Licentiate in Midwifery • light microscopy • linguomesial • longitudinal muscle • light minimum
LMA	left mentoanterior
LMB	Laurence-Moon-Biedl syndrome • left mainstem bronchus
LMC	lymphocyte-mediated cytotoxicity
LMCA	left main coronary artery
LMCL	left midclavicular line
LMD	local medical doctor
LMF	lymphocytic mitogenic factor
LMHC	Licensed Mental Health Counselors
LMHT	licensed mental health technician
LMI	leukocyte migration inhibition
LML	left mediolateral
LMM	lentigo maligna melanoma
LMP	last menstrual period • left mentoposterior
LMS	Licentiate in Medicine and Surgery • labor market survey
LMT	left mentotransverse • leukocyte migration technique • lateral meniscus tear
lmtd	limited
LMW	low molecular weight
LMWD	low molecular weight dextran
LMWH	low molecular weight heparin
LN	lobular neoplasia • lymph node
LNC	lymph-node cells
LNMP	last normal menstrual period

LNPF	lymph node permeability factor
LO	linguo-occlusal
LOA	leave of absence • left occipitoanterior
LOC	laxative of choice • level of care • level of consciousness • loss of consciousness • loss of control
loc cit	in the place cited (*loco citato*)
loc dol	to the painful spot (*loco dolenti*)
LoCHO	low carbohydrate
LoCHol	low cholesterol
LOD	line of duty
log	logarithm
LOH	length of hospitalization
LOINC	Logical Observation Identifiers, Names, and Codes
LOM	limitation of motion • loss of motion
LOMSA	left otitis media suppurative, acute
LOMSCh	left otitis media suppurative, chronic
LoNa$^+$	low sodium
long	longitudinal
LOP	leave on pass • left occipitoposterior
LOQ	lower outer quadrant
LOR	loss of resistance
LOS	length of stay
lot	lotion
LOT	left occipitotransverse
LP	latent period • leukocytic pyrogen • light perception • lipoprotein • low power • low pressure • lumbar puncture • lymphoid predominance
L/P	lactate-pyruvate ratio
LPA	left pulmonary artery

L-PAM	L-phenylalanine mustard
LPCA	Licensed Professional Counseling Association
lpf	low-power field
LPF	leukocytosis-promoting factor • low-power field
LPFB	left posterior fascicular block
LPH	left posterior hemiblock
LPHB	left posterior hemiblock
lpi	lines per inch
LPICA	left posterior internal carotid artery
lpm	lines per minute • liters per minute
LPM	liters per minute
LPN	licensed practical nurse
LPO	left posterior oblique
L POST	left posterior
LPS	Lanterman-Petris-Short • levator palpebrae superioris (muscle) • lipase • lipopolysaccharide
LPV	left portal vein • lymphotropic papovavirus
LQ	left quadrant
Lr	lawrencium
LR	lactated Ringer's • latency relaxation • lateral rectus (muscle)
L-R	left to right
L/R	left/right
LRC	Lipid Research Center
LRCP	Licentiate of the Royal College of Physicians
LRCS	Licentiate of the Royal College of Surgeons
LRD	living related donor
LRE	leukemic reticuloendotheliosis
LRF	liver residue factor • luteinizing hormone-releasing factor

LRH	luteinizing hormone-releasing hormone
LRI	lower respiratory infection
LRQ	lower right quadrant
LRR	labyrinthine righting reflex
LS	lumbosacral
L/S	lecithin-sphingomyelin ratio • liver-spleen
LSA	left sacroanterior • left subclavian artery • Licentiate of the Society of Apothecaries
LSB	left sternal border
LScA	left scapuloanterior
LScP	left scapuloposterior
LSD	least significant digit • lysergic acid diethylamide
LSH	lutein-stimulating hormone • lymphocyte-stimulating hormone
LSK	liver, spleen, kidneys
LSM	lysergic acid morpholide
LSO	left salpingo-oophorectomy • lumbosacral orthosis
LSP	left sacroposterior
LSS	liver-spleen scan • lumbosacral spine
LST	lateral sinus thrombophlebitis • left sacrotransverse
LSU	life-support unit
LSW	left-sided weakness
lt	left • light • low tension
LT	left triceps • leukotriene • locum tenens • lymphocyte transformation • lymphocytic thyroiditis • lymphotoxin • long term
LTA	laryngotrachael anesthesia
LTAC	long-term acute care
LTB	laryngotracheobronchitis
LTC	long-term care

LTCF	long-term care facility
LTCS	low transverse Cesarean section
LTCU	long-term care unit
LTD	limited • long-term disability • long-term disability insurance
LTF	lipotropic factor • lymphocyte transforming factor
LTH	luteotropic hormone
LTM	long-term memory
LTP	L-tryptophan
LTPP	lipothiamide pyrophosphate
LTR	long-terminal repeat
LTT	leucine tolerance test • lymphocyte transformation test
Lu	letetium
LU	left upper
LUCs	large unstained cells
LUE	left upper extremity
LUIS	low-dose urea in invert sugar
LUL	left upper lobe
LUO	left ureteral orifice
LUOQ	left upper outer quadrant
LUQ	left upper quadrant
LV	left ventricle, left ventricular • live vaccine
LVAD	left ventricle assist device
LVD	left ventricular dimension
LVE	left ventricular enlargement
LVEDP	left ventricular end-diastolic pressure
LVEDV	left ventricular end-diastolic volume
LVEF	left ventricular ejection fraction
LVET	left ventricular ejection time

LVFP	left ventricular filling pressure
LVH	large-vessel hematocrit • left ventricular hypertrophy
LVID	left ventricular internal dimension
LVIDP	left ventricular initial diastolic pressure
LVLG	left ventrolateral gluteal
LVN	licensed visiting nurse • licensed vocational nurse
LVO	left ventricular outflow • left ventricular overactivity
LVP	left ventricular pressure
LVR	low vision rehabilitation
LVSW	left ventricular stroke work
LVSWI	left ventricular stroke work index
LW	left ear, warm stimulus
L&W	Lee and White (clotting time) • living and well
LWCT	Lee-White clotting time
LWOP	leave without pay
lx	lux (illuminance unit)
Lx	local irradiation
lym	lymphocyte
LYM	lymphedema
Lys	lysine
lytes	electrolytes
LZM	lysozyme

M

m	handful (*manipulus*) • mass • meter • mili- • minim • minute • molar • morphine • mucoid • murmur • noon (*meridies*)

M	chin (*mentum*) • macerate(d) • male • malignant • married • massage • mature • mean • median • medical • medium • mega- • melts at • membrane • memory • metabolite • meter • method • *Micrococcus* • minim • mitral • mix, mixture • molar • molecular weight • Monday • morgan (unit of chromosome map distance) • morphine • mother • muscle • myeloma • myopia, myopic • noon (*meridies*) • thousand (*mille*)
mμ	millimicro- • millimicron
m^2	square meter
m^3	cubic meter
ma	milliampere
mA	milliampere
MA	mandelic acid • manifest achievement • Master of Arts • medical abbreviation • medical assistant • medical audit • membrane antigen • menstrual age • mental age • meter angle • Miller-Abbott (tube) • milliampere
MAA	macroaggregated albumin
MAB	management of assaultive behavior • monoclonal antibody
MABP	mean arterial blood pressure
mac	macerate
MAC	malignancy associated changes • maximum (maximal) allowable concentration • maximum allowable cost • methotrexate, actinomycin D, cyclophosphamide • mid-arm circumference • minimum alveolar concentration • minimum anesthetic concentration • mitral anular calcium • monitored anesthesia care • Mycobacterium avium complex • membrane attack complex
MACC	methotrexate, doxorubicin, cyclophosphamide, lomustine
MAC INH	membrane attack complex inhibitor
MADC	mean average daily census
MADD	multiple acyl CoA dehydrogenation deficiency
MADRS	Medicare automated data retrieval system
MAE	moves all extremities

MAEW	moves all extremities well
MAF	macrophage activating factor • minimum (minimal) audible field • medical assistance facilities
mag	large (*magnus*) • magnification
Mag	magnesium
MAG	myelin-associated glycoprotein
MAHA	microangiopathic hemolytic anemia
MAI	*Mycobaterium avium* infection • *Mycobacterium avium intracellulare*
MAIC	*Mycobacterium avium intracellulare* complex
mall	malleolus
MALT	mucosa-associated lymphoid tissue
mam	milliampere-minute
M+Am	compound myopic astigmatism
MAMC	mid-arm muscle circumference
man	handful (*manipulus*) • manipulation
mand	mandible, mandibular
manif	manifest, manifested
manip	handful (*manipulus*) • manipulation
man pr	early in the morning (*mane primo*)
MAO	maximal acid output • monoamine oxidase
MAODP	Medic Alert Organ Donor Program
MAOI	monoamine oxidase inhibitor
MAP	mean aortic pressure • mean arterial pressure • medical assistance program • medical audit program • minimum (minimal) audible pressure • monophasic action potential • muscle action potential
MAPS	Make-A-Picture Story (test)
MAR	Medication Administration Record • minimal angle resolution

MARC	Medical Air Rescue Corps
MARS	Mevinolin Atherosclerosis Regression Study
mas	milliampere-second
MaS	milliampere-second
MAS	meconium aspiration syndrome
masc	masculine • mass concentration
MASER	microwave amplification by stimulated emission of radiation
MASH	mobile army surgical hospital • mutual aid and self-help
MASRI	Medication Adherence Self-Report Inventory
mass	massage
mast	mastectomy
mAST	mitochondrial asparate aminotransferase
MAST	Medical Anti-Shock Trousers • Michigan Alcoholism Screening Test • Military Anti-Shock Trousers • Multiple Antigen Simultaneous Testing
Mat	maternity
MAT	manual arts therapy, therapist • motivation analysis test • multifocal atrial tachycardia
matut	in the morning (*matutimus*)
max	maxilla, maxillary • maximal, maximum
mb	mix well (*misce bene*)
Mb	myoglobin
MB	Bachelor of Medicine (*Medicinae Baccalaureus*) • Marsh-Bendall factor • methylene blue
MBA	Master of Business Administration
M-BACOD	methotrexate, bleomycin, Adriamycin, cyclophosphamide, Oncovin, dexamethasone
MBC	maximum (maximal) breathing capacity • minimum (minimal) bactericidal concentration
MBD	minimal brain dysfunction

MBF	meat base formula • myocardial blood flow
MBO	management by objectives • mesiobucco-occlusal
MbO_2	oxymyoglobin
MBP	mean blood pressure • melitensis, bovine, porcine (antigen) • myelin basic protein (assay) • Munchausen's by proxy
MBRT	methylene blue reduction time
MBT	mixed bacterial toxin
mc	millicurie
Mc	megacurie • megacycle
MC	macroglobulinemia • Master of Surgery (*Magister Chirurgiae*) • medical center • medical corps • medullary cystic disease • metacarpal • microencephaly • mineralocorticoid • mixed cellularity • mycelial phase • managed care
M&C	morphine and cocaine
M-C	Magovern-Cromie (prosthesis)
MCA	middle cerebral artery
M-CAF	macrophage colony-stimulating factor
MCAF	monocyte chemotactic and activating factor
MCAH	maternal, child, and adolescent health
MCAR	mixed-cell agglutination reaction
MCAT	Medical College Admission Test
McB	McBurney's point
MCB	membranous cytoplasmic body
MCC	missing in colon carcinoma
MCCU	Mobile Coronary Care Unit
MCD	mean corpuscular diameter • medullary cystic disease • metabolic coronary dilation • mean of consecutive differences
MCE	medical-care evaluation • Medicare Code Editor

MCF	macrophage chemotactic factor • medium corpuscular fragility
mcg	microgram
MCGN	mesangiocapillary glomerulonephritis
mch	millicurie-hour
MCh	Master of Surgery (*Magister Chirurgiae*)
MCH	maternal and child health • mean corpuscular hemoglobin • Microfibrillar Collagen Hemostat
MCHB	Maternal and Child Health Bureau
MCHC	mean corpuscular hemoglobin concentration
MCHS	maternal and child health services
mCi	millicurie
mCid	millicuries destroyed
MCL	maximum containment laboratory • midclavicular line • modified chest lead
MCL^1	modified chest lead
MCLNS	mucocutaneous lymph-node syndrome
MCNS	minimal-change nephrotic syndrome
MCO	managed care organization
mcoul	millicoulomb
MCP	metacarpal • metaclopramide
MCPH	metacarpophalangeal
MCPO-1	monocyte chemotactic peptide-1
mcps	megacycles per second
MCR	metabolic clearance rate
MCT	mean circulation time • medium-chain triglyceride • medullary carcinoma of the thyroid • multiple compressed tablet
MCTD	mixed connective-tissue disease
MCU	maximum care unit

MCV	mean cell volume • mean clinical value • mean corpuscular volume
md	median
Md	mendelevium
MD	Doctor of Medicine (*Medicinae Doctor*) • macular degeneration • mandibular • manic depression • mean deviation • medical department • mentally deficient • mesiodistal • mitral disease • muscular dystrophy
MDA	malonyldialdehyde • manual dilatation of the anus • methylenedioxyamphetamine (hallucinogenic drug) • motor discriminative acuity • Muscular Dystrophy Association • right mentoanterior (*mentodextra anterior*) • physician anesthesiologist
MDC	Major Diagnostic Category
MDD	major depressive disorder • mean daily dose
MDF	myocardial depressant factor
MDH	malate dehydrogenase
MDI	metered dose inhaler • multiple daily injections
m dict	as directed (*more dictu*)
Mdn	median
MDP	right mentoposterior (*mentodextra posterior*) • methylene diphophonate
MDQ	minimal detectable quantity
MDR	minimum (minimal) daily requirement
MDRTP	multi-drug resistant tuberculosis
MDS	Master of Dental Surgery • minimal data sheet • minimal data set
MDSO	mentally disordered sex offender
MDT	right mentotransverse (*mentodextra transversa*)
Me	methyl
ME	maximum effort • medical education • medical examiner • metabolic and electrolyte disorder • middle ear • medical end

M/E	myeloid-erythroid ratio
MEA	multiple endocrine adenomatosis
meas	measure, measured, measuring
MeB	methylene blue
mec	meconium
MEC	medical executive committee • minimum effective concentration
MeCbl	methylcobalomin
MeCCNU	semustine
mech	mechanism
med	median • medicine, medical • medium
MED	median erthyrocyte diameter • minimum (minimal) effective dose • minimum (minimal) erythema dose
MEDLARS	Medical Literature Analysis and Retrieval System
MEDLINE	MEDLARS on-line
MEDPAC	Medicare Payment Advisory Committee
MEDPAR	Medicare Provider Analysis and Review
MEDPRO	Medical Education Resources Program
med-surg	medical-surgical
med tech	medical technician • medical technologist
MEE	methylethyl ether
MEF	maximum (maximal) expiratory flow
MEFR	maximum (maximal) expiratory flow rate
MEFV	maximum (maximal) expiratory flow volume
meg	megacycle • megaloblastic
MEG	mercaptoethylguanidine
MEI	Medicare Economic Index
MEL	murine erythroleukemia

MELAS	mitochondrial encephalopathy, lactic acidosis and stroke-like episodes
mem	member
MEM	macrophage electrophoretic migration • macrophage electrophoretic mobility • minimum (minimal) essential medium
memb	membrane
MEN	multiple endocrine neoplasia
menst	menstrual, menstruate, menstruating
MEOS	microsomal ethanol-oxidizing system
MEP	mean effective pressure • motor end-plate
mEq	milliequivalent
mEq/L	milliequivalent per liter
MER	methanol extraction residue
MERRF	myoclonus with epilepsy and ragged red fibers
MES	maintenance electrolyte solution • morpholino-ethanesoufonic acid
MESH	Medical Subject Headings
met	metal, metallic
Met	methionine
MET	metabolic equivalent • multiple-employer trust
metab	metabolic, metabolism, metabolites
metas	metastasis, metastasize, metastasizing
meth	method
metHb	methemoglobin
methyl-CCNU	semustine
metMb	metmyoglobin
mets	metastasis, metastasize, metastasizing
m et sig	mix and write a label (*misce et signa*)
mev	megaelectron-volt (million electron volts)

meV	megaelectron-volt (million electron volts)
MeV	megaelectron-volt (million electron volts)
MEWA	multiple employer welfare arrangement
mf	microfilaria
mF	millifarad
MF	medium frequency • microscopic factor • mitotic figure • multiplying factor • mycosis fungoides • myelin figure
M/F	male-female ratio
M&F	male and female • mother and father
MFA	methyl fluoracetate
MFAT	multifocal atrial tachycardia
MFB	medial forebrain bundle • metallic foreign body
MFD	maternal-fetal diagnostics • midforceps delivery • minimum (minimal) fatal dose
MFG	modified heat-degraded gelatin
M flac	*membrana flaccida*
MFMER	Mayo Foundation for Medical Education and Research
MFP	monofluorophosphate
MFPVC	multifocal premature ventricular contractions
MFS	medical fee schedule • Medicare Fee Schedule
m ft	let a mixture be made (*mistura fiat*)
MFT	muscle-function test
mg	milligram
mg%	milligrams per 100 cubic centimeters or per 100 grams
Mg	magnesium
MG	membranous glomerulopathy • menopausal gonadotrophin • mesiogingival • myasthenia gravis
MGCRB	Medicare Geographic Classification Review Board
MGD	mixed gonadal dysgenesis

mg-el	milligram-element
MGF	maternal grandfather
mg-hr	milligram-hour
mg/kg	milligrams per kilograms (of body weight)
mgm	milligram
MGM	maternal grandmother
MGN	membranous glomerulonephritis
$MgSO_4$	magnesium sulfate
MH	malignant hyperthermia • marital history • medical history • melanophore hormone • menstrual history • mental health • municipal hospital
MHA	Master in Health Administration • Mental Health Association • microangiopathic hemolytic anemia
MHA-TP	microhemagglutinin-*Treponema pallidum* (test)
MhB	methemoglobin
MHB	maximum (maximal) hospital benefit
MHC	major histocompatibility complex • mental health center • multiphasic health checkup • midhumeral circumference
MHD	maximum (maximal) human dose • minimum (minimal) hemolytic dose
MHI	Mental Health Institute
MHP	maternal health program • mercury hydroxypropane • methoxyhydroxypropane
MHPG	methoxyhydroxyphenylglycol
MHSP	municipal health service demonstration projects
MHW	mental health worker
MHz	megahertz
MI	maturation index • mental illness • mesioincisal • mitral insufficiency • myocardial infarction
M&I	maternal and infant care
MIA	medically indigent adult • missing in action

MIB	Medical Impairment Bureau
MIBG	metaiodobenzene/guanidine
MiC	minocycline
MIC	medical intensive care • microscopic • minimum (minimal) inhibitory concentration • mobile intensive care
MICU	medical intensive care unit • mobile intensive care unit
mid	middle
MID	mesioincisodistal • minimal inhibiting dose • minimum (minimal) infective dose
mid sag	midsagittal
MIF	macrophage-inhibiting factor • melanocyte-inhibiting factor • melanocyte- stimulating hormone-inhibiting factor • merthiolate iodine formalin (solution) • migration-inhibiting factor
MIFR	maximum (maximal) inspiratory flow rate
MII	major IRM investments
mil	milliliter
MILIS	Multicenter Investigation of the Limitation of Infarct Size
min	mineral • minim • minimum • minimal • minute • minor
MIO	minimum (minimal) identifiable odor
MIP	Medicare Integrity Program
MIRD	Medical Internal Radiation Dose (Committee)
MIS	Management Information System • medical information services • minimally invasive solution • minimally invasive surgery
misc	miscarriage • miscellaneous
mist	mixture (*mistura*)
mit	send (*mitte*)
MIT	Metabolic Intolerance Test • monoiodotyrosine
mit insuf	mitral insufficiency

mIU	milli-international unit
mixt	mixture
MJ	marijuana
MJI	mid-joint injury
MK	marked • monkey kidney
MKM	myopic keratomileusis
MKS	meter-kilogram-second (system)
ml	midline • milliliter
mL	milliliter
ML	Licentiate in Medicine • mesiolingual • middle lobe • midline
M/L	medical/legal
MLa	mesiolabial
MLA	left mentoanterior (*mentolaeva anterior*) • Medical Library Association
MLaI	mesiolabioincisal
MLaP	mesiolabiopulpal
MLB	minimum (minimal) lethal concentration • mixed leukocyte culture • mixed lymphocyte culture
MLCR	mixed lymphocyte culture reaction
MLD	masking level differences • median lethal dose • metachromatic leukodystrophy • minimum (minimal) lethal dose • manual lymph drainage
MLEpis	midline episiotomy
MLF	medial longitudinal fasciculus
MLG	mitochondria lipid glucogen
MLI	mesiolinguoincisal
MLNS	mucocutaneous lymph node syndrome
MLO	mesiolinguo-occlusal

MLP	left mentoposterior (*mentolaeva posterior*) • mesiolinguopulpal
MLR	mixed lymphocyte reaction • mixed lymphocyte response
MLS	mean lifespan • median longitudinal section • mucolipidosis
MLT	left mentotransverse (*mentolaeva transversa*) • median lethal time • medical laboratory technician
mm	millimeter • murmur • muscles
mm^2	square millimeter
mm^3	cubic millimeter
mM	millimol (millimole)
MM	medical malleolus • motor meal • mucous membrane • multiple myeloma • myeloid metaplasia • maternity management
M&M	morbidity and mortality
MMA	methylmalonic acid
MMC	migrating myoelectric complex
MMD	mass median diameter
MME	major movable equipment
MMECT	multiple monitored electroconvulsive therapy
MMEF	maximum (maximal) midexpiratory flow
MMEFR	maximum (maximal) midexpiratory flow rate
MMF	maximum (maximal) midexpiratory flow
MMFR	maximum (maximal) midexpiratory flow rate
mmHg	millimeters of mercury
MMI	methimazole (methylmercaptoimidazole) • maximum medical improvement
MMIHS	megacystis-microcolon-intestinal hypoperistalsis syndrome
MMIS	Medicaid Management Information System
MMK	Marshall-Marchetti-Krantz (procedure)

mM/L	millimols (millimoles) per liter
MMP	matrix metalloproteases
MMPI	Minnesota Multiphasic Personality Inventory
mmpp	millimeters partial pressure
MMR	mass miniature radiography • mass miniature roentgenography • maternal mortality rate • measles, mumps, rubella • mouth-to-mouth resuscitation • maximum medical recovery
MMS	methyl methanesulfonate
MMSE	Mini Mental State Examination
MMT	manual muscle test • medial meniscus tear
MMTP	methadone maintenance treatment program
MMWR	Morbidity and Mortality Weekly Report
mn	midnight
mN	millinormal
Mn	manganese
MN	midnight • mononuclear • motor neuron • multinodular • myoneural
MNCV	motor-nerve conduction velocity
MND	minimum (minimal) necrotizing dose • motor neuron disease
MNG	multinodular goiter
MNJ	myoneural junction
MNS	minor blood group system
MNU	methylnitrosourea
Mo	mode • molybdenum
MO	manually operated • medical officer • mesio-occlusal • mineral oil • minute output • mitral orifice • month • months old
MOA	mechanisms of allergy • Memorandum or Agreement
MOAB	monoclonal antibody

MOB	medical office building
mod	moderate, moderately • modified • modulation • module
MOD	mesio-occlusodistal • maturity-onset diabetes mellitus
Mod/Alt	modified or alternative work or duties
mod praesc	as directed (*modo praescripto*)
MODS	multiple organ dysfunction syndrome
MODY	maturity-onset diabetes of youth
MOF	methoxyflurane
MOH	medical officer of health
MOJAC	mood, orientation, judgement, affect, content
mol	molecule, molecular
moll	soft (*mollis*)
mol wt	molecular weight
MOM	milk of magnesia
MoMSV	Moloney murine sarcoma virus
mon	monocyte • month
mono	infectious mononucleosis
monos	monocytes
MOP	medical outpatient program
MOPP	mechlorethamine, Oncovin, procarbazine, prednisone
MOPV	monovalent oral poliovirus vaccine
mor dict	as directed (*more dicto*)
morph	morphology, morphologic
mOs	milliosmol
m osmole	milliosmol
MOTT	mycobacteria other than tubercle
MOU	memorandum of understanding
mp	as directed (*modo praescripto*) • melting point

MP	mechanical percussion , mechanical percussor • menstrual period • mentoposterior • mercaptopurine • mesiopulpal • metacarpophalangeal • methylprednisolone • monophosphate • mucopolysaccharide
6-MP	6-mercaptopurine
MPA	Master of Public Administration • medroxyprogesterone acetate
MPAP	mean pulmonary artery pressure
MPB	male pattern baldness
MPC	maximum (maximal) permissible concentration
MPCWP	mean pulmonary capillary wedge pressure
MPD	maximum (maximal) permissible dose • myofacial pain dysfunction
MPGN	membranoproliferative glomerulonephritis
MPH	Master of Public Health
MPHR	maximum (maximal) predicted heart rate
MPI	Master Patient Index • maximum point of impulse • multiphasic personality inventory
MPN	most probable number
MPO	myeloperoxidase
MPP	maximum (maximal) print position
MPR	mercaptopurine riboside
MPS	macular photocoagulation study • mucopolysaccharide
MPV	mean platelet volume
MQ	memory quotient
mr	milliroentgen
mR	milliroentgen
MR	magnetic resonance • may repeat • measles, rubella • medial rectus • medical record • mental retardation, mentally retarded • metabolic rate • methyl red • milk-ring (test) • mitral reflux • mitral regurgitation • mixed respiratory • Medical Review

MRA	magnetic resonance angiography • Medical Record Administrator
mrad	millirad
MRAN	medical resident admitting note
MRC	Medical Research Council • Medical Reserve Corps
MRCP	Member, Royal College of Physicians
MRCS	Member, Royal College of Surgeons
MRD	minimum (minimal) reacting dose
MRDM	malnutrition-related diabetes mellitus
MRE	maximum (maximal) restrictive exercise
mrem	millirem
MRF	melanocyte-releasing factor • melanocyte-stimulating hormone-releasing factor
MRFIT	multiple risk factor intervention trial
MRH	melanocyte-releasing hormone
MRHD	maximum (maximal) recommended human dose
MRHFP	Medicare Rural Hospital Flexibility Program
mrhm	milliroentgens per hour at one meter
MRI	magnetic resonance imaging • mortality risk index
MRIH	melanocyte release-inhibiting hormone
MRL	minimal response level
mRNA	messenger ribonucleic acid
MRQ	medical review questionnaire
MRR	marrow release rate
MRS	methicillin-resistant *staphylococcus aureus*
MRSA	methicillin-resistant *staphylococcus aureus*
MRT	major role therapy
MRU	minimum (minimal) reproductive units
MRxi	may repeat one time

ms	millisecond
MS	mass spectrometry • Master of Science • Master of Surgery • medical-surgical • mental status • mitral stenosis • morphine sulfate • multiple sclerosis • muscle strength • musculoskeletal
MSA	Medical Services Administration • Medical Services Association • multiplication stimulating activity • medical savings account • Medicare savings account
MSAFP	maternal serum α - fetoprotein
MSC	mandatory settlement conference
MSD	Master of Science in Dentistry • midsleep disturbance • mild sickle-cell disease • most significant digit • multiple sulfatase deficiency
MSDS	material safety data sheets
MSE	mental status examination
msec	millisecond
MSG	monosodium glutamate
MSH	melanocyte-stimulating hormone • melanophore-stimulating hormone
MSHCA	Master of Science in Health Care Administration
MSHIF	melanocyte-stimulating hormone-inhibiting factor
MSHRF	melanocyte-stimulating hormone-releasing factor
MSIS	Medicaid Statistical Information System
MSL	midsternal line
MSLA	multisample Luer adapter
MSLT	multiple sleep latency test
MSN	Master of Science in Nursing
MSO	management services organization
MSP	Medicare as secondary payor
MSPH	Master of Science in Public Health
MSRPP	Multidimensional Scale for Rating Psychiatric Patients

mss	massage
MSS	medical social services • mental status schedule • metabolic support service • minor surgery suite
MST	median survival time
MSTA	mumps skin test antigen
MSTh	mesothorium
MSU	medical-surgical unit • midstream urine
MSUA	midstream urinalysis
MSUD	maple syrup urine disease
MSV	Moloney's sarcoma virus • murine sarcoma virus
MSW	Master of Social Welfare • Master of Social Work • Medical Social Worker
MT	empty • medial thickening • mediastinal tube • medical technologist, medical technology • metatarsal • music therapy • tympanic membrane (*membrana tympani*) • multiple trauma
MT6	mercaptomerin
MT (ASCP)	Registered Medical Technologist (American Society of Clinical Pathologists)
MTBF	mean time between (equipment) failures
MTBI	mild traumatic brain injury
MTC	medullary thyroid carcinoma
MTD	maximum (maximal) tolerated dose • metastatic trophoblastic disease
mtDNA	mitochondrial DNA
MTF	military treatment facility • modulation transfer function
MTM	modified Thayer-Martin (agar)
MTP	metatarsophalangeal
MTR	Meinicke turbidity reaction
MTS	Medicare Transaction System
MTT	mean transit time

MTU	methylthiouracil
MTV	mammary tumor virus
MTX	methotrexate
mu	mouse unit
mU	milliunit
Mu	Mache unit
MUAP	motor unit action potential
MUGA	multiple-gated acquisition scanning
mult	multiplication, multiply
multip	multipara
MUO	myocardiopathy of unknown origin
MUP	motor unit potential
musc	muscular, muscle
MUST	medical unit, self-contained and transportable
muu	mouse uterine unit
mv	millivolt
mV	millivolt
MV	mechanical ventilation • megavolt • minute volume • mitral valve
MVA	mitral-valve area • motor vehicle accident
MVB	mixed venous blood
MVC	maximum (maximal) vital capacity
MVD	microvascular decompression
MVE	maximum voluntary effort • Murray Valley encephalitis
MVI	multivitamin infusion
MVO_2	myocardial oxygen consumption • oxygen content of mixed venous blood
MVO_2R	myocardial oxygen consumption rate
MVP	mitral valve prolapse

MVPP	Mustargen, vinblastine, procarbazine, prednisone
MVPS	Medical Volume Performance Standard
MVRI	mixed vaccine, respiratory infection
mV-sec	millivolt-second
MVV	maximum (maximal) ventilatory volume • maximum (maximal) voluntary ventilation
MVVPP	Mustargen, vincristine, vinblastine, procarbazine, prednisone
mw	microwave
mW	milliwatt
MW	molecular weight
M-W	Mallory-Weiss syndrome • men and women
MWIA	Medical Women's International Association
MWt	molecular weight
Mx	mastectomy • maxillary • multiple • myringotomy
My	myopia
myco	mycobacterium
myel	myelin • myelogram
myelo	myelocyte
MyG	myasthenia gravis
myo	myocardial, myocardium
MZ	monozygotic, monozygous

N

n	born (*nee*) • nano- (one-billionth) • normal • nostril • number • symbol for index of refraction • neutron
N	nasal • negative • *Neisseria* • nerve • neurologist, neurology • neuter • neutron dosage unit • newton • nitrogen • nodal • nonmalignant • normal • normal concentration • number
Na	sodium (*natrium*)

NA	Narcotics Anonymous • neutralizing antibody • nicotinic acid • *Nomina Anatomica* (nomenclature) • noradrenalin (norepinephrine) • not applicable • not available • nuclear antigen • nucleic acid • numeric aperture • nurse anesthetist • nurse's aide • nursing assistant
NAA	no apparent abnormalities
NAACOG	Nurses Association of the American College of Obstetricians and Gynecologists
NAATP	National Association of Addiction Treatment Providers
NAB	neutralizing antibodies
NaBr	sodium bromide
NAC	*N*-acetylcysteine • Nursing Audit Committee
NACA	National Advisory Council on Aging
NaCl	sodium chloride
NAD	National Association of the Deaf • nicotinamide adenine dinucleotide • nicotonic acid dehydrogenase • no acute distress • no apparent distress • no appreciable disease • nothing abnormal detected
NADEP	National Association of Disability Evaluatory Professionals
NADH	nicotinamide adenine dinucleotide, reduced form
NADONA/LTC	National Association of Directors of Nursing Administration in Long Term Care
NADP	nicotinamide adenine dinucleotide phosphate
NADPH	nicotinamide adenine dinucleotide phosphate, reduced form
NAET	Nambrudripad Allergy Elimination Technique
NaF	sodium fluoride
NAG	nonagglutinable vibrios
NAHC	National Association for Home Care
NaHCO$_3$	sodium bicarbonate
NAHMOR	National Association of HMO Regulators
NAHQ	National Association for Healthcare Quality
NAI	non-accidental injury

Nal (TI)	thallium-activated sodium iodide (scintillation detector)
NALGHC	National Alliance of Lesbian and Gay Health Clinics
NAME	nevi, atrial myxoma and neurofibroma ephelides
NAMH	National Association for Mental Health
NAN	N-acetylneuraminic acid
NANA	*N*-acetylneuraminic acid
NANAD	National Association of Anorexia Nervosa and Related Disorders
NANB	non-A, non-B (viral hepatitis)
NANBV	non-A, non-B virus
NANDA	North American Nursing Diagnosis Association
NAP	nonacute profile
NAPA	*N*-acetyl-*p*-aminophenol (acetaminiphen) • *N*-acetylprocainamide
NAPCA	National Air Pollution Control Administration
NAPNAP	National Association of Pediatric Nurse Associates and Practitioners
NAPNES	National Association of Practical Nurse Education and Service
NAPPH	National Association of Private Psychiatric Hospitals
NAPS	National Auxiliary Publications Service
NAPT	National Association of Physical Therapists
NAQAP	National Association of Quality Assurance Professionals
NAR	nasal airway resistance
NARC	narcotic • narcotics officer • National Association for Retarded Children
NARIC	National Rehabilitation Information Center
NARPPS	National Association of Rehabilitation Professionals in the Private Sector
NAS	nasal • National Academy of Sciences • no added salt
NASA	National Aeronautics and Space Administration

NASCD	National Association for Sickle Cell Disease
NAS-NRC	National Academy of Sciences-National Research Council
NASTAD	National Alliance of State and Territorial AIDS Directors
NASW	National Association of Social Workers
nat	national • native • nature, natural
NATCO	North American Transplant Coordinators Organization
Nb	niobium
NB	Negri bodies • newborn • normoblast • note well (*nota bene*)
NBC	nuclear, biological, chemical
NBI	no bone injury
NBM	nothing by mouth
NBME	National Board of Medical Examiners
NBN	Newborn Nursery
NBO	nonbed occupancy
NBR	Nursing Boards Review
NBS	National Bureau of Standards
NBT	nitroblue tetrazolium
NBTE	nonbacterial thrombotic endocarditis
NBTNF	newborn, term, normal, female
NBTNM	newborn, term, normal, male
nc	nanocurie
NC	nasal canal • no change • noncontributory • nurse corps
N/C	no complaints
NCA	National Certification Agency • National Council on Alcoholism • neurocirculatory asthenia • nonspecific cross-reacting antigen
NCAI	National Coalition for Adult Immunization
NcAMP	nephrogenous cyclic adenosine monophosphate

NCB	no code blue
NCCAM	National Center for Complimentary and Alternative Medicine
NCCLS	National Committee for Clinical Laboratory Standards
NCCMHC	National Council of Community Mental Health Centers
NCD	not considered disabling
NCF	night care facility • neutrophil chemotactic factor
NCHCA	National Committee for Health Certifying Agencies
NCHS	National Center for Health Statistics
NCHSR	National Center for Health Services Research
nCi	nanocurie
NCI	naphthalene creosote, iodoform (powder) • National Cancer Institute
NCLEX	National Council Licensure Examination for Nurses
NCME	Network for Continuing Medical Education
NCN	National Council of Nurses
NCNC	normochromic, normocytic (erythrocyte)
NCNR	National Center for Nursing Research
NCOA	National Council on the Aging
NCP	National Cancer Program • nursing care plan
NCQA	National Council for Quality Assurance
NCR	neurologic/circulatory/range of motion
NCRP	National Council on Radiation Protection and Measurements
NCS	noncoronary sinus
NCSH	National Clearinghouse for Smoking and Health
NCSNNE	National Commission for the Study of Nursing and Nursing Education
NCV	noncholera vibrio • nerve conduction velocity
NCVS	nerve conduction velocity studies
n_D	refractive index

Nd	neodymium
ND	Doctor of Nursing • natural death • neoplastic disease • neutral density • New Drugs (AMA publication) • normal delivery • not diagnosed • not done
NDA	National Dental Association • New Drug Application
NDC	National Drug Code (number)
NDCD	New Drug Code Directory
NDE	near-death experience
NDF	no disease found
NDGA	nordihydroguaiaretic acid
NDI	nephrogenic diabetes insipidus
NDM	N-desmethylmethsuximide
nDNA	nuclear DNA
NDT	Neurological Development Therapy • non-destructive testing
NDTI	National Disease and Therapeutic Index
NDV	Newcastle Disease Virus
NDx	nondiagnostic
Nd:YAG	neodymium: yttrium aluminum garnet (laser)
Ne	neon
NE	neurological examination • no ectopy • norepinephrine • not enlarged • not examined • nursing educator
NEAA	nonessential amino acids
neb	nebulizer
NEC	necrotizing enterocolitis • not elsewhere classified
NED	no evidence of disease • normal equivalent deviation
NEEP	negative end-expiratory pressure
NEF	Nurses Educational Fund
NEFA	nonesterified fatty acid
neg	negative

NEISS	National Electronic Injury Surveillance System
neo	neoarsphenamine
NEP	negative expiratory pressure
NER	nonionizing electromagnetic radiation
nerv	nervous
neuro	neurologic
NF	National Formulary • none found • nonfunction • normal flow
NFCA	National Family Caregivers Association
NFCC	neighborhood family-care center
NFIC	National Foundation for Ileitis and Colitis
NFLPN	National Federation for Licensed Practical Nurses
NFP	natural family planning • not for profit
NFPA	National Fire Protection Association
NFSID	National Foundation for Sudden Infant Death
NFTD	normal, full-term delivery
ng	nanogram
NG	nasogastic • new growth • no good
NGF	nerve growth factor
NGR	narrow gauze roll
NGS	National Geriatrics Society
NGT	nasogastric tube
NGU	nongonococcal urethritis
NH	nodal-His • nodular and histiocytic • nursing home
NH_3	ammonia
NH_4+	ammonium ion
NH_4Cl	ammonium chloride
NHF	National Hemophilia Foundation

NHI	national health insurance • National Heart Institute
NHIF	National Head Injury Foundation
NHL	non-Hodgkin's lymphoma
NHLBI	National Heart, Lung and Blood Institute
NHLI	National Heart and Lung Institute
NHPCO	National Hospice and Palliative Care Organization
NHPP	normal human pooled plasma
NHS	National Health Service Corps
Ni	nickel
NIA	National Institute on Aging • no information available
NIAA	National Institute on Alcohol Abuse and Alcoholism
NIADDK	National Institute of Arthritis, Diabetes and Digestive Kidney Diseases
NIAID	National Institute of Allergy and Infectious Diseases
NIAMD	National Institute of Arthritis and Metabolic Diseases
NIAMS	National Institute of Arthritis and Musculoskeletal and Skin Diseases
NICHE	Nurses Improving Care to the Hospitalized Elderly
NICHHD	National Institute of Child Health and Human Development
NICU	neonatal intensive care unit • newborn intensive care unit
NIDA	National Institute on Drug Abuse
NIDCD	National Institute on Deafness and Other Communication Disorders
NIDDKD	National Institute of Diabetes, Digestive & Kidney Diseases
NIDDM	noninsulin-dependent diabetes mellitus
NIDR	National Institute of Dental Research
NIDRR	National Institute on Disability and Rehabilitation Research
NIEHS	National Institute of Environmental Health Services
NiF	negative inspiratory force

NIGMS	National Institute of General Medical Sciences
NIH	National Institutes of Health
NIHD	noise-induced hearing damage
NIMH	National Institute of Mental Health
NINCDS	National Institute of Neurological and Communicative Disorders and Stroke
NINDB	National Institute of Neurological Diseases and Blindness
NINDS	National Institute of Neurological Diseases and Stroke
NIOSH-CDC	National Institute for Occupational Safety and Health - Centers for Disease Control
NIP	National Inpatient Profile • Nurse Intervention Program
NIRMP	National Interns and Residents Matching Program
NIRR	noninsulin-requiring remission
NIT	nasointestinal tube
nit ox	nitrous oxide
NJPC	National Joint Practice Commission
NK	natural killer (cells)
NKA	no known allergies
NKDA	no known drug allergies
NKF	National Kidney Foundation
nl	nanoliter
NL	normal
NLA	neuroleptanalgesia
NLM	National Library of Medicine
NLN	National League for Nursing
NLP	neurolinguistic program • no light perception
NLT	no later than • no less than
nm	nanometer

NM	neuromuscular • night and morning • nitrogen mustard • nodular and mixed (lymphocytic-histiocytic) • nuclear medicine
NMC	nodular, mixed-cell (lymphoma) • Nurse Managed Center
NMHA	National Mental Health Association
NMI	no middle initial
NMM	nodular malignant melanoma
NMN	nicotinamide mononucleotide • no middle name
nmol	nanomol (nanomole)
NMR	nuclear magnetic resonance
NMRI	Naval Medical Research Institute
NMRS	National Registry of Medical Secretaries
NMS	neuroleptic malignant syndrome
NMSS	National Multiple Sclerosis Society
nn	nerves
NN	nurses' notes
N:N	azo group (chemical group with two nitrogen atoms)
NND	neonatal death • New and Nonofficial Drugs (AMA publication)
NNE	neonatal necrotizing enterocolitis
NNN	Nicolle-Novy-MacNeal (medium)
NNP	neonatal nurse practitioner
NNR	New and Nonofficial Remedies
NNS	non-nutritive sucking
no	number (*numero*)
No	nobelium
NO	nitric oxide • nitroso- • nursing office
N_2O	nitrous oxide
NOA	notice of admission

NOAADN	National Organization for the Advancement of Associate Degree Nursing
noc	night (*nox*)
NOCA	National Organization for Competency Assurance
noct	at night (*nocte*)
noct maneq	at night and in the morning (*nocte maneque*)
NODMAR	Notice of Discharge Medicare Appeal Rights
NODSS	nasal/oral discriminate sampling system
NOFTT	nonorganic failure to thrive
NOMI	nonocclusive mesenteric infarction
NONC	Notice of Non-Coverage
non rep	do not repeat (*non repetatur*)
NOP	National Outpatient Profile
NOPE	notice of possible entitlements
NOPHN	National Organization for Public Health Nursing
norm	normal
normet	normetanephrine
NOS	not otherwise specified
NOTT	nocturnal oxygen therapy trial
Np	neptunium
NP	neuropeptide • neuropsychiatric • not otherwise provided for • nucleoplasmic index • nucleoprotein • nurse-practitioner • nursing procedure
NPA	National Perinatal Association • near point of accommodation • no previous admission
NPC	nasopharyngeal carcinoma • near point of convergence • nodal premature contraction • nonproductive cough • no previous complaint
NPCN	National Poison Center Network
NPD	Niemann-Pick disease • nonprescription drugs
NPDB	National Practitioner Data Bank

NPDR	nonproliferative diabetic retinopathy
NPH	neutral protamine Hagedorn (insulin) • no previous history • normal-pressure hydrocephalus
NPJT	nonparoxysmal junctional tachycardia
NPL	nasopharyngolaryngoscopy
NPN	nonprotein nitrogen
npo	nothing by mouth (*nulla per os*)
npo/hs	nothing by mouth at bedtime (*nulla per os hora somni*)
NPP	non-physician provider • nurse in private practice
NPR	Notice of Program Reimbursement
NPRM	notice of proposed rule-making
NPSG	nocturnal polysomnogram
NPSRC	National Professional Standards Review Council
NPT	normal pressure and temperature • neuro-psychological testing • nocturnal penile tumescence
NQWMI	non-Q wave myocardial infarction
nr	do not repeat (*non repetatur*)
NR	nerve root • neutral red • nonreactive • non-rebreathing • no refill • normal range • normal record
NRB	non-reportable birth
NRBC	nucleated red blood cells
NRC	National Research Council • noise reduction coeffecient • normal retinal correspondence • Nuclear Regulatory Commission
NRC-NAS	National Research Council - National Academy of Sciences
NREM	nonrapid eye movement, non-REM sleep
NRMC	Naval Regional Medical Center
NRMS	National Registry of Medical Secretaries
nRNA	nuclear ribonucleic acid
NRS	normal rabbit serum

ns	nanosecond • no sequelae • nylon suture
NS	nephrotic syndrome • nervous system • neurosurgery, neurosurgical, neurosurgeon • nodular sclerosis • normal saline • normal serum • not significant • not stated • Nursing Services
1/2 NS	half-normal saline
NSA	Neurological Society of America • normal serum albumin • no significant abnormality • nursing service administration
NSABP	National Surgical Adjuvant Breast Project
NSAC	National Society for Autistic Children
NSAIA	nonsteroidal anti-inflammatory analgesic
NSAID	nonsteroidal anti-inflammatory drug
NSC	non service-connected • National Safety Council
NSCC	National Society for Crippled Children
NSCIF	National Spinal Cord Injury Foundation
NSCLC	non-small cell lung cancer
NS/CST	nipple stimulation/contraction stress test
NSD	nitrogen-specific detector • nominal standard dose • normal spontaneous delivery • no significant defect • no significant deficiency
nsec	nanosecond
NSF	National Science Foundation
NSFTD	normal spontaneous full-term delivery
nsg	nursing
NSGCT	nonsiminomatous germ cell tumors
NSHD	nodular sclerosing Hodgkin's disease
NSIDSF	National Sudden Infant Death Syndrome Foundation
NSILA	nonsuppressible insulin-like activity
NSILP	nonsuppressible insulin-like protein
NSNA	National Student Nurses' Association
NSP	not specified

NSPB	National Society for the Prevention of Blindness
NSR	normal sinus rhythm
NSS	normal saline solution • nutritional support services
NSST	Northwestern Syntax Screening Test
NST	nasotracheal • nonstress test • not sooner than • nutrition support team
NSU	nonspecific urethritis
NSVD	normal spontaneous vaginal delivery
nsy	nursery
NT	nasotracheal • neutralization test • not tested
N&T	nose and throat
NTA	Narcotics Treatment Administration • National Tuberculosis Association
N/TBC	nontuberculosis
NTBR	not to be resuscitated
NTD	neural tube defect
NTG	nitroglycerin
NTM	non-TB mycobacterium
NTMI	nontransmural myocardial infarction
NTP	nitropaste • normal temperature and pressure
NTV	nervous tissue vaccine
nU	nanounit
nuc	nucleated
nucl	nuclear
NUD	nonulcer dyspepsia
NUG	necrotizing ulcerative gingivitis
Nullip	nulliparous
num	numerator
NUN	non-urea nitrogen

NV	naked vision • near vision • next visit • nonvaccinated • nonvenereal • non-volatile
N&V	nausea and vomiting
NVD	nausea, vomiting, diarrhea • neck-venous distention • nonvalvular (heart) disease • no venous distention
NVWSC	nonvolatile whole-smoke condensate
NW	naked weight
NWB	nonweight-bearing
NWHRC	National Women's Health Resource Center
NYD	not yet diagnosed
NYHA	New York Heart Association (classification)
NYP	not yet published
nyst	nystagmus
NZB	New Zealand black (mouse)
NZW	New Zealand white (mouse)

O

o	ortho
O	doctor's office • eye (*oculus*) • none • occiput, occipital • oral, orally • orthopedic • other • output • oxygen • pint (*octarius*) • orthotics
O	without
O$_2$	both eyes • oxygen
O$_3$	ozone
OA	occiput anterior • ocular albinism • old age • orotic acid • osteoarthritis • oxalic acid • oxaloacetic acid
OAA	Old Age Assistance • oxaloacetic acid
OAAD	ovarian ascorbic acid depletion (test)
OAE	otoacoustic emissions test
OAF	open air factor • osteoclast-activating factor • osteocyte-activating factor

OALF	organic acid-labile fluoride
OAP	ophthalmic artery pressure
OASDHI	Old Age-Survivors Disability and Health Insurance
OASI	Old Age and Survivors Insurance
OASP	organic acid-soluble phosphorus
OAVD	oculoauriculovertebral dysplasia
OB	obstetric(s), obstetrician • occult blood
OBAE	Office of Benefit Assistance and Enforcement
OBD	Office of Benefit Determination
OBG	obstetrician-gynecologist • obstetrics and gynecology
OB/GYN	obstetrician-gynecologist • obstetrics and gynecology
obl	oblique
OBRA	Omnibus Budget Reconciliation Act of 1993
OBS	organic brain syndrome
obsd	observed
obst	obstetric(s), obstetrician • obstruction
OC	occlusocervical • office call • only child • oral contraceptive • oxygen consumed
O&C	onset and course
OCA	oral contraceptive agent
O_2Cap	oxygen capacity
occ	occasional • occiput, occipital
occas	occasional, occasionally
OCD	obsessive-compulsive disorder • ovarian cholesterol depletion
OCE	other controllable expenses
OCG	oral cholecystogram
OCN	Oncology Certified Nurse
O_2Con	oxygen concentration • oxygen content

OCP	oral contraceptive pills • ova, cysts and parasites
OCT	oral contraceptive therapy • ornithine carbamoyltransferase • oxytocin challenge test
O_2CT	oxygen content
OCU	observation care unit • outpatient care unit
OCV	ordinary conversational voice
od	every day (*omni die*)
OD	Doctor of Optometry • occupational disease • Officer of the Day • once daily • open drop • optical density • outside diameter • overdose • right eye (*oculus dexter*)
ODA	right occipitoanterior (*occipitodextra anterior*)
ODC	oxygen dissociation curve • oxyhemoglobin dissociation curve
ODD	oculodentodigital dysplasia • oppositional defiant disorder
ODP	right occipitoposterior (*occipitodextra posterior*)
ODT	right occipitotransverse (*occipitodextra transversa*)
OE	on examination • otitis externa • Overeaters Anonymous
OEE	outer enamel epithelium
O&E	observation and examination
O/E	ratio of observed to expected
OEM	open-end marriage
OEO	Office of Economic Opportunity
OER	oxygen-enhancement ratio
OERR	order entry and results reporting
OF	occipitofrontal • other facility
OFD	object-to-film distance • occipitofrontal diameter • oral-facial-digital (syndrome)
off	official
OFS	Office of Medical Fee Schedule
OFTT	organic failure to thrive

OG	orogastric
OGA	orogastric aspirate
OGTT	oral glucose tolerance test
oh	every hour (*omni hora*)
OH	hydroxyl group • occupational health • open-heart • orthostatic hypotension • out-patient hospital
OHA	oral hypoglycemic agents
OHC	outer hair cell
OH-cbl	hydroxocobalamin
OHCS	hydroxycorticosteroid
OHD	organic heart disease
OHF	Omsk hemorrhagic fever • overhead frame
OHFA	hydroxy fatty acids
OHI	ocular hypertension indicator
ohm-cm	ohm-centimeter
OHP	hydroxyproline • oxygen under high pressure
OHS	occupational health service • open-heart surgery
OHT	over-head trapeze
OI	opportunistic infection • opsonic index • osteogenesis imperfecta • oxygen intake
OIC	osteogenesis imperfecta congenita
OIG	Office of the Inspector General
OIH	ortho-iodohippurate • ovulation-inducing hormone
oint	ointment
OIP	occupational injury program
OJ	orange juice
OJT	on-the-job training
OKN	optokinetic nystagmus
Ol	oil

OL	left eye (*oculus laevus*)
OLA	left occipitoanterior (*occipitolaeva anterior*)
OLB	open lung biopsy
Ol oliv	olive oil (*oleum olivae*)
OLP	left occipitoposterior (*occipitolaeva posterior*)
OLT	left occipitotransverse (*occipitolaeva transversa*) • orthotopic liver transplantation
om	every morning (*omni mane*)
OM	occipitomental (diameter of head) • Occupational Medicine • osteomyelitis • otitis media
OMA	Office of Medical Affairs
OMB	Office of Management and Budget
OME	otitis media with effusion
OML	orbitomeatal line
omn bih	every two hours (*omni bihora*)
omn hor	every hour (*omni hora*)
omn noct	every night (*omni nocte*)
OMPA	octamethyl pyrophosphoramide
OMVI	operating a motor vehicle intoxicated
on	every night (*omni nocte*)
ON	optic neuritis
onco	oncology
OND	other neurological disease
ONP	operating nursing procedure
OOA	out-of-area
OOB	out of bed
OOF	owned and operated facility
OOLR	ophthalmology, otology, laryngology, and rhinology
OOT	out of town

OP	occipitoparietal • occipitoposterior • opening pressure • operative procedure • orthopedic condition • osmotic pressure • outpatient
O&P	ova and parasites
OPA	organ procurement agency
OPB	outpatient basis
OPC	outpatient clinic
op cit	in the work cited (*opere citato*)
OPD	optical path difference • outpatient department • outpatient dispensary
opg	opening
OPG	oculoplethysmography
Oph	ophthalmology • ophthalmoscope
Ophth	ophthalmology • ophthalmoscope
OpMi	operating microscope
OPO	organ procurement organization
opp	opposite • opposed
OPRT	orotate phosphoribosyltransferase
OPS	outpatient section • outpatient service • outpatient surgery
OPSC	outpatient surgery center
OPSR	Office of Professional Standards Review
opt	optical, optician, optics • optimal
OPT	outpatient
OPV	oral poliovirus vaccine
OQS	Office of Quality Standards
o/r	oxidation/reduction
OR	occupancy rate • oil retention enema • operating room • organ recovery • orienting reflex
O-R	oxidation-reduction

ORC	order/results/communication • oxidized regenerated cellulose
ord	orderly • ordinate
ORD	optical rotatory dispersion
OREF	open reduction external fixation
OR en	oil retention enema
org	organic • organism
ORG	optimal recovery guidelines
ORH	Office of Rural Health
ORIF	open reduction internal fixation
orig	origin, original
ORL	otorhinolaryngology
ORN	Operating Room Nurse
ORS	Orthopedic Research Society • orthopedic surgery
ORT	operating room technician • orthopedics
orth	orthopedics
ortho	orthopedics
ORx	oriented
os	mouth (*os*)
Os	osmium
OS	left eye (*oculus sinister*) • Osgood-Schlatter's disease • osteogenic sarcoma
OSA	obstructive sleep apnea
OSAS	obstructive sleep apnea syndrome
O_2Sat	oxygen saturation
osc	oscillate
OSC	Organized System of Care
OSD	overside drainage
OSHA	Occupational Safety and Health Administration

osm	osmol
OSMF	oral submucous fibrosis
OST	Office of Science and Technology
osteo	osteomyelitis
OT	objective test • occipitotransverse • occupational therapist, occupational therapy • old terminology • old tuberculin • oral thrush • orotracheal • otolaryngology, otolaryngologist
OTA	Office of Technology Assessment
OTC	ornithine transcarbamylase • over-the-counter • oxytetracycline
OTCD	over-the-counter drug
OTCRx	over-the-counter drug
OTD	organ tolerance dose
oto	otology, otologist
otol	otology, otologist
OTR	Registered Occupational Therapist
OTSG	Office of the Surgeon General
OU	both eyes (*oculi unitas*) • each eye (*oculus uterque*) • observation unit
ov	egg (*ovum*) • ovary
OV	obvious • office visit
OVD	occlusal vertical dimension
OW	out-of-wedlock
O/W	oil in water
OWCP	Office of Workers' Compensation Program
oxidn	oxidation
OXT	oxytocin
oz	ounce (*onza*)
oz. ap.	ounces apothecary's
oz. av.	ounces avoirdupois

P

p	after (*post*) • by weight (*pondere*) • handful (*pugillus*) • near (*proximum*) • papilla • para- • partial pressure • pico- • probable error • pupil
P	by weight (*pondere*) • para- • parenteral • part • partial pressure • pharmacopeia • phenolphthalein • phosphorus • pico- • pint • plasma • pole • population • position • positive • posterior • postpartum • presbyopia • pressure • probable error • protein • psoralen • psychiatrist, psychiatry • pulse • pupil
p	after (*post*) • mean pressure (gas)
P_1	first parental generation • pulmonic first sound
P_2	pulmonic second sound
^{32}P	radioactive phosphorus • radiophosphorus
Pa	Pascal (unit of pressure) • protactinium
PA	panic attack • paralysis agitans • parietal cell antibody • pathology • permeability area • pernicious anemia • phosphoarginine • physician advisor • physician's assistant • plasminogen activator • posteroanterior • primary amenorrhea • primary anemia • procainamide • professional association • protrusio acetabuli • psychoanalysis, psychoanalyst • pulmonary artery • pulpoaxial
P&A	percussion and auscultation
PAB	para-aminobenzoic (acid) • peripheral androgen blockade • premature atrial beat
PABA	para-aminobenzoic acid
PAC	papular acrodermatitis of childhood • parent-adult-child • phenacetin, aspirin, caffeine • pre-admission certification • premature atrial contraction
PACE	performance and cost efficiency • program of all-inclusive care for the elderly
$PaCO_2$	arterial carbon dioxide partial pressure • partial pressure of carbon dioxide
$PACO_2$	alveolar carbon dioxide partial pressure
PACU	Post-Anesthesia Care Unit

PAD	per adjusted discharge • phenacetin, aspirin, desocyephedrine • peripheral artery disease
p ae	in equal parts (*partes aequales*)
PAEDP	pulmonary artery end-diastolic pressure
PAF	platelet-activating factor • platelet-aggregating factor • pulmonary arteriovenous fistula
PAFS	periarticular fiber system
PAGE	polyacrylamide gel electrophoresis
PAH	para-aminohippuric (acid)
PAHA	para-aminohippuric acid
PAHM	Professional Academy for Healthcare Management
PAI	plasminogen activator inhibitor
PAIg	platelet-associated immunoglobulin
PAL	pediatric advanced life support • posterior axillary line
palp	palpable
PALS	periarteriolar lymphocyte sheaths
PA-LS-ID	pernicious anemia-like syndrome and immunoglobulin deficiency
Palv	alveolar pressure
PAM	crystalline penicillin G in aluminum monostearate • phenylalanine mustard • pralidoxime • pulmonary alveolar microlithiasis
PAMP	pulmonary artery mean pressure
PAN	perarteritis nodosa • peroxyacetyl nitrate • polyarteritis nodosa • pancreat, pancreatic
PAO	patient assessment office • peak acid output • psychiatric admitting office
PaO_2	arterial oxygen partial pressure • partial pressure of oxygen
PAO_2	alveolar oxygen partial pressure • oxygen content of pulmonary artery blood
PAOP	pulmonary artery occlusion pressure

pap	papilla
Pap	Papanicolaou (smear, stain, test)
PAP	patient assessment procedure • peroxidase- antiperoxidase (method) • primary atypical pneumonia • private ambulatory patient • prostatic acid phosphatase • pulmonary alveolar proteinosis • pulmonary artery pressure
par	parallel
PAr	polyarteritis
PAR	postanesthesia recovery • postanesthesia room • problem-analysis report
para	a woman who has given birth • number of pregnancies producing viable offspring: para-0, para-I, para-II, etc.
paradox	paradoxical
par aff	part affected
PARP	poly-ADP-ribose polymerase
PARS	Personal Adjustment and Role Skills Scale
part aeq	in equal parts (*partes aequales*)
part vic	in divided doses (*partitis vicibus*)
PARU	postanesthesia recovery unit
Pas	pascal (unit of pressure)
PAS	para-aminosalicylic (acid) • patient appointment and scheduling • performance appraisal system • periodic acid-Schiff (method, reaction, stain, technique, test) • pre-admission screening • pregnancy advisory service • professional activities study • physician-assisted suicide
PASA	para-aminosalicylic acid
PAS-C	para-aminosalicylic acid crystallized with ascorbic acid
PASG	pneumatic anti-shock garment
PASP	pulmonary artery systolic pressure
Past	*Pasteurella*
pat	patent • patient

PAT	paroxysmal atrial tachycardia • pre-admission testing • pregnancy at term
path	pathologist, pathology, pathologic
PATH	Partnership Approach to Health
PAVe	procarbazine, melphalen, vinblastine
PAWP	pulmonary artery wedge pressure
Pb	lead (*plumbum*) • presbyopia
PB	Paul-Bunnell (antibodies test) • peripheral blood • Pharmacopoeia Britannica • phonetically balanced • pinch biopsy • pressure breathing
PBA	percutaneous bladder aspiration
PBB	polybrominated biphenyl
PBC	point of basal convergence • primary biliary cirrhosis
PBCTN	percutaneous balloon compression of the trigeminal nerve
PBE	a form of tuberculin (*Perlsucht bacillen emulsion*)
PBG	porphobilinogen
PBI	protein-bound iodine
PBL	peripheral-blood lymphocytes
PBP	porphyrin biosynthetic pathway • progressive bulbar palsy
PBS	peripheral-blood smear • phosphate-buffered saline • polybrominated salicylanilides
PBSC	peripheral blood stem cell
PBSCT	peripheral-blood stem cell transplantation
PBV	pulmonary blood volume
PBW	posterior bite wing
PBZ	Pyribenzamine
pc	after meals (*post cibos*) • per cent • picocurie

PC	avoirdupois weight (*pondus civile*) • packed cells • parent cell • parent to child • personal computer • phosphatidylcholine • phosphocreatine • platelet concentrate • platelet count • pneumotoxic center • presenting complaint • professional corporation • pubococcygeus • pulmonary capillary
PCA	patient controlled analgesia • passive cutaneous anaphylaxis • personal care attendant
PCAST	President's Committee of Advisors on Science and Technology
Pcb	near point of convergence to the intercentral baseline
PCB	paracervical block
PCBs	polychlorinated biphenyls
PCc	periscopic concave
PCC	patient-care coordinator • pheochromocytoma • phosphate-carrier compound • Poison Control Center
PCCM	Primary Care Case Managers
PCD	polycystic disease
PCE	physical capacities evaluation
PCF	Patient Compensation Fund • pharyngoconjunctival fever • prothrombin conversion factor
PCG	phonocardiogram, phonocardiography • primary care giver
PCH	paroxysmal cold hemoglobinuria
PCi	picocurie
PCI	pneumatosis cystoides intestinorum
PCK	polycystic kidney (disease)
PCL	posterior cruciate ligament
PCLN	psychiatric consultation liaison nurse
PCM	patient case manager • protein-calorie malnutrition
PCMR	President's Committee on Mental Retardation
PCN	penicillin • primary care network, nurse
PCNG	penicillin-G

PCNL	percutaneous nephrostolithotomy
PCO	patient complains of • polycystic ovary
PCOS	polycystic ovarian syndrome
pCO_2	partial pressure of carbon dioxide
PCO_2	partial pressure of carbon dioxide
PCP	peripheral coronary pressure • phenylcyclidine (hallucinogenic drug) • *Pneumocystis carinii* pneumonia • Primary Care Physician • Psilcybin
PCPA	para-chlorophenylalanine
pcpt	perception
PCr	phosphocreatine
PCR	polymerase chain reaction • probable cause relationship
pcs	preconscious
PCS	patient-care standards • patient-care systems • patient classification system • primary C-section • perimortem cesarean section
PCT	plasmacrit test • porcine calcitonin • porphyria cutanea tarda • prothrombin consumption test • proximal convoluted tubule
PCU	patient care unit (of cost) • progressive care unit
p cut	percutaneous
PCV	packed-cell volume • parietal-cell vagotomy • polycythemia vera
PCW	pulmonary capillary wedge
PCWP	pulmonary capillary wedge pressure
PCx	periscopic convex
PCXR	portable chest x-ray
pd	papilla diameter • prism diopter • pupillary distance

PD	Doctor of Pharmacy • interpupillary distance • paralyzing dose • Parkinsonian dementia • Parkinsons' disease • pediatrics • peritoneal dialysis • postural drainage • potential difference • pressor dose • prism diopter • provocation dose • psychotic dementia • psychotic depression • pulmonary disease
PD_{50}	median paralyzing dose
PDA	patent ductus arteriosus • pediatric allergy • permanent disability advance • personal digital assistant • posterior descending (coronary) artery
PDB	para-dichlorobenzene
PDC	pediatric cardiology • physical dependence capacity • private diagnostic clinic • pulmonary diffusion capacity
PDD	pervasive developmental disorder
PDE	paroxysmal dyspnea on exertion • prenatally drug exposed
PDF	probability density function
PDGF	platelet-derived growth factor
PDH	packaged disaster hospital • past dental history
PDLL	poorly differentiated lymphocytic lymphoma
PDM	polymyositis and dermatomyositis
PDN	private duty nurse
PDPP	pre-deductible payment percentage
PDQ	Prescreening Development Questionnaire
pdr	powder
PDR	Physicians' Desk Reference
PDS	pain dysfunction syndrome • polydiaxone sutures
PDT	phenyldimethyltriazine • photodynamic therapy
PDW	platelet distribution width
Pe	perylene • pressure on expiration

PE	paper electrophoresis • pharyngoesophageal • phenylephrine • phosphatidylethanolamine • physical examination • physical exercise • plasma exchange • polyethylene • probable error • pulmonary embolism
PEA	pulseless electrical activity
PEC	patient education coordinator • peritoneal exudate cells
Pecho	prostatic echogram
PED	pediatrics, pediatrician
Peds	pediatrics
PEEP	positive end-expiratory pressure • protein electrophoresis
PEF	peak expiratory flow
PEFR	peak expiratory flow rate
PEFV	partial expiratory flow volume
PEG	percutaneous endoscopic gastrostomy • pneumoencephalogram, pneumoencephalography • polyethylene glycol
PEI	phosphorous excretion index
Pel	elastic recoil pressure of lung
PEL	permissible exposure limits
PEM	protein-energy malnutrition
PEMA	phenylethylmalonamide
pen	penetrating • penicillin
PEN	parenteral and enteral nutrition • professional excellence in nursing
PENG	photoelectric nystagmography
Pent	Pentothal
PEP	Performance Evaluation Procedure • phosphoenolpyruvate • polyestradiol phosphate • pre-ejection period • pre-ejection phase
PEP/LVET	pre-ejection period/left ventricular ejection time
PEPR	precision encoder and pattern recognizer

per	periodic • person • through, by (*per*)
PER	pediatric emergency room
perf	perforation, perforating
perim	perimeter
periph	peripheral
PERL	pupils equal and react to light
perm	permanent
perp	perpendicular
PERRLA	pupils equal, round, react to light and accommodation
pers	personal
PERS	Personal Emergency Response System
PERT	Program Evaluation Review Technique
pes	foot (*pes*)
PET	positron emission tomography • pre-eclamptic toxemia • Psychiatric Emergency Team
PETN	pentaerythritol tetranitrate
PETT	positron emission transaxial tomography
pev	peak electron-volts
peV	peak electron-volts
pf	power factor
Pf	permeability factor
PF	physicians' forum • platelet factor • precursor fluid
PFC	persistent fetal circulation • plaque-forming cells
PFFD	proximal femur focal deficiency
PFG	peak-flow gauge
PFK	phosphofructokinase
PFM	peak flowmeter
PFO	patent foramen ovale

PFR	peak flow rate • pericardial friction rub
PFT	pulmonary function test
PFU	plaque-forming unit
pg	picogram
Pg	pregnant
PG	paregoric • pepsinogen • phosphatidylglycerol • pituitary gonadotropin • plasma gastrin • postgraduate • prostaglandin
2-PG	2-phosphoglycerate
3-PG	3-phosphoglycerate
PGA	pteroylglumatic acid
PG-AC	phenylglycine acid chloride
PGB	prostaglandin B
PGE_2	prostaglandin E2
PGF	paternal grandfather
$PGF_2\alpha$	prostaglandin $F_{2\alpha}$
PGH	pituitary growth hormone • plasma growth hormone
PGI_2	prostacyclin (prostaglandin I2)
PGM	paternal grandmother
PGO	pontogeniculo-occipital
PGR	psychogalvanic response • percutaneous glycerol rhizotomy
PGU	postgonococcal urethritis
PGY	postgraduate year
ph	phase
pH	measure of hydrogen ion concentration (degrees of alkalinity or acidity)
Ph	pharmacopoeia • phenanthrene • phenyl • Philadelphia chromosome • phosphate
Ph[1]	Philadelphia chromosome

PH	past history • perianal herpes simplex virus infection • personal history • Pharmaceutical Services • pinhole • previous history • public health • pulmonary hypertension
PHA	passive hemagglutination • phenylalanine • phytohemagglutinin
pahr	pharmacy, pharmaceutical, pharmacist, pharmacopeia
pharm	pharmacy, pharmaceutical, pharmacist, pharmacopeia
pharmacol	pharmacologic
Pharm B	Bachelor of Pharmacy (*Pharmaciae Baccalaureus*)
Pharm C	Pharmaceutical Chemist
Pharm D	Doctor of Pharmacy (*Pharmaciae Doctor*)
Pharm G	Graduate in Pharmacy
Pharm M	Master of Pharmacy (*Pharmaciae Magister*)
Ph B	Pharmacopoeia Britannica
PHC	post-hospital care • premolar aplasia, hyperhydrosis and premature cavities • primary hepatocellular carcinoma
PHCC	Prehospital Care Coordinator
PhD	doctoral degree (Doctor of Philosophy)
PHDD	personal history of depressive disorders
Phe	phenylalanine
PHE	periodic health examination
PHF	paired helical filaments
PhG	German Pharmacopeia • Graduate in Pharmacy
pHi	gastric intramural pH
PHI	protected health information
phial	bottle (*phiala*)
PHKC	postmortem human kidney cells
PHLA	post-heparin lipolytic activity
PHN	public health nurse • public health nursing

PHO	physician-hospital organization
phos	phosphatase • phosphate
PHP	phosphorus • prepaid health plan • pseudohypoparathyroidism
PHPPD	productive hours per patient day
PHS	Public Health Service
PHT	peroxide hemolysis test • phenytoin
PHTN	portal hypertension
phy	phytohemagglutinin
phys	physical • physician
physio	physiologic
Pi.	pressure of inspiration
PI	parainfluenza (virus) • paternity index • performance indicator • present illness • pressure on inspiration • protamine insulin • protease inhibitor
PICC	peripherally inserted central catheter
PICU	pediatric intensive care unit • pulmonary intensive care unit
PID	pelvic inflammatory disease • prolapsed intervertebral disc
PIE	pulmonary infiltration with eosinophilia • pulmonary interstitial emphysema
PIF	peak inspiratory flow • prolactin-inhibiting (inhibitory) factor • proliferation inhibitory factor
PIFR	peak inspiratory flow rate
PIGPA	pyruvate, inosine, glucose, phosphate, adenine
PIH	pregnancy-induced hypertension
pil	pill (*pilula*)
PIN	personal identification number
PINS	person in need of supervision
PINV	post-imperative negativity (reaction)

PIP	peak inspiratory pressure • periodic interim payment • personal injury protection • proximal interphalangeal
PI-PB	performance versus intensity function for phonetically balanced words
pit	pituitary
PIT	plasma iron turnover
PITR	plasma iron turnover rate
PIV	parainfluenza virus
PIVKA	protein in vitamin K absence
PJC	premature junctional contraction
PJRT	permanent junctional reciprocating tachycardia
PJS	Peutz-Jeghers syndrome
PJT	paroxysmal junctional tachycardia
PJVT	paroxysmal junctional-ventricular tachycardia
pK	dissociation constant
PK	Prausnitz-Küstner (reaction) • psychokineses • pyruvate kinase
pKa	measure of acid strength
PKD	polycystic kidney disease
PKF	phagocytosis and killing function
PKS	pharmacokinetic service
PKU	phenylketonuria
Pl	plasma
PL	perception of light • phospholipid • platelet
P_L	transpulmonary pressure
PLA	peroxidase-labeled antibodies (test) • pulpolinguoaxial
Plat	platelet
PLDH	plasma lactic dehydrogenase
PLE	polymorphous light eruption

PLED	periodic lateralized epileptiform discharge
PLG	plasminogen
PLIF	posterolumbar interbody fusion
PLISSIT	Permission, Limited Information, Specific Suggestions, Intensive Therapy
PLL	prolymphocytic leukemia
PLM	polarized-light microscope
PLN	posterior lymph node
PLS	primary lateral sclerosis
PLT	platelet • psittascosis-lymphogranuloma venereum-trachoma • primed lymphocyte typing
plx	plexus
pm	after noon (*post meridiem*) • picometer
pM	picomolar
Pm	promethium
PM	after noon (*post meridiem*) • pacemaker • peritoneal macrophage • petit mal (epilepsy) • physical medicine • pneumo-mediastinum • polymyositis • postmortem • presystolic murmur • preventive medicine • pulpomesial • purple membrane • pain management
P/M	parent-metabolite ratio
PMA	papillary, marginal, attached • paramethoxyamphetamine (hallucinogenic drug) • Primary Mental Abilities (test) • progressive muscular atrophy
PMB	polymorphonuclear basophilic (leukocytes) • postmenopausal bleeding
PMC	Patient Management Categories • pseudomembranous colitis
PMD	private medical doctor
PME	polymorphonuclear eosinophilic (leukocyte)
PMF	progressive massive fibrosis
PMH	past medical history • public mental hospital

PMI	past medical illness • patient medication instruction (sheets) • point of maximum (maximal) impulse • point of maximum (maximal) intensity • previous medical illness
PML	progressive multifocal leukoencephalopathy
PMLE	polymorphous light eruption
PMM	pentamethylmelamine
PMMA	polymethyl methacrylate
PMN	polymorphonuclear neutrophilic (leukocytes) • polymorphonuclear neutrophils
PMNR	periadenitis mucosa necrotica recurrens
PMP	previous menstrual period • pain management program
PMPM	per member per month
PMR	physical medicine and rehabilitation • polymyalgia rheumatica • proportionate mortality ratio • proton magnetic resonance
PM&R	physical medicine and rehabilitation
PMS	postmenopausal syndrome • pregnant mare serum • premenstrual syndrome
PMSG	pregnant mare serum gonadotropin
PMT	premenstrual tension • pelvic muscle training
PMVL	posterior mitral-valve leaflet
PN	parenteral nutrition • percussion note • periarteritis nodosa • peripheral nerve • peripheral neuropathy • plaque neutralizing • practical nurse • progress note • psychiatry-neurology • psychoneurology • psychoneurotic, psychoneurosis • pulmonary disease
P&N	psychiatry and neurology
PNA	pentosenucleic acid • peptide nucleic acid
PNC	penicillin • peripheral nucleated cell • premature nodal contraction
PNCM	professional nurse case manager
PND	paroxysmal nocturnal dyspnea • postnasal drip
PNET	peripheral neuroectodermal tumor

PNF	proprioceptive neuromuscular facilitation
PNH	paroxysmal nocturnal hemoglobinuria
PNI	peripheral nerve injury • postnatal infection • psychoneuroimmunology
PNMT	phenylethanolamine N-methyltransferase
PNP	paranitriphenol • pediatric nurse practitioner • platelet neutralization procedure • psychogenic nocturnal polydipsia
PNPR	positive-negative pressure respiration
PNRS	premature nursery
PNS	parasympathetic nervous system • peripheral nervous system • peripheral nerve stimulation
PNT	percutaneous nephrostomy tube
Pnx	pneumothorax
po	by mouth (*per os*)
pO_2	partial pressure of oxygen
Po	ponomium
PO	parieto-occipital • phone order • postoperative • predominating organism
P & O	prosthetics and orthotics
PO_2	partial pressure of oxygen
PO_4	phosphate
POA	pancreatic oncofetal antigen • primary optic atrophy
POB	penicillin in oil and beeswax • place of birth
POC	post-operative care • products of conception
pocul	cup (*poculum*)
POD	place of death • postoperative day • post-ovulatory day
Pod D	Doctor of Podiatry
PODx	pre-operative diagnosis
POF	pyruvate oxidation factor

pois	poison
polio	poliomyelitis
POLY	polymorphonuclear leukocyte
POMC	pro-opiomelanocortin
POMP	purinethol, Oncovin, methotrexate, prednisone
POMR	problem-oriented medical record
pop	popliteal
POP	2,5-diphenyloxazole • plasma osmotic pressure • Plaster of Paris • postoperative
POPOP	1,4-bis-(5-phenoxazole) benzene
POR	problem-oriented record
PORR	postoperative recovery room
pos	position • positive
POS	Point of Service (health insurance plan)
POSC	problem-oriented system of charting
POSM	patient-operated selector of mechanism
poss	possible
post	posterior • postmortem
POST	posterior
postgangl	postganglionic
post-op	postoperative
pot	potassium • potion
PotAGT	potential abnormality of glucose tolerance
poten	potential
POU	placenta, ovary, uterus
POW	prisoner of war
pp	polyphosphate • private patient

PP	near point of accomodation (*punctum proximum*) • partial pressure • pellagra preventive • Planned Parenthood • posterior pituitary • postpartum • postprandial • Preferred Provider • private patient • private practice • protoporphyrin • pulse pressure • pyrophosphate • placenta previa
P&P	prothrombin and proconvertin
ppa	after shaking the bottle (*phiala prius agitate*)
PPA	Planned Parenthood Association • Pittsburgh pneumonia agent • post-pill amenorrhea • preferred provider agreement • prudent purchase arrangement
ppb	parts per billion
PPB	positive-pressure breathing
PPBS	postprandial blood sugar
PPC	pooled platelet concentrate • progressive patient care
PPD	percussion and postural drainage • permanent partial disability • per patient day • postprandial • prepaid • purified protein derivative (tuberculin) • post-partum depression
PPD-B	purified protein derivative—Battey
PPD-S	purified protein derivative—standard
PPE	partial plasma exchange • personal protective equipment
PPEC	prescribed pediatric extended care
PPF	pellagra-preventive factor • phagocytosis-promoting factor • plasma protein fraction • purified protein fraction
ppg	picopicogram
PPG	photoplethysmograph, photoplethysmography • physician practice group
PPH	persistent pulmonary hypertension • postpartum hemorrhage • primary pulmonary hypertension
PPHx	previous psychiatric history
PPI	patient package insert • Plan Position Indication • proton pump inhibitors
Ppl	pleural pressure

PPLO	pleuropneumonia-like organism
ppm	parts per million • pulses per minute
PPM	permanent pacemaker
PPMM	postpolycythemia myeloid metaplasia
PPNG	penicillinase-producing *Neisseria gonorrhoeae*
PPO	pleuropneumonia organisms • preferred provider organization
PPP	pentose phosphate pathway • platelet-poor plasma • post-partum psychosis
PPPPP	pain, pallor, pulse loss, paresthesia, paralysis
PPR	Price's precipitation reaction
PPS	post-partum sterilization • prospective payment system • prospective pricing system • protein plasma substitute • post-polio syndrome
PPSH	pseudodovaginal peritoneoscrotal hypospadias
ppt	precipitate
PPT	partial prothrombin time
pptd	precipitated
PPTL	post-partum tubal ligation
pptn	precipitation
PPVT	Peabody Picture Vocabulary Test
PQ	permeability quotient • Physician's Questionnaire
pr	pair • per rectum
Pr	praseodymium • presbyopia • prism
PR	far point of accomodation (*punctum remotum*) • partial remission • partial response • peer review • percentile rank • peripheral resistance • phenol red • physician reviewer • pityriasis rosea • pressoreceptor • proctologist • progesterone receptor • public relations • pulmonary rehabilitation • pulse rate
PRA	plasma renin activity
PRAC	practical • practice

PRAS	prereduced, anaerobically sterilized
PRBC	packed red blood cells
PRC	peer review committee • plasma renin concentration
PRD	paired domain • partial reaction of degeneration
PRE	physical reconditioning exercise • progressive resistive exercise
precip	precipitation
pref	preference
preg	pregnancy, pregnant
PREG	pregnenolone
pregn	pregnancy, pregnant
prelim	preliminary
pre-op	preoperative
prep	preparation, prepare
prev	prevention, preventive • previous
PrevAGT	previous abnormality of glucose tolerance
PRF	progressive renal failure • prolactin-releasing factor
PRFA	plasma-recognition-factor activity
PRH	prolactin-releasing hormone
PRICE	Protection, Rest, Ice, Compression, Elevation
primip	primipara
PRIST	paper radioimmunosorbent test
priv	private
PRK	photorefractive keratectomy
PRL	prolactin
prn	as needed (*pro re nata*)
PRN	pain resource nurse
pro	protein

Pro	proline
PRO	peer review organization • professional review organization • prolapse
prob	probable, probability • problem
proc	procedure
proct	proctology, proctologist
prod	produce, produced, product, production
PROEF	post-operative regimen for early oral feeding
prof	profession, professional • professor
prog	prognosis
PROG	progesterone
progn	prognosis
progr	progress
PROM	passive range of motion • premature rupture of membranes • prolonged rupture of membranes
PROPAC	Prospective Payment Assessment Commission
prostat	prostatic
pro Time	prothrombin time
PROWOA	Personal Responsibility and Work Opportunity Act of 1996
prox	proximal
prox luc	the day before (*proxima luce*)
PRP	platelet-rich plasma • polyribose ribitol phosphate • pressure-rate product
PRPP	phosphoribosylpyrophosphate
PRRB	Provider Reimbursement Review Board
PRT	phosphoribosyltransferase • photoradiation therapy
PRTase	phosphoribosyltransferase
PRU	peripheral resistance unit
PRVR	peak-to-resting-velocity ratio

ps	per second • picosecond
Ps	prescription • *Pseudomonas*
PS	chloropicrin • paradoxical sleep • paraseptal • pathologic stage • phosphatidylserine • physical status • plastic surgery • pregnancy serum • programmed symbols • pulmonary stenosis • pyloric stenosis
P/S	ratio of polyunsaturated to saturated fat
P&S	paracentesis and suction • permanent and stationary
PsA	psoriatic arthritis
PSA	prostate-specific antigen
PSAGN	poststreptococcal acute glomerulonephritis
PsAn	psychoanalysis, psychoanalyst
PSAP	prostate-specific acid phosphatase
PSBO	partial small bowel obstruction
PSC	posterior subcapsular cataract • primary sclerosing cholangitis
PSD	peptone-starch-dextrose (agar) • posterior sagittal diameter
PSDA	Patient Self-Determination Act
PSE	partial systemic encephalopathy • point of subjective equality
PSG	pilot study group
PSGN	poststreptococcal glomerulonephritis
PSH	postspinal headache
psi	pounds per square inch
PSI	personnel security index • posterior sagittal index
psia	pounds per square inch absolute
psig	pounds per square inch gauge
PSIS	posterior superior iliac spine
PSL	potassium, sodium chloride, sodium lactate (solution)
PSLT	Picture-Story Language Test

PSM	presystolic murmur
PSMA	progressive spinal muscular atrophy
PSMF	protein-sparing modified fast
PSO	provider-sponsored organization
PSP	phenolsulfonphthalein • progressive supra-nuclear palsy
PSR	problem status report • percutaneous stereotactic radiofrequency thermal rhizotomy
PSRBOW	premature spontaneous rupture of bag of waters
PSRO	professional standards review organization
PSS	physiologic saline solution • progressive systemic sclerosis (systemic scleroderma)
PST	pancreatic suppression test • paroxysmal supraventricular tachycardia • penicillin, strepomycin, tetracycline
PSTF	preventive services task force
PSVER	pattern-shift visual evoked response
PSVT	paroxysmal supraventricular tachycardia
PSW	psychiatric social worker
psy	psychiatry, psychology
psych	psychiatry, psychology
pt	part • patient • pint • point
Pt	platinum
PT	physical therapist, physical therapy • posterior tibial (pulse) • prothrombin time
PTA	percutaneous transluminal angioplasty • Physical Therapy Assistant • plasma thromboplastin antecedent • post-traumatic amnesia • prior to admission
PTAF	policy target adjustment factor
P-TAG	target-attaching globulin precursor
PTAP	purified diphtheria toxoid—alum precipitated
PTB	patellar tendon bearing • prior to birth

PTC	percutaneous transhepatic cholangiography • phenylthiocarbamide • plasma thromboplastin component • pseudotumor cerebri
PTCA	percutaneous transluminal coronary angioplasty
PTD	permanent and total disability
PTE	parathyroid extract • post-traumatic endophthalmitis • pretibial edema • pulmonary thromboembolism
PTEN	pentaerythrital tetranitrate
PTF	plasma thromboplastin factor • post-transfusion fever
PTFD	part-time, full duty
PTFE	polytetrafluoroethylene (graft, paste)
PTH	parathormone (parathyroid hormone) • phenylthiohydantoin • post-transfusion hepatitis
PTLD	post-transplant lymphoproliferative disease
PTN	provider telecommunication network
PTP	posterior tibial pulse
pts	patients
PTS	painful tonic seizure • permanent threshold shift • provider training sessions
PTSD	post-traumatic stress disorder
PTT	partial thromboplastin time
PTU	propylthiouracil
PTX	picrotoxin • pneuomothorax
Pu	plutonium
PU	peptic ulcer • pregnancy urine
PUBS	percutaneous umbilical blood sampling
PuD	pulmonary disease
PUD	peptic ulcer disease
PUF	public use files
PUFA	polyunsaturated fatty acid

PUH	pregnancy urine hormone
pul	pulmonary
PULHES	Physical profile : general Physical, Upper extremities, Lower extremities, Hearing, Eyes, pSychiatric
pulm	gruel (*pulmentum*) • pulmonary, pulmonix
pulv	powder (*pulvis*)
PUN	plasma urea nitrogen
PUO	pyrexia of undetermined origin • pyrexia of unknown origin
PUPPP	pruritic urticarial papules and plaques of pregnancy
purg	purgative
PUVA	psoralen (oral) with long-wavelength ultraviolet light
PUVD	pulsed ultrasonic (blood) velocity detector
PUW	pick-up walker
PV	peripheral vascular • peripheral vein • plasma viscosity • plasma volume • polycythemia vera • portal vein • predictive value • pulmonary vein
PVA	polyvinyl alcohol
PVB	premature ventricular beat
PVC	polyvinyl chloride • post-voiding cystogram • premature ventricular contraction • pulmonary venous congestion
$PVCO_2$	mixed venous carbon dioxide pressure
PVD	peripheral vascular disease • premature ventricular depolarization
PVE	premature ventricular extrasystole
PVH	primary voluntary hospital
PVM	pneumonia virus of mice
PVO_2	mixed venous oxygen pressure
PVOD	peripheral vascular occlusive disease
PVP	povidone (polyvinylpyrrolidone)
PVP-I	povidone (polyvinylpyrrolidone) iodine

PVR	peripheral vascular resistance • pulmonary vascular resistance • post-void residual
PVRI	peripheral vascular resistance index • pulmonary vascular resistance index
PVS	persistent vegetative state
PVSG	Polycythemia Vera Study Group
pvt	private
PVT	paroxysmal ventricular tachycardia • pressure, volume, temperature
P-W	Prader-Willi (syndrome)
PWA	person (s) with AIDS
PWB	partial weight-bearing
PWC	physical work capacity
PWCI	personal watercraft injury
PWLV	posterior wall of left ventricle
PWM	pokewood mitogen
PWOS	post-workout syncope
PWP	pulmonary wedge pressure
PWS	port-wine stain
Px	past history • pneumothorax • prognosis
PX	physical examination
PXE	pseudoxanthoma elasticum
Py	pyrene
PY	pack-year (cigarette use)
P/Y	pack-year (cigarette use)
pyr	pyridine
PZ	pancreozymin
PZA	pyrazinamide
PZI	protamine zinc insulin
PZP	pregnancy zone protein

Q

q	each, every (*quaque*) • four (*quattuor*) • quantity • quart • quartile • volume
Q	coulomb (electrical unit) • perfusion flow • quotient
Q°	perfusion (flow) rate
QA	quality assessment • quality assurance
QAC	Quality Assessment Committee • Quality Assessment Coordinator • Quality Assurance Committee • Quality Assurance Coordinator
QAD	Quality Assessment Director
qam	every morning
QAM	quality assurance monitoring
QAP	quality assurance program • quinine, atabrine, plasmoquine
QA/RM	quality assurance / risk management
QAT	quality action team
QA/UR	quality assurance / utilization review
QBCA	quantitative buffy-coat analysis
Q_C	pulmonary capillary blood flow (perfusion)
QC	quality control
QCIM	Quarterly Cumulative Index Medicus
Qco_2	number of microliters of CO2 given off per mg. dry weight of tissue per hour
qd	every day (*quaque die*)
QEP	quality evaluation program
QES	quality education system
qh	every hour (*quaque hora*)
q2h	every two hours
q3h	every three hours
QI	quality improvement

qid	four times a day (*quater in die*)
QIP	quality improvement plan • quality improvement process • quality intervention plan
QISMC	Quality Improvement System for Managed Care
QIW	qualified injured worker
ql	as much as desired (*quantum libet*)
qm	each morning (*quaque mane*)
QM	quinacrine mustard
QMB	qualified Medicare beneficiary (beneficiaries)
QME	Qualified Medical Exam • Qualified Medical Examiner
qn	every night (*quaque nocte*)
QNS	quantity not sufficient
QO_2	oxygen consumption • oxygen quotient
$Q°O_2$	oxygen consumption rate (microliters per milligram per hour)
qod	every other day
qoh	every other hour
QOL	quality of life
qon	every other night
qp	at will, as much as desired (*quantum placeat*)
QP	quanti-Pirquet (reaction)
qpm	every night
QP/QS	ratio of pulmonary to systemic circulation
qq	each (*quaque, quoque*)
qqh	every four hours (*quaque quarta hora*)
qq hor	every hour
QRN	quality review nurse
QRR	Qualified Rehabilitation Representative
QRS	principle deflection in ECG

qs	quadriceps setting • quantity sufficient (*quantum satis*)
qt	quart • quiet
Qt	Quick's test
quad	quadrant • quadriceps • quadriplegia, quadriplegic
qual	qualitative • quality
qual anal	qualitative analysis
quant	quantitative
quant anal	quantitative analysis
quart	fourth (*quartus*)
quat	four (*quattor*)
quats	quaternary ammonium compounds
quinq	five (*quinque*)
quint	fifth (*quintus*) • quintuplet
quot	daily (*quotide*)
qv	as much as desired (*quantum vis*) • which see (*quod vide*)

R

r	far, remote (*remotum*) • rate • ring chromosome • roentgen
R	Behnken's unit (of roentgen-ray exposure) • organic radical • rad • radioactive • radiology, radiologist • range • Rankine (scale) • rate • Reaumur (scale) • rectal • red • reference • registered trade mark • regression coefficient • resistance (electrical) • respiration • respiratory • exchange ratio • response • reticulocyte • review • *Rickettsia* • right • Rinne's test (hearing) • roentgen
-R	Rinne's test negative
+R	Rinne's test positive
Ra	radium

RA	Radiation Oncology Services • Remittance Advice • renin activity • repeat action • residual air • rheumatoid arthritis • right angle • right arm • right atrial (pressure) • right atrium • right auricle • room air
RAA	renin-angiotensin-aldosterone (system) • right atrial abnormality
RA-ABG	room air arterial blood gases
rac	racemic
RAC	Recombinant DNA Advisory Committee • right atrial catheter
rad	radian • radius • root (*radix*)
RAD	right anterior descending • right axis deviation • reactive attachment disorder
RADA	right acromio-dorso-anterior
RADCA	right anterior descending coronary artery
RADT	Radiation Therapy • registration, admission, discharge, transfer (system)
RAE	right atrial enlargement
RAEB	refractory anemia with excess of blasts
RAH	right anterior hemiblock • right atrial hypertrophy
RAHB	right anterior hemiblock
RAHTG	rabbit antihuman thymocyte globulin
RAI	radioactive iodine • right atrial involvement
RAIU	radioactive iodine uptake
RAM	random access memory
RAMC	Royal Army Medical Corps
RAMI	Risk Adjusted Mortality Index
RAN	resident's admission note
RANT	right anterior
RAO	right anterior oblique

RAP	Radiologists, Anesthesiologists, Pathologists • rheumatoid arthritis precipitin • right atrial pressure • resident assessment protocols • risk analyzer program
RAR	right arm recumbent
ras	scrapings (*rasurae*)
RAS	regular analysts' sessions • reticular activating system
RAST	radioallergosorbent test • right anterior superior thorax
RAT	repeat action tablet • right anterior thorax
RAV	Rous-associated virus
RAW	airway resistance
Rb	rubidium
RB	Rehabilitation Bureau
R&B	right and below
RBA	relative binding activity
RBB	right breast biopsy • right bundle branch
RBBB	right bundle branch block
RBBsB	right bundle branch system block
RBBX	right breast biopsy examination
RBC	red blood cell • red blood (cell) count
RBC-ADA	red-blood-cell adenosine deaminase
RBCD	right border of cardiac dullness
RBC frag	erythrocyte (red-blood-cell) fragility
RBD	regular blood donor • right-border dullness • Reducing Benefit Duration
RBE	relative biologic effectiveness
RBF	regional blood flow • renal blood flow
RBKA	right below-knee amputation
RBKLA	right below-knee leg amputation
RBOW	rupture of bag of waters

RBP	retinol-binding protein • right (arm) blood pressure
RBRVS	resource based relative value study
RC	radial-carpal • red cell • Red Cross • referred care • resource consumption • respirations ceased • respiratory center • right ear, cold stimulus
RCA	red-cell agglutination • Refugee Cash Assistance Program • right coronary artery
RCal	relative calories
rCBF	regional cerebral blood flow
RCC	ratio of costs to charges
RCCA	right common carotid artery
RCD	relative cardiac dullness
RCDR	relative corrected death rate
RCF	red-cell folate • relative centrifugal force
RCL	right coronary lesion
RCM	red-cell mass • right costal margin • Rehabilitation Case Management
RCMP	Royal Canadian Mounted Police
RCP	resource consumption profile • Royal College of Physicians
RCPT	Registered Cardiopulmonary Technician
RCR	rotator cuff repair
RCS	repeat cesarean section • reticulum-cell sarcoma • Royal College of Surgeons
RCT	random controlled trial • red cell toxin • Rorschach content test
RCU	red cell utilization • refined carbohydrate unit • renal care unit • respiratory care unit
RCV	red-cell volume
rd	rutherford (unit of radioactivity)
RD	Raynaud's disease • reaction of degeneration • registered dietitian • respiratory disease • retinal detachment • right deltoid • rubber dam

R&D	research and development
RdA	reading age
RDA	recommended dietary allowance • right dorsoanterior
RDC	Research Diagnostic Criteria
RDE	receptor-destroying enzyme
RDFS	ratio of decayed and filled surfaces (teeth)
RDFT	ratio of decayed and filled teeth
RDP	radiopharmaceutical drug product
RdQ	reading quotient
RDRC	Radioactive Drug Research Committee
RDS	respiratory distress syndrome • reticuloendothelial depressing substance
RDT	regular dialysis treatment
RDW	red (cell) distribution width
re	concerning
Re	rhenium
RE	radium emanation • regional enteritis • reticuloendothelial • retinol equivalent • right extremity • right eye
react	reaction
readm	readmission
rec	fresh (*recens*) • recommendation • record • recreation • recurrent
REC	radioelectrocomplexing
RECA	right external carotid artery
Rec Asst	recreation assistant
RECG	radioelectrocardiography
recip	recipient • reciprocal
Recon	petition for reconsideration
recond	recondition

reconstr	reconstruction
recryst	recrystallize
RECS	Rehabilitation Engineering/Custom Seating
Rec Spec	recreation specialist
rect	rectal • rectified
Rec Tech	recreation technician
red	reduce, reducing, reduction
redn	reduction
REE	resting energy expenditure
REEGT	Registered Electroencephalographic Technician
REEP	role exchange/education practice
ref	refer, referred • reference
REF	renal erythropoietic factor
ref doc	referring doctor
refl	reflex
reg	region • regular
Reg	registered
REG	radioencephalogram • rapid exchange grip
regen	regenerate, regeneration
reg umb	umbilical region
regurg	regurgitate
rehab	rehabilitation
rel	related, relative
REL	rate of energy loss
rem	roentgen equivalent man (unit of radiation exposure)
REM	rapid eye movement (sleep)
rep	let it be repeated (*repetatur*) • roentgen equivalent physical
REP	repeat • report

rept	repeat • report
req	required
res	research • reserve • residence • resident • residue
RES	electrical resistance • reticuloendothelial system
resc	resuscitation
RESDAC	research data assistance center
resp	respective, respectively • respiration, respiratory • responsible
ret	retired
retic	reticulocyte
rev	reverse • review • revolution
rev/min	revolutions per minute
rf	radiofrequency
Rf	retardation factor
RF	Reitland-Franklin (unit) • relative flow (rate) • releasing factor • rheumatic fever • rheumatoid factor
RFA	right femoral artery • right forearm • right frontoanterior
RFFIT	rapid fluorescent focus inhibition test
RFL	right frontolateral
RFLP	restriction fragment length polymorphism
RFP	right frontoposterior • request for proposal
RFR	refraction
RFT	right frontotransverse
RG	right gluteal, right gluteus
RGE	relative gas expansion
Rh	rhesus (blood factor) • rhodium • rhonchi
RH	radiant heat • Rehabilitation Services • relative humidity • releasing hormone • right hand

RHC	regional heart center • respirations have ceased • rural health clinic
RHD	relative hepatic dullness • rheumatic heart disease • rural healthcare delivery
rheum	rheumatic
RHF	right heart failure
RHG	relative hemoglobin
RHH	right homonymous hemianopsia
Rhig	Rh immunoglobulin
rhin	rhinology, rhinologist • rhinorrhea
rhm	roentgens per hour at one meter
RHP	regional health planning • right hemiparesis • right hemiplegia
RHV	right hepatic vein
RI	input resistors • refractive index • respiratory illness • retroactive inhibition
RIA	radioimmunoassay
RIA-DA	radioimmunoassay - double antibody
Rib	ribose
RIC	right iliac crest • right internal capsule • right internal carotid
RICA	right internal carotid artery
RICE	rest, ice, compression, elevation
RICM	right intercostal space
RICU	respiratory intensive-care unit
RID	radial immunodiffusion
RIF	rifampin • right iliac fossa
RIG	rabies immune globulin
RIH	right inguinal hernia
RIHSA	radioiodinated human serum albumin

RIMA	right internal mammary artery
RIND	reversible ischemic neurologic deficit
RIPA	radioimmunoprecipitation assay
RISA	radioiodinated serum albumin
RIST	radioimmunosorbent test
RIVS	ruptured interventricular septum
RK	radial keratotomy • right kidney
RKY	roentgen kymography
rl	fine rales
Rl	medium rales
RL	coarse rales • right lateral • right leg • right lower • right lung • Ringer's lactate • residential living
R-L	right to left
R/L	right to left
R Lat	right lateral
R LAT	right lateral
RLBCD	right lower border of cardiac dullness
RLC	residual lung capacity
RLD	related living donor • right lateral decubitus (position) • ruptured lumbar disc
RLE	right lower extremity
RLF	retrolental fibroplasia • right lateral femoral
rll	right lower lid
RLL	right lower lobe
RLQ	right lower quadrant
RLR	right lateral rectus
RLS	restless legs syndrome
RLSB	right lower sternal border
RLT	right lateral thigh

RLV	Rauscher leukemia virus
RM	radical mastectomy • range of motion • respiratory movement • risk management
RMA	right mentoanterior
RMB	right main-stem bronchus
RMCA	right main coronary artery
RMCL	right midclavicular line
RMD	retromanubrial dullness
RMK	rhesus monkey kidney
RML	right mediolateral • right middle lobe
RMLS	right middle lobe syndrome
RMP	regional medical program • resting membrane potential • right mentoposterior
RMPS	regional medical program service
RMR	resting metabolic rate • right medial rectus
RMS	square foot of mean square
RMSF	Rocky Mountain spotted fever
RMT	right mentotransverse
RMV	respiratory minute volume
Rn	radon
RN	registered nurse • renal disease • Rehabilitation Nursing
RNA	ribonucleic acid
RNase	ribonuclease
RN, C	Registered Nurse, Certified
RN, CM	Registered Nurse Case Manager
RN, CNAA	Registered Nurse, Certified in Nursing Administration, Advanced
RN, CS	Registered Nurse, Certified Specialist
RNICU	regional neonatal intensive-care unit

RNIP	Registered Nurse, Interim Permit
RNMS	registered nurse of the mentally subnormal
RNP	registered nurse-practitioner • ribonucleoprotein
RNS	reference normal serum
Rnt	roentgenology, roentgenologist
RNV	radionuclide venography
RNY	Roux-en-Y gastric bypass
RO	routine order • regional office
R/O	rule out
ROA	right occipitoanterior
ROC	receiver operating characteristic
ROE	return on equity
ROI	return on investment
ROL	right occipitolateral
ROM	range of motion • read-only memory • rupture of membranes
ROP	retinopathy of prematurity • right occipitoposterior
ROS	Radiation Oncology Services • review of systems
rot	rotate, rotated, rotation, rotating
ROT	remedial occupational therapy • right occipitotransverse
ROW	Rendu-Osler-Weber syndrome
RP	radial pulse • Raynaud's phenomenon • refractory period • Respiratory Care Services • retinitis pigmentosa • relapsing polychondritis
RPA	right pulmonary artery
RPCF	Reiter protein complement fixation (test)
RPCH	rural primary case hospitals
RPF	relaxed pelvic floor • renal plasma flow
RPG	radiation protection guide

RPGN	rapidly progressive glomerulonephritis
RPHA	reverse passive hemagglutination
RPI	reticulocyte production index
RPICA	right posterior internal carotid artery
RPLND	retroperitoneal lymph node dissection
rpm	revolutions per minute
RPO	right posterior oblique
R POST	right posterior
RPP	retropubic prostatectomy
RPR	rapid plasma reagin (test)
rps	revolutions per second
RPS	renal pressor substance • review per screen • renal pressor substance
rpt	repeat • report
RPT	registered physical therapist • right posterior thorax
RPV	right portal vein
RQ	recovery quotient • respiratory quotient
RR	radiation response • recovery room • regular respirations • relative risk • respiratory rate
R&R	rate and rhythm • rest and relaxation
RRA	radioreceptor assay • Registered Record Administrator
RRC	recruitment and retention committee
RRE	radiation-related eosinophilia
RR&E	round, regular, and equil (pupils)
RRMS	relapsing-remitting multiple sclerosis
rRNA	ribosomal ribonucleic acid
RRP	Refugee Resettlement Program • relative refractory period
RRR	regular rate and rhythm (heart)
RRRN	round, regular, react normally

RRT	registered respiratory therapist
RRTW	released to return to work
RRV	rhesus rotavirus vaccine
RRx	radiation prescription
Rs	respond, response
RS	*Rauwolfia serpentina* • reinforcing stimulus • Reiter's syndrome • respiratory system • review of systems • Reye's syndrome • Ringer's solution
R-S	reticulated siderocytes
RSA	right sacroanterior • right subclavian artery
RSB	right sternal border
RScA	right scapuloanterior
RScP	right scapuloposterior
RSD	reflex sympathetic dysfunction • reflex sympathetic dystrophy • relative standard deviation
RSI	rapid sequence intubation • repetitive strain injury • repetitive stress injury
R-SICU	respiratory-surgical intensive-care unit
RSIVP	rapid sequence intravenous pyelogram
RSNA	Radiological Society of North America
RSO	radiation safety officer • right salpingo-oophorectomy
RSP	right sacroposterior
RSR	regular sinus rhythm
RSSE	Russian spring-summer encephalitis
RST	radiosensitivity test • rapid surfactant test • reagin screen test • right sacrotransverse
RS v	respiratory syncytial virus
RSV	Rous sarcoma virus • respiratory syncytial virus
RSW	right-sided weakness
rt	right

RT	radiologic technician, technologist • radiotherapy • radium therapy • reaction time • reading time • reciprocating tachycardia • recreational therapy, therapist • registered technician, technologist • respiratory therapy, therapist • right triceps • room temperature
RTA	renal tubular acidosis
RTC	residential treatment center • return to clinic
RTD	resubmission turnaround documents
RTech	radiology technologist, technician
RTF	residential treatment facility • resistance transfer factor • respiratory tract fluid
RTI	Rehabilitation Training Institute
rtn	return
RTN	Registered Technologist, Nuclear Medicine • routine
RTO	return to office
RTR	Registered Technologist, Radiography
RTT	Radiation Therapy Technician
RT_3U	resin T3 (triiodothyronine) uptake (test)
RTUS	real time ultrasonography
RTW	return to work
Ru	ruthenium
RU	radioulnar • rat unit • rectourethral • residual urine • retrograde urogram • roentgen unit
RUA	right upper arm
rub	red (*ruber*)
RUE	right upper extremity
RUG	Resource Utilization Group
rul	right upper lid
RUL	right upper leg • right upper lobe
RUO	right ureteral orifice

rupt	rupture
RUQ	right upper quadrant
RURTI	recurrent upper respiratory tract infection
RV	residual volume • retroversion • right ventricle, ventricular • rubella vaccine
RVA	right ventricular abnormality • rabies vaccine absorbed
RVAD	right ventricular assist device
RVD	relative vertebral density • rest vertical dimension • right ventricular dimension
RVDO	right ventricular diastolic overload
RVE	right ventricular enlargement
RVEDP	right ventricular end-diastolic pressure
RVEDV	right ventricular end-diastolic volume
RVET	right ventricular ejection time
RVF	Rift Valley Fever
RVFP	right ventricular filling pressure
RVG	radionuclide ventriculogram, ventriculography
RVH	renovascular hypertension • right ventricular hypertrophy
RVID	right ventricular internal dimension
RVIDP	right ventricular initial diastolic pressure
RVLG	right ventrolateral gluteal
RVO	relaxed vaginal outlet • right ventricular outflow • right ventricular overactivity
RVP	right ventricular pressure
RVR	renal vein renin
RVS	Relative Value Scale • Relative Value Schedule • Relative Value Studies
RVSW	right ventricular stroke work
RVSWI	right ventricular stroke work index
RVU	relative value units

RVV	rubella vaccine virus
RW	right ear, warm stimulus
Rx	prescription • take (*recipe*) • treatment

S

s̄	without (*sine*) • without spectacles
S	half (*semis*) • left (*sinister*) • mark (*signa*) • sacral (nerve, vertebra) • saline • saturation • second • section • sedimentation coefficient • sensation • sensitive • serum • siderocyte • single • smooth (bacterial colony) • soft (diet) • soluble • son • spherical (lens) • stimulus • subject • sulfur • supravergence • surgery, surgical, surgeon • Svedberg unit
S1-S5	sacral vertebrae 1 through 5
SA	salicylic acid • short-acting • sialoadenectomy • sinoatrial • specific activity • Stokes-Adams (disease) • suicide awareness • surface area • surgeon's assistant • sustained-action • spontaneous abortion
S/A	sugar and acetone
SAARD	slow-acting antirheumatic drug
SAB	sequential androgen blockade • Society of American Bacteriologists • spontaneous abortion
SAC	short arm cast
sacc	cogwheel (respiration)
SACD	subacute combined degeneration
SACE	serum angiotensin-converting enzyme
SACH	solid ankle, cushion heel (foot prosthesis)
SACT	sinoatrial conduction time
SAD	seasonal affective disorder • Self-Assessment Depression Scale • sugar, acetone, diacetic acid (test)
SADBE	squaric acid dibutylester
SADS	Schedule for Affective Disorders and Schizophrenia
SAECG	signal-averaged electrocardiogram

SAED	selected area electron diffraction
SAFA	soluble-antigen fluorescent antibody (test)
SAFE	stationary attachment, flexible endoskeleton (foot prosthesis)
SAH	subarachnoid hemorrhage
SAID	sexually acquired immunodeficiency syndrome • steroidal anti-inflammatory drugs
Sal	*Salmonella*
SAM	self-administered medication • systolic anterior motion
SAN	sinoatrial node
sanit	sanitarium • sanitary, sanitation
SAO	Southeast Asian ovalocytosis
SAO_2	arterial blood oxygen saturation
sap	saponify, saponification
SAP	serum alkaline phosphate
SAPD	self-administration of psychotropic drugs
SAPMS	short arm posterior molded splint
sapon	saponify, saponification
SAQ	short-arc quadriceps test
SART	sinoatrial recovery time
SAS	space-adaptation syndrome • sterile aqueous suspension • subarachnoid space
sat	saturate, saturated
SAT	Scholastic Aptitude Test
satis	satisfactory
SATL	surgical Achilles tendon lengthening
Sb	antimony (*stibium*) • strabismus
SB	Sengstaken-Blakemore (tube) • sideroblast • sinus bradycardia • small bowel • spina bifida • Stanford-Binet (test) • stillbirth, stillborn • suction biopsy

+SB	wearing seatbelts
SBA	stand-by assistance
SBB	specialist in blood bank
SBE	shortness of breath on exertion • subacute bacterial endocarditis
SBFT	small bowel follow-through
SBGM	self blood-glucose monitoring
SBJ	skin, bones, joints
SBMPL	simultaneous binaural midplace localization
SBN_2	single-breath nitrogen (test)
SBO	small bowel obstruction
SBOD	scleral buckle, right eye
SBOS	scleral buckle, left eye
SBP	spontaneous bacterial peritonitis • systolic blood pressure
SBR	strict bed rest
SBS	small bowel series • staff burn-out scale
SBTI	soybean trypsin inhibitor
SBSM	self blood sugar monitoring
Sc	scandium
SC	sacrococcygeal • secretory coil • self care • semilunar (valves) • closure • service-connected • sickle cell • stimulus, conditioned • subcorneal • subcutaneous • sugar-coated • supportive care
S/C	supraclavicular
SCAN	Senior Care Action Network • suspected child abuse and neglect
SCAT	sheep-cell agglutination test • sickle-cell anemia test
SCB	strictly confined to bed
SCC	squamous cell carcinoma
ScD	Doctor of Science

SCD	service-connected disability • sudden cardiac death
ScDA	right scapuloanterior (*scapulodextra anterior*)
ScDP	right scapuloposterior (*scapulodextra posterior*)
SCE	sister-chromatid exchange
SCF	single conversion factor
SCG	sodium cromoglycate
SCH	sole community hospital
sched	schedule
SCHIP	State Children's Health Insurance Program
SCHNC	squamous cell head and neck cancer
SCHP	State Child Health Plan
sci	science • scientific
SCI	spinal cord injury
SCID	severe combined immunodeficiency disease
SCIF	State Compensation Insurance Fund
SCIPP	sacrococcygeal to inferior pubic point
SCIU	spinal cord injury unit
SCIWORA	spinal cord injury without radiological abnormality
SCL	scleroderma • serum copper level • soft contact lens
ScLA	left scapuloanterior (*scapulolaeva anterior*)
SCLC	small-cell lung carcinoma
ScLP	left scapuloposterior (*scapulolaeva posterior*)
SCM	state-certified midwife • sternocleidomastoid muscle
SCN	self-care needs
SCO	supportive care only
scop	scopolamine
SCP	single-celled protein • specialty care physician
SCPK	serum creatine phosphokinase

Scr	scruple • serum creatinine
SCR	spondylitic caudal radiculopathy
SCRAP	Simple Complex Reaction-Time Apparatus
SCS	spinal cord stenosis • spinal cord stimulation
SCT	salmon calcitonin • sentence-completion test • sickle-cell trait • staphylococcal clumping test • sugar-coated tablet
SCU	Special Care Unit
SCUBA	self-contained underwater breathing apparatus
SCUF	slow continuous ultrafiltration
SCV	smooth, capsulated, virulent (bacteria)
SD	senile dementia • septal defect • serologically defined (antigen) • skin dose • spontaneous delivery • standard deviation • sterile dressing • straight drainage • streptodornase • sudden death • shoulder dystocia
SDA	right sacroanterior (*sacrodextra anterior*) • specific dynamic action • succinate dehydrogenase activity
SDAT	senile dementia of the Alzheimer's type
SDE	specific dynamic effect
SDH	sorbitol dehydrogenase • subdural hematoma • succinate dehydrogenase
SDL	self-directed learning
SDLRS	self-directed-learning readiness scale
SDM	standard deviation of the mean
SDP	right sacroposterior (*sacrodextra posterior*) • single-donor platelets
SDS	same-day surgery • sodium dodecyl sulfate
SDT	right sacrotransverse (*sacrodextra transversa*)
Se	selenium
SE	saline enema • *Salmonella enteridities* • spherical equivalent • spin echo • standard error (of the mean) • sphenoethmoidal suture
S-E	Starr-Edwards (prosthesis)

SEA	sheep erythrocyte agglutination (test) • Southeast Asia • spontaneous electrical activity
SEAL	Southeast Asian learners
SEAR	Southeast Asian refugees
sec	second • secondary
SEC	soft elastic capsules • squamous epithelial cells
SECOP	second opinion
sect	section
sed	stool (*sedes*)
SED	skin erythema dose
SEER	surveillance, epidemiology and end results
sed rate	(erythrocyte) sedimentation rate
seg	segment, segmented • segmented cell
SEG	sonoencephalogram, sonoencephalography
sem	semen
SEM	scanning electron microscope • standard error of the mean • systolic ejection murmur
semih	half an hour (*semihora*)
SENA	sympathetic efferent nerve activity
SENIC	Study on the Efficacy of Nosocomial Infection Control
sens	sensitivity
SENTAC	Society for Ear, Nose and Throat Advances in Children
SEO	surgical emergency officer
sep	separately
SEP	sensory evoked potential • somatosensory evoked potential • systolic ejection period
seq	that which follows (*sequela*)
seq luce	the following day (*sequenti luce*)
ser	series • service

Ser	serine
SER	somatosensory evoked response • systolic ejection rate
sero	serology
serv	keep (*serva*) • preserve
SES	socioeconomic status
SET	skin endpoint titration
sev	severe • severed
SeXO	serum xanthine oxidase
Sf	Svedberg flotation unit
SF	salt-free • scarlet fever • slow initial function • spinal fluid • stress formula • synovial fluid
SFA	serum folate • superficial femoral angioplasty
SFC	spinal fluid count
SFD	skin-to-film distance • small-for-dates
SFEMG	single-fiber electromyography
SFP	screen-filtration resistance
SG	signs • skin graft • soluble gelatin • specific gravity • Surgeon General • surgery • survey group • Swan-Ganz (catheter)
S-G	Sachs-Georgi (test)
SGA	small for gestational age
SGAW	specific airway conductance
SGE	significant glandular enlargement • suitable gainful employment
SGF	skeletal growth factor
SGGT	serum gamma-glutamyltransferase
SGO	Surgeon General's Office
SGOT	serum glutamic-pyruvic transaminase
SGR	Sustainable Growth Rate

sh	shoulder
Sh	*Shigella* • short
SH	serum hepatitis • social history • somatotropic hormone • sulfhydryl • surgical history
SHARE	Siblings Helping Persons with Autism through Resources and Energy
SHBD	serum hydroxybutyrate dehydrogenase
SHBG	sex-hormone binding globulin
SHCC	Statewide Health Coordinating Council
SHHH	Self Help for Hard of Hearing People
shld	shoulder
SHMOS	Social Health Maintenance Organization
SHP	Schonlein-Henoch purpura
SHPDA	State Health Planning and Development Agency
SHSWD	Society for Hospital Social Work Directors
Si	silicon
SI	sacroiliac • saturation index • seriously ill • serum iron • soluble insulin • special intervention • stroke index • *Systeme International d'Unites*
SIADH	syndrome of inappropriate secretion of antidiuretic hormone
sib	sibling
SICU	surgical intensive-care unit
SID	Society for Investigative Dermatology
SIDS	sudden infant death syndrome
SIE	stroke in evolution • subacute infective endocarditis
SIECUS	Sex Information and Education Council for the United States
sig	let it be labeled (*signetur*) • signal • significant
SIg	surface immunoglobulin
SIG	sigmoidoscope, sigmoidoscopy
sig n pro	label with the proper name (*signa nomine proprio*)

SI/IS	severity of illness/intensity of services
SIJ	sacroiliac joint
SIMS	surgical indication monitoring system
simul	simultaneously
SIMV	synchronous intermittent mandatory ventilation
sin	without (*sine*)
sing	of each (*singulorum*)
si op sit	if it is necessary (*si opus sit*)
SIP	sickness impact profile • self-imposed penalty
SIRS	Seriousness of Illness Rating Scale • systematic inflammatory response syndrome
SISI	short (small)-increment sensitivity index
SIW	self-inflicted wound
S-J	Stevens-Johnson syndrome
SK	streptokinase
SKIP	Sick Kids Need Involved People • State Kids Insurance Program
SKSD	streptokinase-streptodornase
sl	slight
SL	sensation level • slit lamp • staphage lysate • sublingual
SLA	left sacroanterior (*sacrolaeva anterior*) • slide latex agglutination
SLAC	superior labrum, anterior cuff
SLAP	superior labrum, anterior and posterior
SLB	short leg brace
SLC	short leg cast
SLCVC	single-lumen central venous catheter
SLE	St. Louis encephalitis • systemic lupus erythematosus
SLFIA	substrate-labeled fluorescent immunoassay • substrate-linked fluorescent immunoassay

SLM	spatial light modulator
SLMB	specified low-income Medicare beneficiary
SLO	streptolysin-O
SLP	left sacroposterior (*sacrolaeva posterior*) • Speech/Language Pathology
SLPMS	short leg posterior molded splint
SLR	straight-leg-raising (test)
SLT	left sacrotransverse (*sacrolaeva transversa*)
SLWC	short leg walking cast
sm	small
Sm	samarium • symptoms
SM	smooth muscle • streptomycin • systolic murmur
SMA	schedule of maximum allowance • Sequential Multiple Analyzer • smooth muscle antibody • spinal muscular atrophy • superior mesenteric artery
SMAC	Sequential Multiple Analyzer with Computer
SMAF	specific macrophage arming factor
SMART	Strategies for Management of Anti-Retroviral Therapies
SMBG	self-monitored blood glucose
SMC	selenomethylnorcholesterol
SMD	senile macular degeneration • submanubrial dullness
sm-FeSV	McDonough feline sarcoma virus
SMH	state mental hospital
SMI	Supplementary (Medicare) Insurance Program
SMO	school medical office, officer • senior medical officer
SMON	subacute myelo-opticoneuropathy
SMR	somnolent metabolic rate • Standardized Mortality Rate, Ratio • submucous resection
SMT	stress management training • student medical technologist

SMX	sulfamethoxazole
Sn	tin (*stannum*)
SN	according to nature (*secundum naturam*) • school of nursing • serum neutralization, serum neutralizing • staff nurse • student nurse
S/N	sample-to-negative control ratio • signal-to-noise ratio
SNA	Student Nurses' Association • systems network architecture
SNAB	Staff Nurse Advisory Board
SNAP	sensory nerve action potential
SNCV	sensory-nerve conduction velocity
SNDO	Standard Nomenclature of Diseases and Operations
SNE	subacute necrotizing encephalomyopathy
SNEC	Staff Nurse Executive Committee
SNF	skilled nursing facility
SNF/MR	skilled nursing facility for the mentally retarded
SNGFR	single-nephron glomerular filtration rate
SNM	Society of Nuclear Medicine
SNO	substantive negative outcome
SNOMED	Standardized Nomenclature of Pathology
SNRI	serotonin and norepinephrine reuptake inhibitors
SNS	Society of Neurological Surgeons • sympathetic nervous system
SO	salpingo-oophorectomy • significant other • Social Work Services • suicidal observation • superior oblique • supraoptic • spheno-occipital
sO_2	blood oxygen saturation
SO_2	blood oxygen saturation
SOAF	Statement of Accepted Facts
SOAP	Subjective, Objective, Assessment, Plan (problem-oriented record)

SOAPS	suction, oxygen, apparatus, pharmaceuticals, saline
SOB	shortness of breath • suboccipitobregmatic
soc	social • society
SOC	standard of care
SOI	severity of illness
sol	soluble • solution
SOL	space-occupying lesion • statute of limitations
soln	solution
solu	solute
solv	dissolve (*solve*) • solvent
SOM	serous otitis media
SOMI	sternal-occipital-mandibular immobilizer
SONP	soft organs not palpable
SOP	standard operating procedure
s op s	if necessary (*si opus sit*)
SOTT	synthetic-medium old tuberculin, trichloroacetic acid-precipitated
SOW	scope of work
sp	space • species • specific • spine, spinal • spirit (alcohol)
s/p	status post
Sp	sacropubic
SP	special care services • sulfapyridine • suprapubic • systolic pressure
SPA	salt-poor albumin • spondyloarthropathy
span.	spansule
SPBI	serum protein-bound iodine
SPBT	suprapubic bladder tap
SPC	single point care
SPCA	serum prothrombin conversion accelerator

SPCC	statistical process control chart
SPD	salmon-poisoning disease • sterile processing department
SPDT	single-pole double-throw (switch)
SPE	serum protein electrophoresis
spec	specimen
SPECT	single photon emission computed tomography
SPEP	serum protein electrophoresis
SPF	specific pathogen-free • sun protection (protective) factor
SPFC	suprapubic Foley catheter
sp fl	spinal fluid
SPG	specific gravity • sucrose-phosphate-glutamate
sp gr	specific gravity
sph	spherical • spherical lens
SPI	serum-precipitable iodine
spkr	speaker
SPLK	simultaneous pancreas and living kidney (transplant)
SPMA	spinal progressive muscular atrophy
SP-MS	secondary progressive multiple sclerosis
SPN	student practical nurse
spon	spontaneous
spont	spontaneous
spp	species
SPP	suprapubic prostatectomy
SPPS	stable plasma-protein solution
SPS	systemic progressive sclerosis
SPST	single-pole, single-throw (switch)
SPT	skin prick test
SPU	short procedure unit

SPV	slow-phase velocity
sq	square
SQ	subcutaneous
SQC	semiquantitative culture • statistical quality control
SqCCA	squamous-cell carcinoma of the lung
sq cm	square centimeter
sq ft	square foot
SQUID	Superconducting Quantum Interference Devices
sq m	square meter
sq mm	square millimeter
Sr	strontium
SR	sarcoplasmic reticulum • saturation-recovery • secretion rate • sedimentation rate • senior • sensitization response • sex ratio • side rails • sinus rhythm • stimulus-response • stomach rumble • sustained release • systems review • subacute rehabilitation
SRAW	specific airway resistance
SRBC	sheep red blood cells
SRBOW	spontaneous rupture of bag of waters
SRE	Schedule of Recent Experience
SRF	skin reactive factor • slow-reacting factor • somatotropin-releasing factor
SRF-A	slow-reacting factor of anaphylaxis
SRFC	sheep red-cell rosette-forming cells
SRH	single radial hemolysis • spontaneously resolving hyperthyroidism • stigmata of recent hemorrhage
SRIF	somatotropin release-inhibiting factor
SRMC	single room maternity care
sRNA	soluble ribonucleic acid
SR/NE	sinus rhythm, no ectopy

SROM	spontaneous rupture of membranes
SRP	sacrum right posterior
SRR	surgical recovery room
SRRS	Social Readjustment Rating Scale
SRS	slow-reacting substance • Social Rehabilitation Service
SRS-A	slow-reacting substance of anaphylaxis
SRT	sedimentation rate test • speech reception threshold
SRU	side rails up
ss	one-half (*semis*)
SS	saline soak • saliva sample • saturated solution • sea sickness • serum sickness • Sézary syndrome • siblings • side to side • single-stranded (DNA) • soapsuds • social services • standard score • sterile solution • steroid sulfurylation • suction socket • sulfasalazine • somatostatin
S/S	signs and symptoms • Social Security
SSA	*Salmonella-Shigella* agent • skin-sensitizing antibody • Social Security Administration • Social Security Act
SSD	source-to-skin distance • sudden sniffing death
SSDI	Social Security Disability Income
SSE	soapsuds enema
SSEP	somato-sensory evoked potential
SSI	segmental sequential irradiation • Supplemental Security Income
SSKI	saturated solution of potassium iodide
SSM	superficial spreading melanoma
SSN	Social Security Number
SSO	second surgical opinion
SSOP	Second Surgical Opinion Program
SSPE	subacute sclerosing panencephalitis
SSR	surgical supply room

SSRI	selective serotonin re-uptake inhibitor
SSPL	saturation sound pressure level
sss	layer upon layer (*stratum super stratum*)
SSS	sick sinus syndrome • specific soluble substance • sterile saline soak • strong soap solution
SSSS	staphylococcal scalded-skin syndrome
SSSV	superior sagittal sinus-blood velocity
SST	Sleep Studies
SSU	Saybolt seconds universal
ssv	under a poison label (*sub signo veneni*)
SSV	simian sarcoma virus
st	let it stand (*stet*) • straight
St	subtype
ST	sedimentation time • serum transferrin • sinus tachycardia • skin test • slight trace • standardized test • sublingual tablet • surface tension • surgical technologist • survival time • stroke
STA	serum thrombotic accelerator • spine team assessment
staph	staphylococcus, staphylococcal
stat	immediately (*statim*)
STAT	signal transduction-activated transcription (factors)
stb	stillborn
STB	silicotuberculosis
STC	stroke treatment center
std	standard
STD	sexually transmitted disease • short-term disability • skin-test dose • sodium tetradecyl sulfate • standard test dose
STET	submaximal treadmill exercise test
STF	specialized treatment facility

ST-FeSv	Snyder-Thielen feline sarcoma virus
STH	somatotropic hormone
S-Thal	hemoglobin S and thalassemia
stim	stimulation
stip	stipulation with request for award
STK	streptokinase
STM	short-term memory • streptomycin
STP	dimethoxymethylamphetamine (hallucinogenic drug) • standard temperature and pressure
STPD	standard temperature and pressure-dry
str	*Streptococcus*
strep	*Streptococcus*
struct	structure
STS	serologic test for syphilis • Society of Thoracic Surgeons • standard test for syphilis • sugar-tong splint
STSG	split-thickness skin graft
STU	skin-test unit
su	let him take (*sumat*)
SU	sensation unit • strontium unit
S & U	supine and upright
SUA	serum uric acid
subcu	subcutaneous
subq	subcutaneous
Subro	subrogation
subst	substance
SUD	skin unit dose • sudden unexpected death
SUDS	single-unit delivery system • sudden unexpected death syndrome
SUID	sudden unexplained infant death

sum	let him take (*sumat*) • summation
SUN	serum urea nitrogen
sup	superficial • superior • supervision, supervisor
supp	support • suppository
surg	surgeon, surgery, surgical
susp	suspension
sv	alcoholic spirit (*spiritus vini*) • single vibration
SV	simian virus • sinus venosus • spoken voice • spontaneous ventilation • stroke volume
SV40	simian vacuolating virus 40
SVC	slow vital capacity • superior ven cava • suprahepatic vena cava
SVCS	superior vena cava syndrome
SVE	sterile vaginal examination • supracentricular ectopy
SVG	saphenous-vein graft
SVI	stroke volume index
SVPB	supraventricular premature beat
SVR	systemic vascular resistance
SVRI	systemic vascular resistance index
SVT	supraventricular tachycardia
sw	switch
SW	social worker
S & W	serious and willful
SWB	salaries, wages, benefits
SWD	short-wave diathermy
SWI	stroke work index • surgical wound infection
SWR	serum Wassermann reaction
SWS	slow-wave sleep
Sx	signs • symptoms

sym	symmetrical
symp	symptoms
syn	syndrome
sync	synchronous
synch	synchronous
synth	synthetic
Syph	syphilis
syr	syringe • syrup
sys	system, systemic
syst	systemic, systolic
Sz	seizure

T

t	life (time) • temporal • three • times (ter) • ton (metric) • translocation (in genetics)
T	life (time) • obtained under test conditions • temperature • tension (pressure) • tera- • tesla (unit of magnetic flux density) • thoracic (nerve, vertebra) • thymine • tidal (volume) • tocopherol • tonometer reading • topical (medication) • total • transition point • transverse • *Treponema* • tritium
T-	decreased tension (pressure)
T+	increased tension (pressure)
t1/2	half-life (time)
T1/2	half-life (time)
T_1	monoiodotyrosine
T_2	diiodotyrosine
T_3	triiodothyronine
T_4	tetraiodothyronine (thyroxine)
T1-T12	thoracic vertebra 1 through 12
Ta	tantalum

TA	temperature, axillary • thyroglobulin autoprecipitation • toxin-antitoxin • transactional analysis • transaldolase • transantral • tryptophan-acid (reaction)
T & A	tonsillectomy and adenoidectomy
TAA	tumor-associated antigen
tab	tablet
TAB	therapeutic abortion • typhoid, parathyroid A, parathyroid B
TAC	tetracaine, adrenaline, and cocaine
TACE	chlorotrianisene (trianisylchloroethylene)
tachy	tachycardia
TAD	transverse abdominal diameter
TAF	tissue angiogenesis factor • tumor angiogenesis factor
TAG	target-attaching globulin
TAH	total abdominal hysterectomy • total artificial heart
tal	such (talis)
TAM	toxin-antitoxin mixture • toxoid-antitoxoid mixture • treat arrhythmias medically
TAME	tosyl-L-arginine methyl ester
tan	tangent
TANI	total axial (lymph) node irradiation
TAO	thromboangiitis obliterans • toleandomycin (triacetyloleandomycin)
TAPVC	total anomalous pulmonary venous connection
TAPVD	total anomalous pulmonary venous drainage
TAQW	transient abnormal Q waves
TAR	thrombocytopenia-absent radius (syndrome) • treatment authorization request
TARA	tumor-associated rejection antigen
TAT	tetanus antitoxin • Thematic Apperception Test • toxin-antitoxin • turnaround time • tyrosine aminotransferase

t_b	biologic half-life
Tb	terbium • tubercule bacillus
TB	thymol blue • toluidine blue • total body • tuberculosis
TBA	tertiary butylacetate • thiobarbituric acid • to be admitted • tumor-bearing animal
TBC	tuberculosis, tuberculous
TBG	testosterone-binding globulin • thyroxine-binding globulin
TBI	total-body irritation • traumatic brain injury
TBII	TSH-binding inhibitory immunoglobulin
TBIL	total bilirubin
TBili	total bilirubin
TBLC	term birth, live child
TBM	tuberculous meningitis
TBN	tubular basement membrane • total body nitrogen
TBNA	total-body neutron activation
TBP	bithionol (thiobisdichlorophenol) • thyroxine-binding protein
TBR	total bed rest
TBS	tribromsalan (tribromosalicylanilide)
TBSA	total burn surface area
tbsp	tablespoonful
Tb-T	tracheobronchial toilet
TBT	transcervical balloon tuboplasty
TBV	total blood volume
TBW	total body water
^{99m}Tc	technetium metastable radionuclide used in diagnostic scanning
Tc	technetium

TC	tetracycline • therapeutic concentrate • throat culture • tissue culture • to contain • transplant center • treatment completed • tuberculosis, contagious • tubocurarine • transcutaneous
T & C	turn and cough • type and crossmatch
TCA	tricarboxylic acid • trichloroacetate • trichloroacetic acid • tricyclic amine • tricyclic antidepressant
TCAP	trimethylcetylammonium pentachlorophenate
TCB	to call back
TCBS	thiosulfate-citrate-bile salts-sucrose (agar)
TCC	transitional cell carcinoma
TCD	tissue culture dose
TCD_{50}	median tissue culture dose
TCDB	turn, cough, deep breath
TCE	trichloroethylene
T-cells	thymus-dependent cells (lymphocytes)
TCGF	T-cell growth factor
TCI	tricuspid insufficiency
TCID	tissue culture infective dose
$TCID_{50}$	median tissue culture infective dose
TCM	tissue culture medium
TCMI	T-cell-mediated immunity
TCN	transcultural nursing
$TcPO_2$	transcutaneous PO_2 monitor
TCR	T-cell receptor
TCT	thrombin clotting time
TD	tardive dyskinesia • thoracic duct • time disintegration • to deliver • torsion dystonia • total disability • transverse diameter • tumor dose • typhoid dysentery • temporary disability
T_4D	thyroxine displacement (assay)

TDA	therapeutic drug assay • thyroid-stimulating hormone-displacing antibody • tryptophan deaminase agar
TDB	temporary disability benefits
TDD	thoracic-duct drainage • total digitalizing dose
TDI	toluene diisocyanate • Temporary Disability Insurance
TDL	thoracic-duct lymphocytes
TDM	therapeutic drug monitoring
TDN	totally digestible nutrients
tds	to be taken three times a day (*ter die sumendum*)
TdT	terminal deoxynucleotidyl transferase
TDT	tone decay test
t_e	effective half-life
Te	tellurium • tetanus
TE	tracheoesophageal • trial and error
T & E	trial and error
TEA	tetraethylammonium
TEAB	tetraethylammonium bromide
TEAC	tetraethylammonium chloride
TEAE	triethylaminoethyl
TeBG	testosterone-binding globulin
TEC	total eosinophil count
tech	technical • technique
TED	threshold erythema dose • thrombo-embolic deterrent
TEDS	thromboembolus deterrent stocking
TEE	thermal effect of exercise • transesophageal echocardiogram • total energy expenditure
TEF	thermal effect of food
t_{eff}	effective half-life
TEFRA	Tax Equity and Fiscal Responsibility Act

TEG	thromboelastography
TEL	tetraethyl lead
TEM	transmission electron microscope • triethylenemelamine
temp	temperature • temporary
temp dext	to the right temple (*tempori dextro*)
temp sinst	to the left temple (*tempori sinistro*)
TEN	total enteral nutrition • toxic epidermal necrolysis
TENS	transcutaneous electrical nerve stimulator
TEPA	triethylenephosphoramide
TEPP	tetraethyl pyrophosphate
ter	rub (*tere*)
Terb	terbutaline
term	terminal
tert	tertiary
TERT	Total End-Range Time
TES	treatment of emergent symptom
TET	treadmill exercise test
TETD	disulfiram (tetraethylthiuram disulfide)
TETRAC	tetraiodothyroacetic acid
tet tox	tetanus toxoid
tf	to follow • tuning fork
Tf	transferrin
TF	transfer factor
TFA	total fatty acids
TFB	trifascicular feminization syndrome
TFT	thyroid function test
tg	type genus
Tg	thyroglobulin

TG	thioguanine • thyroglobulin • toxic goiter • triglyceride • type genus
TGA	transient global amnesia
TGF	transforming growth factor(s)
TGF-α	type alpha-transforming growth factor
TGF-β	transforming growth factor - beta
TGE	transmissible gastroenteritis • tryptone glucose extract
TGFA	triglyceride fatty acid
TGT	thromboplastin generation test • thromboplastin generation time
TGV	thoracic gas volume
th	thoracic
Th	thorium
TH	tube holder
THA	tetrahydroaminoacridine • total hip arthroplasty • total hydroxyapatite • Texas Hospital Association
THAM	tris(hydroxymethyl)aminomethane
THC	tetrahydrocannabinol (marijuana) • tanshepatic cholangiogram, cholangiography
ther	therapeutic • therapy
Ther Ex	therapeutic exercise
therm	thermometer
THF	tetrahydrofluorenone • tetrahydrofolate • tetrahydrofuran
THFA	tetrahydrofolic acid
Thg	thyroglobulin
THI	trihydroxyindole
thor	thorax, thoracic
Thr	threonine
THR	total hip replacement

throm	thrombosis
THS	terahydro-compound S • tetrahydrodeoxycortisol • Traditional Health Services
THU	tetrahydrouridine
Ti	titanium
TI	transverse diameter between ischia • tricuspid incompetence • tricuspid insufficiency
TIA	transient ischemic attack
TIBC	total iron-building capacity
tib-fib	tibia and fibula
TIC	trypsin inhibitory capacity
tid	three times a day (*ter in die*)
TID	titrated initial dose
TIG	tetanus immune globulin
TIMI	thrombolysis in myocardial infarction
tin	three times a night (*ter in nocte*)
TIN	tubulinterstitial nephropathy
tinct	tincture
TIP	Terbutaline infusion pump
TIPS	transjugular intrahepatic portasystemic shunt
TIR	terminal innervation ratio
TIRI	total immunoreactive insulin
TIS	Titanium Interbody Spacer
TISS	Therapeutic Intervention Scoring System
Title XVII	Medicare
Title XIX	Medicaid
tiwk	three times a week
TJ	triceps jerk
TK	through the knee • tourniquet • transketolase

TKA	total knee arthroplasty
TKD	tokodynamometer
TKG	tokodynagraph
TKO	to keep open
TI	thallium
TL	team leader • tubal ligation
T/L	terminal latency (EMG)
TLC	tender loving care • thin-layer chromatography • total lung capacity • total lymphocyte count
TLCVC	triple-lumen central venous catheter
TLD	thermoluminescent dosimeter • transluminescent dosimeter
TLE	thin-layer electrophoresis
TLI	total lymphoid irradiation
TLR	tonic labyrinthine reflex • Traditional Living Residence
TLSO	thoracolumbosacral orthosis
TLV	threshold limit value • total lung volume
Tm	maximum (maximal) tubular excretory capacity • thulium
TM	temporomandibular • Thayer-Martin (medium) • trademark • Transcendental Meditation • transport mechanism • trimester • tympanic membrane
TMA	trimellitic anhydride • trimethylamine
TMB	too many birthdays
TmG	maximum (maximal) tubular glucose reabsorption rate
TMI	threatened myocardial infarction • transmandibular implant
TMJ	temporomandibular joint (syndrome)
TML	tetramethyl lead
TMP	thymidine monophosphate • trimethoprim • trimethylpsoralen
TMP-SMX	trimethoprim-sulfamethoxazole

TMP-SMZ	trimethoprim-sulfamethoxazole
TMP-SMZ-DS	trimethoprim-sulfamethoxazole-double strength
TMST	treadmill stress test
TMT	tympanic membrane thermometer
TMV	tobacco mosaic virus
Tn	normal intraocular tension
TN	true-negative • trigeminal neuralgia
TNA	Texas Nurses Association
TNBP	tri(n-butyl) phosphate
TNCC	trauma nursing core course
TNF	tumor necrosis factor
TNF-α	tumor necrosis factor alpha
TNG	nitroglycerin (trinitroglycerol)
TNI	total nodal irradiation
TNM	tumor, nodes, metastases
TNPM	transient neonatal pustular melanosis
TNS	transcutaneous electrical nerve stimulator
TNT	trinitrotoluene
TNTC	too numerous to count
TO	original tuberculin • target organ • telephone order • temperature, oral • Theiler's Original (virus) • tincture of opium
TOA	time of arrival • tubo-ovarian abscess
TOCP	triorthocresyl phosphate
tol	tolerance
tomo	tomogram, tomography
tonoc	tonight
top	topical, topically
TOP	termination of pregnancy

TOPS	Total Ozone Portable Spectrometer
TOPV	trivalent oral poliovirus vaccine
TORCH	*Toxoplasma*, rubella, cytomegalovirus, herpes simplex (screen)
TORP	total ossicular replacement prosthesis
TOTAL-C	total cholesterol
tourn	tourniquet
tox	toxic, toxicity, toxicology
t_p	physical half-life
TP	toilet paper • total protein • *Treponema pallidum* • true-positive
tPA	tissue plasminogen activator
TPA	third party administrator • tissue plasminogen activator
TPC	thromboplastic plasma component
TPCF	*Treponema pallidum* complement fixation (test)
TPD	temporary partial disability
TPE	therapeutic plasma exchange (plasmapheresis)
TPH	thromboembolic pulmonary hypertension
TPHA	*Treponema pallidum* hemagglutination (test)
TPi	*Treponema pallidum* immobilization (test)
TPIA	*Treponema pallidum* immune adherence
TPM	temporary pacemaker
TPN	total parenteral nutrition • triphospyridine nucleotide
TPNH	triphospyridine nucleotide reduced form
TPO	tryptophan peroxidase
TPP	thiamine pyrophosphate
TPR	temperature, pulse and respiration • testosterone production rate • total peripheral resistance • total pulmonary resistance
TPVR	total peripheral vascular resistance

TQM	total quality management
t_r	radiologic half-life
tr	tincture • trace • traction • treatment • tremor
TR	new tuberculin (tuberculin residue) • severe trauma • temperature, rectal • therapeutic radiology • tricuspid regurgitation • tubular resorption • turbidity-reducing • Therapeutic Recreation
trach	trachea • tracheostomy
TRAM	transverse rectus abdominis myocutaneous
trans	transverse
transm	transmission
traspl	transplant
trans sect	transverse section
TRAP	tartrate-resistant leukocyte acid phosphatase
TRBF	total renal blood flow
TRC	tanned red cell
treat	treatment
Trend	Trendelenburg (position, cannula, etc.)
Trep	*Treponema*
TRF	T-cell replacing factor • thyrotropin-releasing factor
TRH	thyrotropin-releasing hormone
TRI	total response index • trifocal
TRIC	trachoma-inclusion conjunctivitis
Trich	*Trichomonas*
trid	three days (*tridium*)
Trig	triglycerides
TRIS	tris (hydroxymethyl) aminomethane
TRIT	triturate
tRNA	transfer ribonucleic acid

TRO	temporary restraining order
Trp	tryptophan
TRP	tubular resorption of phosphate
TRS	tuboreticular structures
TRT	treatment • testosterone replacement therapy
TRU	turbidity-reducing unit
T_3RU	triiodothyronine resin uptake
TRUS	transrectal ultrasound
Tryp	tryptophan
TS	terminal sensation • test solution • thoracic surgery • tracheal sound • tricuspid stenosis • triple-strength • tubular sound • Tourette's Syndrome
T/S	thyroid-serum iodide ratio
TSA	trypticase soy agar • tumor-specific antigen
TSBB	transtracheal selective bronchial brushing
TSD	target-to-skin distance • Tay-Sachs disease
TSF	thrombopoietic-stimulating factor • triceps skin fold
TSG	tumor supression gene
TSH	thyroid-stimulating hormone-releasing factor
TSI	thyroid-stimulating immunoglobulin • triple sugar iron (agar)
TSIA	triple sugar iron agar
tsp	teaspoon
TSP	total serum protein
T-spica	thumb spica (bandage, cast)
T-spine	thoracic spine
TSR	transfer • total shoulder replacement
TSS	toxic shock syndrome
TST	tumor skin test
TSTA	tumor-specific transplantation antigen

TT	tetanus toxoid • therapeutic touch • thrombin time • thymol turbidity (test) • transit time (blood through heart)
TT_4	total (serum) thyroxine
TTA	transtracheal aspirates
TTC	triphenyltetrazolium chloride
TTD	temporary total disability
TTH	thyrotropic hormone
TTI	tension-time index • tissue thromboplastin inhibition (test) • temporary total impairment
TTM	transtelephonic ECG monitoring
TTN	transient tachypnea of the newborn
TTNB	transient tachypnea of the newborn
TTP	therapeutic touch practitioner • thrombotic thrombocytopenic purpura • thymidine triphosphate
TTS	temporary threshold shift
TU	toxin unit • transmission unit • tuberculin unit
T_3U	triiodothyronine resin uptake (test)
tuberc	tuberculosis, tuberculous
TUR	transurethral resection
T_3UR	triiodothyronine uptake ratio
turb	turbidity
TURB	transurethral resection of the bladder
TURBTs	transurethral resection of the bladder tumors
TURP	transurethral resection of the prostrate
tus	cough (*tussis*)
tv	transvenous
TV	television • tetrazolium violet • tidal volume • total volume • trial visit • *Trichomonas vaginalis*
TVC	timed vital capacity • true vocal chord
TVH	total vaginal hysterectomy

TVR	tonic vibration reflex
TW	thin-walled
TWB	touch weight-bearing
TWE	tap-water enema
TWZ	triangular working zone
Tx	traction • transplant • treatment
TXA_2	thromboxane A_2
TXB_2	thromboxane B_2
Ty	type
Tyr	tyrosine
TZD	thiazolidinediones

U

U	unit • upper • uracil • uranium • urine • urology, urologist
U100	100 units per millimeter
ua	up to, as far as (*usque ad*)
UA	uric acid • urinalysis • urocanic acid • unstable angina
U/A	urinalysis • uterine activity
UAC	umbilical artery catheter
UAGA	Uniform Anatomical Gift Act
UAI	uterine activity integral
UAL	up (out of bed) as tolerated
UB	Unna's boot
UB-82	Uniform Billing Form of 1982
UBA	undenatured bacterial antigen
UBE	upper body exercise
UBG	urobilinogen
UBI	ultraviolet blood irradiation

UC	ulcerative colitis • Uldall catheter • unchanged • unit coordinator • urea clearance • urinary catheter • usual care • uterine contractions
U & C	usual and customary
UCA	unit communications assistant • unadjusted copayment amount
UCC	urgent care center
UCD	usual childhood diseases • unemployment compensation disability
UCE	urea cycle enzymopathy
UCG	urinary chorionic gonadotropin
UCHD	usual childhood diseases
UCL	uncomfortable loudness level • urea clearance • upper control limits
UCNT	undifferentiated carcinoma of the nasopharyngeal type
UCPA	United Cerebral Palsy Associations
UCR	unconditioned reflex • unconditioned response • usual, customary and reasonable
UCR/PACE	usual, customary and reasonable/performance and cost efficiency
UCS	unconditioned stimulus
UCV	uncontrolled variable
UCVA	uncorrected visual acuity
ud	as directed (*ut dictum*)
UD	unipolar depression • urethral discharge • uridine diphosphate
UDC	usual diseases of childhood
UDCA	ursodeoxycholic acid
UDO	undetermined origin
UDP	uridine diphosphate
UDPG	uridine diphosphoglucose

UDPGA	uridine disphosphoglucuronic acid
UDPGT	uridine diphosphoglucuronyltransferase
UE	upper extremity
UEF	Uninsured Employers Fund
UES	upper esophageal sphincter
UF	ultrafiltration
UFA	unesterified fatty acids
UG	urogenital
UGA	under general anesthesia
UGDP	University Group Diabetes Program
UGH	uveitis, glaucoma, hyphema
UGI	upper gastrointestinal
UGI-SBFT	upper gastrointestinal with small bowel follow-through (x-ray)
UHDDS	Uniform Hospital Discharge Data Set
UHF	ultrahigh frequency
UHV	ultrahigh voltage
UI	uroporphyrin isomerase
UIBC	unsaturated iron-binding capacity
UK	urokinase
UKPDS	United Kingdom Prospective Diabetes Study
U/L	upper and lower
ULQ	upper left quadrant
ult	ultimate, ultimately
ult praes	at last prescribed (*ultimum praescriptus*)
UM	upper motor (neuron) • uracil mustard • uterine monitor • Utilization Management
umb	umbilical, umbilicus
UMP	uridine monophosphate

UN	urea nitrogen
U_{NA}	urine sodium
uncomp	uncompensated
uncond	unconditioned
uncond ref	unconditioned reflex
uncor	uncorrected
unCS	unconditioned stimulus
ung	ointment (*unguentum*)
unilat	unilateral, unilaterally
univ	university
unk	unknown
UNOS	United Network for Organ Sharing
UnS	unconditioned stimulus
UNSCEAR	United Nations Scientific Committee on the Effects of Atomic Radiation
UOP	urinary output
UOQ	upper outer quadrant
UOS	unit of service
UP	ureteropelvic • uteroplacental
U/P	ratio of urine concentration to plasma concentration
up ad lib	up (out of bed) as desired (*ad libitum*)
UPDRS	Unified Parkinson's Disease Rating Scale
UPI	uteroplacental insufficiency
UPJ	ureteropelvic junction
UPP	urethral pressure profilometry
UPPP	uvulopalatal pharyngoplasty
UPRR	unit peer recognition and reward
UQ	upper quadrant

ur	urine
UR	unconditioned reflex • unconditioned response • unrelated • upper respiratory • utilization review
URC	utilization review committee • utilization review coordinator
Urd	uridine
URI	upper respiratory infection
Urol	urology, urologist
URQ	upper right quadrant
URTI	upper respiratory tract infection
US	ultrasonic, ultrasonography, ultrasound • unconditioned stimulus • unit secretary
U/S	ultrasound
USAEC	United States Atomic Energy Commission
USAMRID	United States Army Medical Research Institute of Infectious Disease
USAN	United States Adopted Name
USD	United States Dispensatory
USN	ultrasonic nebulization, nebulizer • United States Navy
USNH	United States Naval Hospital
USP	United States Pharmacopeia
USPC	United States Pharmacopeial Convention
USPHS	United States Public Health Service
USPSTF	United States Preventive Services Task Force
USR	unheated serum reagin
USRDA	United States Recommended Dietary Allowance
UTBG	unbound thyroxine-binding globulin
ut dict	as directed (*ut dictum*)
utend	to be used (*utendus*)
UTI	urinary tract infection

UTP	uridine triphosphate
UTZ	ultrasound
UU	urine urobilinogen
UUN	urine urea nitrogen
UV	ultraviolet
UVA	long-wavelength ultraviolet light (320-400 nm)
UVB	medium-wavelength ultraviolet light (290-320 nm)
UVC	short-wavelength ultraviolet light (less than 290 nm)
UVJ	ureterovesical junction
UVL	ultraviolet light
UVR	ultraviolet radiation
UWS	underwater seal (drainage)
UZ	ultrasound

V

v	see (*vide*) • vein • velocity • venous blood • volt
V	unipolar ECG chest lead (V1, V2...V6) • vanadium • vein • velocity • venous blood • ventilation • verbal • vertex • *Vibrio* • viral, virus • virulence • vision • visual acuity • visual capacity • voice • volt • volume
V°	gas volume per unit of time
va	volt-ampere
Va	arterial gas volume
VA	alveolar gas volume • vacuum aspiration • ventroculoatrial • Veterans Administration • visual acuity • volt-ampere • videoarthroscopy • volume adjustment
vac	vacuum
VAC	vincristine, actinomycin D, cyclophosphamide • vacuum-assisted closure
vacc	vaccination

VACTERL	vertebral, anal, cardiac, tracheoesophageal, renal, limb (syndrome)
VAD	ventricular assistive device • vincristine, adriamycin, dexamethasone
VAE	venous air embolism
VAERS	Vaccine Adverse Event Reporting System
vag	vagina, vaginal
Vag Hyst	vaginal hysterectomy
VAH	Veterans Administration Hospital
VAHS	virus-associated hemophagocytic syndrome
val	valine • valve
VAMC	Veterans Administration Medical Center
VAMP	vincristine, amethopterin, 6-mercaptopurine, prednisone
VAP	ventilator-associated pneumonia
V°a/Q°c	ratio of ventilation (alveolar) to perfusion (pulmonary capillary)
var	variation, variety
VAS	visceral analog scores
vasc	vascular
VASC	Verbal Auditory Screen for Children
vasodil	vasodilation
VAT	ventricular pacing, atrial sensing, triggered mode (pacemaker)
VATER	vertebral, anal, tracheoesophageal fistula, and radial or renal (deficiencies)
VATH	vinblastine, adriamycin, thiotepa, halotestin
VATS	video-assisted thoracoscopic surgery
VB	vinblastine
VBAC	vaginal birth after cesarean
VBG	venoaortocoronary artery bypass graft • vertical banded gastroplasty

VBI	vertebrobasilar insufficiency
VBM	vinblastine, bleomycin, methotrexate
V_c	pulmonary capillary gas volume
VC	acuity of color vision • capillary volume • vena cava • venous capacitance • ventilatory capacity • vincristine • vital capacity • vocal cord
VCA	viral capsid antigen
V_{CF}	mean fiber-shortening rate
VCF	vertebral body compression fracture
VCG	vectorcardiogram
VCM	vinyl chloride monomer
VCO_2	carbon dioxide output
$V°CO_2$	carbon dioxide output rate
VCR	vincristine
VCU	voiding cystourethrogram
vd	double vibrations
V_D	dead-space gas volume
VD	venereal disease
VDA	venous digital angiogram • visual discriminatory acuity
VDC	vasodilator center
VDEL	Venereal Disease Experimental Laboratory
VDG	venereal disease - gonorrhea
VDH	valvular disease of the heart
VDM	vasodepressor material
VDRL	Venereal Disease Research Laboratory (test)
VDS	vasodilator substance • venereal disease - syphilis
VDT	video display terminal
VDU	visual display unit
V_D/V_T	ratio of dead-space gas volume to tidal gas volume

V_E	volume of expired gas
VE	vesicular exanthem • visual examination • vocational evaluation
VEA	ventricular ectopic arrhythmia
vect	vector
VEE	Venezuelan equine encephalitis • Venezuelan equine encephalomyelitis
VEGF	vascular endothelial growth factor
vel	velocity
VEM	vasoexcitor material • vasoexcitor mechanism
vent	ventilation, ventilator • ventral • ventricle, ventricular
vent fib	ventricular fibrillation
VEP	visual evoked potential
VER	visual evoked response
vert	vertebra • vertical
ves	bladder (*vesica*) • vesicular
vesic	bladder (*vesica*)
VESID	Vocational and Educational Services for Individuals with Disabilities
VETS	Veterans Adjustment Scale
VF	ventricular fibrillation • ventricular flutter • video frequency • visual field • vocal fremitus
VFC	ventricular function curve
VFD	visual feed-back display
VFib	ventricular fibrillation
VFl	ventricular flutter
v flutter	ventricular flutter
VFT	vestibular function tests
VF/VT	ventricular fibrillation and ventricular tachycardia

VG	vein graft • ventricular gallop • very good
VH	vaginal hysterectomy • veterans hospital • viral hepatitis
VHA	volunteer health agency
VHCA	Virginia Healthcare Association
VHDL	very high density lipoprotein
VHF	very high frequency • viral hemorrhagic fever
VHL	Von Hippel-Lindau disease
V_I	volume of inspired gas
VI	volume index
VIA	virus-inactivating agent
vib	vibration
VIC	vasoinhibitory center
vid	see (*vide*)
VIG	vaccinia immune globulin
vin	wine (*vinum*)
VIP	vasoactive intestinal polypeptide • very important person
VIQ	Verbal Intelligence Quotient
vis	vision • visiting, visitor
VIS	vaginal irrigation smear
visc	visceral • viscous, viscosity
vit	vital • vitamin
vitel	yolk (*vitellus*)
viz	that is, namely (*videlicet*)
VLA	very late activation (antigen)
VLBW	very low birth weight
VLCD	very low density lipoprotein
VLDL-TG	very low density lipoprotein - triglyceride
VLF	very low frequency

VLM	visceral larva migrans
VLP	ventriculolumbar perfusion
VM	Venturi mask • viomycin • voltmeter
VMA	vanillylmandelic acid
V_{max}	maximum velocity, rate
VMO	vastus medialis oblique
VNA	Visiting Nursing Association
VNS	Visiting Nurse Service
VO	verbal order
VO_2	oxygen consumption
$V°O_2$	oxygen consumption rate
VOC	volatile organic compounds
VOD	vision, right eye (*oculus dexter*)
vol	volume
VOO	ventricular pacing, no sensing, no other function (pacemaker)
VOS	vision, left eye (*oculus sinister*)
VOT	Visual Organization Test
vp	vapor pressure
VP	variegate porphyria • vasopressin • venipuncture • venous pressure • ventriculo-peritoneal shunt • Voges-Proskauer reaction
V&P	vagotomy and pyloroplasty
VPA	valproic acid
VPB	ventricular premature beat
VPC	ventricular premature contraction
VPD	ventricular premature depolarization
VPI	velopharyngeal insufficiency
VPN	Vice-President, Nursing
$V°/Q°$	ventilation-perfusion ratio

VR	right vision • variable ratio • venous return • ventilation rate • ventral root (of spinal nerves) • ventricular response • vocal resonance • vocational rehabilitation
VRA	Vocational Rehabilitation Administration • Visual Response Audiometry
VR&E	vocational rehabilitation and education
VRI	viral respiratory infection
VRMA	Vocational Rehabilitation Maintenance Allowance
VRIN	variable response inconsistency scale
VRIS	variable response inconsistency scale
VRP	very reliable product
VRT	voice-recognition technology
VRTD	Vocational Rehabilitation Maintenance Benefit
VRV	ventricular residual volume
vs	single vibrations • versus • vibration-second
VS	ventricular septum • vesicular sound • vesicular stomatitis • vital signs • volumetric solution
VSD	ventricular septal defect

W

w	watt • week • wife • with
W	tungsten (*wolfram*) • water • watt • weber (unit of magnetic flux) • wehnelt unit • weight • white cell • widow, widowed, widower • width • word fluency
WA	when awake
WAIS	Wechsler Adult Intelligence Scale
WAIS-R	Wechsler Adult Intelligence Scale - Revised
WAN	wide area network
WAP	wandering atrial pacemaker
Wass	Wassermann test
Wb	weber (unit of magnetic flux)

WB	washable base • water bottle • Wechsler-Bellevue (scale) • weight-bearing • wet-bulb • whole blood
WBAT	weight-bearing as tolerated
WBC	white blood cell • while blood (cell) count
WBCT	whole-blood clotting time
WBH	whole-body hematocrit
WBPTT	whole-blood partial thromboplastin time
WBR	whole body radiation
WBS	whole body scan
WBT	wet-bulb temperature
w/c	wheelchair
WC	ward clerk • water closet (bathroom) • wheelchair • whooping cough • worker's compensation
WCAB	Worker's Compensation Appeals Board
WCHPO	Worker's Compensation Healthcare Provider Organization
WCGS	Western Collaborative Group Study
WCJ	worker's compensation judge
WCR	Walthard's cell rests
wd	ward • wound
WD	well-developed • well-differentiated • wet dressing • Wilson's disease • wrist disarticulation
w/d	warm and dry • well-developed
WDHA	watery diarrhea, hypokalmeia, achlorhydria
WDHH	watery diarrhea, hypokalemia, hypochlorhydria
WD/WN	well-developed, well-nourished
W/E	week-end
WEE	Western equine encephalitis • Western equine encephalomyelitis
wf	white female

WFC	Work Fitness Center
WFL	within functional limits
wh	whisper, whispered • white
WH	well-healed • well-hydrated • Work Hardening
WHO	World Health Organization
w-hr	watt-hour
WHVP	wedged hepatic venous pressure
WIA	wounded in action
WIC	Welfare and Institution Code • women, infants and children
wid	widow, widowed, widower
WIMP	Workers in Modified Productivity
WISC	Wechsler Intelligence Scale for Children
WISC-R	Wechsler Intelligence Scale for Children - Revised
wk	weak • week
WK	Wernicke-Korsakoff (syndrome)
/wk	per week
WL	waiting list • wavelength • work load
WLM	working-level month
WLS	weight loss surgery
wm	white male
WM	wall motion • wet mount • whole milk • whole mount
WMA	World Medical Association
WMS	wall-motion study • Wechsler Memory Scale
Wms. Flex. Ex.	Williams flexion exercises
w/n	well-nourished
WN	well-nourished
wnd	wound
WNL	within normal limits

wo	weeks old
w/o	without
W/O	water in oil
WOR	Weber-Osler-Rondu (syndrome)
WOU	women's outpatient unit
w/p	whirlpool
WP	wet pack • working point
WPPSI	Wechsler Preschool and Primary Scale of Intelligence
WPW	Wolf-Parkinson-White (syndrome)
WR	Wassermann reaction • work rate • wedge resection
WRAT	Wide-Range Achievement Test
ws	watt second
WS	ward secretary • water-soluble
WSD	water seal drainage
wt	weight
w/u	work-up
w/v	weight (of solute) per volume (of solvent)
WV	whispered voice
w/w	weight (of solute) per weight (of solvent)

X

x	axis • multiplied by • times
X	cross • cross section • Kienböck's unit (of X-ray exposure) • multiplied by • times • transverse section • unknown
x̄	mean
X	except
Xa	chiasma
Xao	xanthosine
XC	excretory cystogram

XD	X-linked dominant
XDP	xeroderma pigmentosum
Xe	xenon
Xfmr	transformer
XGP	xanthogranulomatous pyelonephritis
XLP	X-linked lymphoproliferative (disorder)
X-match	crossmatch
XMP	xanthosine monophosphate
XO	xanthine oxidase
XOAN	x-linked ocular albinism
XP	exophoria • xeroderma pigmentosum
XR	x-linked recessive • x-ray
XRT	X-ray therapy
XT	exotropia, exotropic
XU	excretory urogram
XUV	extreme ultraviolet
XX	normal female sex chromosome type
XY	normal male sex chromosome type
Xyl	xylose
Xylo	Xylocaine

Y

y	yield
Y	young • yttrium
YACP	young adult chronic patient
YAG	yttrium-aluminum-garnet (laser)
Yb	ytterbium
yd	yard

YE	yellow enzyme
yel	yellow
YF	yellow fever
y/o	years old
YOB	year of birth
YP	yeast phase • yield pressure
yr	year
ys	yellow spot
YS	yolk sac
YTD	year-to-date
Y2K	Year 2000

Z

Z	no effect • symbol for atomic number • zero • zone
Z, Z′, Z″	increasing degrees of contraction
ZDV	zidovudine
ZE	Zollinger-Ellison (syndrome)
ZES	Zollinger-Ellison syndrome
ZIG	zoster immune globulin
ZIP	zoster immune plasma
Zn	zinc
Zn fl	zinc flocculation (test)
ZPG	zero population growth
Zr	zirconium
ZSR	zeta sedimentation rate • zinc sedimentation rate
Zz	ginger (*zingiber*)

EPONYMS

Aaron's sign	Pain in the epigastric or precordial region in appendicitis.
Aarskog syndrome	Faciogenital dysphasia.
Abadie's sign	Spasm of the levator palpebrae superioris in thyrotoxicosis.
Abbe's flap	A triangular portion of the lower lip used to repair a defect in the upper lip.
Abbe's operation	Using a triangular portion of the lower lip to repair a defect in the upper lip.
Abbott's method	Treatment of scoliosis by pulling the spine into the proper position and then applying a plaster cast to hold in place.
Abderhalden-Kauffman-Lignac syndrome	Renal rickets with cystinosis.
Abernethy's fascia	Fascia iliaca.
Abraham's sign	A percussive sound heard over the lung with early tuberculosis.
Abrams' heart reflex	Contraction of the myocardium when the precordial region is irritated.
Abrikosov's tumor	Granular cell tumor.
Achard's syndrome	Arachnodactyly associated with a receding mandible and joint laxity in the hands and feet.
Achard-Thiers syndrome	Women with diabetes and aspects of both adrenogenital syndrome and Cushing syndrome including masculinization and menstrual disorders.
Achilles tendon	Tendon attaching the gastrocnemius to the calcaneus.
Ackerman tumor	Verrucous carcinoma of the larynx.
Acosta disease	Hypoxic disease caused by high elevation.
Adair Dighton's syndrome	Osteogenesis imperfecta.
Adams Stokes syndrome	Episodic cardiac arrest and syncope.
Addison disease	Syndrome caused by insufficient hormone production by the adrenal glands.

Adson test	Test for thoracic outlet syndrome.
Albee lumbar fusion	Fusion of the spine using grafts across the spinous processes in spondylolisthesis.
Alber-Schönberg disease	Osteoporosis.
Albrecht's bone	Basiotic bone.
Albright's syndrome	Inherited hypoparathyroidism associated with skeletal defects; polyostotic fibrous dysplasia.
Alcock canal	Tunnel enclosing pudendal vessels and nerves.
Alpers disease	Progressive cerebral poliodystrophy.
Alzheimer's disease	Irreversible degenerative senile dementia.
Ames test	Test for carcinogens using strains of Salmonella typhinium that will mutate if carcinogens are present.
Anders disease	Adiposa tuberosa simplex.
Andersen disease	Type IV glycogenosis.
Andersen's syndrome	Cystic fibrosis of the pancreas, bronchiectasis and vitamin A deficiency.
Andrade's syndrome	Familial amyloid polyneuropathy.
Apert's syndrome	Acrocephalosyndactyly, type I.
Apert-Crouzon disease	Acrocephalosyndactyly, type I.
Apgar score	Numerical score evaluating the condition of an infant at birth.
Aran-Duchenne disease	Spinal muscular atrophy.
Argyll Robertson pupil	Miotic pupil which reacts to accommodation but does not react to light.
Arnold ganglion	Otic ganglion, situated below the foramen ovale, medial to the mandibular nerve.
Arnold-Chiari deformity (malformation/syndrome)	Congenital anomaly of the cerebellum and medulla oblongata.
Arnold Pick disease (atrophy)	Circumscribed cerebral atrophy.
Ascheim-Zondek test	Pregnancy test performed by injecting the woman's urine into immature female mice.
Aschoff bodies (nodules)	Granuloma specific for rheumatic fever.
Ashman phenomenon	Aberrant arrhythmia of atrial fibrillation.
Asperger's syndrome	Idiot savant.

Auer bodies	Faulty granule formations in myeloblastic and monoblastic leukemia.
Auerbach plexus	Esophageal autonomic nerve plexus.
Austin Flint murmur	Diastolic mitral valve murmur.
Ayerza disease (syndrome)	Type of polycythemia vera.
Baastrup disease	"Kissing spine" – false joint of the lumbar spine.
Baastrup syndrome	Kissing spines.
Babès-Ernst granules (bodies)	Metachromatic granules present in bacterial cells, yeasts, fungi and protozoa.
Babington disease	Hereditary telangiectasia.
Babinsku reflex (sign)	Dorsiflexion of the great toe upon plantar stimulation, considered indicative of pyramidal tract disturbance.
B.A.D.S. syndrome	Oculocutaneous albinism.
Baghdad boil	Lesion occurring in the cutaneous leishmaniasis.
Baker cyst	Enlarged popiteal bursa associated with degenerative disease of the knee.
Balser fatty necrosis	Gangrenous pancreatitis with omental bursitis and disseminated patches of necrosis of the fatty tissues.
Bamberger-Marie disease	Hypertrophic pulmonary osteoarthropathy.
Banks-Dervin rod	Multiple level rod that is fixed with the oblique spinous process to contralateral lamina screws.
Bannwarth's syndrome	European term for menengopolyneuritis found with Lyme disease.
Banti disease (syndrome)	Portal hypertension with congestive splenomegaly.
Barlow disease	Infantile scurvy.
Barlow syndrome	Mitral valve prolapse syndrome.
Barr body	Sex chromatin.
Barrett's esophagus (syndrome)	Chronic peptic ulcer of the lower esophagus.
Bartholin cyst	Retention cyst of the major vestibular or Bartholin gland.
Bartholin gland	Greater vestibular gland; vulvovaginal gland

Barton fracture	Fracture of the distal radius into the wrist joint.
Bartter syndrome	Juxtaglomerular cell hyperplasia with hypokalemic alkalosis and hyperaldosteronism.
Basedow disease	Graves' disease; a form of hyperthyroidism characterized by thyrotoxicosis with diffuse hyperplasia, exophthalmos of pretibial myxedema.
Bassen-Kornzweig syndrome	Abetalipoproteinemia.
Battle sign	Discoloration near the tip of the mastoid process which is seen in basilar skull fractures.
Bearn-Kunkel syndrome	Lupoid hepatitis.
Beau lines	Transverse grooves on fingernails after serious illness or trauma.
Behçet's syndrome	Chronic inflammatory disorder involving ulcerations of mucous membranes in the mouth, genitals and eyes, and frequently arthritis.
Bell's palsy	Paralysis of the facial nerve.
Bence Jones protein	Abnormal protein found in the urine of patients with multiple myeloma.
Benedict solution	Aqueous solution of sodium citrate, sodium carbonate and copper sulfate that is used to test for the presence of glucose in the urine.
Berger disease	Glomerulonephritis.
Bernheim syndrome	Right venticular failure with left ventricular hypertrophy.
Bezold's abscess	Abscess in the neck following a bout of mastoiditis.
Billroth gastrectomy (operation)	Resection of the stomach with anastomosis to the duodenum (Billroth I) or to the jejunum (Billroth II).
Blackfan-Diamond anemia	Congenital hypoplastic anemia.
Blalock-Taussig operation	Surgery to repair the congenital cardiac defect known as the tetralogy of Fallot.
Bohman fusion	Posterior triple spinous process wiring technique in the cervical spine to secure bone graft.
Bosworth lumbar fusion	A fusion using an H-shaped bone graft in spondylolisthesis.

Bradford procedure	Staged anterior and posterior approach for interbody fusion and correction of deformity.
Brattstrom fusion	Use of acrylic cement for C-1 to C-2 fusion.
Braxton-Hicks contractions	Light, painless uterine contractions during pregnancy.
Bright disease	Chronic nonsuppurative nephritis.
Briquet's syndrome	Somatization disorder.
Brissaud-Marie syndrome	Hysterical glossolabial hemispasm.
Broca's aphasia	Also termed ataxic, expressive or motor aphasia; patients with Broca's aphasia have difficulty with verbal expression and articulation, but may write or sign well.
Brock's operation	Transventricular valvotomy.
Brompton solution (cocktail)	Analgesic cocktail usually of morphine and cocaine often given to the terminally ill.
Brooks and Jenkins fusion	Loops of wire around lamina of C-1 and C-2 to hold bone graft between lamina.
Brunner glands	Duodenal glands.
Budd-Chiari syndrome	Hepatosplenomegaly, jaundice, ascites and portal hypertension caused by hepatic vein occlusion.
Burkitt's lymphoma	Malignant lymphoma usually found in Africa, but also seen elsewhere including the United States, that may involve the facial bones, ovaries, or abdominal lymph nodes.
Callahan fusion	Individual wire fixation of a strut bone graft to involved facets.
Capner procedure	Draining of thoracic spinal abscess through an anterolateral approach.
Chadwick sign	Blue discoloration of vaginal mucosa that indicates pregnancy.
Charcot's syndrome	Amyotrophic lateral sclerosis.
Charcot-Marie-Tooth disease	Peroneal muscular atrophy.
Cheyne-Stokes respirations	Recurrent episodes of rapid breathing alternating with apnea, often seen in coma resulting from affection of the nervous centers.
Chopart's amputation	Transtarsal amputation of the forefoot.

Christmas disease	Hemophilia B; also called Factor IX deficiency (hemophilia); caused by hereditary deficiency of Factor IX.
Chvostek's sign	Spasm of the facial muscles caused by tapping the facial nerve near the parotid gland.
Colles fracture	Fractured distal radius with posterior displacement.
Conn's syndrome	Primary aldosteronism.
Coombs test	Antiglobulin test.
Cotrell-Dobousset instrumentation	Posterior fixation device for spinal deformity, fracture, tumor, and degenerative conditions.
Cowper cyst	Retention cyst of the bulbourethral glands.
Crohn's disease	Regional ileitis or enteritis.
Cronkite-Canada syndrome	Juvenile polyposis and ectodermal lesions.
Cushing syndrome	Hyperadrenocorticism; also called Cushing's basophilism or pituitary basophilism.
Dakin solution (fluid)	Antiseptic of diluted sodium hypochlorite used to irrigate wounds.
Dandy-Walker syndrome	A form of hydrocephalus.
de Andrade and McNab fusion	Anterior approach for cervical occipital fusion.
Delmege's sign	Flattening of the deltoid muscles seen as an early sign of tuberculosis.
Donohue's syndrome	Leprechaunism.
Douglas' abscess	Abscess in the rectouterine pouch.
Down syndrome	Syndrome of mental retardation caused by chromosomal abnormality where chromosome 21 appears three times instead of twice in some or all cells. Also called trisomy 21; formerly called mongoloidism.
Dressler's syndrome	Post-myocardial infarction syndrome.
Dubois' abscess	Abscess of the thymus in congenital syphilis.
Duchenne paralysis	(1) Progressive bulbar paralysis; (2) pseudohypertrophic muscular dystrophy.
Dunn procedure	Use of a conturing L-rod for posterior stabilization with myelomeningocele spinal deformity.

Dupuytren's contracture	Flexure of the 4th and 5th fingers due to contracture of palmar fascia.
Dwyer instrumentation	Anteriorly placed screws and band device for correction of spinal deformities.
Dwyer-Hartsill procedure	Pedicle screws wired to a rectangular frame along with posterolateral fusion.
Eddowes disease (syndrome)	Osteogenesis imperfecta.
Edwards instrumentation	Posterior rod and sleeve device used in destabilization of traumatic spinal conditions.
Ehlers-Danlos syndrome	Cutis hyperelastica; a group of inherited connective tissue disorders producing overelasticity and friability of the skin, excessive extensibility of the joints, and fragility of the cutaneous blood vessels, due to deficient quality or quantity of collagen.
Epstein's anomaly	Rare congenital heart defect in which an abnormal tricuspid valve prevents backward blood flow from the right ventricle to the right atrium.
Epstein's syndrome	Nephrotic syndrome.
Epstein-Barr virus	Virus found in infectious mononucleosis and Burkitt's lymphoma; human herpesvirus 4.
Erb-Goldflam disease	Myasthenia gravis.
Ewing sarcoma	Malignant bone tumor usually found in children.
Faber's syndrome	Hypochronic anemia.
Fabere's sign	The hip is rotated internally and externally then placed in an external position with the foot resting on the opposite knee. Pain denotes hip disease rather than lumbar disc pathology.
Fallot tetralogy	Ventricular-septal defect, pulmonary stenosis, right ventricular hypertrophy and dextraposition of the aorta occurring as a congenital anomaly.
Forestier disease	Ankylosing spinal hyperostosis.
Franco's operation	Suprapubic cystotomy.
Friedländer bacillus	*Klebsiella pneumoniae.*
Friedreich ataxia	Hereditary spinal ataxia; an autosomal recessive disease usually beginning in childhood with sclerosis of the posterior and lateral columns of

the spinal cord and ataxia of the lower extremities, followed by paralysis and contractures.

Fuller's operation	Perineal incision and drainage of the seminal vesicles.
Gallie fusion	Wire around lamina of C-1 and C-2.
Getty procedure	Excision of lamina and a portion of the facet for decompression of lumbar spinal stenosis.
Gifford sign	Inability to evert the upper eyelid in Graves' disease (hyperthyroidism).
Gill lumbar fusion	Removal of the posterior spinal arch in spondylolisthesis.
Goodpasture syndrome	Acute glomerulonephritis with intrapulmonary hemorrhage, hemoptysis and anemia, usually progressing to renal failure.
Graves' disease	Hyperthyroidism characterized by diffuse goiter, often seen with exophthalmos.
Guillain-Barré syndrome	Acute idiopathic polyneuritis; rapidly progressing ascending motor neuron paralysis usually beginning with the feet and spreading to the legs, arms, trunk and face.
Gull disease	Atrophy of the thyroid with myxedema (hypothyroidism).
Halifax fusion	Clamp across lamina of C-1 and C-2.
Hand-Schüller-Christian disease	Chronic idiopathic histiocytosis.
Hansen disease	Leprosy.
Harrington rod	Instrumentation and fusion using a straight, stiff rod for distraction or compression; associated with a posterior spinal fusion in the thoracic or thoracolumbar spine for scoliosis or trauma.
Hartmann pouch	Abnormal pouch formed at the neck of the gallbladder.
Hartmann's procedure	Colon resection.
Hartmann solution	Intravenous lactated Ringer's solution.
Hashimoto disease	Autoimmune thyroiditis.
Heberden nodes	Bony prominence and flexion deformities of the finger joints associated with osteoarthritis.

Heimlich maneuver	Method of dislodging a foreign body from the airway by applying quick thrust pressure to the subdiaphragmatic area.
Henoch-Schonlein purpura	Allergic or anaphylactic purpura (an inflammation of small blood vessels of the skin, joint, gastrointestinal tract and kidneys).
Hey's hernia	An encysted hernia.
Hibbs spinal fusion	Lumbar spinal fusion that includes fusing the spinous process, lamina, and facet for stabilization.
Hirschberg sign	Adduction reflex of the foot.
Hirschsprung's disease	Congenital megacolon.
Hodgkin's disease	Common malignant lymphoma marked by chronic enlargement of the lymph nodes together with enlargement of the spleen and often liver.
Hodgson disease	Uniform aneurysmal dilation of the aorta associated with insufficiency of the aortic valve, often accompanied by dilation or hypertrophy of the heart.
Hodgson procedure	Anterior approach to C-1 and C-2 area for drainage of tuberculous abscess.
Holter monitor	Device for recording an ambulatory electrocardiogram.
Homan's sign	Pain upon passive dorsiflexion of the foot as a positive sign for deep venous thrombus.
Horton syndrome (cephalalgia)	Histaminic or cluster headache.
Huntington chorea	Hereditary chorea; autosomal dominant disease characterized by irregular, spasmodic movements in the face and extremities, accompanied by progressive mental deterioration ending in dementia.
Hurler disease (syndrome)	Mucopolusaccharidosis IH.
Ishihara test	Test for color blindness that utilizes plates upon which figures are formed from round dots of various colors.
Isola instrumentation	Posterior fixation device.
Jacobs locking hook	Thick, threaded rods for fixation of various spinal deformities.

Jakob-Creutzfeldt disease	Spastic pseudoparalysis; a rare, usually fatal, transmissible spongiform encephalopathy characterized by progressive dementia, myoclonus and ataxia.
Jarcho-Levin syndrome	Defects of the spine associated with a small, stiff thorax and pulmonary compromise.
Kaneda device	Anteriorly placed fixation device for spinal deformities.
Kawasaki syndrome (disease)	Febrile mucocutaneous lymph node disease.
Kaposi sarcoma	Multiple idiopathic hemorrhagic sarcoma; multifocal malignant neoplasm characterized by reddish-purple cutaneous lesions, usually seen in men over 60 years of age and as an opportunistic infection in AIDS patients.
K-B technique	Kleihauer-Betke, a procedure done to diagnose fetomaternal hemorrhage.
Kernig sign	Flexion of hip and extension of leg while recumbent causes pain; a positive sign for meningitis.
Killian's operation	Excision of the anterior wall of the frontal sinus.
Kirschner wire (apparatus)	Steel wire used for skeletal fixation of, and obtaining skeletal traction in, fractures.
Klinefelter's syndrome	XXY syndrome; feminization of males due to extra X chromosomes combined with one Y chromosome, resulting in small testes and infertility.
Knodt distraction rod	Device used for distraction stabilization of the thoracic and lumbar spine.
Koenig syndrome (König)	Diarrhea alternating with constipation, seen with abdominal pain, meteorism and gurgling sounds on the right iliac fossa, symptomatic of cecal tuberculosis.
Kostmann's syndrome	Infantile genetic agranulocytosis.
Kostuick-Harrington instrumentation	Anteriorly placed device for spinal deformity correction.
Krebs cycle	Citric acid or trocarboxylic acid cycle; a basic metabolic mechanism involving the oxidation of acetic acid for energy stored in phosphate bonds.
Krönlein's hernia	Inguinoproperitoneal hernia.

Kussmaul disease	Polyarteritis nodosa; necrosis of the small and medium-sized arteries.
Kussmal respirations	Rapid, deep respiration due to diabetic ketoacidosis.
Lachman test	Test used to confirm anterior or posterior cruciate instability.
Laënnec cirrhosis	Alcoholic micronodular cirrhosis in which normal liver nodules are replaced by small regeneration nodules, sometimes containing fat.
Landry's syndrome	Acute idiopathic polyneuritis.
Langerhans adenoma	Islet cell adenoma of the pancreas; insulinoma.
Langerhans, isles of	Pancreatic insulin- and glucagon-producing cell clusters or islets
LaVeen shunt	Peritoneal-jugular shunt.
Leeds procedure	Segmental wiring of a contoured square-ended Harrington rod for scoliosis.
LeFort's fracture	Bilateral horizontal fracture of the maxilla.
Legg-Calvé-Perthes disease	Osteochondritis deformans juvenilis; necrosis of the upper end of the femur.
Lhermitte sign	Flexing the neck forward causes electric-shock-like pain in the extremities as a sign of multiple sclerosis or compression and other disorders of the cervical cord.
Lightwood's syndrome	Renal tubular acidosis.
Lobstein's syndrome	Osteogenesis imperfecta.
Localio procedure	Method of partial excision of the sacrum for sacral tumors.
Long Beach pedicle screw	Posterolateral fusion screw and rod device.
Loughheed and White procedure	Coccygectomy and drainage from space anterior to sacrum for drainage of lower abdominal abscesses.
Luque ISF	Pedicle screw and plate device used for posterolateral fusion fixation.
Lyme disease	Recurrent multisystemic disorder caused by a tick-borne spirochete characterized by erythema chronicum migrans lesions, fever, malaise, headache and stiff neck, followed by arthritic pain in the large joints.

MacCarthy procedure	Method of excision of the sacrum for sacral tumors.
Mageri fusion	Wire looped around lamina of C-1 and C-2.
Magerl fusion	Transarticular facet screw fusion for posterior C-1 on C-2 with the use of bilateral screws directed from inferior posterior lateral mass to anterior superior C-1.
Mallory-Weiss tear (lesion)	An esophageal or gastric tear, often due to prolonged or forceful vomiting, as seen in Mallory-Weiss syndrome.
Marfan disease (syndrome)	Autosomal-dominant congenital disorder of collagen and elastic connective tissues characterized by abnormal length of extremities, subluxation of the lens, and cardiovascular abnormalities.
Marie-Bamberger disease	Hypertrophic pulmonary osteoarthropathy; a disorder usually affecting the long bones of the arms and legs, often secondary to chronic pulmonary and heart disease.
Marie's sign	Tremor of the extremities seen in Graves' Disease.
Marie-Strümpell disease	Rheumatoid inflammation of the spine.
Marshall-Marchetti-Krant z operation	Surgery to relieve stress incontinence where the anterior portion of the urethra, vesical neck, and bladder are sutured to the posterior surface of the pubic bone.
McAffee fusion	Anterior retropharyngeal approach to upper cervical spine; often used for fusion, allowing excision of tumor.
McBurney's point	Spot on the abdomen overlying the normal position of the base of the appendix—this is a point of tenderness in acute appendicitis.
McConckey cocktail	Cod liver oil and tomato juice.
McDonald's operation	Using a purse-string suture to close the cervical os as a treatment for incompetent cervix.
McMurray test	Forcefully rotating the knee to assess for a tear of the meniscus.
Meckel's diverticulum	Abnormal sac or pouch near the ileum due to remains of the embryonic sac.
Ménière syndrome (disease)	Nausea, vomiting, tinnitus, vertigo and hearing loss caused by disease of the labyrinth.

Meyer fusion	Posterior fusion using vertical strut grafts and wires.
Millard-Gubler syndrome	Gubler hemiplegia or paralysis; 6th and 7th nerve palsy with contralateral hemiplegia affecting limbs on one side of the body and the face on the other, together with paralysis of outward movement of the eye, caused by infarction of the pons.
Milroy's disease	Congenital hereditary lymphedema.
Montgomery glands	Sweat glands located in the areola of the nipple.
Moore's syndrome	Abdominal epilepsy; producing paroxysmal abdominal pain as a sign of abnormal neuronal discharge from the brain.
Moro reflex	Startle reflex; contraction of the limb and neck muscles in infants when startled by a sudden noise, jolt or a short drop.
Morton's neuroma	Benign tumor of the tissue that surrounds the digital nerve leading to the toes.
Morvan's syndrome	Syringomyelia.
Moynahan syndrome	Progressive cardiomyopathic lentiginosis.
Munchausen syndrome	Repeated presentation to a physician and/or hospital with claims of an acute illness that is false, for the purpose of gaining medical attention.
Naffziger syndrome	Scalenusanticus syndrome.
Newman fusion	C-1 to C-2 posterior fusion without fixation.
Niemann-Pick disease	Sphingolipidosis; autosomal-recessive inherited lipid histiocytosis with accumulation of phispholipid (sphingomyelin) in histiocytes in the liver, spleen, lymph nodes and bone marrow.
Nissen operation	Fundoplication.
Osgood-Schlatter disease	Osteochondrosis of the tibial tuberosity as seen in adolescents.
Osler disease	Polycythemia vera or erythemia; chronic disease characterized by bone marrow hyperplasia, increase in blood volume as well as in number of red cells, redness of the skin, and splenomegaly.
Overton fusion	Dowel graft that is applied across facet joints.

Paget disease	(1) Osteitis deformans; (2) intraductal carcinoma of the breast; (3) neoplasm of the vulva.
Pancoast's tumor	Adenocarcinoma of the lung involving pain in the shoulder and arm due to 8th cervical and 1st thoracic nerve involvement.
Parkinson's disease	Paralysis agitans; a neurological disorder characterized by a reduction in dopamine levels, hypokinesia, tremors, and muscular rigidity.
Patau syndrome	Trisomy 13 syndrome; a chromosomal abnormality in which an extra chromosome 13 causes defects of the central nervous system, mental retardation, with cleft palate, polydactyly and cardiac problems, among others.
Patey's operation	Modified radical mastectomy.
Pel-Epstein fever	Cyclic fever common with Hodgkin disease featuring intermittent febrile episodes lasting for several days.
Pepper syndrome	Neuroblastoma of the adrenal gland with metastases in the liver.
Phalen's sign	Procedure to assess for possible carpal tunnel syndrome: wrists are flexed and held for one minute, if positive, there will be numbness in the fingers.
Pick's adenoma	Androblastoma.
Pickwickian syndrome	Name derived from the overweight boy in Charles Dickens' *Pickwick Papers*; obesity, somnolence and hypoxia with carbon dioxide retention.
Pott's disease	Tuberculosis of the spine.
Pott's fracture	Fracture of the lower fibula and injury of the lower tibial articulation, producing outward displacement of the foot.
Prinzmetal angina	Angina pectoris in which attacks occur during rest and for longer duration, accompanied by an ST segment elevation.
Raynaud's phenomenon	Intermittent ischemia of the fingers or toes marked by severe pallor and often accompanied by paralysis or pain, precipitated by exposure to the cold.

Reiter syndrome (disease)	Urethritis, arthritis and conjunctivitis, sometimes with diarrhea.
Rendu-Osler-Weber syndrome	Hereditary hemorrhagic telangiectasia.
Rett syndrome	Cerebroatrophic hyperammonemia.
Reye syndrome	Rare, often fatal, disease of children following an acute febrile illness such as influenza or varicella infection, characterized by recurrent vomiting, encephalopathy, hepatomegaly and fatty degeneration of the viscera.
Riley fusion	Extensive anterior approach for fusion of C-1 to C-3 or lower.
Ritter disease	Staphylococcal scalded skin syndrome; usually seen in infants where large areas of skin peel off, as in a second-degree burn, as a result of upper respiratory staphylococcal infection.
Rivers cocktail	Philadelphia cocktail; dextrose in saline with thiamine and insulin given intravenously to detoxify alcoholics.
Roaf, Kirkaldy-Willis and Cattero procedure	Drainage of a thoracic spinal abscess through dorsolateral approach.
Robinson and Rieux's hernia	Retrocecal hernia.
Rogozinki instrumentation	Combined anteroposterior device used in correction of spinal deformities.
Romberg sign	Increased unsteadiness when a standing patient closes the eyes indicating a loss of proprioceptive control.
Roux-en-Y anastomosis (operation)	Y-shaped anastomosis which includes the small intestine.
Roy-Camille fusion	Posterior bone graft with wire and parallel vertical screw plate fixation from occiput to C-3.
Roy-Camille instrumentation	Posterior pedicle screw and plate device for spinal stabilization.
Sabin vaccine	Live oral attenuated poliovirus vaccine.
St. Vitus' dance	Involuntary movement disorder now referred to as Syndenham's chorea.
Salk vaccine	Original poliovirus vaccine containing inactivated strains of the poliomyelitis virus.

Scheuermann disease	Inflammation of the anterior cartilage of the thoracic and lumbar spine.
Schmorl nodes	Extension of the invertebral disk into the vertebral bodies.
Scholiner costoplasty	Multiple rib partial excisions for rib deformity.
Scott procedure	Use of cross-wire fixation transverse process to inferior pedicle in stabilization of spondylolysis fusion.
Seddon procedure	Drainage of thoracic spinal abscess through anterolateral approach with partial resection of rib.
Shy-Dager syndrome	Chronic idiopathic orthostatic hypotension.
Simmons fusion	Use of keystone-shaped graft in anterior fusion.
Simmons procedure	Posterior osteotomy.
Sjögren syndrome	Keratoconjunctivitis sicca, xerostomia and rheumatoid arthritis, usually seen in menopausal women.
Skene glands	Paraurethral glands; mucous glands located in the wall of the female urethra.
Smith Peterson procedure	Lumbar spine osteotomy for correction of kyphotic deformity in ankylosing spondylitis.
Speed procedure (Kellogg Speed)	Spinal fusion and anterior interbody fusion by using tibial cortical grafts.
Spetzler fusion	Approach to anterior C-1 to C-3 by using a transoral approach for fusion following excision of tumor.
Steffee plate	Plate and screw device for posterolateral fusion fixation.
Stein-Leventhal syndrome	Polycystic ovary syndrome; sclerocystic disease of the ovaries commonly characterized by hirsutism, obesity, amenorrhea, infertility and enlarged ovaries.
Stevens-Johnson syndrome	Severe, sometimes fatal, bullous form of erythema multiforme involving the mucous membranes.
Stokes-Adams syndrome	Condition caused by heart block with sudden attacks of unconsciousness and seizures.
Strümpell-Marie disease	Ankylosing or rheumatoid spondylitis; arthritis of the spine resembling rheumatoid arthritis usually affecting young males.

Swan-Ganz catheter	Flexible, flow-directed cardiac catheter featuring a balloon tip to measure pressure in the pulmonary artery.
Syme's amputation	Modified disarticulation through the ankle joint.
Tay-Sachs disease	Cerebral sphingolipidosis, infantile type; amaurotic familial idiocy (obsolete); an inherited disease appearing at 3 to 6 months of age, characterized by doll-like facies, cherry-red macular spot, loss of vision and progressive spastic paralysis.
Tinel's sign	Procedure done to assess for a lesion or beginning regeneration of a nerve. Perscussion is made over the site of a divided nerve and tingling is felt in the distal end of the limb.
Tommaselli syndrome (disease)	Fever and hematuria due to quinine overdose.
Tornwaldt abscess	Abscess of the adenoids.
Treacher Collins syndrome	Mandibulofacial dystosis limited to the orbit and malar regions.
Tsuli procedure	Expansive, multiple laminectomy for severe cervical spondylosis.
Turner sign	Discoloration of the groin following acute pancreatitis.
Unna boot	Zinc oxide and gelatin paste used to treat vericose ulcers.
Unschuld's sign	Cramping in the calves of the legs, as seen in early diabetes mellitus.
van Hook's operation	Ureteroureterostomy.
Vermont (Krag) instrumentation	Posteriorly placed internal fixation device.
Vincent disease (gingivitis)	Necrotizing ulcerative gingivitis; trench mouth; characterized by gingival erythema and pain, fetid odor, and necrosis and sloughing giving rise to a gray pseudomembrane.
von Hippel-Lindau disease	Hereditary phakomatosis characterized by retinal and cerebral aniomas.
von Recklinghausen disease	Neurofibromatosis characterized by café au lait spots, intertriginous freckling, iris hamartomas and other neurofibromas.

von Willebrand's disease	Hereditary bleeding disorder also known as angiohemophilia or vascular hemophilia; characterized by a deficiency of coagulating Factor VIII with a tendency to bleed from mucous membranes for a prolonged period of time.
Warren shunt	Distal splenorenal shunt.
Wenckebach phenomenon	Cardiac arrhythmia where the P-R interval grows progressively longer until a beat is dropped.
Wertheim Bohlman fusion	Use of iliac crest graft and wire fixation from occiput to C-2 for occipital cervical fusion.
Whipple operation	Pancreaticoderodenectomy.
Whipple's disease	Intestinal lipodystrophy.
Whitecloud and Larocca fusion	Anterior technique for cervical spine fusion using fibular graft.
Wilks syndrome	Myasthenia gravis.
Wiltse plate	Screw plate device for posterior spinal stabilization.
Wiltse procedure	Bilateral lateral spine fusion for spondylolisthesis.
Wisconsin (Drummond) interspinous instrumentation	Series of wires, rods, and buttons for multisegmental spine stabilization.
Wolff-Parkinson-White syndrome	Paroxysmal tachycardia (or atrial fibrillation) and pre-excitation in which the electrocardiogram displays a short P-R interval and a wide QRS complex.
Zenker diverticulum	Pharyngoesophageal diverticulum; the most common diverticulum at the junction of the esophagus and the pharynx.
Zollinger-Ellison syndrome	Multiple endocrine neoplasia featuring peptic ulceration, gastric hyperacidity and pancreatic gastrin-secreting non-beta cell tumors.

CPT & HCPCS CODING

This chapter deals with one of the most important parts of the reimbursement puzzle: how to use the CPT and HCPCS coding systems to code properly for the procedures and services you perform and the supplies and materials you use or distribute. Selection of the proper coding system and the proper code has a tremendous impact on your reimbursement. This requires a fundamental understanding of the CPT and HCPCS coding systems, including format and conventions. Steps for accurate and precise coding are defined along with critical coding and billing issues, such as the use of modifiers, levels of service, multiple procedures, etc. Following the general discussion of the CPT and HCPCS coding systems, a discussion of each of the specialty sections appears.

CPT

CPT is an acronym for Current Procedural Terminology. *Physicians' Current Procedural Terminology* (CPT) is a listing of over 7,000 codes and descriptions used to report medical services and procedures performed by physicians and other medical professionals. The purpose of the CPT coding system is to provide a uniform language that accurately describes medical, surgical, and diagnostic services and to provide an effective means for reliable nationwide communication among physicians, hospitals, and health insurance companies.

CPT codes and terminology serve a variety of important functions in the field of medical nomenclature for the reporting of physician procedures and services under government and private health insurance programs. CPT is also used for administrative management purposes such as claims processing and for the development of guidelines for medical care review.

Medical nomenclature and procedural coding is a rapidly changing field. As new procedures are developed, old procedures become obsolete, and existing procedures are modified to reflect changes in medical practice. The American Medical Association (AMA) revises and publishes CPT on an annual basis. The changes that appear in each revision are prepared by the CPT Editorial Panel with the assistance of physicians representing all specialties of medicine.

A thorough understanding of the CPT coding system is vital to protecting and maximizing your reimbursement. All government health insurance programs, such as CHAMPUS, Medicare, Medicaid, and the Federal Employees Health Plan (FEHP) programs mandate use of CPT codes. With few exceptions, most commercial health insurance companies also mandate the use of CPT codes. The few exceptions to the mandatory use of CPT codes are typically found in the processing of workers' compensation claims.

HCPCS

HCPCS is an acronym for Healthcare Common Procedure Coding System. The HCPCS coding system was developed in 1983 by the Health Care Financing Administration (now known as CMS) for the purpose of standardizing the coding systems used to process Medicare claims on a national basis.

HCPCS is a two-level coding system incorporating CPT codes as Level I and nationally mandated codes designated as HCPCS Level II. HCPCS codes must be used when billing Medicare carriers and, in some states, Medicaid carriers. Some private health insurance companies allow or mandate the use of HCPCS codes, mostly those processing Medicare claims.

The HCPCS Level II codes are used to bill Medicare for ambulance services, durable medical equipment, orthotics, prosthetics, supplies, materials, and injections. HCPCS Level II may also include codes for certain procedures and services that are not defined in the current edition of the CPT code book.

KEY POINTS REGARDING CPT AND HCPCS

- CPT codes describe procedures, services, and supplies.

- CPT codes are five-digit, numeric or alphanumeric codes.

- CPT codes are accepted or required by all third-party payers.

- CPT codes are self-definitive. With the exception of a few codes that contain the term *specify* in the description, each code has only one meaning.

- CPT codes are revised each fall and become effective January 1. Hundreds of CPT codes are added, changed, or deleted each year. You need to purchase a new copy of the CPT code book each year.

- HCPCS codes describe supplies, materials, and services provided by medical professionals.

- HCPCS codes are five-digit, alphanumeric codes. The first digit is a letter between A and Z, and the second through fifth digits are numbers.

- The HCPCS coding system includes two-digit modifiers at the national level and may be alphabetic or alphanumeric.

- The HCPCS coding system is a two-level system consisting of CPT Level I and HCPCS Level II national codes.

- HCPCS codes are mandatory for billing Medicare carriers and some Medicaid carriers as well.

- HCPCS codes are revised annually each fall and become effective January 1. Typically, hundreds of codes are added, changed, or deleted. You need to purchase a copy of the revised codes each year.

- HCPCS codes follow a specific hierarchy of selection and use. HCPCS National Level II takes precedence over HCPCS Level I (CPT).

- Accurate HCPCS coding may make a significant difference in your reimbursement from Medicare carriers.

- Accurate CPT and HCPCS coding puts you in control of the reimbursement process.

STRUCTURE OF THE CPT CODING SYSTEM

The CPT coding system is a systematic method for coding procedures and services performed by physicians and other health care professionals. Each procedure or service is identified with a five-digit numeric code. The use of CPT codes simplifies the reporting of services. With this coding and recording system, the procedure or service rendered by the physicians is accurately identified.

The CPT code book is divided into code sections. Within each section are subsections with anatomic, procedural, condition, or descriptor subheadings. The procedures and services with their identifying codes are presented in numeric order except for codes found in the Evaluation and Management section (99200-99499). These codes are located at the beginning of the CPT code book because they are used by all medical professionals and they are the most frequently used codes. The sections of the CPT code book are:

Evaluation and Management	99200-99499
Anesthesia	00100-01999
Surgery	10000-69999
Radiology	70000-79999
Pathology and Laboratory	80000-89999
Medicine	90000-99199
Category II Codes	0001F-0011F
Category III Codes	0001T-0061T

STRUCTURE OF THE HCPCS CODING SYSTEM

HCPCS is a systematic method for coding supplies, materials, injections, and services performed by physicians and other health care professionals. Each supply, material, injection, or service is identified with a five-digit alphanumeric code. With the HCPCS coding system, the supplies, materials, injections, and services rendered to Medicare patients may be accurately identified. There are three levels of codes within the HCPCS coding system.

HCPCS LEVEL I: CPT

The major portion of the HCPCS coding system, referred to as HCPCS Level I, is CPT. Most of the procedures and services provided by health care professionals, including those provided to Medicare patients, are reported with CPT codes. However, one of the shortcomings of the CPT coding system is the limited CPT codes available to describe supplies, materials, and injections, which led to the development of HCPCS Level II codes as a supplement to the CPT coding system.

HCPCS LEVEL II: NATIONAL CODES

HCPCS Level II codes are alphanumeric codes that start with a letter followed by four numbers. The range of HCPCS Level II codes is from A0000 through V0000. There are also HCPCS Level II modifier codes. HCPCS Level II codes are defined and maintained by CMS and are uniform in description throughout the United States when describing covered services to Medicare intermediaries. However, due to what is known as "carrier discretion," the processing and reimbursement of HCPCS Level II codes are not necessarily uniform.

There are over 2,400 HCPCS Level II codes covering supplies, materials, injections, and services. A fundamental understanding of how and when to use HCPCS codes may have a significant impact on your Medicare reimbursement. Most health care professionals will use HCPCS Level II codes only from the Medical and Surgical Supplies section and Drugs Administered by Other Than Oral Method, commonly referred to as "A" codes and "J" codes.

HCPCS SECTIONS

The main body of HCPCS Level II codes is divided into 18 sections. The supplies, materials, injections, and services are presented in numeric order. The 18 major sections of HCPCS Level II are:

Transportation Services	A0000-A0999
Chiropractic Services	A2000-A2999
Medical and Surgical Supplies	A4000-A4999
Miscellaneous and Experimental	A9000-A9999
Enteral and Parenteral Therapy	B4000-B9999
Dental Procedures	D0000-D9999
Durable Medical Equipment (DME)	E0000-E9999
Rehabilitative Services	H5000-H6000
Drugs Administered Other Than Oral Method (Injections)	J0000-J8999
Chemotherapy Drugs	J9000-J9999
Orthotic Procedures	L0000-L4999
Prosthetic Procedures	L5000-L9999
Medical Services	M0000-M9999
Pathology and Laboratory	P0000-P9999
Temporary Codes	Q0000-Q0099
Diagnostic Radiology Services	R0000-R5999
Vision Services	V0000-V2799
Hearing Services	V5000-V5999

HOW TO USE THE CPT CODING SYSTEM

A health care professional using CPT for coding selects the name and associated code of the procedure or service that most accurately identifies and describes the service(s) performed. In surgery, this may be an operation; in medicine, an office visit, hospital visit, consultation, or diagnostic procedure; in radiology, an x-ray. The professional selects names and codes for additional services or procedures and, when necessary, selects and adds modifiers for additional or reduced services or for extenuating circumstances. Any services or procedures coded in this manner are also documented in the patient's medical record.

It is important to recognize that the listing of a service or procedure and its code number in a specific section of the CPT code book does not restrict its use to a specific specialty group. Any procedure or service in any section of the CPT code book may be used to designate the services rendered by any qualified physician or other medical professional.

The codes and descriptions listed in the CPT code book are those that are generally consistent with contemporary medical practice and being performed by medical professionals in clinical practice. Inclusion in CPT does not represent endorsement by the American Medical Association of any particular diagnostic or therapeutic procedure. Inclusion or exclusion of a procedure does not imply any health insurance coverage or reimbursement policy.

FORMAT AND CONVENTIONS

CPT procedure terminologies have been developed as stand-alone descriptions of medical procedures. However, some of the procedures in CPT are not printed in their entirety but refer back to a common portion of the procedure listed in a preceding entry. This is evident when an entry is followed by one or more indentations. Any terminology after the semicolon has a subordinate status, as do the subsequent indented entries. For example:

25100   Arthrotomy, wrist joint; with biopsy

25105   with synovectomy

Note that the common part of code 25100, the part before the semicolon, is considered to be part of code 25105.

GUIDELINES

Specific "Guidelines" are presented at the beginning of each of the six sections of the CPT code book. The guidelines define items that are necessary to interpret and report the procedures and services contained in that section. CPT guidelines also provide explanations regarding terms that apply only to a particular section.

MODIFIERS

A CPT modifier provides the means to report that a service or procedure has been altered or modified by some specific circumstance but not changed in its definition or code. The proper use of modifiers reduces the need for separate procedure listings to describe the modifying circumstance. Modifiers are typically used to indicate that:

- A service or procedure has both a professional and technical component.

- A service or procedure was performed by more than one physician and/or in more than one location.

- A service or procedure has been increased or reduced.

- Only part of a service was performed.

- An adjunctive service was performed.

- A bilateral procedure was performed.

- A service or procedure was provided more than once.

- Unusual events occurred.

A complete listing of CPT modifiers is found in Appendix A of the CPT code book. In addition, a list of modifiers common to each of the six sections described above is located in the Guidelines of each section.

APPENDICES

Following the six main sections listing the CPT codes and descriptors, the CPT code book includes several appendices and an alphabetical index.

Appendix A: Modifiers

Appendix A of the CPT code book is a complete list of all CPT modifiers and definitions.

Appendix B: Summary of Additions, Deletions, and Revisions

Appendix B of the CPT code book is a summary listing of all additions, deletions, and revisions contained in the current edition. Appendix B of the CPT code book will help you to quickly identify new CPT codes, deleted CPT codes, and changes to CPT code definitions that may affect your practice.

Appendix C: Clinical Examples Supplement

Appendix C of the CPT code book is the Clinical Examples Supplement to CPT. The supplement includes clinical examples that describe the services and medical conditions that illustrate various levels of E/M services.

Appendix D: Summary of CPT Add-on Codes

Appendix D of the CPT code book is a listing of CPT add-on codes, procedures listed in the Surgery section of the CPT code book are commonly performed in addition to the primary procedure. These procedures are designated as "add-on" codes with a + symbol appearing to the left of the CPT code.

Appendix E: Summary of Codes Exempt From Modifier -51

Appendix E of the CPT code book is a listing of CPT codes that are exempt from the use of the multiple-procedure modifier -51 but have not been designated as CPT add-on procedures or services. The modifier -51 exempt codes are identified in the CPT code book with a Ø symbol appearing to the left of the CPT code.

Appendix F: Summary of Codes Exempt From Modifier -63

Appendix F of the CPT code book is a listing of CPT codes that are exempt from the use of the low weight for neonates and infants modifier - 63.

Appendix G: Summary of CPT Codes That Include Conscious Sedation

Appendix G of the CPT code book is a listing of CPT codes that include conscious sedation as an inherent part of providing the procedure.

Appendix H: Alphabetic Index of Performance Measures by Clinical Condition or Topic

Appendix H of the CPT code book provides an index to performance measures and sources for Category II CPT codes.

Appendix I: Genetic Testing Code Modifiers

Appendix I of the CPT code book provides a list of modifiers used in reporting molecular laboratory procedures related to genetic testing.

Appendix J: Electrodiagnostic Medicine Listing of Sensory, Motor and Mixed Nerves

Appendix J of the CPT codes book assigns each sensory, motor and mixed nerve with its appropropriate nerve conduction study code, i.e. 95900, 99503 or 99504.

Appendix K: Product Pending FDA Approval

Appendix K of the CPT code book is a list of CPT Category I codes pending future FDA approval.

Appendix L: Vascular Families

Appendix L of the CPT code book lists the assignment of branches to first, second, and third order assuming the starting point is catheterization of the aorta.

Appendix M: Crosswalk to Deleted CPT Codes

A summary list of deleted CPT codes and descriptions cross-walked to current CPT codes.

CPT INDEX

A complete alphabetical index is found in the back of the CPT code book. The index includes listings by procedure and anatomic site. Procedures and services commonly known by their eponyms or other designations are also included.

How to Use the Alphabetical Index

When you are using the alphabetical index to locate CPT codes, always use the following search sequence:

1) Look for the procedure or service performed.

2) Look for the organ involved.

3) Look for the condition treated.

4) Look for synonyms, eponyms, or abbreviations.

When using the CPT alphabetical index, it is important to understand how entries to the index have been made. Generally, index entries will fall into one or more of the categories described below.

Main Terms

1) Procedure or Service
Pin
Prophylactic

Femur	27187, 27495
Humerus	24498

Note that in the above example, the procedure/service was listed as the heading and a "range" of codes followed. The range of codes directs the coder to the appropriate section of the CPT where additional information on procedures may be obtained.

2) Organ
Bile duct

Cyst	47715
Repair	47716

3) Condition
Tumor
(SEE ALSO Lesion)

Abdomen	49200, 49201
Abdominal wall	22900
Acetabulum	27076
Ankle	27615-27619

4) Synonyms, Eponyms, and Abbreviations
EEG
(SEE electroencephalogram)

HAI Test
(SEE Hemagglutination Inhibition Test)

Mitchell procedure
(SEE Repair, Toe, Bunion

Modifying Terms

A main term may be followed by a series of up to three indented terms that modify the main term. When modifying terms appear, they should be reviewed carefully, as these subterms do have an effect on code selection.

Cross-References

Cross-references direct the user to review additional information. There are two types of cross-references used in the CPT index.

1) "SEE"—Directs the user to refer to the term listed after the word "SEE." This type of reference is used primarily for synonyms, eponyms and abbreviations.

2) "SEE ALSO"—Directs the user to look under another main term if the procedure is not listed under the first main entry.

HOW TO USE THE HCPCS CODING SYSTEM

HCPCS Level II codes must be used when coding and billing supplies, materials, injections, and certain services provided to Medicare patients. For health care professionals, the most commonly used HCPCS Level II codes are for medical/surgical supplies and injections. Many of the HCPCS Level II codes describe equipment sold or rented as durable medical equipment and/or medical/surgical appliances.

The listing of a supply, material, injection, or service and its code number in a specific section of HCPCS Level II does not usually restrict its use to a specific profession or specialty group. However, there are some HCPCS Level II codes that are, by definition, profession or specialty specific.

The codes and descriptions listed in HCPCS Level II are generally consistent with contemporary medical practice as defined by CMS. Inclusion in HCPCS Level II does not represent endorsement by any medical association of any particular supply, material, injection, or service. Inclusion of a supply, material, injection, or service does not imply any health insurance coverage or reimbursement policy. HCPCS Level II codes are intended by CMS to be implemented identically on a national basis. However, as CMS also allows some "carrier discretion" with respect to administering the Medicare program, there are variations on a national level in terms of acceptance and reimbursement of these codes.

FORMAT AND CONVENTIONS

HCPCS procedure terminologies have been developed as stand-alone descriptions of medical supplies, materials, injections, and services by CMS. HCPCS Level II codes are published by many different publishers. The HCPCS published annually by PMIC follows the format and conventions of the CPT coding system exactly, which allows the user to easily switch back and forth from one system to another.

GUIDELINES

There are no "official" coding guidelines provided by CMS for HCPCS Level II. Information regarding the appropriate use of HCPCS Level II codes may be obtained from Medicare bulletins published by Medicare intermediaries, books on Medicare rules and regulations, and books on coding such as this one. There are extensive guidelines in the version of HCPCS Level II codes published by PMIC.

HCPCS LEVEL II MODIFIERS

In addition to the specific uses of modifiers as described previously, HCPCS Level II modifiers include the following additional uses:

- A service was supervised by an anesthesiologist.

- A service was performed by a specific medical professional, for example, a clinical psychologist, clinical social worker, nurse practitioner, or physician assistant.

- A service was provided as part of a specific government program.

- A service was provided to a specific side of the body.

- Equipment was purchased or rented.

- Single or multiple patients were seen during nursing home visits.

It is important to note that HCPCS Level II modifiers may be combined with CPT codes when reporting services to Medicare.

CODING RULES FOR HCPCS

Both levels of the HCPCS coding system must be considered when providing services to Medicare patients. Improper coding on Medicare claims may result in denial, reduced payments, or delayed payments plus the possibility of audits and fines. CPT codes cover the majority of procedures and services provided by most health care professionals, but there are specific instances in which HCPCS Level II codes must be used for maximum reimbursement.

MEDICAL AND SURGICAL SUPPLIES

One of the most important uses for HCPCS Level II codes is to report the provision of medical and surgical supplies to Medicare patients. CPT lists very few codes for medical and surgical supplies, usually with instructions to specify. HCPCS Level II includes codes with specific definitions for hundreds of medical and surgical supplies.

HCPCS CODE OVERLAP

You may occasionally encounter a coding situation in which there is an overlap of the CPT and HCPCS coding systems. For example, you may provide a service that may be reported by either a CPT code or a HCPCS National Level II code. How do you know which to choose?

The following rules represent how such coding situations should be handled:

1) HCPCS Level II codes always have the highest priority. If there is a choice between a HCPCS Level II code and a CPT code, use the HCPCS Level II code.

2) For CPT supply, materials, or injection codes that contain the instruction *specify*, try to find a HCPCS Level II code that describes the specific supply, material, or injection.

FORMAT OF HCPCS CODES

All HCPCS Level II codes begin with a letter followed by four numbers. HCPCS Level II codes fall into the range of A0000 through V5999.

GENERAL CODING & BILLING ISSUES

Most billing, coding, and reporting issues involving CPT and/or HCPCS apply generally to all medical specialties and professions. However, there are some specialty-specific issues defined in each of the sections of the CPT code book that apply only to the particular medical specialty.

SUPPORTING DOCUMENTATION

One of the most important billing, coding and reporting issues is that you should have medical record support for the procedures, services, and supplies that you are reporting on health insurance claims. Most medical chart reviewers take the position that if something is not documented in the medical record, then the service or procedure didn't happen and is therefore not subject to reimbursement.

If your practice is selected for an audit by Medicare or other health insurance company, the accuracy and completeness of the documentation of your medical records, or lack thereof, will have a significant impact on the outcome of the audit. The current emphasis on "fraud" and "abuse" by Medicare, Medicaid, and private health insurance companies necessitates a review of documentation by all medical professionals.

Use the following list to review the documentation policies, procedures, and standards of your medical practice:

- Are your medical records maintained in a current, uniform, legible, and consistent manner?

- Do all entries include the date, provider name, chief complaint, clinical findings, diagnosis or impression, tests and medications ordered, procedures performed, and instructions given to the patient?

- Are all entries signed or countersigned by the responsible provider?

- Are all laboratory, x-ray, and other test results recorded properly?

- Are the consultations and advice given to patients by telephone documented accurately and consistently?

- Do your entries clearly document the need for the level of service you are billing?

- Does the working diagnosis clearly support the need for the procedures or services provided?

SPECIAL MEDICARE CONSIDERATIONS

To satisfy Medicare requirements, there must be sufficient documentation in the medical record to verify the services billed and the level of care required. Section 1833(e) of Title XVIII of the Social Security Act requires "available information that documents a claim." If there is no documentation to justify the services or level of care, the claim cannot be considered for Medicare benefits.

If there is insufficient documentation to support claims that have already been paid by Medicare, the reimbursement will be considered an overpayment and a refund will be requested by Medicare. Medicare has the authority to review any information, including medical records, when such information pertains to a Medicare claim.

BILATERAL MODIFIER USAGE

With the exception of the Radiology section, all procedure codes that defined bilateral procedures were deleted from the 1990 edition of the CPT code book. This was the stated intent of the AMA for several previous editions of the CPT code book. The modifier -50 had been previously added to CPT for the purpose of reporting bilateral procedures.

21. DIAGNOSIS OR NATURE OF ILLNESS OR INJURY. (RELATE ITEMS 1,2,3 OR 4 TO ITEM 24E BY LINE)

1. L____ . __   3. L____ . __

2. L____ . __   4. L____ . __

24.	A DATE(S) OF SERVICE						B Place of Service	C Type of Service	D PROCEDURES, SERVICES, OR SUPPLIES (Explain Unusual Circumstances)		E DIAGNOSIS CODE
	From MM	DD	YY	To MM	DD	YY			CPT/HCPCS	MODIFIER	
1	05	15	07				21		20680		
2	05	15	07				21		20680	50	
3											
4											

Providers who have been using bilateral procedure codes need to revise their code listings and superbills to reflect the deletion of these codes and start using modifier -50 as indicated in the claim example that follows. Note that what you could previously bill with a single line on a claim form now requires two separate lines as defined in the CPT.

UNLISTED PROCEDURES OR SERVICES

The AMA and CMS recognize that there may be services or procedures performed by medical professionals that are not found in CPT or HCPCS. Therefore, a number of specific code numbers have been included for reporting unlisted procedures. When an unlisted procedure code is used, the service or procedure must be described and a report describing the service or procedure must be submitted with the health insurance claim.

The unlisted procedure codes are frequently overused because 1) it is easier to use an unlisted procedure code than locate a specific code and 2) the medical practice is using outdated copies of the CPT or HCPCS and is unaware that specific procedure codes do exist for the procedures or services they are providing. Using unlisted procedure codes increases the practice workload, as detailed reports must be submitted to explain to health insurance companies what services were actually provided. This in turn delays reimbursement, as the carriers must process these claims manually instead of through their normal claim-processing system.

Avoid the use of unlisted procedure codes whenever possible. Make sure you obtain a new copy of the CPT and HCPCS annually to make sure you are using the most current codes. HCPCS Level II contains numerous codes defined as unlisted supplies, materials, and services. Services for these codes are usually not allowed or paid. Consult your local Medicare intermediary before using any of these codes.

CPT CHANGES, ADDITIONS, AND DELETIONS

Every year, hundreds of codes are added, changed, or deleted from the CPT code book. A summary of these changes is found in Appendix B of your CPT code book and provides a quick reference for coding review. In addition to appearing in CPT's Appendix B, these modifications are identified throughout the CPT code book. It is imperative that you purchase a new copy of the CPT code book every year in order to make sure that you are using the most current codes. Using current CPT codes is important for two reasons:

1. Since coding directly affects reimbursement, using out-of-date codes may result in lower payments.

2. Using out-of-date codes may expose you to audit liability, with the potential for monetary fines and other penalties, particularly with the Medicare program.

ADDITIONS TO CPT

CPT codes new to the current edition are identified with a small black circle placed to the left of the code number. Examples of CPT codes that are new to the CPT 2007 book include:

- **27326** Neurectomy, popliteal (gastrocnemius)

- **54865** Exploration of epididymis, with or without biopsy

This special identification of new codes appears only in the current CPT code book. In the following edition, these CPT codes will no longer have a small black circle to the left of the code number.

CHANGES TO CPT CODE DEFINITIONS

CPT code definitions changed in the current edition are identified with a small black triangle placed to the left of the code number. Examples of CPT code definitions that were changed in the CPT 2007 book include:

▲ 19361 Breast reconstruction with latissimus dorsi flap, without prosthetic implant

▲ 76645 Ultrasound, breast(s) (unilateral or bilateral), real time other than adjustable gastric band (separate procedure)

The only way to determine exactly what part of the definition has been changed is to compare the current changed definition with the definition from the previous edition of the CPT code book. This special identification of changed definitions appears only in the current CPT code book. In the following edition, these CPT codes will no longer have a small black triangle to the left of the code number.

DELETIONS FROM CPT

CPT codes deleted from the current CPT code book are enclosed within parentheses; deleted codes usually include a reference to replacement codes. Examples of CPT codes that are identified in the 2007 edition as deleted from the CPT 2007 book include:

(25611 has been deleted. To report, use 25606)

(92573 has been been deleted. To report the Lombard test use 92700)

HCPCS CHANGES, ADDITIONS, AND DELETIONS

Every year, hundreds of codes are added, deleted, or changed from HCPCS Level II. As there is no standardized format for HCPCS Level II, your awareness of these changes will depend on, first, having a copy of the current HCPCS codes and, second, the reporting format chosen by the publisher of the HCPCS Level II you use.

The HCPCS Level II code book published annually by PMIC uses the same symbol notation system as that of the CPT code book, namely, black circles, black triangles, and parentheses to identify new HCPCS codes, changes to HCPCS code definitions, and HCPCS code deletions. It is mandatory that you purchase a new copy of HCPCS Level II each year in order to make sure you are using the most current codes. Using current HCPCS Level II codes is important for two reasons:

1. Using out-of-date HCPCS Level II codes may result in a delay, reduction, or denial of your Medicare claims.

2. Using out-of-date HCPCS Level II codes may result in noncompliance with Medicare rules and regulations, exposing you to possible fines and penalties.

ADDITIONS TO HCPCS

HCPCS codes new to the current edition are identified with a small black circle placed to the left of the code number. Examples of HCPCS codes that are new to the HCPCS 2007 book include:

- **A4461** Surgical dressing holder non-reusable, each

- **J0129** Injection abatacept, 10 mg

This special identification of new codes appears only in the current HCPCS book. In the following edition, these HCPCS codes will no longer have a small black circle to the left of the code number.

CHANGES TO HCPCS CODE DEFINITIONS

HCPCS code definitions changed in the current edition are identified with a small black triangle placed to the left of the code number. Examples of code definitions that were changed in the HCPCS 2007 book include the following:

▲ C2620 Pacemaker, single chamber non rate-responsive (implantable)

▲ E2209 Arm trough, with or with hand support, each

The only way to determine exactly what part of the definition has been changed is to compare the current changed definition with the definition from the previous edition of the HCPCS book. This special identification of changed definitions appears only in the current HCPCS book. In the following edition, these HCPCS codes will no longer have a small black triangle to the left of the code number.

DELETIONS FROM HCPCS

HCPCS codes deleted from the current HCPCS book are enclosed within parentheses and usually include a reference to replacement codes. Examples of HCPCS codes identified as deleted from the HCPCS 2007 book include the following:

(**J7320** Code deleted 12/31/2006)

(**L6865** Code deleted 12/31/2006)

In the HCPCS book published by PMIC, this special identification of deleted HCPCS codes with the year of deletion appears in subsequent editions.

STARRED PROCEDURES

The "starred procedure" designation, formerly an asterisk (*) following the CPT code, was eliminated effective with the 2004 edition of the CPT code book.

DEFINITION OF NEW VERSUS ESTABLISHED PATIENT

CPT E/M service codes 99200-99499 require that you distinguish between new patients and established patients. The designation of new or established does not preclude the use of a specific level of service.

NEW PATIENT OR INITIAL VISIT

A *new* patient is defined in the current edition of the CPT code book as "one who has not received any professional services from the physician or another physician of the same specialty who belongs to the same group practice, within the past three years."

When a physician is on call or covering for another physician, the patient's visit is classified as it would have been by the physician who is not available. No distinction is made between new and established patients in the emergency department.

ESTABLISHED PATIENT OR FOLLOW-UP VISITS

An *established* patient is defined in the current edition of the CPT code book as "one who has received professional services from the physician or another physician of the same specialty who belongs to the same group practice, within the past three years."

As previously stated, on-call physicians should classify patients the same as the physician for whom they are covering. No distinction is made between new and established patients in the emergency department.

PLACE (LOCATION) OF SERVICE

CPT makes specific distinctions for place (location) of service for codes in the E/M service codes. HCPCS Level II also includes codes that refer to specific locations of service. The place of service may have considerable impact on reimbursement. The following list defines CPT and HCPCS Level II code ranges for specific places of service:

Office [and Other Outpatient]	99201-99215
Home Services	99341-99353
Hospital [Inpatient]	99221-99238

Consultations	99241-99245, 99251-99255, 99261-99263
SNF, ICF, Long-Term Care	99301-99315
Nursing Home, Custodial Care, Etc.	99321-99333
Emergency Room [Assigned Physician]	99281-99288

HOSPITAL CARE

Reporting of hospital visits frequently causes reimbursement problems for health care professionals. The three most common coding errors are:

- More than one physician submits an initial hospital care code for the same patient.

- Follow-up hospital visits are coded and billed incorrectly.

- Concurrent care visits by multiple specialists are not coded and billed properly.

If more than one physician is involved in the process of hospitalizing a patient, for example, surgeon and internist, the physicians must decide which one is going to actually admit the patient and bill for the admission. If both do, the first health insurance claim to arrive will be processed and paid, and the second will be rejected.

There are valid reasons for visiting a patient more than once daily while hospitalized, however, many physicians and even some health insurance billers do not know that subsequent hospital visit codes are for "daily" services. When a physician visits the patient twice in one day, providing a brief level of service each time, the physician or biller may incorrectly report two hospital visit services for the same day, instead of a higher-level code incorporating both visits.

Reporting multiple hospital visits provided on the same day separately on the health insurance claim form usually results in either the entire claim being returned for clarification or the second visit being denied as an apparent duplication. Unfortunately, health insurance billers who are unclear on the proper coding of same-day hospital visits may simply accept the rejection without question and write off the unpaid visit as uncollectible.

The CPT code book clearly defines subsequent hospital care as "per day," meaning daily services. If you visit the patient twice in one day, providing the equivalent of "brief" services each time, report the service using the appropriate E/M service code that defines the cumulative level of service provided.

HOSPITAL DISCHARGE

The CPT code for hospital discharge services is E/M service code 99238, defined as Hospital discharge day management. Hospital discharge services include final examination of the patient, discussion of the hospital stay, instructions for continuing care, and preparation of discharge records. Many health insurance companies do not recognize and/or do not reimburse this CPT code.

Options for the use of code 99238 include the use of one of the other hospital daily services codes from the E/M series 99231-99233 and perhaps using a code that has a higher value than your routine hospital visit.

REFERRAL

A referral is the transfer of the total care or specific portion of care of a patient from one physician to another. A referral is not a request for consultation. If a patient is referred to you for total care or a portion of his/her care, use E/M visit codes to report your services. If a patient is sent to you for a consultation, use E/M consultation codes to report your services.

SEPARATE OR MULTIPLE PROCEDURES

It is appropriate to designate multiple procedures that are rendered on the same date by separate entries. For example, if a proctosigmoidoscopy was performed in addition to a hospital visit, the proctosigmoidoscopy would be considered a *separate* procedure and listed in addition to the hospital visit on the claim form. Another example would be individual medical psychotherapy rendered in addition to a brief subsequent hospital service. In this instance, both services would be reported.

MULTIPLE SURGICAL PROCEDURES

It is common for several surgical procedures to be performed at the same operative session. When multiple procedures are performed on the same day or at the same session, the "major" procedure or service is listed first followed by secondary, additional, or "lesser" procedures or services. Modifier -51 is added to all procedures following the first one.

CONSULTATIONS

A consultation includes services rendered by a physician whose opinion or advice is requested by a physician or other appropriate source for the further evaluation and/or management of the patient. When the consulting physician assumes responsibility for the continuing care of the patient, the service is no longer considered a consultation. Any services rendered at subsequent visits are reported using E/M service codes.

Consultation follow-up visits provided in an office or other outpatient location are reported with the established patient E/M visit codes.

CONFIRMATORY CONSULTATIONS

Confirmatory consultation codes are used when the consultation is requested by the patient or other agency. Typically, the consultation will involve a second or third opinion on the necessity or appropriateness of a medical treatment or surgical procedure recommended by another physician. If the second opinion is mandated by a professional review organization, add CPT modifier -32 if the patient *is not* a Medicare patient but add HCPCS Level II modifier -SF if the patient *is* a Medicare patient.

EMERGENCY SERVICES

Proper coding for services performed in the emergency department depends on whether or not the physician is assigned to the emergency department. If the physician is assigned to the emergency department, emergency services would be coded from the E/M service codes 99281-99285. For services performed in the emergency department at the request of or for the convenience of the patient or physician, use E/M service codes 99201-99215 to report.

SUPPLIES AND MATERIALS PROVIDED BY THE PHYSICIAN

The CPT coding system includes specific codes for identifying certain supplies and materials provided by the physician. The HCPCS Level II coding system provides over 2,000 specific codes for identifying supplies, materials, and equipment on Medicare claims. These codes are used to bill for supplies and materials that are not included in the definition of the basic service.

CPT CODES FOR SUPPLIES AND MATERIALS

78990 & 79900 These codes, found in the Nuclear Medicine subsection of the Radiology section of the CPT code book, are used to report diagnostic and therapeutic radio-pharmaceuticals when provided by the physician.

92390-92396 These codes are used to bill for the supply of spectacles, contact lenses, low-vision aids, and ocular prostheses.

95144-95170 Provision of antigens for allergen immunotherapy. These codes are used to bill for antigens provided to the patient.

96545 Provision of chemotherapy agent. CPT codes 96400-96530 are used to bill for administration. These codes include preparation of chemotherapy agent(s) and administration but do not include supply of the specific agent.

99070 Supplies and materials provided by the physician. This global code is used to identify virtually all other materials and supplies, such as sterile trays, drugs, cast or strap materials, etc., over and above those usually included with the office visit or service rendered.

This code is valid only for private health insurance companies and some Medicaid carriers. This code may not be used to bill Medicare carriers for materials and supplies. Use the appropriate HCPCS Level II code to bill Medicare.

99071 Educational supplies, such as books, tapes, and pamphlets, provided by the physician for the patient's education at cost to physician.

Educational materials are normally supplied at no charge to the patient. Most practices provide this type of material as a service to their patients. It is also an important component of the practice's marketing program.

78990 & 79900 These codes, found in the Nuclear Medicine subsection of the Radiology section of the CPT code book, are used to report diagnostic and therapeutic radio-pharmaceuticals when provided by the physician.

HCPCS CODES FOR SUPPLIES AND MATERIALS

A4000-A4999   Medical and surgical supplies such as bandages, syringes, catheters, urinary supplies, ostomy supplies, surgical trays, and various miscellaneous supplies commonly provided to patients.

B4000-B9999   Enteral and parenteral therapy supplies such as feeding kits, formulae, and infusion pumps.

E0000-E9999   Durable medical equipment such as ambulation devices, commodes, decubitus care equipment, heat/cold application equipment, bath and toilet aids, hospital beds and accessories, oxygen and related respiratory equipment, TENS, wheelchairs and accessories, oxygen supplies and equipment, and artificial kidney machines and accessories.

L0000-L4999   Orthotic supplies, materials, and devices such as cervical collars, body jackets, surgical supports, correction pads, and orthopedic footwear.

L5000-L9999   Prosthetic supplies, materials, devices, and fittings such as artificial limbs, terminal devices (hooks, hands, gloves), externally powered devices, batteries, breast prostheses, elastic supports.

V2000-V2900   Vision supplies, materials, and devices such as spectacles, contact lenses, and eye prostheses.

V5000-V5399   Hearing services, materials, and supplies such as audiologic assessment, fitting, and/or repair of hearing aids, and supply of hearing aids.

Some private health insurance companies, mostly those that are also Medicare carriers, allow or require use of HCPCS codes when billing for supplies and materials for patients. If you are having reimbursement problems with a private carrier for supplies and materials, contact its provider relations department and inquire about the use of HCPCS codes on private claims.

Some Medicaid carriers require HCPCS codes for billing supplies, but it is not unusual to find a completely different carrier-defined coding system for Medicaid claims. Check with your local Medicaid carrier if you are unsure.

PROCEDURE DOWN-CODING

Down-coding occurs when a health insurance claims examiner or a claims processing computer system changes the procedure code you reported on a health insurance claim form to another procedure code with a lesser reimbursement value. While described by health insurance payers as simply a correction process, down-coding provides the health insurance company with an opportunity to delay or reduce payment or even deny health insurance claims. Down-coding costs medical professionals and their patients millions of dollars annually.

DOWN-CODING DUE TO DIAGNOSIS CODE

As health insurance companies continue to improve the sophistication of their claims-processing systems, including implementation of automated pre- and postpayment review, expect to see more claims denied, returned, questioned, or down-coded due to incorrect, incomplete, or inadequate diagnosis coding.

The four major coding issues related to the relationship of ICD-9-CM and CPT codes are:

1. ICD-9-CM diagnosis codes must support the CPT services and procedures provided and reported.

2. ICD-9-CM diagnosis codes must support the need for the place (location) of service where the CPT procedures were performed or services provided.

3. ICD-9-CM diagnosis codes must support the level of care reported.

4. ICD-9-CM diagnosis codes must support the frequency of services reported.

DOWN-CODING DUE TO LACK OF DOCUMENTATION

The CPT coding system provides concise definitions of the key components required to report E/M service codes. Your documentation must clearly support the E/M service codes reported for the visit. Each E/M service code description consists of key components, contributory factors, and time. The performance of key components, either three of three or two of three, must be documented for every service.

Of the contributory factors, which include counseling, coordination, and nature of the presenting problem, only the last must be documented for every service. Counseling and/or coordination of care is not necessarily provided at every encounter and needs to be documented only if actually provided.

The time spent either face to face with the patient and/or family or as unit/floor time for hospital care and hospital consultations should be noted for every service. This is particularly important in a situation in which counseling and/or coordination of care takes up more than 50 percent of the face-to-face physician time. In this situation, time is considered the key or controlling factor, and the extent of counseling and/or coordination of care must be documented in the medical record.

Consider that in an eight- or nine-hour workday, there are a limited number of time units that can be allocated to E/M services. Obviously, the collective time reported, as reflected in the choice of E/M service codes, cannot exceed the amount of time available in the workday.

For example, E/M code 99255, the highest level of inpatient consultation in the CPT code book, has an average time of 110 minutes. In an eight-hour day, only four of these services could be reported by one individual, and that is only if he or she did not take lunch or breaks or spend time doing anything else.

PURCHASED DIAGNOSTIC SERVICES

It is common for physicians to bill patients and health insurance companies for diagnostic services that were procured or ordered on behalf of the patient but not actually provided by the ordering physician. It is also common for the ordering physician to "mark-up" the fee for the purchased service prior to billing. This is referred to as *global billing*.

Medical equipment companies, particularly those offering electrocardiography, pulmonary diagnostic equipment, and other diagnostic equipment, have used this global billing concept in the past as a method of selling physicians a new "profit center" for their practice. Some even provided technicians, who were not employees of the practice, to perform the diagnostic tests in the physician's office. OBRA 1987 placed severe restrictions on global billing of certain diagnostic tests as of March 1, 1988.

The Medicare regulations apply to diagnostic tests other than clinical laboratory tests, including, but not limited to: EKGs, EEGs, cardiac monitoring, x-rays, and ultrasound. Global billing is allowed only when the billing physician personally performs or supervises the diagnostic procedure. To qualify under the supervision definition, the person performing the test must be an employee of the physician or group. Ownership interest in an outside supplier does not meet the supervision requirement.

Billing for purchased services under the new requirement is complicated. You must provide the supplier's name, address, provider number, and net charge on your claim form. In addition, you must typically include a HCPCS modifier to indicate that the service was purchased. Billing for global services usually will also require a HCPCS modifier to indicate that the service was not purchased. This requirement does not apply to the professional component of these services if provided separately. You may continue to bill for this service using modifier -26.

We strongly recommend that you discontinue billing for the technical component of diagnostic services that you did not provide or supervise as defined in this regulation. You are no longer making any profit on the procedures, and you are increasing your costs due to the increased reporting requirements. In addition, you are increasing your audit liability risk if you are not properly billing these services.

CPT MODIFIERS

A complete understanding of CPT modifiers, including how and when to report them, is vital to the reimbursement management process. The incorrect use of CPT modifiers may result in claim delays or claim denials. Using certain CPT modifiers too frequently may increase your audit liability, while the proper and judicious use of CPT modifiers may result in higher reimbursement.

Appendix A of the CPT code book lists all CPT modifiers. In addition, pertinent modifiers are repeated in each section of the CPT. Following is a list of the CPT modifiers along with a brief description and billing considerations when appropriate.

-21 Prolonged evaluation and management services

When the E/M service(s) provided is (are) prolonged or otherwise greater than that usually required for the highest level of E/M service within a given category, the prolonged E/M service(s) may be identified by adding a modifier -21 to the E/M service code number. A report may also be appropriate.

-22 Unusual procedural services

When the service(s) provided is (are) greater than that usually required.

Modifier -22 is one of the most frequently abused and misused modifiers. Many health care professionals routinely add modifier -22 to CPT procedure codes with the expectation that higher reimbursement will be forthcoming. Most health insurance companies routinely ignore an undocumented modifier -22 on health insurance claims for the same reason.

Most of the time, it is more appropriate to choose a CPT code of a higher value than to use modifier -22. If you do report this modifier with your services, you must include documentation in the form of a cover letter or report with your health insurance claim to explain the situation or circumstances that make your procedure unusual.

-23   Unusual anesthesia

Modifier -23 is used to report a procedure was performed under general anesthesia that is normally performed with no anesthesia.

-24   Unrelated evaluation and management service by the same physician during a postoperative period

The physician may need to indicate that an E/M service was performed during a postoperative period for a reason or reasons unrelated to the original procedure. This circumstance may be reported by adding the modifier -24 to the appropriate level of E/M service, or the separate five-digit modifier 09924 may be used.

-25   Significant, separately identifiable evaluation and service by the same physician on the same day of a procedure

The physician may need to indicate that on the day a procedure or service identified by a CPT code was performed, the patient's condition required a significant, separately identifiable E/M service above and beyond the usual preoperative and postoperative care associated with the procedure that was performed. This circumstance may be reported by adding the modifier -25 to the appropriate level of E/M service, or the separate five-digit modifier 09925 may be used.

-26   Professional component

Used to report the physician component of a procedure that consists of a technical and a professional component. These are typically diagnostic procedures.

This modifier became more important with the implementation of the Medicare purchased diagnostic services regulations.

-27   Multiple outpatient hospital E/M encounters on the same date

Occasionally a patient may be seen in the hospital outpatient setting more than once in a single day by different providers. For example, a patient is first seen in the emergency room and then referred to the clinic or vice versa. This circumstance is reported by adding modifier -27 to the appropriate outpatient and/or emergency service E/M codes.

Note: This modifier may not be used for reporting multiple E/M services by the same physician on the same date.

-32   Mandated services

This modifier is reported to identify services that were mandated by a third party, such as a peer review organization or health insurance company.

HCPCS modifier -SF is reported instead of CPT modifier -32 if the patient is a Medicare patient.

-47   Anesthesia by surgeon

This modifier is reported when regional or general anesthesia is provided by the surgeon. Modifier -47 is not used for reporting local anesthesia and also is not used with codes from the Anesthesia section of the CPT code book.

-50   Bilateral procedure

This modifier is reported when bilateral procedures requiring a separate incision are performed during the *same* operative session. Proper reporting of this modifier on the CMS1500 health insurance claim form requires the CPT procedure code to be listed two times: first with no modifier, and the second time with modifier -50.

-51   Multiple procedures

When multiple surgical procedures are performed at the same operative session, all secondary, additional, or lesser procedures are listed after the primary procedure with the addition of the modifier -51. Modifier -51 must be used properly and carefully, because it has a tremendous impact on reimbursement.

-52   Reduced services

Modifier -52 is reported when a service or procedure is partially reduced or eliminated. The intended use of this modifier is to report the reduction of a service without affecting the provider profiles maintained by health insurance companies.

Modifier -52 is another frequently misused modifier. Many medical practices mistakenly use modifier -52 to mean "reduced fee" and use it as a discounting method. Not only is this incorrect, you may be seriously damaging your profile with health insurance companies.

The proper use for modifier -52 is to report that a service was not completed or that some part of a multiple-part service was not performed. A fee reduction may be in order as well; however that is not the primary purpose of the modifier.

-53   Discontinued procedure

Modifier -53 is used to report the elective termination of a surgical or diagnostic procedure. Occasionally, it may be necessary for the physician to terminate a surgical or diagnostic procedure that threatens the well being of the patient. This circumstance is reported by adding modifier -53 to the CPT code reported by the physician for the discontinued procedure.

-54   Surgical care only

This modifier is reported when one physician performs a surgical procedure and another provides preoperative and/or postoperative care.

-55   Postoperative management only

This modifier is reported when one physician performs the postoperative care after another physician has performed the surgical procedure.

-56   Preoperative management only

This modifier is reported when one physician performs preoperative care and evaluation prior to another physician performing the surgical procedure.

-57   Decision for surgery

This modifier is reported to identify an E/M service that resulted in the initial decision to perform surgery.

-58   Staged or related procedure or service by the same physician during the postoperative period

Modifier -58 is reported when a physician needs to indicate that a procedure or service performed during the postoperative period was: a) planned prospectively at the time of the original procedure (staged); b) more extensive than the original procedure; or c) for therapy following a diagnostic surgical procedure.

Modifier -58 is not used to report the treatment of a problem that requires a return to the operating room.

-59 Distinct procedural service

Reported when a physician needs to indicate that a procedure or service was distinct or independent of other services performed on the same day.

-62 Two surgeons

Modifier -62 is reported when the skills of two surgeons, usually with different skills, are required in the management of a specific surgical procedure.

-63 Procedure performed on infants less than 4 kg

Procedures performed on neonates and infants up to a present body weight of 4 kg may involve significantly increased complexity and physician work. This circumstance is reported by adding the modifier -63 to the procedure code.

-66 Surgical team

Modifier -66 is reported when highly complex procedures require the services of several physicians at the same time.

-73 Discontinued out-patient hospital/ambulatory surgery center (ASC) procedure *prior to* the administration of anesthesia

Extenuating circumstances or those that threaten the well being of the patient may necessitate cancellation of a surgical or diagnostic procedure scheduled for the out-patient hospital or ASC setting. If this cancellation occurs *prior to* the administration of anesthesia, the discontinued procedure is reported with the addition of modifier -73.

Note: If the cancellation was elective, the service should not be reported.

-74 Discontinued out-patient hospital/ambulatory surgery center (ASC) procedure *after* the administration of anesthesia

Extenuating circumstances or those that threaten the well being of the patient may necessitate cancellation of a surgical or diagnostic procedure scheduled for the out-patient hospital or ASC setting. If this cancellation occurs *after* the administration of anesthesia, the discontinued procedure is reported with the addition of modifier -73.

-76 Repeat procedure by same physician

This modifier is reported when a procedure or service is repeated by the same physician.

-77   Repeat procedure by another physician

This modifier is reported when a procedure is performed that was previously performed by another physician.

-78   Return to the operating room for a related procedure during the postoperative period

The physician may need to indicate that another procedure was performed during the postoperative period of the initial procedure. When this subsequent procedure is related to the first and requires the use of the operating room, it is reported by adding modifier -78 to the related procedure. (For repeat procedures on the same day, see -76.)

-79   Unrelated procedure or service by the same physician during the postoperative period

The physician may need to indicate that the performance of a procedure or service during the postoperative period was unrelated to the original procedure. This circumstance may be reported by adding the modifier -79 to the procedure or service. (For repeat procedures on the same day, see -76.)

-80   Assistant surgeon

This modifier is used to report surgical assistant services provided by the first assistant surgeon.

-81   Minimum assistant surgeon

This modifier is reported to report minimal services provided by a second assistant surgeon.

-82   Assistant surgeon (qualified resident not available)

This modifier is used to report assistant surgeon services provided at teaching hospitals when a qualified resident surgeon was not available to assist.

-90   Reference (outside) laboratory

When laboratory procedures billed on a health insurance claim are performed by an outside laboratory, add modifier -90.

-91   Repeat clinical diagnostic laboratory test

It may occasionally be necessary to repeat the same laboratory test on the same day to obtain subsequent (multiple) test results. This is reported by adding the modifier -91 to the CPT code for the subsequent test(s). Note: This modifier may not be used for tests that are repeated to confirm initial results, due to problems with specimens or equipment, or for any other reason when a normal, one-time, reportable result is all that is necessary.

-99   Multiple modifiers

Occasionally, two or more modifiers may be necessary to completely describe a service. In this situation, modifier -99 should be added to the basic procedure, and other applicable modifiers may be listed as part of the description of the service.

HCPCS MODIFIERS

The HCPCS coding system includes modifiers at two levels. HCPCS Level I modifiers are the same as CPT modifiers. HCPCS Level II modifiers are either one- or two-digit codes in either alpha or alphanumeric format. HCPCS modifiers may be added, deleted, or changed in each new edition of the HCPCS book. These changes are frequent, and it is very important that you review this section of the new HCPCS book each year.

HCPCS LEVEL II MODIFIERS

Following is the complete list of HCPCS Level II modifiers and descriptions:

-A1   Dressing for one wound

-A2   Dressing for two wounds

-A3   Dressing for three wounds

-A4   Dressing for four wounds

-A5   Dressing for five wounds

-A6   Dressing for six wounds

-A7   Dressing for seven wounds

-A8   Dressing for eight wounds

-A9   Dressing for nine or more wounds

-AA   Anesthesia services performed personally by anesthesiologist

-AD Medical supervision by a physician: more than four concurrent anesthesia procedures

-AE Registered dietician

-AF Specialty physician

-AG Primary physician

-AH Clinical psychologist

-AJ Clinical social worker

-AK Non-participating physician

-AM Physician, team member service

-AP Determination of refractive state was not performed in the course of diagnostic ophthalmological examination

-AQ Physician providing a service in an unlisted health professional shortage area (HPSA)

-AS Physician assistant, nurse practitioner, or clinical nurse specialist services for assistant at surgery

-AT Acute treatment

This modifier should be used when reporting Chiropractic Manipulation codes 98940, 98941, 98942.

-AU Item furnished in conjunction with a urological, ostomy, or tracheostomy supply

-AV Item furnished in conjunction with a prosthetic device, prosthetic, or orthotic

-AW Item furnished in conjunction with a surgical dressing

-AX Item furnished in conjunction with dialysis services

-BA Item furnished in conjunction with parenteral enteral nutrition (PEN) services

-BL Special acquisition of blood and blood products

-BO Orally administered nutrition, not by feeding tube

-BP The beneficiary has been informed of the purchase and rental options and has elected to purchase the item

-BR The beneficiary has been informed of the purchase and rental options and has elected to rent the item

-BU The beneficiary has been informed of the purchase and rental options and after 30 days has not informed the supplier

-CA Procedure payable only in the inpatient setting when performed emergently on an outpatient who expires prior to admission

-CB Service ordered by a renal dialysis facility (RDF) physician as part of the ESRD beneficiary's dialysis benefit, is not part of the composite rate, and is separately reimbursable

-CC Procedure code change

Use modifier -CC when the procedure code submitted was changed either for administrative reasons or because an incorrect code was filed.

-CD AMCC test has been ordered by an ESRD facility or MCP physician that is part of the composite rate and is not separately billable

-CE AMCC test has been ordered by an ESRD facility or MCP physician that is a composite rate test but is beyond the normal frequency covered under the rate and is separately reimbursable based on medical necessity

-CF AMCC test has been ordered by an ESRD facility or MCP physician that is not part of the composite rate and is separately billable

-CG Innovator drug dispensed

-CR Catastrophe/disaster related

-E1 Upper left, eyelid

-E2 Lower left, eyelid

-E3 Upper right, eyelid

-E4 Lower right, eyelid

-EJ Subsequent claims for a defined course of therapy (e.g., EPO, sodium hyaluronate, infliximab)

-EM Emergency reserve supply (For ESRD benefit only)

-EP Service provided as part of Medicaid early periodic screening diagnosis and treatment (EPSDT) program

-ET Emergency services

-EY No physician or other licensed health care provider order for this item or service

-F1 Left hand, second digit

-F2 Left hand, third digit

-F3 Left hand, fourth digit

-F4 Left hand, fifth digit

-F5 Right hand, thumb

-F6 Right hand, second digit

-F7 Right hand, third digit

-F8 Right hand, fourth digit

-F9 Right hand, fifth digit

-FA Left hand, thumb

-FB Item provided without cost to provider, supplier or practitioner or credit received for replaced device (examples, but note limited to: covered under warranty, replaced due to defect, free samples)

-FP Service provided as part of Medicaid family planning program

-G1 Most recent URR reading of less than 60

-G2 Most recent URR reading of 60 to 64.9

-G3 Most recent URR reading of 65 to 69.9

-G4 Most recent URR reading of 70 to 74.9

-G5 Most recent URR reading of 75 or greater

-G6 ESRD patient for whom fewer than six dialysis sessions have been provided in a month

-G7 Pregnancy resulted from rape or incest or pregnancy certified by physician as life threatening

-G8 Monitored anesthesia care (MAC) for deep complex, complicated, or markedly invasive surgical procedure

-G9 Monitored anesthesia care for patient who has a history of severe cardiopulmonary condition

-GA Waiver of liability statement on file

-GB Claim being resubmitted for payment because it is no longer covered under a global payment demonstration

-GC This service has been performed in part by a resident under the direction of a teaching physician

-GE This service has been performed by a resident without the presence of a teaching physician under the primary care exception

-GF Nonphysician services in a critical care hospital

Used when services are provided in a critical care hospital by a Nurse Practitioner (NP), certified registered nurse anesthetist (CRNA), certified registered nurse (CRN), clinical nurse specialist (CNS), or physician assistant (PA).

-GG Performance and payment of a screening mammogram and diagnostic mammogram on the same patient, same day

-GH Diagnostic mammogram converted from screening mammogram on same day

-GJ Opt-out physician or practitioner emergency or urgent service

-GK Actual item/service ordered by physician, item associated with -GA or -GZ modifier

-GL Medically unnecessary upgrade provided instead of standard item, no charge, no advance beneficiary notice (ABN)

-GM Multiple patients on one ambulance trip

-GN Services delivered under an outpatient speech language pathology plan of care

-GO Services delivered under an outpatient occupational therapy plan of care

-GP Services delivered under an outpatient physical therapy plan of care

-GQ Via asynchronous telecommunications system

-GR This service was performed in whole or in part by a resident in a department of veterans affairs medical center or clinic, supervised in accordance with VA policy

-GS Dosage of EPO or darbepoietin alfa has been reduced and maintained in response

-GT Via interactive audio and video telecommunication systems

-GV Attending physician not employed or paid under arrangement by the patient's hospice provider

-GW Service not related to the hospice patient's terminal condition

-GY Item or service statutorily excluded or does not meet the definition of any Medicare benefit

-GZ Item or service expected to be denied as not reasonable and necessary

-H9 Court-ordered

-HA Child/adolescent program

-HB Adult program, non-geriatric

-HC Adult program, geriatric

-HD Pregnant/parenting women's program

-HE Mental health program

-HF Substance abuse program

-HG Opioid addiction treatment program

-HH Integrated mental health/substance abuse

-HI Integrated mental health and mental retardation and developmental disabilities program

-HJ Employee assistance program

-HK Specialized mental health programs for high-risk populations

-HL Intern

-HM Less than bachelor degree level

-HN Bachelor's degree level

-HO Master's degree level

-HP Doctoral level

-HQ Group setting

-HR Family/couple with client present

-HS   Family/couple without client present

-HT   Multidisciplinary team

-HU   Funded by child welfare agency

-HV   Funded state addictions agency

-HW   Funded by state mental health agency

-HX   Funded by county/local agency

-HY   Funded by juvenile justice agency

-HZ   Funded by criminal justice agency

-J1   Competitive acquisition program no-pay submission for a prescription number

-J2   Competitive acquisition program, restocking of emergency drugs after emergency administration

-J3   Competitive acquisition program (CAP), drug not available through CAP as written, reimbursed under average sales price methodology

-JW   Drug amount discarded/not administered to any patient

-K0   Lower-extremity prosthesis functional level 0

Patient does not have the ability or potential to ambulate or transfer safely with or without assistance and a prosthesis does not enhance the quality of life or mobility.

-K1   Lower-extremity prosthesis functional level 1

Patient has the ability or potential to use a prosthesis for transfers or ambulation on level surfaces at fixed cadence. Typical of the limited and unlimited household ambulator.

-K2   Lower-extremity prosthesis functional level 2

Patient has the ability or potential for ambulation with the ability to traverse low-level environmental barriers such as curbs, stairs, or uneven surfaces. Typical of the limited community ambulator.

-K3   Lower-extremity prosthesis functional level 3

Patient has the ability or potential for ambulation with variable cadence. Typical of the community ambulator who has the ability to traverse most environmental barriers and may have vocational, therapeutic, or exercise activity that demands prosthetic utilization beyond simple locomotion.

-K4 Lower-extremity prosthesis functional level 4

Patient has the ability or potential for prosthetic ambulation that exceeds the basic ambulation skills, exhibiting high-impact, stress, or energy levels typical of the prosthetic demands of the child, active adult, or athlete.

-KA Add-on option/accessory for wheelchair

-KB Beneficiary-requested upgrade for ABN, more than four modifiers identified on claim

-KC Replacement of special power wheelchair interface

-KD Drug or biological infused through DME

-KF Item designated by FDA as class III device

-KH DMEPOS item, initial claim, purchase or first-month rental

-KI DMEPOS item, second- or third-month rental

-KJ DMEPOS item, parenteral enteral nutrition (PEN) pump or capped rental, months four to 15

-KM Replacement of facial prosthesis including new impression/moulage

-KN Replacement of facial prosthesis using previous master model

-KO Single drug unit dose formulation

-KP First drug of a multiple drug unit dose formulation

-KQ Second or subsequent drug of a multiple drug unit dose formulation

-KR Rental item, billing for partial month

-KS Glucose monitor supply for diabetic beneficiary not treated with insulin

-KX Specific required documentation on file

-KZ New coverage not implemented by managed

-LC Left circumflex coronary artery

-LD Left anterior descending coronary artery

-LL Lease/rental

Use the -LL modifier when DME equipment rental is to be applied against the purchase price.

-LR Laboratory round trip

-LS FDA-monitored intraocular lens implant

-LT Left side

Used to identify procedures performed on the left side of the body.

-MS Six-month maintenance and servicing fee for reasonable and necessary parts and labor that are not covered under any manufacturer or supplier warranty

-NR New when rented (use the -NR modifier when DME that was new at the time of rental is subsequently purchased)

-NU New equipment

-P1 A normal healthy patient

-P2 A patient with mild systemic disease

-P3 A patient with severe systemic disease

-P4 A patient with severe systemic disease that is a constant threat to life

-P5 A moribund patient who is not expected to survive without the operation

-P6 A declared brain-dead patient whose organs are being removed for donor purposes

-PL Progressive addition lenses

-Q2 HCFA/ORD demonstration project procedure/service

-Q3 Live kidney donor surgery and related services

-Q4 Service for ordering/referring physician qualifies as a service exemption

-Q5 Service furnished by a substitute physician under a reciprocal billing arrangement

-Q6 Service furnished by a locum tenens physician

-Q7 One class A finding

-Q8 Two class B findings

-Q9 One class B and two class C findings

-QA FDA investigational device exemption

-QC Single-channel monitoring

-QD Recording and storage in solid-state memory by a digital recorder

-QE Prescribed amount of oxygen is less than one liter per minute (LPM)

-QF Prescribed amount of oxygen exceeds four liters per minute (LPM) and portable oxygen is prescribed

-QG Prescribed amount of oxygen is greater than four liters per minute (LPM)

-QH Oxygen-conserving device is being used with an oxygen delivery system

-QJ Services/items provided to a prisoner or patient in state or local custody, however the state or local government, as applicable, meets the requirements in 42 cfr 4114(B)

-QK Medical direction of two, three, or four concurrent anesthesia procedures involving qualified individuals

-QL Patient pronounced dead after ambulance called

-QM Ambulance service provided under arrangement by a provider of services

-QN Ambulance service furnished directly by a provider of services

-QP Documentation is on file showing that the laboratory test(s) was ordered individually or ordered as a CPT-recognized panel other than automated profile codes 80002-80019, G0058, G0059, and G0060

-QR Item or service provided in a Medicare specified study

-QS Monitored anesthesia care service

-QT Recording and storage on tape by an analog tape recorder

-QV Item or service provided as routine care in a Medicare qualifying clinical trial

-QW CLIA waived test

-QX CRNA service: with medical direction by a physician

-QY Medical direction of one certified registered nurse anesthetist (CRNA) by an anesthesiologist

-QZ CRNA service: without medical direction by a physician

-RC Right coronary artery

-RD Drug provided to beneficiary, but not administered incident-to

-RP Replacement and repair

Modifier -RP may be used to indicate replacement of DME, orthotic and prosthetic devices that have been in use for some time. The claim shows the code for the part, followed by the -RP modifier and the charge for the part.

-RR Rental

Use the -RR modifier when DME is to be rented.

-RT Right side
Used to identify procedures performed on the right side of the body.

-SA Nurse practitioner rendering service in collaboration with a physician

-SB Nurse midwife

-SC Medically necessary service or supply

-SD Services provided by registered nurse with specialized, highly technical home infusion training

-SE State and/or federally funded programs/services

-SF Second opinion ordered by a professional review organization (PRO) per section 9401, PL 99-272 (100% reimbursement—no Medicare deductible or coinsurance)

-SG Ambulatory surgical center (ASC) facility service

-SH Second concurrently administered infusion therapy

-SJ Third or more concurrently administered infusion therapy

-SK Member of high-risk population (use only with codes for immunization)

-SL State-supplied vaccine

-SM Second surgical opinion

-SN Third surgical opinion

-SQ Item ordered by home health

-ST Related to trauma or injury

-SU Procedure performed in physician's office (to denote use of facility and equipment)

-SV Pharmaceuticals delivered to patient's home but not utilized

-SW Services provided by a certified diabetic educator

-SY Persons who are in close contact with member of high-risk population (use only with codes for immunization)

-T1 Left foot, second digit

-T2 Left foot, third digit

-T3 Left foot, fourth digit

-T4 Left foot, fifth digit

-T5 Right foot, great toe

-T6 Right foot, second digit

-T7 Right foot, third digit

-T8 Right foot, fourth digit

-T9 Right foot, fifth digit

-TA Left foot, great toe

-TC Technical component

Under certain circumstances, a charge may be made for the technical component alone. Under those circumstances, the technical component charge is identified by adding modifier -TC to the usual procedure number. Technical component charges are institutional charges and not billed separately by physicians. However, portable x-ray suppliers bill only for technical component and should utilize modifier -TC. The charge data from portable x-ray suppliers will then be used to build customary and prevailing profiles.

-TD RN

-TE LPN/LVN

-TF Intermediate level of care

-TG   Complex/high-tech level of care

-TH   Obstetrical treatment/services, prenatal or postpartum

-TJ   Program group, child and/or adolescent

-TK   Extra patient or passenger, non-ambulance

-TL   Early intervention/individualized family service plan (IFSP)

-TM   Individualized education program

-TN   Rural/outside providers' customary service area

-TP   Medical transport, unloaded vehicle

-TQ   Basic life support transport by a volunteer ambulance provider

-TR   School-based individualized education program (IEP) services provided outside the public school district responsible for the student

-TS   Follow-up service

-TT   Individualized service provided to more than one patient in same setting

-TU   Special payment rate, overtime

-TV   Special payment rates, holidays/weekends

-TW   Back-up equipment

-U1   Medicaid level of care 1, as defined by each state

-U2   Medicaid level of care 2, as defined by each state

-U3   Medicaid level of care 3, as defined by each state

-U4   Medicaid level of care 4, as defined by each state

-U5   Medicaid level of care 5, as defined by each state

-U6   Medicaid level of care 6, as defined by each state

-U7   Medicaid level of care 7, as defined by each state

-U8   Medicaid level of care 8, as defined by each state

-U9   Medicaid level of care 9, as defined by each state

-UA Medicaid level of care 10, as defined by each state

-UB Medicaid level of care 11, as defined by each state

-UC Medicaid level of care 12, as defined by each state

-UD Medicaid level of care 13, as defined by each state

-UE Used durable medical equipment

-UF Services provided in the morning

-UG Services provided in the afternoon

-UH Services provided in the evening

-UJ Services provided at night

-UK Services provided on behalf of the client to someone other than the client (collateral relationship)

-UN Two patients served

-UP Three patients served

-UQ Four patients served

-UR Five patients served

-US Six or more patients served

-VP Aphakic patient

AMBULANCE SERVICE MODIFIERS

Origin and destination modifiers

-D Diagnostic or therapeutic site other than -P or -H

-E Residential, domiciliary, custodial facility (nursing home, not skilled nursing facility)

-G Hospital-based dialysis facility (hospital or hospital-related)

-H Hospital

-I Site of transfer (for example, airport or helicopter pad between types of ambulance)

-J Non-hospital-based dialysis facility

-N   Skilled nursing facility (SNF)

-P   Physician's office (includes HMO non-hospital facility, clinic)

-R   Residence

-S   Scene of accident or acute event

-X   Intermediate stop at physician's office en route to the hospital
Includes HMO non-hospital facility, clinic. Note: Modifier -X can be used as a designation code only in the second position of a modifier.

The above single-letter ambulance service modifiers are used in combination on the claim form to indicate the origin and destination of the ambulance trip. The first letter indicates the transport's place of origin; the second letter indicates the destination. Following are several examples of origin/destination modifier combinations.

-EE   Ambulance trip from an ECF or nursing home to another ECF or nursing home

-EH   Ambulance trip from an ECF or nursing home to a hospital

-EP   Ambulance trip from an ECF or nursing home to a physician's office

-ER   Ambulance trip from an ECF or nursing home to a patient's residence

-HE   Ambulance trip from a hospital to an ECF or nursing home

-HH   Ambulance trip for discharge/transfer from one hospital to another hospital

-HR   Ambulance trip from a hospital to a patient's residence

-PH   Ambulance trip from a physician's office to a hospital

-RA   Ambulance trip from the patient's residence to a physician's office

-RE   Ambulance trip from the patient's residence to an ECF or nursing home

-RH   Ambulance trip from the patient's residence to a hospital

-SH   Ambulance trip from the scene of an accident

PET SCAN MODIFIERS

The following single-digit characters are used in combination as a two-digit modifier to indicate the results of a current and previous PET scan.

-N Negative

-E Equivocal

-P Positive, but not suggestive of extensive ischemia

-S Positive and suggestive of extensive ischemia (>20 percent of the left ventricle)

EVALUATION & MANAGEMENT SERVICES

The evaluation and management codes, commonly referred to as E/M service codes, were developed by a special CPT editorial panel working in conjunction with the Physician Payment Review Committee (PPRC). The use of these codes was mandated by law for all Medicare claims for services rendered on or after January 1, 1992. Private carriers were not required to adopt or use these new codes; however, the historical trend is that new policies and procedures mandated by Medicare are followed shortly by Medicaid and private health insurance.

CLASSIFICATION OF EVALUATION AND MANAGEMENT SERVICES

The Evaluation and Management section of the CPT code book includes codes for reporting visits, consultations, prolonged service, case management services, preventive medicine services, newborn care, and special services. The section is divided into categories such as office visits, hospital visits, and consultations. Most of the categories are further divided into two or more subcategories.

The subcategories for E/M services are further classified into levels of service that are identified by specific codes. The level of service classification is important, because the physician work required to provide the service varies by the type of service, the place of service, and the patient's clinical status.

The basic format of the E/M service codes and definitions is the same for most categories.

- A unique five-digit CPT code number is listed.

- The *place* and/or *type* of service is specified, for example, "office consultation."

- The *content* of the service is defined, for example, "comprehensive history and comprehensive examination."

- The *nature* of the presenting problem(s) usually associated with a given level is described.

- The *time* typically required to provide the service is specified.

SUBSECTION INFORMATION

The Evaluation and Management section of the CPT code book is divided into 19 subsections, namely:

Office or Other Outpatient Services	99201-99215
Hospital Observation Discharge Services	99217
Hospital Observation Services	99218-99220
Hospital Inpatient Services	99221-99238
Consultations	99241-99275
Emergency Department Services	99281-99288
Pediatric Patient Transport	99289-99290
Critical Care Services	99291-99292
Continuing Intensive Care Services	99298-99300
Neonatal Intensive Care	99295-99297
Nursing Facility Services	99301-99313
Custodial Care Services	99321-99333
Domiciliary, Resth Home, or Home Care Oversight Services	99339-99340
Home Services	99341-99353
Prolonged Services	99354-99359
Standby Services	99360
Case Management Services	99361-99373
Care Plan Oversight Services	99375-99376
Preventive Medicine Services	99381-99249
Newborn Care	99431-99440
Special E/M Services	99450-99456
Other E/M Services	99499

All subsections within the Evaluation and Management section have extensive notes that should be reviewed carefully prior to selecting codes for services located within the section.

MATERIALS SUPPLIED BY THE PHYSICIAN

Supplies and materials provided by the physician over and above those usually included with the E/M or other services rendered may be listed separately. List all drugs, trays, supplies, and materials provided.

DEFINITIONS OF COMMONLY USED TERMS

Certain key words and phrases are used throughout the Evaluation and Management section. The following definitions are intended to reduce the potential for differing interpretations and to increase the consistency of reporting by physicians in differing specialties.

NEW AND ESTABLISHED PATIENTS

E/M services are further classified depending upon the relationship of the patient to the physician. *New* patients typically require more physician work and more time than *established* patients, a fact that is acknowledged by the relative values of the E/M service codes.

In the CPT code book, a *new patient* is defined as "one who has not received any professional services from the physician, or another physician of the same specialty who belongs to the same group practice, within the past three years."

An *established patient* is defined as "one who has received professional services from the physician, or another physician of the same specialty who belongs to the same group practice, within the past three years."

If the physician is on call or providing coverage for another physician, the patient's encounter is classified as "new" or "established" exactly as it would have been by the original physician.

There is no distinction made between new and established patients in the emergency department. E/M services in the emergency category may be reported for any new or established patient who presents for treatment in the emergency department.

CHIEF COMPLAINT

Provide a concise statement describing the symptom, problem, condition, diagnosis, or other factor that is the reason for the encounter with the patient. This is usually stated in the patient's own words.

CONCURRENT CARE

Concurrent care is the provision of similar services, for example hospital visits, to the same patient by more than one physician on the same day. When concurrent care is provided, no special reporting is required. However, in order to distinguish your services from those of another physician on the same date, it is important that you carefully record the diagnostic codes that made the visit necessary.

COUNSELING

Counseling is defined in the CPT code book as "a discussion with a patient and/or family" concerning one or more of the following:

- diagnostic results, impressions, and/or recommended diagnostic studies

- the prognosis

- the risks and benefits of treatment options

- instructions for treatment and/or follow-up

- the importance of compliance with treatment options

- risk factor reduction

- patient and family education

Counseling is listed as one of the seven components of E/M services; however, there are no specified measurements included in the definition of the services.

HISTORY

Family History

The family history includes a review of medical events in the patient's family that includes: 1) significant information about the health status or cause of death of parents, siblings, and children, 2) specific diseases related to problems identified in the chief complaint or history of the present illness or system review, and 3) diseases of family members that may be hereditary or place the patient at risk.

History of the Present Illness

Provide a chronological description of the development of the patient's present illness from the first sign and/or symptom to the present. This includes a description of location, quality, severity, timing, context, modifying factors, and associated signs and symptoms significantly related to the presenting problem.

Past History

The past history includes a review of the patient's past experiences with illnesses, injuries, and treatments that includes significant information about: 1) prior major illnesses and injuries, 2) prior operations, 3) prior hospitalizations, 4) current medications, 5) allergies, 6) age-appropriate immunization status, and 7) age-appropriate feeding/dietary status.

Social History

The social history includes an age-appropriate review of past and current activities that includes significant information about: 1) marital status and/or living arrangements, 2) current employment, 3) occupational history, 4) use of drugs, alcohol, and tobacco, 5) level of education, 6) sexual history, and 7) other relevant social factors.

SYSTEM REVIEW (REVIEW OF SYSTEMS)

A system review, or review of systems, is defined in the CPT code book as an inventory of body systems obtained by asking questions to identify signs and/or symptoms that the patient may be experiencing or has experienced.

The review of systems helps to define the problem, clarify the differential diagnosis, and identify needed testing and also serves as baseline data on other systems that might be affected by any possible management options.

A system review or review of systems as defined in the CPT code book includes the following elements: 1) constitutional symptoms (fever, weight loss, etc.), 2) eyes, 3) ears, nose, mouth, and throat, 4) cardiovascular system, 5) respiratory system, 6) gastrointestinal system, 7) genitourinary system, 8) musculoskeletal system, 9) integumentary (skin and/or breast) system, 10) neurological system, 11) psychiatric evaluation, 12) endocrine system, 13) hematologic and lymphatic systems, and 14) allergic/immunologic situations.

LEVELS OF EVALUATION AND MANAGEMENT SERVICES

Within each category or subcategory of E/M service, there are three to five levels of services available for reporting purposes. Levels of E/M services are not interchangeable among the different categories or subcategories of service. For example, the first level of E/M services in the subcategory of office visit, new patient, does not have the same definition as the first level of E/M services in the subcategory of office visit, established patient.

The levels of E/M services include examinations, evaluations, treatments, conferences with or concerning patients, preventive pediatric and adult health supervision, and similar medical services. The levels of E/M services encompass the wide variations in skill, effort, time, responsibility, and medical knowledge required for the prevention or diagnosis and treatment of illness or injury and the promotion of optimal health. Each level of E/M services may be used by all physicians.

Each E/M service code is defined by a combination of up to seven components: 1) the history, 2) the physical examination, 3) the amount of medical decision making, 4) the amount of counseling needed, 5) the amount of coordination of care, 6) the nature of the presenting problem, and 7) the amount of time spent face to face with the patient or in the hospital unit.

KEY COMPONENTS

The first three of these components (history, examination, and medical decision making) are considered as the key components when selecting a level of E/M services.

HISTORY

There are four types of history used to define specific E/M services:

Problem Focused

- Chief complaint;

- Brief history of present illness or problem.

Expanded Problem Focused

- Chief complaint;

- Brief history of present illness;

- Problem pertinent system review.

Detailed

- Chief complaint;

- Extended history of present illness;

- Extended system review;

- Pertinent past;

- Family and/or social history.

Comprehensive

- Chief complaint;

- Extended history of present illness;

- Complete system review; complete past;

- Family and social history.

In the definition of some E/M services, you may see the term "interval" used to describe a history that is a component of follow-up hospital care.

EXAMINATION

There are four types of examination used to define E/M service codes:

Problem Focused

A *Problem Focused* examination is defined as an examination that is limited to the affected body area or organ system.

Expanded Problem Focused

An *Expanded Problem Focused* examination is defined as an examination of the affected body area or organ system and other symptomatic or related organ systems.

Detailed

A *Detailed* examination is defined as an extended examination of the affected body area(s) and other symptomatic or related organ system(s).

Comprehensive

A *Comprehensive* examination is defined as a general multisystem examination or a complete single-system specialty examination. The comprehensive examination performed as part of the preventive medicine E/M service is multisystem, but its extent is based on age and risk factors identified.

For the purposes of these CPT definitions, the following body areas are recognized:

- Head, including the face
- Neck
- Chest, including breasts and axilla
- Abdomen
- Genitalia, groin, buttocks
- Back
- Each extremity

For the purposes of these CPT definitions, the following organ systems are recognized:

- Eyes
- Ears, Nose, Mouth, and Throat
- Cardiovascular
- Respiratory
- Gastrointestinal
- Genitourinary
- Musculoskeletal
- Skin
- Neurologic
- Psychiatric
- Hematologic/Lymphatic/Immunologic

You will also see the term "interval" used to describe an examination that is a component of follow-up hospital care.

MEDICAL DECISION MAKING

Medical decision making refers to the complexity of establishing a diagnosis and/or selecting a management option as measured by:

1. the number of possible diagnoses and/or the number of management options considered;

2. the amount and/or complexity of medical records, diagnostic tests, and/or other information that must be obtained and analyzed;

3. the risk of significant complications, morbidity, and/or mortality, as well as comorbidities, associated with the patient's presenting problem(s), the diagnostic procedure(s), and/or the possible management options.

Four types of medical decision making are defined in CPT: straightforward, low complexity, moderate complexity, and high complexity. In addition, some codes include choices or ranges of medical decision making, for example "straightforward or low" and "low to moderate."

Straightforward

*   Minimal number of diagnoses or management options

*   Minimal or no data to be reviewed

*   Minimal risk of complications and/or morbidity or mortality

Low Complexity

*   Limited number of diagnoses or management options

*   Limited amount and/or complexity of data to be reviewed

*   Low risk of complications and/or morbidity or mortality

Moderate Complexity

*   Multiple diagnoses or management options

*   Moderate amount and/or complexity of data to be reviewed

- Moderate risk of complications and/or morbidity or mortality

High Complexity

- Extensive diagnoses or management options

- Extensive amount and/or complexity of data to be reviewed

- High risk of complications and/or morbidity or mortality

Combinations

Note that combinations of the above may also be found in the descriptions of some E/M service codes. For example, you will find codes for which the level of medical decision making is defined as "straightforward or low" or "low to moderate complexity."

CONTRIBUTORY COMPONENTS

The next three components—counseling, coordination of care, and the nature of the presenting problem—are considered *contributory* factors in the majority of encounters. Although counseling and coordination of care are important components of E/M services, it is not required that either or both be provided at every patient encounter.

COORDINATION OF CARE

There is no definition of coordination of care provided in the CPT. The only statement made is: "Coordination of care with other providers or agencies without a patient encounter on that day is reported using the case management codes."

In the case in which counseling and/or coordination of care dominates (more than 50%) the face-to-face physician/patient encounter, then *time* is considered the key or controlling factor to qualify for a particular level of E/M services. The extent of counseling and/or coordination of care must be documented in the medical record.

NATURE OF THE PRESENTING PROBLEM

A presenting problem is a disease, condition, illness, injury, symptom, sign, finding, complaint, or other reason for encounter, with or without a diagnosis being established at the time of the encounter. There are five types of presenting problems that are used in defining the E/M service codes:

Minimal

A problem that may not require the presence of the physician, but service is provided under the physician's supervision.

Self-limited or Minor

A problem that runs a definite and prescribed course, is transient in nature, and is not likely to permanently alter health status *or* has a good prognosis with management and/or compliance.

Low Severity

A problem for which the risk of morbidity without treatment is low; there is little to no risk of mortality without treatment; full recovery without functional impairment is expected.

Moderate Severity

A problem for which the risk of morbidity without treatment is moderate; there is moderate risk of mortality without treatment; uncertain prognosis *or* increased probability of prolonged functional impairment.

High Severity

A problem for which the risk of morbidity without treatment is high to extreme; there is a moderate to high risk of mortality without treatment *or* high probability of severe, prolonged functional impairment.

Combinations

Note that combinations of the above may also be found in the code descriptions. For example, you will find codes for which the presenting problem(s) are defined as "moderate severity" or "high severity" or "moderate to high severity."

Other Definitions of Nature of the Presenting Problem

In addition to the above five specific definitions found in CPT, there are other definitions found in the E/M service codes used to report Subsequent Hospital Care and Follow-up Inpatient Consultations. See the following table for these additional definitions.

E/MCodes	Nature of Presenting Problem(s)	Equivalent To
99231 or 99261	Stable, recovering or improving	Self-limited or minor
99232 or 99262	Inadequate response or minor complication	Low to moderate severity
99233 or 99263	Significant complication or new problem	Moderate to high severity

TIME

Most E/M service codes include specific or typical time units as part of the definition. The times expressed in the E/M visit code definitions are averages and therefore represent a range of times that may be higher or lower, depending on actual clinical circumstances.

Time is not a component for the emergency department levels of E/M services, because emergency department services are typically provided on a variable-intensity basis, often involving multiple encounters with several patients over an extended period of time. Therefore, it is difficult for physicians to provide accurate estimates of the time spent face to face with the patient.

FACE-TO-FACE TIME

For office visits and office consultations, the phrase "face-to-face time" is used. For coding purposes, face-to-face time is defined as only that time that the physician spends face to face with the patient and/or family. This includes the time during which the physician performs such tasks as obtaining a history, performing an examination, and counseling the patient.

UNIT/FLOOR TIME

For inpatient hospital care, initial and follow-up hospital consultations, and nursing facility assessments, the phrase "unit/floor time" is used. Unit/floor time includes the time that the physician is present on the patient's hospital unit and at the bedside rendering services for that patient. This includes the time the physician spends establishing or reviewing the patient's chart, examining the patient, writing notes, and communicating with other professionals and the patient's family.

DIAGNOSTIC TESTS OR STUDIES

The performance of diagnostic tests or studies for which specific CPT codes are available is not included in the levels of E/M services. Any diagnostic tests or studies performed by the physician for which specific CPT codes are available should be reported separately, in addition to the appropriate E/M service code.

UNLISTED SERVICES

An E/M service may be provided that is not listed in the E/M section of the CPT code book. When reporting such a service, the appropriate "Unlisted" code may be used to indicate the service, identifying it by "Special Report." The "Unlisted Services" and accompanying codes for the E/M section are:

99249   Unlisted preventive medicine service

99499   Unlisted E/M service

SPECIAL REPORT

An unlisted service or one that is unusual, variable, or new may require a special report demonstrating the medical appropriateness of the service. Pertinent information should include an adequate definition or description of the nature, extent, and need for the procedure plus the time, effort, and equipment necessary to provide the service. Additional items that may be included are complexity of the symptoms, final diagnosis, pertinent physical findings, diagnostic and therapeutic procedures, concurrent problems, and follow-up care.

CLINICAL EXAMPLES

Clinical examples of the codes for E/M services are provided to assist physicians and other health care professionals in understanding the meaning of the descriptors and selecting the correct code. The clinical examples printed in each edition of the CPT code book are developed by physicians in the listed specialties.

The clinical examples, when used in conjunction with the revised E/M descriptions and time guidelines, provide a comprehensive and powerful new tool for physicians to report the services provided to their patients.

MODIFIERS

Listed services may be modified under certain circumstances. When applicable, the modifying circumstance against general guidelines should be identified by the addition of the appropriate modifier code, which may be reported in either of two ways. The modifier may be reported by a two-digit number placed after the procedure code. Modifiers that may be used with E/M service codes are:

-21 Prolonged E/M services

-24 Unrelated E/M service by the same physician during a postoperative period

-25 Significant, separately identifiable E/M service by the same physician on the day of a procedure

-32 Mandated services

-52 Reduced services

-57 Decision for surgery

CHOOSING EVALUATION AND MANAGEMENT CODES

Choosing the correct E/M service code to report is a nine-step process. The most important steps, in terms of both reimbursement and audit liability, are verifying compliance and documentation.

1. Identify the Category of Service

❑ Office or Other Outpatient Services
❑ Hospital Observation Services
❑ Hospital Inpatient Services
❑ Consultations
❑ Emergency Department Services
❑ Critical Care Services
❑ Neonatal Intensive Care
❑ Nursing Facility Services
❑ Domiciliary, Rest Home, or Custodial Care Services
❑ Home Services

❑ Prolonged Services
❑ Standby Services
❑ Case Management Services
❑ Preventive Medicine Services
❑ Newborn Care
❑ Special or Other E/M Services

2. **Identify the Subcategory of Service**

❑ New Patient
❑ Established Patient
❑ Initial Care
❑ Subsequent Care
❑ Follow-up

3. **Determine the Extent of History Obtained**

❑ Problem Focused
❑ Expanded Problem Focused
❑ Detailed
❑ Comprehensive

4. **Determine the Extent of Examination Performed**

❑ Problem Focused
❑ Expanded Problem Focused
❑ Detailed
❑ Comprehensive

5. Determine the Complexity of Medical Decision Making

❑ Straightforward
❑ Low Complexity
❑ Moderate Complexity
❑ High Complexity

6. Record the Approximate Amount of Time

❑ Face-to-face time for office visits and consults
❑ Unit or floor time for hospital care, hospital consults, and nursing facilities

If counseling and/or coordination of care exceeds 50 percent of the total face-to-face physician/patient encounter, then *time* is considered to be the key or controlling factor that qualifies the choice of a particular level of E/M service. The extent of counseling and/or coordination of care must be documented in the medical record.

7. Verify Compliance With Reporting Requirements

All Three Key Components Required

To report services to new patients, initial care, office or confirmatory consultations, emergency department services, and comprehensive nursing facility assessments, all three key components must meet or exceed the stated requirements.

❑ History component met or exceeded
❑ Examination component met or exceeded
❑ Medical decision-making component met or exceeded

<u>Two of Three Key Components Required</u>

To report services to established patients, subsequent or follow-up care, two of the three key components must meet or exceed the stated requirements.

❑ History component met or exceeded; and/or

❑ Examination component met or exceeded; and/or

❑ Medical decision-making component met or exceeded

8. Verify Documentation

Make sure that the medical record includes proper documentation of the history, examination, medical decision making, the nature of the problem(s), the approximate amount of time, and, when appropriate, the extent of counseling and/or coordination of care.

9. Assign the Code

Below is an example of the code selection process.

EXAMPLE OF THE CODE SELECTION PROCESS

1.	Category of Service	*Office*
2.	Subcategory	*New patient*
3.	History	*Problem focused*
4.	Examination	*Problem focused*
5.	Medical Decision Making	*Straightforward*
6.	Intra-service Time	*10 minutes*
7.	Key Components	*Met or exceeded*
8.	Documentation	*Met or exceeded*
9.	Assign the Code	***99201***

OFFICE AND OTHER OUTPATIENT SERVICES

E/M service codes 99201-99215 are used to report services provided to new and established patients in the office or other outpatient facility, including the emergency department when the physician is not assigned to the emergency department. The key coding issues are the extent of history obtained, the extent of examination performed, and the complexity of medical decision making. Additional reporting issues include counseling and/or coordination of care, the nature of presenting problem(s), and the face-to-face time spent with the patient and/or family.

CODING RULES

1) A patient is considered an outpatient until inpatient admission to a health care facility occurs.

2) If outpatient E/M services are provided in conjunction with or result in an inpatient admission, the service is reported using the codes for initial hospital care.

3) The codes in this section may also be used to report the services provided by a physician to a patient in an observation area of a hospital.

CORRECT CODING ISSUES FOR E/M SERVICES

CPT codes for evaluation and management services are principally included in the group of CPT codes 99201-99499. The codes are divided into groups to describe the place of service (e.g., office, hospital, home, nursing facility, emergency department, critical care, etc.), the type of service (e.g., new or initial encounter, follow-up or subsequent encounter, consultation, etc.), and various miscellaneous services (e.g., prolonged physician service, care plan oversight service, etc.). Because of the nature of evaluation and management services, which mostly represent cognitive services (medical decision making) based on history and examination, correct coding primarily involves determination of the level of history, examination, and medical decision making that was performed rather than reporting multiple codes. Only one evaluation and management service code may be reported per day.

The prolonged physician service with direct face-to-face patient contact (CPT codes 99354 and 99355) represents an exception and may be used in conjunction with another evaluation and management code. Other services that are described by codes based on the duration of the encounter, such as critical care services, must be reported alone and not with the prolonged-service codes.

Evaluation and management services, in general, are cognitive services, and significant procedural services are not included in the evaluation and management services. Certain procedural services that arise directly from the evaluation and management service are included as part of the evaluation and management service. Cleansing of traumatic lesions, closure of lacerations with adhesive strips, dressings, counseling and educational services, among other services are included in evaluation and management services.

Because of the intensive nature of caring for critically ill patients, certain services beyond patient history, examination, and medical decision making are included in the overall evaluation and management associated with critical care. By CPT definition, services including the interpretation of cardiac output measurements (CPT codes 93561 and 93562), chest x-rays (CPT codes 71010 and 71020), blood gases, data stored in computers (EKGs, blood pressures, hematologic data), gastric intubation (CPT code 91105), temporary transcutaneous monitoring (CPT code 92953), ventilator management (CPT codes 94656, 94657, 94660, 94662), and vascular access procedures (HCPCS/CPT codes 36000, 36410, 36600) are included in critical care services.

Certain sections of CPT codes have incorporated codes describing specialty-specific services that primarily involve evaluation and management. When codes for these services are reported, a separate evaluation and management service described by the series of CPT codes 99201-99499 is not to be reported on the same date. Examples of these codes include general and special ophthalmologic services, general and special diagnostic and therapeutic psychiatric services, among others. Procedural services involve some degree of physician involvement or supervision that is integral to the service; separate evaluation and management services are not reported unless a significant, separately identifiable service is provided. Examples of such procedures include allergy testing and immunotherapy, osteopathic manipulative treatment, physical therapy services, and neurologic and vascular testing procedures.

HOSPITAL OBSERVATION SERVICES

Occasionally, a physician wishes to "observe" or watch a patient for a period of time to determine if an inpatient admission is necessary. An example is a pregnant woman may be admitted to an observation area with early signs of labor. As the labor may turn out to be false, admission to the observation area allows the patient to be observed without being admitted as an inpatient. The patient may be subsequently discharged from the observation area or admitted as an inpatient.

E/M service codes 99217-99220 are used to report services provided to patients designated or admitted under "observation status" in a hospital. It is not necessary that the patient actually be located in an observation area designated by the hospital. However, if such an area does exist in a hospital as a separate unit, for example in the emergency area, the hospital observation codes should be reported if the patient is placed in such as area.

CODING RULES

1. All Observation Care codes are "per day" and should be reported only once per date of service.

2. When a patient is designated as on "observation status" in the course of an encounter in another site of service, such as the emergency department, doctor's office, or nursing facility, all E/M services provided by the supervising physician in conjunction with initiating "observation status" are considered part of the initial observation care when performed on the same date.

3. E/M services on the same date provided in sites that are related to initiating "observation status" should not be reported separately.

4. Observation Care codes should not be used for postoperative recovery services if the procedure is considered part of the surgical package.

5. CPT code 99217, Observation care discharge day management, is used to report all services provided on discharge from "observation status" if the discharge is on other than the initial date of "observation status." If the patient is admitted and discharged from "observation status" on the same day, use Observation Care or Inpatient Care codes as appropriate.

HOSPITAL INPATIENT SERVICES

Hospital services refer to hospital visits during the course of an inpatient hospital stay. The services may be provided by the patient's primary physician and/or other physicians in the event of multiple illnesses or injuries. E/M service codes 99221-99239 are used to report services provided in the hospital. The key coding issues are the extent of history obtained, the extent of examination performed, and the complexity of medical decision making. Additional reporting issues include counseling and/or coordination of care, the nature of presenting problem(s), and the time spent at the bedside and on the patient's facility floor or unit.

CODING RULES

1. The codes defined as Initial Hospital Care are used to report the first hospital inpatient encounter with the patient by the admitting physician.

2. For initial inpatient encounters by physicians other than the admitting physician, use codes from the inpatient consultation or subsequent hospital care series as appropriate.

3. When the patient is admitted to the hospital in the course of an encounter in another location, for example, office or hospital emergency department, all E/M services provided by the reporting physician in conjunction with the admission are considered part of the initial hospital care when performed on the same date of service.

4. The admitting physician should report all service related to the admission provided in all other locations.

5. E/M services provided on the same date of service in locations other than the hospital that are related to the admission are not reported separately.

6. For observation care or inpatient hospital care services provided to patients who are admitted and discharged on the same date, report with codes 99234-99236 from the Observation or Inpatient Care services subsections.

CONSULTATIONS

A consultation is the process of taking a history, performing a physical examination, and ordering and interpreting appropriate diagnostic tests for the purpose of rendering an expert opinion about a patient's illness and/or injury. E/M service codes 99241-99275 are used to report office, inpatient, and confirmatory consultation services provided to new or established patients. The key coding issues are the location of the service, the extent of history obtained, the extent of examination performed, and the complexity of medical decision making. Additional reporting issues include counseling and/or coordination of care, the nature of presenting problem(s), and the time, depending on location, spent either face to face with the patient and/or family or at the bedside and on the patient's facility floor or unit.

CODING RULES

1. The request for a consultation from the attending physician or other appropriate source and the need for a consultation must be documented in the patient's medical record.

2. The consultant's opinion and any services that were ordered or performed must be documented in the patient's medical record and communicated to the requesting physician or source.

3. Consultations that are initiated by request from the patient and/or family may be reported using codes for confirmatory consultations or office services as appropriate.

4. If a confirmatory consultation is required by a third party, such as a Peer Review Organization (PRO), modifier -32 should be added to the basic service.

5. Any specifically identifiable procedure performed on or subsequent to the date of the initial consultation is reported separately.

6. If the consultant subsequently assumes responsibility for management of all or a portion of the patient's condition(s), then either hospital services or office services are used as appropriate.

EMERGENCY SERVICES

E/M service codes 99281-99288 are used to report services provided to new or established patients in the emergency department. An emergency department is defined as an organized, hospital-based facility for the provision of unscheduled episodic services to patients who present for immediate medical attention. The emergency department facility must be available 24 hours a day.

The key coding issues of E/M emergency services are the extent of history obtained, the extent of examination performed, and the complexity of medical decision making. Additional reporting issues include counseling and/or coordination of care and the nature of presenting problem(s).

Time is not a descriptive component for E/M services provided in the emergency department. These services are typically provided on a variable-intensity basis, often involving multiple encounters with several patients over an extended period of time. Therefore, it is difficult for physicians to provide accurate estimates of the time spent face to face with the patient in the emergency department.

CODING RULES

1. No distinction is made between new and established patients in the emergency department.

2. If the emergency department is used for observation or inpatient care services, report using codes from the Observation Care services subsection of the CPT code book.

3. For critical care services provided in the emergency department, use the appropriate codes from the Critical Care subsection of the CPT code book.

CRITICAL CARE SERVICES

Critical care includes the care of critically ill patients in a variety of medical emergencies that requires the constant attention of the physician. Cardiac arrest, shock, bleeding, respiratory failure, postoperative complications, and a critically ill neonate are examples of medical emergencies defined in CPT. Critical care is usually, but not always given in a critical area, such as the coronary care unit, intensive care unit, respiratory care unit, or the emergency care facility.

The codes listed in this section of the CPT code book are intended to include cardiopulmonary resuscitation (CPR) and the variety of services commonly employed with this procedure as well as other acute emergency situations. Other services, such as catheter placement, cardiac output measurement, dialysis management, control of gastrointestinal hemorrhage, cardioversion, etc., are considered to be included when billing critical care services under these time-based codes.

E/M service codes 99291-99292 are used to report services for specific conditions (usually) provided in a critical care area. Critical care is defined in the new E/M section identically to the previous visit definition provided above. Key coding issues include the condition of the patient (supported by diagnostic coding), the service(s) provided, and the amount of time spent. Follow-up critical care services may be reported using E/M service codes from this section or hospital E/M service codes from the series 99231-99233.

CODING RULES

1. The critical care codes are used to report the total duration of time spent by a physician providing constant attention to a critically ill patient.

2. Critical care code 99291 is used to report the first hour of critical care on a given day. It may be reported only once per day even if the time spent is not continuous on that day.

3. Critical care 99292 is used to report each additional 30 minutes beyond the first hour.

4. Other procedures that are not considered included in the critical care services, for example, suturing of lacerations, setting of fractures, reduction of joint dislocations, lumbar puncture, peritoneal lavage, and bladder tap, are reported separately.

NEONATAL INTENSIVE CARE

Neonatal intensive care refers to services provided to a critically ill newborn or infant, usually in the neonatal intensive care unit (NICU). The services include management, monitoring, and treatment of the patient; parent counseling; case management services; and personal direct supervision of the health care team. E/M service codes 99295-99297 are used to report services provided by a physician directing the provision of these services.

CODING RULES

1. Neonatal intensive care services start with the date of admission and are reported only once per day, per patient.

2. Once the neonate is no longer considered to be critically ill, report with codes for subsequent hospital care instead of neonatal intensive care.

3. Neonatal intensive care codes are reported in addition to physician standby code 99360 or newborn resuscitation code 99440 when the physician is present for the delivery and newborn resuscitation is required.

NURSING FACILITY SERVICE

A patient may be transferred from an inpatient hospital to a nursing facility for supervised care when the patient no longer requires the skill levels of the inpatient hospital. E/M service codes 99301-99313 are used to report services provided in nursing facilities. The key coding issues are the extent of history obtained, the extent of examination performed, and the complexity of medical decision making. Additional reporting issues include counseling and/or coordination of care, the nature of presenting problem(s), and the time spent at the bedside and on the patient's facility floor or unit.

These codes are also used to report E/M services provided to a patient in a psychiatric residential treatment center. If procedures such as medical psychotherapy are provided in addition to E/M services, these are reported in addition to the E/M services.

Nursing facilities included in this category are required to conduct assessments of each patient's functional capacity. Physicians have the primary responsibility for assuring that all patients receive thorough assessments and that medical care plans are instituted and/or revised as appropriate.

Codes in this section apply to Comprehensive Nursing Facility Assessments and Subsequent Nursing Facility care. Both subcategories apply to new and established patients. Comprehensive Assessments may be performed at one or more sites during the assessment process, including the hospital, the office, a nursing facility, a domiciliary facility, and/or the patient's home.

CODING RULES

1. When a patient is admitted to the nursing facility in the course of an encounter in another location, for example, the office or hospital emergency department, all E/M services provided by the physician in conjunction with that admission are considered part of the initial nursing facility care when performed on the same date as the admission.

2. The nursing facility care level of service reported by the admitting physician should include the services related to the admission the physician provided in the other location(s).

3. With the exception of hospital discharge services, E/M service on the same date provided in locations other than the nursing facility that are related to the admission should not be reported separately.

4. More than one comprehensive assessment may be necessary during an inpatient confinement.

5. When reporting these codes to Medicare, include the HCPCS Level II modifier -SP or -MP.

DOMICILIARY, REST HOME, OR CUSTODIAL SERVICES

E/M service codes 99321-99333 are used to report services provided to new and established patients in domiciliary, rest home, or custodial care facilities. The key coding issues are the extent of history obtained, the extent of examination performed, and the complexity of medical decision making. Additional reporting issues include counseling and/or coordination of care and the nature of presenting problem(s).

When reporting these codes to Medicare, include HCPCS Level II modifier -SP or -MP to indicate single or multiple patients seen during the visit. Consult your local Medicare intermediary before using these modifiers.

HOME MEDICAL SERVICES

E/M home visit codes 99341-99353 are used to report services provided to new and established patients in the patient's home. The key coding issues are the extent of history obtained, the extent of examination performed, and the complexity of medical decision making. Additional reporting issues include counseling and/or coordination of care and the nature of presenting problem(s).

PROLONGED SERVICES

E/M service codes 99354-99360 are used to report inpatient or outpatient services that include prolonged service or physician standby service that is beyond the usual service. The key coding issues are the location of the service, whether the service is direct (face to face) or not direct, and the total duration of the prolonged service.

CODING RULES

1. Prolonged services are reported in addition to other physician services.

2. Prolonged services involving direct (face-to-face) time is reported as cumulative time on a given date, even if the time is not continuous.

3. If the total duration of prolonged services is less than 30 minutes, the prolonged service is not reported.

CASE MANAGEMENT SERVICES

Case management is a process in which a physician is responsible for direct care of a patient and for coordinating and controlling other health care services needed by the patient. Case management services may be provided during medical conferences or by telephone. E/M service codes 99361-99373 are used to report case management services. The key coding issues are the type of service, the amount of time spent, and the level of service provided.

CARE PLAN OVERSIGHT SERVICES

Care plans prepared and/or reviewed by a physician are frequently required for patients under the care of home health agencies, in hospices, or residing in nursing facilities. E/M service codes 99374-99380 are used to report care plan oversight services. The key coding issues are the location of service, the complexity of the plan, and the amount of physician time provided within a 30-day period.

CODING RULES

1. Care plan oversight services are reported separately from office, hospital, home, or nursing facility services, unless the work involved is infrequent or of low intensity.

2. Only one physician may report care plan oversight services for a patient for a specific period of time.

3. Care plan oversight codes should not be used to report supervision of patients in nursing facilities or under the care of home health agencies unless they require recurrent supervision or therapy.

PREVENTIVE MEDICINE SERVICES

E/M service codes 99381-99429 are used to report routine E/M of adults and children in the absence of patient complaints or counseling and/or risk factor reduction intervention services to healthy individuals. The key coding issues are whether the patient is a new patient or established patient, the age of the patient, the circumstances of the examination, and the nature of any abnormalities encountered. The key coding issues for counseling services are whether the service was provided to an individual or to a group and the amount of time spent counseling.

CODING RULES

1. The extent and focus of the preventive medicine service, and the code chosen to report it, depend largely on the age of the patient.

2. If an abnormality is found during the course of providing a preventive medicine service, or if a preexisting problem is addressed during the service, and the problem or abnormality requires additional work, then an E/M service code from the Office/Outpatient service subsection should be reported. Modifier -25 should be added to the E/M Office/Outpatient code to indicate that significant, separately identifiable E/M service was provided on the same day as the preventive medicine service.

3. Immunizations and diagnostic studies involving laboratory, radiology, or other procedures are not included in the preventive medicine service and should be reported separately.

NEWBORN CARE

E/M service codes 99341-99440 are used to report services provided to newborns in several different settings. The key coding issues are the location of the service and the level of service(s) provided.

CODING RULES

1. Newborn care code 99436, Attendance at delivery, may be reported in addition to Newborn care code 99431, History and examination of the normal newborn infant, when the attendance at the delivery is requested by the delivering physician.

2. If the newborn is assessed and discharged on the same day, report with code 99425. If the discharge date occurs on a date subsequent to the admission date, report with code 99238.

SPECIAL SERVICES AND REPORTS

There are several codes listed in this category of the Medicine section of the CPT code book that may be reported in addition to basic E/M services. The proper use of Special Services codes may result in a significant increase in reimbursement. Most of the codes in the Special Services and Reports section are "add-on" codes. This means that they are reported in addition to whatever other codes describe the procedures or services performed. Specific codes from this section that may be used with or in place of E/M service codes include:

MISCELLANEOUS SERVICES

99000-   Handling and/or conveyance of specimen

99002

99024   Postoperative follow-up visit, included in global service

This code is used to track no-charge postoperative visits. See the Surgery section Guidelines.

SERVICES RENDERED AFTER REGULAR OFFICE HOURS

99050   Services requested after office hours in addition to basic service

99052   Services requested between 10:00 PM and 8:00 AM in addition to basic service

99054   Services requested on Sundays and holidays in addition to basic service

Note that codes 99050, 99052, and 99054 are reported in addition to the basic E/M services code.

SERVICES RENDERED AT SPECIAL LOCATION

99056   Services provided at request of patient in a location other than physician's office

Note that code 99056 is reported in addition to the basic E/M service code.

OFFICE EMERGENCY SERVICES

99058   Office services provided on an emergency basis

The diagnostic codes used to bill for this service must clearly justify the nature of the emergency.

99082   Unusual travel (e.g., transportation and escort of patient)

DOCUMENTATION GUIDELINES

Documentation in the medical records of all services provided is critical in terms of reimbursement and audit liability. From the point of view of Medicare or private health insurance company claims auditors, if you billed a service or procedure but did not document it or did not document it completely in the patient's medical records, you did not perform it and you can't bill for it.

Every year, millions of dollars are reclaimed by Medicare and private health insurance carriers from physicians and other health care professionals because the medical record documentation does not support the services and procedures billed. You can protect your practice from audit liability by following the most current documentation guidelines published by CMS.

The following guidelines for E/M services were developed jointly by the American Medical Association (AMA) and CMS. The goal of CMS in publishing these guidelines is to provide physicians and claims reviewers with advice about preparing or reviewing documentation for E/M services.

In developing and testing the validity of these guidelines, special emphasis was placed on assuring that they:

- are consistent with the clinical descriptors and definitions contained in CPT,

- would be widely accepted by clinicians and minimize any changes in record-keeping practices, and

- would be interpreted and applied uniformly by users across the country.

WHAT IS DOCUMENTATION AND WHY IS IT IMPORTANT?

Medical record documentation is required to record pertinent facts, findings, and observations about an individual's health history, including past and present illnesses, examinations, tests, treatments, and outcomes. The medical record chronologically documents the care of the patient and is an important element contributing to high-quality care. The medical record facilitates:

- the ability of the physician and other health care professionals to evaluate and plan the patient's immediate treatment and to monitor the patient's health care over time;

- communication and continuity of care among physicians and other health care professionals involved in the patient's care;

- accurate and timely claims review and payment;

- appropriate utilization review and quality of care evaluations; and

- collection of data that may be useful for research and education.

An appropriately documented medical record can reduce many of the hassles associated with claims processing and may serve as a legal document to verify the care provided, if necessary.

WHAT DO PAYERS WANT AND WHY?

Because payers have a contractual obligation to enrollees, they may require reasonable documentation that services are consistent with the health insurance coverage provided. They may request information to validate:

- the site of service;

- the medical necessity and appropriateness of the diagnostic and/or therapeutic services provided; and/or

- that services provided have been accurately reported.

GENERAL PRINCIPLES OF MEDICAL RECORD DOCUMENTATION

The principles of documentation listed below are applicable to all types of medical and surgical services in all settings. For E/M services, the nature and amount of physician work and documentation vary by type of service, place of service, and the patient's status. The general principles listed below may be modified to account for these variable circumstances in providing E/M services.

1. The medical record should be complete and legible.

2. The documentation of each patient encounter should include:

a. reason for the encounter and relevant history, physical examination findings, and prior diagnostic test results;

b. assessment, clinical impression, or diagnosis;

c. plan for care; and

d. date and legible identity of the observer.

3. If not documented, the rationale for ordering diagnostic and other ancillary services should be easily inferred.

4. Past and present diagnoses should be accessible to the treating and/or consulting physician.

5. Appropriate health risk factors should be identified.

6. The patient's progress, response to, and changes in treatment and any revision of diagnosis should be documented.

7. The CPT and ICD-9-CM codes reported on the health insurance claim form or billing statement should be supported by the documentation in the medical record.

DOCUMENTATION OF E/M SERVICES

This section provides definitions and documentation guidelines for the three key components of E/M services and for visits that consist predominately of counseling or coordination of care. The three *key* components—history, examination, and medical decision making—appear in the descriptors for office and other outpatient services, hospital observation services, hospital inpatient services, consultations, emergency department services, nursing facility services, domiciliary care services, and home services. Note that documentation guidelines are identified by the symbol •*DG*.

The descriptors for the levels of E/M services recognize seven components that are used in defining the levels of E/M services. These components are:

- history

- examination

- medical decision making

- counseling

- coordination of care

- nature of presenting problem

- time

The first three of these components (i.e., history, examination, and medical decision making) are the key components in selecting the level of E/M services. In the case of visits that consist predominantly of counseling or coordination of care, time is the key or controlling factor to qualify for a particular level of E/M service.

Because the level of E/M service is dependent on two or three key components, performance and documentation of only one component (e.g., examination) at the highest level does not necessarily mean that the encounter in its entirety qualifies for the highest level of E/M service.

These documentation guidelines for E/M services reflect the needs of the typical adult population. For certain groups of patients, the recorded information may vary slightly from that described here. Specifically, the medical records of infants, children, adolescents, and pregnant women may have additional or modified information recorded in each history and examination area.

As an example, newborn records may include under history of the present illness the details of mother's pregnancy and the infant's status at birth; social history will focus on family structure; and family history will focus on congenital anomalies and hereditary disorders in the family. In addition, the content of a pediatric examination will vary with the age and development of the child. Although not specifically defined in these documentation guidelines, these patient group variations of history and examination are appropriate.

DOCUMENTATION OF HISTORY

The levels of E/M services are based on four types of history (Problem Focused, Expanded Problem Focused, Detailed, and Comprehensive). Each type of history includes some or all of the following elements:

- Chief complaint

- History of present illness

- Review of systems

- Past, family, and/or social history

The extent of history of present illness; the review of systems; and the past, family, and/or social history obtained and documented is dependent upon clinical judgment and the nature of the presenting problem(s).

The following table shows the progression of the elements required for each type of history. To qualify for a given type of history, *all three elements* in the table must be met. (A chief complaint is indicated at all levels.)

Present History	Review of Systems	Past, Family or Social History	Type of History
Brief	N/A	N/A	Problem Focused
Brief	Problem Focused	N/A	Expanded Problem Focused
Extended	Extended	Pertinent	Detailed
Extended	Complete	Complete	Comprehensive

- *DG:* The chief complaint; review of systems; and past, family, and/or social history may be listed as separate elements of history or they may be included in the description of the history of the present illness.

- *DG:* A review of systems and/or a past, family, and/or social history obtained during an earlier encounter does not need to be re-recorded if there is evidence that the physician reviewed and updated the previous information. This may occur when a physician updates his or her own record or in an institutional setting or group practice where many physicians use a common record. The review and update may be documented by:

  o describing any new review of systems and/or past, family, and/or social history information or noting there has been no change in the information; and

  o noting the date and location of the earlier review of systems and/or past, family, and/or social history.

- *DG:*   The review of systems and/or past, family, and/or social history may be recorded by ancillary staff or on a form completed by the patient. To document that the physician reviewed the information, there must be a notation supplementing or confirming the information recorded by others.

- *DG:*   If the physician is unable to obtain a history from the patient or other source, the record should describe the patient's condition or other circumstance that precludes obtaining a history.

Definitions and specific documentation guidelines for each of the elements of history are listed below.

CHIEF COMPLAINT

The chief complaint is a concise statement describing the symptom, problem, condition, diagnosis, physician-recommended return, or other factor that is the reason for the encounter, usually stated in the patient's words.

- *DG:*   The medical record should clearly reflect the chief complaint.

HISTORY OF PRESENT ILLNESS

The history of present illness is a chronological description of the development of the patient's present illness from the first sign and/or symptom or from the previous encounter to the present. It includes the following elements:

- location

- quality

- severity

- duration

- timing

- context

- modifying factors

- associated signs and symptoms

Brief and *extended* history of present illnesses are distinguished by the amount of detail needed to accurately characterize the clinical problem(s). A *brief* history of present illness consists of one to three elements of the history of present illness.

- *DG:*   *The medical record should describe one to three elements of the present illness (history of present illness).*

An *extended* history of present illness consists of at least four elements of the history of present illness or the status of at least three chronic or inactive conditions.

- *DG:*   *Medical record should describe at least four elements of the present illness (history of present illness) or the status of at least three chronic or inactive conditions.*

REVIEW OF SYSTEMS

A review of systems is an inventory of body systems obtained through a series of questions seeking to identify signs and/or symptoms that the patient may be experiencing or has experienced. For purposes of review of systems, the following systems are recognized:

- Constitutional symptoms (e.g., fever, weight loss)
- Eyes
- Ears, Nose, Mouth, Throat
- Cardiovascular
- Respiratory
- Gastrointestinal
- Genitourinary
- Musculoskeletal
- Integumentary (skin and/or breast)
- Neurological
- Psychiatric
- Endocrine

- Hematologic/Lymphatic

- Allergic/Immunologic

A *problem pertinent* review of systems inquires about the system directly related to the problem(s) identified in the history of present illness.

- *DG:*   *The patient's positive responses and pertinent negatives for the system related to the problem should be documented.*

An *extended* review of systems inquires about the system directly related to the problem(s) identified in the history of present illness and a limited number of additional systems.

- *DG:*   *The patient's positive responses and pertinent negatives for two to nine systems should be documented.*

A *complete* review of systems inquires about the system(s) directly related to the problem(s) identified in the history of present illness plus all additional body systems.

- *DG:*   *At least 10 organ systems must be reviewed. Those systems with positive or pertinent negative responses must be individually documented. For the remaining systems, a notation indicating all other systems are negative is permissible. In the absence of such a notation, at least 10 systems must be individually documented.*

PAST, FAMILY, AND/OR SOCIAL HISTORY

The past, family, and/or social history consists of a review of three areas:

- past history (the patient's past experiences with illnesses, operations, injuries, and treatments);

- family history (a review of medical events in the patient's family, including diseases that may be hereditary or place the patient at risk); and

- social history (an age-appropriate review of past and current activities).

For certain categories of E/M services that include only an interval history, it is not necessary to record information about the past, family, and/or social history. Those categories are subsequent hospital care, follow-up inpatient consultations, and subsequent nursing facility care.

A *pertinent* past, family, and/or social history is a review of the history area(s) directly related to the problem(s) identified in the history of present illness.

- *DG:*   *At least one specific item from **any** of the three history areas must be documented for a pertinent past, family, and/or social history.*

A *complete* past, family, and/or social history is a review of two or all three of the past, family, and/or social history areas, depending on the category of the E/M service. A review of all three history areas is required for services that by their nature include a comprehensive assessment or reassessment of the patient. A review of two of the three history areas is sufficient for other services.

- *DG:*   *At least one specific item from **two** of the three history areas must be documented for a complete past, family, and/or social history for the following categories of E/M services: office or other outpatient services, established patient; emergency department; domiciliary care, established patient; and home care, established patient.*

- *DG:*   *At least one specific item from **each** of the three history areas must be documented for a complete past, family, and/or social history for the following categories of E/M services: office or other outpatient services, new patient; hospital observation services; hospital inpatient services, initial care; consultations; comprehensive nursing facility assessments; domiciliary care, new patient; and home care, new patient.*

DOCUMENTATION OF EXAMINATION

The levels of Evaluation and Management services are based on four types of examination:

- **Problem Focused:** a limited examination of the affected body area or organ system.

- **Expanded Problem Focused:** a limited examination of the affected body area or organ system and any other symptomatic or related body area(s) or organ system(s).

- **Detailed:** an extended examination of the affected body area(s) or organ system(s) and any other symptomatic or related body area(s) or organ system(s).

- **Comprehensive:** a general multisystem examination or a complete examination of a single organ system and other symptomatic or related body area(s) or organ system(s).

These types of examinations have been defined for a general multisystem examination and the following single-organ systems:

- Cardiovascular

- Ears, Nose, Mouth, and Throat

- Eyes

- Genitourinary (Female)

- Genitourinary (Male)

- Hematologic/Lymphatic/Immunologic

- Musculoskeletal

- Neurological

- Psychiatric

- Respiratory

- Skin

A general multisystem examination or a single-organ system examination may be performed by any physician regardless of specialty. The type (general multisystem or single-organ system) and content of examination are selected by the examining physician and are based upon clinical judgment, the patient's history, and the nature of the presenting problem(s).

The content and documentation requirements for each type and level of examination are summarized below and then described in detail in tables that follow. In the tables, organ systems and body areas recognized by CPT for purposes of describing examinations are shown in the left column. The contents, or individual elements, of the examination pertaining to that body area or organ system are identified by bullets (•) in the right column.

Parenthetical examples, "(e.g., ...)," have been used for clarification and to provide guidance regarding documentation. Documentation for each element must satisfy any numeric requirements (such as "Measurement of *any three of the following seven...*") included in the description of the element. Elements with multiple components but with no specific numeric requirement (such as "Examination of *liver* and *spleen*") require documentation of at least one component. It is possible for a given examination to be expanded beyond what is defined here. When that occurs, findings related to the additional systems and/or areas should be documented.

- *DG:*   *Specific abnormal and relevant negative findings of the examination of the affected or symptomatic body area(s) or organ system(s) should be documented. A notation of "abnormal" without elaboration is insufficient.*

- *DG:*   *Abnormal or unexpected findings of the examination of any asymptomatic body area(s) or organ system(s) should be described.*

- *DG:*   *A brief statement or notation indicating "negative" or "normal" is sufficient to document normal findings related to unaffected area(s) or asymptomatic organ system(s).*

GENERAL MULTISYSTEM EXAMINATIONS

General multisystem examinations are described in detail below. To qualify for a given level of multisystem examination, the following content and documentation requirements should be met:

- **Problem Focused Examination**—should include performance and documentation of *one to five elements* identified by a bullet (•) in one or more organ system(s) or body area(s).

- **Expanded Problem Focused Examination**—should include performance and documentation of *at least six elements* identified by a bullet (•) in one or more organ system(s) or body area(s).

- **Detailed Examination**—should include *at least six organ systems or body areas*. For each system/area selected, performance and documentation of *at least two elements* identified by a bullet (•) are expected. Alternatively, a detailed examination may include performance and documentation of *at least 12 elements* identified by a bullet (•) in two or more organ systems or body areas.

- **Comprehensive Examination**—should include *at least nine organ systems or body areas*. For each system/area selected, *all elements* of the examination identified by a bullet (•) should be performed, unless specific directions limit the content of the examination. For each area/system, documentation of *at least two elements* identified by a bullet is expected.

SINGLE-ORGAN SYSTEM EXAMINATIONS

The single-organ system examinations recognized by CPT are described in detail next. Variations among these examinations in the organ systems and body areas identified in the left columns and in the elements of the examinations described in the right columns reflect differing emphases among specialties. To qualify for a given level of single-organ system examination, the following content and documentation requirements should be met:

- *Problem Focused Examination*—should include performance and documentation of *one to five elements* identified by a bullet (•), whether in a box with a shaded or unshaded background.

- *Expanded Problem Focused Examination*—should include performance and documentation of *at least six elements* identified by a bullet (•), whether in a box with a shaded or unshaded background.

- *Detailed Examination*—examinations other than the eye and psychiatric examinations should include performance and documentation of *at least 12 elements* identified by a bullet (•), whether in box with a shaded or unshaded background.

  Eye and **psychiatric** examinations should include the performance and documentation of *at least nine elements* identified by a bullet (•), whether in a box with a shaded or unshaded background.

- *Comprehensive Examination*—should include performance of *all elements* identified by a bullet (•), whether in a box with a shaded or unshaded background.

Documentation of every element in each box with a shaded background and at least one element in each box with an unshaded background is expected.

GENERAL MULTI-SYSTEM EXAMINATION

SYSTEM/BODY AREA	ELEMENTS OF EXAMINATION
Constitutional	• Measurement of **any three of the following seven** vital signs: 1) sitting or standing blood pressure, 2) supine blood pressure, 3) pulse rate and regularity, 4) respiration, 5) temperature, 6) height, 7) weight (May be measured and recorded by ancillary staff)
	• General appearance of patient (e.g., development, nutrition, body habitus, deformities, attention to grooming)
Eyes	• Inspection of conjunctivae and lids
	• Examination of pupils and irises (e.g., reaction to light and accommodation, size and symmetry)
	• Ophthalmoscopic examination of optic discs (e.g., size, C/D ratio, appearance) and posterior segments (e.g., vessel changes, exudates, hemorrhages)
Ears, Nose, Mouth, Throat	• External inspection of ears and nose (e.g., overall and appearance, scars, lesions, masses)
	• Otoscopic examination of external auditory canals and tympanic membranes
	• Assessment of hearing (e.g., whispered voice, finger rub, tuning fork)
	• Inspection of nasal mucosa, septum and turbinates
	• Inspection of lips, teeth and gums
	• Examination of oropharynx: oral mucosa, salivary glands, hard and soft palates, tongue, tonsils and posterior pharynx
Neck	• Examination of neck (e.g., masses, overall appearance, symmetry, tracheal position, crepitus)
	• Examination of thyroid (e.g., enlargement, tenderness, mass)

Respiratory	• Assessment of respiratory effort (e.g., intercostal retractions, use of accessory muscles, diaphragmatic movement)
	• Percussion of chest (e.g., dullness, flatness, hyperresonance)
	• Palpation of chest (e.g., tactile fremitus)
	• Auscultation of lungs (e.g., breath sounds, adventitious sounds, rubs)
Cardiovascular	• Palpation of heart (e.g., location, size, thrills)
	• Auscultation of heart with notation of abnormal sounds and murmurs
	Examination of:
	• Carotid arteries (e.g., pulse amplitude, bruits)
	• Abdominal aorta (e.g., size, dbruits)
	• Femoral arteries (e.g., pulse amplitude, bruits)
	• Pedal pulses (e.g., pulse amplitude)
	• Extremities for edema and/or varicosities
Chest (Breasts)	• Inspection of breasts (e.g., symmetry, nipple discharge)
	• Palpation of breasts and axillae (e.g., masses or lumps, tenderness)
Gastrointestinal (Abdomen)	• Examination of abdomen with notation of presence of masses or tenderness
	• Examination of liver and spleen
	• Examination for presence or absence of hernia
	• Examination (when indicated) of anus, perineum and rectum, including sphincter tone, presence of hemorrhoids, rectal masses
	• Obtain stool sample for occult blood test when indicated
Genitourinary Male	• Examination of the scrotal contents (e.g., hydrocele, spermatocele, tenderness of cord, testicular mass) *continued*

- Examination of the penis

- Digital rectal examination of prostate gland (e.g., size, symmetry, nodularity, tenderness)

Genitourinary Female

- Pelvic examination (with or without specimen collection for smears and cultures), including

- Examination of external genitalia (e.g., general appearance, hair distribution, lesions) and vagina (e.g., general appearance, estrogen effect, discharge, lesions, pelvic support, cystocele, rectocele)

- Examination of urethra (e.g., masses, tenderness, scarring)

- Examination of bladder (e.g., fullness, masses, tenderness)

- Cervix (e.g., general appearance, lesions, discharge)

- Uterus (e.g., size, contour, position, mobility, tenderness, consistency, descent or support)

- Adnexa/parametria (e.g., masses, tenderness, organomegaly, nodularity)

Lymphatic

Palpation of lymph nodes in **two or more** areas:

- Neck

- Axillae

- Groin

- Other

Musculoskeletal

- Examination of gait and station

- Inspection and/or palpation of digits and nails (eg clubbing, cyanosis, inflammatory conditions, petechiae, ischemia, infections, nodes)

- Examination of joints, bones and muscles of **one or more of the following six** areas: 1) head and neck; 2) spine, ribs and pelvis; 3) right upper extremity; 4) left upper extremity; 5) right lower extremity; and 6) left lower extremity. The examination of a given area includes:

- Inspection and/or palpation with notation of presence of any misalignment, asymmetry, crepitation, defects, tenderness, masses, effusions

- Assessment of range of motion with notation of any pain, crepitation or contracture

- Assessment of stability with notation of any dislocation (luxation), subluxation or laxity

- Assessment of muscle strength and tone (e.g., flaccid, cog wheel, spastic) with notation of any atrophy or abnormal movements

Skin

- Inspection of skin and subcutaneous tissue (e.g., rashes, lesions, ulcers)

- Palpation of skin and subcutaneous tissue (e.g., induration, subcutaneous nodules, tightening)

Neurologic

- Test cranial nerves with notation of any deficits

- Examination of deep tendon reflexes with notation of pathological reflexes (e.g., Babinski)

- Examination of sensation (e.g., by touch, pin, vibration, proprioception)

Psychiatric

- Description of patient's judgment and insight

Brief assessment of mental status including:

- Orientation to time, place and person

- Recent and remote memory

- Mood and affect (e.g., depression, anxiety, agitation)

CONTENT AND DOCUMENTATION REQUIREMENTS

Level of Exam	Perform and Document:
Problem Focused	**One to five** elements identified by a bullet.
Expanded Problem Focused	**At least six** elements identified by a bullet.
Detailed	**At least two** elements identified by a bullet **from each of six areas/systems** OR **at least twelve** elements identified by a bullet in **two or more areas/systems**.
Comprehensive	Perform **all elements** identified by a bullet in **at least nine** organ systems or body areas and document **at least two** elements identified by a bullet **from each of nine areas/systems**.

CARDIOVASCULAR EXAMINATION

SYSTEM/BODY AREA	ELEMENTS OF EXAMINATION
Constitutional	• Measurement of any **three of the following seven** vital signs: 1) sitting or standing blood pressure, 2) supine blood pressure, 3) pulse rate and regularity, 4) respiration, 5) temperature, 6) height, 7) weight (May be measured and recorded by ancillary staff) • General appearance of patient (e.g., development, nutrition, body habitus, deformities, attention to grooming)
Head and Face	
Eyes	• Inspection of conjunctivae and lids (e.g., xanthelasma)
Ears, Nose, Mouth and Throat	• Inspection of teeth, gums and palate • Inspection of oral mucosa with notation of presence of pallor or cyanosis
Neck	• Examination of jugular veins (e.g., distension; a, v or cannon a waves) • Examination of thyroid (e.g., enlargement, tenderness, mass)
Respiratory	• Assessment of respiratory effort (e.g., intercostal retractions, use of accessory muscles, diaphragmatic movement) • Auscultation of lungs (e.g., breath sounds, adventitious sounds, rubs)
Cardiovascular	• Palpation of heart (e.g., location, size and forcefulness of the point of maximal impact; thrills; lifts; palpable S3 or S4) • Auscultation of heart including sounds, abnormal sounds and murmurs

continued

- Measurement of blood pressure in two or more extremities when indicated (e.g., aortic dissection, coarctation)

Examination of:

- Carotid arteries (e.g., waveform, pulse amplitude, bruits, apical-carotid delay)

- Abdominal aorta (e.g., size, bruits)

- Femoral arteries (e.g., pulse amplitude, bruits)

- Pedal pulses (e.g., pulse amplitude)

- Extremities for peripheral edema and/or varicosities

Chest (Breasts)

Gastrointestinal (Abdomen)
- Examination of abdomen with notation of presence of masses or tenderness

- Examination of liver and spleen

- Obtain stool sample for occult blood from patients who are being considered for thrombolytic or anticoagulant therapy

Genitourinary (Abdomen)

Lymphatic

Musculoskeletal
- Examination of the back with notation of kyphosis or scoliosis

- Examination of gait with notation of ability to undergo exercise testing and/or participation in exercise programs

- Assessment of muscle strength and tone (e.g., flaccid, cog wheel, spastic) with notation of any atrophy and abnormal movements

Extremities	• Inspection and palpation of digits and nails (e.g., clubbing, cyanosis, inflammation, petechiae, ischemia, infections, Osler's nodes)
Skin	• Inspection and/or palpation of skin and subcutaneous tissue (e.g., stasis dermatitis, ulcers, scars, xanthomas)
Neurological/Psychiatric	Brief assessment of mental status including: • Orientation to time, place and person • Mood and affect (e.g., depression, anxiety, agitation)

CONTENT AND DOCUMENTATION REQUIREMENTS

Level of Exam	Perform and Document:
Problem Focused	**One to five** elements identified by a bullet.
Expanded Problem Focused	**At least six** elements identified by a bullet.
Detailed	**At least twelve** elements identified by a bullet.
Comprehensive	Perform **all** elements identified by a bullet; document every element in each box with a shaded border and at least one element in each box with an unshaded border.

EAR, NOSE AND THROAT EXAMINATION

SYSTEM/BODY AREA	ELEMENTS OF EXAMINATION
Constitutional	• Measurement of **any three of the following seven** vital signs: 1) sitting or standing blood pressure, 2) supine blood pressure, 3) pulse rate and regularity, 4) respiration, 5) temperature, 6) height, 7) weight (May be measured and recorded by ancillary staff)
	• General appearance of patient (e.g., development, nutrition, body habitus, deformities, attention to grooming)
	• Assessment of ability to communicate (e.g., use of sign language or other communication aids) and quality of voice
Head and Face	• Inspection of head and face (e.g., overall appearance, scars, lesions and masses)
	• Palpation and/or percussion of face with notation of presence or absence of sinus tenderness
	• Examination of salivary glands
	• Assessment of facial strength
Eyes	• Test ocular motility including primary gaze alignment
Ears, Nose, Mouth and Throat	• Otoscopic examination of external auditory canals and tympanic membranes including pneumo-otoscopy with notation of mobility of membranes
	• Assessment of hearing with tuning forks and clinical speech reception thresholds (e.g., whispered voice, finger rub)
	• External inspection of ears and nose (e.g., overall appearance, scars, lesions and masses)
	• Inspection of nasal mucosa, septum and turbinates

continued

487

	• Examination of oropharynx: oral mucosa; inspection of lips, teeth and gums; hard and soft palates; tongue; tonsils; and posterior pharynx (e.g., asymmetry, lesions, hydration of mucosal surfaces)
	• Inspection of pharyngeal walls and pyriform sinuses (e.g., pooling of saliva, asymmetry, lesions)
	• Examination by mirror of larynx including the condition of the epiglottis, false vocal cords, true vocal cords and mobility of larynx (Use of mirror not required in children)
	• Examination by mirror of nasopharynx including appearance of the mucosa, adenoids, posterior choanae and eustachian tubes (Use of mirror not required in children)
Neck	• Examination of neck (e.g., masses, overall appearance, symmetry, tracheal position, crepitus)
	• Examination of thyroid (e.g., enlargement, tenderness, mass)
Respiratory	• Inspection of chest including symmetry, expansion and/or assessment of respiratory effort (e.g., intercostal retractions, use of accessory muscles, diaphragmatic movement)
	• Auscultation of lungs (e.g., breath sounds, adventitious sounds, rubs)
Cardiovascular	• Auscultation of heart with notation of abnormal sounds and murmurs
	• Examination of peripheral vascular system by observation (e.g., swelling, varicosities) and palpation (e.g., pulses, temperature, edema, tenderness)
Chest (Breasts)	
Gastrointestinal (Abdomen)	
Genitourinary	

Lymphatic	• Palpation of lymph nodes in neck, axillae, groin and/or other location
Musculoskeletal	
Extremities	
Skin	
Neurological/Psychiatric	• Test cranial nerves with notation of any deficits Brief assessment of mental status including: • Orientation to time, place and person • Mood and affect (e.g., depression, anxiety, agitation)

CONTENT AND DOCUMENTATION REQUIREMENTS

Level of Exam	Perform and Document:
Problem Focused	**One to five** elements identified by a bullet.
Expanded Problem Focused	**At least six** elements identified by a bullet.
Detailed	**At least twelve** elements identified by a bullet.
Comprehensive	Perform **all** elements identified by a bullet; document every element in each box with a shaded border and at least one element in each box with an unshaded border.

EYE EXAMINATION

SYSTEM/BODY AREA	ELEMENTS OF EXAMINATION
Constitutional	

Head and Face

Eyes	• Test visual acuity (Does not include determination of refractive error)
	• Gross visual field testing by confrontation
	• Test ocular motility including primary gaze alignment
	• Inspection of bulbar and palpebral conjunctivae
	• Examination of ocular adnexae including lids (e.g., ptosis or lagophthalmos), lacrimal glands, lacrimal drainage, orbits and preauricular lymph nodes
	• Examination of pupils and irises including shape, direct and consensual reaction (afferent pupil), size (e.g., anisocoria) and morphology
	• Slit lamp examination of the corneas including epithelium, stroma, endothelium, and tear film
	• Slit lamp examination of the anterior chambers including depth, cells, and flare
	• Slit lamp examination of the lenses including clarity, anterior and posterior capsule, cortex, and nucleus
	• Measurement of intraocular pressures (except in children and patients with trauma or infectious disease)
	• Ophthalmoscopic examination through dilated pupils (unless contraindicated) of
	• Optic discs including size, C/D ratio, appearance (e.g., atrophy, cupping, tumor elevation) and nerve fiber layer
	• Posterior segments including retina and vessels (e.g., exudates and hemorrhages)

Ears, Nose, Mouth and Throat

Neck

Respiratory

Cardiovascular

Chest (Breasts)

Gastrointestinal (Abdomen)

Genitourinary

Lymphatic

Musculoskeletal

Extremities

Skin

Neurological/Psychiatric	Brief assessment of mental status including:
	• Orientation to time, place and person
	• Mood and affect (e.g., depression, anxiety, agitation)

CONTENT AND DOCUMENTATION REQUIREMENTS

Level of Exam	Perform and Document:
Problem Focused	**One to five** elements identified by a bullet.
Expanded Problem Focused	**At least six** elements identified by a bullet.
Detailed	**At least nine** elements identified by a bullet.
Comprehensive	Perform **all** elements identified by a bullet; document every element in each box with a shaded border and at least one element in each box with an unshaded border.

GENITOURINARY EXAMINATION

SYSTEM/BODY AREA	ELEMENTS OF EXAMINATION
Constitutional	• Measurement of **any three of the following seven** vital signs: 1) sitting or standing blood pressure, 2) supine blood pressure, 3) pulse rate and regularity, 4) respiration, 5) temperature, 6) height, 7) weight (May be measured and recorded by ancillary staff) • General appearance of patient (e.g., development, nutrition, body habitus, deformities, attention to grooming)
Head and Face	
Eyes	
Ears, Nose, Mouth and Throat	
Neck	• Examination of neck (e.g., masses, overall appearance, symmetry, tracheal position, crepitus) • Examination of thyroid (e.g., enlargement, tenderness, mass)
Respiratory	• Assessment of respiratory effort (e.g., intercostal retractions, use of accessory muscles, diaphragmatic movement) • Auscultation of lungs (e.g., breath sounds, adventitious sounds, rubs)
Cardiovascular	• Auscultation of heart with notation of abnormal sounds and murmurs • Examination of peripheral vascular system by observation (e.g., swelling, varicosities) and palpation (e.g., pulses, temperature, edema, tenderness)
Chest (Breasts)	[See genitourinary (female)]

Gastrointestinal (Abdomen)	• Examination of abdomen with notation of presence of masses or tenderness
	• Examination for presence or absence of hernia
	• Examination of liver and spleen
	• Obtain stool sample for occult blood test when indicated

Genitourinary (male)	• Inspection of anus and perineum
	Examination (with or without specimen collection for smears and cultures) of genitalia including:
	• Scrotum (e.g., lesions, cysts, rashes)
	• Epididymides (e.g., size, symmetry, masses)
	• Testes (e.g., size, symmetry, masses)
	• Urethral meatus (e.g., size, location, lesions, discharge)
	• Penis (e.g., lesions, presence or absence of foreskin, foreskin retractability, plaque, masses, scarring, deformities)
	Digital rectal examination including:
	• Prostate gland (e.g., size, symmetry, nodularity, tenderness)
	• Seminal vesicles (e.g., symmetry, tenderness, masses, enlargement)
	• Sphincter tone, presence of hemorrhoids, rectal masses

Genitourinary (female)	Includes **at least seven of the following eleven** elements identified by bullets:
	• Inspection and palpation of breasts (e.g., masses or lumps, tenderness, symmetry, nipple discharge)
	• Digital rectal examination including sphincter tone, presence of hemorrhoids, rectal masses
	Pelvic examination (with or without specimen collection for smears and cultures) including:

- External genitalia (e.g., general appearance, hair distribution, lesions)

- Urethral meatus (e.g., size, location, lesions, prolapse)

- Urethra (e.g., masses, tenderness, scarring)

- Bladder (e.g., fullness, masses, tenderness)

- Vagina (e.g., general appearance, estrogen effect, discharge, lesions, pelvic support, cystocele, rectocele)

- Cervix (e.g., general appearance, lesions, discharge)

- Uterus (e.g., size, contour, position, mobility, tenderness, consistency, descent or support)

- Adnexa/parametria (e.g., masses, tenderness, organomegaly, nodularity)

- Anus and perineum

Lymphatic

- Palpation of lymph nodes in neck, axillae, groin and/or other location

Musculoskeletal

Extremities

Skin

- Inspection and/or palpation of skin and subcutaneous tissue (e.g., rashes, lesions, ulcers)

Neurological/Psychiatric

Brief assessment of mental status including:

- Orientation (e.g., time, place and person) and

- Mood and affect (e.g., depression, anxiety, agitation)

CONTENT AND DOCUMENTATION REQUIREMENTS

Level of Exam	Perform and Document:
Problem Focused	**One to five** elements identified by a bullet.
Expanded Problem Focused	**At least six** elements identified by a bullet.
Detailed	**At least twelve** elements identified by a bullet.
Comprehensive	Perform **all** elements identified by a bullet; document every element in each box with a shaded border and at least one element in each box with an unshaded border.

HEMATOLOGIC, LYMPHATIC, AND/OR IMMUNOLOGIC EXAMINATION

SYSTEM/BODY AREA	ELEMENTS OF EXAMINATION
Constitutional	• Measurement of **any three of the following seven** vital signs: 1) sitting or standing blood pressure, 2) supine blood pressure, 3) pulse rate and regularity, 4) respiration, 5) temperature, 6) height, 7) weight (May be measured and recorded by ancillary staff) • General appearance of patient (e.g., development, nutrition, body habitus, deformities, attention to grooming)
Head and Face	• Palpation and/or percussion of face with notation of presence or absence of sinus tenderness
Eyes	• Inspection of conjunctivae and lids
Ears, Nose, Mouth and Throat	• Otoscopic examination of external auditory canals and tympanic membranes • Inspection of nasal mucosa, septum and turbinates • Inspection of teeth and gums • Examination of oropharynx (e.g., oral mucosa, hard and soft palates, tongue, tonsils, posterior pharynx)
Neck	• Examination of neck (e.g., masses, overall appearance, symmetry, tracheal position, crepitus) • Examination of thyroid (e.g., enlargement, tenderness, mass)
Respiratory	• Assessment of respiratory effort (e.g., intercostal retractions, use of accessory muscles, diaphragmatic movement) • Auscultation of lungs (e.g., breath sounds, adventitious sounds, rubs)

| **Cardiovascular** | • Auscultation of heart with notation of abnormal sounds and murmurs |
| | • Examination of peripheral vascular system by observation (e.g., swelling, varicosities) and palpation (e.g., pulses, temperature, edema, tenderness) |

Chest (Breasts)

| **Gastrointestinal (Abdomen)** | • Examination of abdomen with notation of presence of masses or tenderness |
| | • Examination of liver and spleen |

Genitourinary

| **Lymphatic** | • Palpation of lymph nodes in neck, axillae, groin, and/or other location |

Musculoskeletal

| **Extremities** | • Inspection and palpation of digits and nails (e.g., clubbing, cyanosis, inflammation, petechiae, ischemia, infections, nodes) |

| **Skin** | • Inspection and/or palpation of skin and subcutaneous tissue (e.g., rashes, lesions, ulcers, ecchymoses, bruises) |

Neurological/Psychiatric	Brief assessment of mental status including:
	• Orientation to time, place and person
	• Mood and affect (e.g., depression, anxiety, agitation)

CONTENT AND DOCUMENTATION REQUIREMENTS

Level of Exam	Perform and Document:
Problem Focused	**One to five** elements identified by a bullet.
Expanded Problem Focused	**At least six** elements identified by a bullet.
Detailed	**At least twelve** elements identified by a bullet.
Comprehensive	Perform **all** elements identified by a bullet; document every element in each box with a shaded border and at least one element in each box with an unshaded border.

MUSCULOSKELETAL EXAMINATION

SYSTEM/BODY AREA	ELEMENTS OF EXAMINATION
Constitutional	• Measurement of **any three of the following seven** vital signs: 1) sitting or standing blood pressure, 2) supine blood pressure, 3) pulse rate and regularity, 4) respiration, 5) temperature, 6) height, 7) weight (May be measured and recorded by ancillary staff) • General appearance of patient (e.g., development, nutrition, body habitus, deformities, attention to grooming)
Head and Face	
Eyes	
Ears, Nose, Mouth and Throat	
Neck	
Respiratory	
Cardiovascular	• Examination of peripheral vascular system by observation (e.g., swelling, varicosities) and palpation (e.g., pulses, temperature, edema, tenderness)
Chest (Breasts)	
Gastrointestinal (Abdomen)	
Genitourinary	
Lymphatic	• Palpation of lymph nodes in neck, axillae, groin and/or other location

Musculoskeletal	• Examination of gait and station
	• Examination of joint(s), bone(s) and muscle(s)/tendon(s) of **four of the following six** areas: 1) head and neck; 2) spine, ribs and pelvis; 3) right upper extremity; 4) left upper extremity; 5) right lower extremity; and 6) left lower extremity. The examination of a given area includes:
	• Inspection, percussion and/or palpation with notation of any misalignment, asymmetry, crepitation, defects, tenderness, masses or effusions
	• Assessment of range of motion with notation of any pain (e.g., straight leg raising), crepitation or contracture
	• Assessment of stability with notation of any dislocation (luxation), subluxation or laxity
	• Assessment of muscle strength and tone (e.g., flaccid, cog wheel, spastic) with notation of any atrophy or abnormal movements

NOTE: For the comprehensive level of examination, all four of the elements identified by a bullet must be performed and documented for each of four anatomic areas. For the three lower levels of examination, each element is counted separately for each body area. For example, assessing range of motion in two extremities constitutes two elements.

Extremities	[See musculoskeletal and skin]

Skin	• Inspection and/or palpation of skin and subcutaneous tissue (e.g., scars, rashes, lesions, cafe-au-lait spots, ulcers) in **four of the following six** areas: 1) head and neck; 2) trunk; 3) right upper extremity; 4) left upper extremity; 5) right lower extremity; and 6) left lower extremity.

NOTE: For the comprehensive level, all four areas must be examined and documented. For the three lower levels, each body area is counted separately. For example, inspection and/or palpation of the skin and subcutaneous tissue of two extremities constitutes two elements.

Neurological/Psychiatric	• Test coordination (e.g., finger/nose, heel/knee/shin, rapid alternating movements in the upper and lower extremities, evaluation of fine motor coordination in young children)
	• Examination of deep tendon reflexes and/or nerve stretch test with notation of pathological reflexes (e.g., Babinski)
	• Examination of sensation (e.g., by touch, pin, vibration, proprioception)
	Brief assessment of mental status including
	• Orientation to time, place and person
	• Mood and affect (e.g., depression, anxiety, agitation)

CONTENT AND DOCUMENTATION REQUIREMENTS

Level of Exam	Perform and Document:
Problem Focused	**One to five** elements identified by a bullet.
Expanded Problem Focused	**At least six** elements identified by a bullet.
Detailed	**At least twelve** elements identified by a bullet.
Comprehensive	Perform **all** elements identified by a bullet; document every element in each box with a shaded border and at least one element in each box with an unshaded border.

NEUROLOGICAL EXAMINATION

SYSTEM/BODY AREA	ELEMENTS OF EXAMINATION
Constitutional	• Measurement of **any three of the following seven** vital signs: 1) sitting or standing blood pressure, 2) supine blood pressure, 3) pulse rate and regularity, 4) respiration, 5) temperature, 6) height, 7) weight (May be measured and recorded by ancillary staff) • General appearance of patient (e.g., development, nutrition, body habitus, deformities, attention to grooming)
Head and Face	
Eyes	• Ophthalmoscopic examination of optic discs (e.g., size, C/D ratio, appearance) and posterior segments (e.g., vessel changes, exudates, hemorrhages)
Ears, Nose, Mouth and Throat	
Neck	
Respiratory	
Cardiovascular	• Examination of carotid arteries (e.g., pulse amplitude, bruits) • Auscultation of heart with notation of abnormal sounds and murmurs • Examination of peripheral vascular system by observation (e.g., swelling, varicosities) and palpation (e.g., pulses, temperature, edema, tenderness)
Chest (Breasts)	
Gastrointestinal (Abdomen)	
Genitourinary	
Lymphatic	

Musculoskeletal	• Examination of gait and station
	Assessment of motor function including:
	• Muscle strength in upper and lower extremities
	• Muscle tone in upper and lower extremities (e.g., flaccid, cog wheel, spastic) with notation of any atrophy or abnormal movements (e.g., fasciculation, tardive dyskinesia)

| **Extremities** | [See musculoskeletal] |

Skin

Neurological/Psychiatric	Evaluation of higher integrative functions including:
	• Orientation to time, place and person
	• Recent and remote memory
	• Attention span and concentration
	• Language (e.g., naming objects, repeating phrases, spontaneous speech)
	• Fund of knowledge (e.g., awareness of current events, past history, vocabulary)
	Test the following cranial nerves:
	• 2nd cranial nerve (e.g., visual acuity, visual fields, fundi)
	• 3rd, 4th and 6th cranial nerves (e.g., pupils, eye movements)
	• 5th cranial nerve (e.g., facial sensation, corneal reflexes)
	• 7th cranial nerve (e.g., facial symmetry, strength)
	• 8th cranial nerve (e.g., hearing with tuning fork, whispered voice and/or finger rub)
	• 9th cranial nerve (e.g., spontaneous or reflex palate movement)

continued

- 11th cranial nerve (e.g., shoulder shrug strength)

- 12th cranial nerve (e.g., tongue protrusion)

- Examination of sensation (e.g., by touch, pin, vibration, proprioception)

- Examination of deep tendon reflexes in upper and lower extremities with notation of pathological reflexes (e.g., Babinski)

- Test coordination (e.g., finger/nose, heel/knee/shin, rapid alternating movements in the upper and lower extremities, evaluation of fine motor coordination in young children)

Psychiatric

CONTENT AND DOCUMENTATION REQUIREMENTS

Level of Exam	Perform and Document:
Problem Focused	**One to five** elements identified by a bullet.
Expanded Problem Focused	**At least six** elements identified by a bullet.
Detailed	**At least twelve** elements identified by a bullet.
Comprehensive	Perform **all** elements identified by a bullet; document every element in each box with a shaded border and at least one element in each box with an unshaded border.

PSYCHIATRIC EXAMINATION

SYSTEM/BODY AREA	ELEMENTS OF EXAMINATION
Constitutional	• Measurement of **any three of the following seven** vital signs: 1) sitting or standing blood pressure, 2) supine blood pressure, 3) pulse rate and regularity, 4) respiration, 5) temperature, 6) height, 7) weight (May be measured and recorded by ancillary staff) • General appearance of patient (e.g., development, nutrition, body habitus, deformities, attention to grooming)
Head and Face	
Eyes	
Ears, Nose, Mouth and Throat	
Neck	
Respiratory	
Cardiovascular	
Chest (Breasts)	
Gastrointestinal (Abdomen)	
Genitourinary	
Lymphatic	
Musculoskeletal	• Assessment of muscle strength and tone (e.g., flaccid, cog wheel, spastic) with notation of any atrophy and abnormal movements • Examination of gait and station
Extremities	
Skin	

Neurological

Psychiatric	• Description of speech including: rate; volume; articulation; coherence; and spontaneity with notation of abnormalities (e.g., perseveration, paucity of language)
	• Description of thought processes including: rate of thoughts; content of thoughts (e.g., logical vs. illogical, tangential); abstract reasoning; and computation
	• Description of associations (e.g., loose, tangential, circumstantial, intact)
	• Description of abnormal or psychotic thoughts including: hallucinations; delusions; preoccupation with violence; homicidal or suicidal ideation; and obsessions
	• Description of the patient's judgment (e.g., concerning everyday activities and social situations) and insight (e.g., concerning psychiatric condition)
	Complete mental status examination including:
	• Orientation to time, place and person
	• Recent and remote memory
	• Attention span and concentration
	• Language (e.g., naming objects, repeating phrases)
	• Fund of knowledge (e.g., awareness of current events, past history, vocabulary)
	• Mood and affect (e.g., depression, anxiety, agitation, hypomania, lability)

CONTENT AND DOCUMENTATION REQUIREMENTS

Level of Exam	Perform and Document:
Problem Focused	One to five elements identified by a bullet.
Expanded Problem Focused	At least six elements identified by a bullet.
Detailed	At least nine elements identified by a bullet.
Comprehensive	Perform all elements identified by a bullet; document every element in each box with a shaded border and at least one element in each box with an unshaded border.

RESPIRATORY EXAMINATION

SYSTEM/BODY AREA	ELEMENTS OF EXAMINATION
Constitutional	• Measurement of **any three of the following seven** vital signs: 1) sitting or standing blood pressure, 2) supine blood pressure, 3) pulse rate and regularity, 4) respiration, 5) temperature, 6) height, 7) weight (May be measured and recorded by ancillary staff) • General appearance of patient (e.g., development, nutrition, body habitus, deformities, attention to grooming)
Head and Face	
Eyes	
Ears, Nose, Mouth and Throat	• Inspection of nasal mucosa, septum and turbinates • Inspection of teeth and gums • Examination of oropharynx (e.g., oral mucosa, hard and soft palates, tongue, tonsils and posterior pharynx)
Neck	• Examination of neck (e.g., masses, overall appearance, symmetry, tracheal position, crepitus) • Examination of thyroid (e.g., enlargement, tenderness, mass) • Examination of jugular veins (e.g., distension; a, v or cannon a waves)
Respiratory	• Inspection of chest with notation of symmetry and expansion • Assessment of respiratory effort (e.g., intercostal retractions, use of accessory muscles, diaphragmatic movement) • Percussion of chest (e.g., dullness, flatness, hyperresonance) *continued*

	• Palpation of chest (e.g., tactile fremitus)
	• Auscultation of lungs (e.g., breath sounds, adventitious sounds, rubs)
Cardiovascular	• Auscultation of heart including sounds, abnormal sounds and murmurs
	• Examination of peripheral vascular system by observation (e.g., swelling, varicosities) and palpation (e.g., pulses, temperature, edema, tenderness)
Chest (Breasts)	
Gastrointestinal (Abdomen)	• Examination of abdomen with notation of presence of masses or tenderness
	• Examination of liver and spleen
Genitourinary	
Lymphatic	• Palpation of lymph nodes in neck, axillae, groin and/or other location
Musculoskeletal	• Assessment of muscle strength and tone (e.g., flaccid, cog wheel, spastic) with notation of any atrophy and abnormal movements
	• Examination of gait and station
Extremities	• Inspection and palpation of digits and nails (e.g., clubbing, cyanosis, inflammation, petechiae, ischemia, infections, nodes)
Skin	• Inspection and/or palpation of skin and subcutaneous tissue (e.g., rashes, lesions, ulcers)
Neurological/Psychiatric	Brief assessment of mental status including:
	• Orientation to time, place and person
	• Mood and affect (e.g., depression, anxiety, agitation)

CONTENT AND DOCUMENTATION REQUIREMENTS

Level of Exam	Perform and Document:
Problem Focused	**One to five** elements identified by a bullet.
Expanded Problem Focused	**At least six** elements identified by a bullet.
Detailed	**At least twelve** elements identified by a bullet.
Comprehensive	Perform **all** elements identified by a bullet; document every element in each box with a shaded border and at least one element in each box with an unshaded border.

SKIN EXAMINATION

SYSTEM/BODY AREA	ELEMENTS OF EXAMINATION
Constitutional	• Measurement of **any three of the following seven** vital signs: 1) sitting or standing blood pressure, 2) supine blood pressure, 3) pulse rate and regularity, 4) respiration, 5) temperature, 6) height, 7) weight (May be measured and recorded by ancillary staff) • General appearance of patient (e.g., development, nutrition, body habitus, deformities, attention to grooming)
Head and Face	
Eyes	• Inspection of conjunctivae and lids
Ears, Nose, Mouth and Throat	• Inspection of lips, teeth and gums • Examination of oropharynx (e.g., oral mucosa, hard and soft palates, tongue, tonsils, posterior pharynx)
Neck	• Examination of thyroid (e.g., enlargement, tenderness, mass)
Respiratory	
Cardiovascular	• Examination of peripheral vascular system by observation (e.g., swelling, varicosities) and palpation (e.g., pulses, temperature, edema, tenderness)
Chest (Breasts)	
Gastrointestinal (Abdomen)	• Examination of liver and spleen • Examination of anus for condyloma and other lesions
Genitourinary	

Lymphatic
- Palpation of lymph nodes in neck, axillae, groin and/or other location

Musculoskeletal

Extremities
- Inspection and palpation of digits and nails (e.g., clubbing, cyanosis, inflammation, petechiae, ischemia, infections, nodes)

Skin
- Palpation of scalp and inspection of hair of scalp, eyebrows, face, chest, pubic area (when indicated) and extremities

  Inspection and/or palpation of skin and subcutaneous tissue (e.g., rashes, lesions, ulcers, susceptibility to and presence of photo damage) in **eight of the following ten** areas:

- Head, including the face and
- Neck
- Chest, including breasts and axillae
- Abdomen
- Genitalia, groin, buttocks
- Back
- Right upper extremity
- Left upper extremity
- Right lower extremity
- Left lower extremity

NOTE: For the comprehensive level, the examination of at least eight anatomic areas must be performed and documented. For the three lower levels of examination, each body area is counted separately. For example, inspection and/or palpation of the skin and subcutaneous tissue of the right upper extremity and the left upper extremity constitutes two elements.

- Inspection of eccrine and apocrine glands of skin and subcutaneous tissue with identification and location of any hyperhidrosis, chromhidroses or bromhidrosis

Neurological/Psychiatric   Brief assessment of mental status including:

- Orientation to time, place and person

- Mood and affect (e.g., depression, anxiety, agitation)

CONTENT AND DOCUMENTATION REQUIREMENTS

Level of Exam	Perform and Document:
Problem Focused	**One to five** elements identified by a bullet.
Expanded Problem Focused	**At least six** elements identified by a bullet.
Detailed	**At least twelve** elements identified by a bullet.
Comprehensive	Perform **all** elements identified by a bullet; document every element in each box with a shaded border and at least one element in each box with an unshaded border.

DOCUMENTATION OF THE COMPLEXITY OF MEDICAL DECISION MAKING

The levels of E/M services recognize four types of medical decision making (straightforward, low complexity, moderate complexity, and high complexity). Medical decision making refers to the complexity of establishing a diagnosis and/or selecting a management option as measured by:

- the number of possible diagnoses and/or the number of management options that must be considered;

- the amount and/or complexity of medical records, diagnostic tests, and/or other information that must be obtained, reviewed, and analyzed; and

- the risk of significant complications, morbidity, and/or mortality, as well as comorbidities, associated with the patient's presenting problem(s), the diagnostic procedure(s), and/or the possible management options.

The table below shows the progression of the elements required for each level of medical decision making. To qualify for a given type of decision making, *two of the three elements in the table must be either met or exceeded.*

Number of Diagnoses	Amount of Data to Review	Risk of Complication	Type of Decision Making
Minimal	Minimal or None	Minimal	Straightforward
Limited	Limited	Low	Low Complexity
Multiple	Moderate	Moderate	Moderate Complexity
Extensive	Extensive	High	High Complexity

Each of the elements of medical decision making is described below.

NUMBER OF DIAGNOSES OR MANAGEMENT OPTIONS

The number of possible diagnoses and/or the number of management options that must be considered is based on the number and types of problems addressed during the encounter, the complexity of establishing a diagnosis, and the management decisions that are made by the physician.

Generally, decision making with respect to a diagnosed problem is easier than that for an identified but undiagnosed problem. The number and type of diagnostic tests employed may be an indicator of the number of possible diagnoses. Problems that are improving or resolving are less complex than those that are worsening or failing to change as expected. The need to seek advice from others is another indicator of complexity of diagnostic or management problems.

- *DG:*   *For each encounter, an assessment, clinical impression, or diagnosis should be documented. It may be explicitly stated or implied in documented decisions regarding management plans and/or further evaluation.*

-     *For a presenting problem with an established diagnosis, the record should reflect whether the problem is: a) improved, well controlled, resolving, or resolved or b) inadequately controlled, worsening, or failing to change as expected.*

-     *For a presenting problem without an established diagnosis, the assessment or clinical impression may be stated in the form of differential diagnoses or as a "possible," "probable," or "rule out" (R/O) diagnosis.*

- *DG:*   *The initiation of, or changes in, treatment should be documented. Treatment includes a wide range of management options, including patient instructions, nursing instructions, therapies, and medications.*

- *DG:*   *If referrals are made, consultations requested, or advice sought, the record should indicate to whom or where the referral or consultation is made or from whom the advice is requested.*

AMOUNT AND/OR COMPLEXITY OF DATA TO BE REVIEWED

The amount and complexity of data to be reviewed are based on the types of diagnostic testing ordered or reviewed. A decision to obtain and review old medical records and/or obtain history from sources other than the patient increases the amount and complexity of data to be reviewed.

Discussion of contradictory or unexpected test results with the physician who performed or interpreted the test is an indication of the complexity of data being reviewed. On occasion, the physician who ordered a test may personally review the image, tracing, or specimen to supplement information from the physician who prepared the test report or interpretation; this is another indication of the complexity of data being reviewed.

- *DG:*   *If a diagnostic service (test or procedure) is ordered, planned, scheduled, or performed at the time of the E/M encounter, the type of service, e.g., lab or x-ray, should be documented.*

- *DG:*   *The review of lab, radiology, and/or other diagnostic tests should be documented. A simple notation such as "WBC elevated" or "chest x-ray unremarkable" is acceptable. Alternatively, the review may be documented by initialing and dating the report containing the test results.*

- *DG:*   *A decision to obtain old records or decision to obtain additional history from the family, caretaker, or other source to supplement that obtained from the patient should be documented.*

- *DG:*   *Relevant findings from the review of old records and/or the receipt of additional history from the family, caretaker, or other source to supplement that obtained from the patient should be documented. If there is no relevant information beyond that already obtained, that fact should be documented. A notation of "old records reviewed" or "additional history obtained from family" without elaboration is insufficient.*

- *DG:*   *The results of discussion of laboratory, radiology, or other diagnostic tests with the physician who performed or interpreted the study should be documented.*

• *DG:*   *The direct visualization and independent interpretation of an image, tracing, or specimen previously or subsequently interpreted by another physician should be documented.*

RISK OF SIGNIFICANT COMPLICATIONS, MORBIDITY, AND/OR MORTALITY

The risk of significant complications, morbidity, and/or mortality is based on the risks associated with the presenting problem(s), the diagnostic procedure(s), and the possible management options.

• *DG:*   *Comorbidities/underlying diseases or other factors that increase the complexity of medical decision making by increasing the risk of complications, morbidity, and/or mortality should be documented.*

• *DG:*   *If a surgical or invasive diagnostic procedure is ordered, planned, or scheduled at the time of the E/M encounter, the type of procedure, e.g., laparoscopy, should be documented.*

• *DG:*   *If a surgical or invasive diagnostic procedure is performed at the time of the E/M encounter, the specific procedure should be documented.*

• *DG:*   *The referral for or decision to perform a surgical or invasive diagnostic procedure on an urgent basis should be documented or implied.*

The Table of Risk later in this section may be used to help determine whether the risk of significant complications, morbidity, and/or mortality is *minimal, low, moderate,* or *high.* Because the determination of risk is complex and not readily quantifiable, the table includes common clinical examples rather than absolute measures of risk. The assessment of risk of the presenting problem(s) is based on the risk related to the disease process anticipated between the present encounter and the next one. The assessment of risk of selecting diagnostic procedures and management options is based on the risk during and immediately following any procedures or treatment. *The highest level of risk in any one category (presenting problem(s), diagnostic procedure(s), or management options) determines the overall risk.*

DOCUMENTATION OF AN ENCOUNTER DOMINATED BY COUNSELING OR COORDINATION OF CARE

In the case in which counseling and/or coordination of care dominates (more than 50% of) the physician/patient and/or physician/family encounter (face-to-face time in the office or other outpatient setting, floor/unit time in the hospital, or floor/unit time in the nursing facility), time is considered the key or controlling factor to qualify for a particular level of E/M services.

• **DG:**   *If the physician elects to report the level of service based on counseling and/or coordination of care, the total length of time of the encounter (face-to-face or floor time, as appropriate) should be documented and the record should describe the counseling and/or activities to coordinate care.*

TABLE OF RISK

LEVEL OF RISK	PRESENTING PROBLEM(S)	DIAGNOSTIC PROCEDURES	MANAGEMENT OPTIONS
Minimal	• One self-limited or minor problem, e.g., cold, insect bite, tinea corporis	• Laboratory tests requiring venipuncture • Chest x-rays • EKG/EEG • Urinalysis • Ultrasound, e.g., echocardiography • KOH prep	• Rest • Gargles • Elastic bandages • Superficial dressings
Low	• Two or more self-limited or minor problems • One stable chronic illness, e.g., well controlled hypertension, non-insulin dependent diabetes, cataract, BPH • Acute uncomplicated illness or injury, e.g., cystitis, allergic rhinitis, simple sprain	• Physiologic tests not under stress, e.g., pulmonary function tests • Non-cardiovascular imaging studies with contrast, e.g., barium enema • Superficial needle biopsies • Clinical laboratory tests requiring arterial puncture • Skin biopsies	• Over-the-counter drugs • Minor surgery with no identified risk factors • Physical therapy • Occupational therapy • IV fluids without additives
Moderate	• One or more chronic illnesses with mild exacerbation, progression, or side effects of treatment • Two or more stable chronic illnesses • Undiagnosed new problem with uncertain prognosis, e.g., lump in breast • Acute illness with systemic symptoms, e.g., pyelonephritis, pneumonitis, colitis • Acute complicated injury, e.g., head injury with brief loss of consciousness	• Physiologic tests under stress, e.g., cardiac stress test, fetal contraction stress test • Diagnostic endoscopies with no identified risk factors • Deep needle or incisional biopsy • Cardiovascular imaging studies with contrast and no identified risk factors, e.g., arteriogram, cardiac catheterization • Obtain fluid from body cavity, e.g. lumbar puncture, thoracentesis, culdocentesis	• Minor surgery with identified risk factors • Elective major surgery (open, percutaneous or endoscopic) with no identified risk factors • Prescription drug management • Therapeutic nuclear medicine • IV fluids with additives • Closed treatment of fracture or dislocation without manipulation

continued

TABLE OF RISK *(continued)*

LEVEL OF RISK	PRESENTING PROBLEM(S)	DIAGNOSTIC PROCEDURES	MANAGEMENT OPTIONS
High	• One or more chronic illnesses with severe exacerbation, progression, or side effects of treatment • Acute or chronic illnesses or injuries that pose a threat to life or bodily function, e.g., multiple trauma, acute MI, pulmonary embolus, severe respiratory distress, progressive severe rheumatoid arthritis, psychiatric illness with potential threat to self or others, peritonitis, acute renal failure • An abrupt change in neuro • logic status, e.g., seizure, TIA, weakness, sensory loss	• Cardiovascular imaging studies with contrast with identified risk factors • Cardiac electrophysiological tests • Diagnostic endoscopies with identified risk factors • Discography	• Elective major surgery (open, percutaneous or endoscopic) with identified risk factors • Emergency major surgery (open, percutaneous or endoscopic) • Parenteral controlled substances • Drug therapy requiring intensive monitoring for toxicity • Decision not to resuscitate or to de-escalate care because of poor prognosis

NATIONAL CORRECT CODING POLICY

In December 1989, the Omnibus Budget Reconciliation Act of 1989 (P.L. 101-239) was enacted. Section 6102 of P.L. 101-239 amended Title XVIII of the Social Security Act (the Act) by adding a new section 1848, Payment for Physicians' Services. This section of the Act provided for replacing the previous reasonable charge mechanism of actual, customary, and prevailing charges with a resource-based relative-value scale (RBRVS) fee schedule that began in 1992.

With the implementation of the Medicare Fee Schedule, it was increasingly important to assure that uniform payment policies and procedures were followed by all carriers so that when the same service is rendered in various carrier jurisdictions, it is paid for in the same way. In addition, accurate coding and reporting of services by physicians were major concerns to guarantee proper payment.

PURPOSE

The Centers for Medicare and Medicaid Services (CMS) developed the National Correct Coding Initiative to promote national correct coding methodologies and to control improper coding that leads to inappropriate payment in Part B claims. The coding policies developed are based on coding conventions defined in the American Medical Association's CPT code book, national and local policies and edits, coding guidelines developed by national societies, analysis of standard medical and surgical practice, and review of current coding practice.

WHAT IS CORRECT CODING?

Procedures should be reported with the HCPCS/CPT codes that most comprehensively describe the services performed. Unbundling occurs when multiple procedure codes are billed for a group of procedures that are covered by a single comprehensive code.

Two types of practices lead to unbundling. The first is unintentional and results from a misunderstanding of coding. The second is intentional and is used by providers to manipulate coding in order to maximize payment.

Correct coding requires reporting a group of procedures with the appropriate comprehensive code. Examples of unbundling are described below:

- Fragmenting one service into component parts and coding each component part as if it were a separate service. For example, the correct CPT comprehensive code to use for upper gastrointestinal endoscopy with biopsy of stomach is CPT code 43239. Separating the service into two component parts, using CPT code 43235 for upper gastrointestinal endoscopy and CPT code 43600 for biopsy of stomach, is inappropriate.

- Reporting separate codes for related services when one comprehensive code includes all related services. An example of this type is coding a total abdominal hysterectomy with or without removal of tubes, with or without removal of ovaries (CPT code 58150) plus salpingectomy (CPT code 58700) plus oophorectomy (CPT code 58940) rather than using the comprehensive CPT code 58150 for all three related services.

- Breaking out bilateral procedures when one code is appropriate. For example, bilateral mammography is coded correctly using CPT code 76091 rather than incorrectly submitting CPT code 76090-RT for right mammography and CPT code 76090-LT for left mammography.

- Down-coding a service in order to use an additional code when one higher-level, more-comprehensive code is appropriate. A laboratory should bill CPT code 80048 (Basic metabolic panel) when coding for calcium, carbon dioxide, chloride, creatinine, glucose, potassium, sodium, and urea nitrogen performed as automated multichannel tests. It would be inappropriate to report CPT codes 82310, 82374, 82435, 82565, 82947, 84132, 84295, and/or 84520 in addition to the CPT code 80048 unless one of these laboratory tests was performed at a different time of day to obtain follow-up results, in which case a -91 modifier would be utilized.

- Separating a surgical approach from a major surgical service. For example, a provider should not bill CPT code 49000 for exploratory laparotomy and CPT code 44150 for total abdominal colectomy for the same operation, because the exploration of the surgical field is included in the CPT code 44150.

GENERAL CORRECT CODING POLICIES

The Physicians' Current Procedural Terminology (CPT) developed by the American Medical Association and HCPCS Level II codes developed by the Centers for Medicare and Medicaid Services (CMS) are listings of descriptive terms and identifying codes for reporting medical services and procedures performed by physicians. The codes in the CPT code book are copyrighted by the AMA and updated annually by the CPT Editorial Panel based on input from the AMA Advisory Committee, which serves as a channel for requests from various providers and specialty societies. The purpose of both coding systems and annual updates is to communicate specific services rendered by physicians and other providers, usually for the purpose of claim submission to third-party (insurance) carriers. A multitude of codes is necessary because of the wide spectrum of services provided by various medical care providers. Because many medical services can be rendered by different methods and combinations of various procedures, multiple codes describing similar services are frequently necessary to accurately reflect what service a physician performs. While often only one procedure is performed at a patient encounter, multiple procedures are performed at the same session at other times. In the latter case, the preprocedure and postprocedure work does not have to be repeated. Therefore, a comprehensive code, describing the multiple services commonly performed together, can be defined.

Third-party payers have adopted the CPT coding system for use by providers to communicate payable services. It therefore becomes more important to identify the various potential combinations of services to accurately adjudicate claims.

There are two sets of Correct Coding Initiative (CCI) tables, correct coding (also known as comprehensive/component) edits, and mutually exclusive edits. All edits consist of code pairs that are arranged in column 1 and column 2 of the tables. All edits are included in the first table except those meeting the criteria for mutually exclusive code edits (Chapter I, Section R). Edits based on the criteria for "Gender-Specific Procedures" (formerly "Designation of Sex") (Chapter I, Section S) are also included in the mutually exclusive code edit tables. The column 2 code in both tables is not payable with the column 1 code unless the edit permits use of a modifier associated with CCI (Chapter I, Section H). The correct coding edit table contains many edits in which the column 2 code is a component of the column 1 comprehensive code. However, this table also contains many edits for which there is no comprehensive/component relationship, but the column 1 code and column 2 code should not be reported together for other reasons. The following policies encompass general issues/coding principles that are to be applied in all subsequent chapters. Specific examples are stated to clarify the policy but do not represent the only code or service that is included in the policy.

CODING BASED ON STANDARDS OF MEDICAL/SURGICAL PRACTICE

In order for this system to be effective, it is essential that the coding description accurately describe what actually transpired at the patient encounter. Because many physician activities are so integral to a procedure, it is impractical and unnecessary to list every event common to all procedures of a similar nature as part of the narrative description for a code. Many of these common activities reflect simple normal principles of medical/surgical care. These "generic" activities are assumed to be included as acceptable medical/surgical practice, and, while they could be performed separately, they should not be considered as such when a code descriptor is defined. Accordingly, all services integral to accomplishing a procedure will be considered included in that procedure.

Many of these generic activities are common to virtually all procedures. On other occasions, some are integral to only a certain group of procedures but are still essential to accomplish these particular procedures. Accordingly, it would be inappropriate to separately code these services based on standard medical and surgical principles.

Some examples of generic services integral to standard of medical/surgical services include:

- Cleansing, shaving, and prepping of skin

- Draping of patient

- Positioning of patient

- Insertion of intravenous access for medication

- Sedative administration by the physician performing the procedure (see Chapter II, Anesthesia section, for the separate policy)

- Local, topical, or regional anesthetic administered by physician performing procedure

- Surgical approach, including identification of anatomical landmarks, incision, evaluation of the surgical field, simple debridement of traumatized tissue, lysis of simple adhesions, isolation of neurovascular, muscular (including stimulation for identification), bony, or other structures limiting access to surgical field

- Surgical cultures

- Wound irrigation

- Insertion and removal of drains, suction devices, dressings, pumps into same site

- Surgical closure

- Application, management, and removal of postoperative dressings, including analgesic devices (peri-incisional TENS unit, institution of Patient Controlled Analgesia)

- Preoperative, intraoperative, and postoperative documentation, including photographs, drawings, dictation, transcription as necessary to document the services provided

- Surgical supplies, unless excepted by existing CMS policy

In the case of individual services, there are numerous specific services that may typically be involved in order to accomplish a column 1 procedure. Generally, performance of these services represents the standard of practice for a more-comprehensive procedure, and the services are therefore to be included in that service.

Because many of these services are unique to individual CPT coding sections, the rationale for correct coding will be described in that particular section. The principle of the policy to include these services into the column 1 procedure remains the same as the principle applied to the generic service list noted above. Specifically, these principles include:

1. The service represents the standard of care in accomplishing the overall procedure.

2. The service is necessary to successfully accomplish the column 1 procedure; failure to perform the service may compromise the success of the procedure.

3. The service does not represent a separately identifiable procedure unrelated to the column 1 procedure planned.

Specific examples consist of:

Medical:

1. Procurement of a rhythm strip in conjunction with an electrocardiogram. The rhythm strip would not be separately reported if it was procured by the same physician performing the interpretation, since it is an integral component of the interpretation.

2. Procurement of upper-extremity (brachial) Doppler study in addition to lower-extremity Doppler study in order to obtain an "ankle-brachial index" (ABI). The upper-extremity Doppler would not be separately reported.

3. Procurement of an electrocardiogram as part of a cardiac stress test. The electrocardiogram would not be separately reported if procured as a routine serial EKG typically performed before, during, and after a cardiac stress test.

Surgical:

1. Removal of a cerumen impaction prior to myringotomy. The cerumen impaction is precluding access to the tympanic membrane, and its removal is necessary for the successful completion of the myringotomy.

2. Performance of a bronchoscopy prior to a thoracic surgery (e.g., thoracotomy and lobectomy). Assuming that a diagnostic bronchoscopy has already been performed for diagnosis and biopsy and the surgeon is simply evaluating for anatomic assessment for sleeve or more-complex resection, the bronchoscopy would not be separately reported. Essentially, this "scout" endoscopy represents a part of the assessment of the surgical field to establish anatomical landmarks, extent of disease, etc. If an endoscopic procedure is done as part of an open procedure, it is not separately reported. However, if an endoscopy is performed for purposes of an initial diagnosis on the same day as the open procedure, the endoscopy is separately reported. In the case in which the procedure is performed for diagnostic purposes immediately prior to a more-definitive procedure, the -58 modifier may be utilized to indicate that these procedures are staged or planned services. Additionally, if endoscopic procedures are performed on distinct, separate areas at the same session, these procedures would be reported separately. For example, a thoracoscopy and mediastinoscopy, being separate endoscopic procedures, would be separately reported. On the other hand, a cursory evaluation of the upper airway as part of a bronchoscopic procedure would not be separately reported as a laryngoscopy, sinus endoscopy, etc.

3. Lysis of adhesions and exploratory laparotomy reported with colon resection or other abdominal surgery. These procedures represent gaining access to the organ system of interest and are not separately reported.

MEDICAL/SURGICAL PACKAGE

As a result of the variety of surgical, diagnostic, and therapeutic nonsurgical procedures commonly performed in medical practice, the extent of the CPT code book has grown. The need for precise definitions for the various combinations of services is further warranted because of the dependence of providers on CPT coding for reporting to third-party payers. When a Resource-Based

Relative-Value System (RBRVS) is used in conjunction with CPT coding, the necessity for accurate coding is amplified.

In general, most services have preprocedure and postprocedure work associated with them; when performed at a single patient encounter, the preprocedure and postprocedure work does not change proportionately when multiple services are performed. Additionally, the nature of the preprocedure and postprocedure work is reasonably consistent across the spectrum of procedures.

In keeping with the policy that the work typically associated with a standard surgical or medical service is included in the CPT code book's code description of the service, some general guidelines can be developed. With few exceptions, these guidelines transcend a majority of CPT descriptions, irrespective of whether the service is limited or comprehensive.

1. A majority of invasive procedures require the availability of vascular and/or airway access; accordingly, the work associated with obtaining this access is included in the preprocedure services, and returning a patient to the appropriate postprocedure state is included in the procedural services. Intravenous access and airway access (e.g., HCPCS/CPT codes 36000, 36400, 36410) are frequently necessary; therefore, CPT codes describing these services are not separately reported when performed in conjunction with a column 1 procedure. Airway access is associated with general anesthesia, and no CPT code is available for elective intubation. The CPT code 31500 is not to be reported for elective intubation in anticipation of performing a procedure, as this represents a code for providing the service of emergency intubation.

    Furthermore, CPT codes describing services to gain visualization of the airway (nasal endoscopy, laryngoscopy, bronchoscopy) were created for the purpose of coding a diagnostic or therapeutic service and are not to be reported as a part of intubation services.

    When vascular access is obtained, the access generally requires maintenance of an infusion or use of an anticoagulant (heparin lock injection) (e.g., CPT codes 90780-90784). These services are necessary for the maintenance of the access and are not to be separately reported. Additionally, use of an anticoagulant for access maintenance cannot be separately reported (e.g., CPT code 37201).

    In some situations, more-invasive access services (central venous access, pulmonary artery access) are performed with a specific type of procedure. Because this is not typically the case, the codes referable to these services may be separately reported.

Placement of central access devices (central lines, pulmonary artery catheters, etc.) involves passage of catheters through central vessels and, in the case of PA catheters, through the right ventricle; additionally, these services often require the use of fluoroscopic support. Separate reporting of CPT codes for right heart catheterization, first-order venous catheter placement, or other services that represent a separate procedure is not appropriate when the CPT code that describes the access service is reported. General fluoroscopic services necessary to accomplish routine central vascular access or endoscopy cannot be separately reported unless a specific CPT code has been defined for this service.

2. When anesthesia is provided by the physician performing the primary service, the anesthesia services are included in the primary procedure (CMS Global Surgery Policy). If it is medically necessary for a separate provider (anesthesiologist/anesthetist) to provide the anesthesia services (e.g., monitored anesthesia care), a separate service may be reported.

3. Most procedures require cardiopulmonary monitoring, either by the physician performing the procedure or an anesthesiologist/certified registered nurse anesthetist. Because these services are integral and routine, they are not to be separately reported. This may include cardiac monitoring, intermittent EKG procurement, oximetry, or ventilation management (e.g., CPT codes 93000, 93005, 93040, 93041, 94656, 94760, 94761, 94770). These services, when integral to the monitoring service, are not to be separately reported.

When, in the course of a procedure, a nondiagnostic biopsy is obtained and subsequently excision, removal, destruction, or other elimination of the biopsied lesion is accomplished, a separate service cannot be reported for the biopsy procurement, as this represents part of the removal. When a single lesion is biopsied multiple times, only one biopsy removal service should be reported. When multiple distinct lesions are nonendoscopically biopsied, a biopsy removal service may be reported for each lesion separately with a modifier, indicating a different service was performed or a different site was biopsied (see Section H of Chapter I for definition of the -59 modifier). The medical record (e.g., operative report) should indicate the distinct nature of this service. However, for endoscopic biopsies of lesions, multiple biopsies of multiple lesions are reported with one unit of service regardless of how many biopsies are taken. If separate biopsy removal services are performed on separate lesions and it is felt to be medically necessary to submit pathologic specimens separately, the medical record should identify the precise location of each biopsy site. If the decision to perform a more-comprehensive procedure is based on the biopsy result, the biopsy is diagnostic, and the biopsy service may be separately reported.

5. In the performance of a surgical procedure, it is routine to explore the surgical field to determine the anatomic nature of the field and evaluate for anomalies. Accordingly, codes describing exploratory procedures (e.g., CPT code 49000) cannot be separately reported. If a finding requires extension of the surgical field and it is followed by another procedure unrelated to the primary procedure, this service may be separately reported using the appropriate CPT code and modifiers.

6. When a definitive surgical procedure requires access through abnormal tissue (e.g., diseased skin, abscess, hematoma, seroma, etc.), separate services for this access (e.g., debridement, incision, and drainage) are not reported. For example, if a patient presents with a pilonidal cyst and it is determined that it is medically necessary to excise this cyst, it would be appropriate to submit a bill for CPT code 11770 (excision of pilonidal cyst); it would not, however, be appropriate to also report CPT code 10080 (incision and drainage of pilonidal cyst), as it was necessary to perform the latter to accomplish the primary procedure.

7. When excision and removal are performed ("-ectomy" code), the approach generally involves incision and opening of the organ ("-otomy" code). The incision and opening of the organ or lesion cannot be separately reported when the primary service is the removal of the organ or lesion.

8. There are frequently multiple approaches to various procedures, and there are often clusters of CPT codes describing the various approaches (e.g., vaginal hysterectomy as opposed to abdominal hysterectomy). These approaches are generally mutually exclusive of one another and, therefore, not to be reported together for a given encounter. Only the definitive, or most comprehensive, service performed can be reported. Endoscopic procedures are often performed as a prelude to, or as a part of, open surgical procedures. When an endoscopy represents a distinct diagnostic service prior to an open surgical service and the decision to perform surgery is made on the basis of the endoscopy, a separate service for the endoscopy may be reported. The -58 modifier may be used to indicate that the diagnostic endoscopy and the open surgical service are staged or planned procedures.

9. When an endoscopic service is performed to establish the location of a lesion, confirm the presence of a lesion, establish anatomic landmarks, or define the extent of a lesion, the endoscopic service is not separately reported, as it is a medically necessary part of the overall surgical service. Additionally, when an endoscopic service is attempted and fails and another

surgical service is necessary, only the successful service is reported. For example, if a laparoscopic cholecystectomy is attempted and fails and an open cholecystectomy is performed, only the open cholecystectomy can be reported; if appropriate, a -22 modifier may be added to indicate unusual procedural services.

10. A number of CPT codes describe services necessary to address the treatment of complications of the primary procedure (e.g., bleeding or hemorrhage). When the services described by CPT codes as complications of a primary procedure require a return to the operating room, they may be reported separately; generally, due to global surgery policy, they should be reported with the -78 modifier, indicating that the service necessary to treat the complication required a return to the operating room during the postoperative period. When a complication described by codes defining complications arises during an operative session, however, a separate service for treating the complication is not to be reported. An operative session ends upon release from the operating or procedure suite (as defined in MCM 4821).

EVALUATION AND MANAGEMENT SERVICES

All CPT and HCPCS Level II codes have a global surgery indicator. The separate payment for Evaluation and Management (E & M) services provided on the same day of service as procedures with a global surgery indicator of 000, 010, or 090 is covered by global surgery rules.

Procedures with a global surgery indicator of XXX are not covered by these rules. Many of these XXX procedures are performed by physicians and have inherent preprocedure, intraprocedure, and postprocedure work usually performed each time the procedure is completed. This work should never be reported as a separate E & M code. Other XXX procedures are not usually performed by a physician and have no physician work relative-value units associated with them. A physician should never report a separate E & M code with these procedures for the supervision of others performing the procedure or for the interpretation of the procedure. With most XXX procedures, the physician may, however, perform a significant and separately identifiable E & M service on the same day of service, which may be reported by appending the modifier -25 to the E & M code. This E & M service may be related to the same diagnosis necessitating performance of the XXX procedure but cannot include any work inherent in the XXX procedure, supervision of others performing the XXX procedure, or time for interpreting the result of the XXX procedure. Appending the modifier -25 to a significant, separately identifiable E & M service when performed on the same date of service as an XXX procedure is correct coding.

STANDARD PREPARATION/MONITORING SERVICES

Anesthesia services require certain other services to prepare a patient prior to the administration of anesthesia and to monitor a patient during the course of anesthesia. The advances in technology allow for intraoperative monitoring of a variety of physiological parameters. Additionally, when monitored anesthesia care is provided, the attention devoted to patient monitoring is of a similar level of intensity so that general anesthesia may be established if need be. The specific services necessary to prepare and monitor a patient vary among procedures, based on the extent of the surgical procedure, the type of anesthesia (general, MAC, regional, local, etc.), and the surgical risk. Although a determination as to medical necessity and appropriateness must be made by the physician performing the anesthesia, when these services are performed, they are included in the anesthesia service. Because it is recognized that many of these services may occur on the same date of surgery but are not performed in the course of and as part of the anesthesia provision for the day, in some cases these codes will be separately paid by appending the -59 modifier, indicating that the service rendered was independent of the anesthesia service.

ANESTHESIA SERVICE INCLUDED IN SURGICAL PROCEDURE

Under the National Global Surgical Policy, Medicare does not allow separate payment for the anesthesia services performed by the physician who also furnishes the medical or surgical service. In this case, payment for the anesthesia service is made through the payment for the medical or surgical service. For example, separate payment is not allowed for the surgeon's performance of a local or surgical anesthesia if the surgeon also performs the surgical procedure. CPT codes describing anesthesia services or services that are bundled into anesthesia should not be reported in addition to the basic procedure requiring the anesthesia services if performed by the same physician.

CODING SERVICES SUPPLEMENTAL TO A PRINCIPAL PROCEDURE (ADD-ON CODES)

The CPT coding system identifies certain codes that are to be submitted in addition to other codes. Generally, these are identified with the statement "list separately in addition to code for primary procedure" in parentheses, and other times the supplemental code is to be used only with certain primary codes that are parenthetically identified. The basis for these CPT codes is to enable providers to separately identify a service that is performed in certain situations as an additional service or a commonly performed supplemental service complementary to the primary procedure. Incidental services that are necessary to accomplish the primary procedure (e.g., lysis of adhesions in the course of an open cholecystectomy) are not separately reported. Certain complications with an inherent potential to occur in an invasive procedure are, likewise, not separately reported unless resulting in the necessity for a significant separate procedure to be performed. For example, control of bleeding during a procedure is considered part of the procedure and is not separately reported.

Supplemental codes frequently specify codes or ranges of codes with which they are to be used. It would be inappropriate to use these with codes other than those specified. On occasion, a procedure described by a CPT code is modified or enhanced, due to either the unique nature of the clinical situation or advances in technology since the code was first published. When CPT codes are not labeled as supplemental codes in the manner described above, they are not to be reported unless the actual procedure is, in fact, performed. Using nonsupplemental codes that approximate part of a more-comprehensive procedure but do not describe a separately identifiable service is not appropriate.

Example: If, in the course of interpreting an echocardiogram, an ejection fraction is estimated, it would be inappropriate to code a cardiac blood pool imaging with ejection fraction determination (CPT code 78472) in addition to an echocardiography code (CPT code 93307). Although the cardiac blood pool imaging does determine an ejection fraction, it does so by nuclear gaiting techniques that are not used in an echocardiogram.

In other cases, codes are interpreted as being supplemental to a primary code without an explicit statement in the CPT code book that the code is supplemental. Unless the code is explicitly identified in such a fashion, it would be improper as a coding convention to submit a primary procedure code as a supplemental code.

MODIFIERS

In order to expand the information provided by CPT codes, a number of modifiers have been created by the AMA and the CMS. These modifiers, in the form of two characters, either numbers, letters, or a combination of each, are intended to transfer specific information regarding a certain procedure or service. Modifiers are attached to the end of a HCPCS/CPT code and give the physician a mechanism to indicate that a service or procedure has been modified by some circumstance but is still described by the code definition.

Like CPT codes, the use of modifiers (either AMA- or CMS-defined modifiers) requires explicit understanding of the purpose of each modifier. It is also important to identify when the purpose of a modifier has been expanded or restricted by a third-party payer. It is essential to understand the specific meaning of the modifier by the payer to which a claim is being submitted before using it.

There are modifiers created by either the AMA or the CMS that have been designated specifically for use with the correct coding and mutually exclusive code pairs. These modifiers are -E1 through -E4, -FA, -F1 through -F9, -LC, -LD, -LT, -RC, -RT, -TA, -T1 through -T9, -25, -58, -59, -78, -79, and -91. When one of these modifiers is used, it identifies the circumstances for which both services rendered to the same beneficiary, on the same date of service, by the same provider should be allowed separately because one service was performed at a different site, in a different session, or as a distinct service. The -59 modifier will be explained in greater detail in this section. In addition, pertinent information about three other modifiers (-22, -25, and -58) is provided.

1. **-22 Modifier:** The -22 modifier is identified in the CPT code book as unusual procedural services. By definition, this modifier would be used in *unusual* circumstances; routine use of the modifier is inappropriate, as this practice would suggest cases routinely have unusual circumstances. When an unusual or extensive service is provided, it is more appropriate to utilize the -22 modifier than to report a separate code that does not accurately describe the service provided.

2. **-25 Modifier:** The -25 modifier is identified in the CPT code book as a significant, separately identifiable evaluation and management service by the same physician on the same day of the procedure or other service. This modifier may be appended to an evaluation and management (E & M) code reported with another procedure on the same day of service. CCI includes edits bundling E & M codes into various procedures not covered by global surgery rules. If, in addition to the procedure, the physician performs a significant and separately identifiable E & M service beyond the usual preprocedure, intraprocedure, and postprocedure physician work, the E & M may be reported with the -25 modifier appended. The E & M and procedure(s) may be related to the same or different diagnoses.

3. **-58 Modifier:** The -58 modifier is described as a staged or related procedure or service by the same physician during the postoperative period. It indicates that a procedure was followed by another procedure or service during the postoperative period. This may be because it was planned prospectively, because it was more extensive than the original procedure, or because it represents therapy after a diagnostic procedural service. When an endoscopic procedure is performed for diagnostic purposes at the time of a

more-comprehensive therapeutic procedure and the endoscopic procedure does not represent endoscopy, the -58 modifier may be appropriately used to signify that the endoscopic procedure and the more-comprehensive therapeutic procedure are staged or planned procedures. From the National Correct Coding Initiative perspective, this action would result in the allowance and reporting of both services as separate and distinct.

4. **-59 Modifier:** The -59 modifier has been established for use when several procedures are performed on different anatomical sites or at different sessions (on the same day). The specific language according to the CPT manual is:

> **-59 Modifier:** Distinct procedural service: Under certain circumstances, the physician may need to indicate that a procedure or service was distinct or independent from other services performed on the same day. Modifier -59 is used to identify procedures/services that are not normally reported together but are appropriate under the circumstances. This may represent a different session or patient encounter, different procedure or surgery, different site or organ system, separate incision/excision, separate lesion, or separate injury (or area of injury in extensive injuries) not ordinarily encountered or performed on the same day by the same physician.
>
> When certain services are reported together on a patient by the same physician on the same date of service, there may be a perception of unbundling, when, in fact, the services were performed under circumstances that did not involve this practice at all. Because carriers cannot identify this based simply on CPT coding on either electronic or paper claims, the -59 modifier was established to permit services of such a nature to bypass correct coding edits if the modifier is present. The -59 modifier indicates that the procedure represents a distinct service from others reported on the same date of service. This may represent a different session, different surgery, different site, different lesion, different injury, or different area of injury (in extensive injuries). Frequently, another, already established modifier has been defined that describes this situation more specifically. In the event that a more-descriptive modifier is available, it should be used in preference to the -59 modifier.
>
> Example: If a patient requires placement of a flow-directed pulmonary artery catheter for hemodynamic monitoring via the subclavian vein, it would be appropriate to submit the CPT code 93503 (Insertion and placement of flow-directed catheter, e.g., Swan-Ganz, for monitoring purposes) for the service. If, later in the day, the catheter must be removed and a central venous catheter is inserted through the femoral

vein, the appropriate code for this service would be CPT code 36010 (Introduction of catheter, superior or inferior vena cava). Because the pulmonary artery (PA) catheter requires passage through the vena cava, it may appear that the service for the PA catheter was being "unbundled" if both services were reported on the same day. Accordingly, the central venous catheter code should be reported with the -59 modifier (CPT code 36010-59), indicating that this catheter was placed in a different site as a different service on the same day.

Other examples of the appropriate use of the -59 modifier are contained in the individual chapter policies.

The -59 modifier is often misused. The two codes in a code pair edit often, by definition, represent different procedures. The provider cannot use the -59 modifier for such an edit based on the two codes being different procedures. However, if the two procedures are performed at separate sites or at separate patient encounters on the same date of service, the -59 modifier may be appended. Additionally, the -59 modifier cannot be used with E & M services (CPT codes 99201-99499) or radiation treatment management (CPT code 77427).

Example: The column 1/column 2 code edit with column 1 code 38221 (bone marrow biopsy) and column 2 code 38220 (bone marrow, aspiration only) are two separate procedures when performed at separate anatomic sites or separate patient encounters. In these circumstances, it would be acceptable to use the -59 modifier. However, if both 38221 and 38220 are performed at the same site at the same patient encounter, which is the usual practice, the -59 modifier should not be used. Although 38221 and 38220 are different procedures, they are bundled when performed at the same site and same patient encounter.

HCPCS/CPT PROCEDURE CODE DEFINITION

The format of the CPT manual includes descriptions of procedures that are, in order to conserve space, not listed in their entirety for all procedures. The partial description is indented under the main entry and constitutes what is always followed by a semicolon in the main entry. The main entry then encompasses the portion of the description preceding the semicolon. The main entry applies to and is a part of all indented entries that follow with their codes. An example is:

70120   Radiologic examination, mastoids; less than three views per side

70130   complete minimum of three views per side

The common portion of the description is "radiologic examination, mastoids," and this description is considered a part of both codes. The distinguishing part of each of these codes is what follows the semicolon.

In some procedure descriptions, the code definition specifies other procedures that are included in this comprehensive code. CPT procedure code 29855 is an example. Since the code description for CPT code 29855 states that the code includes arthroscopy, it follows that the surgical knee arthroscopy (CPT code 29871) cannot be reported with CPT code 29855.

In addition, a code description may define a correct coding relationship in which one code is a part of another based on the language used in the descriptor. Some examples of this type of correct coding by code definition are:

1. "Partial" and "complete" CPT codes are reported. The partial procedure is included in the complete procedure.

2. "Partial" and "total" CPT codes are reported. The partial procedure is included in the total procedure.

3. "Unilateral" and "bilateral" CPT codes are reported. The unilateral procedure is included in the bilateral procedure.

4. "Single" and "multiple" CPT codes are reported. The single procedure is included in the multiple procedure.

HCPCS/CPT CODING MANUAL INSTRUCTION/GUIDELINE

Each of the six major sections of the CPT code book and several of the major subsections include guidelines that are unique to that section. These directions are not all-inclusive or limited to definitions of terms, modifiers, unlisted procedures or services, special or written reports, details about reporting separate, multiple, or starred procedures and qualifying circumstances. These instructions appear in various places and are found at the beginning of each major section, at the beginning of subsections, and before or after a series of codes or individual codes. They define items or provide explanations that are necessary to appropriately interpret and report the procedures or services and to define terms that apply to a particular section. Notations are made in parentheses when CPT codes are deleted or cross-referenced to another similar code so that the provider has better guidance in the appropriate assignment of a CPT code for the service.

SEPARATE PROCEDURE

The narrative for many CPT codes includes a parenthetical statement that the procedure represents a "separate procedure." The inclusion of this statement indicates that the procedure can be performed separately but should not be reported when a related service is performed. The "separate procedure" designation is used with codes in the surgery (CPT codes 10000-69999), radiology (CPT codes 70000-79999), and medicine (CPT codes 90000-99199) sections. When a related procedure is performed, a code with the designation of "separate procedure" is not to be reported with the primary procedure.

Example: If the code identified as a "separate procedure" is reported with a related procedure code, such as when a sesamoidectomy, thumb or finger (CPT code 26185) is reported with an excision or curettage of a bone cyst or benign tumor of the proximal, middle, or distal phalanx of the finger with autograft (CPT code 26215), then the sesamoidectomy (separate procedure) should not be reported. By definition, the "separate procedure" is commonly performed as integral and part of a larger service and usually represents a procedure that the physician performs through the same incision or orifice, at the same site, or using the same approach.

In the case in which a separate procedure is performed on the same day but at a different session or at an anatomically unrelated site, the "separate procedure" code may be reported in addition to a code for a procedure that would be related if performed at the same patient encounter or at an anatomically related site. Modifier -59 should be included, indicating that this service was, in fact, a separate service.

In other sections of the CPT code book, the word "separate" is used in a phrase identified as "separate or multiple procedures" with a different meaning.

FAMILY OF CODES

In a family of codes, there are two or more component codes that are not reported separately because they are included in a more-comprehensive code as members of the code family. Comprehensive codes include certain services that are separately identifiable by other component codes. The component codes as members of the comprehensive code family represent parts of the procedure that should not be listed separately when the complete procedure is done. However, the component codes are considered individually if performed independently of the complete procedure and if not all the services listed in the comprehensive codes were rendered to make up the total service. If all multiple services described by a comprehensive code are performed, the comprehensive code should be reported. It is not appropriate to report the separate component codes individually. It is also not appropriate to report the component code(s) with the comprehensive code.

MORE-EXTENSIVE PROCEDURES

When procedures are performed together that are basically the same, or performed on the same site but are qualified by an increased level of complexity, the less-extensive procedure is included in the more-extensive procedure. In the following situations, the procedure viewed as the more complex would be reported:

1. "Simple" and "complex" CPT codes reported; the simple procedure is included in the complex procedure on the same site.

2. "Limited" and "complete" CPT codes reported; the limited procedure is included in the complete procedure on the same site.

3. "Simple" and "complicated" CPT codes reported; the simple procedure is included in the complicated procedure on the same site.

4. "Superficial" and "deep" CPT codes reported; the superficial procedure is included in the deep procedure on the same site.

5. "Intermediate" and "comprehensive" CPT codes reported; the intermediate procedure is included in the comprehensive procedure on the same site.

6. "Incomplete" and "complete" CPT codes reported; the incomplete procedure is included in the complete procedure on the same site.

7. "External" and "internal" CPT codes reported; the external procedure is included in the internal procedure on the same site.

SEQUENTIAL PROCEDURES

An initial approach to a procedure may be followed at the same encounter by a second, usually more-invasive approach. There may be separate CPT codes describing each service. The second procedure is usually performed because the initial approach was unsuccessful in accomplishing the medically necessary service; these procedures are considered "sequential procedures." Only the CPT code for one of the services, generally the more-invasive service, should be reported. An example of this situation is a failed laparoscopic cholecystectomy followed by an open cholecystectomy at the same session. Only the code for the successful procedure, in this case the open cholecystectomy, should be reported.

"WITH" VERSUS "WITHOUT" PROCEDURES

In the CPT code book, there are various procedures that have been separated into two codes with the definitional difference being "with" versus "without" (e.g., with and without contrast). Both procedure codes cannot be reported. When done together, the "without" procedure is included in the "with" procedure. An example would be a closed treatment of a fracture with manipulation and without manipulation. The CPT code without manipulation is included in the code with manipulation. Another example is a procedure described as under or requiring "anesthesia" and "without anesthesia." The "without anesthesia" procedure code is included in the "under" or "requiring anesthesia" procedure code.

LABORATORY PANEL

When all component tests of a specific organ- or disease-oriented laboratory panel (e.g., CPT codes 80074, 80061) are reported separately, they should be reported in the comprehensive panel code that includes the multiple component tests. The individual tests that make up a panel are not to be separately reported.

Example: CPT code 80090 (TORCH antibody panel) includes the following tests:

CPT code 86644: Antibody—cytomegalovirus

CPT code 86694: Antibody—herpes simplex

CPT code 86762: Antibody—rubella

CPT code 86777: Antibody—toxoplasma

When all four tests are performed, the panel test (CPT code 80090) should be reported in place of the individual tests.

MUTUALLY EXCLUSIVE PROCEDURES

There are numerous procedure codes that are not to be reported together because they are mutually exclusive. Mutually exclusive codes are those codes that cannot reasonably be done in the same session. An example of a mutually exclusive situation is when the repair of the organ can be performed by two different methods. One repair method must be chosen to repair the organ and must be reported. A second example is the reporting of an "initial" service and a "subsequent" service. It is contradictory for a service to be classified as an initial and a subsequent service at the same time.

CPT codes that are mutually exclusive based on either the CPT definition or the medical impossibility/improbability that the procedures could be performed at the same session can be identified as code pairs. These codes are not necessarily linked to one another with one code narrative describing a more-comprehensive procedure compared to the component code, but can be identified as code pairs that should not be reported together.

In order to identify these code pairs, an independent table of mutually exclusive codes has been developed as part of the CCI. This table differs from the correct coding table of column 1 and column 2 codes. Although the codes are listed as column 1 and column 2 codes, the column 2 code is not a component or part of the column 1 comprehensive code. Rather, the two codes cannot be reported at the same time. In the processing of the code pair when reported together, in general the procedure with the lower work relative-value unit will be allowed. Accordingly, the code for this procedure has been placed in column 1. In cases in which the work relative-value unit is 0 for one or both of the procedures or the procedure(s) is (are) not paid according to the physicians' fee schedule, the code with the lowest Medicare allowance in general has been inserted in column 1.

GENDER-SPECIFIC PROCEDURES

Many procedure codes have a gender-specific classification within their narrative. These codes are not reported with codes having the opposite-gender designation, because this would reflect a conflict in gender classification by either the definition of the code descriptions themselves (as they appear in the CPT code book) or the fact that the performance of these procedures on the same patient would be anatomically impossible.

The sections that this policy pertains to are the male and female genital procedures. Other codes indicate in their definition that a particular gender classification is required for the use of that particular code. An example of this situation would be CPT code 53210 for total urethrectomy including cystostomy in a female as opposed to CPT code 53215 for the male. Both of these procedures are not to be reported together. Some other examples of these code pairs are: 53210/53250, 52275/52270, and 57260/53620. These specific edits have been included in the Mutually Exclusive Table because both procedures of a code pair edit cannot be performed on a patient.

EXCLUDED SERVICES

Because some procedures are identified as excluded from coverage under the Medicare program as "excluded services," there is no need to address the issue of correct coding with these codes. In the development of National Correct Coding Policy and Correct Coding Edits, these excluded services have been ignored.

UNLISTED SERVICES OR PROCEDURES

The codes listed after each section and/or subsection that end in -99 (or -9 in a few cases) are used to report a service that is not described in any code listed elsewhere in the CPT code book. Because of advances in technology or physician expertise with new procedures, a code may not be assigned to a procedure when the procedure is first introduced as accepted treatment. The unlisted service or procedure codes are then necessary to code the service. Every effort should be made to find the appropriate code to describe the service, and frequent use of these unlisted codes instead of the proper codes is not appropriate. Correct code assignment would occur after the documentation has been reviewed, and bundling of code pairs would then take place based on the changed code or correctly submitted code. The unlisted service or procedure codes have not been included in the Correct Coding Policy or Edits because of the multiple procedures that can be assigned to these codes.

ANESTHESIA SERVICES

GUIDELINES

Proper reporting and billing of anesthesia services depend on the health insurance carrier involved. As of April 1, 1989, anesthesia services covered under Medicare are reported and billed using CPT codes from the Anesthesia section of the CPT code book. For most other health insurance carriers, anesthesia services are billed using CPT codes from the Surgery section of the CPT code book to describe the major surgical procedure.

The reporting of anesthesia services is appropriate by or under the responsible supervision of a physician. These services may include general, regional, supplementation of local anesthesia, or other supportive services.

Following is a sample health insurance claim illustrating how anesthesia for a TURP is billed to a group or private health insurance carrier.

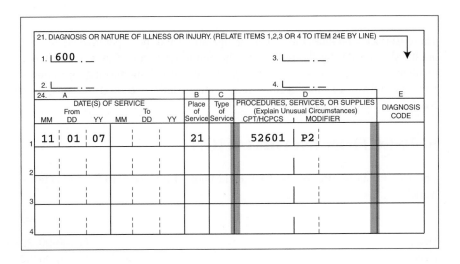

The same service provided to a Medicare beneficiary is billed as illustrated in the following sample claim form:

21. DIAGNOSIS OR NATURE OF ILLNESS OR INJURY. (RELATE ITEMS 1,2,3 OR 4 TO ITEM 24E BY LINE)							

1. |600|.__   3. |___|.__

2. |___|.__   4. |___|.__

24. A DATE(S) OF SERVICE						B Place of Service	C Type of Service	D PROCEDURES, SERVICES, OR SUPPLIES (Explain Unusual Circumstances) CPT/HCPCS | MODIFIER		E DIAGNOSIS CODE
From MM	DD	YY	To MM	DD	YY			CPT/HCPCS	MODIFIER	
1	11	01	07				21		00914	P2	
2											
3											
4											

These services include the usual preoperative and postoperative visits, the anesthesia care during the procedure, the administration of fluids and/or blood incident to the anesthesia or surgery, and the usual monitoring procedures. Unusual forms of monitoring (e.g., intra-arterial, central venous, and Swan-Ganz) are not included.

SUBSECTION INFORMATION

The Anesthesia section of the CPT code book is divided into 16 subsections, namely:

Head	00100-00222
Neck	00300-00352
Thorax (Chest Wall and Shoulder Girdle)	00400-00474
Intrathoracic	00500-00580
Spine and Spinal Cord	00600-00670
Upper Abdomen	00700-00796
Lower Abdomen	00800-00884
Perineum	00900-00955

Pelvis (Except Hip)	01000-01190
Upper Leg (Except Knee)	01200-01274
Knee and Popliteal Area	01300-01444
Lower Leg (Below Knee)	01460-01682
Upper Arm and Elbow	01700-01784
Forearm, Wrist, and Hand	01800-01860
Radiological Procedures	01900-01922
Miscellaneous Procedure(s)	01990-01999

TIME REPORTING

Time for anesthesia procedures may be reported as is customary in the local area. Anesthesia time begins when the anesthesiologist starts to prepare the patient for the induction of anesthesia in the operating room or in an equivalent area and ends when the anesthesiologist is no longer in personal attendance, that is, when the patient may be safely placed under postoperative supervision.

PHYSICIANS' SERVICES

Services rendered by anesthesiologists rendered in the office, home, or hospital and consultation and other medical services are coded from the E/M section.

MATERIALS SUPPLIED BY PHYSICIAN

Supplies and materials provided by the physician over and above those usually included with the office visit or other services rendered may be listed separately.

SEPARATE OR MULTIPLE PROCEDURES

It is appropriate to indicate multiple procedures that are rendered on the same day by separate entries.

SPECIAL REPORT

A service that is rarely provided, unusual, variable, or new may require a special report to help determine medical appropriateness of the service. This simply means that you may need to provide additional documentation either routinely, as when billing unlisted procedure codes or using modifier -22, or when requested to do so by a health insurance carrier.

ANESTHESIA MODIFIERS

All anesthesia services are reported by use of the appropriate Surgery or Anesthesia code plus the addition of a physical status modifier. The use of other optional modifiers may be appropriate.

PHYSICAL STATUS MODIFIERS

Physical Status modifiers are represented by the initial letter P followed by a single digit from 1 to 6 as defined below:

-P1   A normal healthy patient.

-P2   A patient with a mild systemic disease.

-P3   A patient with severe systemic disease.

-P4   A patient with severe systemic disease that is a constant threat to life.

-P5   A moribund patient who is not expected to survive without the operation.

-P6   A declared brain-dead patient whose organs are being removed for donor purposes.

The above six levels are consistent with the American Society of Anesthesiologists' (ASA) ranking of patient status. Physical status is included to distinguish between various levels of complexity of the service provided.

OTHER MODIFIERS

Under certain circumstances, medical services and procedures may need to be further modified. Other modifiers commonly used in Anesthesia include:

-22   Unusual services

-23   Unusual anesthesia

-32   Mandated services

-51   Multiple procedures

-AA   Anesthesia by anesthesiologist

-AB   Four or fewer concurrent services by CRNA or AA employed by anesthesiologist

-AC   Four or fewer concurrent services by CRNA not employed by anesthesiologist

-AD   Supervision of more than four concurrent anesthesia services by anesthesiologist

-AF   Anesthesia complicated by total body hypothermia

-AG   Anesthesia for emergency surgery on a patient who is moribund or who has an incapacitating systemic disease that is a constant threat to life

-QI   Medical direction of own employees by anesthesiologist (three concurrent procedures)

-OJ   Medical direction of own employees by anesthesiologist (four concurrent procedures)

-QK   Medical direction of other than own employees by anesthesiologist (two concurrent procedures)

-QL   Medical direction of other than own employees by anesthesiologist (three concurrent procedures)

-QM   Medical direction of other than own employees by anesthesiologist (four concurrent procedures)

QUALIFYING CIRCUMSTANCES FOR ANESTHESIA

Many anesthesia services are provided under particularly difficult circumstances, depending on factors such as extraordinary condition of patient, notable operative conditions, and unusual risk factors. This section includes a list of important qualifying circumstances that significantly impact on the character of the anesthetic service provided. These procedures are not reported alone but would be reported as additional procedure codes. More than one code may be selected.

99100 Anesthesia for patient of extreme age, under one year and over 70

99116 Anesthesia complicated by utilization of total-body hypothermia

99135 Anesthesia complicated by utilization of controlled hypotension

99140 Anesthesia complicated by emergency conditions (specify)

In addition to the previous guidelines, it is common for anesthesia to be administered by Certified Registered Nurse Anesthetists either providing services independently or under the supervision of a physician.

CORRECT CODING ISSUES FOR ANESTHESIA SERVICES

General Issues

Anesthesia care conventionally includes all services associated with the administration of analgesia/anesthesia provided by an anesthesiologist and/or certified registered nurse anesthetist (CRNA) to a patient undergoing a surgical or other invasive procedure so that intervention can be undertaken. This may involve local, regional, epidural, general anesthesia, or monitored anesthesia care (MAC) and usually involves administration of anxiolytics or amnesia-inducing medications. Additionally, anesthesia care includes evaluating preoperatively the patient with a sufficient history and physical examination so that the risk of adverse reactions can be minimized, planning alternative approaches to accomplishing anesthesia, and answering all questions regarding the anesthesia procedure asked by the patient.

The anesthesiologist assumes responsibility for the postanesthesia recovery period, which is included in the anesthesia care package. It encompasses all care until the patient is released to the surgeon or another physician; this point of release generally occurs at the time of release from the postanesthesia recovery area.

Standard Anesthesia Coding

The following policies reflect national Medicare correct coding guidelines for anesthesia services:

1. Principles of Medicare coding for Anesthesia services involving administration of anesthesia are reported by the use of the anesthesia five-digit CPT procedure codes (00100-01860). These codes specify "Anesthesia for" followed by a general area of surgical intervention. Subsequent CPT codes (01905-01933) are unique to anesthesia for interventional radiology. Several CPT codes (01990-01999) describe miscellaneous anesthesia services.
   Anesthesia services are provided by or under the supervision of a physician. These services may include, but are not limited to general or regional anesthesia and monitoring of physiological parameters during

local or peripheral block anesthesia with sedation (when medically necessary) or other supportive services in order to afford the patient anesthesia care deemed optimal by the anesthesiologist during any procedure.

Anesthesia codes describe a general anatomic area or service that usually relates to a number of surgical procedures, often from multiple sections of the CPT code book. For Medicare purposes, only one anesthesia code is reported unless the anesthesia code is an add-on code. In this case, both the code for the primary anesthesia service and the anesthesia add-on code are reported according to CPT code book instructions. It is acceptable to bill the code that accurately describes the anesthesia for the procedure that has the highest basic unit value.

2.   Another unique characteristic of anesthesia coding is the reporting of time units for time spent delivering anesthesia. In contrast to some evaluation and management services which can be coded based on time, payment for anesthesia services varies with or increases with increments of time. In addition to billing a basic unit value for an anesthesia service, the units of service reflecting the time of anesthesia attendance are reported. Anesthesia time involves the continuous actual presence of the anesthesiologist and starts when the anesthesiologist begins to prepare the patient for anesthesia care in the operating room or equivalent area and ends when the anesthesiologist is no longer in personal attendance, i.e., when the patient may be safely placed under postoperative supervision. Non-monitored interval time may not be considered for calculation of time units.

Example: A patient who undergoes a cataract extraction may require monitored anesthesia care (see below). This may require administration of a sedative in conjunction with a peri/retrobulbar injection for regional block anesthesia. Subsequently, an interval of 30 minutes or more may transpire during which time the patient does not require monitoring by an anesthesiologist/certified registered nurse anesthetist. After this period, monitoring will commence again for the cataract extraction, and ultimately the patient will be released to the surgeon's care or to recovery. The time that may be reported would include the time for the monitoring during the block and during the procedure. The interval time and the recovery time are not to be included in the time unit calculation. Also, if unusual services that are not bundled into the anesthesia service are required, the time spent delivering these services before anesthesia time begins or after it ends may not be included as reportable anesthesia time.

However, if it is medically necessary for the anesthesiologist/CRNA to be in direct one-to-one observation monitoring the patient during the interval time and is not billing any other service, the time can be included.

3. It is standard medical practice for an anesthesiologist/CRNA to provide a patient examination and evaluation prior to surgery. This is considered part of the anesthesia service. The time spent in performing the evaluation is included in the base unit of the code and therefore is not included as anesthesia time. If surgery is canceled, either because of other circumstances or because of findings on the preoperative evaluation by the anesthesiologist and cancellation occurs subsequent to the preoperative evaluation, payment may be allowed to the anesthesiologist for an evaluation and management service, and the appropriate E & M code (usually a consultation code) may be reported.

Similarly, routine postoperative evaluation is included in the basic unit for the anesthesia service. Additional time units would be inappropriate, and evaluation and management codes are not to be used in addition to the anesthesia code. Postoperative evaluation and management services related to the surgery are not separately payable to the anesthesiologist except in the circumstance during which the anesthesiologist is providing significant, separately identifiable services such as ongoing critical care services, postoperative pain management services, or extensive unrelated ventilator management. Management of epidural or subarachnoid drug administration (CPT code 01996) is separately payable on dates of service subsequent to surgery but not on the date of surgery. If the only service provided is management of epidural/subarachnoid drug administration, then an evaluation and management service is not appropriate in addition to CPT code 01996. Payment for management of epidural/subarachnoid drug administration is limited to one unit of service per postoperative day irrespective of the number of visits necessary to manage the catheter per postoperative day (CPT definition). While an anesthesiologist or CRNA may be able to bill for this service, only one payment will be made per day. Postoperative pain management services are generally provided by the surgeon, who is reimbursed under a global payment policy related to the procedure, and shall not be reported by the anesthesiologist unless separate, medically necessary services are required that cannot be rendered by the surgeon. The surgeon is responsible to document in the medical record the reason care is being referred to the anesthesiologist.

In certain circumstances, critical care services are provided by the anesthesiologist. It is currently national CMS policy that CRNAs cannot be reimbursed for evaluation and management services in the critical care area. In the case of anesthesiologists, the routine immediate postoperative care is not separately reported except as described above.

Procedural services such as placement of lines, emergency intubation (outside of the operating suite), etc. are payable to anesthesiologists as well as CRNAs if these procedures are furnished within the parameters of appropriate state licensing laws.

4. One principle of CPT coding is that if a service is usually provided as part of a more-comprehensive service, then it should be included in and be considered part of the service. The advances in technology allow for intraoperative monitoring of a variety of physiological parameters. The following preparation/monitoring services are integral to anesthesia services in general and are not to be separately reported:

- Transporting, positioning, prepping, and draping of the patient for satisfactory anesthesia induction/surgical procedures.

- Placement of external devices necessary for cardiac monitoring, oximetry, capnography, temperature, EEG, CNS evoked responses (e.g., BSER), Doppler flow.

- Placement of peripheral intravenous lines necessary for fluid and medication administration.

- Placement of airway (endotracheal tube, orotracheal tube, etc.).

- Laryngoscopy (direct or endoscopically) for placement of airway (endotracheal tube, etc.).

- Placement of nasogastric or orogastric tube.

- Intraoperative interpretation of monitored functions (blood pressure, heart rate, respirations, oximetry, capnography, temperature, EEG, BSER, Doppler flow, CNS pressure).

- Interpretation of laboratory determinations (arterial blood gases such as Ph, PO_2, PCO_2, bicarbonate, hematology, blood chemistries, lactate, etc.) by the anesthesiologist/CRNA.

- Nerve stimulation for determination of level of paralysis or localization of nerve(s). Codes for EMG services are for diagnostic purposes for nerve dysfunction; to report these codes, a complete report must be present in the medical record.

- When the following CPT codes are reported with an anesthesia code, it is assumed that these services are being reported as part of the anesthesia service and so will not be paid in addition to the anesthesia code. Because it is recognized that many of these procedures may occur on the same date of surgery but are not performed in the course of and as part of the anesthesia provision for the day, these codes will be separately paid only if the -59 modifier is appended to the code, indicating that the service rendered was independent of the anesthesia service.

- CPT codes describing services that, when performed as part of the anesthesia service, would be considered included in the anesthesia code include the following partial list:

> 31505, 31515, 31527 (Laryngoscopy) (Laryngoscopy codes are for diagnostic or surgical services)

> 31622, 31645, 31646 (Bronchoscopy)

> 36000-36015 (Introduction of needle or catheter)

> 36400-36440 (Venipuncture and transfusion)

> Blood sample procurement through existing lines or requiring only venipuncture or arterial puncture

> 62310-62311, 62318-62319 (Injection of diagnostic or therapeutic substance):

CPT codes 62310-62311 and 62318-62319 may be reported on the date of surgery if performed for postoperative pain relief rather than as the means for providing the regional block for the surgical procedure. If a narcotic or other analgesic is injected through the same catheter as the anesthetic, CPT codes 62311 and 62319 should not be billed. The -59 modifier will indicate that the injection was performed for postoperative pain relief, but a procedure note should be included in the medical record.

Example: A patient has an epidural block with sedation and monitoring for arthroscopic knee surgery. The anesthesiologist bills for CPT code 01382 for "Anesthesia for arthroscopic procedures of knee joint." The epidural catheter is left in place for postoperative pain management. The anesthesiologist may not also bill for CPT codes 62311 (injection of diagnostic or therapeutic substance) or 01996 (daily management of epidural) on the date of surgery. The CPT code 01996 may be reported with one unit of service per day on subsequent days until the catheter is removed. On the other hand, if the anesthesiologist performed general anesthesia and bills for CPT code 01382 and reasonably believes that postoperative pain is likely to be sufficient to warrant an epidural catheter, the CPT code 62319-59 may be reported, indicating that this is a separate service from the anesthesia service. In this instance, the service is separately payable whether the catheter is placed before, during, or after the surgery. If the epidural catheter was placed on a different date from the surgery, then the -59 modifier would not be necessary. The CPT code 01996 may not be reported on dates subsequent to reporting 62319. Evaluation and management codes are used to report daily hospital management of continuous epidural or subarachnoid drug administration performed in conjunction with 62318-62319.

64400-64565 (Nerve blocks)

67500 (Retrobulbar injection)

81000-81015, 82013, 82205, 82270, 82273 (Performance and interpretation of laboratory tests)

90780-90788 (IV infusion—injections)

91000, 91055, 91105 (Esophageal, gastric intubation)

92511-92520, 92543 (Special otorhinolaryngologic services)

92950 (Cardiopulmonary resuscitation)

92953 (Temporary transcutaneous pacemaker)

92960 (Cardioversion)

93000-93010 (Electrocardiography)

93015-93018 (Cardiovascular stress tests)

93040-93042 (Electrocardiography)

93307-93314 (Echocardiography when displayed for monitoring purposes) When performed for diagnostic purposes with documentation of a formal report, this will be considered a significant, separately identifiable, and separately payable service.

93315-93317 (Transesophageal echocardiography). When performed for diagnostic purposes with documentation of a formal report, this will be considered a significant, separately identifiable, and separately payable service.

93318 (Transesophageal echocardiography for monitoring purposes)

93922-93981 (Extremity arterial venous studies) When performed diagnostically with a formal report, this will be considered a significant, separately identifiable, and, if medically necessary, a payable service.

94640, 94650, 94651 (Inhalation/IPPB treatments)

94656, 94660-94662 (Ventilation management/CPAP services) If performed as management for maintenance ventilation during a surgical procedure, this is part of the anesthesia service. This is separately payable if performed as an ongoing service after transfer out of the operating room or postanesthesia recovery to a hospital unit/ICU. The -59 modifier would be necessary to signify that this was a separate service.

94664-94665 (Inhalations)

94680-94690 (Expired gas analysis)

94760-94770 (Oximetry)

99201-99499 (Evaluation and management)

(This is not a comprehensive list of all services included in anesthesia services.)

When a physician performs a procedure and, incidentally, provides the anesthesia, the anesthesia for the procedure is not reported. (The anesthesia for a procedure, if provided by the surgeon, is included in the global surgery package.)

Radiologic Anesthesia Coding

In keeping with standard anesthesia billing guidelines for Medicare, only one anesthesia code may be reported for anesthesia services provided in conjunction with radiological procedures. Radiological supervision and interpretation codes will usually be applicable to radiological procedures being performed.

The appropriate supervision and interpretation code may be reported by the appropriate provider (radiologist, cardiologist, neurosurgeon, radiation oncologist, etc.). Accordingly, S & I codes are not included in anesthesia codes referable to these procedures; only the appropriate provider, however, may bill for supervision and interpretation services.

CPT code 01920 (Anesthesia for cardiac catheterization including coronary angiography and ventriculography) (not to include Swan-Ganz catheter) can be reported for monitored anesthesia care (MAC) in patients who are critically ill or critically unstable. If the physician performing the radiologic service places a catheter as part of that service and, through the same site, a catheter is left and used for monitoring purposes, it is inappropriate for either the anesthesiologist/certified registered nurse anesthetist or the physician performing the radiologic procedure to bill for placement of the monitoring catheter (e.g., CPT codes 36488-36500).

Monitored Anesthesia Care (MAC)

There has been a shift to providing more surgical and diagnostic services in an ambulatory, outpatient, or office setting. Accompanying this, there has also been a change in the provision of anesthesia services from traditional general anesthetic to a combination of local or regional anesthetic with certain conscious-altering drugs. This type of anesthesia is referred to as monitored anesthesia care if provided directly by a physician or an anesthesiologist or by a medically directed CRNA. In essence, MAC involves patient monitoring sufficient to anticipate the potential need to administer general anesthesia during a surgical or other procedure. MAC requires careful and continuous evaluation of various vital physiologic functions and the recognition and treatment of any adverse changes. CMS recognizes this type of anesthesia service as a payable service if medically necessary and reasonable.

Because MAC requires at least the same level of monitoring as that of general anesthesia, it is treated the same as general anesthesia except that the appropriate modifiers must be used for payment purposes. The guidelines as promulgated previously apply equally to MAC. It is particularly important to note that Medicare policy allows only one anesthesia CPT code to be reported, and the time units reported represent only the time when the patient was continuously monitored by a physician or anesthesiologist (personally) or by a CRNA. Preoperative and postoperative assessments follow standard anesthesia billing guidelines.

Anesthesiologists and CRNAs

CMS recognizes the services of anesthesiologists as providers and physicians in a supervisory capacity. Anesthesiologists personally performing anesthesia services bill in a standard fashion, in accordance with CMS regulations as outlined in the Medicare Carriers' Manual (e.g., Sections 4137, 4830, 15018). CMS also recognizes CRNAs and anesthesiologists' assistants practicing under the medical direction of anesthesiologists or practicing independently of anesthesiologists. Billing instructions and regulations regarding this arrangement are outlined in the Medicare Carriers' Manual as noted above and in Section 16003.

SURGERY SERVICES

GUIDELINES

In addition to the common issues relevant to all physicians discussed in the Introduction to CPT, the Surgery section contains definitions and items unique to that section.

PHYSICIANS' SERVICES

Visits rendered by surgeons in the office, home, or hospital plus consultations and other medical services are reported using E/M services codes. In addition, codes in the series 99000-99199, found in the category Special Services and Reports in the Medicine section, are also frequently used by surgeons.

LISTED SURGICAL PROCEDURES

The procedures listed in the Surgery section include the operation, local, metacarpal/digital block or topical anesthesia when used, and normal, uncomplicated follow-up care. This concept is referred to as a Package for surgical procedures.

FOLLOW-UP CARE

FOR DIAGNOSTIC PROCEDURES

The follow-up care for diagnostic procedures such as endoscopy and injection procedures for radiography includes only that care related to recovery from the diagnostic procedure itself. Care of the condition for which the diagnostic procedure was performed or of other concomitant conditions is not included and should be listed separately.

FOR THERAPEUTIC SURGICAL PROCEDURES

The follow-up care for therapeutic surgical procedures includes only the care that is usually a part of the surgical service. Complications, exacerbations, recurrence of the presence of other diseases, or injuries requiring additional services should be reported with the identification of appropriate procedures.

MATERIALS SUPPLIED BY PHYSICIAN

Supplies and materials provided by the physician over and above those usually included with the office visit or other services rendered should be listed separately. HCPCS Level II codes should be used when appropriate.

MULTIPLE SURGICAL PROCEDURES

It is common for several surgical procedures to be performed at the same operative session. When multiple procedures are performed on the same day or at the same session, the "major" procedure or service is listed first followed by secondary, additional, or "lesser" procedures or services. CPT modifier -51 is added to all procedures following the first one.

Billing multiple procedures incorrectly can have a serious impact on your reimbursement. An inexperienced biller may simply list the procedures on the health insurance claim in the order dictated or described in the operative report.

There are two critical decisions related to billing multiple surgical procedures, namely: 1) the order in which the procedures are listed on the claim form and 2) whether or not to bill additional procedures at full or reduced fees.

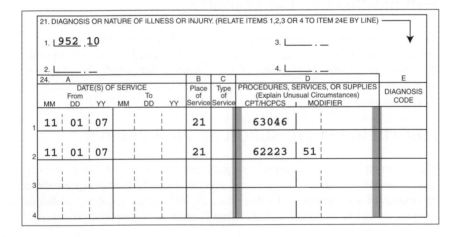

ORDER OF LISTING

The first procedure to be listed when billing under the multiple-procedure rule is the procedure with the highest fee. Additional procedures should be listed in descending order by fee. Modifier -51 should be added to each additional procedure.

All health insurance carriers will reduce the allowance for the additional procedures, typically by 50 percent for the second procedure and 50 to 75 percent for the third and subsequent procedures. Listing the procedures in descending order by fee minimizes the possibility of an incorrect reduction.

BILLING FULL VERSUS REDUCED FEES

We recommend that you list your full fee for each procedure billed as part of multiple surgical procedures. This does not mean that you should expect to be reimbursed the full amount that you list as the total of all the multiple procedures. Our reasoning on this matter is simple. First, health insurance carriers *will* reduce the allowances for the additional procedures. Listing full fees in descending order will result in the maximum allowable reimbursement for you or your patient. Second, there is no easy way to inform the health insurance carrier that you have already reduced your fees.

At this time, the only way to inform the health insurance carrier that you have reduced your fees for additional procedures is to include a statement to that effect somewhere on your claim form. Considering the circumstances under which your claim is processed, this method is very risky, often resulting in double reductions and delayed or lost reimbursement.

This method of billing is not designed to *increase* your reimbursement but rather to *maximize* it. We also recommend that after you have received the maximum benefits from the health insurance carrier, that the balance remaining, less any patient coinsurance or deductible requirements, be written off. We recognize that billing practices vary in different areas of the country, and you should continue to use the method that is recommended or required by the health insurance carriers in your area.

SEPARATE PROCEDURE

Some of the listed procedures are commonly carried out as an integral part of a total service and, as such, do not warrant a separate identification. When, however, such a procedure is performed independently of and is not immediately related to other services, it may be listed as a "separate procedure." Thus, when a procedure that is ordinarily a component of a larger procedure is performed alone for a specific purpose, it may be considered to be a separate procedure.

SUBSECTION INFORMATION

The Surgery section of the CPT code book is divided into 16 subsections, namely:

Integumentary System	10040-19499
Musculoskeletal System	20000-29999
Respiratory System	30000-32999
Cardiovascular System	33000-37799
Hemic and Lymphatic Systems	38000-38999
Mediastinum and Diaphragm	39000-39599
Digestive System	40000-49999
Urinary System	50000-53899
Male Genital System	54000-55899
Intersex Surgery	55970-55980
Female Genital Surgery	56000-58999
Maternity Care and Delivery	59000-59899
Endocrine System	60000-60699
Nervous System	61000-64999
Eye and Ocular Adnexa	65000-68899
Auditory System	69000-69999

Each subsection of the Surgery section of the CPT code book is divided into organs, then into procedures involving anatomic sites. Each anatomic site is further separated into surgical processes such as Incision, Excision, Repair, Removal, Amputation, etc.

The following subsections within the Surgery section have Notes that should be reviewed carefully prior to selecting codes for services located within the section:

Musculoskeletal	20000-29999
Vascular Injection Procedures	33000-37799
Laparoscopy/Peritoneoscopy/Hysteroscopy	56300-56399
Maternity Care and Delivery	59000-59899

UNLISTED SERVICE OR PROCEDURE

A service or procedure may be provided that is not listed in the current CPT code book. When reporting such a service, you may use the appropriate Unlisted Procedure code. You must include a report that clearly explains the service or procedure you are reporting.

SPECIAL REPORT

A service that is rarely provided, unusual, variable, or new may require a special report in determining medical appropriateness of the service. This simply means that you may need to provide additional documentation either routinely, as when billing unlisted procedure codes or using modifier -22, or when requested to do so by a health insurance carrier.

When preparing reports to accompany health insurance claims, you should include a description of the nature, extent, and need for the procedure and the time, effort, and equipment necessary to provide the service. Try to keep these reports as brief and simple as possible. Additional items that may need to be included are:

* complexity of symptoms

* final diagnosis

* pertinent physical findings

* diagnostic and therapeutic procedures

* concurrent problems

* follow-up care

MODIFIERS

Listed surgical services and procedures may be modified under certain circumstances. When applicable, the modifying circumstance is identified by adding the appropriate two-digit modifier to the base procedure code(s). Virtually all of the 22 modifiers listed in Appendix A of the CPT may be applied to surgical procedures.

-20   Microsurgery

-22   Unusual Procedural Services

-26   Professional Component

-32   Mandated Services

-47   Anesthesia by Surgeon

-50   Bilateral Procedure

-51   Multiple Procedures

-52   Reduced Services

-54   Surgical Care Only

-55   Postoperative Management Only

-56   Preoperative Management Only

-57   Decision for Surgery

-58   Staged or Related Procedure or Service by the Same Physician During the Postoperative Period

-62   Two Surgeons

-66   Surgical Team

-76   Repeat Procedure by Same Physician

-77   Repeat Procedure by Another Physician

-78   Return to the Operating Room for a Related Procedure During the Postoperative Period

-79   Unrelated Procedure or Service by the Same Physician During the Postoperative Period

-80   Assistant Surgeon

-81   Minimum Assistant Surgeon

-82   Assistant Surgeon (When Qualified Resident not Available)

-90   Reference (Outside) Laboratory

-99   Multiple Modifiers

-LT   Procedure Performed on Left Side of Body

-RT   Procedure Performed on Right Side of Body

ADD-ON CODES

Some of the procedures listed in the Surgery section of the CPT code book are commonly performed in addition to the primary procedure. These additional or supplemental procedures are designated as "add-on" codes.

CPT codes defined as add-on codes are identified by a black plus sign placed to the left of the code number. In addition, add-on codes include phrases such as "each additional" within the definition or "(List separately in addition to primary procedure)" following the definition. Examples of CPT codes identified as add-on codes in the CPT 2007 book include:

+11001 Debridement of extensive eczematous or infected skin; up to 10% of body surface, each additional 10% of the body surface (List separately in addition to code for primary procedure)

+33530 Reoperation, coronary artery bypass procedure or valve procedure, more than one month after original operation (List separately in addition to code for primary procedure)

STARRED PROCEDURES

The "starred procedure" designation, formerly an asterisk (*) following the CPT code, was eliminated effective with the 2004 edition of the CPT code book.

SURGICAL DESTRUCTION

Surgical destruction is considered a part of a surgical procedure, and the different methods of destruction are not usually listed separately unless the technique substantially alters the standard management of a problem or condition. Exceptions under these special circumstances are provided for by the addition of separate procedure codes.

INTEGUMENTARY SYSTEM

CORRECT CODING ISSUES FOR THE INTEGUMENTARY SYSTEM

CPT coding of the integumentary system includes coding narrative for services performed by a number of specialties. While the coding system is oriented toward dermatological procedures, the dermatological aspects of the practice of plastic surgery are covered as are the dermatologic elements (particularly closure, tissue transfer, grafts, and adjacent and distant flaps) of multiple surgical procedures, especially radical or mutilative surgical procedures. Integumentary procedures are also often performed in staged fashions due to the sophistication of services rendered.

Generally, integumentary procedures include incision, biopsy, removal, paring/curettement, shaving, destruction (multiple methodologies), excision, repair, adjacent tissue rearrangement, grafts, flaps, and specialized services such as burn management and Mohs' Micrographic Surgery.

When a column 1 code describes other column 2 codes, all of which were performed, the column 1 code should be used rather than listing the individual column 2 codes. Additionally, because of the technical advances and changes in technology, standard medical practice should be reflected as accurately as possible in CPT coding. The CPT code should reflect what transpires in a standard surgical setting. Necessary services performed in order to accomplish a more-comprehensive service are included in the CPT code describing the more-complex service.

Evaluation and Management

Evaluation and Management (E & M) of integumentary disorders may represent a separately identifiable service, serve as a prelude to a decision to perform a service, or be performed in follow-up of previously performed procedures. Policies referable to the appropriateness of reporting evaluation and management codes in conjunction with surgical procedures are well-established in the standard CMS Global Surgery Policy. In essence, if the evaluation and management service provided is for the purpose of deciding that a major surgical procedure is to be performed, this service is a significant, separately identifiable service and may be reported separately by attaching modifier -57 to the appropriate level of evaluation and management service code. Surgical procedures have a "global period" following surgery (generally 0, 10, or 90 days); during this time, E & M services provided in the follow-up of the surgical procedure have been calculated into the relative-value units for the surgery and are not to be separately reported. On the occasion when a separate condition is evaluated and a significant, separately identifiable service for a different problem is provided postoperatively, a separate E & M code may be reported and indicated with the -24 modifier.

Surgical dressings, supplies, and local anesthetics used for a procedure are not to be separately reported as routine. There are some exceptions to this policy (e.g., surgical tray used for some office procedures). Wound closures using adhesive strips, topical skin adhesive, or tape alone do not represent a separately identifiable surgical procedure and are, therefore, included in the appropriate E & M service.

Anesthesia

Anesthesia for dermatologic procedures, when provided by the physician performing the procedure, is considered part of the procedure. This would include local infiltration, regional block, sedation, etc. performed by the physician doing the procedure. Local anesthesia or local anesthesia with sedation is often accomplished by the physician providing the primary services. General anesthesia or monitored anesthesia care may be required for more-extensive dermatologic procedures (extensive debridement, flaps, grafts, etc.). In these cases, if anesthesia services are performed by another provider, the different physician may bill separately for his/her services. Billing for "anesthesia" services rendered by a nurse or other office personnel (unless the nurse is an independent certified nurse anesthetist, CRNA, etc.) is inappropriate, as these services are incident to the physician's services.

Use of injection codes for therapeutic injection or aspiration of lesions is inappropriate if the injection is administered for local anesthesia for a specific procedure. CPT codes such as 10160 (puncture aspiration), 20500-20501 (injection of sinus), 20550 (injection of tendon sheath, etc.), and 20600-20610 (arthrocentesis) are not to be reported separately if they are used to reflect local anesthetic techniques for another procedure.

In the postoperative state, patients treated with epidural or subarachnoid drug administration will require adjustment/management of the catheter, dosage, etc. (CPT code 01996). This service may be coded by the anesthesiologist for payment. The management of postoperative pain by the surgeon, including epidural or subarachnoid drug administration, is included in the global period associated with the operative procedure. If no surgery is performed but a catheter is placed for pain control (e.g., burn injury not requiring surgery), CPT code 01996 (daily management of epidural or subarachnoid drug administration) is appropriately reported by the managing physician.

Incision and Drainage

Incision and drainage services, as related to the integumentary system, generally involve cutaneous or subcutaneous drainage of cysts, pustules, infections, hematomas, seromas, or fluid collections. In cases in which, in the course of an excision of a lesion, an area of involvement is identified that requires drainage, either as a part of the procedure or in order to gain access to the area of interest, coding/billing for incision and drainage of this fluid collection would be inappropriate if the excision or other procedure is performed in the same session.

Example: A patient who presents with a pilonidal cyst may require simple incision/drainage or may require an extensive excision. In the former case, the appropriate CPT coding is 10080 (or 10081 if complicated). If the pilonidal cyst is excised, while it is obvious that drainage from the cyst will occur in the course of its excision, the appropriate coding is CPT code 11770 (or 11771 or 11772, depending on the complexity), not CPT codes 10080 *and* 11770. If it is evident that an extensive cellulitis is present around the cyst that prevents the complete procedure from being accomplished, it may be reasonable to bill for CPT code 10080. Then, after perhaps a week of antibiotic therapy, you may complete the procedure using code 11770-78 (Return to the operating room for a related procedure during the postoperative period). The nature of the treatment should be driven by medical decision making rather than by coding conventions.

A. Procedure codes such as incision and drainage of hematomas (e.g., CPT code 10140) are not to be reported during the same session or at the same site as an excision, repair, destruction, removal, etc.

B. Codes describing services necessary to address complications, such as CPT code 10180 (incision and drainage, complex, postoperative wound infection), should not be submitted for services rendered at the same surgical session that resulted in the complication. If performed in conjunction with the primary procedure, it would be included in the primary, column 1, procedure. For example, if a patient has undergone a thoracotomy and a necrotizing pneumonia with empyema develops, it may be necessary to perform a lobectomy through the previous incision. The reason for the surgery is to perform the lobectomy; therefore the lobectomy code should be reported. Since the drainage of the empyema is necessary to accomplish the lobectomy, it would be inappropriate to bill for CPT code 10180 (incision and drainage). On the other hand, if the patient would require only drainage of a thoracotomy wound infection (without lobectomy) and it is determined to be medically necessary to place a gastrostomy tube at the same time, the CPT code 10180 could be reported with the appropriate gastrostomy tube placement code.

Lesion Removal

For a given lesion, only one type of removal is reported, whether it is destruction (e.g., laser, freezing), debridement, paring, curettement, shaving, or excision. CPT definition describes the nature of each of these forms of removal. CPT definition also defines the lesions (specifically full-thickness excision) by lesion diameter. In the case in which an initial attempt using a less-invasive procedure is followed by a more-invasive lesion removal, the more-complex procedure used would be appropriately reported, but not both procedures. Additionally, multiple codes describing destruction of a lesion are not to be reported for a given lesion; if multiple distinct lesions are removed using different methods, an anatomic modifier or the -59 modifier would be used to indicate a different site, a different method, or a different lesion. The distinct location of the lesions should be reflected in the medical record.

A lesion biopsy represents a partial removal of a lesion and is frequently performed as a part of a lesion excision, for example, in order to procure a pathological specimen. Generally, a part of or the entire lesion is submitted for biopsy. When a biopsy is performed as part of a lesion removal, it is part of the overall procedure and is not to be considered as a separate procedure.

If a biopsy is performed on a separate date at a separate session and subsequently a definitive procedure is performed, the biopsy code may be reported followed by a separate removal code, indicating the different dates of service.

Tissues removed are often submitted for surgical pathological evaluation; in some cases, physicians qualified in dermatopathology may perform these evaluations. These codes generally include CPT codes 88300-88309 (surgical pathology). Additionally, when the physician is asked to review slides obtained from another physician's excision and subsequently performs additional removal/biopsy, a separate code for review of outside slides is not reported, i.e., CPT code 88321, in addition to an evaluation and management service. The decision to perform surgery is generally based on an evaluation and management service that includes review of prior records, including tissues, slides, etc. The dermatopathology evaluation must be medically necessary and reasonable. When lesions of like nature (e.g., multiple seborrheic keratoses) are encountered, removal of multiple lesions is frequently accomplished at the same operative session. If it is determined to be medically necessary to separately submit the lesions for pathologic evaluation, documentation of the precise location of each separately submitted lesion must be present. If multiple lesion specimens are submitted as a collective group without documentation specifying locations sufficient to differentiate the source of each specimen, then the surgical pathology code should be submitted as one specimen (one unit of service) even if the specimens were subsequently separated.

Lesions or margins obtained during Mohs' Micrographic Surgery should not be coded under the surgical pathology codes. The definition of Mohs' Micrographic Surgery includes the services defined by the surgical pathology codes (CPT codes 88300-88309) and excision codes (CPT codes 11600-11646 and 17260-17286). These procedure codes are part of the Mohs' Micrographic Surgery CPT codes (17304-17310). Billing separately for one of the above pathology codes and/or one of the excision codes is inappropriate. It is recognized that a Mohs' surgeon may find it necessary to obtain a diagnostic biopsy in order to make the decision to perform surgery. When a diagnostic biopsy is necessary, it may be reported separately. The -58 modifier may be utilized to indicate that the diagnostic biopsy and Mohs' Micrographic Surgery are staged or planned procedures.

Lesion removal, by whatever method (usually excisional), may require simple, intermediate, or complex closure and, in unusual circumstances, tissue transfer procedures. When the lesion removal requires only bandaging, strip closure, or simple closure (see CPT definition of simple closure), this is included in the lesion excision and is not to be reported separately.

Accordingly, CPT codes 12001-12021 (simple repairs) are considered part of the lesion removal codes. Intermediate and complex closures, when medically necessary, may be coded separately. In the case of Mohs' Micrographic Surgery (CPT codes 17304-17310), all necessary repairs may be coded.

In the course of destruction, excision, incision, removal, repair, or closure, debridement of nonviable tissue surrounding a lesion, injury, or incision is often necessary to accomplish the primary service. The debridement codes (CPT codes 11000-11042) are not to be reported separately, as this service is necessary as a part of the total procedure according to standard medical practice.

CPT codes describing intralesional chemotherapy (CPT Codes 96405, 96406) refer to injection of chemotherapeutic agents into one or multiple lesions. CPT codes 11900 and 11901 describe nonspecific intralesional injection(s) into one or more lesions. While one or the other code may be appropriate for a given service, both lesion injection codes are not to be reported together (unless separate lesions are injected with different agents, in which case the -59 modifier should be attached to the intralesional injection code). The CPT codes 11900 and 11901 (injection, intralesional) are not to be used for local anesthetic injection in anticipation of chemotherapy or any other definitive service performed on a lesion or group of lesions. Local anesthesia is considered a part of the definitive procedure. These intralesional CPT injection codes (96405, 96406, 11900, and 11901) are included in the following list of CPT codes if the injection represents local anesthesia:

11200-11201 (Removal of skin tags)
11300-11313 (Shaving of lesions)
11400-11471 (Excision of lesions, benign)
11600-11646 (Excision of lesions, malignant)
12001-12018 (Repair—simple)
12020-12021 (Treatment of wound dehiscence)
12031-12057 (Repair—intermediate)
13100-13160 (Repair—complex)
11719-11762 (Trimming, debridement, and excision of nails)
11770-11772 (Excision of pilonidal cysts)
11765   (Wedge excision)

Repair and Tissue Transfer

When lesional excision is of such an extent that closure cannot be accomplished by simple, intermediate, or complex closure, then other methodology must be employed. Frequently, adjacent-tissue transfer or tissue rearrangement is employed (Z-plasty, W-plasty, flaps, etc.). This family of codes (CPT codes 14000-14350) involves excision with adjacent-tissue transfer and correlates to excision codes. Excision CPT codes (11400-11646) and repair CPT codes (12001-13160) are not to be separately reported when CPT codes 14000-14350 are reported. On the other hand, skin grafting performed in conjunction with these codes may be separately reported if it is not included in the specific code definition. In the case of closure of traumatic wounds, these codes are appropriate only when the closure requires the surgeon to develop a specific adjacent-tissue transfer; lacerations that coincidentally are approximated using a tissue transfer technique (e.g., Z-plasty or W-plasty) should be reported with the more-simple closure code. Debridement necessary to accomplish these tissue transfer procedures is part of the column 1 procedure performed. Separate debridement CPT codes (11000-11042) or repair CPT codes (12001-13160) would be inappropriately reported with these CPT codes (14000-14350) for the same lesion/injury. Procurement of cultures or tissue samples as a part of a closure are included in the closure code and are not to be separately reported.

Grafts and Flaps

Free-skin grafts are coded by type (split or full), location, and size. For a specific location, a primary code is defined and followed by a supplemental code for additional coverage area. As a result of this coding scheme, for a given area of involvement, the initial code is limited to one unit of service; the supplemental code may have multiple units of service, depending on the area to be covered. Because only one type of skin graft is typically applied for a specific area, the primary free-skin graft CPT codes (15100, 15120, 15200, 15220, 15240, 15260) are mutually exclusive. If multiple areas require different grafts, a modifier indicating different sites should be used (anatomic or -59 modifier).

Generally, debridement of nonintact skin (CPT codes 11000-11042) in anticipation of a skin graft is necessary prior to application of the skin graft and is included in the skin graft (CPT codes 15050-15400). When skin is intact, however, and the graft is being performed after excisional preparation of intact skin, the CPT code 15000 (Excisional preparation) is separately reported. CPT code 15000 is not to be used to describe debridement of nonintact, necrotic, or infected skin, and its use is not indicated with other lesion removal codes.

A. CPT codes 15350 (application of allograft) and 15400 (application of xenograft) are part of all other graft codes and are not to be separately reported with other grafts (CPT codes 15050-15261) for graft placement on the same site.

B. The CPT code 67911 describes the "Correction of lid retraction." A parenthetical notation is added advising that if autogenous graft materials are used, tissue graft codes 20920, 20922, or 20926 can be reported. Accordingly, all other procedures necessary to accomplish the service are included.

C. Flap grafts (CPT codes 15570-15576) include excision of lesions at the same site (CPT codes 11400-11646).

Breast (Incision, Excision, Introduction, Repair, and Reconstruction)

Because of the unique nature of procedures developed to address breast disease, a section of CPT (19000-19499) is set aside for such services.

Fine-needle aspiration biopsies, core biopsies, open incisional or excisional biopsies, and related procedures performed to procure tissue from a lesion for which an established diagnosis exists are not to be reported separately at the time of a lesion excision unless performed on a different lesion or on the contralateral breast. However, if a diagnosis is not established, and the decision to perform the excision or mastectomy is dependent on the results of the biopsy, then the biopsy is separately reported. The -58 modifier may be used appropriately to indicate that the biopsy and the excision or mastectomy are staged or planned procedures.

Because excision of lesions occurs in the course of performing a mastectomy, breast excisions are not separately reported from a mastectomy unless performed to establish the malignant diagnosis before proceeding to the mastectomy.

Specifically, CPT codes 19110-19126 (breast excision) are in general included in all mastectomy CPT codes 19140-19240 of the same side. However, if the excision is performed to obtain tissue to determine pathologic diagnosis of malignancy prior to proceeding to a mastectomy, the excision is separately reportable with the mastectomy. The -58 modifier should be utilized in this situation.

Use of other integumentary codes for incision and closure are included in the codes describing various breast excision or mastectomy codes. Because of the frequent need to biopsy lymph nodes or remove muscle tissue in conjunction with mastectomies, these procedures have been included in the CPT coding for mastectomy. It would be inappropriate to separately bill for ipsilateral lymph node dissection in conjunction with the appropriate mastectomy codes. In the circumstance in which a breast lesion is identified and treated and it is determined to be medically necessary to biopsy the contralateral nodes, use of the biopsy or lymph node dissection codes (using the appropriate anatomic modifier, -LT or -RT for left or right, to indicate this) would be acceptable. Additionally, breast reconstruction codes that include the insertion of a prosthetic implant are not to be reported with CPT codes that describe the insertion of a breast prosthesis only.

The CPT coding for breast procedures generally refers to unilateral procedures; when performed bilaterally, the -50 modifier would be appropriate. This is identified parenthetically, when appropriate, in the CPT narrative.

General Policy Statements

A. Repair/closure of a surgical incision, CPT codes 12001-12018, is not separately reported from other surgical procedures. The closure is an intricate part of the surgical procedure performed. As noted previously, simple closure of dermatologic excisions is included in the dermatologic procedure.

B. CPT codes 15851-15852 refer to suture removal and dressing change under anesthesia. These codes are not to be reported when a patient requires a general anesthesia for a related procedure (e.g., a return to the operating room for complications when an incision is reopened, necessitating removal of sutures and redressing). Additionally, these codes, particularly CPT code 15852, are not to be reported with a primary procedure performed under general anesthesia.

There are a number of supplemental CPT codes defined in the CPT code book. The following is a listing of supplemental codes present in the integumentary section of the CPT code book. Although not all-inclusive, the supplemental code must be used in combination with the primary CPT code, or else the supplemental code cannot be reported.

Primary CPT code	Supplemental CPT code
11000 (Debridement up to 10%)	11001 (Each additional 10%)
11200 (Removal of skin tags, up to 15 lesions)	11201 (Each additional 10 lesions)
11730 (Avulsion of nail plate)	11732 (Each additional nail plate)
15100 (Split graft, 100 cm^2 or less)	15101 (Each additional 100 cm^2)
15240 (Full-thickness graft 20 cm^2 or less)	15241 (Each additional 20 cm^2)

WOUND REPAIR

The repair of wounds is classified in CPT as simple, intermediate, or complex.

SIMPLE REPAIR

Simple repair codes are reported when the wound is superficial, for example, involving skin and/or subcutaneous tissues, without significant involvement of deeper structures, and requiring simple suturing. For closure with adhesive strips, list appropriate visit only.

INTERMEDIATE REPAIR

Intermediate repair codes are used to report the repair of wounds that, in addition to the above, require layer closure. Such wounds usually involve deeper layers, such as fascia or muscle, to the extent that at least one of the layers requires separate closure.

COMPLEX REPAIR

Complex repair codes include the repair of wounds requiring reconstructive surgery, complicated wound closures, skin grafts, or unusual and time-consuming techniques of repair to obtain the maximum functional and cosmetic result. It may include creation of the defect and necessary preparation for repairs or the debridement and repair of complicated lacerations or avulsions.

STEPS FOR CODING WOUND REPAIRS

There are four steps required for the accurate reporting of wound repair codes.

1) The repaired wound(s) should be measured and recorded in centimeters, whether curved, angular, or stellate.

2) When multiple wounds are repaired, add together the lengths of those in the same classification (see above) and report as a single item. When more than one classification of wounds is repaired, list the more complicated as the primary procedure and the less complicated as the secondary procedure, using modifier -51.

3) Decontamination and/or debridement is considered a separate procedure only when gross contamination requires prolonged cleansing, when appreciable amounts of devitalized or contaminated tissue are removed, or when debridement is carried out separately without immediate primary closure.

4) If the wound repair involves nerves, blood vessels, and/or tendons, choose codes from the appropriate subsection of the Surgery section (Nervous, Cardiovascular, Musculoskeletal) for repair of these structures.

The repair of these associated wounds is included in the primary procedure unless it qualifies as a complex wound, in which case modifier -51 applies. Simple ligation of vessels in an open wound is considered as part of an open wound closure. Simple "exploration" of nerves, blood vessels, or tendons exposed in an open wound is also considered part of the essential treatment of the wound and is not a separate procedure unless appreciable dissection is required.

HCPCS Level II codes for medical and surgical supplies, A4000-A4999, may be used to report supplies and materials provided to Medicare patients if the supplies and materials are not considered to be included with or part of the basic service(s) or procedure(s).

FREE-SKIN GRAFTS

When coding free-skin grafts, the choice of codes is based on the size and location of the defect (recipient area) and the type of graft to be used. The graft codes include simple debridement of granulations or recent avulsion.

When a primary procedure such as orbitectomy, radical mastectomy, or deep-tumor removal requires skin graft for definite closure, use codes from the appropriate anatomical subsection for the primary procedure and codes from the series 15000-15416 for the skin graft. Note that the repair of a donor site requiring skin graft or local flaps should be coded as an additional procedure.

HCPCS Level II codes for medical and surgical supplies, A4000-A4999, may be used to report supplies and materials provided to Medicare patients if the supplies and materials are not considered to be included with or part of the basic service(s) or procedure(s).

MUSCULOSKELETAL SYSTEM

The procedures and services listed in this section of the CPT code book include the application and removal of the first cast or traction device only. Subsequent replacement of the cast and/or traction device may be coded using the cast and strapping procedure codes appearing at the end of the section.

Most bone, cartilage, and fascia graft procedures include obtaining of the graft by the operating surgeon. When a surgical associate obtains the graft for the operating surgeon, the additional service should be coded and reported separately using codes from the 20900-20926 range. In addition, a surgical modifier for assistant surgeon or cosurgeon should be included when billing the associate's services.

When coding the re-reduction of a fracture and/or dislocation performed by the primary physician, add modifier -76 to the procedure code. If the re-reduction is performed by another physician, then modifier -77 would be added to the procedure code.

HCPCS Level II codes for medical and surgical supplies, A4000-A4999, may be used to report supplies and materials provided to Medicare patients if the supplies and materials are not considered to be included with or part of the basic service(s) or procedure(s).

CORRECT CODING ISSUES FOR THE MUSCULOSKELETAL SYSTEM

The general guidelines regarding correct coding apply to the CPT codes in the range of 20000-29999. Specific issues unique to this section of CPT are clarified in the following guidelines.

Anesthesia

Anesthesia administered by a physician performing a procedure is included in the procedure. Accordingly, injections of local anesthesia for musculoskeletal procedures (surgical or manipulative) are not to be separately reported.

Specifically, the CPT code 20550 (Injection tendon, ligament...) is not to be used as an injection code to provide local anesthesia for a surgical, closed, manipulative, or other procedure; this is not the intent of the CPT code. Many code pair edits are included in the Correct Coding Initiative based on this policy. When separate anatomic areas are being treated, the appropriate anatomic modifier or the -59 modifier should be used to indicate this situation.

Biopsy

In accordance with the sequential procedure policy, when a biopsy is performed in conjunction with any excision, destruction, removal, repair, or internal fixation procedure, the biopsy procedure is not to be separately coded, assuming a diagnosis has already been established that makes the excision, destruction, removal, repair, or fixation procedure medically necessary. If the biopsy is performed at a different site and represents a significant, separately identifiable service, a biopsy service can be reported. For example, if a patient presents with an upper-extremity fracture and, during an internal fixation procedure, it is determined to be medically reasonable to perform a bone biopsy of the iliac crest while under the same anesthetic, a separate service for a bone biopsy, with the -59 modifier, could be reported. If, however, through the same incision, a biopsy of the humerus was obtained, this service is not to be separately reported. In the circumstance in which the decision to perform the more-comprehensive procedure (excision, destruction, removal, repair, or fixation procedure) is dependent on the results of the biopsy procedure, the biopsy procedure may be separately reported.

Additionally, in accordance with the sequential procedure policy, when an arthroscopic procedure is followed by an open procedure at the same session, only the column 1 service is reported; generally, this would be the open procedure. If an arthroscopic service is performed at one site and an open procedure is performed at another, the arthroscopic service is reported with a modifier indicating that these services were performed at different anatomic sites (e.g., -RT or -LT modifier, -59 modifier, etc.)

Fractures

A. In general, the application of external immobilization devices (including casts) at the time of a procedure also includes removal services during (or after) the postprocedure period. CPT codes have been included for removal and modification of external fixation devices by a physician other than the physician who initially applied the device. These codes are not to be reported by the same entity (physician, practice, group, etc.) that performed the initial application service. When the initial service includes only an evaluation and management service and does not include a definitive procedure (e.g., surgical repair, reduction of a fracture, or joint dislocation), the cast/strapping may be separately reported from the evaluation and management service. When the only service rendered at a visit is cast or strapping application, a separate evaluation and management service should not be reported unless separate evaluation/management services are performed that satisfy the evaluation and management guidelines. CPT codes describing modification or removal of casts (e.g., 29700-29750) are not to be reported when these modifications are performed at the same session as the primary (open or closed) procedure.

B. Different codes have been created for removal of internal fixation devices as a separate procedure and modification/removal of these devices in conjunction with other procedures. When a superficial or deep implant (buried wire, pin, rod) requires a surgical procedure to remove it (e.g., CPT code 20670) and it is performed as a separate procedure, this service may be reported. On the other hand, when the service is necessary to accomplish another procedure involving the same area, it is not to be reported separately.

C. In accordance with the general policy on most extensive procedures, when a fracture requires closed reduction followed by open reduction at the same patient encounter (e.g., inability to accomplish the closed reduction), only the open reduction service is reported.

D. When interdental wiring (e.g., CPT code 21497) is necessary in the treatment of facial (or other) fractures or as part of a facial reconstructive surgery or arthroplasty, it is included as part of the service; accordingly, a separate service using the CPT code 21497 is not reported. If reported with other head and neck procedure codes, it should be coded with the -59 modifier, indicating a separate distinct service was performed. The medical record should reflect the nature of the separately identifiable service.

E. When it is necessary to perform skeletal/joint manipulation under anesthesia to assess range of motion or accomplish fracture reduction as part of another related procedure, the corresponding manipulation code (e.g., CPT codes 22505, 23700, 27275, 27570, and 27860) is not to be separately reported.

F. CPT codes 22840-22848 and 22851 (spinal instrumentation) are to be reported only with CPT codes 22325, 22326, 22327, and 22548-22812 for fracture, dislocation, or arthrodesis of the spine.

General Policy Statements

A. When a tissue transfer procedure (e.g., graft) is described in the principle procedure code, a separate service is not reported for performing the tissue transfer service necessary to complete the procedure.

B. In situations in which monitoring of interstitial fluid pressure is routinely performed as part of the postoperative care (e.g., distal lower-extremity procedures with risk of anterior compartment compression), a separate code for monitoring of interstitial fluid pressure (e.g., CPT code 20950) should not be reported.

C. When electrical stimulation is used to aid bone healing, the appropriate bone stimulation codes (CPT codes 20974-20975) should be reported; the codes for nerve stimulation (CPT codes 64550-64595) are inappropriate for this service. If a neurostimulator is medically necessary for other indications (e.g., pain control), a separate service is reported; however, the -59 modifier should be attached, indicating that this service is distinct in that it represents treatment of different symptoms; accordingly, the medical record should reflect the indication for the nerve stimulator. In addition, CPT codes 97014 and 97032 (physical medicine for electrical stimulation) are not to be reported in conjunction with the above-listed codes by the surgeon.

D. Routinely, exploration of the surgical field is performed during a surgical session; codes describing independent exploratory services are not to be reported when a more-comprehensive procedure is being performed in the same area. Specifically, an exploration code such as CPT code 22830 (exploration of spinal fusion) is not reported with other procedures involving the spine unless performed at a different site/different incision from the other procedure(s). If, for example, a cervical spine procedure was being performed and, at the same operative session, a lumbar fusion was explored through a separate incision, the CPT code 22830-59 could be reported, assuming the requirement for medical necessity was satisfied.

E. Debridements (CPT codes 11040-11042 and 11720-11721) are included in the surgical procedures conducted on the musculoskeletal system when debridement of tissue is in the immediate surgical field of other than fractures and dislocations. If, however, tissue debridement is necessary for a more-extensive area (e.g., concurrent soft-tissue damage due to trauma), the debridement codes can be reported. In open fractures and/or dislocations, debridement of tissue due to the fracture should be separately reported using the CPT codes 11010-11012.

F. Grafts, such as CPT codes 20900-20924, are to be separately reported only if the major procedure code description does not include graft in its definition.

G. The CPT code 20926 is a general code for tissue grafting (e.g., paratenon, fat, dermis) to be used when the primary procedure does not include grafting and when another graft code does not more accurately describe the nature of the grafting procedure being performed. Accordingly, it should not be used with codes in which the graft is already listed as a part of the procedure or with other grafting codes (see Chapter III for other graft codes).

GRAFTS OR IMPLANTS

Codes for obtaining autogenous bone, cartilage, tendon, fascia lata grafts, or other tissues through separate incisions are to be used only when a graft is not already listed as part of the basic procedure.

RECONSTRUCTION OF ORAL AND FACIAL DEFORMITIES

Codes 21079-21089 describe professional services for the rehabilitation of patients with oral, facial, or other anatomical deformities by means of prostheses (such as an artificial eye, ear, or nose) or intraoral obturator to close a cleft. These codes should be used only when the physician, not an outside laboratory, actually designs and prepares the prosthesis.

CAST APPLICATION

Codes in this section are used only when the cast application or strapping is a replacement procedure performed during or after the period of follow-up care. An additional visit code, dependent on location, is reportable only if significant identifiable other services are provided at the time of the cast application or strapping.

For coding cast or strap application in situations not involving surgery, for example, casting of a sprained ankle or knee, use the appropriate level of visit code plus code 99070 or equivalent HCPCS Level II code to bill for casting materials.

HCPCS Level II codes for medical and surgical supplies, A4000-A4999, may be used to report supplies and materials provided to Medicare patients if the supplies and materials are not considered to be included with or part of the basic service(s) or procedure(s).

ARTHROSCOPY

Per CPT definition, surgical arthroscopy *always* includes a diagnostic arthroscopy and would therefore never be coded and billed in addition to the surgical procedure. However, there are several arthroscopy procedures defined as separate procedures, indicating that the codes may be used for reporting and billing if the diagnostic arthroscopy is the only procedure performed.

RESPIRATORY SYSTEM

Codes from this section of the CPT code book are used to report invasive and surgical procedures performed on the nose; sinuses; larynx; trachea and bronchi; and the lungs and pleura. When coding endoscopic procedures from this section of the CPT code book, code the appropriate endoscopy of each anatomic site examined.

CORRECT CODING ISSUES FOR THE RESPIRATORY SYSTEM

1. Because the upper airway is bordered by a mucocutaneous margin, several CPT codes may define services involving biopsy, destruction, excision, removal, revision, etc. of lesions of this margin, specifically the nasal and oral surfaces. When billing a CPT code for these services, only the one CPT code that most accurately describes the service performed should be coded, generally from the CPT section describing either integumentary services (CPT codes 10040-19499) or respiratory services (CPT codes 30000-32999). When the narrative accompanying the CPT codes from the respiratory system section includes tissue transfer (grafts, flaps, etc.), individual tissue transfer/graft/flap codes (e.g., CPT codes 14000-15770) are not to be separately coded.

2. In keeping with the general guidelines previously promulgated, when a biopsy of an established lesion of the respiratory system is obtained as part of an excision, destruction, or other type of removal, either endoscopically or surgically, at the same session, a biopsy code is not to be reported by the surgeon in addition to the removal code. In the case of multiple similar or identical lesions, the biopsy code is not separately reported even if performed in a different area. As noted previously, in the circumstance in which the decision to perform the more-comprehensive procedure (excision,

destruction, or other type of removal) is dependent on the results of the biopsy, the procedure may be separately reported. If, at the same session, a biopsy is necessary to establish the need for surgery, the -58 modifier would be used to indicate this.

Example: If a patient presents with nasal obstruction, sinus obstruction, and multiple nasal polyps, it may be reasonable to perform a biopsy prior to, or in conjunction with, polypectomy and ethmoidectomy. In this case, a separate code (e.g., CPT code 31237 for nasal/sinus endoscopy) is not to be reported with the column 1 nasal/sinus endoscopy code (e.g., CPT code 31255) even though the latter code does not specifically list a biopsy in its CPT narrative because the biopsy tissue is procured as part of the surgery, not to establish the need for surgery.

3. When a diagnostic endoscopy of the respiratory system is performed, it is routine to evaluate the access regions as part of the medically necessary service; a separate service for this evaluation is not to be reported. For example, if an anterior ethmoidectomy is endoscopically performed, it is inappropriate to bill a diagnostic nasal endoscopy simply because the approach to the sinus was transnasal. As another example, fiberoptic bronchoscopy services routinely involve a limited inspection of the nasal cavity, the pharynx, and the larynx. Only the bronchoscopic code is reported, but not with the nasal endoscopy, laryngoscopy, etc. for this service, as this service is routine and incidental to the bronchoscopy.

If a diagnostic endoscopy is performed and this results in a decision to perform a (nonendoscopic) surgical procedure, then this endoscopy could be separately reported, indicating that this represented a distinct diagnostic service. The -58 modifier may be used to denote that the diagnostic endoscopy and the nonendoscopic surgical procedure are staged or planned procedures. Diagnostic endoscopy of the respiratory system (e.g., sinus endoscopy, laryngoscopy, bronchoscopy, pleuroscopy, etc.) performed at the same encounter as a surgical endoscopy is included in the surgical endoscopy according to CPT code book guidelines. Additionally, when an open surgical procedure is performed and, at the same session, is preceded by a "scout" endoscopy to evaluate the surgical field, the endoscopy code is not reported separately. This policy applies either if the endoscopic procedure is to confirm the anatomical nature of the patient's respiratory system and adequacy of the surgical procedure (e.g., tracheostomy, etc.) or if an attempt to perform an endoscopic procedure fails and is converted to an open procedure.

Example: If a patient presents with aspiration of a foreign body and a bronchoscopy is performed indicating a lobar foreign body obstruction, an attempt may be made to remove this bronchoscopically. It would be inappropriate to code and bill for CPT codes 31622 (bronchoscopy—diagnostic) and 31635 (surgical bronchoscopy); only the "surgical" endoscopy, CPT code 31635, would be appropriate. In this example, if the endoscopic effort was unsuccessful and a thoracotomy is planned, the diagnostic bronchoscopy could be separately coded in addition to the thoracotomy. The -58 modifier may be used to indicate that the diagnostic bronchoscopy and the thoracotomy are staged or planned procedures. If the surgeon decided to repeat the bronchoscopy after induction of general anesthesia to confirm the surgical approach to the foreign body, billing a service for this confirmatory bronchoscopy is inappropriate, although the initial diagnostic bronchoscopy could still be reported.

4. When a sinusotomy is performed in conjunction with a sinus endoscopy, only one service is reported. If the medically necessary service was the sinusotomy and the endoscopy was performed to evaluate adequacy or visualize the sinus cavity for disease, then the primary procedure would be best represented by the appropriate sinusotomy CPT procedure code. On the other hand, as a sinusotomy is usually required to accomplish a medically necessary diagnostic (or surgical) sinus endoscopy, the sinus endoscopy would be the primary (medically necessary) service and should be reported. CPT code book narrative indicates that a surgical sinus endoscopy always includes a sinusotomy and diagnostic endoscopy.

5. Control of bleeding during a procedure is an integral part of endoscopic procedures and is not separately reported (e.g., CPT code 30901 for control of nasal hemorrhage is not to be reported with CPT code 31235 for nasal/sinus endoscopy, etc.). If bleeding is a late complication and requires a significant, separately identifiable service after the patient has been released from the endoscopic procedure, a separate service may be reported with the -78 modifier, indicating that a related procedure was performed to treat a complication during the postoperative period.

6. When endoscopic procedures are performed, the most-comprehensive code describing the service rendered is reported. If multiple procedures are performed and not adequately described by a single CPT procedure code, more than one code may be reported; however, the multiple-procedure modifier -51 is attached to the appropriate secondary service CPT codes. Additionally, only medically necessary services are reported; incidental examination of other areas is not to be separately reported.

7. When laryngoscopy is required for placement of an endotracheal tube (e.g., CPT code 31500), a laryngoscopy code is not to be separately coded. Additionally, when a laryngoscopy is used to place an endotracheal tube for nonemergent reasons (e.g., general anesthesia, bronchoscopy, etc.), a

separate service is not to be reported for the laryngoscopy. The CPT code 31500 refers only to endotracheal intubation as an emergency procedure and is not reported when an elective intubation is performed. When intubation is performed in the setting of a rapidly deteriorating patient who will require mechanical ventilation, a separate service may be reported with adequate documentation of the reasons for intubation.

8.   When tracheostomy is performed as an essential part of laryngeal surgery, in accordance with the separate procedure policy, the CPT code 31600 is not separately reported. This would include laryngotomy, laryngectomy, laryngoplasty codes, or other codes that routinely require placement of a tracheostomy.

9.   If a laryngoscopy is required for the placement of a tracheostomy, the tracheostomy (CPT codes 31603-31614) is reported and not the laryngoscopy.

10. CPT code 92511 (nasopharyngoscopy with endoscopy) should not be reported as a distinct service when performed as a cursory inspection with other respiratory endoscopic procedures.

11. A surgical thoracoscopy is included in and not to be separately reported from an open thoracotomy when performed at the same session; the thoracotomy would represent the most extensive procedure successfully accomplished. If, however, the thoracoscopy was performed for purposes of an initial diagnosis and the decision to perform surgery is based on the results of the thoracoscopy, then it is separately reported. The -58 modifier may be used to indicate that the diagnostic thoracoscopy and the thoracotomy are staged or planned procedures.

VASCULAR INJECTION PROCEDURES

When using codes from this section, note that the listed procedures include local anesthesia, introduction of needles or catheter, injection of contrast medium with or without automatic power injection, and pre- and postinjection care specifically related to the injection procedure.

The most common code used in this section is code 36410, which is used to code for routine venipuncture for collection of specimen(s). Note that catheters, drugs, and contrast media are not included in the codes contained in this section. These should be coded using CPT code 99070 or the appropriate HCPCS Level II code for Medicare patients.

The codes listed in this section do not cover radiological vascular injections, injection procedures for cardiac catheterization, or chemotherapy. Refer to the Radiology or Medicine sections of the CPT code book for the appropriate codes for these procedures.

HCPCS Level II codes for medical and surgical supplies, A4000-A4999, may be used to report supplies and materials provided to Medicare patients if the supplies and materials are not considered to be included with or part of the basic service(s) or procedure(s).

HEMIC AND LYMPHATIC SYSTEMS

Codes from this section of the CPT code book are used to report invasive and surgical procedures performed on the spleen and lymph nodes. Bone marrow transplants are reported using codes 38230-38241 from this section.

When bone marrow aspiration is performed alone, the appropriate code to report is CPT code 38220. When a bone marrow biopsy is performed, the appropriate code is CPT code 38221 (bone marrow biopsy); this code cannot be reported with CPT code 20220 (bone biopsy). CPT codes 38220 and 38221 may be reported together only if the two procedures are performed at separate sites or at separate patient encounters. When both a bone marrow biopsy (CPT code 38221) and bone marrow aspiration (CPT code 38220) are performed at the same site through the same incision, only the bone marrow biopsy (CPT 38221) should be reported.

MEDIASTINUM AND DIAPHRAGM

Codes from this section of the CPT code book are used to report invasive and surgical procedures performed on the mediastinum and the diaphragm.

DIGESTIVE SYSTEM

Codes from this section of the CPT code book are used for invasive and surgical procedures performed on the lips; mouth; tongue; dentoalveolar structures; palate; salivary gland; pharynx, adenoids and tonsils; esophagus; stomach; intestines; rectum; anus; liver; biliary tract; pancreas; and the abdomen, peritoneum, and omentum. When coding esophagoscopy procedures, code the appropriate endoscopy of each anatomic site examined.

CORRECT CODING ISSUES FOR THE DIGESTIVE SYSTEM

The general policy statements defined previously also apply to procedures described by the CPT range of codes that deal with the digestive system (40490-49999). The nature of services identified in this section requires specific clarification in relation to these general policy statements.

Endoscopic Services

Endoscopic services are performed in many settings, e.g., office, outpatient, and ambulatory surgical centers (ASCs). Procedures that are performed as an integral part of an endoscopic procedure are considered part of the endoscopic procedure. Services such as venous access (e.g., CPT code 36000) and/or injection (e.g., CPT codes 90780-90784), noninvasive oximetry (e.g., CPT codes 94760 and 94761), anesthesia provided by the surgeon, etc. are included in the endoscopic procedure code. These column 2 codes are not to be reported separately.

1. When a diagnostic endoscopy is performed in conjunction with endoscopic therapeutic services, the appropriate CPT code to use is the most-comprehensive endoscopy code describing the service performed. If the same therapeutic endoscopy service is performed repeatedly (e.g., polyp removal) in the same area described by the CPT narrative, only one CPT code is reported with one unit of service. If different therapeutic services are performed and are not adequately described by a more-comprehensive CPT code, the appropriate codes can be designated in accordance with the multiple GI endoscopy rules previously established by CMS.

2. When a diagnostic endoscopy is followed by a surgical endoscopy, the diagnostic endoscopy is considered part of the surgical endoscopy (per CPT definition) and is not to be separately reported.

3. Gastroenterologic tests included in CPT codes 91000-91299 are frequently complementary to endoscopic procedures. Esophageal and gastric washings for cytology are described as part of an upper endoscopy (CPT code 43235), therefore CPT codes 91000 (esophageal intubation) and 91055 (gastric intubation) should not be separately reported when performed as part of an upper-endoscopic procedure. Provocative testing (CPT code 91052) can be expedited during gastrointestinal endoscopy (procurement of gastric specimens); when performed at the same time as GI endoscopy, CPT code 91052 should be coded with the -52 modifier, indicating a reduced level of service was performed.

4. When a small intestinal endoscopy or enteroscopy is performed as a necessary part of a procedure, only the most-comprehensive (column 1) code describing the service performed is to be reported. When services described by the range of CPT codes 44360-44386 (small-intestinal endoscopies) are performed as part of another service (e.g., surgical repair or creation of enterostomy, etc.), these codes are not separately reported. As noted previously, when an endoscopic procedure is confirmatory or is performed to establish anatomical landmarks ("scout" endoscopy), the endoscopic procedure is not separately reported. In the case in which the endoscopic procedure is performed as a diagnostic procedure upon which the decision to perform a more-extensive (open) procedure is made, the endoscopic procedure may be separately reported. The -58 modifier may be used to indicate that the diagnostic endoscopy and the more-extensive, open procedure are staged or planned services.

5. When endoscopic esophageal dilation is performed, the appropriate endoscopic esophageal dilation code is to be reported. The CPT codes 43450-43458 (dilation of esophagus) are not used in addition (even if attempted unsuccessfully prior to endoscopic dilation); in such a case, the -22 modifier can be used to indicate an unusual endoscopic dilation procedure.

6. When it is necessary to perform diagnostic endoscopy of the hepatic/biliary/pancreatic system using separate approaches (e.g., biliary T-tube endoscopy with ERCP, etc.), the appropriate CPT codes for both may be reported. However, the code should include the -51 modifier, indicating multiple procedures were performed at the same session.

7. When intubation of the GI tract is performed (e.g., percutaneous G-tube placement, etc.), it is not appropriate to bill a separate code for tube removal. Specifically, the CPT code 43247 (endoscopic removal of foreign body) is not to be reported for routine removal of therapeutic devices previously placed.

8. When an endoscopic or open procedure is performed and a biopsy is also performed followed by excision, destruction, or removal of the biopsied lesion, the biopsy is not separately reported. Additionally, when bleeding results from an endoscopic or surgical service, the control of bleeding at the time of the service is included in the endoscopic procedure. Separate procedure codes for control of bleeding are not to be coded. In the case of endoscopy, if it is necessary to repeat the endoscopy at a later time during the same day to control bleeding, a procedure code for endoscopic control of bleeding may be reported with the -78 modifier, indicating that this service represents a return to the endoscopy suite or operating room for a related procedure during the postoperative period. In the case of open

surgical services, the appropriate complication codes may be reported if a return to the operating room is necessary, but the complication code should not be reported if the complication described by the CPT code occurred during the same operative session.

9. Only the most-extensive endoscopic procedure is reported for a session. For example, if a sigmoidoscopy is completed and the physician performs a colonoscopy during the same session, then only the colonoscopy is coded. It is, however, acceptable to bill for multiple services provided during an endoscopic procedure (with the exception of treating bleeding induced by the procedure); these services would be reimbursed under the multiple-endoscopic payment rules for gastrointestinal endoscopy.

10. When a transabdominal colonoscopy (via colotomy) (CPT code 45355) and/or standard sigmoidoscopy or colonoscopy is performed as a necessary part of an open procedure (e.g., colectomy), the endoscopic procedure(s) is (are) not separately reported. On the other hand, if either endoscopic procedure is performed as a diagnostic procedure upon which the decision to perform the open procedure is made, then the procedure(s) may be reported separately. The -58 modifier may be used to indicate that the diagnostic endoscopy and the open procedure are staged or planned services.

Abdominal Procedures

When any open abdominal procedure is performed, an exploration of the surgical field is routinely performed to identify anatomic structures or any anomalies that may be present. Accordingly, an exploratory laparotomy (CPT code 49000) is not separately reported with any open abdominal procedure. If routine exploration of the abdomen during an open abdominal procedure identifies abnormalities requiring a more-extensive surgical field that makes the procedure unusual, the -22 modifier may be reported with supporting documentation in the medical record, indicating that an unusual procedural service was performed.

When, in the course of a hepatectomy a cholecystectomy is necessary in order to successfully perform the hepatectomy, a separate procedure code is not coded for the cholecystectomy; component column 2 procedures necessary to perform a more-comprehensive column 1 procedure are included in the column 1 code describing the more-comprehensive service.

Appendectomies are commonly performed incidentally during many abdominal procedures. The appendectomy is to be reported separately only if it is medically necessary. If done incidental to another procedure, the appendectomy would be included in the major procedure performed.

When in the course of an open abdominal procedure a hernia repair is performed, a service is reported only if the hernia repair is medically necessary at a different incisional site. Incidental hernia repair in the course of an abdominal procedure that is not medically necessary should not be reported. The medical record should document the medical necessity of the service if it is reported.

When a recurrent hernia requires repair, the appropriate recurrent-hernia repair code is reported. A code for incisional hernia repair is not to be reported in addition to the recurrent-hernia repair unless a medically necessary incisional hernia repair is performed at a different site. In this case, the -59 modifier should be attached to the incisional hernia repair code.

General Policy Statements

1. When a vagotomy is performed in conjunction with esophageal or gastric surgery, the appropriate CPT code describing the comprehensive column 1 coded service is reported. The range of CPT codes 64752-64760 includes services described by the vagotomy codes performed as separate procedures and are not reported in addition to esophageal or gastric surgical CPT codes (e.g., 43635-43641) that include vagotomy as part of the service.

2. When a closure of an enterostomy or enterovesical fistula requires the resection and anastomosis of a segment of bowel, the CPT codes 44626 and 44661 include the anastomosis or the enteric resection. Accordingly, additional enteric resection codes are not to be reported.

3. In accordance with the sequential procedure policy, only one code for hemorrhoidectomy is reported; the most-extensive procedure necessary to successfully accomplish the hemorrhoidectomy would be appropriate. Additionally, if in the course of a hemorrhoidectomy an abscess is identified and drained, a separate procedure code is not reported for the incision and drainage, as this was performed in the course of the hemorrhoidectomy. If the incision and drainage of the abscess occurred at a different site than the hemorrhoidectomy, then this procedure could appropriately be reported with a -59 modifier.

4. A number of groups of codes describe surgical procedures of a progressively more-comprehensive nature or with different approaches to accomplish similar services. In general, these groups of codes are not to be reported together (see mutually exclusive policy). While a number of these groups of codes exist in CPT, several specific examples include CPT codes 45110-45123 for proctectomies, CPT codes 44140-44160 for colectomies, CPT codes 43620-43639 for gastrectomies, and CPT codes 48140-48180 for pancreatectomies.

5.   When it is necessary to create or revise an enterostomy or to remove or excise a section of bowel due to fistula formation, a separate enterostomy closure code or fistula closure code is not reported. In the case of creating or revising an enterostomy, the closure is mutually exclusive; and in the case of fistula excision, the closure is included in the excision procedure.

6.   Because the digestive tract is bordered by a mucocutaneous margin, several CPT codes may define services involving biopsy, destruction, excision, removal, etc. of lesions of this margin. When a lesion involving this margin is identified and it is medically necessary to remove it, only one code that most accurately describes the service performed should be submitted, generally from the CPT section describing either integumentary services (10040-19499) or digestive services (40490-49999). For example, if a patient presents with a benign lip lesion and it is removed with a wedge excision, it would be acceptable to bill the CPT code 40510 (excision of lip) or the appropriate code from CPT codes 11440-11446 (excision of lesions); billing a code from both sections would be inappropriate.

7.   Laparoscopic procedures performed in place of an open procedure are subject to the standard surgical practice guidelines.

URINARY SYSTEM

Codes from this section of the CPT code book are used to report invasive and surgical procedures performed on the kidney, ureter, bladder, prostate (resection), and urethra. The general policies previously promulgated regarding CPT-defined services apply to the urinary tract. Because of the contiguous nature of the urinary tract and the accessibility of the urinary tract to endoscopic intervention, several specific issues require emphasis.

CORRECT CODING ISSUES FOR THE URINARY SYSTEM

1.   Many procedures involving the female and male urinary systems include the placement of a urethral catheter for postoperative drainage. Because this is integral to the service and represents the standard of medical practice, placement of a urinary catheter is not separately coded. In addition, catheterizations (e.g., CPT codes 53670 and 53675) are not separately reported when done at the time of or just prior to a surgical procedure.

2.   Many lesions of the genitourinary tract that require biopsy, excision, or destruction involve the mucocutaneous border, and several CPT codes may generally describe the nature of the biopsy obtained. For a biopsy of a lesion

or group of similar lesions, one unit of service for the CPT code that most accurately describes the service rendered is reported. As noted in the general policies in Chapter I, when a biopsy is followed by an excision or destruction during the same session, only the most-extensive service is reported. Additionally, separate codes (e.g., integumentary and genitourinary excision codes) are not to be reported unless the biopsy, excision, destruction, etc. service involves completely separate lesions; in these cases, the -59 modifier will indicate that separate lesions were removed. The medical record should reflect accurately the precise location of the lesions removed, particularly if it is medically necessary to submit each lesion as a separate specimen for pathological evaluation.

3. Policies regarding injections and infusions (e.g., HCPCS/CPT codes 36000, 36410, 90780, and 90781) as part of more-extensive procedures have previously been defined and apply to the genitourinary family of codes. When irrigation procedures or drainage procedures are necessary and are integral to successfully accomplish a genitourinary (or any other) procedure, only the more-extensive service is reported.

4. Unless otherwise defined by CPT code book instructions, the repair and closure of surgical procedures are included in the CPT code for the more-extensive procedure and are not to be separately reported. In many genitourinary services, hernia repair is included in the CPT code book descriptor for the service; accordingly, a hernia repair is not separately reported. If the hernia repair performed is at a different site, this can be separately reported with the -59 modifier, indicating that this service occurred at a different site (i.e., via a different incision).

5. In general, multiple methods of accomplishing a procedure (e.g., prostatectomy) are not performed at the same session (see general policy on mutually exclusive services); therefore, only one method of accomplishing a given procedure can be reported. In the event that an initial approach is unsuccessful and an alternative approach is undertaken, the approach that successfully accomplishes the procedure becomes the medically necessary service and is reported; if appropriate, a -22 modifier may be appended to the procedure code for the successful approach.

6. When an endoscopic procedure is performed as an integral part of an open procedure, only the open procedure is reported. If the endoscopy is only confirmatory ("scout endoscopy"), the endoscopy does not represent a diagnostic or surgical endoscopy, but represents exploration of the surgical field and should not be separately reported under the diagnostic or surgical endoscopy codes. When an endoscopic procedure is attempted unsuccessfully and converted to an open procedure, only the open procedure is reported (see general policy on sequential procedures). If the endoscopy

is performed for diagnostic purposes and a subsequent therapeutic service can be performed at the same session, the procedure is coded at the highest level of specificity; if the CPT code book narrative includes endoscopy, then the endoscopy is not separately coded. If the narrative does not include endoscopy and a separate endoscopy is necessary as a diagnostic procedure, this can be reported separately. The -58 modifier may be used to indicate that the diagnostic endoscopy and the subsequent therapeutic service are staged or planned procedures. The medical record must describe the intent and findings of the diagnostic endoscopy in these cases.

7. When multiple endoscopic procedures are performed at the same session, the most-comprehensive code accurately describing the service performed is reported; if several procedures are performed at the same endoscopic session, the -51 modifier is attached. (For example, if a renal endoscopy is performed through an established nephrostomy, a biopsy is performed, a lesion is fulgurated, and a foreign body (calculus) is removed, then the appropriate CPT coding would be CPT codes 50557 and 50561-51, *not* CPT codes 50551, 50555, 50557, and 50561.) This policy applies to endoscopic procedures in general and specifically to endoscopic procedures of the genitourinary system.

8. When bladder irrigation is performed as part of a more-comprehensive procedure or in order to accomplish access or visualization of the urinary system, the bladder irrigation (CPT code 51700) is not to be reported. This code is to be used for irrigation with therapeutic agents or for irrigation as an independent therapeutic service.

9. When electromyography (EMG) is performed as part of a biofeedback session, neither CPT code 51784 nor 51785 is to be reported unless a significant, separately identifiable diagnostic EMG service is provided. If either the CPT code 51784 or the CPT code 51785 is to be used for a diagnostic electromyogram, then a separate report must be available in the medical record to indicate this service was performed for diagnostic purposes.

10. When endoscopic visualization of the urinary system involves several regions (e.g., kidney, renal pelvis, calyx, and ureter), the appropriate CPT code is defined by the approach (e.g., nephrostomy, pyelostomy, ureterostomy, etc.) as indicated in the CPT descriptor. When multiple endoscopic approaches are simultaneously necessary to accomplish a medically necessary service (e.g., renal endoscopy through a nephrostomy and cystourethroscopy performed at the same session), they may be separately coded with the multiple-procedure modifier -51 on the less-extensive codes. When multiple endoscopic approaches are necessary

to accomplish the same procedure, the successful endoscopic approach should be reported.

11. When urethral catheterization or urethral dilation (e.g., CPT codes 53600-53675) is necessary to accomplish a more-extensive procedure, the urethral catheterization/dilation is not to be separately reported.

12. Multiple ureteral anastomosis procedures are defined by CPT codes 50740-50810 and 50860. In general, they represent mutually exclusive procedures and are not to be reported together. If one anastomosis is performed on one ureter and a different anastomosis is performed on a contralateral ureter, the appropriate modifier (e.g., -LT, -RT) is used with the appropriate CPT code to describe the service performed on the respective ureter.

13. CPT code 50860 (ureterostomy, transplantation of ureter to skin) is mutually exclusive of CPT codes 50800-50830 (e.g., ureterostomy, ureterocolon conduit, urinary undiversion) unless performed at different locations, in which case an anatomic modifier should be used.

14. The CPT codes 53502-53515 describe urethral repair codes for urethral wounds or injuries (urethrorrhaphy). When a urethroplasty is performed, codes for urethrorrhaphy should not be reported in addition, since "suture to repair wound or injury" is included in the urethroplasty service.

URODYNAMICS

The codes in this section may be used separately or in various combinations. When multiple procedures are performed in the same session, modifier -51 should be added to the second and all subsequent codes. Procedures in this section are performed by or under the direct supervision of a physician.

In addition, all materials and supplies used in the provision of these services (such as instruments, equipment, fluids, gases, probes, catheters, technician's fees, medications, gloves, trays, tubing, and other sterile supplies) are considered to be included in the base code. Use modifier -26 to code and bill for interpretation of results or operation of equipment only.

CYSTOSCOPY, URETHROSCOPY, AND CYSTOURETHROSCOPY

The descriptions of codes in this section are listed so that the main procedure can be identified without having to list all of the minor related procedures performed at the same time. For example:

52601   Transurethral resection of prostate, including control of postoperative bleeding, complete (vasectomy, meatotomy, cystourethroscopy, urethral calibration and/or dilation, and internal urethrotomy are included)

All of the secondary procedures are included in the single code 52601. If any of the secondary procedures requires significant additional time and effort to the point of making the procedure "unusual," modifier -22 should be added with an appropriate increase in fee and a report explaining what made the procedure unusual.

MALE GENITAL SYSTEM

Codes from this section of the CPT code book are used to report invasive and surgical procedures performed on the penis, testis, epididymis, scrotum, spermatic cord, and prostate.

CORRECT CODING ISSUES FOR THE MALE GENITAL SYSTEM

1. Transurethral drainage of a prostatic abscess (e.g., CPT code 52700) is included in male transurethral prostatic procedures and is not reported separately.

2. Urethral catheterization (e.g., CPT codes 53670 and 53675), when medically necessary to successfully accomplish a procedure, should not be separately reported.

3. The puncture aspiration of a hydrocele (e.g., CPT code 55000) is included in services involving the tunica vaginalis and proximate anatomy (scrotum, vas deferens) and in inguinal hernia repairs.

4. A number of codes describe surgical procedures of a progressively more-comprehensive nature or with different approaches to accomplish similar services. In general, these groups of codes are not to be reported together (see mutually exclusive policy). While a number of these groups of codes exist in CPT, a specific example includes the series of codes describing prostate procedures (CPT codes 55801-55845). In addition, all prostatectomy procedures (e.g., CPT codes 52601-52648 and 55801-55845) are also mutually exclusive.

FEMALE GENITAL SYSTEM

Codes from this section of the CPT code book are used to report invasive and surgical procedures performed on the perineum, vulva and introitus, vagina, cervix uteri, corpus uteri, oviduct, and ovarium. In vitro fertilization is also reported using codes 58970-58976 from this section.

CORRECT CODING ISSUES FOR THE FEMALE GENITAL SYSTEM

1. When a pelvic examination is performed in conjunction with a gynecologic procedure, either as a necessary part of the procedure or as a confirmatory examination, the pelvic examination is not separately reported. A diagnostic pelvic examination may be performed for the purposes of deciding to perform a procedure; however, this examination is included in the evaluation and management service at the time the decision to perform the procedure is made.

2. All surgical laparoscopic, hysteroscopic, and peritoneoscopic procedures include diagnostic procedures. Therefore, CPT code 49320 is included in 38120, 38570-38572, 43280, 43651-43653, 44200-44202, 44970, 47560-47570, 49321-49323, 49650-49651, 54690-54692, 55550, 58550-58551, 58660-58673, and 60650; and code 58555 is included in 58558-58563.

3. Lysis of adhesions (CPT code 58660) is not to be reported separately when done in conjunction with other surgical laparoscopic procedures.

4. Pelvic exam under anesthesia indicated by CPT code 57410 is included in all major and most minor gynecological procedures and is not to be reported separately. This procedure represents routine evaluation of the surgical field.

5. Dilation of vagina or cervix (CPT codes 57400 or 57800), when done in conjunction with vaginal approach procedures, is not to be reported separately unless the CPT code manual description states "without cervical dilation."

6. Administration of anesthesia, when necessary, is included in every surgical procedure code when performed by the surgeon.

LAPAROSCOPY—HYSTEROSCOPY

The descriptions of codes in this section are listed so that the main procedure can be identified without having to list all of the minor related procedures performed at the same time. For example:

58558   Hysteroscopy, surgical; with sampling (biopsy) of endometrium and/or polypectomy, with or without D & C

The secondary procedure(s) is (are) included in the single code 58558. If any of the secondary procedures requires significant additional time and effort to the point of making the procedure "unusual," modifier -22 should be added with an appropriate increase in fee and a report explaining why the procedure was unusual.

MATERNITY CARE AND DELIVERY

Codes from this section of the CPT code book are used to report routine maternity care and invasive and surgical procedures performed as part of prenatal, delivery, and postpartum care. The services normally provided in uncomplicated maternity cases include antepartum care, delivery, and postpartum care.

ANTEPARTUM CARE

The definition of antepartum care for coding purposes includes the initial and subsequent history; physical examinations; recording of weight, blood pressures, and fetal heart tones; routine chemical urinalysis; and routine visits.

Routine antepartum visits are defined as:

* Monthly visits up to 28 weeks' gestation,

* Biweekly visits up to 36 weeks' gestation, and

* Weekly visits until delivery.

Any other visits or services provided within this time period should be coded separately. Using six to eight weeks' gestation as the typical starting point, the above definition translates into between nine and 11 routine visits per patient.

DELIVERY

Delivery services are defined as including hospital admission, the admission history and physical examination, management of uncomplicated labor, and vaginal or cesarean delivery.

- The definition of delivery services *includes* the hospital admission, admission history, and physical.

- Resuscitation of newborn infants when necessary, defined in previous editions, is not included in the delivery services. If the delivering physician has to resuscitate the newborn infant, the physician may code this service as a separate procedure.

- Medical problems "complicating labor and delivery management" may require additional resources and should be reported using E/M service codes.

POSTPARTUM CARE

Postpartum care is defined as hospital and office visits following vaginal or cesarean delivery. No number of visits is defined by CPT; however, the typical fee for total obstetrical care includes a single office follow-up visit six weeks postpartum.

COMPLICATIONS OF PREGNANCY

The services defined previously are for normal, uncomplicated maternity care. For medical complications of pregnancy, for example, cardiac problems, neurological problems, diabetes, hypertension, toxemia, hyperemesis, preterm labor, and premature rupture of membranes, use E/M service codes.

For surgical complications of pregnancy, such as appendectomy, hernia, ovarian cyst, Bartholin cysts, etc., use codes from the Surgery section of the CPT code book. Note that in either case, complications are not considered to be part of routine maternity care and should be coded and billed in addition to maternity codes.

PARTIAL MATERNITY SERVICES

Occasionally, a physician may provide all or part of the antepartum and/or postpartum care but does not perform the actual delivery due to termination of the pregnancy by abortion or referral to another physician for delivery. In this circumstance, the physician has the option of using the inclusive codes 59420 or

59430 from the Maternity Care and Delivery section or to code and bill for each visit using E/M service codes 99201-99215.

CORRECT CODING ISSUES FOR MATERNITY SERVICES

The majority of procedures in this section (CPT codes 59000-59899) include only what is described by the code in the CPT definition. Additional procedures performed on the same day would be reported separately. The few exceptions to this rule consist of:

1. CPT codes 59050 (fetal monitoring during labor), 59300 (episiotomy), and 59414 (delivery of placenta) are included in CPT codes 59400 (routine obstetric care), 59409 (vaginal delivery only), 59410 (vaginal delivery and postpartum care), 59510 (routine obstetric care), 59514 (cesarean delivery), and 59515 (cesarean delivery and postpartum care). They are not to be separately reported.

2. The total obstetrical packages (e.g., CPT codes 59400 and 59510) include antepartum care, the delivery, and postpartum care. They do not include, among other services, ultrasound, amniocentesis, special screening tests for genetic conditions, visits for unrelated conditions (incidental to pregnancy), or additional and frequent visits due to high-risk conditions.

ENDOCRINE SYSTEM

Codes from this section of the CPT code book are used to report invasive and surgical procedures performed on the thyroid gland, parathyroid, thymus, adrenal glands, and carotid body.

NERVOUS SYSTEM

Codes from this section of the CPT code book are used to report invasive and surgical procedures on the skull; meninges and brain; spine and spinal cord; and the extracranial nerves, peripheral nerves, and autonomic nervous system.

CORRECT CODING ISSUES FOR THE NERVOUS SYSTEM

1. A burr hole is often necessary in anticipation of intracranial surgery (e.g., craniotomy, craniectomy) to gain access to intracranial contents, to alleviate pressure in anticipation of further surgery, or to place an intracranial

pressure-monitoring device as part of the surgery. As these services are integral to the performance of the subsequent services, codes representing these services are not to be separately reported if performed at the same session; if performed prior to the comprehensive procedure, the -58 modifier can be used to indicate that the burr hole and the intracranial surgery are staged or planned services.

In addition, taps, punctures, or burr holes accompanied by drainage procedures (e.g., hematoma, abscess, cyst, etc.) followed by other procedures are not separately reported unless performed as staged procedures. The -58 modifier may be used to indicate staged or planned services. Many intracranial procedures include bone grafts by CPT definition, and these grafts should not be reported separately.

2. Biopsies performed in the course of central nervous system (CNS) surgery should not be reported as separate procedures.

3. Craniotomies and craniectomies always include a general exploration of the accessible field; accordingly, it is not appropriate to code an exploratory surgery (e.g., CPT codes 61304, 61305) when another procedure is performed at the same session.

4. When services are performed at the same session but represent different types of services or are being performed at different sites (see example below), the -59 modifier should be added. This modifier indicates that this service was a distinct, separate service and should not be included in the column 1 code.

Example: A patient with an open head injury and a contra-coup subdural hematoma requires a craniectomy for the open head injury and a burr hole drainage on the opposite side for the subdural hematoma. The performance of a burr hole at the time of the craniectomy would be considered part of the craniectomy. However, the contralateral burr hole would be considered a separate service not integral to the craniectomy. To correctly code the burr hole for the contralateral subdural hematoma and the column 1 coded service (the craniectomy), the burr hole should be coded with the appropriate modifier (-59, -RT, -LT, etc.). In this example, the correct coding would be CPT codes 61304 with one unit of service and 61154-59 with one unit of service.

5. The use of general intravascular access devices (e.g., intravenous lines, etc.), cardiac monitoring, oximetry, laboratory sample procurement, and other routine monitoring for patient safety has been addressed in the previous policy for general anesthesia or monitored anesthesia care (MAC). These policies also apply for procedures that do not require the presence of an anesthesiologist or certified registered nurse anesthetist. As an example,

if a physician is performing a spinal puncture for intrathecal injection and administers an anxiolytic agent, but the procedure does not require the presence of an anesthesiologist or certified registered nurse anesthetist, the vascular access and any appropriate monitoring necessary are considered part of the spinal puncture procedure and are not to be reported separately.

6. When a spinal puncture is performed, the local anesthesia necessary to perform the spinal puncture is included in the procedure itself. The submission of nerve block or facet block codes for local anesthesia for a diagnostic or therapeutic lumbar puncture is inappropriate when there is no independent medical necessity of the administration of local anesthetic except for the lumbar puncture. Separate codes are not to be reported. In comparison, if in the course of a nerve or other anesthetic block procedure cerebrospinal fluid is withdrawn, it is inappropriate to bill for a diagnostic lumbar puncture; only the nerve (or other) block should be reported; the CSF procurement is not for diagnostic purposes.

7. The appropriate code for the open treatment of median nerve compression at the wrist (carpal tunnel syndrome) is CPT code 64721; according to CPT manual definition, this includes the open release of the transverse carpal ligament. Additionally, if an arthroscopic procedure (CPT code 29848) fails and must be followed by an open procedure (CPT code 64721), only the open, or successful, procedure can be reported, if necessary with a -22 modifier.

8. Nerve repairs by suture or neurorrhaphies (CPT codes 64831-64876) include suture and anastomosis of nerves when performed to correct traumatic injury to or anastomosis of nerves that are proximally associated (e.g., facial-spinal, facial-hypoglossal, etc.). When neurorrhaphy is performed in conjunction with a nerve graft (CPT codes 64885-64907), a neuroplasty, transection, excision, neurectomy, excision of neuroma, etc., then a separate service is not reported for the primary nerve suture.

9. In the same area of the cortex, neurostimulator electrodes can be implanted in only one fashion; accordingly, the CPT code 61850 (burr hole) is included in the CPT code 61860 (craniectomy). Codes describing craniotomy procedures (e.g., CPT codes 62100-62121) are generally bundled into craniectomy codes (e.g., CPT codes 61860-61875).

10. Because procedures necessary to accomplish a column 1 procedure are included in the column 1 procedure, CPT codes such as 62310-62311 and 62318-62319 (injection of diagnostic or therapeutic substances) are included in the codes describing more-invasive back procedures. Additionally, at the same site, codes describing laminotomy procedures are included in laminectomy codes. CPT codes 22100-22116 (partial excision

of vertebral components) represent distinct procedures and, accordingly, are not reported with laminotomy/laminectomy procedures unless the services are performed as described in the codes.

11. CPT codes describing the performance of a tracheostomy are not to be reported with the CPT code 61576 (transoral approach to skull base including tracheostomy), as this service is included in the descriptor for the code.

EYE AND OCULAR ADNEXA

Codes from this section of the CPT code book are used to report invasive and surgical procedures performed on the eyeball, cornea, anterior segment, posterior segment, and ocular adnexa.

CORRECT CODING ISSUES FOR OPHTHALMOLOGY

1. When a subconjunctival injection (e.g., CPT code 68200) with a local anesthetic is performed as part of a more-extensive anesthetic procedure (e.g., peribulbar or retrobulbar block), a separate service for this procedure is not to be reported. This is a routine part of the anesthetic procedure and does not represent a separate service.

2. Iridectomy, trabeculectomy, and anterior vitrectomy may be performed in conjunction with cataract removal. When an iridectomy is performed in order to accomplish the cataract extraction, it is an integral part of the procedure; it does not represent a separate service and is not separately reported. Similarly, the minimal vitreous loss occurring during routine cataract extraction does not represent a vitrectomy and is not to be separately reported unless it is medically necessary for a different diagnosis. While a trabeculectomy is not performed as a part of a cataract extraction, it may be performed to control glaucoma at the same time as a cataract extraction.

If the procedure is medically necessary at the same time as a cataract extraction, it can be reported under a different diagnosis (e.g., glaucoma). The codes describing iridectomies, trabeculectomies, and anterior vitrectomies, when performed with a cataract extraction under a separate diagnosis, must be reported with the -59 modifier. This indicates that the procedure was performed as a different service for a separate situation. The medical record should reflect the medical necessity of the service if separately reported. For example, if a patient presents with a cataract and has evidence of glaucoma (i.e., elevated intraocular pressure preoperatively) and a trabeculectomy represents the appropriate treatment for the glaucoma, a separate service for the trabeculectomy would be separately reported. Performance of a trabeculectomy as a preventive service for an expected transient increase in intraocular pressure postoperatively, without other evidence for glaucoma, is not to be separately reported.

3. The various approaches to removing a cataract are mutually exclusive when performed on the same eye.

4. Some retinal detachment repair procedures include some vitreous procedures (e.g., CPT code 67108 includes 67015, 67025, 67028, 67031, 67036, 67039, and 67040). Certain retinal detachment repairs are mutually exclusive of anterior procedures, such as focal endolaser photocoagulation (e.g., CPT codes 67110 and 67112 are mutually exclusive of CPT code 67108).

5. CPT codes 68020-68200 (incision, drainage, excision of the conjunctiva) are included in all conjunctivoplasties (CPT codes 68320-68362).

6. CPT code 67950 (canthoplasty) is included in repair procedures such as blepharoplasties (CPT codes 67917, 67924, 67961, 67966).

7. Correction of lid retraction (CPT code 67911) includes full-thickness graft (e.g., CPT code 15260) as part of the total service performed.

8. In the circumstance that it is medically necessary and reasonable to inject sclerosing agents in the same session as surgery to correct glaucoma, the service is included in the glaucoma surgery. Accordingly, codes such as CPT codes 67500, 67515, and 68200 for injection of sclerosing agents (e.g., 5-FU, HCPCS/CPT code J9190) should not be reported with other pressure-reducing or glaucoma procedures.

AUDITORY SYSTEM

Codes from this section of the CPT code book are used to report invasive and surgical procedures performed on the external ear, middle ear, inner ear, and temporal bone.

CORRECT CODING ISSUES FOR THE AUDITORY SYSTEM

1. When a mastoidectomy is included in the description of an auditory procedure (e.g., CPT codes 69530, 69802, and 69910), separate codes describing mastoidectomy are not reported.

2. Myringotomies (e.g., CPT codes 69420 and 69421) are included in tympanoplasties and tympanostomies.

RADIOLOGY SERVICES

GUIDELINES

General guidelines applicable to all physicians for reporting of medical services and procedures are defined in the Introduction to the CPT code book. Some of the general guidelines are repeated in this section. Definitions and items unique to radiology services, including nuclear medicine and diagnostic ultrasound, are also listed.

SUBJECT LISTINGS

The codes in this section apply to radiological services performed by or under the responsible supervision of a physician.

SEPARATE OR MULTIPLE PROCEDURES

It is appropriate to designate multiple procedures that are rendered on the same date by separate entries.

SUBSECTION INFORMATION

The Radiology section of the CPT code book is divided into four subsections, namely:

Diagnostic Radiology (Diagnostic Imaging)	70000-76499
Diagnostic Ultrasound	76500-76999
Radiation Oncology	77261-77999
Nuclear Medicine	78000-79999

Several of the subheadings or subsections have special needs or instructions unique to that section. The following subsections of the Radiology section have Notes that should be reviewed carefully before choosing codes from the section:

Diagnostic Ultrasound	76500-76999
Therapeutic Radiology	77261-77799
Nuclear Medicine	78000-79999

COMPLETE PROCEDURES

Interventional radiologic procedures or diagnostic studies involving injection of contrast media include all usual preinjection and postinjection services, for example, necessary local anesthesia, placement of needle or catheter, injection of contrast media, supervision of the study, and interpretation of results. When one of these procedures is performed in full by a single physician, it is designated as a "complete procedure."

SUPERVISION AND INTERPRETATION ONLY

When a procedure is performed by a radiologist-clinician team, it is designated as "supervision and interpretation only," and the separate injection procedure is listed in the appropriate section of the Surgery section of the CPT code book. These codes are used only when a procedure is performed by more than one physician, for example, a radiologist-clinician team.

MODIFIERS

Listed surgical services and procedures may be modified under certain circumstances. When applicable, the modifying circumstance is identified by adding the appropriate two-digit modifier to the base procedure code(s). Modifiers commonly used to report Radiology services include:

-22   Unusual services

-26   Professional component

-32   Mandated services

-51   Multiple procedures

-52   Reduced services

-62   Two surgeons

-66   Surgical team

-76   Repeat procedure by same physician

-77   Repeat procedure by another physician

-78   Return to the operating room for a related procedure during the postoperative period

-79   Unrelated procedure or service by the same physician during the postoperative period

-80   Assistant surgeon

-90   Reference (outside) laboratory

-99   Multiple modifiers

-LT   Left side of body

-RT   Right side of body

BILATERAL PROCEDURE CODES

The Radiology section includes some CPT codes that include the term "bilateral" in the definition. When reporting these services, do not add the modifier -50, because the procedure is already defined as "bilateral."

SPECIAL MEDICARE CONSIDERATIONS

Most of the codes in this section fall under the Medicare Purchased Diagnostic Services guidelines. Coding and reporting should be as instructed by your local Medicare carrier.

CORRECT CODING ISSUES FOR RADIOLOGY

Introduction

The CPT code book includes codes related to diagnostic radiology (imaging), ultrasound, radiation oncology, and nuclear medicine. The diagnostic imaging section includes noninvasive and invasive diagnostic and therapeutic (interventional) procedures, as well as computerized tomography and magnetic resonance imaging. Most correct coding issues are defined by CPT coding convention.

Noninterventional Diagnostic Imaging

Noninvasive/interventional diagnostic imaging includes standard radiographs, single or multiple views, contrast studies, computerized tomography, and magnetic resonance imaging. The CPT code book allows for various combinations of codes to address the number and type of radiographic views. For a given radiographic series, the procedure code that most accurately describes what was performed is appropriate. Because of the number of combinations of views necessary to obtain medically useful information, a complete review of CPT coding options for a given radiographic session is important to assure accurate coding with the most-comprehensive code that describes the services performed rather than billing multiple codes to describe the service.

In the event that radiographs have to be repeated in the course of a radiographic encounter due to substandard quality, only one unit of service for the code can be reported. Additionally, if after reviewing initial films the radiologist elects to obtain additional views in order to render an interpretation, the Medicare policy on the ordering of diagnostic tests should be followed and the CPT code describing the total service is reported, even if the patient was released from the radiology suite and had to return for additional services. The CPT descriptor for many of these services refers to a *minimum* number of views. Accordingly, if more than the minimum number specified is necessary and no other more-specific CPT code is available, only that service should be billed. On the other hand, if additional films are necessary due to a change in the patient's condition, separate billing would be appropriate.

CPT code descriptors that specify a minimum number of views should be reported when the minimum number of views or if more than the minimum number of views must be obtained in order to satisfactorily complete the radiographic study. For example, if three views of the shoulder are obtained, CPT code 73030, one unit of service, should be reported, not 73020 and 73030.

When limited comparative radiographic studies are performed (e.g., postreduction radiographs, postintubation, postcatheter placement, etc.), the CPT code for a comprehensive radiographic series should be reported with a -52 modifier, indicating that a reduced level of interpretive service was provided.

Studies may be performed without contrast, with contrast, or both with and without contrast. There are separate codes available to describe all of these combinations of contrast usage. When studies require contrast, there is not generally an established number of radiographs to be obtained because of patient variation. Accordingly, all radiographs necessary to complete a study are included in the CPT code description. Unless specifically noted, fluoroscopy necessary to complete a procedure and obtain the necessary permanent radiographic record is included in the major procedure performed.

Preliminary "scout" radiographs obtained prior to contrast administration or delayed imaging radiographs are often performed; when a separate CPT code is available to include these radiographs, it should be used. If there is no separate CPT code including additional views, it is assumed that these are included in the basic procedure.

Interventional/Invasive Diagnostic Imaging

When contrast can be administered orally (upper GI) or rectally (barium enema), the administration is included as part of the procedure, and no administration service is reported. When contrast material is parenterally administered, whether or not the timing of the injection has to correlate with the procedure (e.g., IVP, CT scans, gadolinium), the administration and the injection (e.g., HCPCS/CPT codes 36000, 36406, 36410, and 90782-90784) are included in the contrast studies.

When a contrast study is performed in which there is direct correlation of the timing of the study to the injection or administration (e.g., angiography) and different providers perform separate parts of the procedure, each provider would bill the service he/she rendered. The procedural aspect of the service is coded from outside the CPT 70000 series, and the radiographic supervision and interpretation (S & I) service is coded from the 70000 series of codes.

The individual CPT codes in the 70000 section identify which injection or administration code is appropriate for a given procedure; in the absence of a parenthetical CPT note, it is not appropriate to submit an administration component. When an intravenous line is placed (e.g., CPT code 36000) simply for access in the event of a problem with the procedure or for administration of contrast, it is considered part of the procedure. A separate code (e.g., CPT code 36005) is available for the injection procedure for contrast venography and includes the introduction of a needle or an intracatheter (e.g., CPT code 36000).

In the case of urologic procedures and other surgeries, insertion of a urethral catheter (e.g., CPT code 53670) is part of the procedure and is not to be separately reported.

The CPT codes 90783 and 90784 are for intra-arterial and intravenous therapeutic or diagnostic injections. Injections for contrast procedures are included in the procedure; CPT codes 90783 and 90784 cannot be separately reported with radiographic, CT, MRI, or nuclear imaging codes to represent part of the injection procedure.

Evaluation and Management

When physician interaction with a patient is necessary to accomplish a radiographic procedure, typically occurring in invasive or interventional radiology, the interaction generally involves limited pertinent historical inquiry about reasons for the examination, the presence of allergies, acquisition of informed consent, discussion of follow-up, and the review of the medical record. In this setting, a separate evaluation and management service is not reported. As a rule, if the medical decision making that evolves from the procurement of the information from the patient is limited to whether or not the procedure should be performed, whether comorbidity may impact the procedure, or discussion and education with the patient, then an evaluation/management code is not reported separately. If a significant, separately identifiable service is rendered, involving taking a history, performing an exam, and making medical decisions distinct from the procedure, the appropriate evaluation and management service can be reported. The appropriate evaluation and management service code is chosen based on the type of service rendered that satisfies the Evaluation and Management guidelines developed by the AMA and CMS.

In radiation oncology, evaluation and management services would not be separately reported with the exception of an initial consultation, at which time a decision is made whether to proceed with the treatment. Radiation oncology includes clinical treatment planning, simulation, medical radiation physics, dosimetry treatment devices, special services, and clinical treatment management procedures in teletherapy and brachytherapy.

The categories of procedures in this subsection are well-defined according to levels of intensity for clinical treatment planning, devices, delivery, and management.

General Policy Statements

1. Any abdominal radiology procedure that has a radiological supervision and interpretation code (e.g., CPT code 75625 for abdominal aortogram) would also include abdominal x-rays (e.g., CPT codes 74000-74022) as part of the total service.

2. Xeroradiography (e.g., CPT code 76150) is not to be reported with any mammography studies based on CPT coding instruction.

3. Codes for guidance for placement of radiation fields by computerized tomography or ultrasound (CPT codes 76370 or 76950) for the same anatomical area are mutually exclusive.

4. Ultrasound guidance services and diagnostic echography should be reported only when both procedures are performed. Ultrasound guidance services alone do not represent diagnostic echography.

5. CPT code 76970 (ultrasound study, follow-up) cannot be reported with any other echocardiographic or ultrasound guidance procedures because it represents a follow-up procedure on the same day.

6. CPT code 77790 (supervision, handling, loading of radiation source) is not to be reported with any of the remote afterloading brachytherapy codes

(e.g., CPT codes 77781-77784), since these procedures inherently include the supervision of the radioelement.

7. Bone studies such as CPT codes 76020-76065 require a series of radiographs; billing separately for bone studies and individual radiographs obtained in the course of the bone study is inappropriate.

DIAGNOSTIC ULTRASOUND

The following definitions are important when choosing codes for diagnostic ultrasound services and procedures:

A-MODE   Implies a one-dimensional ultrasonic measurement procedure.

M-MODE   Implies a one-dimensional ultrasonic measurement procedure with movement of the trace to record amplitude and velocity of moving echo-producing structures.

B-SCAN   Implies a two-dimensional ultrasonic scanning procedure with a two-dimensional display.

REAL-TIME   Implies a two-dimensional ultrasonic scanning procedure with display of both two-dimensional structure and motion with time.

RADIATION ONCOLOGY

Services defined in this section of the CPT code book include teletherapy and brachytherapy. To report Radiation Oncology services, the following must be performed and documented:

• The initial consultation

• Clinical treatment planning with/without simulation

• Medical radiation physics, dosimetry, treatment devices, and special services

• Clinical treatment management procedures

• Normal follow-up care during treatment and for three months following completion of treatment

CONSULTATION OR CLINICAL MANAGEMENT

Preliminary consultations, evaluation of the patient prior to a decision to treat, or the provision of full medical care (in addition to treatment management) is reported using appropriate E/M service codes.

CLINICAL TREATMENT PLANNING

The clinical treatment planning process is a complex service including interpretation of special testing, tumor localization, treatment volume determination, treatment time/dosage determination, choice of treatment modality, determination of number and size of treatment ports, selection of appropriate treatment devices, and other procedures.

CPT defines three distinct levels of clinical treatment planning: simple, intermediate, and complex. Review this section of the CPT code book for detailed definitions of these levels of service.

CLINICAL TREATMENT MANAGEMENT

Codes in this section presume treatment on a daily basis (four or five fractions per week) with the use of megavoltage photon or high-energy particle sources. Daily and weekly clinical treatment management are mutually exclusive for the same dates. CPT defines three distinct levels of clinical treatment management: simple, intermediate, and complex. Review this section of the CPT code book for detailed definitions of these levels of service.

NUCLEAR MEDICINE

Nuclear medicine procedures may be performed independently or in the course of overall medical care. If the physician providing nuclear medicine services is also responsible for the diagnostic work-up and/or follow-up care of the patient, E/M service codes should be reported in addition to the nuclear medicine procedures.

Radioimmunoassay tests are located in the clinical pathology section, code series 82000-84999. These codes can be used by any specialist performing such tests in a laboratory licensed and/or certified for radioimmunoassays. The reporting of these tests is not confined to clinical pathology laboratories alone.

Note that the services listed in this section do not include the provision of radium or other elements. When those materials are supplied by the physician, they should be listed as separate procedures using code 78990 for diagnostic radionuclide(s) and 79900 for therapeutic radionuclide.

The general policies promulgated above apply to nuclear medicine as well as standard diagnostic imaging. Several issues specific to the practice of nuclear medicine require comment.

The injection of the radionuclide is included as part of the procedure; separate injection codes (e.g., 36000, 90783) should not be reported.

Single-photon emission-computed tomography (SPECT) studies represent an enhanced methodology over standard planar nuclear imaging. When a limited anatomic area is studied, there is no additional information procured by obtaining both planar and SPECT studies. While both represent medically acceptable imaging studies, when a SPECT study of a limited area is performed, a planar study is not to be separately reported. When vascular flow studies are obtained using planar technology in addition to SPECT studies, the appropriate CPT code for the vascular flow study should be reported, not the flow, planar, and SPECT studies. In cases in which planar images must be procured because of the extent of the scanned area (e.g., bone imaging), both planar and SPECT scans may be necessary and reported separately.

HCPCS EQUIPMENT TRANSPORTATION CODES

HCPCS contains three codes (R0070, R0075, and R0076) to report transportation of portable x-ray equipment and personnel to home or nursing home. Consult your local Medicare intermediary before using these codes.

LABORATORY SERVICES

GUIDELINES

Items used by all physicians in reporting their services are presented in the Introduction. Some of the commonalities are repeated here for the convenience of those physicians referring to this section on Pathology and Laboratory. Other definitions and items unique to Pathology and Laboratory are also listed.

SERVICES IN PATHOLOGY AND LABORATORY

The procedures listed in this section of the CPT code book are provided by a pathologist or by technologists who are under the responsible supervision of a physician.

SUBSECTION INFORMATION

The Pathology and Laboratory section of the CPT code book is divided into 16 subsections:

Organ- or Disease-Oriented Panels	80048-80090
Drug Testing	80100-80103
Therapeutic Drug Assays	80150-80299
Evocative/Suppression Testing	80400-80440
Consultations (Clinical Pathology)	80500-80502
Urinalysis	81000-81999
Chemistry	82000-84999
Hematology and Coagulation	85000-85999
Immunology	86000-86849
Transfusion Medicine	86850-86999
Microbiology	87000-87999
Anatomic Pathology	88000-88099
Cytopathology	88100-88199
Cytogenetic Studies	88200-88299
Surgical Pathology	88300-88399
Other Procedures	89000-89399

Several of the subheadings or subsections have special needs or instructions unique to that section. The following subsections of the Pathology and Laboratory section contain Notes that should be reviewed carefully prior to choosing codes from those subsections:

Organ- or Disease-Oriented Panels	80048-80090
Drug Testing	80100-80103
Therapeutic Drug Assays	80150-80299
Evocative/Suppression Testing	80400-80440
Consultations (Clinical Pathology)	80500-80502
Urinalysis	81000-81999
Chemistry	82000-84999
Molecular Diagnostics	83890-83912, 87470-87799
Infectious Agent Antibodies	86602-86804
Microbiology Infectious Agent Detection	87260-87799
Anatomic Pathology	88000-88099
Cytopathology	88141-88167
Surgical Pathology	88300-88399

MODIFIERS

Pathology and laboratory services and procedures may be modified under certain circumstances. When applicable, the modifying circumstances should be identified by adding the appropriate modifier to the basic service code. The addition of modifier -22 requires a special report. Modifiers commonly used to report Pathology and Laboratory procedures include:

-22   unusual services

-26   professional component

-32   mandated services

-52   reduced services

-90   reference (outside) laboratory

ORGAN OR DISEASE PANELS

Codes for organ- or disease-oriented panels were included in CPT due to the increased use of general screening programs by physicians, clinics, hospitals, and other health care facilities. Other codes in this section define profiles that combine laboratory tests under a problem-oriented classification.

There is a list of specific laboratory tests under each of the panel codes that defines the components of each panel. However, each laboratory typically establishes its own profile and provides a listing of the components of that panel performed by the laboratory with test results.

PATHOLOGY CONSULTATIONS

To be considered a clinical pathology consultation, the following components must be present:

- The consultation must be requested from an attending physician.

- The service must require additional medical interpretive judgment by the pathologist.

- The pathologist must render a written report.

Reporting of a test result(s) without medical interpretive judgment *is not* considered a clinical pathology consultation.

SURGICAL PATHOLOGY

Surgical pathology procedure codes include accession, handling, and reporting. The unit of service for codes 88300 through 88309 is the specimen. A specimen is defined as "tissue or tissues that is (are) submitted for individual and separate attention, requiring individual examination and pathologic diagnosis."

CORRECT CODING ISSUES FOR PATHOLOGY AND LABORATORY

Pathology and laboratory CPT coding includes services primarily reported to evaluate specimens obtained from patients (body fluids, cytological specimens, or tissue specimens obtained by invasive/surgical procedures) in order to provide information to the treating physician. This information, coupled with information obtained from history and examination findings and other data, provides the physician with the background upon which medical decision making is established.

Generally, pathology and laboratory specimens are prepared and/or screened by laboratory personnel with a pathologist assuming responsibility for the integrity of the results generated by the laboratory. Certain types of specimens and tests are reviewed personally by the pathologist. CPT coding for this section includes few codes requiring patient contact or evaluation and management services rendered directly by the pathologist. On the occasion that a pathologist provides evaluation and management services (significant, separately identifiable patient care services that satisfy the criteria set forth in the E & M guidelines developed by CMS, formerly HCFA and the AMA), appropriate coding should be rendered from the Evaluation and Management section of the CPT code book.

If, after a test is ordered and performed, additional related procedures are necessary to provide or confirm the result, these would be considered part of the ordered test. For example, if a patient with leukemia has a thrombocytopenia and a manual platelet count (CPT code 85590) is performed in addition to the performance of an automated hemogram with automated platelet count (e.g., CPT code 85025), it would be inappropriate to report CPT codes 85590 and 85025, because the former provides a confirmatory test for the automated hemogram and platelet count (CPT code 85025). As another example, if a patient has an abnormal test result and repeat performance of the test is done to verify the result, the test is reported as one unit of service rather than two.

Organ- or Disease-Oriented Panels

The CPT code book assigns CPT codes to organ- or disease-oriented panels consisting of a group of specified tests. If *all* tests of a CPT-defined panel are performed, the provider may bill the panel code or the individual component test codes. The panel codes may be used when the tests are ordered as that panel or if the individual component tests of a panel are ordered separately. For example, if the individually ordered tests are cholesterol (CPT code 82465), triglycerides (CPT code 84478), and HDL cholesterol (CPT code 83718), the service could be billed as a lipid panel (CPT code 80061).

Evocative/Suppression Testing

Evocative/suppression testing involves administration of agents to determine a patient's response to those agents (CPT codes 80400-80440 are to be used for reporting the laboratory components of the testing). When the test requires physician administration of the evocative/suppression agent as described by CPT codes 90780-90784 (therapeutic/diagnostic injections/infusions), these codes can be separately reported. However, when physician attendance is not required and the agent is administered by ancillary personnel, these codes are not to be separately reported. In the inpatient setting, these codes are reported only if the physician performs the service personally. In the office setting, the service can be reported when performed by office personnel if the physician is directly supervising the service. While supplies necessary to perform the testing are included in the testing, the appropriate HCPCS J codes for the drugs can be separately reported for the diagnostic agents. Separate evaluation and management services are not to be reported, including prolonged services (in the case of prolonged infusions), unless a significant, separately identifiable service is provided and documented. If separate evaluation and management services are provided and reported, the injection procedure is included in this service and is not separately reported.

General Policy Statements

1. Multiple CPT codes are descriptive of services performed for bone and bone marrow evaluation. When a biopsy is performed for evaluation of bone matrix structure, the appropriate code to bill is CPT code 20220 for the biopsy and CPT code 88307 for the surgical pathology evaluation.

    When a bone marrow aspiration is performed alone, the appropriate coding is CPT code 38220. Appropriate coding for the interpretation is CPT code 85097 when the only service provided is the interpretation of the bone marrow smear. When both are performed by the same provider, both CPT codes may be reported. The pathological interpretations (CPT code 88300-88309) are not reported in addition to CPT code 85097 unless separate specimens are processed.

    When it is medically necessary to evaluate both bone structure and bone marrow and both services can be provided with one biopsy, only one code (CPT code 38221 or CPT code 20220) can be reported. If two separate biopsies are necessary, then both can be reported using the -59 modifier on one of the codes. Pathological interpretation codes 88300-88309 may be separately reported for multiple separately submitted specimens. If only one specimen is submitted, only one code can be reported regardless of whether or not the report includes evaluation of both bone structure and bone marrow morphology.

2. The family of CPT codes 87040-87158 refers to microbial culture studies. The type of culture is coded to the highest level of specificity regarding source, type, etc. When a culture is processed by a commercial kit, report the code that describes the test to its highest level of specificity. A screening culture and culture for definitive identification are not performed on the same day on the same specimen and therefore are not reported together.

3. When cytopathology codes are reported, the appropriate CPT code to bill is that which describes, to the highest level of specificity, what services were rendered. Accordingly, for a given specimen, only one code from a family of related codes describing a group of services that could be performed on a specimen with the same end result (e.g., 88104-88108, 88142-88145, 88150-88154, 88164-88167, etc.) is to be reported. If multiple services (separate specimens) are reported, the -59 modifier should be used to indicate that different levels of service were provided for different

specimens. This should be reflected in the cytopathologic reports. Cytopathology smears obtained from fluids are to be reported using the family of CPT codes 88104-88108; it is inappropriate to use the CPT codes 88160-88162 in addition, because the preparation of smears is included in the codes referable to fluids.

4. The CPT codes 80500 and 80502 are used to indicate that a pathologist has reviewed and interpreted, with a subsequent written report, a clinical pathology test. These codes additionally are not to be used with any other pathology service that includes a physician interpretation (e.g., surgical pathology). If an evaluation and management service (face-to-face contact with the patient) takes place by the pathologist, then the appropriate Evaluation and Management code is reported, rather than the clinical pathology consultation codes, even if, as part of the evaluation and management service, review of the test result is performed. Procurement of these services (CPT 80500 and 80502) requires the written order of another physician.

5. The CPT codes 88321-88325 are to be used to review slides, tissues, or other material obtained and prepared at a different location and referred to a pathologist for a second opinion. (These codes should not be reported by pathologists reporting a second opinion on slides, tissue, or material also examined and reported by another pathologist in the same provider group.) Medicare generally does not pay twice for an interpretation of a given technical service (e.g., EKGs, radiographs, etc.). However, it is recognized that there are times that this service is indicated. These codes are not to be used for a face-to-face evaluation of a patient. In the event that a physician provides an evaluation and management service to a patient and, in the course of this service, specimens obtained elsewhere are reviewed as well, this is part of the evaluation and management service and is not to be reported separately. Only the evaluation and management service would be reported.

6. Multiple tests to identify the same analyte marker or infectious agent should not be reported separately. For example, it would not be appropriate to report both direct-probe and amplified-probe technique tests for the same infectious agent.

MEDICINE SERVICES

GUIDELINES

Medicine services include immunizations, therapeutic or diagnostic injections, psychiatric services, dialysis, ophthalmology services, specialty-specific diagnostic services, chemotherapy administration, physical medicine and rehabilitation services, and osteopathic and chiropractic services. In addition to the standard definitions and general instructions found in the Introduction to the CPT code book, the Medicine section of the CPT code book includes specific items that are unique to that section.

MULTIPLE PROCEDURES

Multiple medical procedures provided on the same date should be reported separately. For example, if a physician provides individual psychotherapy in addition to a hospital visit, the psychotherapy should be reported separately from the hospital visit.

SEPARATE PROCEDURES

Some of the procedures listed in the Medicine section are commonly performed or included as an integral part of a total service and therefore do not require or justify separate reporting. However, when such a procedure is provided without performing the basic service and is not directly related to other services, it may be reported as a "separate procedure."

SUBSECTION INFORMATION

The Medicine section of the CPT code book is divided into 27 subsections:

Immune Globulins	90281-90399
Immunization Administration for Vaccines/Toxoids	90465-90474
Vaccines, Toxoids	90476-90749
Therapeutic or Diagnostic Infusions (excluding chemotherapy)	90780-90781
Therapeutic, Prophylactic, or Diagnostic Injections	90782-90799
Psychiatry	90801-90899
Biofeedback	90901-90911
Dialysis	90935-90999

Gastroenterology	91000-91299
Ophthalmology	92002-92499
Special Otorhinolaryngologic Services	92502-92700
Cardiovascular	92950-93799
Noninvasive Vascular Diagnostic Studies	93875-93990
Pulmonary	94010-94799
Allergy and Clinical Immunology	95004-95199
Neurology and Neuromuscular Procedures	95805-95999
Central Nervous System Assessments/Tests	96100-96117
Chemotherapy Administration	96400-96549
Photodynamic Therapy	96567-96571
Special Dermatological Procedures	96900-96999
Physical Medicine and Rehabilitation	97001-97799
Osteopathic Manipulative Treatment	98925-98929
Chiropractic Manipulative Treatment	98940-98943
Special Services, Procedures, and Reports	99000-99091
Qualifying Circumstances for Anesthesia	99100-99140
Sedation With or Without Analgesia	99141-99142
Other Services and Procedures	99170-99199

Most of the subsections have special needs or instructions unique to that section that should be reviewed carefully before reporting.

UNLISTED SERVICE OR PROCEDURE

A Medicine service or procedure may be provided that is not listed in the current edition of the CPT code book. If a specific CPT code cannot be found to report such a service, the appropriate "unlisted procedure" code may be used to report the service. A report that describes the unlisted service or procedure should be filed with the health insurance claim form.

MODIFIERS

Medicine services and procedures may be modified under certain circumstances. When applicable, the modifying circumstance is identified by the addition of the appropriate modifier code. The following modifiers are frequently used with Medicine services:

-22   Unusual services

-26   Professional component

-51   Multiple procedures

This modifier may be used to report multiple medical procedures performed at the same session, as well as a combination of medical and surgical procedures.

-52   Reduced services

-76   Repeat procedure by same physician

-77   Repeat procedure by another physician

-90   Reference (outside) laboratory

-99   Multiple modifiers

SPECIAL REPORT

A Medicine service that is unlisted in the CPT code book, rarely provided, unusual, variable, or new may require a special report in determining medical appropriateness of the service. When providing such services, you may need to provide additional documentation either routinely, for example, when reporting unlisted procedure codes or using modifier -22, or upon request from the health insurance carrier.

MATERIALS SUPPLIED BY PHYSICIAN

Supplies and materials provided by the physician over and above those usually included with the office visit or other services rendered may be listed separately. List all drugs, trays, supplies, and materials provided. HCPCS Level II codes must be used instead of CPT codes when reporting supplies, materials, and/or injections provided to Medicare patients.

IMMUNE GLOBULINS

Immune globulins are administered to provide protection from hepatitis B, diphtheria, rabies, respiratory viruses, tetanus, and other diseases. Immune globulin codes 90281-90399 identify the immune globulin product only and must be reported in addition to immunization administration codes.

IMMUNIZATION ADMINISTRATION FOR VACCINES/TOXOIDS

Immunization is the administration of a vaccine or toxoid to stimulate the immune system to provide protection against disease. Immunizations are usually given in conjunction with an E/M service. When an immunization is the only service performed, a minimal E/M service code may be listed in addition to the injection code.

Coding Rules

1) When an immunization is the only service provided, E/M service code 99221, Minimal service, may be reported in addition to the immunization.

2) Immunization administration codes must be reported in addition to the vaccine and toxoid codes.

3) Supplies or equipment used to inject the vaccine or toxoid are not reported separately.

VACCINES, TOXOIDS

Vaccines and toxoids are administered to provide protection from hepatitis, influenza, typhoid, measles, mumps, polio, and other diseases. Vaccine and toxoid codes 90476-90749 identify the vaccine or toxoid only and must be reported in addition to immunization administration codes.

THERAPEUTIC OR DIAGNOSTIC INFUSIONS

Infusion is the therapeutic introduction of a fluid other than blood into a vein. An infusion flows in by gravity, whereas an injection is forced in by a syringe. Infusion therapy codes are used to report prolonged intravenous injections requiring the presence of a physician during the infusion. These codes are time-specific codes covering the first hour and each additional hour of therapy up to eight hours.

Coding Rules

1) Presence of the physician during the infusion is required.

2) Infusion codes may not be used for chemotherapy infusions.

3) Infusion codes may not be used for intradermal, subcutaneous, intramuscular, or routine intravenous drug injections.

4) Infusion codes may not be reported in addition to prolonged services codes.

THERAPEUTIC, PROPHYLACTIC, OR DIAGNOSTIC INJECTIONS

An injection is the process of forcing a liquid, usually via a needle and syringe, into the skin, muscles, arteries, or veins. Therapeutic or diagnostic injection codes are used for reporting therapeutic injections of medication, via subcutaneous, intramuscular, intra-arterial, or intravenous routes and for reporting intramuscular injection of antibiotics.

Coding Rules

1) When reporting therapeutic or diagnostic injection codes, the injected material should be specified.

2) Therapeutic or diagnostic injection codes may not be used for allergen immunotherapy.

3) Use CPT therapeutic or diagnostic injection codes when reporting injections to commercial health insurance companies, unless otherwise instructed by specific companies.

4) Use HCPCS Level II codes instead of CPT codes to report therapeutic or diagnostic injections on health insurance claims to Medicare.

Therapeutic or Diagnostic Infusions/Injections

The CPT codes 90780-90799 describe services involving therapeutic or diagnostic injections and infusions. The CPT codes 96400-96549 describe administration of chemotherapeutic (primarily antineoplastic) agents; issues referable to chemotherapy administration will be discussed in this section due to the frequent similarities in administration.

Because the placement of peripheral vascular access devices is integral to vascular (intravenous, intra-arterial) infusions and injections, the CPT codes for placement of these devices are not to be separately reported. Accordingly, routine insertion of an intravenous catheter (e.g., CPT codes 36000, 36410) for intravenous infusion, injection, or chemotherapy administration (e.g., CPT codes 90780, 90781, 90784, 96408-96412) would be inappropriate. Insertion of central venous access is not routinely necessary to accomplish these services and, therefore, could be separately reported. Because intra-arterial infusion usually involves selective catheterization of an arterial supply to a specific organ, there is no routine arterial catheterization common to all arterial infusions; selective arterial catheterization codes could be separately reported.

The administration of drugs (such as growth factors, saline, and diuretics) and other than antineoplastic drugs is reported with CPT codes 90780-90784. When the sole purpose of fluid administration (e.g., saline, D5W, etc.) is to maintain patency of the access device, the infusion is neither diagnostic nor therapeutic; therefore, the injection, infusion, or chemotherapy administration codes are not to be separately reported. In the case of transfusion of blood or blood products, the insertion of a peripheral IV (e.g., CPT codes 36000, 36410) is routinely necessary and is not separately reported. Administration of fluid in the course of transfusions to maintain line patency or between units of blood products is, likewise, not to be separately reported. If fluid administration is medically necessary for therapeutic reasons (e.g., to correct dehydration, to prevent nephrotoxicity, etc.) in the course of a transfusion or chemotherapy, this could be separately reported with the -59 modifier, as this is being administered as medically necessary for a different diagnosis.

DRUGS ADMINISTERED OTHER THAN ORAL METHOD

HCPCS Level II includes over 400 codes that describe specific therapeutic injections, miscellaneous drugs and solutions, stinging insect venoms, and immunosuppressive drugs. HCPCS codes must be used when reporting therapeutic injections provided to Medicare beneficiaries. Using a CPT code instead of a HCPCS code to report therapeutic injections will result in processing delays, reduced payment, or denial of your health insurance claim.

PSYCHIATRY

Psychiatry is the study, treatment, and prevention of mental disorders. Psychiatric services include diagnostic and therapeutic services in the hospital, office, or other outpatient setting. Psychiatric service codes are used to report general psychiatry, clinical psychiatry, and psychiatric therapeutic services and procedures. Key coding issues include the type of psychotherapy, the place of service, the face-to-face time spent with the patient during psychotherapy, and whether E/M services are furnished on the same date of service as psychotherapy.

Coding Rules

1) Attending physicians reporting hospital care services in treating a psychiatric inpatient may use the full range of hospital E/M service codes.

2) If the physician is active in the leadership or direction of a treatment team, a code may be selected based upon the services provided that day using Case Management codes from E/M services codes 99361-99362.

3) All procedures performed in addition to hospital care, such as electroconvulsive therapy or medical psychotherapy, should be listed in addition to hospital care.

4) Psychiatric care may be reported without time dimensions, using the codes 90841 or 90845, or with time dimensions, using codes 90843 or 90844, based upon practices customary in the local area.

5) The modifiers -52 (reduced service) or -22 (unusual service) may be used to bill for services that were less or more lengthy than the time-specified codes define.

PSYCHIATRIC CONSULTATIONS

Consultation for psychiatric evaluation of a patient includes examination of a patient and exchange of information with the primary physician and others, such as nurses or family members, and preparation of a report.

Consultation services provided by psychiatrists are reported with E/M consultation codes. Psychiatric consultation services are limited to initial or follow-up evaluation and do not involve psychiatric treatment.

CORRECT CODING ISSUES FOR PSYCHIATRY

CPT codes for psychiatric services include general and special diagnostic services as well as a variety of therapeutic services. By CPT code book definition, therapeutic services (e.g., HCPCS/CPT codes 90804-90829) include psychotherapy and continuing medical diagnostic evaluation; therefore, CPT codes 90801 and 90802 are not reported with these services.

Interactive services (diagnostic or therapeutic) are distinct forms of services for a patient who has not yet developed or has lost the expressive language communication skills to explain his/her symptoms and response to treatment. Accordingly, noninteractive services would not be possible at the same session as interactive services and are not to be reported together with interactive services.

Drug management is included in some therapeutic services (e.g., HCPCS/CPT codes 90801-90829, 90845, 90847-90853, 90865-90870), and therefore CPT code 90862 (pharmacologic management) is not to be reported with these codes.

When medical services, other than psychiatric services, are provided in addition to psychiatric services, separate evaluation and management codes cannot be reported. The psychiatric service includes the evaluation and management services provided according to CMS policy.

DIALYSIS

Dialysis is the process of passing body fluids through a membrane to remove harmful substances. Dialysis is used in the treatment of kidney failure. Key coding issues include the type of dialysis and the location of the service.

Coding Rules

1) All E/M services related to the patient's end-stage renal disease (ESRD) that are rendered on a day when dialysis is performed and all other patient care services that are rendered during the dialysis procedure are included in the dialysis procedure codes.

2) All E/M services unrelated to the dialysis procedure that cannot be rendered during the dialysis session may be reported in addition to the dialysis procedure.

3) Supplies provided to dialysis patients not considered to be included with the dialysis service or procedure are reported using CPT code 99070 or HCPCS codes E1500-E1699 for DME and A4650-A5149 for supplies for ESRD.

GASTROENTEROLOGY

Gastroenterology is the study and treatment of diseases of the stomach and digestive system. The codes listed in this subsection are used to report diagnostic services of the esophagus and/or stomach contents and therapeutic services such as gastric intubation and lavage. Gastroenterology services are usually performed in conjunction with an E/M service, such as a consultation or visit, and should be reported separately in addition to the E/M service.

CORRECT CODING ISSUES FOR GASTROENTEROLOGY

Gastroenterological tests included in CPT codes 91000-91299 are frequently complementary to endoscopic procedures. Esophageal and gastric washings for cytology are described as part of upper endoscopy (e.g., CPT code 43235); therefore, CPT codes 91000 (esophageal intubation) and 91055 (gastric intubation) are not separately reported when performed as part of an upper endoscopy. Provocative testing (CPT code 91052) can be expedited during GI endoscopy (procurement of gastric specimens). When performed at the same time as GI endoscopy, CPT code 91052 is reported with the -52 modifier, indicating that a reduced level of service was performed.

OPHTHALMOLOGY

Ophthalmology is the study and treatment of diseases of the eye. Ophthalmological diagnostic and treatment services are reported using CPT Medicine codes 92002-92499.

Coding Rules

1) Minimal, brief, and limited office services and hospital, home, extended care, emergency department, and consultations are reported using appropriate E/M service codes.

2) Surgical procedures on the eye(s) are reported using codes from the Eye and Ocular Adnexa subsection of the Surgery section of the CPT code book.

3) To report *intermediate* ophthalmological services, the following must be performed and documented: a) evaluation of new or existing condition, b) complications of new diagnostic or management problems (not necessarily related to the primary diagnosis), c) history, d) general medical observation, e) external ocular and adnexal examination, f) other diagnostic procedures as indicated, and g) may include the use of mydriasis

   Intermediate ophthalmological services do not usually include determination of refractive state but may in an established patient under continuing active treatment

4) To report *comprehensive* ophthalmological services, the following must be performed and documented: a) billed as a single service but may be performed at more than one session, b) history, c) general medical observation, d) external and ophthalmoscopic examination, e) gross visual fields, f) basic sensorimotor examination, g) may include, as indicated,

biomicroscopy, examination with cycloplegia or mydriasis and tonometry, h) always includes initiation of diagnostic and treatment programs.

5) For both intermediate and comprehensive ophthalmological services, service components, such as slip lamp examination, keratoscopy, ophthalmoscopy, retinoscopy, tonometry, and motor evaluation, are not reported separately.

SPECIAL OPHTHALMOLOGICAL SERVICES

Special ophthalmological services are defined as a level of service in which a special evaluation of part of the visual system is made that goes beyond the services usually included under general ophthalmological services or in which special treatment is given. Fluorescein angioscopy, quantitative visual field examination, or extended color vision examination should be specifically reported as special ophthalmological services.

CONTACT LENS SERVICES

The prescription of contact lens is defined as specification of optical and physical characteristics, such as power, size, curvature, flexibility, and gas-permeability. It is not considered a part of the general ophthalmological services.

The fitting of contact lens includes instruction and training of the wearer and incidental revision of the lens during the training period. Follow-up of successfully fitted, extended-wear lenses is considered as part of a general ophthalmological service.

The supply of contact lenses may be included as part of the service or fitting or may be billed separately using codes 92391 or 92396.

If contact lenses are included as part of the fitting code, use modifier -26 to indicate the service of fitting without supply. If the prescription and fitting are for only one eye, use modifier -52 to indicate reduced service.

SPECTACLE SERVICES (INCLUDING PROSTHESIS FOR APHAKIA)

Prescription of spectacles, when required, is an integral part of general ophthalmological services and is not reported separately. However, fitting of spectacles is a separate service when provided by the physician and is reported using CPT codes 92340-92371. Presence of physician is not required during the fitting.

Supply of materials including spectacles, contact lenses, low vision aids, and ocular prostheses are not considered part of the service of fitting spectacles and should be reported separately using CPT codes 92390-92396.

CORRECT CODING ISSUES FOR OPHTHALMOLOGY

General ophthalmologic services (e.g., CPT codes 92002-92014) describe components of the ophthalmologic examination. When evaluation and management codes are reported, these general ophthalmologic service codes (e.g., CPT codes 92002-92014) are not to be reported; the same services would be represented by both series of codes.

Special ophthalmologic services represent specific services that are not described as part of a general or routine ophthalmologic examination. Special ophthalmologic services are recognized as significant, separately identifiable services.

For procedures requiring intravenous injection of dye or other diagnostic agent, insertion of an intravenous catheter and dye injection are necessary to accomplish the procedure and are included in the procedure. Accordingly, HCPCS/CPT codes 36000 (introduction of a needle or catheter), 36410 (venipuncture), 90780 (IV infusion), and 90784 (IV injection) as well as selective vascular catheterization codes are not to be separately reported with services requiring intravenous injection (e.g., CPT codes 92230, 92235, 92240, 92287, for angioscopy and angiography).

CPT codes 92230 and 92235 (fluorescein angioscopy and angiography) include injection procedures for angiography.

HCPCS LEVEL II CODES FOR VISION SERVICES

HCPCS Level II includes codes V0000-V2799 for spectacles, contact lenses, and eye prostheses. However; with the exception of postcataract lenses used as a prosthetic device, these services are generally not covered by Medicare. Therefore you would not bill Medicare for these services or use the HCPCS codes to bill any other carrier for these services.

OTORHINOLARYNGOLOGIC SERVICES

Otorhinolaryngology is the study and treatment of diseases of the head and neck, including the ears, nose, and throat. Diagnostic or treatment procedures usually included in a comprehensive otorhinolaryngologic evaluation or office visit are reported as an integrated medical service, using CPT E/M service codes.

Coding Rules

1) Component procedures, such as otoscopy, rhinoscopy, and tuning fork test, that may be provided as part of a comprehensive service are not reported separately.

2) Special otorhinolaryngologic diagnostic or treatment services not usually included in a comprehensive otorhinolaryngologic evaluation or office visit are reported separately.

3) All otorhinolaryngologic services include medical diagnostic evaluation. Technical procedures, which may or may not be performed by the physician personally, are often part of the service, but should not be mistaken to constitute the service itself.

AUDIOLOGIC FUNCTION TESTS

Audiometry is the process of measuring hearing using a machine called an audiometer. Audiometric tests described in this section of the CPT code book presume the use of calibrated electronic equipment. Other hearing tests, such as whispered voice, tuning fork, etc., are considered part of the general otorhinolaryngologic services and are not reported separately. All codes in this section refer to testing of both ears. Use the modifier -52 "Reduced Service" if a test is applied to one ear instead of to two ears. Note that all codes, with the exception of 92559, apply to the testing of individuals. For testing of groups, use code 92559 and specify testing used.

CORRECT CODING ISSUES FOR OTORHINOLARYNGOLOGIC SERVICES

CPT coding for otorhinolaryngologic services involves a number of tests that can be performed qualitatively by confrontation during physical examination or quantitatively with electrical recording equipment. CPT definition specifies which is the case for each code. CPT codes 92552-92557 and 92561-92589 can be performed qualitatively or quantitatively, but according to CPT definition, these can be reported only if calibrated electronic equipment is used. Confrontational estimation of these tests by the physician is part of the evaluation and management service.

HCPCS LEVEL II CODES FOR HEARING SERVICES

HCPCS Level II includes codes V5000-V5999 that describe hearing services such as audiometric exam, hearing aids, etc. Not one of these services is covered by Medicare, therefore Medicare should not be billed for these services, and the HCPCS codes should not be used (unless otherwise instructed) to bill any other carrier.

CARDIOVASCULAR SERVICES

Cardiovascular services refers to the study and treatment of diseases of the heart and vascular (arteries and veins) system. Cardiovascular services codes are used to report therapeutic services such as cardiopulmonary resuscitation (CPR), cardioversion, and percutaneous transluminal coronary angioplasty (PTCA) and also diagnostic procedures such as electrocardiography, echocardiography, and cardiac catheterization.

Coding Rules

1) Cardiovascular services are usually performed in addition to E/M services, such as a consultation or visit, and should be reported in addition to the E/M service.

2) Many cardiovascular services fall under the Medicare Purchased Diagnostic Services guidelines, therefore reporting should be as instructed by your local Medicare carrier.

CORRECT CODING ISSUES FOR CARDIOVASCULAR SERVICES

Cardiovascular medicine services include noninvasive and invasive diagnostic testing (including intracardiac testing) as well as therapeutic services (e.g., electrophysiological procedures). Several unique issues arise due to the spectrum of cardiovascular codes included in this section.

1. When cardiopulmonary resuscitation is performed without other evaluation and management services (e.g., a physician responds to a "code blue" and directs cardiopulmonary resuscitation with the patient's attending physician and then resumes the care of the patient after the patient has been revived), only the CPT code 92950 for CPR should be reported. Levels of critical care services and prolonged management services are determined by time; when CPT code 92950 is reported, the time required to perform CPR is not included in critical care or other timed evaluation and management services.

2. In keeping with the policies outlined previously, procedures routinely performed as part of a comprehensive service are included in the comprehensive service and not separately reported. A number of therapeutic and diagnostic cardiovascular procedures (e.g., CPT codes 92950-92998, 93501-93545, 93600-93624, 93640-93652) routinely utilize intravenous or intra-arterial vascular access, routinely require electrocardiographic monitoring, and frequently require agents administered by injection or infusion techniques. Accordingly, separate codes for routine access, monitoring, injection, or infusion services are not to be reported. Fluoroscopic guidance procedures are integral to invasive intravascular procedures and are included in those services. In unique circumstances, when these services are performed not as an integral part of the procedure, then the appropriate code can be separately reported with the -59 modifier. When supervision and interpretation codes are identified in the CPT code book for a given procedure, these can be separately reported.

3. Cardiac output measurement (e.g., CPT codes 93561-93562) is routinely performed during cardiac catheterization procedures per CPT definition. Therefore, CPT codes 93561-93562 are not to be reported with cardiac catheterization codes.

4. CPT codes 93797 and 93798 describe comprehensive services provided by a physician for cardiac rehabilitation. As this includes all services referable to cardiac rehabilitation, it would be inappropriate to bill a separate evaluation and management service code unless an unrelated, separately identifiable service is performed and documented in the medical record.

5. When a physician who is in attendance for a cardiac stress test obtains a history and performs a limited examination referable specifically to the cardiac stress test, a separate evaluation and management service is not reported unless a significant, separately identifiable service is performed unrelated to the performance of the cardiac stress test and in accordance with the Evaluation and Management section guidelines. The evaluation and management service would be reported with the -25 modifier in this instance.

6. Routine monitoring of EKG rhythm and review of daily hemodynamics, including cardiac outputs, are a part of critical care evaluation and management. Separate billing for review of EKG rhythm strips and cardiac output measurements (e.g., CPT codes 93040-93042, 93561, 93562) and critical care services is inappropriate. An exception to this may include a sudden change in patient status associated with a change in cardiac rhythm that requires a return to the ICU or telephonic transmission to review a rhythm strip. If reported separately, time included for this service is not included in the critical care time calculated for the critical care service.

7. Angioplasty procedures include insertion of a needle and/or catheter, infusion fluoroscopy, and EKG strips (e.g., CPT codes 36000, 36120, 36140, 36160, 36200-36248, 36410, 90780-90784, 76000-76001, and 93040-93042). All are components of performing an angioplasty.

8. Cardiovascular stress tests include insertion of needle and/or catheter, infusion (pharmacologic stress tests), and EKG strips (e.g., CPT codes 36000, 36410, 90780-90784, 93000-93010, and 93040-93042).

9. Ventilation management and continuous positive airway pressure (CPAP) ventilation initiation and management services are mutually exclusive of evaluation and management services with the exception of critical care services. Critical care services (CPT codes 99291-99292) include ventilation management (CPT codes 94656-94657) and CPAP management (CPT codes 94660, 94662).

10. Cardiac catheterization procedures may require procurement of EKG tracings during the procedure to assess chest pain during catheterization and angioplasty; when performed in this fashion, these EKG tracings are not separately reported. EKGs procured prior to or after the procedure may be separately reported with the -59 modifier.

11. CPT codes 93539-93545 (cardiac catheterization) include CPT codes 71034, 76000, and 76001 (fluoroscopy).

NONINVASIVE VASCULAR STUDIES

Vascular studies refers to diagnostic procedures performed to determine blood flow and/or the condition of arteries and/or veins. Vascular studies include patient care required to perform the studies, supervision of the studies, and interpretation of the study results with copies for patient records of hard copy output with analysis of all data, including bidirectional vascular flow or imaging when provided.

The use of a simple hand-held or other Doppler device that does not produce hard copy output or that produces a record that does not permit analysis of bidirectional vascular flow is considered to be part of the physical examination of the vascular system and is not reported separately. To report unilateral noninvasive diagnostic studies, add modifier -52 to the basic code.

A Duplex Scan is defined as "An ultrasonic scanning procedure with display of both two-dimensional structure and motion with time and Doppler ultrasonic signal documentation with spectral analysis and/or color flow velocity mapping or imaging."

Coding Rules

1) Noninvasive vascular studies are usually performed in addition to E/M service, such as a consultation or visit, and should be reported separately in addition to the E/M service.

2) All of the noninvasive vascular services fall under the Medicare Purchased Diagnostic Services guidelines; therefore, reporting should be as instructed by your local Medicare carrier.

PULMONARY SERVICES

Pulmonary services refer to diagnostic procedures performed to determine air flow, blood gases, and the condition of the lungs and respiratory system. Pulmonary services include the laboratory procedure(s), interpretation, and physician's services (except surgical and anesthesia services) unless otherwise stated. It is common for pulmonologists to provide interpretation services only, under contract to medical facilities.

Coding Rules

1) Pulmonary services are usually performed in addition to E/M service, such as a consultation or visit, and should be reported separately in addition to the E/M service.

2) When reporting physician interpretation only for pulmonary services, include the modifier -26 "Professional Component."

3) Most of the pulmonary services fall under the Medicare Purchased Diagnostic Services guidelines; therefore reporting should be as instructed by your local Medicare carrier.

CORRECT CODING ISSUES FOR PULMONARY SERVICES

CPT coding for pulmonary function tests includes both comprehensive and component codes to accommodate variation among pulmonary function laboratories. As a result of these code combinations, several issues are addressed in this policy section.

1. Alternate methods of reporting data obtained during a spirometry or other pulmonary function session cannot be separately reported. Specifically, the flow volume loop is an alternative method of calculating a standard spirometric parameter. The CPT code 94375 is included in standard spirometry (rest and exercise) studies.

2. When a physician who is in attendance for a pulmonary function study obtains a limited history and performs a limited examination referable specifically to the pulmonary function testing, separately coding for an evaluation and management service is not appropriate. If a significant, separately identifiable service is performed unrelated to the technical performance of the pulmonary function test, then an evaluation and management service may be reported.

3. When multiple spirometric determinations are necessary (e.g., CPT code 94070) to complete the service described in the CPT code, only one unit of service is reported.

4. Pulmonary stress testing (e.g., CPT code 94620) is a comprehensive stress test with a number of component tests separately defined in the CPT code book. It is inappropriate to separately code venous access; EKG monitoring; spirometric parameters performed before, during, and after exercise; oximetry; O_2 consumption; CO_2 production; rebreathing cardiac output calculations; etc. when performed as part of a progressive pulmonary exercise test. It is also inappropriate to bill for a cardiac stress test and the component codes used to perform a routine pulmonary stress test when a comprehensive pulmonary stress test was performed. If using a standard exercise protocol, serial electrocardiograms are obtained, and a separate report describing a cardiac stress test (professional component) is included in the medical record, both a cardiac and pulmonary stress test could be reported. The -59 modifier should be reported with the secondary procedure. In addition, if both tests are reported, both tests must satisfy the requirement for medical necessity.

ALLERGY AND IMMUNOLOGY

Allergy and Immunology refers to diagnostic services performed to determine a patient's sensitivity to specific substances, the treatment of patients with allergens by the administration of allergenic extracts, and/or medical conference services.

Coding Rules

1) Allergy and immunology services are usually performed in addition to E/M service, such as a consultation or visit, and should be reported separately in addition to the E/M service.

2) Summary or therapeutic conferences following completion of the diagnostic workup (including discussion, avoidance, elimination, symptomatic treatment, and immunotherapy) should be reported with E/M service codes 99241-99245.

3) Prolonged conferences should be reported with E/M Case Management codes.

ALLERGEN IMMUNOTHERAPY

Allergen immunotherapy codes include the professional services necessary for allergen immunotherapy. E/M service codes may be reported in addition to allergen immunotherapy if and only if other identifiable services are provided at that time. HCPCS includes two codes, J7010 and J7020, to report provision of allergy vaccine to Medicare patients.

CORRECT CODING ISSUES FOR ALLERGEN IMMUNOTHERAPY

The CPT code book divides allergy and clinical immunology into testing and immunotherapy. Immunotherapy is divided into codes that include preparation of the antigen when it is administered at the same session and when it is prepared but delivered for immunotherapy by a different physician. Several specific issues are identified regarding allergy testing and immunotherapy.

1. If a local carrier provides coverage for skin end-point titration and standard testing is performed on the same day for the same allergen, only the code for skin end-point titration is reported. Additionally, the relative-value unit of this test has been determined on the basis of one unit of service for one titration/one allergen. Accordingly, this code should be reported as one unit of service for each antigen, regardless of the number of injections necessary to complete the titration.

2. When photo patch tests (e.g., CPT code 95052) are performed (same antigen/same session) with patch or application tests, only the photo patch testing should be reported. Additionally, if photo testing is performed including application or patch testing, the code for photo patch testing (CPT

code 95052) is to be reported, not CPT code 95044 (patch or application tests) and CPT code 95056 (photo tests).

3. Evaluation and management codes reported with allergy testing or allergy immunotherapy are appropriate only if a significant, separately identifiable service is administered. Obtaining informed consent is included in the immunotherapy. If Evaluation and Management services are reported, medical documentation of the separately identifiable service should be in the medical record.

4. Allergy testing is not performed on the same day as allergy immunotherapy in standard medical practice. These codes should, therefore, not be reported together. Additionally, the testing becomes an integral part to rapid desensitization kits (CPT code 95180) and would therefore not be reported separately.

NEUROLOGY AND NEUROMUSCULAR PROCEDURES

Neurology refers to the study and treatment of the nervous system. Neurology services are usually performed in conjunction with a medical consultation. The consultation should be reported separately using the appropriate E/M consultation code.

Coding Rules

1) All EEG services listed include the tracing, interpretation, and report.

2) For interpretation of EEG only, add modifier -26 to the basic procedure code.

3) Most of the neurology and neuromuscular procedures fall under the Medicare Purchased Diagnostic Services guidelines; therefore, reporting should be as instructed by your local Medicare carrier.

CORRECT CODING ISSUES FOR NEUROMUSCULAR PROCEDURES

The CPT code book defines codes for neuromuscular diagnostic/therapeutic services not requiring surgical procedures. Sleep testing, nerve and muscle testing, and electroencephalographic procedures are included. The CPT code book guidelines regarding sleep testing are very precise and should be reviewed carefully before billing for these services.

1. Sleep testing differs from polysomnography in that the latter requires the presence of sleep staging. Sleep staging includes a qualitative and quantitative assessment of sleep as determined by standard sleep scoring techniques. Accordingly, at the same session, a "sleep study" and "polysomnography" are not reported together.

2. Polysomnography requires at least one central and usually several other EEG electrodes. EEG procurement for polysomnography (sleep staging) differs greatly from that required for diagnostic EEG testing (i.e., speed of paper, number of channels, etc.). Accordingly, EEG testing is not to be reported with polysomnography unless performed separately; the EEG tests, if rendered with a separate report, are to be reported with the -59 modifier, indicating that this represents a different session from the sleep study.

3. Continuous electroencephalographic monitoring services (CPT codes 95950-95962) represent different services than those provided during sleep testing; accordingly, these codes are to be reported only when a separately identifiable service is performed and documented. Additionally, billing standard EEG services would be appropriate only if a significant, separately identifiable service is provided. These codes are to be reported with the -59 modifier to indicate that a different service is clearly documented.

4. When nerve testing (EMG, nerve conduction velocity, etc.) is performed to assess the level of paralysis during anesthesia or during mechanical ventilation, the series of CPT codes 95851-95937 are not to be separately reported; these codes reflect significant, separately identifiable diagnostic services requiring a formal report in the medical record. Additionally, electrical stimulation used to identify or locate nerves as part of a procedure involving treatment of a cranial or peripheral nerve (e.g., nerve block, nerve destruction, neuroplasty, transection, excision, repair, etc.) is part of the primary procedure.

CHEMOTHERAPY ADMINISTRATION

Chemotherapy is the process of treating cancer with chemicals formulated to harm or destroy the cancer cells. Chemotherapy agents are administered via intravenous or infusion methods. Chemotherapy administration may be coded when administered by a physician or a qualified assistant under the supervision of a physician, excluding chemotherapy administered by hospital or home health agency personnel.

Coding Rules

1) Chemotherapy administration is independent of the patient's office visit.

2) The injection procedures may occur independently or on the same day as an office visit.

3) Visit services should be reported using the appropriate E/M service code in addition to the chemotherapy administration code.

4) Regional (isolation) chemotherapy perfusion should be reported using existing codes for arterial infusion.

5) Placement of the intra-arterial catheter should be reported using the appropriate code from the Cardiovascular Surgery section.

Chemotherapy Drugs

Chemotherapy administration codes do not include provision of the chemotherapy agent. CPT code 96545 is used to report and bill for provision of the chemotherapy agent for non-Medicare patients. For Medicare patients, choose HCPCS codes from the series J9000-J9999 to bill for chemotherapy drugs. See the following page for an example of how to bill this service properly.

Preparation of chemotherapy agent(s) is included in the service for administration of the agent. Report separate codes for each parenteral method of administration employed when chemotherapy is administered by different techniques.

CORRECT CODING ISSUES FOR CHEMOTHERAPY

1. Chemotherapy administration codes include codes for the administration of chemotherapeutic agents by multiple routes, the most common being the intravenous route. Separate payment is allowed for chemotherapy administration by push and by infusion technique on the same day, but only one push administration is allowed on a single day. It is recognized that combination chemotherapy is frequently provided by different routes at the same session. The -59 modifier can be appropriately used when two different modes of chemotherapy administration are used. The -59 modifier is used in this situation to indicate that two separate procedures are utilized to administer chemotherapeutic drug(s), not to indicate that two separate drugs are administered. (See MCM Section 15400.)

2. When infusion of saline, an antiemetic, or any other nonchemotherapy drug is required under CPT codes 90780-90781 and administered at the same time as the chemotherapeutic agents, the former infusions are not separately payable; however, the drugs are payable. If the hydration and/or infusion of antiemetics or any other nonchemotherapy drugs is administered on the same day but sequentially to rather than at the same time as the administration of the chemotherapeutic agents, these infusions are payable with CPT codes 90780-90781 using the -59 modifier to indicate that the infusions were administered at different time intervals.

3. In circumstances in which a physician has no face-to-face contact with the patient, a physician may report and be paid for *incident to* services in addition to the chemotherapy administration if these services are furnished by one of the physician's employees, under direct supervision in the office by one of the physician's employees, and the medical records reflect that the physician has actively participated in and managed the patient's course of treatment. The *incident to* A services in this situation are reported with the evaluation and management code 99211.

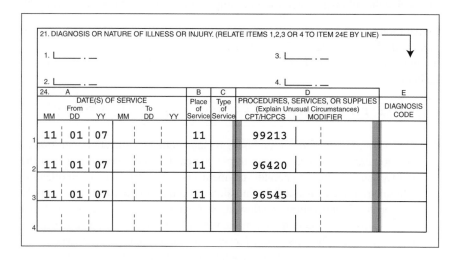

4. Flushing of a vascular access port prior to the administration of chemotherapeutic agents is integral to the chemotherapy administration and therefore is not separately reportable.

PHYSICAL MEDICINE AND REHABILITATION

Physical medicine is the diagnosis, treatment, and prevention of disease with the aid of physical agents such as light, heat, cold, water, or electricity or with mechanical devices. Physical medicine services may be provided by physicians or physical therapists. Physical medicine and rehabilitation codes are divided into three sections: Modalities, Procedures, and Tests and Measurements. Other services performed by medical professionals specializing in physical medicine and/or physical therapy include: muscle testing, range of joint motion, electromyography, biofeedback training by EMG, and transcutaneous nerve stimulation (TNS).

Coding Rules

1) The physician or therapist is required to be in constant attendance when reporting codes for modalities and procedures.

2) The physical medicine procedure codes specify treatment to one area, for the initial 30 minutes, and provide codes to report each additional 15 minutes of treatment.

SPECIAL PHYSICAL MEDICINE CODING ISSUES

Many worker's compensation and casualty health insurance companies use pre-CPT coding systems, such as CRVS, and do not use any form of diagnostic coding, relying instead on special reports to justify the procedures performed and services provided. As the majority of physical medicine services are performed for accidents and injuries, many that are work-related, the medical professionals performing these services must be informed of the specific reporting requirements in the areas that they practice.

MEDICAL NUTRITION THERAPY

Medical Nutrition Therapy (MNT) includes nutritional diagnostic, therapeutic, and counseling services provided by a registered dietitian. Medicare beneficiaries with diabetes and some types of kidney disease may be eligible for medical nutrition therapy to help manage their disease and improve their health. The CPT code book includes three codes that may be used for reporting MNT.

ACUPUNCTURE

Acupuncture is an alternative medicine service wherein stainless steel needles are inserted into various areas of the body. A low-frequency current may be applied to the needles to produce greater stimulation. In keeping with its policy of providing CPT codes for recognized alternative medicine services, the American Medical Association added codes for acupuncture services to the CPT code book in the 2005 edition.

Coding Rules

1) Acupuncture services are reported based on 15-minute increments of personal (face-to-face) contact with the patient, not the duration of acupuncture needle(s) placement.

2) CPT code selection for initial acupuncture services is dependent upon whether electrical stimulation is or is not used.

OSTEOPATHIC SERVICES

Osteopathic medicine is a system of therapy based on the theory that the body is capable of making its own remedies against disease and other toxic conditions when it is in normal structural relationship and has favorable environmental conditions and adequate nutrition. Osteopathic manipulative treatment (OMT) is a form of manual treatment applied by a physician to eliminate or alleviate somatic dysfunction and related disorders. This treatment may be accomplished by a variety of techniques.

Coding Rules

1) E/M services may be reported separately if and only if the patient's condition requires a significant separately identifiable E/M service above and beyond the usual preservice and postservice work associated with the osteopathic manipulation.

2) The codes in this section are used to report OMT services provided in any location.

CHIROPRACTIC SERVICES

Chiropractic medicine is a system of diagnosis and treatment based on the theory that irritation of the nervous system by mechanical, chemical, or psychic factors is the cause of disease. Chiropractic services may include office visits, diagnostic tests, physical therapy, and/or chiropractic manipulation. Chiropractic manipulation treatment (CMT) is a form of manual treatment applied by a chiropractic physician to eliminate or alleviate somatic dysfunction and related disorders.

Coding Rules

1) Chiropractic manipulation treatment includes a premanipulation patient assessment.

2) E/M services provided in conjunction with CMT may be reported separately with the addition of CPT modifier -25, along with any diagnostic tests or other therapy provided.

REPORTING CHIROPRACTIC MANIPULATION TO MEDICARE

Medicare restricts the number of times the CMT code may be reported, provides a maximum reimbursement amount per year, and requires extensive supporting documentation as described below.

Documentation of Treatment Phase

Proper documentation of the treatment phase is extremely important when submitting claims for chiropractic services to Medicare. The treatment phase consists of the date the course of treatment was initiated and the number of treatments rendered to date. Proper documentation enables Medicare to process your claims quickly and accurately. For payment of chiropractic claims, the following information must be on the CMS1500 claim form:

1) The service must be manual manipulation of the spine. This service is reported by CPT codes 98940-98943.

2) The primary diagnosis must be subluxation of the spine, either so stated or identified by a term descriptive of the subluxation. The following diagnoses are acceptable because they would always involve a subluxation:

intervertebral disc disorders	722.0-722.9
curvatures of the spine	737.0-737.9
spondylolisthesis	738.4, 756.12
nonallopathic lesions	739.1-739.4
spondylolysis	756.11

3) The level of subluxation must be stated.

4) The symptoms related to the level of subluxation must be given.

5) The date of the confirming x-ray must be on the claim. Note that the x-ray must have been taken within 12 months prior to or three months after the course of treatment was initiated.

6) The date this course of treatment was initiated and the number of treatments rendered since the start of this course must be on the claim.

Special Situations

If a patient returns with a new condition or injury, this represents a new treatment phase. The treatment phase information should reflect when you first saw the patient for this condition. Do not use the date you first saw the patient for an earlier course of treatment. Note on your CMS-1500 claim form that this is a new condition. Remember that a new documenting x-ray may be required.

In the case of chronic conditions, an x-ray older than 12 months may be acceptable. For coverage of chronic conditions such as scoliosis, spondylolysis, and spondylolisthesis, there must be a reasonable expectation that there is a restorative potential. Remember that maintenance care is not covered by Medicare.

SPECIAL SERVICES AND REPORTS

The Medicine section of the CPT code book includes the subsection Special Services and Reports, with CPT codes 99000-99090, which provides the reporting physician with a means of identifying the completion of special reports and services that are an adjunct to the basic services rendered. The specific special services code reported indicates the special circumstances under which a basic procedure is performed.

The proper use of Special Services codes can result in a significant increase in reimbursement. Most of the codes in this section are "add-on" codes, which means that they are used in addition to whatever other codes describe the procedures or services performed.

SPECIMEN HANDLING

99000   Handling and/or conveyance of specimen transfer from the physician's office to a laboratory

99001   Handling and/or conveyance of specimen for transfer from the patient in other than a physician's office to a laboratory (distance may be indicated)

99002   Handling, conveyance, and/or any other service in connection with the implementation of an order involving devices (e.g., designing, fitting, packaging, handling, delivery, or mailing) when devices such as orthotics, protectives, or prosthetics are fabricated by an outside laboratory or shop but which items have been designed and are to be fitted and adjusted by the attending physician

For routine collection of venous blood, report CPT code 36415.

SPECIAL VISIT CODES

99024   Postoperative follow-up visit, included in global service

                 This code is used to track no-charge postoperative visits. As a component of a surgical package, review the Guidelines of the Surgery section.

SERVICES RENDERED AFTER REGULAR OFFICE HOURS

99050   Services requested after office hours in addition to basic service

99052   Services requested between 10:00 PM and 8:00 AM in addition to basic service

99054   Services requested on Sundays and holidays in addition to basic service

                 Note that codes 99050-99054 are reported in addition to the E/M service code used to report the basic service(s).

SERVICES RENDERED AT SPECIAL LOCATION

99056   Services provided at request of patient in a location other than physician's office

Note that code 99056 is reported in addition to the E/M service code used to report the basic service(s).

OFFICE EMERGENCY SERVICES

99058   Office services provided on an emergency basis

The diagnostic codes used to bill for this service must clearly justify the nature of the emergency.

SUPPLIES AND MATERIALS

99070   Supplies and materials (except spectacles), provided by the physician over and above those usually included with the office visit or other services rendered (list drugs, trays, supplies, or materials provided). For spectacles, use codes 92390-92395.

Note that HCPCS Level II codes are *always* used instead of CPT code 99070 when reporting supplies, materials, and drugs to Medicare.

99071   Educational supplies, such as books, tapes, and pamphlets, provided by the physician for the patient's education at cost to physician

99075   Medical testimony

This code may be used to report medical testimony provided as part of malpractice, worker's compensation, and casualty cases. If you appear as an expert witness, negotiate appearance and stand-by fees with the attorneys up-front. Demand payment prior to appearance.

99078   Physician educational services rendered to patients in a group setting, for example, prenatal, obesity, or diabetic instructions

SPECIAL REPORTS

99080 Special reports such as health insurance forms or the review of medical data to clarify a patient's status—more than the information conveyed in the usual medical communications or standard report form

     This code is used frequently to report review of medical records in worker's compensation and casualty cases.

99082 Unusual travel (e.g., transportation and escort of patient)

     This code may also be used to report travel associated with medical testimony.

99090 Analysis of information data stored in computers (e.g., ECGs, blood pressures, hematologic data)

HOME HEALTH PROCEDURES/SERVICES

CPT codes for home health procedures/services are used by nonphysician providers to report services provided in a patient's residence. The term "residence" includes assisted-living apartments, group homes, custodial care facilities, or schools.

Nonphysician providers authorized to report E & M home visit codes may report home health procedures/services codes in addition to the visit codes in the event both services are performed.

CPT CATEGORY II CODES

This section of the CPT code book includes a set of supplemental tracking codes that can be used for performance measurement. All Category II codes end with the letter F. These codes are designed to facilitate data collection about the quality of care. The use of these codes is optional. These codes are not required for correct coding and should not be used on health insurance claim forms.

CPT CATEGORY III CODES

This section of the CPT code book includes a set of temporary codes to describe emerging technology, services, and procedures. All Category III codes end with the letter T. The codes in this section should be used instead of unlisted codes from other sections of the CPT code book if they correctly describe an unlisted procedure.

TRANSPORTATION SERVICES

CPT includes only one code to report transportation services. If the medical professional accompanied the patient on a long hospital transfer by ambulance, air ambulance, or long distance by common carrier, CPT code 99082 is reported in addition to any other services provided.

HCPCS Level II codes A0000-A0999 cover emergency ambulance service using surface, air, or water transport, plus nonemergency transportation services. There are also specific Ambulance Service Modifiers and a waiting-time table to be used with these codes.

MISCELLANEOUS AND EXPERIMENTAL SERVICES

HCPCS Level II includes codes that may be used to report miscellaneous and experimental services or procedures. Most of the codes in this section begin with the term "noncovered." As Medicare will not reimburse noncovered services, there is no reason to report these codes unless specifically instructed to do so by your local Medicare intermediary.

DENTAL PROCEDURES

There are no CPT codes to report dental services. Most dental procedures are reported using Current Dental Terminology (CDT) published by the American Dental Association. There are HCPCS Level II codes that describe dental services and procedures; however, these codes are generally noncovered by Medicare.

REHABILITATIVE SERVICES

The codes listed in this section of the HCPCS Level II book describe residential care, group psychotherapy, special classes, and other services that are generally noncovered by Medicare.

TEMPORARY CODES

Temporary codes are HCPCS Level II codes assigned by CMS on a temporary basis. These codes change frequently and may be deleted or replaced completely from one year to the next.

CPT ANATOMICAL ILLUSTRATIONS

A fundamental knowledge and understanding of basic human anatomy and physiology is a prerequisite for accurate CPT procedure coding. While a comprehensive treatment of anatomy and physiology is beyond the scope of this text, the large scale, full color anatomical illustrations on the following pages are designed to facilitate the procedure coding process for both beginning and experienced coders.

The illustrations provide an anatomical perspective of procedure coding by providing a side-by-side view of the major systems of the human body and a corresponding list of the most common CPT procedural categories used to report medical, surgical and diagnostic services performed on the illustrated system.

The CPT procedural categories listed on the left facing page of each anatomical illustration are code ranges only and should not be used for coding. These categories are provided as "pointers" to the appropriate section of CPT, where the definitive code may be found.

CPT
ANATOMICAL
ILLUSTRATIONS

PLATE 1. SKIN AND SUBCUTANEOUS TISSUE-MALE

Skin, Subcutaneous and Accessory Structures

Incision and Drainage	10040-10180
Excision-Debridement	11000-11044
Paring or Cutting	11055-11057
Biopsy	11100-11101
Removal of Skin Tags	11200-11201
Shaving of Epidermal or Dermal Lesions	11300-11313
Excision-Benign Lesions	11400-11471
Excision-Malignant Lesions	11600-11646

Nails   11719-11765

Repair (Closure)

Repair-Simple	12001-12021
Repair-Intermediate	12031-12057
Repair-Complex	13100-13160
Adjacent Tissue Transfer	14000-14350
Free Skin Grafts	15000-15400
Flaps (Skin and/or Deep Tissues)	15570-15738
Other Flaps and Grafts	15740-15776
Other Procedures	15780-15879
Pressure Ulcers (Decubitus Ulcers)	15920-15999
Burns	16000-16036

Destruction

Destruction, Benign or Premalignant Lesions	17000-17250
Destruction, Malignant Lesions	17260-17286
Mohs' Micrographic Surgery	17304-17310
Other Destruction Procedures	17340-17999

Laboratory Services

Skin Tests, Immunology	86485-86586
Skin Tests, Allergy	95010-95199

Visit and Medicine Services

E/M Services	99201-99499
Special Dermatological Procedures	96900-96999

Male Figure
(Anterior View)

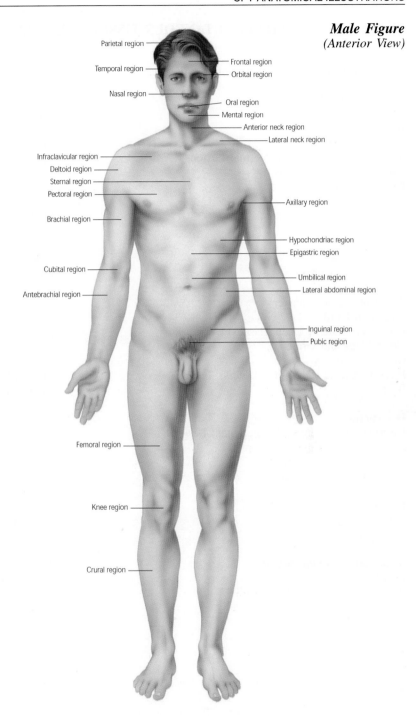

Parietal region

Temporal region

Nasal region

Frontal region

Orbital region

Oral region

Mental region

Anterior neck region

Lateral neck region

Infraclavicular region

Deltoid region

Sternal region

Pectoral region

Brachial region

Axillary region

Hypochondriac region

Epigastric region

Cubital region

Umbilical region

Antebrachial region

Lateral abdominal region

Inguinal region

Pubic region

Femoral region

Knee region

Crural region

PLATE 2. SKIN AND SUBCUTANEOUS TISSUE - FEMALE

Skin, Subcutaneous and Accessory Structures

Incision and Drainage	10040-10180
Excision-Debridement	11000-11044
Paring or Cutting	11055-11057
Biopsy	11100-11101
Removal of Skin Tags	11200-11201
Shaving of Epidermal or Dermal Lesions	11300-11313
Excision-Benign Lesions	11400-11471
Excision-Malignant Lesions	11600-11646

Nails   11719-11765

Repair (Closure)

Repair-Simple	12001-12021
Repair-Intermediate	12031-12057
Repair-Complex	13100-13160
Adjacent Tissue Transfer	14000-14350
Free Skin Grafts	15000-15400
Flaps (Skin and/or Deep Tissues)	15570-15738
Other Flaps and Grafts	15740-15776
Other Procedures	15780-15879
Pressure Ulcers (Decubitus Ulcers)	15920-15999
Burns	16000-16036

Destruction

Destruction, Benign or Premalignant Lesions	17000-17250
Destruction, Malignant Lesions	17260-17286
Mohs' Micrographic Surgery	17304-17310
Other Destruction Procedures	17340-17999

Laboratory Services

Skin Tests, Immunology	86485-86586
Skin Tests, Allergy	95010-95199

Visit and Medicine Services

E/M Services	99201-99499
Special Dermatological Procedures	96900-96999

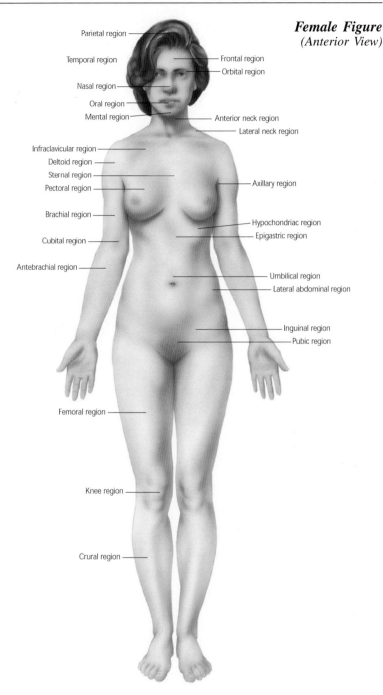

Female Figure
(Anterior View)

Parietal region

Temporal region

Nasal region

Oral region

Mental region

Frontal region

Orbital region

Anterior neck region

Lateral neck region

Infraclavicular region

Deltoid region

Sternal region

Pectoral region

Axillary region

Brachial region

Cubital region

Hypochondriac region

Epigastric region

Antebrachial region

Umbilical region

Lateral abdominal region

Inguinal region

Pubic region

Femoral region

Knee region

Crural region

© Practice Management Information Corp., Los Angeles, CA

PLATE 3. FEMALE BREAST

Breast

Incision	19000-19030
Excision	19100-19272
Introduction	19290-19295
Repair and/or Reconstruction	19316-19396
Other Procedures	19499

Radiology Services

Magnetic Resonance Imaging (MRI)	76093-76094
Stereotactic Localization	76095
Ultrasound	76645
Mammogram	76082-76092

E/M Services   99201-99499

Female Breast

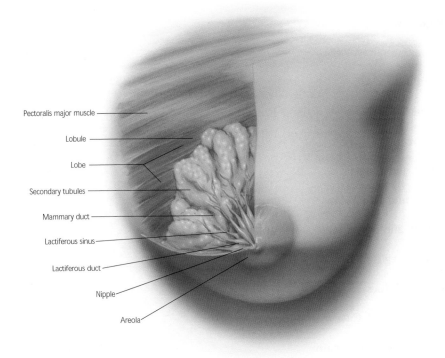

Pectoralis major muscle

Lobule

Lobe

Secondary tubules

Mammary duct

Lactiferous sinus

Lactiferous duct

Nipple

Areola

PLATE 4. MUSCULAR SYSTEM AND CONNECTIVE TISSUE - ANTERIOR VIEW

General	20000-20999
Head	21010-21499
Neck (Soft Tissues) and Thorax	21501-21899
Back and Flank	21920-21935
Spine (Vertebral Column)	22100-22899
Abdomen	22900-22999
Shoulder	23000-23929
Humerous (Upper Arm) and Elbow	23930-24999
Forearm and Wrist	25000-25999
Hand and Fingers	26010-26989
Pelvis and Hip Joint	26990-27299
Femur and Knee Joint	27301-27599
Lower Leg and Ankle Joint	27600-27899
Foot and Toes	28001-28899
Application of Casts/Strapping	29000-29799
Endoscopy/Arthroscopy	29800-29999
E/M Services	99201-99499

Muscular System
(Anterior View)

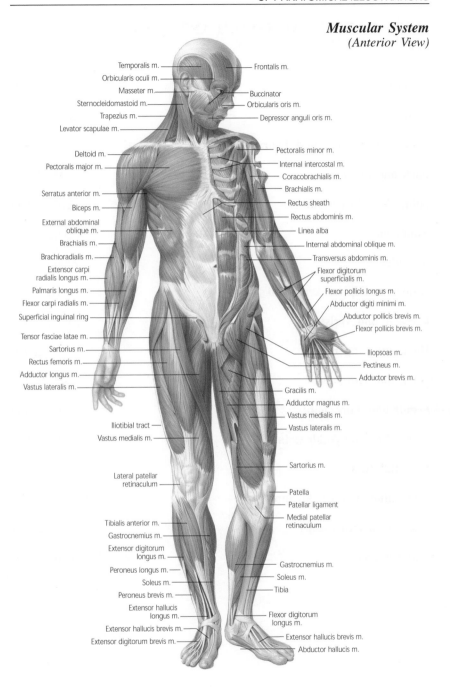

Temporalis m. — — Frontalis m.
Orbicularis oculi m.
Masseter m.
Sternocleidomastoid m. — Buccinator
Trapezius m. — Orbicularis oris m.
Levator scapulae m. — Depressor anguli oris m.

Deltoid m. — — Pectoralis minor m.
Pectoralis major m. — Internal intercostal m.
— Coracobrachialis m.
Serratus anterior m. — Brachialis m.
Biceps m. — Rectus sheath
External abdominal — Rectus abdominis m.
oblique m. — Linea alba
Brachialis m. — Internal abdominal oblique m.
Brachioradialis m. — Transversus abdominis m.
Extensor carpi
radialis longus m. — Flexor digitorum
superficialis m.
Palmaris longus m. — Flexor pollicis longus m.
Flexor carpi radialis m. — Abductor digiti minimi m.
Superficial inguinal ring — Abductor pollicis brevis m.
— Flexor pollicis brevis m.
Tensor fasciae latae m. — Iliopsoas m.
Sartorius m. — Pectineus m.
Rectus femoris m. — Adductor brevis m.
Adductor longus m.
Vastus lateralis m. — Gracilis m.
— Adductor magnus m.
— Vastus medialis m.
— Vastus lateralis m.
Iliotibial tract —
Vastus medialis m. — Sartorius m.

Lateral patellar
retinaculum — Patella
— Patellar ligament
— Medial patellar
retinaculum
Tibialis anterior m. —
Gastrocnemius m. —
Extensor digitorum
longus m. — Gastrocnemius m.
Peroneus longus m. — Soleus m.
Soleus m. — Tibia
Peroneus brevis m. —
Extensor hallucis
longus m. — Flexor digitorum
longus m.
Extensor hallucis brevis m. — Extensor hallucis brevis m.
Extensor digitorum brevis m. — Abductor hallucis m.

PLATE 5. MUSCULAR SYSTEM AND CONNECTIVE TISSUE - POSTERIOR VIEW

General	20000-20999
Head	21010-21499
Neck (Soft Tissues) and Thorax	21501-21899
Back and Flank	21920-21935
Spine (Vertebral Column)	22100-22899
Abdomen	22900-22999
Shoulder	23000-23929
Humerous (Upper Arm) and Elbow	23930-24999
Forearm and Wrist	25000-25999
Hand and Fingers	26010-26989
Pelvis and Hip Joint	26990-27299
Femur and Knee Joint	27301-27599
Lower Leg and Ankle Joint	27600-27899
Foot and Toes	28001-28899
Application of Casts/Strapping	29000-29799
Endoscopy/Arthroscopy	29800-29999
E/M Services	99201-99499

Muscular System
(Posterior View)

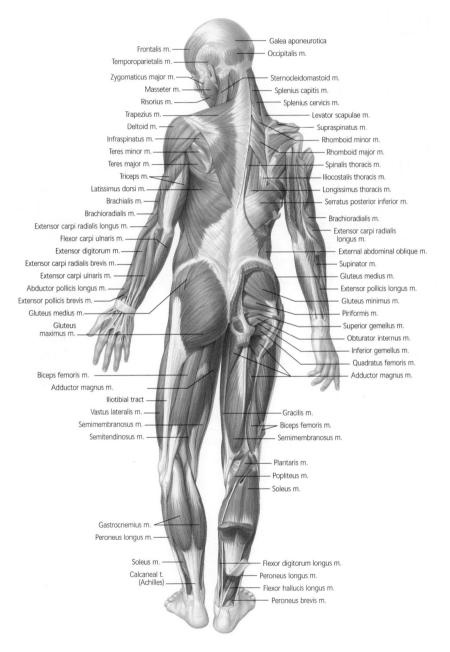

Frontalis m.
Temporoparietalis m.
Zygomaticus major m.
Masseter m.
Risorius m.
Trapezius m.
Deltoid m.
Infraspinatus m.
Teres minor m.
Teres major m.
Triceps m.
Latissimus dorsi m.
Brachialis m.
Brachioradialis m.
Extensor carpi radialis longus m.
Flexor carpi ulnaris m.
Extensor digitorum m.
Extensor carpi radialis brevis m.
Extensor carpi ulnaris m.
Abductor pollicis longus m.
Extensor pollicis brevis m.
Gluteus medius m.
Gluteus maximus m.
Biceps femoris m.
Adductor magnus m.
Iliotibial tract
Vastus lateralis m.
Semimembranosus m.
Semitendinosus m.
Gastrocnemius m.
Peroneus longus m.
Soleus m.
Calcaneal t. (Achilles)

Galea aponeurotica
Occipitalis m.
Sternocleidomastoid m.
Splenius capitis m.
Splenius cervicis m.
Levator scapulae m.
Supraspinatus m.
Rhomboid minor m.
Rhomboid major m.
Spinalis thoracis m.
Iliocostalis thoracis m.
Longissimus thoracis m.
Serratus posterior inferior m.
Brachioradialis m.
Extensor carpi radialis longus m.
External abdominal oblique m.
Supinator m.
Gluteus medius m.
Extensor pollicis longus m.
Gluteus minimus m.
Piriformis m.
Superior gemellus m.
Obturator internus m.
Inferior gemellus m.
Quadratus femoris m.
Adductor magnus m.
Gracilis m.
Biceps femoris m.
Semimembranosus m.
Plantaris m.
Popliteus m.
Soleus m.
Flexor digitorum longus m.
Peroneus longus m.
Flexor hallucis longus m.
Peroneus brevis m.

PLATE 6. MUSCULAR SYSTEM - SHOULDER AND ELBOW

General
Wound exploration - Trauma	20100-20103
Excision	20150-20251
Introduction or Removal	20500-20694
Replantation	20802-20838
Grafts of Implants	20900-20938
Other	20950-20999

Shoulder
Incision	23000-23044
Excision	23065-23222
Introduction or Removal	23330-23350
Fracture and/or Dislocation	23500-23680
Manipulation	23700
Arthrodesis	23800-23802
Amputation	23900-23921
Other	23929

Humerous (Upper Arm) and Elbow
Incision	23930-24006
Excision	24065-24155
Introduction or Removal	24160-24220
Repair, Revision and/or Reconstruction	24300-24498
Fracture and/or Dislocation	24500-24685
Arthrodesis	24800-24802
Amputation	24900-24940
Other	24999

Application of Casts/Strapping
Body and Upper Extremity Casts and Strapping	29000-29280
Removal or Repair	29700-29750
Other	29799

Endoscopy/Arthroscopy
29805-29838

Radiology Services
73000-73225

E/M Services
99201-99499

Shoulder and Elbow
(Anterior View)

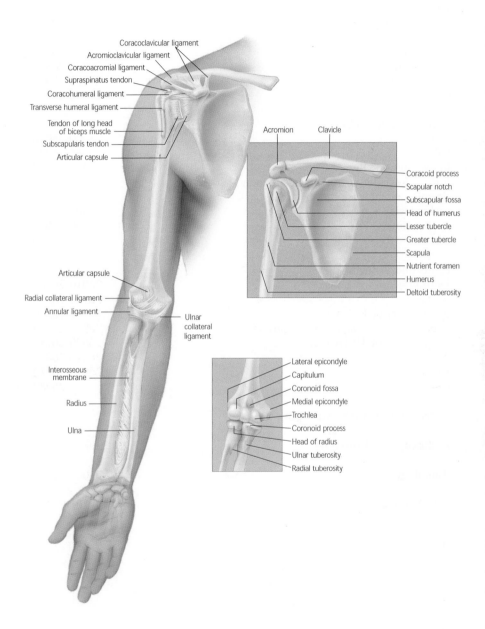

Coracoclavicular ligament
Acromioclavicular ligament
Coracoacromial ligament
Supraspinatus tendon
Coracohumeral ligament
Transverse humeral ligament
Tendon of long head of biceps muscle
Subscapularis tendon
Articular capsule

Acromion
Clavicle

Coracoid process
Scapular notch
Subscapular fossa
Head of humerus
Lesser tubercle
Greater tubercle
Scapula
Nutrient foramen
Humerus
Deltoid tuberosity

Articular capsule
Radial collateral ligament
Annular ligament
Ulnar collateral ligament

Interosseous membrane
Radius
Ulna

Lateral epicondyle
Capitulum
Coronoid fossa
Medial epicondyle
Trochlea
Coronoid process
Head of radius
Ulnar tuberosity
Radial tuberosity

PLATE 7. MUSCULAR SYSTEM - HAND AND WRIST

General

Wound exploration - Trauma	20100-20103
Excision	20105-20251
Introduction or Removal	20500-20694
Replantation	20802-20838
Grafts of Implants	20900-20938
Other	20950-20999

Forearm and Wrist

Incision	25000-25040
Excision	25065-25240
Introduction or Removal	25246-25259
Repair, Revision and/or Reconstruction	25260-25492
Fracture and/or Dislocation	25500-25695
Arthrodesis	25800-25830
Amputation	25900-25931
Other	25999

Hand and Fingers

Incision	26010-26080
Excision	26100-26262
Introduction or Removal	26320
Repair, Revision, and/or Reconstruction	26340-26596
Fracture and/or Dislocation	26600-26785
Arthrodesis	26820-26863
Amputation	26910-26952
Other	26989

Application of Casts/Strapping

29000-29280

Endoscopy/Arthroscopy

29840-29848

Radiology Services

73000-73225

E/M Services

99201-99499

Hand and Wrist

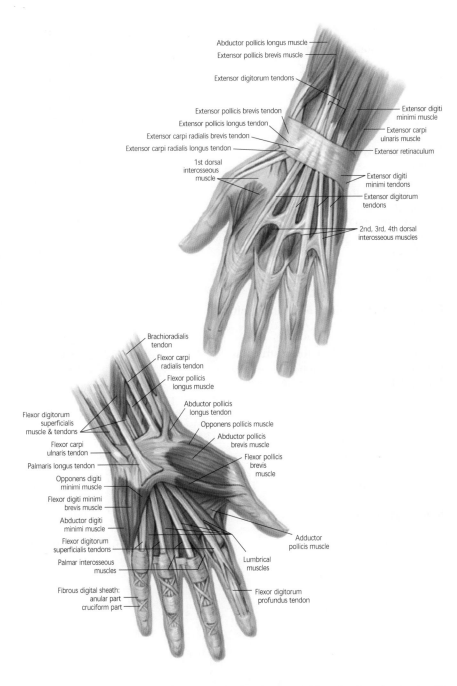

Abductor pollicis longus muscle

Extensor pollicis brevis muscle

Extensor digitorum tendons

Extensor pollicis brevis tendon

Extensor pollicis longus tendon

Extensor carpi radialis brevis tendon

Extensor carpi radialis longus tendon

1st dorsal interosseous muscle

Extensor digiti minimi muscle

Extensor carpi ulnaris muscle

Extensor retinaculum

Extensor digiti minimi tendons

Extensor digitorum tendons

2nd, 3rd, 4th dorsal interosseous muscles

Brachioradialis tendon

Flexor carpi radialis tendon

Flexor pollicis longus muscle

Abductor pollicis longus tendon

Flexor digitorum superficialis muscle & tendons

Opponens pollicis muscle

Abductor pollicis brevis muscle

Flexor carpi ulnaris tendon

Flexor pollicis brevis muscle

Palmaris longus tendon

Opponens digiti minimi muscle

Flexor digiti minimi brevis muscle

Abductor digiti minimi muscle

Adductor pollicis muscle

Flexor digitorum superficialis tendons

Palmar interosseous muscles

Lumbrical muscles

Fibrous digital sheath: anular part cruciform part

Flexor digitorum profundus tendon

PLATE 8. MUSCULOSKELETAL SYSTEM - HIP AND KNEE

General

Wound Exploration - Trauma	20100-20103
Excision	20150-20251
Introduction or Removal	20500-20694
Replantation	20802-20838
Grafts of Implants	20900-20938
Other	20950-20999

Pelvis and Hip Joint

Incision	26990-27036
Excision	27040-27080
Introduction or Removal	27086-27096
Repair, Revision, and/or Reconstruction	27097-27187
Fracture and/or Dislocation	27193-27266
Manipulation	27275
Arthrodesis	27280-27286
Amputation	27290-27295
Other	27299

Femur (Thigh Region) and Knee Joint

Incision	27301-27320
Excision	27323-27365
Repair, Revision, and/or Reconstruction	27380-27499
Fracture and/or Dislocation	27500-27566
Manipulation	27570
Arthrodesis	27580
Amputation	27590-27598
Other	27599

Application of Casts/Strapping	29005-29590
Endoscopy/Arthroscopy	29850-29899
Radiology Services	73500-73725
E/M Services	99201-99499

Hip and Knee
(Anterior View)

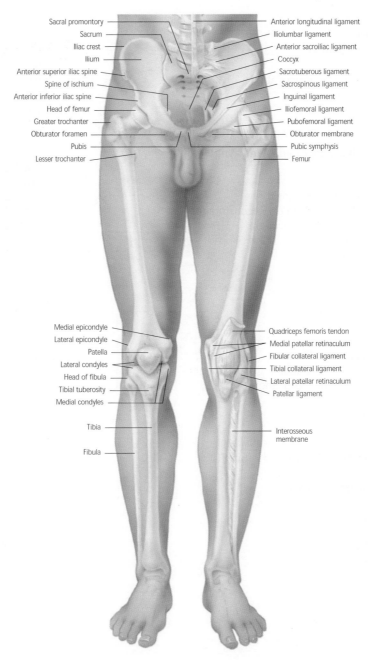

Sacral promontory
Sacrum
Iliac crest
Ilium
Anterior superior iliac spine
Spine of ischium
Anterior inferior iliac spine
Head of femur
Greater trochanter
Obturator foramen
Pubis
Lesser trochanter

Anterior longitudinal ligament
Iliolumbar ligament
Anterior sacroiliac ligament
Coccyx
Sacrotuberous ligament
Sacrospinous ligament
Inguinal ligament
Iliofemoral ligament
Pubofemoral ligament
Obturator membrane
Pubic symphysis
Femur

Medial epicondyle
Lateral epicondyle
Patella
Lateral condyles
Head of fibula
Tibial tuberosity
Medial condyles

Tibia

Fibula

Quadriceps femoris tendon
Medial patellar retinaculum
Fibular collateral ligament
Tibial collateral ligament
Lateral patellar retinaculum
Patellar ligament

Interosseous
membrane

PLATE 9. MUSCULOSKELETAL SYSTEM - FOOT AND ANKLE

General

Wound Exploration - Trauma	20100-20103
Excision	20150-20251
Introduction or Removal	20500-20694
Replantation	20802-20838
Grafts of Implants	20900-20938
Other	20950-20999

Leg (Tibia and Fibula) and Ankle Joint

Incision	27600-27612
Excision	27613-27647
Introduction or Removal	27648
Repair, Revision and/or Reconstruction	27650-27745
Fracture and/or Dislocation	27750-27848
Manipulation	27860
Arthrodesis	27870-27871
Amputation	27880-27889
Other	27892-27899

Foot and Toes

Incision	28001-28035
Excision	28043-28175
Introduction or Removal	28190-28193
Repair, Revision, and/or Reconstruction	28200-28360
Fracture and/or Dislocation	28400-28675
Arthrodesis	28705-28760
Amputation	28800-28825
Other	28899

Application of Casts/Strapping	29305-29590
Endoscopy/Arthroscopy	29891-29999
Radiology Services	73500-73725
E/M Services	99201-99499

Foot and Ankle

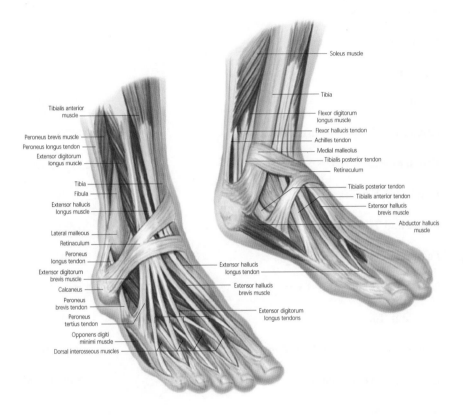

Soleus muscle

Tibia

Tibialis anterior muscle

Flexor digitorum longus muscle

Flexor hallucis tendon

Peroneus brevis muscle

Peroneus longus tendon

Achilles tendon

Extensor digitorum longus muscle

Medial malleolus

Tibialis posterior tendon

Retinaculum

Tibia

Fibula

Tibialis posterior tendon

Tibialis anterior tendon

Extensor hallucis longus muscle

Extensor hallucis brevis muscle

Abductor hallucis muscle

Lateral malleous

Retinaculum

Peroneus longus tendon

Extensor hallucis longus tendon

Extensor digitorum brevis muscle

Calcaneus

Extensor hallucis brevis muscle

Peroneus brevis tendon

Peroneus tertius tendon

Extensor digitorum longus tendons

Opponens digiti minimi muscle

Dorsal interosseous muscles

PLATE 10. SKELETAL SYSTEM - ANTERIOR VIEW

General	20100-20999
Head	21010-21499
Neck (Soft Tissues) and Thorax	21501-21899
Back and Flank	21920-21935
Spine (Vertebral Column)	22100-22899
Abdomen	22900-22999
Shoulder	23000-23929
Humerous (Upper Arm) and Elbow	23930-24999
Forearm and Wrist	25000-25999
Hand and Fingers	26010-26989
Pelvis and Hip Joint	26990-27299
Femur and Knee Joint	27301-27599
Lower Leg and Ankle Joint	27600-27899
Foot and Toes	28001-28899
Application of Casts/Strapping	29000-29799
Endoscopy/Arthroscopy	29800-29999
Radiology Services	70010-73725
E/M Services	99201-99499

Skeletal System
(Anterior View)

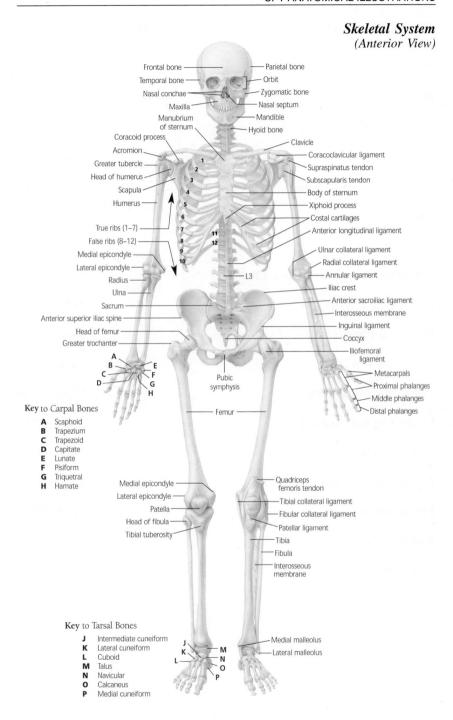

Frontal bone — — Parietal bone
Temporal bone — — Orbit
Nasal conchae — — Zygomatic bone
Maxilla — — Nasal septum
Manubrium of sternum — — Mandible
— Hyoid bone
Coracoid process — — Clavicle
Acromion — — Coracoclavicular ligament
Greater tubercle — — Supraspinatus tendon
Head of humerus — — Subscapularis tendon
Scapula — — Body of sternum
Humerus — — Xiphoid process
— Costal cartilages
True ribs (1–7) — — Anterior longitudinal ligament
False ribs (8–12) —
Medial epicondyle — — Ulnar collateral ligament
Lateral epicondyle — — Radial collateral ligament
Radius — — Annular ligament
Ulna — L3 — Iliac crest
Sacrum — — Anterior sacroiliac ligament
Anterior superior iliac spine — — Interosseous membrane
Head of femur — — Inguinal ligament
Greater trochanter — — Coccyx
— Iliofemoral ligament
A — E
B — F — Metacarpals
C — G — Proximal phalanges
D — H — Middle phalanges
Pubic symphysis — Distal phalanges
— Femur

Key to Carpal Bones
- **A** Scaphoid
- **B** Trapezium
- **C** Trapezoid
- **D** Capitate
- **E** Lunate
- **F** Pisiform
- **G** Triquetral
- **H** Hamate

Medial epicondyle — — Quadriceps femoris tendon
Lateral epicondyle — — Tibial collateral ligament
Patella — — Fibular collateral ligament
Head of fibula — — Patellar ligament
Tibial tuberosity — — Tibia
— Fibula
— Interosseous membrane

Key to Tarsal Bones
- **J** Intermediate cuneiform
- **K** Lateral cuneiform
- **L** Cuboid
- **M** Talus
- **N** Navicular
- **O** Calcaneus
- **P** Medial cuneiform

Medial malleolus
Lateral malleolus

©Scientific Publishing, Ltd., Rolling Meadows, IL

PLATE 11. SKELETAL SYSTEM - POSTERIOR VIEW

General	20100-20999
Head	21010-21499
Neck (Soft Tissues) and Thorax	21501-21899
Back and Flank	21920-21935
Spine (Vertebral Column)	22100-22899
Abdomen	22900-22999
Shoulder	23000-23929
Humerous (Upper Arm) and Elbow	23930-24999
Forearm and Wrist	25000-25999
Hand and Fingers	26010-26989
Pelvis and Hip Joint	26990-27299
Femur and Knee Joint	27301-27599
Lower Leg and Ankle Joint	27600-27899
Foot and Toes	28001-28899
Application of Casts/Strapping	29000-29799
Endoscopy/Arthroscopy	29800-29999
Radiology Services	70010-73725
E/M Services	99201-99499

Skeletal System
(Posterior View)

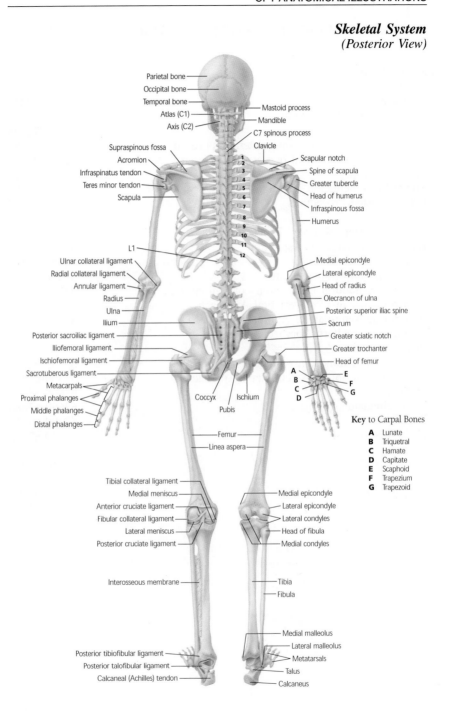

Parietal bone
Occipital bone
Temporal bone
Atlas (C1)
Axis (C2)
Mastoid process
Mandible
C7 spinous process
Clavicle
Supraspinous fossa
Acromion
Infraspinatus tendon
Teres minor tendon
Scapula
Scapular notch
Spine of scapula
Greater tubercle
Head of humerus
Infraspinous fossa
Humerus
L1
Ulnar collateral ligament
Radial collateral ligament
Annular ligament
Radius
Ulna
Ilium
Posterior sacroiliac ligament
Iliofemoral ligament
Ischiofemoral ligament
Sacrotuberous ligament
Metacarpals
Proximal phalanges
Middle phalanges
Distal phalanges
Medial epicondyle
Lateral epicondyle
Head of radius
Olecranon of ulna
Posterior superior iliac spine
Sacrum
Greater sciatic notch
Greater trochanter
Head of femur
Coccyx
Ischium
Pubis
Femur
Linea aspera

Tibial collateral ligament
Medial meniscus
Anterior cruciate ligament
Fibular collateral ligament
Lateral meniscus
Posterior cruciate ligament
Medial epicondyle
Lateral epicondyle
Lateral condyles
Head of fibula
Medial condyles

Interosseous membrane
Tibia
Fibula

Medial malleolus
Lateral malleolus
Metatarsals
Posterior tibiofibular ligament
Posterior talofibular ligament
Calcaneal (Achilles) tendon
Talus
Calcaneus

Key to Carpal Bones

A	Lunate
B	Triquetral
C	Hamate
D	Capitate
E	Scaphoid
F	Trapezium
G	Trapezoid

©Scientific Publishing, Ltd., Rolling Meadows, IL

PLATE 12. SKELETAL SYSTEM - VERTEBRAL COLUMN

Spine (Vertebral Column)

Excision	22100-22116
Osteotomy	22210-22226
Fracture and/or Dislocation	22305-22328
Manipulation	22505
Arthrodesis-Anterior or Anterolateral Approach	22548-22585
Arthrodesis-Posterolateral or Lateral Transverse	22590-22632
Spine Deformity	22800-22819
Spinal Instrumentation	22840-22855
Other/Unlisted Procedures	22899

Nervous System Surgery Procedures

Injection, Drainage, or Aspiration	62263-62319
Catheter Implantation	62350-62355
Reservoir/Pump Implantation	62360-62368
Posterior Extradural Laminotomy or Laminectomy	63001-63048
Transpedicular or Costovertebral Approach	63055-63066
Anterior or Anterolateral Approach	63075-63091
Lateral Extracavitary Approach	63101-63103
Incision	63170-63200
Excision by Laminectomy of Lesion	63250-63290
Excision, Anterior or Anterolateral Approach	63300-63308
Stereotaxis	63600-63615
Neurostimulators (Spinal)	63650-63688
Repair	63700-63710
Shunt, Spinal CSF	63740-63746

Radiology Services

72010-72295

E/M Services

99201-99499

Vertebral Column
(Lateral View)

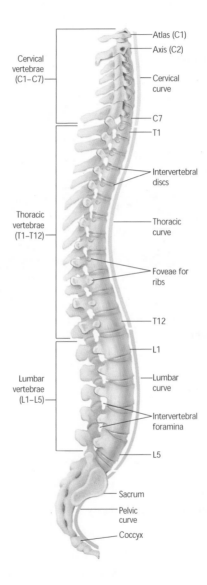

PLATE 13. RESPIRATORY SYSTEM

Nose

Incision	30000-30020
Excision	30100-30160
Introduction	30200-30220
Removal of Foreign Body	30300-30320
Repair	30400-30630
Destruction	30801-30802
Other	30901-30999

Accessory Sinuses

Incision	31000-31090
Excision	31200-31230
Endoscopy	31231-31294
Other	31299

Larynx

Excision	31300-31420
Introduction	31500-31502
Endoscopy	31505-31579
Repair	31580-31590
Destruction	31595
Other	31599

Trachea and Bronchi

Incision	31600-31614
Endoscopy	31615-31656
Introduction	31700-31730
Repair	31750-31830

Lungs and Pleura

Incision	32000-32225
Excision	32310-32540
Endoscopy	32601-32665
Repair	32800-32820
Lung Transplantation	32850-32854
Surgical Collapse Therapy; Thoracoplasty	32900-32960

Radiology Services   71010-71555

E/M Services   99201-99499

Respiratory System

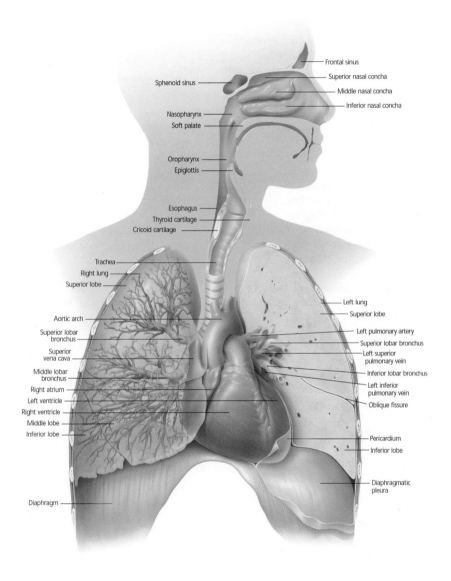

PLATE 14. HEART AND PERICARDIUM

General
Pericardium	33010-33050
Cardiac Tumor	33120-33130
Pacemaker or Defibrillator	33200-33249
Electrophysiologic Operative Procedures	33250-33261
Patient Activated Event Recorder	33282-33284
Wounds of the Heart and Great Vessels	33300-33335

Cardiac Valves
Aortic Valve	33400-33417
Mitral Valve	33420-33430
Tricuspid Valve	33460-33468
Pulmonary Valve	33470-33478

Coronary Artery Bypass
Coronary Artery Anomalies	33500-33506
Venous Grafting for Bypass	33510-33516
Combined Arterial-Venous Grafting	33517-33530
Arterial Grafting for Bypass	33533-33545
Coronary Endarterectomy	33572

Repair of Anomalies and Defects
Single Ventricle/Other Cardiac Anomalies	33600-33619
Septal Defect	33641-33697
Sinus of Valsalva	33702-33722
Total Anomalous Pulmonary Venous Drainage	33730-33732
Shunting Procedures	33735-22767
Transposition of the Great Vessels	33770-33781
Truncus Arteriosus	33786-33788
Aortic Anomalies	33800-33853
Thoracic Aortic Aneurysm	33860-33877
Pulmonary Artery	33910-33924

Heart/Lung Transplant	33930-33945
Cardiac Assist	33960-33980
Radiology Services	75552-75556
E/M Services	99201-99499

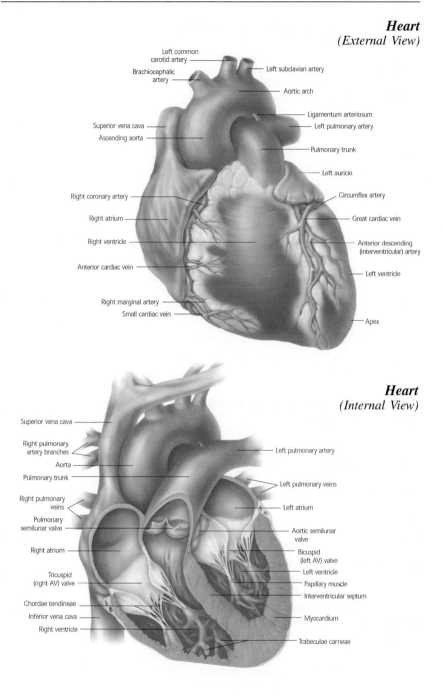

Heart
(External View)

Left common carotid artery
Brachiocephalic artery
Left subclavian artery
Aortic arch
Ligamentum arteriosum
Superior vena cava
Left pulmonary artery
Ascending aorta
Pulmonary trunk
Left auricle
Right coronary artery
Circumflex artery
Right atrium
Great cardiac vein
Right ventricle
Anterior descending (interventricular) artery
Anterior cardiac vein
Left ventricle
Right marginal artery
Small cardiac vein
Apex

Heart
(Internal View)

Superior vena cava
Right pulmonary artery branches
Left pulmonary artery
Aorta
Pulmonary trunk
Left pulmonary veins
Right pulmonary veins
Left atrium
Pulmonary semilunar valve
Aortic semilunar valve
Right atrium
Bicuspid (left AV) valve
Left ventricle
Tricuspid (right AV) valve
Papillary muscle
Interventricular septum
Chordae tendineae
Inferior vena cava
Myocardium
Right ventricle
Trabeculae carneae

©Scientific Publishing, Ltd., Rolling Meadows, IL

PLATE 15. CIRCULATORY SYSTEM

Embolectomy/Thrombectomy
Arterial, With or Without Repair   34001-34203
Venous, Direct or w/Catheter   34401-34490

Venous Reconstruction   34501-34530

Repair
Endovascular Repair of Aneurysm   34800-34900
Direct Repair of Aneurysm   35001-35162
Repair Arteriovenous Fistula   35180-35190
Repair Blood Vessel Other Than for Fistula   35201-35286

Thromboendarterectomy   35301-35390

Transluminal Angioplasty   35450-35476

Transluminal Atherectomy   35480-35495

Bypass Graft
Vein   35500-35572
In-situ Vein   35582-35587
Composite Grafts   35681-35683

Transposition and Exploration/Revision
Arterial Transposition   35691-35697
Exploration/Revision   35700-35907

Vascular Injection Procedures
Intravenous   36000-36015
Intra-Arterial/Intra-Aortic   36100-36299
Venous   36400-36597
Arterial   36600-36660
Intraosseous   36680

Cannulization or Shunt and Other Procedures
Intervascular Cannulization or Shunt   36800-36870
Portal Decompression Procedures   37140-37183
Transcatheter Procedures   37195-37209
Intravascular Ultrasound Services   37250-37251
Ligation and Other Procedures   37565-37799

Radiology Services   75600-75996

E/M Services   99201-99499

Vascular System

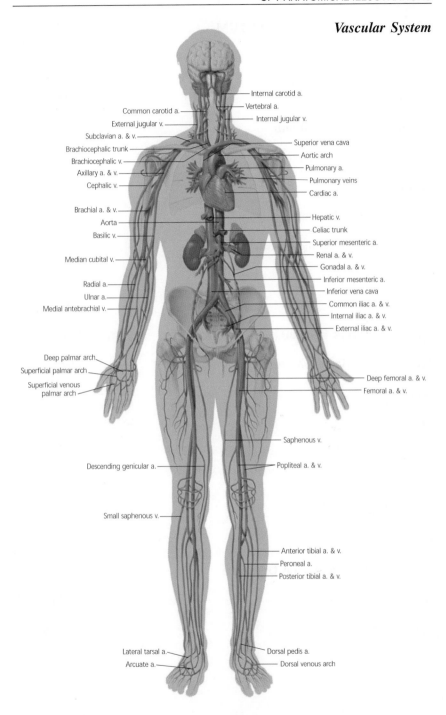

PLATE 16. DIGESTIVE SYSTEM

Lips	40490-40799
Vestibule of Mouth	40800-40899
Tongue and Floor of Mouth	41000-41599
Dentoalveolar Structures	41800-41899
Palate and Uvula	42000-42299
Salivary Gland and Ducts	42300-42699
Pharynx, Adenoids, and Tonsils	42700-42999
Esophagus	43020-43499
Stomach	43500-43999
Intestines (Except Rectum)	44005-44799
Meckel's Diverticulum/Mesentery	44800-44899
Appendix	44900-44979
Rectum	45000-45999
Anus	46020-46999
Liver	47000-47399
Biliary Tract	47400-47999
Pancreas	48000-48999
Abdomen, Peritoneum and Omentum	49000-49999
Radiology Services	74000-74363
E/M Services	99201-99499

Digestive System

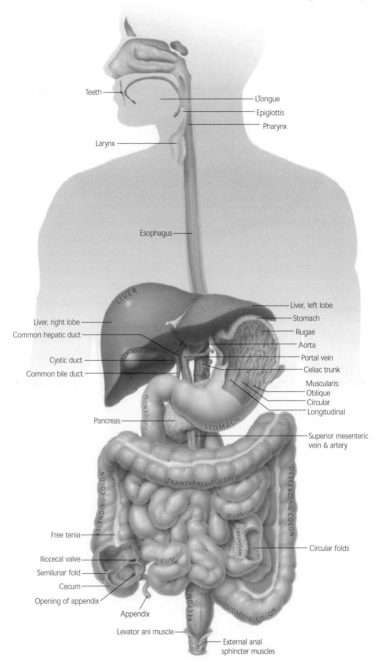

PLATE 17. GENITOURINARY SYSTEM

Kidney

Incision	50010-50135
Excision	50200-50290
Renal Transplantation	50300-50380
Introduction	50390-50398
Repair	50400-50540
Endoscopy/Laparoscopy	50541-50580

Ureter

Incision	50600-50630
Excision	50650-50660
Introduction	50684-50690
Repair	50700-50940
Endoscopy/Laparoscopy	50945-50980

Bladder

Incision	51000-51080
Excision	51500-51597
Introduction	51600-51720
Urodynamics	51725-51798
Repair	51800-51980
Laparoscopy	51990-51992

Endoscopy—Cystoscopy—
Urethroscopy—Cystourethroscopy   52000-52010

Transurethral Surgery

Urethra and Bladder	52204-52318
Ureter and Pelvis	52320-52355
Vesical Neck and Prostate	52400-52700

Urethra

Incision	53000-53085
Excision	53200-53275
Repair	53400-53520
Manipulation	53600-53665

Radiology Services   74400-74485

E/M Services   99201-99499

Urinary System

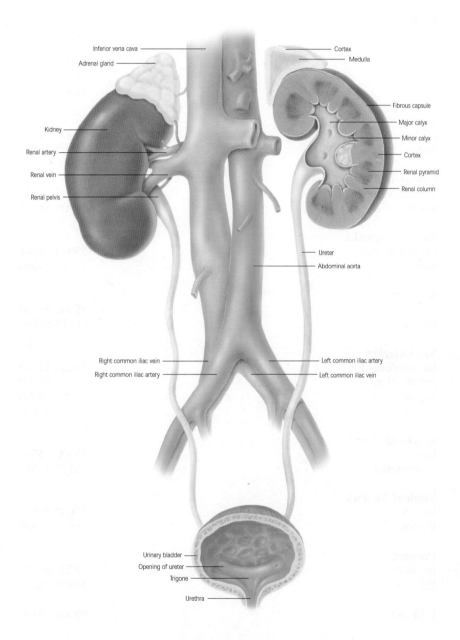

PLATE 18. MALE REPRODUCTIVE SYSTEM

Penis

Incision	54000-54015
Destruction	54050-54065
Excision	54100-54164
Introduction	54200-54250
Repair	54300-54440

Testis

Excision	54500-54560
Repair	54600-54680

Epididymis

Incision/Excision	54700-54861
Repair	54900-54901

Tunica Vaginalis

Incision/Excision	55000-55041
Repair	55060

Scrotum

Incision/Excision	55100-55150
Repair	55175-55180

Vas Deferens

Incision/Excision	55200-55250
Introduction	55300
Repair	55400
Suture	55450

Spermatic Cord

Excision	55500-55540
Laparoscopy	55550-55559

Seminal Vesicles

Incision	55600-55605
Excision	55650-55680

Prostate

Incision	55700-55725
Excision	55801-55865

E/M Services 99201-99499

Male Reproductive System

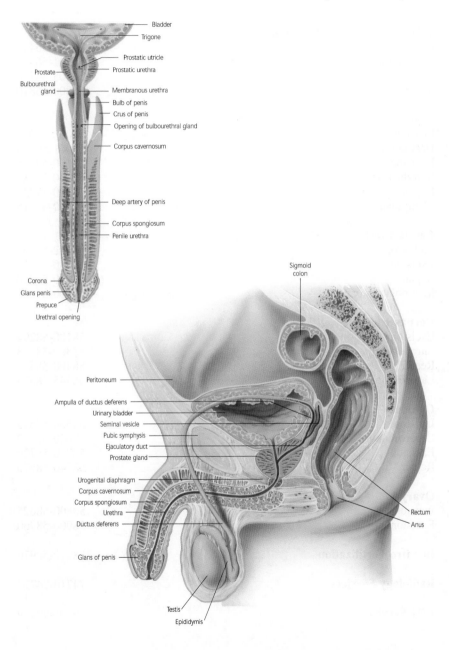

PLATE 19. FEMALE REPRODUCTIVE SYSTEM

Vulva, Perineum and Introitus

Incision	56405-56441
Destruction	56501-56515
Excision	56605-56740
Repair	56800-56810

Vagina

Incision	57000-57023
Destruction	57061-57065
Excision	57100-57135
Introduction	57150-57180
Repair	57200-57335
Manipulation	57400-57415

Cervix Uteri

Endoscopy	57452-57461
Excision	57500-57556
Repair	57700-57720
Manipulation	57800-57820

Corpus Uteri

Excision	58100-58294
Introduction	58300-58353
Repair	58400-58540
Laparoscopy/Hysteroscopy	58545-58579

Oviduct

Incision	58600-58615
Laparoscopy	58660-68679
Excision	58700-58720
Repair	58740-58770

Ovary

Incision	58800-58825
Excision	58900-58960

In Vitro Fertilization   58970-58976

Radiology Services   74710-74775

E/M Services   99201-99499

Female Reproductive System

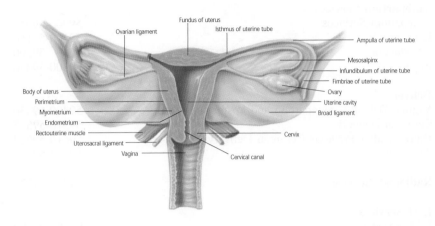

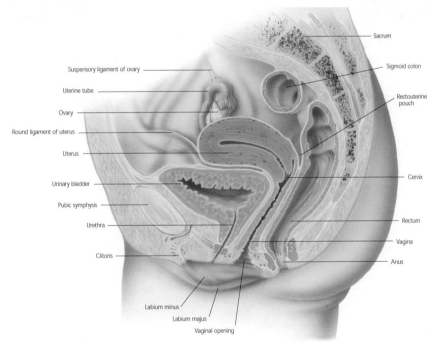

PLATE 20. PREGNANCY, CHILDBIRTH AND THE PUERPERIUM

Antepartum Services

Antepartum Services	59000-59051
Excision	59100-59160
Introduction	59200
Repair	59300-59350

Delivery

Vaginal Delivery, Antepartum and Postpartum Care	59400-59430
Cesarean Delivery	59510-59525
Delivery after Previous Cesarean Delivery	59610-59622
Abortion	59812-59857

Radiology Services

74710-74775

E/M Services

E/M Services	99201-99499
Newborn Care	99431-99440

Female Reproductive System: Pregnancy
(Lateral View)

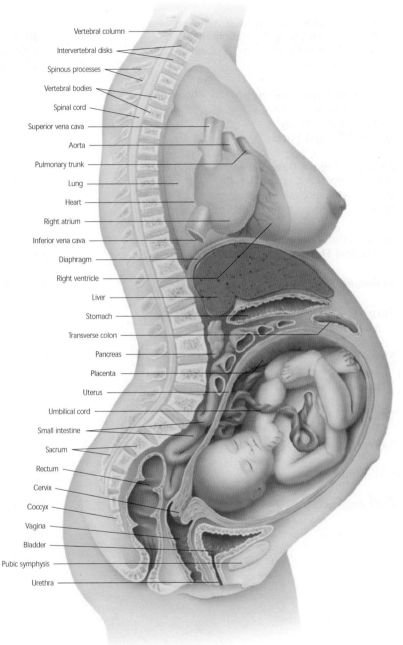

Vertebral column
Intervertebral disks
Spinous processes
Vertebral bodies
Spinal cord
Superior vena cava
Aorta
Pulmonary trunk
Lung
Heart
Right atrium
Inferior vena cava
Diaphragm
Right ventricle
Liver
Stomach
Transverse colon
Pancreas
Placenta
Uterus
Umbilical cord
Small intestine
Sacrum
Rectum
Cervix
Coccyx
Vagina
Bladder
Pubic symphysis
Urethra

PLATE 21. NERVOUS SYSTEM - BRAIN

Skull, Meninges, and Brain
Injection, Drainage, or Aspiration	61000-61070
Twist Drill, Burr Hole(s), or Trephine	61105-61253
Craniectomy or Craniotomy	61304-61576

Surgery of Skull Base Approach Procedures
Anterior Cranial Fossa	61580-61586
Middle Cranial Fossa	61590-61592
Posterior Cranial Fossa	61595-61598

Surgery of Skull Base Definitive Procedures
Base of Anterior Cranial Fossa	61600-61601
Base of Middle Cranial Fossa	61605-61613
Base of Posterior Cranial Fossa	61615-61616

Repair and/or Reconstruction of Surgical Defects of Skull Base
61618-61619

Endovascular Therapy
61623-61626

Surgery for Aneurysm, Arterio-Venous Malformation or Vascular Disease
61680-61711

Stereotaxis
61720-61795

Neurostimulators (Intra-Cranial)
61850-61888

Repair
62000-62148

Neuroendoscopy
62160-62165

CSF Shunt
62180-62258

Radiology Services
70010-70559

E/M Services
99201-99499

Brain
(Base View)

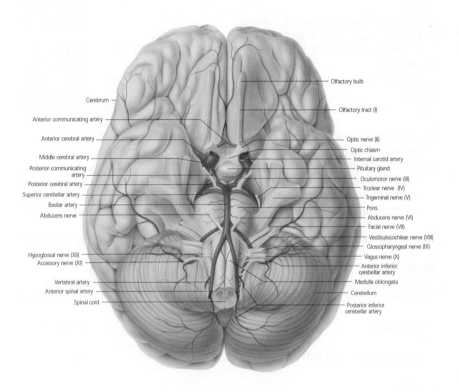

Olfactory bulb

Cerebrum

Olfactory tract (I)

Anterior communicating artery

Anterior cerebral artery

Optic nerve (II)

Optic chiasm

Middle cerebral artery

Internal carotid artery

Posterior communicating artery

Pituitary gland

Posterior cerebral artery

Oculomotor nerve (III)

Superior cerebellar artery

Troclear nerve (IV)

Basilar artery

Trigeminal nerve (V)

Abducens nerve

Pons

Abducens nerve (VI)

Facial nerve (VII)

Vestibulocochlear nerve (VIII)

Glossopharyngeal nerve (IX)

Hypoglossal nerve (XII)

Vagus nerve (X)

Accessory nerve (XI)

Anterior inferior cerebellar artery

Vertebral artery

Medulla oblongata

Anterior spinal artery

Cerebellum

Spinal cord

Posterior inferior cerebellar artery

PLATE 22. NERVOUS SYSTEM

Spine and Spinal Cord

Injection, Drainage or Aspiration	62263-62319
Catheter Implantation	62350-62368
Posterior Extradural Laminotomy or Laminectomy	63001-63048
Transpedicular or Costovertebral Approach	63055-63066
Anterior or Anterolateral Approach	63075-63091
Incision	63170-63200
Excision by Laminectomy of Lesion	63250-63290
Excision, Anterior or Anterolateral Approach Intraspinal Lesion	63300-63308
Stereotaxis	63600-63615
Neurostimulators (Spinal)	63650-63688
Repair	63700-63710
Shunt, Spinal CSF	63740-63746

Extracranial Nerves, Peripheral Nerves and Autonomic Nervous System

Introduction/Injection of Anesthetic Agent Somatic Nerves	64400-64484
Introduction/Injection of Anesthetic Agent Sympathetic Nerves	64505-64530

Neurostimulators

64550-64595

Destruction

Neurolytic Agent Somatic Nerves	64600-64640
Neurolytic Agent Sympathetic Nerves	64680-64681

Neuroplasty

64702-64727

Transection or Avulsion

64732-64772

Excision

Somatic Nerves	64774-64795
Sympathetic Nerves	64802-64823

Neurorrhaphy

Without Nerve Graft	64831-64876
With Nerve Graft	64885-64907

E/M Services

99201-99499

Nervous System

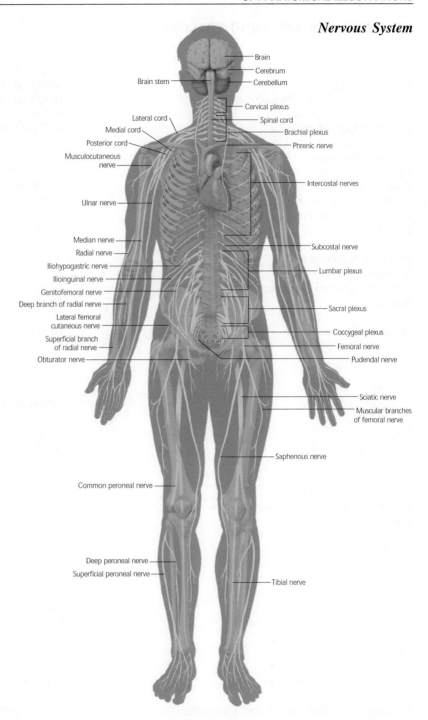

PLATE 23. EYE AND OCULAR ADNEXA

Eyeball

Removal of Eye	65091-65114
Secondary Implant(s) Procedures	65125-65175
Removal of Foreign Body	65205-65265
Repair of Laceration	65270-65290

Anterior Segment

Cornea Procedures	65400-65782
Anterior Chamber Procedures	65800-66030
Anterior Sclera Procedures	66130-66250
Iris, Ciliary Body Procedures	66500-66770
Lens Procedures	66820-66990

Posterior Segment

Vitreous	67005-67040
Retina or Choroid Procedures	67101-67228
Sclera	67250-67255

Ocular Adnexa	67311-67399

Orbit	67400-67599

Eyelids

Incision/Excision	67700-67850
Tarsorrhaphy	67875-67882
Repair	67900-67924
Reconstruction	67930-67975

Conjunctiva

Incision and Drainage	68020-68040
Excision and/or Destruction	68100-68135
Injection	68200
Conjunctivoplasty	68320-68340
Other Procedures	68360-68399

Lacrimal System

Incision/Excision	68400-68550
Repair	68700-68770
Probing and/or Related Procedures	68801-68850

E/M Services	99201-99499

Ophthalmological Services	92002-92287

Contact Lens, Prosthetics and Spectacles	92310-92396

Right Eye
(Horizontal Section)

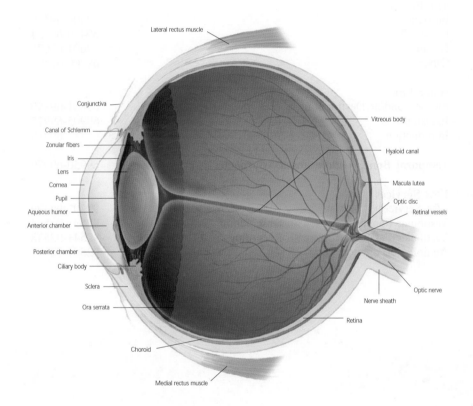

Lateral rectus muscle

Conjunctiva

Canal of Schlemm

Zonular fibers

Iris

Lens

Cornea

Pupil

Aqueous humor

Anterior chamber

Posterior chamber

Ciliary body

Sclera

Ora serrata

Choroid

Medial rectus muscle

Vitreous body

Hyaloid canal

Macula lutea

Optic disc

Retinal vessels

Optic nerve

Nerve sheath

Retina

PLATE 24. AUDITORY SYSTEM

External Ear

Incision	69000-69090
Excision	69100-69155
Removal of Foreign Body	69200-69222
Repair	69300-69320

Middle Ear

Introduction	69400-69410
Incision/Excision	69420-69554
Repair	69601-69676
Other	69700-69799

Inner Ear

Incision and/or Destruction	69801-69840
Excision	69905-69915
Introduction	69930

Temporal Bone, Middle Fossa Approach   69950-69970

E/M Services

E/M Services	99201-99499
Vestibular Function Tests with Observation	92531-92534
Vestibular Function Tests with Recording	92541-92548
Audiologic Function Tests	92551-92597

The Ear

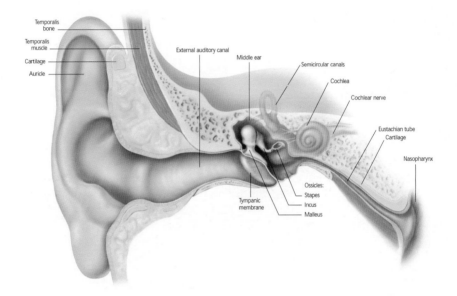

ICD-9-CM CODING

Health care professionals have long used various coding systems such as CPT and HCPCS, to describe procedures, services and supplies. However, most described the reason for the procedure, service or supply with a diagnostic statement, i.e. the diagnosis in words. Of those health care professionals who do code the diagnosis, either due to a requirement for a computer billing system and/or electronic claims filing, many do not code completely or accurately. With the passage of the Medicare Catastrophic Coverage Act of 1988, diagnostic coding using ICD-9-CM became mandatory for Medicare claims. In the area of health care reimbursement rules and regulations, the typical progression is that changes required for Medicare are followed shortly by similar changes for Medicaid and private health insurance carriers.

To some professionals, the requirement to use diagnostic coding may seem a burden or simply another excuse for Medicare intermediaries to delay or deny payment. However, it is important to understand that the proper use of coding systems for both procedures and diagnoses gives the professional absolute control over his or her billing and reimbursement. Accurate diagnosis coding is not easy. It requires a good working knowledge of medical terminology and a fundamental understanding of ICD-9-CM. In addition, the coder must know the rules and regulations required to comply with Medicare requirements for coding.

This chapter provides the information necessary to develop a fundamental understanding of ICD-9-CM coding as well as the steps needed to comply fully with the new Medicare rules and regulations governing ICD-9-CM coding.

KEY POINTS REGARDING ICD-9-CM

1. ICD-9-CM codes are three to five numeric or alphanumeric codes.

2. ICD-9-CM codes describe illnesses, injuries, signs and symptoms, and procedures.

3. With few exceptions, ICD-9-CM codes are accepted or required by all health insurance carriers.

4. Most ICD-9-CM codes have a specific definition; however, some ICD-9-CM codes have more than one definition.

5. ICD-9-CM coding can make a significant difference in your reimbursement.

6. Accurate ICD-9-CM coding puts you in control of the reimbursement process.

MEDICARE REQUIREMENTS FOR ICD-9-CM CODING

The Medicare Catastrophic Coverage Act of 1988 (P.L 100-330) required health care professionals to submit an appropriate diagnosis code (or codes), using the International Classification of Diseases, 9th Revision, Clinical Modification (ICD-9-CM) for each procedure, service, or supply billed under Medicare Part B. Even though the original law was subsequently repealed, the diagnosis coding requirement was maintained.

To comply with the regulations, health care professionals must convert the reason(s) for the procedures, services or supplies, performed or issued, from written diagnostic statements which may include specific diagnoses, signs, symptoms and/or complaints, into ICD-9-CM diagnosis codes. The Health Care Financing Administration originally set the implementation date for this requirement as April 1, 1989, however, it was subsequently delayed twice, until October 1989, at the request of the American Medical Association, to give health care providers additional time to prepare for the change.

CMS GUIDELINES FOR USING ICD-9-CM CODES

The Center for Medicare and Medicaid Services (CMS) has prepared guidelines for using ICD-9-CM codes and instructions on how to report them on claim forms. In addition, CMS has directed your Medicare intermediary to provide you with a written copy of these instructions. The basic CMS guidelines are summarized below. However, it is very important that you obtain a copy of the guidelines from your Medicare intermediary as implementation of CMS requirements varies from one intermediary to another.

1. Indicate on the claim form or itemized statement the appropriate code(s) from the ICD-9-CM code range 001.0 through V82.9 to identify diagnoses, symptoms, conditions, problems, complaints or other reason(s) for the procedure, service or supply provided.

   a. In choosing codes to describe the reason for the encounter, the health care professional will frequently be using codes within the range from 001.0 through 999.9, the section of ICD-9-CM for the classification of diseases and injuries (e.g. infectious and parasitic diseases; neoplasms; signs, symptoms and ill-defined conditions). Codes that describe symptoms, as opposed to diagnoses, are acceptable if this is the highest level of certainty documented by the physician.

b.   ICD-9-CM also provides codes to deal with visits for circumstances other than a disease or injury, such as a visit for a lab test only. These codes are found in the V-code section and range from V01.0 through V82.9.

2.   The ICD-9-CM code for the diagnosis, condition, problem, or other reason for the encounter documented in the medical record as the main reason for the procedure, service or supply provided should be listed first. Additional ICD-9-CM codes that describe any current coexisting conditions are then listed. Do not include codes for conditions that were previously treated and no longer exist.

3.   ICD-9-CM codes should be used at their highest level of specificity.

a.   Assign three digit codes only if there are no four digit codes within the coding category.

b.   Assign four digit codes only if there is no fifth digit subclassification for that category.

c.   Assign the fifth digit subclassification code for those categories where it exists.

Claims submitted with three or four digit codes where four and five digit codes are available may be returned to you by the Medicare intermediary for proper coding. It is recognized that a very specific diagnosis may not be known at the time of the initial encounter. However, that is not an acceptable reason to submit a three digit code when four or five digits are available.

4.   Diagnoses documented as "probable," "suspected," "questionable," or "rule out" should not be coded as if the diagnosis is confirmed. The condition(s) should be coded to the highest degree of certainty for the encounter, such as describing symptoms, signs, abnormal test results, or other reasons for the encounter.

5.   Chronic disease(s) treated on an ongoing basis may be coded and reported as many times as the patient receives treatment and care for the condition(s).

6.   When patients receive ancillary diagnostic services only during an encounter, the appropriate "V code" for the service should be listed first, and the diagnosis or problem for which the diagnostic procedures are being performed should be listed second.

a. V codes will be used frequently by radiologists who perform radiological examinations on referrals. For example, ICD-9-CM code V72.5, Radiological examination, not elsewhere classified, describes the reason for the encounter and should be listed first on the claim form or statement. If the reason for the referral is known, a second ICD-9-CM code which describes the signs or symptoms for which the examination was ordered should be listed.

b. Failure to list a second ICD-9-CM code in addition to the V code may result in claim delays or denials. The ICD-9-CM code V72.5, Radiological examination, not elsewhere classified, includes referrals for routine chest x-rays that are not covered by the Medicare program. Medicare intermediaries may establish screening programs to verify that the referrals were not for routine chest x-rays.

By supplying a second ICD-9-CM code to describe the reason for the referral, these claims can be clearly identified by the Medicare intermediary as referrals to evaluate symptoms, signs or diagnoses. The omission of a second ICD-9-CM code may lead to requests for additional information from Medicare intermediaries prior to processing the claim.

7. For patients receiving only ancillary therapeutic services during an encounter, list the appropriate V code first, followed by the ICD-9-CM code for the diagnosis or problem for which the services are being performed. For example, a patient with multiple sclerosis presenting for rehabilitation services would be coded using code V57.1, Other physical therapy, or code V57.89, Other care involving use of rehabilitation procedures, followed by code 340, multiple sclerosis.

8. For surgical procedures, use the ICD-9-CM code for the diagnosis for which the surgery was performed. If the postoperative diagnosis is known to be different at the time the claim is filed, use the ICD-9-CM code for the post operative diagnosis.

9. Code all documented conditions that coexist at the time of the visit that require or affect patient care, treatment or management. Do not code conditions that were previously treated and no longer exist.

IMPORTANT DIAGNOSIS CODING AND BILLING ISSUES

DIAGNOSES CODES MUST SUPPORT PROCEDURE CODES

Each service/procedure billed for a patient should be supported by a diagnosis that would substantiate those particular services or procedures as necessary in the investigation or treatment of their condition based on currently accepted standards of practice by the medical profession.

PLACE (LOCATION) OF SERVICE

The actual setting that the services are rendered in for particular diagnoses plays an important part in reimbursement. Many people became accustomed to using Emergency Rooms for any type of illness or injury. By utilizing highly specialized places of service for conditions that were not true emergencies, third party payers were being billed with CPT codes indicating emergency services were rendered.

Since the cost of services rendered on an emergency basis is considerably more expensive than those services in an non-emergency situation, third party payers began watching for those claims with diagnoses that did not indicate that a true emergency existed. Payment then was based on what the cost would have been had the patient been treated in the proper setting.

LEVEL OF SERVICE PROVIDED

The patient's condition and the treatment of that condition must be billed according to the criteria, as published by the AMA, for each level of service (i.e., minimal, brief, limited, intermediate, extended, comprehensive). Many practices bill the office visit level that they know will pay better rather than to consider the criteria that must be met to use a particular level of service. Again, the patient's diagnosis enters into this concept as well. As it is often the diagnosis that indicates the complexity of the level of service to be used.

FREQUENCY OF SERVICES

Many times claims are submitted for a patient with the same diagnosis and the same procedure(s) time after time. When the diagnosis indicates a chronic condition and the claims do not indicate any change in the patient's treatment or, gives any indication that the patient's condition has been altered (i.e., exacerbated, other symptomology) the third party payer may deny payment based on the frequency of services for the reported condition.

Currently, statistics are being tabulated from all claims submitted to Medicare or any other third party payer. These statistics will be used in the future as the basis of your fee profile for a prospective payment system. Again, this is why correct reporting by using the most appropriate codes is very important to the financial outlook of a provider.

DOWN CODING

Down-coding is the process of reducing a procedure code from one of a higher value to one of a lower value which results in lowered reimbursement. This process results in the loss of millions of dollars annually by health care professionals and their patients.

With diagnosis coding, the major protection from procedure down coding is that the ICD-9-CM code(s) provide justification for the procedure, service or supply or the level of service provided. For example, if you submit an health insurance claim form listing CPT code 99214, an extended office visit for an established patient, with an ICD-9-CM code of 487.1 defined as Influenza with other respiratory manifestations, the health insurance carrier will almost certainly down code the procedure to a lower level of service such as CPT code 99212 or 99213. A key point to remember is that if there are any current coexisting conditions which may complicate the treatment for the primary condition, it is very important to include the ICD-9-CM codes for the coexisting conditions which will help to justify the level of service provided.

CONCURRENT CARE

Reimbursement problems often arise when a patient is being treated by different professionals, within the same billing entity (medical group or clinic), for different problems at the same time. This is known as concurrent care. For example, a patient may be hospitalized by a clinic's general surgeon for an operation and may also be seen while hospitalized by the group's cardiologist for an unrelated cardiac condition.

If you submit claims for daily hospital visits by both of the above professionals without explanation, most health insurance carriers will reject one daily visit as an apparent "duplication" of service. The ICD-9-CM code becomes the only qualifying factor for justification of concurrent care services.

FORMAT OF ICD-9-CM

The International Classification of Diseases, 9th Revision, Clinical Modification was originally published as a three volume set (2nd edition). Newer versions of ICD-9-CM, Fourth Edition, are available as two separate books (Volume 1 and Volume 2) and as a single book containing Volume 1 and Volume 2, or Volumes 1, 2 and 3 depending on the publisher. The only difference between the newer Fourth Edition of ICD-9-CM and the previous Third Edition, is that the Fourth Edition has the Official Addenda from 1986 through 1991 incorporated in the revised publication.

THE TABULAR LIST (VOLUME 1)

The TABULAR LIST (VOLUME 1) is a numeric listing of diagnosis codes and descriptions consisting of 17 chapters which classify diseases and injuries, two sections containing supplementary codes (V codes and E codes) and six appendices.

The Classification of Diseases and Injuries includes the following 17 chapters:

CHAPTER 1   Infectious and Parasitic Diseases (001-139)

CHAPTER 2   Neoplasms (140-239)

CHAPTER 3   Endocrine, Nutritional and Metabolic Diseases, and Immunity Disorders (240-279)

CHAPTER 4   Diseases of the Blood and Blood-Forming Organs (280-289)

CHAPTER 5   Mental Disorders (290-319)

CHAPTER 6   Diseases of the Nervous System and Sense Organs (320-389)

CHAPTER 7   Diseases of the Circulatory System (340-459)

CHAPTER 8   Diseases of the Respiratory System (460-519)

CHAPTER 9   Diseases of the Digestive System (520-579)

CHAPTER 10   Diseases of the Genitourinary System (580-629)

CHAPTER 11   Complications of Pregnancy, Childbirth, and the Puerperium (630-676)

CHAPTER 12   Diseases of the Skin and Subcutaneous Tissue (680-709)

CHAPTER 13   Diseases of the Musculoskeletal System and Connective Tissue (710-739)

CHAPTER 14   Congenital Anomalies (740-759)

CHAPTER 15   Certain Conditions Originating in the Perinatal Period (760-779)

CHAPTER 16   Symptoms, Signs and Ill-defined Conditions (780-799)

CHAPTER 17   Injury and Poisoning (800-999)

Each chapter of the Tabular List (Volume 1) is structured with the following components:

SECTIONS: groups of three-digit code numbers

CATEGORIES: three-digit code numbers

SUBCATEGORIES: four-digit code numbers

FIFTH-DIGIT SUBCLASSIFICATIONS: five digit code numbers

The two supplementary classifications included in the Tabular List (Volume 1) are:

V CODES   Supplementary Classification of Factors Influencing Health Status and Contact with Health Services (V01-V82)

E CODES   Supplementary Classification of External Causes of Injury and Poisoning (E800-E999)

The six appendices included in the Tabular List (Volume 1) are:

APPENDIX 1   Morphology of Neoplasms

APPENDIX 2   Glossary of Mental Disorders

APPENDIX 3   Classification of Drugs by American Hospital Formulary Service List Number and their ICD-9-CM equivalents

APPENDIX 4   Classification of Industrial Accidents According to Agency

APPENDIX 5   List of Three-Digit Categories

APPENDIX 6   Supplementary Classification of External Causes of Injury and Poisoning

THE ALPHABETICAL INDEX (VOLUME 2)

The Alphabetic Index (Volume 2) of ICD-9-CM consists of an alphabetic list of terms and codes, two supplementary Sections following the alphabetic listing, plus two special tables found within the alphabetic listing.

The Alphabetic Index (Volume 2) is structured as follows:

- Main Terms appear in **BOLDFACE** type

- Subterms are always indented two spaces to the right under main terms

- Carry-Over Lines are always indented more than two spaces from the level of the preceding line

SUPPLEMENTARY SECTIONS

The supplementary sections following the Alphabetic Index (Volume 2) are:

Table of Drugs and Chemicals

This table contains a classification of drugs and other chemical substances to identify poisoning states and external causes of adverse effects.

Index to External Causes of Injuries and Poisonings (E-Codes)

This section contains the index to the codes which classify environmental events, circumstances, and other conditions as the cause of injury and other adverse effects.

SPECIAL TABLES

The two special tables, located within the Alphabetic Index (Volume 2), and found under the main terms as underlined below, are:

- **Hypertension Table**

- **Neoplasm Table**

PROCEDURES: TABULAR LIST AND ALPHABETIC INDEX (VOLUME 3)

The Procedures: Tabular List and Alphabetic Index (Volume 3) consists of two sections of codes which define procedures instead of diagnoses. Frequently used incorrectly by health care professionals, codes from Volume 3 are intended only for use by hospitals. The new U.S. Government Printing Office printing of ICD-9-CM, Fourth Edition, does not include Volume 3.

TABULAR LIST OF PROCEDURES

Includes 16 chapters containing codes and descriptions for surgical procedures and miscellaneous diagnostic and therapeutic procedures.

ALPHABETIC INDEX TO PROCEDURES

Provides an alphabetic index to the Tabular List of Volume 3

ICD-9-CM CODING CONVENTIONS

The ICD-9-CM Tabular List (Volume 1) makes use of certain abbreviations, punctuation, symbols, and other conventions which must be clearly understood. The purpose of these conventions is to first, provide special coding instructions, and second, to conserve space.

INSTRUCTIONAL TERMS

Instructional terms define what is or what is not included in a given subdivision. This is accomplished by using both inclusion and exclusion terms.

INCLUDES: Indicates separate terms, as, modifying adjectives, sites and conditions, entered under a subdivision, such as a category, to further define or give examples of the content of the category.

Excludes Exclusion terms are enclosed in a box and are printed in italics to draw attention to their presence. The importance of this instructional terms is its use as a guideline to direct the coder to the proper code assignment. In other words, all terms following the word EXCLUDES: are to be coded elsewhere as indicated in each instance.

NOTES These are used to define terms and give coding instructions. Often used to list the fifth-digit subclassifications for certain categories.

SEE Acts as a cross reference and, is an explicit direction to look elsewhere. This instructional term must ALWAYS be followed. (Cross references provide the user with other possible modifiers for a term, or, its synonyms.)

SEE   Variation of the instructional term "SEE." This refers the coder to a specific

CATEGORY   category. You must ALWAYS follow this instructional term.

SEE ALSO   A direction given to look elsewhere if the main term or subterm(s) are not sufficient to code the information you have.

CODE FIRST   Identifies those instances where more than one code is required to fully describe a given condition. The notation requires that the underlying disease be coded first.

USE   Adds further information to give a better picture of

ADDITIONAL   ADDITIONAL diagnosis.
CODE

PUNCTUATION MARKS

( )   PARENTHESES are used to enclose supplementary words which may be present or absent in a statement of disease without effecting the code assignment.

[ ]   SQUARE BRACKETS are used to enclose synonyms, alternate wordings or explanatory phrases.

:   COLONS are used after an incomplete phrase or term which requires one or more of the modifiers indented under it to make it assignable to a given category. EXCEPTION to this rule pertains to the abbreviation NOS.

{}   BRACES are used to connect a series of terms to a common stem. Each term on the left of the brace is incomplete and must be completed by a term to the right of the brace.

ABBREVIATIONS

NOS   Not Otherwise Specified - equivalent to Unspecified. This abbreviation refers to a lack of sufficient detail in the statement of diagnosis to be able to assign it to a more specific subdivision within the classification.

NEC   Not Elsewhere Classified - used with ill-defined terms to alert the coder that a specified form of the condition is classified differently. The codes given for such terms should be used only if more precise information is not available. Secondly, NEC is used with terms for which a more specific category is not provided in the TABULAR LIST (VOLUME 1) and, no additional amount of information will alter the code selection.

SYMBOLS

☐   The LOZENGE symbol appearing in the left margin preceding a four-digit code indicates a change in the code number and its content that are not the same as the code number in ICD-9. May be ignored for coding purposes.

RELATED TERMS

AND   Whenever this term appears in a title, it should be interpreted as "and/or."

WITH   When this term is used in a title it indicates a requirement that both parts of the title must be present in the diagnostic statement.

DIAGNOSIS CODING BASICS

Learning and following the basic steps of coding will increase your chances of better and faster reimbursement from third party payers, as well as, establish meaningful profiles for future reimbursement rates. To become a proficient coder, two basic principles must be considered.

- First, it is imperative that you use both the Alphabetic Index (Volume 2) and the Tabular List (Volume 1) when locating and assigning a code number. Attempting to code only from the Alphabetic Index (Volume 2) will cause you to miss any additional information provided only in the Tabular List (Volume 1), such as exclusions, instructions to use additional codes or the need for a fifth-digit.

- Second, the level of specificity is important in all coding situations. So, a three-digit code that has subdivisions indicates you must use the appropriate subdivision code. Also, any time a fifth-digit subclassification is provided, you must use the fifth-digit code.

NINE STEPS FOR ACCURATE AND PRECISE CODING

1. Locate the main term within the diagnostic statement.

2. Locate that main term in the Alphabetic Index (Volume 2). Keep in mind that the primary arrangement for main terms is by condition in the Alphabetic Index (Volume 2); main terms can be referred to in outmoded, ill-defined and lay terms as well as proper medical terms; main terms can be expressed in broad or specific terms, as nouns, adjectives or eponyms and can be with or without modifiers. Certain conditions may be listed under more than one main term.

3. Remember to refer to all notes under the main term. Be guided by the instructions in any notes appearing in a box immediately after the main term.

4. Examine any modifiers appearing in parentheses next to the main term. See if any of these modifiers apply to any of the qualifying terms used in the diagnostic statement.

5. Take note of the subterms indented beneath the main term. Subterms differ from main terms in that they provide greater specificity becoming more specific the further they are indented to the right of the main term in two-space increments and, they provide the anatomical sites affected by the disease or injury.

6. Be sure to follow any cross reference instructions. These instructional terms ("see" or "see also") must be followed to locate the correct code.

7. Confirm the code selection in the Tabular List (Volume 1). Make certain you have selected the appropriate classification in accordance with the diagnosis.

8. Follow instructional terms in the Tabular List (Volume 1). Watch for exclusion terms, notes and fifth-digit instructions that apply to the code number you are verifying.

   NOTE: It is necessary to search not only the selected code number for instructions but also, the category, section and chapter in which the code number is collapsible. Many times the instructional information is located one or more pages preceding the actual page you find the code number on.

9. Finally, assign the code number you have determined to be correct.

ITALICIZED ENTRIES

During the process of designating a code to identify a principal diagnosis it is important to remember that italicized entries or codes in slanted brackets cannot be used. In these instances, it is required that the etiology code be sequenced first and the manifestation code be listed second even if the physician recorded them in the opposite order.

OTHER AND UNSPECIFIED CODES

Subcategories for diagnoses listed as "Other" and "Unspecified" are referred to as residual subcategories. Remember, the subdivisions are arranged in a hierarchy starting with the more specific and ending with the least specific. In the Tabular List (Volume 1), in most instances, the four-digit subcategory ".8" has been reserved for "Other" specified conditions not classifiable elsewhere and the four-digit subcategory ".9" has been reserved for "Unspecified" conditions. Following is an example demonstrating this principle.

005 Other food poisoning (bacterial)

Excludes: salmonella infections (003.0-003.9)
toxic effect of:
food contaminants (989.7)
noxious foodstuffs (988-0-988.9)

005.0   Staphylococcal food poisoning
Staphylococcal toxemia specified as due to food

005.1   Botulism
Food poisoning due to Clostridium botulinum

005.2   Food poisoning due to Clostridium perfringens [C. welchii]
Enteritis necroticans

005.3   Food poisoning due to other Clostridia

005.4   Food poisoning due to Vibrio parahaemolyticus

005.8   Other bacterial food poisoning
Excludes: salmonella food poisoning (003.0-003.9)

005.81   Food poisoning due to Vibrio vulnificus

005.89   Other bacterial food poisoning
Food poisoning due to Bacillus cereus

005.9   Food poisoning, unspecified

As you look at Category 005, note that codes 005.0-005.4 indicate that the food poisoning is related to specific types of organisms. Therefore, subcategories 005.0-005.4 are regarded as more specific than subcategory 005.9. Fifth-digit subclassification 005.89 Other bacterial food poisoning would include other specific types of bacterial food poisoning not classified elsewhere, as well as bacterial food poisoning NOS. Whereas subcategory 005.9 Food poisoning unspecified would be used for a diagnostic statement of "Food poisoning NOS" where the causative organism is not mentioned.

The hierarchy from more specific to less specific is not consistently maintained at the fifth-digit level. The level of specificity at the fifth-digit level is usually (not always) indicated by the use of 0 and 9. The digit 9 identifies the entry for "Other specified" while the digit 0 identifies the "Unspecified" entry. Below is an example.

279 Disorders involving the immune mechanism

279.0 Deficiency of humoral immunity

279.00 Hypogammaglobulinemia, unspecified
Agammaglobulinemia NOS

279.01 Selective IgA immunodeficiency

279.02 Selective IgM immunodeficiency

279.03 Other selective immunoglobulin deficiencies
Selective deficiency of IgG

279.04 Congenital hypogammaglobulinemia
Agammaglobulinemia:
Bruton's type
X-linked

279.05 Immunodeficiency with increased IgM
Immunodeficiency with hyper-IgM:
autosomal recessive
X-linked

279.06 Common variable immunodeficiency
Dysgammaglobulinemia (acquired)
(congenital) (primary)
Hypogammaglobulinemia:
acquired primary
congenital non-sex-linked
sporadic

279.09 Other
Transient hypogammaglobulinemia of infancy

Notice that the fifth-digit 0 identifies "Unspecified" and the fifth-digit 9 identifies "Other specified."

ACUTE AND CHRONIC CODING

Whenever a particular condition is described as both acute and chronic, code according to the subentries in the Alphabetic Index (Volume 2) for the stated condition. The following directions should be considered.

1. If there are separate subentries listed for acute, subacute and chronic, then use both codes, sequencing the code for the acute condition first.

2. If there are no subentries to identify acute, subacute or chronic, ignore these adjectives when selecting the code for the particular condition.

3. If a certain condition is described as a subacute condition and the index does not provide a subentry designating subacute, then code the condition as if it were acute.

CODING SUSPECTED CONDITIONS

Whenever the diagnosis is stated as "questionable," "probable," "likely," or "rule out," it is advisable to code documented symptoms or complaints by the patient. The reason for this is that you do not want an insurance carrier to include a disease code in the patient's history if in fact the "suspected" condition is never proven.

Keep in mind that there are no "rule out" codes per se in the ICD-9-CM coding system. If your diagnostic statement is "Rule out Breast Carcinoma" and you use code 174.9 Malignant neoplasm of female breast, unspecified, the code definition does not state "rule out." Therefore, the insurance carrier processes the code 174.9 as is, which results in the patient having an insurance history of breast cancer.

To avoid what could become a problem for you and your patient (including the potential of litigation), you should use codes for signs and symptoms in these cases. For example, use code 611.72 Lump or mass in breast, or 611.71 Mastodynia (breast pain) if these symptoms exist and this is the highest degree of certainty you can code to.

If the patient is asymptomatic but there is a family history of breast cancer then you should consider using a V-code, such as V16.3 Family history of malignant neoplasm, breast as your diagnosis code. There are also V-codes to indicate screening for a particular illness or disease. In the above example, code V76.1 Special screening for malignant neoplasm, breast could also have been used.

It is important to note that when you use a screening code from the V-code section you should also code signs or symptoms. The reason for doing so is because most health insurance carriers do not provide coverage for routine screening procedures or preventive medicine.

COMBINATION CODES

A combination code is used to fully identify an instance where two diagnoses or a diagnosis with an associated secondary process (manifestation) or complication is included in the description of a single code number. These combination codes are identified by referring to the subterms in the Alphabetic Index (Volume 2) and the inclusion and exclusion terms in the Tabular List (Volume 1).

Examples of commonly used combination codes include 034.0 Streptococcal sore throat and 404 Hypertensive heart and renal disease. Code 034.0 exists because the throat is often infected with Streptococcus and code 404 must be used whenever a patient has both heart and renal disease instead of assigning codes from categories 402 and 403.

Two main terms may be joined together by combination terms listed in the Alphabetic Index (Volume 2) as subterms such as:

> *associated with*
> *complicated (by)*
> *due to*
> *during*
> *following*
> *in*
> *secondary to*
> *with*
> *without*

The listing for the above terms advises the coder to use one or two codes depending on the condition.

MULTIPLE CODING

There are single conditions that require more than one code. "Use additional code" notes are found in the Tabular List at codes that are not part of an etiology/ manifestation pair where a secondary code is useful to fully describe a condition. The sequencing rule is the same: "use additional code" indicates that a secondary code should be added.

For example, for infections that are not included in chapter 1, a secondary code from category 041, Bacterial infection in conditions classified elsewhere and of unspecified site, may be required to identify the bacterial organism causing the infection. A "use additional code" note will normally be found at the infection code and indicates a need for the organism code to be added as the secondary code.

There are also "code first" notes under certain codes that are not specifically manifestation codes but may be due to an underlying cause. When a "code first" note is present and an underlying condition is present, the underlying condition should be sequenced first.

"Code, if applicable, any causal condition first" notes indicate that this code may be assigned as a principal diagnosis when the causal condition is unknown or not applicable. If a causal condition is known, then the code for that condition should be sequenced as the principal or first-listed diagnosis.

Multiple codes may be needed for late effects, complication codes and obstetric codes to more fully describe a condition. See the specific guidelines for these sections for further instruction.

When is multiple coding mandatory? Only if the instructional term "code also" appears in italics under an italicized subdivision in the Tabular List (Volume 1). In this instance, you should interpret mandatory as....requires the use of both codes, and that these codes must be sequenced with the code for the etiology being listed first and the code identifying the manifestation listed second. You will recognize mandatory multiple coding situations by instructional terms used in the Tabular List (Volume 1). Terms to watch for are: "Code also....," "Use additional code...," and "Note:..."

If you turn to Category 330 in the Tabular List (Volume 1), you will notice the instructional term cited: "Use additional code to identify associated mental retardation." The phrase "...identify associated mental retardation" should be interpreted as "...identify associated mental retardation, if stated to be present in the diagnostic statement." With this understood, these diagnostic statements would be coded as below.

Coding Examples

Cerebral degeneration in childhood with mental retardation

330.9   Unspecified cerebral degeneration in childhood

319   Unspecified mental retardation

Cerebral degeneration in childhood

330.9   Unspecified cerebral degeneration in childhood

In the Alphabetic Index (Volume 2), if two codes are listed, the first should be sequenced first with the code in italicized brackets listed second to indicate the additional code. However, the fact that two codes appear after a subterm in the Alphabetic Index does not automatically indicate mandatory multiple coding. It is necessary to verify both code numbers in the Tabular List. If, in the Tabular List, the code number is also in italics as in the Alphabetical Index and, the instructional term "Code also" appears in italics, then both criteria have been met for mandatory multiple coding.

Coding Example

Diabetic neuropathy

250.60   Diabetes with neurological manifestations

357.2   Polyneuropathy in diabetes

In the Alphabetic Index (Volume 2) under "Diabetes," you will find "Neuropathy" listed followed by the codes 250.6 and [357.2] in brackets.

It should also be noted at this point, that even though mandatory multiple coding is always indicated by the presence of the instructional term "Code first" in italics beneath the italicized code number and title for the manifestation, this does not always hold true under the code number for the etiology. Multiple coding is not to be used in those instances when a combination code accurately identifies all of the elements within the diagnostic statement.

CODING LATE EFFECTS

A late effect is the residual effect (condition produced) after the acute phase of an illness or injury has terminated. There is no time limit on when a late effect code can be used. The residual may be apparent early, such as in cerebrovascular accident cases, or it may occur months or years later, such as that due to a previous injury. Coding of late effects generally requires two codes sequenced in the following order: The condition or nature of the late effect first; the late effect code second.

An exception to the above guideline is when the code for late effect is followed by a manifestation code identified in the Tabular List and title, or when the late effect code has been expanded (at the fourth and fifth-digit levels) to include the manifestation(s). The code for the acute phase of an illness or injury that led to the late effect is never used with a code for the late effect.

Coding Example

Hemiplegia due to previous cerebral vascular accident

342.90   Hemiplegia, unspecified, affecting unspecified side

438.20   Late effects of cerebrovascular disease, Hemiplegia affecting unspecified side

The residual for this statement is "Hemiplegia" as it is the long term condition that resulted from a previous acute illness. The cause for this statement is "Cerebral vascular accident" as it is the original illness no longer in its acute phase but which did cause the long term residual condition now present.

How do you recognize when to use late effects coding and when not to? Often, the diagnostic statement will contain key words to help identify a late effects situation. Key words used in defining late effects include:

late

due to an old injury

due to a previous illness/injury

due to an illness/injury occurring one year or more ago

In cases where these key words (phrases) are not included within the diagnostic statement, an effect is considered to be late if sufficient time has elapsed between the occurrence of the acute illness/injury and the development of the residual effect.

Coding Example

Excessive scar tissue due to third degree burn, right leg

709.2   Scar conditions and fibrosis of skin

906.7   Late effect of burn of other extremities

The previous diagnostic statement does not indicate the time element with any modifying terms as "old" or "previous." The fact that enough time has elapsed for the development of scar tissue indicates that the acute phase of the injury has subsided and the scarring should be coded as a late effect.

If a diagnostic statement only specifies the cause of the late effect and does not indicate the residual, then use the code number for the cause.

Coding Example

Residuals of tuberculosis

137   Late effects of tuberculosis

The above statement does not identify the actual residuals, so you would use the code for the cause.

To find the code for such a statement in the Alphabetic Index (Volume 2), refer to the main term "LATE" and the subterm "EFFECTS OF." The only codes available for causes of late effects are:

137   Late effects of tuberculosis

138   Late effects of acute poliomyelitis

139   Late effects of other infectious and parasitic diseases

268.1   Rickets, late effects

326   Late effects of intracranial abscess or pyogenic infection

438   Late effects of cerebrovascular disease

677   Late effects of complication of pregnancy, childbirth and the puerperium

905   Late effects of musculoskeletal and connective tissue injuries

906   Late effects of injuries to skin and subcutaneous tissues

907   Late effects of injuries to the nervous system

908   Late effects of other and unspecified injuries

909   Late effects of other and unspecified external causes

Be sure to distinguish between a late effect and a historical statement in a diagnosis. Whenever the statement uses the terms "effects of old...," "sequela of...," or "residuals of...," then code as late effects. If the diagnosis is expressed in terms as "history of...," these are coded to personal history of the illness or injury and are coded to the V-Codes (V-10 to V-15).

CODING IMPENDING OR THREATENED CONDITIONS

Code any condition described at the time of discharge as impending or threatened as follows:

1. If it did occur, code as confirmed diagnosis.

2. If it did not occur, reference the Alphabetic Index to determine if the condition has a subentry term for impending or threatened and also reference main term entries for Impending and for Threatened.

3. If the subterms are listed, assign the given code.

4. If the subterms are not listed, code the existing underlying condition(s) and not the condition described as impending or threatened.

CODING INJURIES

Injuries comprise a major section of ICD-9-CM. Categories 800-959 include fractures, dislocations, sprains and various other types of injuries. Injuries are classified first according to the general type of injury and within each type there is a further breakdown by anatomical site.

When coding injuries, assign separate codes for each injury unless a combination code is provided, in which case the combination code is assigned. Multiple injury codes are provided in ICD-9-CM, but should not be assigned unless information for a more specific code is not available. These codes are not to be used for normal, healing surgical wounds or to identify complications of surgical wounds.

The code for the most serious injury, as determined by the physician, is sequenced first.

1. Superficial injuries such as abrasions or contusions are not coded when associated with more severe injuries of the same site.

2. When a primary injury results in minor damage to peripheral nerves or blood vessels, the primary injury is sequenced first with additional code(s) from categories 950-957, Injury to nerves and spinal cord, and/ or 900-904, Injury to blood vessels. When the primary injury is to the blood vessels or nerves, that injury should be sequenced first.

In cases where a patient has multiple injuries, the most severe injury is the principal diagnosis. Where multiple sites of injury are specified in the diagnosis, you should interpret the term "with" as indicating involvement of both sites, and interpret the term "and" as indicating involvement of either or both sites. You will also note that fifth-digits are commonly used when coding injuries to provide information regarding level of consciousness, specific anatomical sites and severity of injuries.

CODING FRACTURES

The principles of multiple coding of injuries should be followed in coding fractures. Fractures of specified sites are coded individually by site in accordance with both the provisions within categories 800-829 and the level of detail furnished by medical record content. Combination categories for multiple fractures are provided for use when there is insufficient detail in the medical record (such as trauma cases transferred to another hospital), when the reporting form limits the number of codes that can be used in reporting pertinent clinical data, or when there is insufficient specificity at the fourth-digit or fifth-digit level. More specific guidelines are as follows:

1. Multiple fractures of same limb classifiable to the same three-digit or four-digit category are coded to that category.

2. Multiple unilateral or bilateral fractures of same bone(s) but classified to different fourth-digit subdivisions (bone part) within the same three-digit category are coded individually by site.

3. Multiple fracture categories 819 and 828 classify bilateral fractures of both upper limbs (819) and both lower limbs (828), but without any detail at the fourth-digit level other than open and closed type of fractures.

4. Multiple fractures are sequenced in accordance with the severity of the fracture and the physician should be asked to list the fracture diagnoses in the order of severity.

Some general rules to apply when coding fractures follow. Fractures can either be "open" or "closed." An "open" fracture is when the skin has been broken and there is communication with the bone and the outside of the body. Whereas, with a "closed" fracture the bone does not have contact with the outside of the body.

Note the following descriptions as set forth in the ICD-9-CM at the four-digit subdivision level to help distinguish between an "open" and "closed" fracture.

Closed Fractures

comminuted
linear
fissured
spiral
impacted
elevated
simple
greenstick

depressed
march
fractured nos
slipped epiphysis

Open Fractures

compound
missile
puncture
with foreign body
infected

Anytime that it is not indicated whether a fracture is open or closed, code it as if it were closed. Fracture-dislocations are classified as fractures. Pathological fractures are classified to the condition causing the fracture (i.e. osteoporosis) with the use of an additional code to identify the Pathologic fracture (733.1).

CODING BURNS

Current burns (940-949) are classified by depth, extent and by agent (E code). Burns are classified by depth as first degree (erythema), second degree (blistering), and third degree (full-thickness involvement).

1. Sequence first the code that reflects the highest degree of burn when more than one burn is present.

2. Classify burns of the same local site (three-digit category level, 940-947) but of different degrees to the subcategory identifying the highest degree recorded in the diagnosis.

3. Non-healing burns are coded as acute burns. Necrosis of burned skin should be coded as a non-healed burn.

4. Assign code 958.3, Posttraumatic wound infection, not elsewhere classified, as an additional code for any documented infected burn site.

5. When coding burns, assign separate codes for each burn site. Category 946 Burns of Multiple specified sites, should only be used if the location of the burns are not documented. Category 949, Burn, unspecified, is extremely vague and should rarely be used.

6. Assign codes from category 948, Burns classified according to extent of body surface involved, when the site of the burn is not specified or when there is a need for additional data. It is advisable to use category 948 as additional coding when needed to provide data for evaluating burn mortality, such as that needed by burn units. It is also advisable to use

category 948 as an additional code for reporting purposes when there is mention of a third-degree burn involving 20 percent or more of the body surface.

In assigning a code from category 948:

a. Fourth-digit codes are used to identify the percentage of total body surface involved in a burn (all degree).

b. Fifth-digits are assigned to identify the percentage of body surface involved in third-degree burn.

c. Fifth-digit zero (0) is assigned when less than 10 percent or when no body surface is involved in a third-degree burn.

Category 948 is based on the classic rule of nines in estimating body surface involved: head and neck are assigned nine percent, each arm nine percent, each leg 18 percent, the anterior trunk 18 percent, posterior trunk 18 percent, and genitalia one percent. Physicians may change these percentage assignments where necessary to accommodate infants and children who have proportionately larger heads than adults and patients who have large buttocks, thighs, or abdomen that involve burns.

7. Encounters for the treatment of the late effects of burns (i.e., scars or joint contractures) should be coded to the residual condition (sequelae) followed by the appropriate late effect code (906.5-906.9). A late effect E code may also be used, if desired.

8. When appropriate, both a sequelae with a late effect code, and a current burn code may be assigned on the same record.

Remember when coding burns, code only the most severe degree of burns when the burns are of the same site but of different degrees. In cases of burns where it is noted that there is an infection, assign the code for the burn and also the code for the infection (958.3 Posttraumatic wound infection NEC).

POISONING AND ADVERSE EFFECTS OF DRUGS

There are two different sets of code numbers to use to differentiate between poisoning and adverse reactions to the correct substances properly administered. First, you must make the distinction between poisoning and adverse reaction. Poisoning by drugs includes:

Poisoning

Accidental

1. Given in error during diagnostic or therapeutic procedures.

2. Given in error by one person to another (for example, mother to child).

3. Taken in error by self.

Purposeful

1. Suicide attempt.

2. Homicide attempt.

Adverse Reaction in Spite of Proper Administration of Correct Substance

1. In therapeutic of diagnostic procedure.

2. Taken by self or given to another as prescribed.

3. Accumulative effect (intoxication due to...).

4. Interaction of prescribed drugs.

5. Synergistic reaction (enhancing the effect of another drug).

6. Allergic reaction.

7. Hypersensitivity.

To code poisoning by drugs, use the Alphabetic Index (Volume 2) which contains the Table of Drugs and Chemicals. This table includes one column to identify the poisoning code (960-989) and four columns of External Cause Codes to classify whether the poisoning was an accident, suicide, assault or undetermined.

The column labeled "Therapeutic Use" is not used for poisonings but in coding adverse reactions to correct substances properly administered. The External Cause Codes are optional but may be used if a facility's coding policy requires their use.

Note that in the Alphabetic Index (Volume 2) that the subterm entry "Drug" under the main term of "Poisoning" refers the coder to the Table of Drugs and Chemicals for the code assignment. Because the Table of Drugs and Chemicals is so extensive, it is acceptable to code directly from the Table without verifying the code obtained in Volume 1.

What if the drug which caused the poisoning is not listed in the Table of Drugs and Chemicals?

1. Refer to Appendix C in Volume 1 (American Hospital Formulary Service) and locate the name of the drug.

2. Note the AHFS category number listed.

3. Turn to the Table of Drugs and Chemicals in the Alphabetic Index (Volume 2) of ICD-9-CM.

4. Locate the term "Drug."

5. Refer to the subterm "AHFS List."

6. Look through the list until you find the AHFS Category Number determined in step 2 above. The AHFS Category Numbers are listed in numeric order.

7. Assign the code.

How Do You Identify Poisoning By Drugs?

The statement of diagnosis will usually have descriptive terms that would indicate poisoning. Look for terms such as:

Intoxication
Overdose
Poisoning
Toxic effect
Wrong drug given/taken in error
Wrong dosage given/taken in error

Adverse effects of a medicine taken in combination with alcohol or from taking a prescribed drug in combination with a drug the patient took on his/her own initiative (for example antihistamines) are coded as poisonings. If you wish to code a manifestation of the poisoning as well, this code is always listed second, after listing the code identifying the poison first.

Adverse Effects of Drugs

The World Health Organization (WHO) defines adverse drug reaction as any response to a drug "which is noxious and unintended and which occurs at doses used in man for prophylaxis, diagnosis or therapy." Notice that this definition does not include the terms "overdose" or "poisoning."

Why does ICD-9-CM differentiate between poisoning and adverse drug reaction? Tabulation of statistical data indicates how often a drug reaction occurred because of the drug itself versus how often the drug was either not given or taken properly. Two codes are required when coding adverse drug reactions to the correct substance properly administered. One code is used to identify the manifestation or the nature of the adverse reaction such as urticaria, vertigo, gastritis, etc. This code is assigned from Categories 001-799 in Volume 1.

Refer to the main term identifying the manifestation in the Alphabetic Index (Volume 2). But remember that the Table of Drugs and Chemicals is not used to locate the code for the manifestation, and the code used to identify the manifestation does not identify the drug responsible for the adverse reaction.

A second code is required to identify the drug causing the adverse reaction. In ICD-9-CM, the only codes provided to identify the drug causing an adverse reaction to a substance properly administered are E930 through E949. Anytime a code is selected from the E930-E949 range, it can never be sequenced first or stand as a solo code.

Locating the Proper E Code

How do you locate the proper E code to identify the drug which was responsible for causing an adverse reaction to a correct substance properly administered? Turn to the Table of Drugs and Chemicals in the Alphabetic Index (Volume 2). Earlier we noted that the column labeled "Therapeutic Use" was not used for coding instances involving poisoning. However, for adverse drug reactions to a correct substance properly administered, the "Therapeutic Use" column is used to find the proper code within the range E930 through E949 to identify the drug.

Drug Interactions Between Two or More Drugs

Drug interactions between two or more prescribed drugs are classified as adverse drug reactions to a correct substance properly administered. This holds true regardless of whether the drugs were prescribed by the same physician or different physicians.

Two types of drug interactions should be noted:

1. Synergistic interaction. One drug enhances the action of another drug so that the combined effect is greater than the sum of the effects of each used alone.

2. Antagonistic interaction. One drug represses the action of another drug.

To properly code drug interactions, first code the manifestation. Then code each drug involved in the interaction using the E codes from the column labeled "Therapeutic Use" from the Table of Drugs and Chemicals.

Coding Example

Gastritis due to interaction between Motrin and Procainamide

535.50   Unspecified gastritis and gastroduodenitis

List the manifestation first

E935.8   Other specified analgesics and antipyretics

E942.0   Cardiac rhythm regulators

Coding Example

When a diagnostic statement does not state specifically the manifestation or nature of the adverse reaction, you should use the code provided to identify an adverse drug reaction of unspecified nature, 995.2 Unspecified adverse effect of drug, medicinal and biological substance. For example:

Allergic reaction to Motrin, proper dose

995.2   Unspecified adverse effect of drug medicinal and biological substance

E935.8   Other specified analgesics and antipyretics

Note in the above example that the code indicating the manifestation, although unspecified as to the nature, is listed first followed by the E code to identify the drug. When the drug causing an adverse effect is unknown or unspecified, use code E947.9 Unspecified drug or medicinal substance.

It is very important to remember that codes in the range 960 through 979 are never used in combination with codes in the range E930 through E949 because codes in the range 960-979 identify poisonings and codes in the range E930-E949 identify the external cause of adverse reactions to the correct substance properly administered.

CODING COMPLICATIONS OF MEDICAL AND SURGICAL CARE

A complication is when you have the occurrence of two or more diseases in the same patient. Recent studies have revealed serious deficiencies in properly coding complications for insurance claims processing. Often the complication is never mentioned. Complications are responsible for many of the procedures that are ordered for patients, therefore the complication should be coded and submitted on your insurance claims.

POSTOPERATIVE COMPLICATIONS

Postoperative complications that affect a specific anatomical site or body system are classified to the appropriate chapter 1 through 16 of the Tabular Index (Volume 1). Postoperative complications affecting more than one anatomical site or body system are classified in the chapter on injury and poisoning (Chapter 17, Categories 996-999). If the Alphabetic Index (Volume 2) does not provide a specific main term and subterm to identify a postoperative complication, classify the complication to categories 996-999.

Coding Example

Postcholecystectomy syndrome

576.0   Postcholecystectomy syndrome

The Alphabetic Index (Volume 2) specifically classifies the postoperative condition to one of the categories from 001 through 799. See main term "Complication," subterms "surgical procedure" and "postcholecystectomy syndrome."

Coding Examples

Postoperative wound infection

998.5   Postoperative infection

The Alphabetic Index (Volume 2) has a main term "Infection" and subterms "wound, postoperative" for this condition. Note that this code appears in Chapter 17 within categories 996-999.

Postoperative atelectasis

997.3   Respiratory complications

Refer to the main term "Atelectasis" in the Alphabetic Index (Volume 2). Note there is no subterm for postoperative beneath this main term. Therefore, you must presume this complication is classified to one of the categories in the range 969-999. You may also code 518.0 Pulmonary collapse, to identify the nature of the respiratory complication for statistical purposes; however, the code for the complication must be listed first.

COMPLICATIONS FROM MECHANICAL DEVICES

Subcategories in the range 996.0 through 996.5 are used to identify mechanical complications of devices. Mechanical complications are the result of a malfunction on the part of the internal prosthetic implant or device. What indicates a mechanical complication? Breakdown or obstruction, displacement, leakage, perforation or protrusion of the devices are all forms of mechanical complications.

Coding Examples

Displacement of cardiac pacemaker electrode

996.01   Mechanical complication of cardiac device, implant, and graft due to cardiac pacemaker (electrode)

Protrusion of nail into acetabulum

996.4   Mechanical complication of internal orthopedic device, implant, and graft

Other complications of devices, such as infection or hemorrhage, are due to an abnormal reaction of the body to an otherwise properly functioning device. All complications involving infection are coded to category 996.7 Other complications of internal prosthetic device, implant and graft.

Coding Examples

Infected arteriovenous shunt

996.6   Infection and inflammatory reaction due to internal prosthetic device, implant, and graft

Anterior chamber hemorrhage due to displaced prosthetic lens

996.7   Other complications of internal (biologic) (synthetic) prosthetic device, implant, and graft

CARDIAC COMPLICATIONS

In the case of cardiac complications, ICD-9-CM defines the "immediate postoperative period" as "the period between surgery and the time of discharge from the hospital." This definition is the basis of whether to code cardiac complications under subcategory 997.1 Cardiac complications affecting specified body systems, not elsewhere classified, or under subcategory 429.4 Functional disturbances following cardiac surgery.

Use 997.1 for a cardiac complication that occurs anytime between surgery and hospital discharge from any type of procedure performed. Use subcategory 429.4 to code long-term cardiac complications resulting from cardiac surgery.

It is important to distinguish between complications and aftercare. Aftercare is usually an encounter for something planned in advance (example, removal of Kirshner wire). Aftercare is classified using codes in the range of V51-V58. An encounter for a complication occurs from unforeseen circumstances, such as wound infection, resulting in complication of the patient's condition.

CODING CIRCULATORY DISEASES

Because of the variety of terms and phrases used by physicians to identify diseases of the circulatory system, you will often experience difficulty in coding. To accurately code disorders of the circulatory system, it is imperative that the coder carefully read all inclusion, exclusion and "use additional code" notations contained in the Tabular List (Volume 1).

Fifth digit subclassifications are also frequently used to code combination disorders or to provide further specificity in this section. Even those in specialties other than cardiology will frequently find themselves coding circulatory system diagnoses due to the prevalence of circulatory disorders in this country.

Chapter 7 of the Tabular List (Volume 1), titled Diseases of the Circulatory System, contains the following major sections:

Acute Rheumatic Fever (390-392) Chronic Rheumatic Heart Disease (393-398) Hypertensive Disease (401-405) Ischemic Heart Disease (410-414) Diseases of Pulmonary Circulation (415-417) Other Forms of Heart Disease (420-429) Cerebrovascular Disease (430-438) Diseases of Arteries, Arterioles, and Capillaries (440-448) Diseases of Veins, Lymphatics, and Ohter Diseases of the Circulatory System (451-459)

DISEASES OF MITRAL AND AORTIC VALVES

Certain diseases of the mitral valve of unspecified etiology are presumed to be of rheumatic origin and others are not. None of the disorders of the aortic valve of unspecified etiology are presumed to be of rheumatic origin. When you have disorders involving both the mitral and aortic valves of unspecified etiology, then they are presumed to be of rheumatic origin.

Coding Examples

Mitral valve insufficiency

424.0   Mitral valve disorders

Refer to the main term "Insufficiency" in the Alphabetic Index (Volume 2). Note the subterm "mitral (valve)."

Mitral valve stenosis

394.0   Mitral stenosis

Refer to the main term "Stenosis" and the sub-term "mitral (valve)" in the Alphabetic Index (Volume 2).

Aortic valve insufficiency

424.1   Aortic valve disorders

Aortic valve stenosis

424.1   Aortic valve disorders

Look up the main term "Stenosis" and the subterm "aortic" in the Alphabetic Index (Volume 2). Remember that aortic valve disorders of unspecified etiology are not considered rheumatic in nature or origin.

Insufficiency of mitral and aortic valves

396.3   Mitral valve insufficiency and aortic valve insufficiency

Under the main term "Insufficiency" in the Alphabetic Index (Volume 2) you will find the subterm "aortic." Further review will locate "with," "mitral valve disease," "insufficiency, incompetence or regurgitation" which directs you to code 396.3

Ischemic Heart Disease

In ischemic heart disease, the manifestations are due to a lack of blood flow to the heart rather than to the anatomical lesion of the coronary arteries. The most common cause of coronary heart disease is coronary atherosclerosis. However, ischemic heart disease can be due to non-coronary disease, such as aortic valvular stenosis, as well. There are many synonyms used to indicate ischemic heart disease such as: coronary artery heart disease, ASHD, and coronary ischemia. Categories in the range 410-414, Ischemic Heart Disease, includes that with mention of hypertension. Use an additional code to identify the presence of hypertension.

Coding Examples

Angina pectoris

413.9   Other and unspecified angina pectoris

As no mention of hypertension is made in the diagnostic statement, a single code is all that is required.

Angina pectoris with essential hypertension

413.9   Other and unspecified angina pectoris

401.9   Essential hypertension, unspecified

In this example, the mention of hypertension in the diagnostic statement requires the use of a second code.

MYOCARDIAL INFARCTION

A myocardial infarction is classified as acute if it is either specified as "acute" in the diagnostic statement or with a stated duration of eight weeks or less. When a myocardial infarction is specified as "chronic" or with symptoms after eight weeks from the date of the onset, it should be coded to subcategory 414.8 Other specified forms of chronic ischemic heart disease. If a myocardial infarction is specified as old or healed or has been diagnosed by special investigation (EKG) but is currently not presenting any symptoms, code using category 412 Old myocardial infarction.

Coding Examples

Myocardial infarction three weeks ago

410.92   Acute myocardial infarction, unspecified site

Chronic myocardial infarction with angina

414.8   Other specified forms of chronic ischemic heart disease

413.9   Other and unspecified angina pectoris

Myocardial infarction diagnoses by EKG, symptomatic

412   Old myocardial infarction

ARTERIOSCLEROTIC CARDIOVASCULAR DISEASE (ASCVD)

Arteriosclerotic cardiovascular disease (ASCVD) is classified to subcategory 429.2 Cardiovascular disease, unspecified. You should use an additional code to identify the presence of arteriosclerosis when coding ASCVD. For example, the diagnostic statement "generalized arteriosclerotic cardiovascular disease" should be coded using 429.2 followed by 440.9 Generalized and unspecified atherosclerosis.

"Other forms of heart disease", categories 420-429, are used for multiple coding purposes to fully identify a stated diagnosis. The exception to this rule is if the Alphabetic Index (Volume 2) or Tabular List (Volume 1) specifically instructs you otherwise.

Coding Examples

Arteriosclerotic heart disease with acute pulmonary edema

428.1	Left heart failure
414.00	Coronary atherosclerosis, of unspecified type of vessel, native or graft

Note that the code for ASHD (414.00) is listed second as a possible underlying cause of the acute situation.

Arteriosclerotic heart disease with congestive heart failure

428.0	Congestive heart failure, unspecified
414.00	Coronary atherosclerosis, of unspecified type of vessel, native or graft

CEREBROVASCULAR DISEASE

When coding cerebrovascular disease (codes 430-438), you should code the component parts of the diagnostic statement identifying the cerebrovascular disease, unless specifically instructed to do otherwise in the Alphabetic Index (Volume 2) or Tabular List (Volume 1).

Coding Examples

Cerebrovascular arteriosclerosis with subarachnoid hemorrhage

430   Subarachnoid hemorrhage

437.0   Cerebral atherosclerosis

Cerebrovascular accident secondary to thrombosis

434.00   Cerebral thrombosis, without mention of cerebral infarction

In this example, you use only one code because of the instructions in the Alphabetic Index (Volume 2). When you look up the main term "Accident" with subterm "cerebrovascular," you are instructed to "(see also Disease, cerebrovascular, acute) 436." When you locate the main term "Disease" and subterms "cerebrovascular," "acute" and "thrombotic," you are further instructed to "see Thrombosis, brain". This is where you finally locate the single code for this diagnosis, 434.0. When you look up the code in the Tabular List (Volume 1), you are instructed to add a fifth digit "0" if it is without mention of cerebral infarction, and "1" if it is with cerebral infarction.

Whenever there are conditions resulting from the acute cerebrovascular disease, code them if they are stated to be residual(s). If the resulting condition is stated to be transient, do not code them.

Coding Examples

Cerebrovascular accident with residual aphasia

436   Acute, but ill-defined, cerebrovascular disease

784.3   Aphasia

Cerebrovascular accident with transient hemiparesis

436   Acute, but ill-defined, cerebrovascular disease

LATE EFFECTS OF CEREBROVASCULAR DISEASE

Category 438 is used to indicate conditions classifiable to categories 430-437 as the causes of late effects (neurologic deficits), themselves classified elsewhere. These late effects include neurologic deficits that persist after initial onset of conditions classifiable to 430-437. The neurologic deficits caused by cerebrovascular disease may be present from the onset or may arise at any time after the onset of the condition classifiable to 430-437.

Codes from category 438 may be assigned on a health care record with codes from 430-437, if the patient has a current cerebrovascular accident (CVA) and deficits from an old CVA. Assign code V12.59 (and not a code from category 438) as an additional code for history of cerebrovascular disease when no neurologic deficits are present.

HYPERTENSIVE DISEASE

As demonstrated earlier with ischemic heart disease, conditions that are classified to cerebrovascular disease (codes 430-438) include that with mention of hypertension, but you must identify the hypertension with another code (401-405) and list it second.

Hypertension is frequently the cause of various forms of heart and vascular disease. However, the mention of hypertension with some heart conditions should not be interpreted as a combination resulting in hypertensive heart disease. The combination is only to be made if there is a cause-and-effect relationship between hypertension and a heart condition classified to subcategories 425.8, 428.0-428.9, 429.0-429.3 and 429.8-429.9.

Hypertensive disease is classified to the categories 401-405. The Table of Hypertension (see example next page) is located in the Alphabetic Index (Volume 2) under the main term "Hypertension." This Table contains subterms to identify types of hypertension and complications. It contains a complete listing of all conditions due to or associated with hypertension and classifies them according to malignant, benign, and unspecified.

INDEX TO DISEASES		Hypertension, hypertensive

Hypertension, hypertensive	Malignant	Benign	Unspecified
renal (disease) (see also			
Hypertension, kidney)	403.00	403.10	403.90
renovascular NEC	405.01	405.11	405.91
secondary NEC	405.09	405.19	405.99
due to			
aldosteronism, primary	405.09	405.19	405.99
brain tumor	405.09	405.19	405.99
bulbar poliomyelitis	405.09	405.19	405.99
calculus			
kidney	405.09	405.19	405.99
ureter	405.09	405.19	405.99

1. Hypertension, essential or NOS.

   Assign hypertension (arterial) (essential) (primary) (systemic) (NOS) to category code 401 with the appropriate fourth digit to indicate malignant (.0), benign (.1), or unspecified (.9). Do not use either .0 malignant or .1 benign unless medical record documentation supports such a designation.

2. Hypertension with Heart Disease.

   Heart conditions (425.8, 429.0-429.3, 429.8, 429.9) are assigned to a code from category 402 when a causal relationship is stated (due to hypertension) or implied (hypertensive). Use an additional code from category 428 to identify the type of heart failure in those patients with heart failure. More than one code from category 428 may be assigned if the patient has systolic or diastolic failure and congestive heart failure.

   The same heart conditions (425.8, 428, 429.0-429.3, 429.8, 429.9) with hypertension, but without a stated casual relationship, are coded separately. Sequence according to the circumstances of the admission/encounter.

3. Hypertensive Renal Disease with Chronic Renal Failure

   Assign codes from category 403, Hypertensive renal disease, when conditions classified to categories 585-587 are present. Unlike hypertension with heart disease, ICD-9-CM presumes a cause-and-effect relationship and classifies renal failure with hypertension as hypertensive renal disease.

4. Hypertensive Heart and Renal Disease

   Assign codes from combination category 404, Hypertensive heart and renal disease, when both hypertensive renal disease and hypertensive heart disease are stated in the diagnosis. Assume a relationship between the hypertension and the renal disease, whether or not the condition is so designated. Assign an additional code from category 428 to identify the type of heart failure. More than one code from category 428 may be assigned if the patient has systolic or diastolic failure and congestive heart failure.

5. Hypertensive Cerebrovascular Disease

   First assign codes from 430-438, Cerebrovascular disease, then the appropriate hypertension code from categories 401-405.

6. Hypertensive Retinopathy

   Two codes are necessary to identify the condition. First assign the code from subcategory 362.11, Hypertensive retinopathy, then the appropriate code from categories 401-405 to indicate the type of hypertension.

7. Hypertension, Secondary

Two codes are required: one to identify the underlying etiology and one from category 405 to identify the hypertension. Sequencing of codes is determined by the reason for admission/encounter.

8. Hypertension, Transient

Assign code 796.2, Elevated blood pressure reading without diagnosis of hypertension, unless patient has an established diagnosis of hypertension. Assign code 642.3x for transient hypertension of pregnancy.

9. Hypertension, Controlled

Assign appropriate code from categories 401-405. This diagnostic statement usually refers to an existing state of hypertension under control by therapy.

10. Hypertension, Uncontrolled

Uncontrolled hypertension may refer to untreated hypertension or hypertension not responding to current therapeutic regimen. In either case, assign the appropriate code from categories 401-405 to designate the stage and type of hypertension. Code to the type of hypertension.

11. Elevated Blood Pressure

For a statement of elevated blood pressure without further specificity, assign code 796.2, Elevated blood pressure reading without diagnosis of hypertension, rather than a code from category 401.

First you need to be able to make a distinction between conditions specified as "due to" or "with" hypertension. Keep in mind that the phrase "due to hypertension" and the word "hypertensive" are considered synonymous.

Coding Examples

Hypertensive heart disease

402.90   Hypertensive heart disease, unspecified, without heart failure

Heart disease due to hypertension

402.90   Hypertensive heart disease, unspecified, without heart failure

Each of the above diagnostic statements indicate clearly a cause-and-effect relationship between hypertension and the condition by specifying that the condition is "due to." Therefore, both statements are coded using 402.90.

If the phrase "with hypertension" is stated or, the diagnostic statement mentions the conditions separately, then you code the conditions separately.

Coding Example

Myocarditis with hypertension

> **429.0**   Myocarditis, unspecified
>
> **401.9**   Essential hypertension, unspecified

As a cause-and-effect relationship is not indicated in the diagnostic statement, the conditions are coded separately.

HIGH BLOOD PRESSURE VERSUS ELEVATED BLOOD PRESSURE

With the ICD-9-CM coding system there is a differentiation made between high blood pressure (hypertension) and elevated blood pressure without a diagnosis of hypertension. If the diagnostic statement indicates elevated blood pressure without the diagnosis of hypertension, it is coded to subcategory 796.2 Elevated blood pressure reading without diagnosis of hypertension. If the diagnostic statement indicates high blood pressure or hypertension, it is coded to category 401 Essential hypertension.

DIABETES MELLITUS CODING

In 1980, the American Diabetic Association reclassified the types of diabetes mellitus to signify whether or not the patient is dependent on insulin for survival of life. In 1994, additional classifications were added. Note the revisions (bracketed portions) of the statements below for the fifth-digit subclassification.

0   type II [non-insulin dependent type] [NIDDM type] [adult-onset type] or unspecified type, not stated as uncontrolled

> Fifth digit 0 is for use with type II, adult onset diabetic patients, even if the patient requires insulin

1   type I [insulin dependent type] [IDDM] [juvenile type], not stated as uncontrolled

2   type II [non-insulin dependent type] [NIDDM] [adult-onset type] or unspecified type, uncontrolled

Fifth digit 2 is for use with type II, adult onset diabetic patients, even if the patient requires insulin

3   type I [insulin dependent type][IDDM][juvenile type], uncontrolled

Do not assume a patient has insulin-dependent diabetes simply because the patient is receiving insulin, as some non-dependent diabetics may require temporary use when they encounter stressful situations such as surgery or physical or mental illness.

Anytime diabetes is described as "brittle" or "uncontrolled" you should interpret it as diabetes mellitus complicated and assign code 250.9 with the appropriate fifth-digit, 0, 1, 2 or 3. However, if there is also a specific complication present, then assign the code identifying that specific complication, for example, Diabetes mellitus, brittle, with ketoacidosis would be 250.13.

CODING MENTAL DISORDERS

The Glossary of Mental Disorders found in Appendix B of the Tabular List (Volume 1) is used as a guide to provide a common frame of reference for statistical comparisons. It is an alphabetized listing of mental disorders with definitions. The coder should choose code assignments based on the terminology used by the physician or psychiatrist and not by the coder's impression of the content of the categories and subcategories.

GLOSSARY OF MENTAL DISORDERS

Amnestic syndrome: A syndrome of prominent and lasting reduction of memory span, including striking loss of recent memory, disordered time appreciation, and confabulation. The commonest causes are chronic alcoholism [alcohol amnestic syndrome; Korsakoff's alcoholic psychosis], chronic barbiturate dependence, and malnutrition. An amnestic syndrome may be the predominating disturbance in the early states of presenile and senile dementia, arteriosclerotic dementia, and in encephalitis and other inflammatory and degenerative diseases in which there is particular bilateral involvement of the temporal lobes, and certain temporal lobe tumors.

–alcoholic see alcohol amnestic syndrome under Alcoholic psychoses

Amoral personality–see Personality disorder, antisocial type

INFECTIOUS AND PARASITIC DISEASES

There are two categories for identifying the organism causing diseases classified elsewhere. These codes may be used as either additional codes, or as solo codes depending on the diagnostic statement.

041	Bacterial infection in conditions classified elsewhere and of unspecified site
079	Viral and chlamydial infection in conditions classified elsewhere and of unspecified site

Coding Examples

Acute UTI due to Escherichia coli

599.0	Urinary tract infection, site not specified
041.4	Escherichia coli [E. coli]

Staphylococcus infection

041.11	Staphylococcus aureus

Bacterial infection

041.9	Bacterial infection, unspecified

The basic coding principles regarding combination codes (one code accurately identifies the components of the condition) applies throughout the chapter on Infectious and Parasitic Diseases.

In the Alphabetic Index (Volume 2), a subterm that identifies an infectious organism takes precedence in code assignment over a subterm at the same indentation level that identifies a site or other descriptive term.

Coding Example

Chronic syphilitic cystitis

095.8	Other specified forms of late symptomatic syphilis

Using the Alphabetic Index (Volume 2) to look up the main term "Cystitis (bacillary)," you will note the subterms "chronic 595.2" and "syphilitic 095.8" at the same indentation level under the main term. Therefore, code 095.8 is assigned to this diagnostic statement, as the organism has precedence over other descriptive terms or anatomical sites.

HUMAN IMMUNODEFICIENCY VIRUS (HIV) DISEASE

1. Code only confirmed cases of HIV infection/illness. This is an exception to the hospital inpatient guideline Section II, H.

   In this context, confirmation does not require documentation of positive serology or culture for HIV; the physician' diagnostic statement that the patient is HIV positive, or has an HIV-related illness is sufficient.

2. Selection and sequencing

   a. If a patient is admitted for an HIV-related condition, the principal diagnosis should be 042, followed by additional diagnosis codes for all reported HIV-related conditions.

   b. If a patient with HIV disease is admitted for an unrelated condition (such as a traumatic injury), the code for the unrelated condition (e.g., the nature of injury code) should be the principal diagnosis. Other diagnoses would be 042 followed by additional diagnosis codes for all reported HIV-related conditions.

   c. Whether the patient is newly diagnosed or has had previous admissions/ encounters for HIV conditions is irrelevant to the sequencing decision.

   d. V08 Asymptomatic human immunodeficiency virus [HIV] infection status, is to be applied when the patient without any documentation of symptoms is listed as being HIV positive, known HIV, HIV test positive, or similar terminology. Do not use this code if the term AIDS is used or if the patient is treated for any HIV-related illness or is described as having any condition(s) resulting from his/her HIV positive status; use 042 instead.

   e. Patients with inconclusive HIV serology, but no definitive diagnosis or manifestations of the illness, may be assigned code 795.71, Nonspecific serologic evidence of human immunodeficiency virus [HIV]

   f. Previously diagnosed HIV-related illness: Patients with any known prior diagnosis of an HIV-related illness should be coded to 042. Once a patient had developed an HIV-related illness, the patient should always be assigned code 042 on every subsequent admission/encounter. Patients previously diagnosed with any HIV illness (042) should never be assigned to 795.71 or V08.

   g. HIV Infection in Pregnancy, Childbirth and the Puerperium: During pregnancy, childbirth or the puerperium, a patient admitted (or presenting for a health care encounter) because of an HIV-related illness should receive a principal diagnosis of 647.6X, Other viral diseases in the mother classifiable elsewhere, but complicating the pregnancy, childbirth or the puerperium, followed by 042 and the code(s) for the HIV-related illness(es). Codes from Chapter 11 Pregnancy, Childbirth and the Puerperium always take sequencing priority.

Patients with asymptomatic HIV infection status admitted (or presenting for a health care encounter) during pregnancy, childbirth, or the puerperium should receive codes of 647.6X and V08.

h. Encounters for Testing for HIV: If a patient is being seen to determine his/her HIV status, use code V73.89, Screening for other specified viral disease. Use code V69.8, Other problems related to lifestyle, as a secondary code if an asymptomatic patient is in a known high risk group for HIV. Should a patient with signs or symptoms or illness, or a confirmed HIV related diagnosis be tested for HIV, code the signs and symptoms or the diagnosis. An additional code V65.44 HIV counseling may be used if counseling is provided during the encounter for the test.

When a patient returns to be informed of his/her HIV test results use code V65.44, HIV counseling, if the results of the test are negative.

If the results are positive but the patient is asymptomatic use code V08, Asymptomatic HIV infection. If the results are positive and the patient is symptomatic use code 042, HIV disease, with codes for the HIV related symptoms or diagnosis. The HIV counseling code may also be used if counseling is provided for patients with positive test results.

SEPTICEMIA, SYSTEMIC INFLAMMATORY RESPONSE SYNDROME (SIRS), SEPSIS, SEVERE SEPSIS, AND SEPTIC SHOCK

1. In most cases, it will be a code from category 038 *Septicemia* that will be used in conjunction with a code from subcategory 995.9.

    a. If the documentation in the record states streptococcal sepsis, codes 038.0 and code 995.91 should be used, in that sequence.

    b. If the documentation states streptococcal septicemia, only code 038.0 should be assigned. However, the physician should be queried whether the patient has sepsis, an infection with SIRS.

    c. Either the term sepsis or SIRS must be documented to assign a code from subcategory 995.9.

2. If the terms sepsis, severe sepsis, or SIRS are used with an underlying infection other than septicemia, such as pneumonia, cellulitis or a nonspecified urinary tract infection, code 038.9 should be assigned first, then code 995.91, followed by the code for the initial infection. The use of the terms sepsis or SIRS indicates that the patient's infection has advanced to the point of a systemic infection so the systemic infection should be sequenced before the localized infection. The insturctional note under subcategory 995.9 instructs to assign the underlying condition first.

   Note: The terms urosepsis is a nonspecific term. If that is the only term documented then only code 599.0 should be assigned based on the default for the term in the ICD-9-CM index, in addition to the code for the causal organism if known.

3. For patients with severe sepsis, the code for the systemic infection (038.x) or trauma should be sequenced first, followed by either code 995.92, *Systemic inflammatory response syndrome due to infectious process with organ dysfunction*, or code 995.94, *Systemic inflammatory response syndrome due to noninfectious process with organ dysfunction*. Codes for the specific organ dysfunction should also be assigned.

4. If septic shock is documented, it is necessary to code first the initiating systemic infection or trauma, then either code 995.92 or 995.94, followed by the code 785.52, *Septic shock*.

5. Sepsis and septic shock associated with abortion, ectopic pregnancy, and molar pregnancy are classified to category codes in Chapter 11 (630-639).

6. Negative or inconclusive blood cultures do not preclude a diagnosis of septicemia or sepsis in patients with clinical evidence of the condition, however the physician should be queried.

MANIFESTATIONS

Manifestations are characteristic signs or symptoms of an illness. Signs and symptoms that point rather definitely to a given diagnosis are assigned to the appropriate chapter of ICD-9-CM. For example, hematuria is assigned to the Genitourinary System chapter. However, Chapter 16 Symptoms, Signs and Ill-Defined Conditions (780-799), includes ill-defined conditions and symptoms that may suggest two or more diseases or may point to two or more systems of the body, and are used in cases lacking the necessary study to make a final diagnosis.

Conditions allocated to Chapter 16 include:

1. Cases for which no more specific diagnosis can be made even after all facts bearing on the case have been investigated; for example code 784.0 *Headache.*

2. Signs or symptoms existing at the time of initial encounter that proved to be transient and whose cause could not be determined; for example code 780.2 *Syncope and collapse.*

3. Provisional diagnoses in a patient who failed to return for further investigation or care; for example code 782.4 *Jaundice, unspecified, not of newborn.*

4. Cases referred elsewhere for investigation or treatment before the diagnosis was made; for example code 782.5 *Cyanosis.*

5. Cases in which a more precise diagnosis was not available for any other reason; for example code 780.4 *Dizziness and giddiness.*

6. Certain symptoms which represent important problems in medical care and which it might be desired to classify in addition to a known cause; for example, code 780.01 *Coma.*

In the last case, if the cause of a symptom or sign is stated in the diagnosis, assign the code identifying the cause. An additional code may be assigned to further identify this symptom or sign if there is a need to further identify the symptom or sign. In such cases, the code identifying the cause will ordinarily be listed as the principal diagnosis.

ETIOLOGY/MANIFESTATION CONVENTION

Certain conditions have both an underlying etiology and multiple body system manifestations. For such conditions, the ICD-9-CM has a coding convention that requires the underlying condition be sequenced first followed by the manifestation. Wherever such a combination exists there is a "Use additional code" note at the etiology code, and a "Code first" note at the manifestation code. These instructional notes indicate the proper sequencing order of the codes, etiology followed by manifestation.

In most cases, the manifestation codes will have "in diseases classified elsewhere" in the code title. Such codes are a component of the etiology/manifestation convention. The code title indicates that it is a manifestation code. The "diseases classified elsewhere" codes are never permitted to be used as first listed or principal diagnosis codes. They must be used in conjunction with an underlying condition code and they must be listed following the underlying condition.

There are manifestation codes that do not have "in diseases classified elsewhere" in their title. For such codes a "Use additional code" note will still be present and the rules for sequencing apply. In addition to the notes in the Tabular Listing, these conditions also have a specific index entry structure. In the alphabetical index, both conditions are listed together with the etiology code first followed by the manifestation codes in [brackets]. The code in brackets is always to be sequenced second.

The most commonly used etiology/manifestation combinations are the codes for Diabetes mellitus, category 250. For each code under category 250 there is a "Use additional code" note for the manifestation that is specific for that particular diabetic manifestation. Should a patient have more than one manifestation of diabetes, more than one code from category 250 may be used with as many manifestation codes as are needed to fully describe the patient's complete diabetic condition. The diabetes category 250 codes should be sequenced first, followed by the manifestation codes.

"Code first" and "Use additional code" notes are also used as sequencing rules in the classification for certain codes that are not part of an etiology/ manifestation combination.

CODING OF NEOPLASMS

The coding of neoplasms requires a good understanding of medical terminology. All neoplasms are classified in the Tabular List (Volume 1) in Chapter 2 Neoplasms 140-239 which contains the following broad groups:

140-195	Malignant neoplasms, stated or presumed to be primary, of specified sites, except of lymphatic and hematopoietic tissue
196-198	Malignant neoplasms, stated or presumed to be secondary, of specified sites
199	Malignant neoplasms, without specification of site
200-208	Malignant neoplasms, stated or presumed to be primary of lymphatic and hematopoietic tissue
210-229	Benign neoplasms
230-234	Carcinoma in situ
235-238	Neoplasms of uncertain behavior
239	Neoplasms of unspecified nature

INDEX TO DISEASES					Neoplasm	
	Malignant Primary	Malignant Secondary	Malignant Ca In Situ	Benign	Uncertain	Unspecified
Neoplasm, neoplastic	199.1	199.1	234.9	229.9	238.9	239.9
abdomen, abdominal	195.2	198.89	234.8	229.8	238.8	239.8
cavity	195.2	198.89	234.8	229.8	238.8	239.8
organ	195.2	198.89	234.8	229.8	238.8	239.8
viscera	195.2	198.89	234.8	229.8	238.8	239.8
wall	173.5	198.2	232.5	216.5	238.2	239.2
connective tissue	171.5	198.89	—	215.5	238.1	239.2
abdominopelvic	195.8	198.89	234.8	229.8	238.8	239.8
acoustic nerve	192.0	198.4	—	225.1	237.9	239.7
acromion (process)	170.4	198.5	—	213.4	238.0	239.2
adenoid (pharynx) (tissue)	147.1	198.89	230.0	210.7	235.1	239.0

Table of Neoplasms

The Table of Neoplasms appears in the Alphabetic Index (Volume 2) under the main term "Neoplasms." This table gives the code numbers for neoplasms of anatomical site. For each anatomical site there are six possible code numbers according to whether the neoplasm in questions is either:

Malignant:
>   Primary
>   Secondary
>   Ca in situ
Benign
Of uncertain behavior
Of unspecified nature

Definitions of Site and Behaviors of Neoplasms

Primary   Identifies the stated or presumed site of origin.

Secondary   Identifies site(s) to which the primary site has spread (direct extension) or metastasized by lymphatic spread, invading local blood vessels, or by implantation as tumor cells shed into body cavities.

In-situ   Tumor cells that are undergoing malignant changes but are still confined to the point of origin without invasion of surrounding normal tissue (non-infiltrating, non-invasive or pre-invasive carcinoma).

Benign   Tumor does not invade adjacent structures or spread to distant sites but may displace or exert pressure on adjacent structures.

Uncertain   The pathologist is not able to determine whether the tumor is benign or malignant behavior because some features of each are present.

Unspecified   Neither the behavior nor the histological type of tumors are specified in the diagnostic Nature statement. This type of diagnosis may be encountered when the patient has been treated elsewhere and comes in terminally ill without accompanying information, is referred elsewhere for work-up, or no work-up is performed because of advanced age or poor condition of the patient.

Steps to Coding Neoplasms

1. ICD-9-CM disregards classification of neoplasms by histological type (according to tissue origin) with the exception of lymphatic and hematopoietic neoplasms, malignant melanoma of skin, lipoma, and a few common tumors of bone, uterus, ovary, etc. All other tumors are classified by system, organ or site. The existence of these exceptions makes it necessary to first consult the Alphabetic Index (Volume 2) to determine whether a specific code has been assigned to a specified histological type. For example, Malignant melanoma of skin of scalp is coded 172.4 although the code specified in the "Malignant: Primary Column" of the Neoplasm Table for skin of scalp is 173.4.

2. The General Alphabetical Index (Volume 2) also provides guidance to the appropriate column for neoplasms which are not assigned a specific code by histological type. For example, if you look up Lipomyoma, specified site in the Alphabetic Index (Volume 2), you will find "see Neoplasm, connective tissue, benign."

    The guidance in the Alphabetic Index (Volume 2) can be over-ridden if a descriptor is present. For example, Malignant adenoma of colon is coded as 153.9 and not as 211.3 because the adjective "malignant" overrides the entry "adenoma see also Neoplasm, benign."

3. The Neoplasm Table may be consulted directly if a specific neoplasm diagnosis indicates which column of the table is appropriate but does not delineate a specific type of tumor.

4. Sites marked with an asterisk (*), such as buttock NEC* or calf*, should be classified to malignant neoplasm of skin of these sites if the variety of neoplasm is a squamous cell carcinoma or an epidermoid carcinoma and to benign neoplasm of skin of these sites if the variety of neoplasm is a papilloma (of any type).

5. Primary malignant neoplasms are classified to the site of origin of the neoplasm. In some cases, it may not be possible to identify the site of origin, such as malignant neoplasms originating from contiguous sites.

   Neoplasms with overlapping site boundaries are classified to the fourth-digit subcategory .8 "other." For example, code 151.8 Malignant neoplasm of contiguous or overlapping sites of stomach whose point of origin cannot be determined.

6. Neoplasms which demonstrate functional activity require an additional code to identify the functional activity.

Coding Example

Cushing's syndrome due to malignant pheochromocytoma

194.0   Malignant neoplasm of adrenal gland

255.0   Disorders of adrenal glands; Cushing's syndrome

Code sequencing depends on the circumstances of the encounter.

7. Two categories in the malignant neoplasm section represent departures from the usual principles of classification in that the fourth-digit subdivisions in each case are not mutually exclusive. These categories are 150 Malignant neoplasm of esophagus and 201 Hodgkin's disease. The dual axis is provided to account for differing terminology, for there is no uniform international agreement on the use of these terms.

Coding Example

Malignant neoplasm of the esophagus

150.0   Cervical esophagus

150.1   Thoracic esophagus

150.2   Abdominal esophagus

or using alternate coding

150.3   Upper third of esophagus

150.4   Middle third of esophagus

150.5   Lower third of esophagus

8. When the treatment is directed at the primary site of the malignancy, designate the primary site as the principal diagnosis, except when the encounter or hospital admission is solely for *Radiotherapy* (V58.0) or, for *Chemotherapy* (V58.1).

9. When surgical intervention for removal of a primary site or secondary site malignancy is followed by adjunct chemotherapy or radiotherapy, code the malignancy using codes in the 140-198 series, or, where appropriate, in the 200-203 series as long as chemotherapy or radiotherapy is being actively administered. If the admission is for chemotherapy or radiotherapy, the malignancy code is listed second.

10. When the primary malignancy has been previously excised or eradicated from its site and there is no adjunct treatment directed to that site, and there is no evidence of any remaining malignancy at the primary site, use the appropriate code from the V10 series to indicate the site of the primary malignancy. Any mention of extension, invasion or metastasis to a nearby structure or organ, or to a distant site, is coded as a secondary malignant neoplasm to that site and may be the principal diagnosis in the absence of the primary site.

11. If the patient has no secondary malignancy and if the reason for admission or for the visit is follow-up of the malignancy, two codes are used and sequenced.

Coding Example

Follow-up of breast cancer treated with chemotherapy. No evidence of recurrence.

V67.2   Follow-up examination following chemotherapy

V10.3   Personal history of carcinoma of breast

12. Malignancies of hematopoietic and lymphatic tissue are always coded to the 200.0-208.9 series unless specified as "in remission." If they are in remission, they are coded as V10.60-V10.79.

13. If the primary malignant neoplasm previously excised or eradicated has recurred, code it as primary malignancy of the stated site unless the Alphabetic Index (Volume 2) directs you to do otherwise.

Coding Examples

Recurrence of prostate carcinoma

185   Malignant neoplasm of prostate

Recurrence of breast carcinoma in mastectomy site

198.2   Secondary malignant neoplasm of other specified sites, skin of breast

Make sure to code any mention of secondary site(s).

14. Terminology referring to metastatic cancer is often ambiguous, so when there is doubt as to the meaning intended, the following rules should be used:

   a. Cancer described as metastatic "from" a site should be interpreted as primary of that site.

   b. Cancer described as metastatic "to" a site should be interpreted as secondary of that site.

Coding Examples

Carcinoma in axillary lymph nodes and lungs metastatic from breast

174.9   Malignant neoplasm of breast (female), unspecified

196.3   Secondary and unspecified malignant neoplasm of lymph nodes of axilla and upper limb

197.0   Secondary malignant neoplasm of lung

Adenocarcinoma of colon with extension to peritoneum

153.9   Malignant neoplasm of colon, unspecified

197.6   Secondary malignant neoplasm of retroperitoneum and peritoneum

15. Diagnostic statements when only one site is identified as metastatic:

    a. Code to the category for "primary of unspecified site" for the morphological type concerned UNLESS the code thus obtained is either 199.0 or 199.1.

    b. If the code obtained in the above step is 199.0 or 199.1, then code the site qualified as "metastatic" as for a primary malignant neoplasm of the stated site EXCEPT for the sites listed below, which should always be coded as secondary neoplasm of the state site:

Bone

Brain

Diaphragm

Heart

Liver

Lymph nodes

Mediasinum

Meninges

Peritoneum

Pleura

Retroperitoneum

Spinal cord

Sites classifiable to 195

    c. Also assign the appropriate code for primary or secondary malignant neoplasm of specified or unspecified site, depending on the diagnostic statement you are coding.

Coding Examples

Metastatic renal cell carcinoma of lung

189.0   Malignant neoplasm of kidney, except pelvis

197.0   Secondary malignant neoplasm of lung

Metastatic carcinoma of lung

162.9   Malignant neoplasm of bronchus and lung, unspecified

199.1   Malignant neoplasm without specification of site, other

This code is assigned to identify "secondary neoplasm of unspecified site" per the instructions in step C above.

Metastatic carcinoma of brain

198.3   Secondary malignant neoplasm of other specified sites, brain and spinal cord

199.1   Malignant neoplasm without specification of site, other

In this case, the brain is one of the sites listed in Step B as an exception. So for this diagnostic statement, the code assignment is for secondary neoplasm of the brain and primary malignant neoplasm of unspecified site.

16. When two or more sites are stated in the diagnostic statement and all are qualified to be "metastatic," you should code as for "primary site unknown" and code the stated sites as secondary neoplasms of those sites.

Coding Example

Metastatic melanoma of lung and liver

172.9   Malignant melanoma of skin, site unspecified

197.0   Secondary malignant neoplasm of lung

197.7   Secondary malignant neoplasm of liver, specified as secondary

17. When there is no site specified in the diagnostic statement, but the morphological type is qualified as "metastatic," code as for "primary site unknown." Then assign the code for secondary neoplasms of unspecified site.

Coding Example

Metastatic apocrine adenocarcinoma

173.9   Other malignant neoplasms of skin, site unspecified

199.1   Malignant neoplasm without specification of site, other

18. When two or more sites are stated in the diagnosis and only some are qualified as "metastatic" while others are not, code as for "primary site unknown." However, you should interpret the following sites as secondary neoplasms:

Bone

Brain

Diaphragm

Heart

Liver

Meninges

Peritoneum

Pleura

Retroperitoneum

Spinal Cord

Sites classifiable to category 195

Coding Example

Carcinoma of lung, metastatic, and brain

198.3   Secondary malignant neoplasm of brain and spinal cord

197.0   Secondary malignant neoplasm of lung

199.1   Malignant neoplasm without specification of site, other

PREGNANCY, CHILDBIRTH, AND THE PUERPERIUM

Chapter 11 of the Tabular List (Volume 1) uses fifth-digit subclassifications extensively. In general, the fifth digit is not given in the Alphabetic Index (Volume 2), so each code must be verified in the Tabular List (Volume 1).

GENERAL RULES FOR OBSTETRICS CASES

1. Obstetric cases require codes from Chapter 11, codes in the range 630-677, Complications of Pregnancy, Childbirth, and the Puerperium. Should the physician document that the pregnancy is incidental to the encounter, then code V22.2 should be used in place of any Chapter 11 codes. It is the physician's responsibility to state that the condition being treated is not affecting the pregnancy.

2. Chapter 11 codes have sequencing priority over codes from other chapters. Additional codes from other chapters may be used in conjunction with Chapter 11 codes to further specify conditions. For example, sepsis and septic shock associated with abortion, ectopic pregnancy, and molar pregnancy are classified to category codes in Chapter 11 (630-639) .

3. Chapter 11 codes are to be used only on the maternal record, never on the record of the newborn.

4. Categories 640-648 and 651-676 have required fifth-digits, which indicate whether the encounter is antepartum or postpartum, and whether a delivery has also occurred.

5. The fifth-digits that are appropriate for each code number, are listed in brackets under each code. The fifth-digits on each code should all be consistent with each other. That is, should a delivery occur, all of the fifth-digits should indicate that the delivery occurred.

6. For prenatal outpatient visits for patients with high-risk pregnancies, a code from category V23, Supervision of high-risk pregnancy, should be used as the principal or first-listed diagnosis. Secondary Chapter 11 codes may be used in conjunction with these codes if appropriate. A thorough review of any pertinent "Excludes" note is necessary to be certain that these V codes are being used properly.

7. An "Outcome of delivery" code (V27.0-V27.9) should be included on every maternal record when a delivery has occurred. These codes are not to be used on subsequent records or on the newborn record.

8. For routine outpatient prenatal visits when no complications are present, codes V22.0, Supervision of normal first pregnancy, and V22.1, Supervision of other normal pregnancy, should be used as the first-listed diagnoses. These codes should not be used in conjunction with Chapter 11 codes.

SELECTION OF OBSTETRIC PRINCIPAL OR FIRST-LISTED DIAGNOSIS

1. In episodes when no delivery occurs, the principal diagnosis should correspond to the principal complication of the pregnancy that necessitated the encounter. Should more than one complication exist, all of which are treated or monitored, any of the complication codes may be sequenced first.

2. When a delivery occurs, the principal diagnosis should correspond to the main circumstances or complication of the delivery.

In cases of cesarean delivery, the selection of the principal diagnosis should correspond to the reason the cesarean delivery was performed unless the reason for admission/encounter was unrelated to the condition resulting in the cesarean delivery.

FETAL CONDITIONS AFFECTING THE MANAGEMENT OF THE MOTHER

Codes from category 655, Known or suspected fetal abnormality affecting management of the mother, and category 656, Other fetal and placental problems affecting the management of the mother, are assigned only when the fetal condition is actually responsible for modifying the management of the mother, i.e., by requiring diagnostic studies, additional observation, special care, or termination of pregnancy. The fact that the fetal condition exists does not justify assigning a code from this series to the mother's record.

HIV INFECTION IN PREGNANCY, CHILDBIRTH AND THE PUERPERIUM

During pregnancy, childbirth or the puerperium, a patient admitted because of an HIV-related illness should receive a principal diagnosis of 647.6X, Other viral diseases in the mother classifiable elsewhere, but complicating the pregnancy, childbirth or the puerperium, followed by 042 HIV disease, and the code(s) for the HIV-related illness(es) . This is an exception to the sequencing rule found in above.

Patients with asymptomatic HIV infection status admitted during pregnancy, childbirth, or the puerperium should receive codes of 647.6X and V08.

NORMAL DELIVERY

1. Code 650, Normal delivery, is for use in cases when a woman is admitted for a full-term normal delivery and delivers a single, healthy infant without any complications antepartum, during the delivery, or postpartum during the delivery episode.

2. Code 650 may be used if the patient had a complication at some point during her pregnancy but the complication is not present at the time of the admission for delivery.

3. Code 650 is always a principal diagnosis. It is not to be used if any other code from Chapter 11 is needed to describe a current complication of the antenatal, delivery, or perinatal period. Additional codes from other chapters may be used with code 650 if they are not related to or are in any way complicating the pregnancy.

4. V27.0, Single liveborn, is the only outcome of delivery code appropriate for use with 650.

THE POSTPARTUM PERIOD

1. The postpartum period begins immediately after delivery and continues for six weeks following delivery.

2. A postpartum complication is any complication occurring within the six-week period.

3. Chapter 11 codes may also be used to describe pregnancy-related complications after the six-week period should the physician document that a condition is pregnancy related.

4. Postpartum complications that occur during the same admission as the delivery are identified with a fifth-digit of subsequent admissions/encounters for postpartum complications, should identified with a fifth-digit of "4".

5. When the mother delivers outside the hospital prior to admission and is admitted for routine postpartum care and no complications are noted, code V24.0, Postpartum care and examination immediately after delivery, should be assigned as the principal diagnosis.

6. A delivery diagnosis code should not be used for a woman who has delivered prior to admission to the hospital. Any postpartum procedures should be coded.

LATE EFFECT OF COMPLICATION OF PREGNANCY, CHILDBIRTH, AND THE PUERPERIUM

1. Code 677, Late effect of complication of pregnancy, childbirth, and the puerperium is for use in those cases when an initial complication of a pregnancy develops a sequelae requiring care or treatment at a future date.

2. This code may be used at any time after the initial postpartum period.

3. This code, like all late effect codes, is to be sequenced following the code describing the sequelae of the complication.

ABORTIONS

1. Fifth-digits are required for abortion categories 634-637. Fifth-digit 1, Incomplete, indicates that all of the products of conception have not been expelled from the uterus. Fifth-digit 2, Complete, indicates that all products of conception have been expelled from the uterus prior to the episode of care.

2. A code from categories 640-648 and 651-657 may be used as additional codes with an abortion code to indicate the complication leading to the abortion.

Fifth-digit 3 is assigned with codes from these categories when used with an abortion code because the other fifth-digits will not apply. Codes from the 660-669 series are not to be used for complications of abortion.

3. Code 639, Complications following abortion and ectopic and molar pregnancies, is to be used for all complications following abortion. Code 639 cannot be assigned with codes from categories 634-638.

4. When an attempted termination of pregnancy results in a liveborn fetus, assign code 644.21, Early onset of delivery, with an appropriate code from category V27, Outcome of Delivery. The procedure code for the attempted termination of pregnancy should also be assigned.

5. Subsequent admissions for retained products of conception following a spontaneous or legally induced abortion are assigned the appropriate code from category 634, Abortion, or 635 Legally induced abortion, with a fifth digit of 1, Incomplete. This advice is appropriate even when the patient was discharged previously with a discharge diagnosis of "complete abortion."

Pregnancy Coding Examples

Pregnancy, 3 months gestation complicated by benign essential hypertension

642.03   Benign essential hypertension complicating pregnancy, childbirth, and the puerperium, antepartum condition or complication

Categories 647 and 648 are used for conditions that are usually classified elsewhere, but which have been classified here because they are complications of pregnancy. The interaction of certain conditions with the pregnant state complicates the pregnancy and/or aggravates the non-obstetrical condition (i.e., diabetes mellitus, drug dependence, thyroid dysfunction) and are the main reasons for the obstetrical care provided.

Coding Example

Rubella in woman, 7 months gestation

647.53   Infectious and parasitic conditions in the mother classifiable elsewhere, but complicating pregnancy, childbirth or the puerperium, rubella, antepartum condition or complication

Pregnancy with diabetes mellitus

648.03   Other current conditions in the mother classifiable elsewhere, but complicating pregnancy, childbirth or the puerperium, diabetes mellitus, antepartum condition or complication

If greater detail is needed for the complication, use an additional code to identify the complication more completely.

Coding Example

Pregnancy with pernicious anemia

648.23   Other current conditions in the mother classifiable elsewhere, but complicating pregnancy, childbirth or the puerperium, anemia, antepartum condition or complication

281.0   Pernicious anemia

NEWBORN (PERINATAL) GUIDELINES

For coding and reporting purposes, the perinatal period is defined as birth through the 28th day following birth. The following guidelines are provided for reporting purposes. Hospitals may record other diagnoses as needed for internal data use.

GENERAL PERINATAL RULES

All clinically significant conditions noted on routine newborn examination should be coded. A condition is clinically significant if it requires: clinical evaluation; or therapeutic treatment; or diagnostic procedures; or extended length of hospital stay; or increased nursing care and/or monitoring; or has implications for future health care needs.

Note: The perinatal guidelines listed above are the same as the general coding guidelines for additional diagnoses, except for the final point regarding implications for future health care needs. Whether or not a condition is clinically significant can only be determined by the physician.

USE OF CODES V30-V39

When coding the birth of an infant, assign a code from categories V30-V39, *Liveborn infant according to the type of birth.* A code from this series is assigned as a principal diagnosis, and assigned only once to a newborn at the time of birth.

NEWBORN TRANSFERS

If the newborn is transferred to another institution, the V30 series is not used at the receiving hospital.

USE OF CATEGORY V29

1. Assign a code from category V29, Observation and evaluation of newborns and infants for suspected conditions not found, to identify those instances when a healthy newborn is evaluated for a suspected condition that is determined after study not to be present. Do not use a code from category V29 when the patient has specific signs or symptoms of a suspected problem. In such cases, code the sign or symptom.

2. A V29 code is to be used as a secondary code after V30, Outcome of delivery. It may also be assigned as a principal code for readmissions or encounters when the V30 code no longer applies. It is for use only for healthy newborns and infants for which no condition after study is found to be present.

MATERNAL CAUSES OF PERINATAL MORBIDITY

Codes from categories 760-763, Maternal causes of perinatal morbidity and mortality, are assigned only when the maternal condition has actually affected the fetus or newborn. The fact that the mother has an associated medical condition or experiences some complication of pregnancy, labor or delivery does not justify the routine assignment of codes from these categories to the newborn record.

CONGENITAL ANOMALIES

Assign an appropriate code from categories 740-759, Congenital Anomalies, as an additional diagnosis when a specific abnormality is diagnosed for an infant. Congenital anomalies may also be the principal or first-listed diagnosis for admissions/encounters subsequent to the newborn admission. Such abnormalities may occur as a set of symptoms or multiple malformations. A code should be assigned for each presenting manifestation of the syndrome if the syndrome is not specifically indexed in ICD-9-CM.

CODING OF ADDITIONAL PERINATAL DIAGNOSES

1. Assign codes for conditions that require treatment or further investigation, prolong the length of stay, or require resource utilization.

2. Assign codes for conditions that have been specified by the physician as having implications for future health care needs.

Note: This guideline should not be used for adult patients.

3. Assign a code for Newborn conditions originating in the perinatal period (categories 760-779), as well as complications arising during the current episode of care classified in other chapters, only if the diagnoses have been documented by the responsible physician at the time of transfer or discharge as having affected the fetus or newborn.

PREMATURITY AND FETAL GROWTH RETARDATION

Codes from category 764, Slow fetal growth and fetal malnutrition, and subcategories 765.0, Extreme immaturity, and 765.1, Other preterm infant, should not be assigned based solely on recorded birthweight or estimated gestational age, but on the attending physician's clinical assessment of maturity of the infant. Note: since physicians may utilize different criteria in determining prematurity, do not code the diagnosis of prematurity unless the physician documents this condition.

A code from subcategory 765.2X, Weeks of gestation, should be assigned as an additional code with category 764 and codes 765.0 and 765.1 in order to specify weeks of gestation as documented by the physician.

V CODES: CLASSIFICATION OF FACTORS INFLUENCING HEALTH STATUS AND CONTACT WITH HEALTH SERVICE

ICD-9-CM provides codes to deal with encounters for circumstances other than a disease or injury. The Supplementary Classification of Factors Influencing Health Status and Contact with Health Services (V01.0 -V83.89) is provided to deal with occasions when circumstances other than a disease or injury (codes 001-999) are recorded as a diagnosis or problem.

V codes are used for four primary circumstances:

1. When a person who is not currently sick encounters the health services for some specific reason, such as to act as an organ donor, to receive prophylactic care such as inoculations or health screenings, or to receive counseling on health related issue.

2. When a person with a resolving disease or injury, or a chronic, long-term condition requiring continuous care, encounters the health care system for

specific aftercare of that disease or injury (e.g., dialysis for renal disease, chemotherapy for malignancy, or a cast change). Note: A diagnosis/symptom code should be used whenever a current/acute, diagnosis is being treated or a sign or symptom is being studied.

3. When circumstances or problems influence a person's health status but are not in themselves a current illness or injury.

4. For newborns, to indicate birth status.

V codes are for use in both the inpatient and outpatient setting but are generally more applicable to the outpatient setting. V codes may be used as either a first-listed (principal diagnosis code in the inpatient setting) or secondary code depending on the circumstances of the encounter. Certain V codes may only be used as first listed, and others only as secondary codes.

V Codes indicate a reason for an encounter. They are not procedure codes. A corresponding procedure code must accompany a V code to describe the procedure performed. Key words found in diagnostic statements which may result in selection of a V code include:

Admission for
Aftercare
Attention to
Care (of)
Carrier
Checking/checkup
Contact
Contraception
Counseling
Dialysis
Donor
Examination
Fitting of
follow up
Health or healthy
History (of)
Maintenance
Maladjustment
Observation
Problem (with)
Prophylactic

Replacement (of)

Screening

Status

Supervision (of)

Test

Transplant

Vaccination

CATEGORIES OF V CODES

Contact/Exposure

Category V01 indicates *Contact with or exposure to communicable diseases.* These codes are for patients who do not show any sign or symptom of a disease but have been exposed to it by close personal contact with an infected individual or are in an area where a disease is epidemic. These codes may be used as a first-listed code to explain an encounter for testing, or, more commonly, as a secondary code to identify a potential risk.

Inoculations and Vaccinations

Categories V03-V06 are used for encounters for inoculations and vaccinations. These codes indicate that a patient is being seen to receive a prophylactic inoculation against a disease. The injection itself must be represented by the appropriate procedure code. A code from V03-V06 may be used as a secondary code if the inoculation is given as a routine part of preventive health care, such as well-baby visit.

Status

Status codes indicate that a patient is either a carrier of a disease or has the sequelae or residual of a past disease or condition. This includes such things as the presence of prosthetic or mechanical devices resulting from past treatment. A status code is informative because the status may affect the current course of treatment and its outcome. A status code is distinct from a history code. The history code indicates that the patient no longer has the condition.

Status V codes/categories:

V02   Carrier or suspected carrier of infectious diseases

Carrier status indicates that a person harbors the specific organisms of a disease without manifest symptoms and is capable of transmitting the infection.

V08   Asymptomatic HIV infection status

This code indicates that a patient has tested positive for HIV but has manifested no signs or symptoms of the disease.

V09   Infection with drug-resistant microorganisms

This category indicates that a patient has an infection which is resistant to drug treatment. Sequence the infection code first.

V21   Constitutional states in development

V22.2   Pregnant state, incidental

This code is a secondary code only for use when the pregnancy is in no way complicating the reason for visit. Otherwise, a code from the obstetric chapter is required.

V26.5X   Sterilization status

V42   Organ or tissue replaced by transplant

V43   Organ or tissue replaced by other means

V44   Artificial opening status

V45   Other postprocedural states

V46   Other dependence on machines

V49.6   Upper limb amputation status

V49.7   Lower limb amputation status

V49.81   Asymptomatic postmenopausal status (age-related) (natural)

V49.82   Dental sealant status

V58.6   Long-term (current) drug use

This subcategory indicates a patient's continuous use of a prescribed drug (including such things as aspirin therapy) for *the long-term treatment of a condition or for prophylactic use. It is not for use for patients who have addictions to drugs.*

V83   *Genetic carrier status*

Categories V42-V46, and subcategories V49.6, V49.7 are for use only if there are no complications or malfunctions of the organ or tissue replaced, the amputation site or the equipment on which the patient is dependent. These are always secondary codes.

History (of)

There are two types of history V codes, personal and family. Personal history codes explain a patient's past medical condition that no longer exists and is not receiving any treatment but that has the potential for recurrence, and, therefore, may require continued monitoring. The exceptions to this general rule are category V14, Personal history of allergy to medicinal agents and subcategory V15.0, Allergy, other than to medicinal agents. A person who has had an allergic episode to a substance or food in the past should always be considered allergic to the substance.

Family history codes are used when a patient has a family member who has had a particular disease that causes the patient to be at higher risk of getting the disease.

Personal history codes may be used in conjunction with follow-up codes and family history codes may be used in conjunction with screening codes to explain the need for a test or procedure. History codes are also acceptable on any medical record regardless of the reason for visit. A history of an illness, even if no longer present, is important information that may alter the type of treatment ordered.

History V codes/categories:

V10   *Personal history of malignant neoplasm*

V12   *Personal history of certain other diseases*

V13   *Personal history of other diseases*

Except: V13.4, Personal history of arthritis, and V13.6, Personal history of congenital malformations. These are lifelong conditions so not history codes.

V14   *Personal history of allergy to medicinal agents*

V15	*Other personal history presenting hazards to health*
	Except: V15.7, Personal history of contraception.
V16	*Family history of malignant neoplasm*
V17	*Family history of certain chronic disabling diseases*
V18	*Family history of certain other specific conditions*
V19	*Family history of other conditions*

Screening

Screening is the testing for disease or disease precursors in seemingly well individuals so that early detection and treatment can be provided for those who test positive for the disease. Screenings that are recommended for many subgroups in a population include: routine mammograms for women over 40 or a fecal occult blood test for everyone over 50, because the incidence of breast cancer and colon cancer in these subgroups is higher than in the general population; or an amniocentesis to rule out a fetal anomaly for pregnant women over 35, because the incidence of Down's syndrome is higher in older mothers.

The testing of a person to rule out or confirm a suspected diagnosis because the patient has some sign or symptom is a diagnostic examination, not a screening. In these cases, the sign or symptom is used to explain the reason for the test.

A screening code may be a first-listed code if the reason for the visit is specifically the screening exam. It may also be used as an additional code if the screening is done during an office visit for other health problems. A screening code is not necessary if the screening is inherent to a routine examination, such as a pap smear done during a routine pelvic examination.

Should a condition be discovered during the screening then the code for the condition may be assigned as an additional diagnosis.

The V code indicates that a screening exam is planned. A procedure code is required to confirm that the screening was performed.

Screening V codes/categories:

V28	*Antenatal screening*
V73- *V82*	*Special screening examinations*

Observation

There are two observation V code categories. They are for use in very limited circumstances when a person is being observed for a suspected condition that is ruled out. The observation codes are not for use if an injury or illness or any signs or symptoms related to the suspected condition are present. In such cases the diagnosis/ symptom code is used with the corresponding E code to identify any external cause.

The observation codes are to be used as principal diagnosis only. The only exception to this is when the principal diagnosis is required to be a code from the category V30, Live born infant. Then the V29 observation code is sequenced after the V30 code. Additional codes may be used in addition to the observation code but only if they are unrelated to the suspected condition being observed.

Observation V codes/categories:

V29   *Observation and evaluation of newborns for suspected condition not found*

     A code from category V30 should be sequenced before the V29 code.

V71   *Observation and evaluation for suspected condition(s) not found*

Aftercare

Aftercare visit codes cover situations when the initial treatment of a disease or injury has been performed and the patient requires continued care during the healing or recovery phase, or for the long-term consequences of the disease. The aftercare V code should not be used if treatment is directed at a current, acute disease or injury, the diagnosis code is to be used in these cases. Exceptions to this rule are codes V58.0, Radiotherapy, and V58.1, Chemotherapy. These codes are to be first listed, followed by the diagnosis code when a patient's encounter is solely to receive radiation therapy or chemotherapy for the treatment of a neoplasm. Should a patient receive both chemotherapy and radiation therapy during the same encounter, codes V58.0 and V58.1 may be used together with either one being sequenced first.

The aftercare codes are generally listed first to explain the specific reason for the encounter. An aftercare code may be used as an additional code when some type of aftercare is provided in addition to the reason for admission and no diagnosis code is applicable. An example of this would be the closure of a colostomy during an encounter for treatment of another condition.

Certain aftercare V code categories need a secondary diagnosis code to describe the resolving condition or sequelae. For others, the condition is inherent in the code title. Additional V code aftercare category terms include, "fitting and adjustment," and "attention to artificial openings."

Aftercare V codes/categories:

V52	*Fitting and adjustment of prosthetic device and implant*
V53	*Fitting and adjustment of other device*
V54	*Other orthopedic aftercare*
V55	*Attention to artificial openings*
V56	*Encounter for dialysis and dialysis catheter care*
V57	*Care involving the use of rehabilitation procedures*
V58.0	*Radiotherapy*
V58.1	*Chemotherapy*
V58.3	*Attention to surgical dressings and sutures*
V58.41	*Encounter for planned post-operative wound closure*
V58.42	*Aftercare following surgery for neoplasm*
V58.43	*Aftercare following surgery for injury and trauma*
V58.49	*Other specified aftercare following surgery*
V58.71- V58.78	*Aftercare following surgery to specified body systems NEC*
V58.81	*Fitting and adjustment of vascular catheter*
V58.82	*Fitting and adjustment of non-vascular catheter NEC*
V58.83	*Encounter for therapeutic drug monitoring*
V58.89	*Other specified aftercare*

Follow-Up

The follow-up codes are for use to explain continuing surveillance following completed treatment of a disease, condition, or injury. They infer that the condition has been fully treated and no longer exists. They should not be confused with aftercare codes which explain current treatment for a healing condition or its sequelae.

Follow-up codes may be used in conjunction with history codes to provide the full picture of the healed condition and its treatment. The follow-up code is sequenced first, followed by the history code.

A follow-up code may be used to explain repeated visits. Should a condition be found to have recurred on the follow-up visit, then the diagnosis code should be used in place of the follow-up code.

Follow-up V codes/categories:

V24	*Postpartum care and evaluation*
V67	*Follow-up examination*

Donor

Category V59 is the donor codes. They are for use for living individuals who are donating blood or other body tissue. These codes are only for individuals donating for others, not for self donations. They are not to identify cadaveric donations.

Counseling

Counseling V codes are for use for when a patient or family member receives assistance in the aftermath of an illness or injury, or when support is required in coping with family or social problems. They are not necessary for use in conjunction with a diagnosis code when the counseling component of care is considered integral to standard treatment.

Counseling V codes/categories:

V25.0	*General counseling and advice for contraceptive management*
V26.3	*Genetic counseling and testing*
V26.4	*General counseling and advice for procreative management*
V61	*Other family circumstances*
V65.1	*Person consulting on behalf of another person*
V65.3	*Dietary surveillance and counseling*
V65.4	*Other counseling, not elsewhere classified*

Obstetrics and Related Conditions

See the Obstetrics guidelines for further instruction on the use of these codes. V codes for pregnancy are for use in those circumstances when none of the problems or complications included in the codes from the Obstetrics chapter exist, such as a routine prenatal visit or postpartum care. V22.0, Supervision of normal first pregnancy, and V22.1, Supervision of other normal pregnancy, are always first listed and are not to be used with any other code from the Obstetrics chapter.

Category V27, Outcome of delivery, should be included on all maternal delivery records. It is always a secondary code. V codes for family planning (contraceptive) or procreative management and counseling should be included on an obstetric record either during the pregnancy or the postpartum stage, if applicable.

Obstetrics and related conditions V codes/categories:

V22	*Normal pregnancy*
V23	*Supervision of high-risk pregnancy*

Except: V23.2, Pregnancy with history of abortion. Code 646.3, Habitual aborter, from the OB chapter is required to indicate a history of abortion during a pregnancy.

V24	*Postpartum care and evaluation*
V25	*Encounter for contraceptive management*

Except: V25.0X (See counseling above)

V26   *Procreative management*

Except: V26.5x, Sterilization status, V26.3 and V26.4 (Counseling)

V27	*Outcome of delivery*
V28	*Antenatal screening*

Newborn, Infant and Child

See the Newborn Guidelines for further instruction on the use of these codes.

Newborn V codes/categories:

V20	*Health supervision of infant or child*

V29	*Observation and evaluation of newborns for suspected condition not found*
V30- V39	*Liveborn infant according to type of birth*

Routine and Administrative Examinations

The V codes allow for the description of encounters for routine examinations, such as a general check-up, or examinations for administrative purposes, such as a pre-employment physical. The codes are for use as first-listed codes only and are not to be used if the examination is for diagnosis of a suspected condition or for treatment purposes. In such cases the diagnosis code is used. During a routine exam, should a diagnosis or condition be discovered, it should be coded as an additional code. Pre-existing and chronic conditions, and history codes may also be included as additional codes as long as the examination is for administrative purposes and not focused on any particular condition.

Pre-operative examination V codes are for use only in those situations when a patient is being cleared for surgery and no treatment is given.

Routine and administrative examinations V codes/categories:

V20.2	*Routine infant or child health check*
	Any injections given should have a corresponding procedure code.
V70	*General medical examination*
V72	*Special investigations and examinations*
	Except V72.5 and V72.6

Miscellaneous V Codes

The miscellaneous V codes capture a number of other health care encounters that do not fall into one of the other categories. Certain of these codes identify the reason for the encounter, others are for use as additional codes which provide useful information on circumstances which may affect a patient's care and treatment.

Miscellaneous V codes/categories:

V07	*Need for isolation and other prophylactic measures*

V50	Elective surgery for purposes other than remedying health states
V58.5	Orthodontics
V60	Housing, household, and economic circumstances
V62	Other psychosocial circumstances
V63	Unavailability of other medical facilities for care
V64	Persons encountering health services for specific procedures, not carried out
V66	Convalescence and palliative care
V68	Encounters for administrative purposes
V69	Problems related to lifestyle

Nonspecific V Codes

Certain V codes are so non-specific, or potentially redundant with other codes in the classification, that there can be little justification for their use in the inpatient setting. Their use in the outpatient setting should be limited to those instances when there is no further documentation to permit more precise coding. Otherwise, any sign or symptom, or any other reason for the visit which is captured in another code, should be used instead.

Nonspecific V codes/categories:

V11	Personal history of mental disorder
	A code from the mental disorders chapter, with an in remission fifth-digit, should be used.
V13.4	Personal history of arthritis
V13.6	Personal history of congenital malformations
V15.7	Personal history of contraception
V23.2	Pregnancy with history of abortion
V40	Mental and behavioral problems
V41	Problems with special senses and other special functions
V47	Other problems with internal organs

V48	*Problems with head, neck, and trunk*
V49	*Other conditions influencing health status*

Exceptions: V49.6, Upper limb amputation status, V49.7, Lower limb amputation status, V49.81, Postmenopausal status, and V49.82, Dental sealant status

V51	*Aftercare involving the use of plastic surgery*
V58.2	*Blood transfusion, without reported diagnosis*
V58.9	*Unspecified aftercare*
V72.5	*Radiological examination, NEC*
V72.6	*Laboratory examination*

Codes V72.5 and V72.6 are not to be used if any sign or symptoms, or reason for a test is documented.

V Code Coding Example

Colostomy status with colostomy malfunction

569.60	*Colostomy and enterostomy complications, unspecified*

The code V44.3 Artificial opening status, colostomy would not be used in this case because of the complication.

E CODES: SUPPLEMENTAL CLASSIFICATION OF EXTERNAL CAUSES OF INJURY AND POISONING

E-codes permit the classification of environmental events, circumstances and conditions as the cause of injury, poisoning and other adverse effects. The use of E-codes, together with the code identifying the injury or condition, provides additional information of particular concern to industrial medicine, insurance carriers, national safety programs and public health agencies. External causes of injury and poisoning codes (E codes) are intended to provide data for injury research and evaluation of injury prevention strategies. E codes capture how the injury or poisoning happened (cause), the intent (unintentional or accidental; or intentional, such as suicide or assault), and the place where the event occurred.

The following guidelines are provided for those who are currently collecting E codes in order that there will be standardization in the process. If your institution plans to begin collecting E codes, these guidelines are to be applied. The use of E codes is supplemental to the application of ICD-9-CM diagnosis codes. E codes are never to be recorded as a principal diagnosis (first-listed in non-inpatient setting) and are not required for reporting to CMS.

These guidelines apply for the coding and collection of E codes from records in hospitals, outpatient clinics, emergency departments, other ambulatory care settings and physician offices, and nonacute care settings, except when other specific guidelines apply.

Some major categories of E codes include:

- transport accidents;

- poisoning and adverse effects of drugs, medicinal substances and biologicals;

- accidental falls;

- accidents caused by fire and flames;

- accidents due to natural and environmental factors;

- late effects of accidents, assaults or self injury;

- assaults or purposely inflicted injury;

- suicide or self inflicted injury.

GENERAL E CODE CODING GUIDELINES

1. An E code may be used with any code in the range of 001-V83.89, which indicates an injury, poisoning, or adverse effect due to an external cause.

2. Assign the appropriate E code for all initial treatments of an injury, poisoning, or adverse effect of drugs.

3. Use a late effect E code for subsequent visits when a late effect of the initial injury or poisoning is being treated. There is no late effect E code for adverse effects of drugs.

4. Use the full range of E codes to completely describe the cause, the intent and the place of occurrence, if applicable, for all injuries, poisonings and adverse effects of drugs.

5. Assign as many E codes as necessary to fully explain each cause. If only one E code can be recorded, assign the E code most related to the principal diagnosis.

6. The selection of the appropriate E code is guided by the Index to External Causes, which is located after the alphabetical index to diseases, and by "Inclusion" and "Exclusion" notes in the Tabular List.

7. An E code can never be a principal (first-listed) diagnosis.

PLACE OF OCCURRENCE GUIDELINE

Use an additional code from category E849 to indicate the Place of Occurrence for injuries and poisonings. This describes the place where the event occurred and not the patient's activity at the time of the event.

Note: Do not use E849.9 if the place of occurrence is not stated.

ADVERSE EFFECTS OF DRUGS, MEDICINAL AND BIOLOGICAL SUBSTANCES GUIDELINES

1. Do not code directly from the Table of Drugs and Chemicals. Always refer back to the Tabular List.

2. Use as many codes as necessary to describe completely all drugs, medicinal or biological substances.

3. If the same E code would describe the causative agent for more than one adverse reaction, assign the code only once.

4. If two or more drugs, medicinal or biological substances are reported, code each individually unless the combination code is listed in the Table of Drugs and Chemicals. In that case, assign the E code for the combination.

5. When a reaction results from the interaction of a drug(s) and alcohol, use poisoning codes and E codes for both.

6. If the reporting format limits the number of E codes that can be used in reporting clinical data, code the one most related to the principal diagnosis. Include at least one from each category (cause, intent, place) if possible.

   If there are different fourth-digit codes in the same three-digit category, use the code for Other specified of that category. If there is no Other specified code in that category, use the appropriate Unspecified code in that category.

   If the codes are in different three-digit categories, assign the appropriate E code for other multiple drugs and medicinal substances.

7. Codes from the E930-E949 series must be used to identify the causative substance for an adverse effect of drug, medicinal and biological

substances, correctly prescribed and properly administered. The effect, such as tachycardia, delirium, gastrointestinal hemorrhaging, vomiting, hypokalemia, hepatitis, renal failure, or respiratory failure, etc., is coded and followed by the appropriate code from the E930-E949 series.

MULTIPLE CAUSE CODING GUIDELINES

If two or more events cause separate injuries, an E code should be assigned for each cause. The first-listed E code will be selected in the following order:

1. E codes for child and adult abuse take priority over all other E codes see Child and Adult Abuse Guidelines below.

2. E codes for terrorism events take priority over all other E codes except child and adult abuse.

3. E codes for cataclysmic events take priority over all other E codes except child and adult abuse, and terrorism.

4. E codes for transport accidents take priority over all other E codes except cataclysmic events, and child and adult abuse, and terrorism.

5. The first-listed E code should correspond to the cause of the most serious diagnosis due to an assault, accident or self-harm, following the order of hierarchy listed above.

CHILD AND ADULT ABUSE GUIDELINE

1. When the cause of an injury or neglect is intentional child or adult abuse, the first-listed E code should be assigned from categories E960-E969, Homicide and injury purposely inflicted by other persons, (except category E967). An E code from category E967, Perpetrator of child and adult abuse, should be added as an additional code to identify the perpetrator, if known.

2. In cases of neglect when the intent is determined to be accidental, E code E904.0, Abandonment or neglect of infants and helpless persons, should be the first listed E code.

UNKNOWN OR SUSPECTED INTENT GUIDELINE

1. If the intent (accident, self-harm, assault) of the cause of an injury or poisoning is unknown or unspecified, code the intent as undetermined E980-E989.

2. If the intent (accident, self-harm, assault) of the cause of an injury or poisoning is questionable, probable or suspected, code the intent as undetermined E980-E989.

UNDETERMINED CAUSE GUIDELINES

When the intent of an injury or poisoning is known, but the cause is unknown, use codes: E928.9, Unspecified accident; E958.9, Suicide and self-inflicted injury by unspecified means; or E968.9, Assault by unspecified means.

These E codes should rarely be used, since the documentation in the medical record, in inpatient, outpatient and other setting, should normally provide sufficient detail to determine the cause of the injury.

LATE EFFECTS OF EXTERNAL CAUSE GUIDELINES

1. Late effect E codes exist for injuries and poisonings but not for adverse effects of drugs, misadventures and surgical complications.

2. A late effect E code (E929, E959, E969, E977, E989, or E999.1) should be used with any report of a late effect or sequela resulting from a previous injury or poisoning (905-909).

3. A late effect E code should never be used with a related current "nature of injury" code.

MISADVENTURES AND COMPLICATIONS OF CARE GUIDELINES

1. Assign a code in the range of E870-E876 if misadventures are stated by the physician.

2. Assign a code in the range of E878-E879 if the physician attributes an abnormal reaction or later complication to a surgical or medical procedure, but does not mention misadventure at the time of the procedure as the cause of the reaction.

TERRORISM GUIDELINES

1. When the cause of an injury is identified by the Federal Government (FBI) as terrorism, the first-listed E code should be from category E979, Terrorism. The definition of terrorism employed by the FBI is found at the inclusion note at E979. The terrorism E code is the only E code that should

be assigned. Additional E codes from the assault categories should not be assigned.

2. When the cause of an injury is only suspected to be the result of terrorism, a code from category E979 should not be assigned. Assign an E code based on circumstances in the documentation of intent and mechanism.

3. Assign code E979.9, Terrorism, secondary effects, for conditions occurring subsequent to the terrorist event. This code should not be assigned for conditions that are due to the initial terrorist act.

4. For statistical purposes, these codes will be tabulated within the category for assault, expanding the current category from E960-E969 to include E979 and E999.1.

EXAMPLES USING E CODES

When using E-codes, search the Alphabetic Index (Volume 2) for the main term identifying the cause such as "accident," "fire," "shooting," "fall," or "collision." To find the E-code for an adverse reaction to surgical or medical treatment, use the main term "reaction."

Coding Example

Burns to right arm, occurred while burning trash

943.00   Burn of upper limb, except wrist and hand, unspecified degree

E897   Accident caused by controlled fire not in building or structure

E-codes are important for providing the details of an accident to an insurance carrier to enable them to issue faster and more accurate reimbursement. Most insurance carriers want to be sure they reimburse only for services covered under their policy and not for services covered under worker's compensation, automobile or homeowner's insurance. A clear understanding of the circumstances will eliminate questions from the insurance carrier which cause delays in reimbursements.

Coding Example

Fractured ribs due to fall from ladder at home

807.00   Fracture of ribs, closed, unspecified

E881.0   Fall from ladder

E849.0   Place of occurrence, home

Using the above E-codes to provide important information regarding the circumstances of the injury to the insurance carrier eliminates any doubt about the insurer's responsibility for coverage. When using E-codes always list the E-codes as secondary or supplemental to the code(s) describing the injury.

PRINCIPAL AND ADDITIONAL DIAGNOSIS(ES): GUIDELINES FOR INPATIENT, SHORT-TERM, ACUTE CARE, AND LONG TERM CARE HOSPITAL RECORDS

SELECTING PRINCIPAL DIAGNOSES

The circumstances of inpatient admission always govern the selection of principal diagnosis. The principal diagnosis is defined in the Uniform Hospital Discharge Data Set (UHDDS) as that condition established after study to be chiefly responsible for occasioning the admission of the patient to the hospital for care.

The UHDDS definitions are used by acute care short-term and long term care hospitals to report inpatient data elements in a standardized manner. In determining principal diagnosis, the coding conventions in the ICD-9-CM, Volumes I and II take precedence over these official coding guidelines. (See Section IA).

The importance of consistent, complete documentation in the medical record cannot be overemphasized. Without such documentation the application of all coding guidelines is a difficult, if not impossible, task.

1. Codes for symptoms, signs, and ill-defined conditions

    Codes for symptoms, signs, and ill-defined conditions from Chapter 16 are not to be used as principal diagnosis when a related definitive diagnosis has been established.

2. Two or more interrelated conditions, each potentially meeting the definition for principal diagnosis.

    When there are two or more interrelated conditions (such as diseases in the same ICD-9-CM chapter or manifestations characteristically associated with a certain disease) potentially meeting the definition of principal diagnosis, either condition may be sequenced first, unless the circumstances of the admission, the therapy provided, the Tabular List, or the Alphabetic Index indicate otherwise.

3. Two or more diagnoses that equally meet the definition for principal diagnosis.

   In the unusual instance when two or more diagnoses equally meet the criteria for principal diagnosis as determined by the circumstances of admission, diagnostic workup and/or therapy provided, and the Alphabetic Index, Tabular List, or other coding guideline does not provide sequencing direction, any one of the diagnoses may be sequenced first.

4. Two or more comparative or contrasting conditions.

   In those rare instances when two or more contrasting or comparative diagnoses are documented as either/or (or similar terminology), they are coded as if the diagnoses were confirmed. The diagnoses are sequenced according to the circumstances of the admission. If no further determination can be made as to which diagnosis should be principal, either diagnosis may be sequenced first.

5. Symptom(s) followed by contrasting/comparative diagnoses.

   When a symptom(s) is followed by contrasting/comparative diagnoses, the symptom code is sequenced first. All the contrasting/comparative diagnoses should be coded as additional diagnoses.

6. Original treatment plan not carried out.

   Sequence as the principal diagnosis the condition, which after study occasioned the admission to the hospital, even though treatment may not have been carried out due to unforeseen circumstances.

7. Complications of surgery and other medical care.

   When the admission is for treatment of a complication resulting from surgery or other medical care, the complication code is sequenced as the principal diagnosis. If the complication is classified to the 996-999 series, an additional code for the specific complication may be assigned.

8. Uncertain Diagnosis.

   If the diagnosis documented at the time of discharge is qualified as probable, possible, suspected, likely, questionable, or still to be ruled out, code the condition as if it existed or was established. The bases for these guidelines are the diagnostic workup, arrangements for further workup or observation, and initial therapeutic approach that correspond the closest to the established diagnosis.

RULES FOR REPORTING ADDITIONAL DIAGNOSES

For reporting purposes, the definition for other diagnoses is interpreted as additional conditions that affect patient care in terms of requiring: clinical evaluation; or therapeutic treatment; or diagnostic procedures; or extended length of hospital stay; or increased nursing care and/or monitoring.

The UHDDS item # 11-b defines Other Diagnoses as "all conditions that coexist at the time of admission, that develop subsequently, or that affect the treatment received and/or the length of stay. Diagnoses that relate to an earlier episode which have no bearing on the current hospital stay are to be excluded."

UHDDS definitions apply to inpatients in acute care, short-term, hospital setting. The UHDDS definitions are used by acute care short-term and long term care hospitals to report inpatient data elements in a standardized manner.

The following guidelines are to be applied in designating other diagnoses when neither the Alphabetic Index nor the Tabular List in ICD-9-CM provide direction. The listing of the diagnoses in the patient record is the responsibility of the attending physician.

1. Previous conditions

   If the physician has included a diagnosis in the final diagnostic statement, such as the discharge summary or the face sheet, it should ordinarily be coded. Some physicians include in the diagnostic statement: resolved conditions or diagnoses and status-post procedures from previous admission that have no bearing on the current stay. Such conditions are not to be reported and are coded only if required by hospital policy.

   However, history codes (V10-V19) may be used as secondary codes if the historical condition or family history has an impact on current care or if it influences treatment.

2. Abnormal findings

   Abnormal findings (laboratory, x-ray, pathologic, and other diagnostic results) are not coded and reported unless the physician indicates their clinical significance. If the findings are outside the normal range and the attending physician has ordered other tests to evaluate the condition or prescribed treatment, it is appropriate to ask the physician whether the abnormal finding should be added.

   Note: This differs from the coding practices in the outpatient setting for coding encounters for diagnostic tests that have been interpreted by a physician.

3. Uncertain Diagnosis

    If the diagnosis documented at the time of discharge is qualified as probable, possible, suspected, likely, questionable, or still to be ruled out, code the condition as if it existed or was established. The basis for these guidelines are the diagnostic workup, arrangements for further workup or observation, and initial therapeutic approach that correspond most closely with the established diagnosis.

DIAGNOSTIC CODING AND REPORTING GUIDELINES FOR OUTPATIENT SERVICES

These coding guidelines for outpatient diagnoses have been approved for use by hospitals/physicians in coding and reporting hospital-based outpatient services and physician office visits.

Information about the use of certain abbreviations, punctuation, symbols, and other conventions used in the ICD-9-CM Tabular List (code numbers and titles), can be found under Conventions Used in the Tabular List. Information about the correct sequence to use in finding a code is also described previously in Section I.

The terms "encounter" and "visit" are often used interchangeably in describing outpatient service contacts and, therefore, appear together in these guidelines without distinguishing one from the other.

Though the conventions and general guidelines apply to all settings, coding guidelines for outpatient and physician reporting of diagnoses will vary in a number of instances from those for inpatient/hospital diagnoses, recognizing that:

The Uniform Hospital Discharge Data Set (UHDDS) definition of "principal diagnosis" applies only to inpatients in acute, short-term, general and long term care hospitals.

Coding guidelines for inconclusive diagnoses (probable, suspected, rule out, etc.) were developed for inpatient reporting and do not apply to outpatients.

1. Selection of first-listed condition

    In the outpatient setting, the term "first-listed diagnosis" is used in lieu of "principal diagnosis."

    In determining the first-listed diagnosis, the coding conventions of ICD-9-CM as well as the general and disease-specific guidelines take precedence over the outpatient guidelines.

Diagnoses often are not established at the time of the initial encounter/visit. It may take two or more visits before the diagnosis is confirmed.

The most critical rule involves beginning the search for the correct code assignment through the Alphabetic Index. Never begin searching initially in the Tabular List as this will lead to coding errors.

2. The appropriate code or codes from 001.0 through V83.89 must be used to identify diagnoses, symptoms, conditions, problems, complaints, or other reason(s) for the encounter/visit.

3. For accurate reporting of ICD-9-CM diagnosis codes, the documentation should describe the patient's condition using terminology which includes specific diagnoses as well as symptoms, problems, or reasons for the encounter. There are ICD-9-CM codes to describe all of these.

4. The selection of codes 001.0 through 999.9 will frequently be used to describe the reason for the encounter. These codes are from the section of ICD-9-CM for the classification of diseases and injuries (e.g. infectious and parasitic diseases; neoplasms; symptoms, signs, and ill-defined conditions, etc.).

5. Codes that describe symptoms and signs, as opposed to diagnoses, are acceptable for reporting purposes when a diagnosis has not been established (confirmed) by the physician. Chapter 16 of ICD-9-CM, Symptoms, Signs, and Ill-defined Conditions (codes 780.0 to 799.9) contain many, but not all codes for symptoms.

6. ICD-9-CM provides codes to deal with encounters for circumstances other than a disease or injury. The Supplementary Classification of Factors Influencing Health Status and Contact with Health Services (V01.0-V83.89) is provided to deal with occasions when circumstances other than a disease or injury are recorded as diagnosis or problems.

7. Level of Detail in Coding

   a. ICD-9-CM is composed of codes with either 3, 4, or 5 digits. Codes with three digits are included in ICD-9-CM as the heading of a category of codes that may be further subdivided by the use of fourth and/or fifth digits, which provide greater specificity.

   b. A three-digit code is to be used only if it is not further subdivided. Where fourth-digit subcategories and/or fifth-digit subclassifications are provided, they must be assigned. A code is invalid if it has not been coded to the full number of digits required for that code.

8. List first the ICD-9-CM code for the diagnosis, condition, problem, or other reason for encounter/visit shown in the medical record to be chiefly responsible for the services provided. List additional codes that describe any coexisting conditions.

9. Do not code diagnoses documented as probable, suspected, questionable, rule out, or working diagnosis. Rather, code the condition(s) to the highest degree of certainty for that encounter/visit, such as symptoms, signs, abnormal test results, or other reason for the visit.

   Note: This differs from the coding practices used by hospital medical record departments for coding the diagnosis of acute care, short-term hospital inpatients.

10. Chronic diseases treated on an ongoing basis may be coded and reported as many times as the patient receives treatment and care for the condition(s).

11. Code all documented conditions that coexist at the time of the encounter/visit, and require or affect patient care treatment or management. Do not code conditions that were previously treated and no longer exist. However, history codes (V10-V19) may be used as secondary codes if the historical condition or family history has an impact on current care or influences treatment.

12. For patients receiving diagnostic services only during an encounter/visit, sequence first the diagnosis, condition, problem, or other reason for encounter/ visit shown in the medical record to be chiefly responsible for the outpatient services provided during the encounter/visit. Codes for other diagnoses (e.g., chronic conditions) may be sequenced as additional diagnoses. For outpatient encounters for diagnostic tests that have been interpreted by a physician, and the final report is available at the time of coding, code any confirmed or definitive diagnosis(es) documented in the interpretation. Do not code related signs and symptoms as additional diagnoses.

   Note: This differs from the coding practice in the hospital inpatient setting regarding abnormal findings on test results.

13. For patients receiving therapeutic services only during an encounter/visit, sequence first the diagnosis, condition, problem, or other reason for encounter/ visit shown in the medical record to be chiefly responsible for the outpatient services provided during the encounter/visit. Codes for other diagnoses (e.g., chronic conditions) may be sequenced as additional diagnoses.

The only exception to this rule is that when the primary reason for the admission/encounter is chemotherapy, radiation therapy, or rehabilitation, the appropriate V code for the service is listed first, and the diagnosis or problem for which the service is being performed listed second.

14. For patient's receiving preoperative evaluations only, sequence a code from category V72.8, Other specified examinations, to describe the pre-op consultations. Assign a code for the condition to describe the reason for the surgery as an additional diagnosis. Code also any findings related to the pre-op evaluation.

15. For ambulatory surgery, code the diagnosis for which the surgery was performed. If the postoperative diagnosis is known to be different from the preoperative diagnosis at the time the diagnosis is confirmed, select the postoperative diagnosis for coding, since it is the most definitive.

16. For routine outpatient prenatal visits when no complications are present, codes V22.0, Supervision of normal first pregnancy, and V22.1, Supervision of other normal pregnancy, should be used as principal diagnoses. These codes should not be used in conjunction with Chapter 11 Pregnancy, Childbirth and the Puerperium codes.

A NOTE ABOUT ICD-10

ICD-10 was first published by the World Health Organization (WHO) in 1992. The National Center for Health Statistics (NCHS), the Federal agency responsible for use of the International Statistical Classification of Diseases and Related Health Problems, 10th revision (ICD-10) in the United States, has developed a clinical modification of the classification for morbidity purposes. The ICD-10 is used to code and classify mortality data from death certificates, having replaced ICD-9 for this purpose as of January 1, 1999. ICD-10-CM is planned as the replacement for ICD-9-CM, volumes 1 and 2.

The ICD-10 is copyrighted by the World Health Organization (WHO), which owns and publishes the classification. WHO has authorized the development of an adaptation of ICD-10 for use in the United States for U.S. government purposes. As agreed, all modifications to the ICD-10 must conform to WHO conventions for the ICD. Except in rare instances, no modifications have been made to existing three-digit categories and four-digit codes, with the exception of title changes that did not change the meaning of the category or code.

ICD-10-CM was developed following a thorough evaluation by a Technical Advisory Panel and extensive additional consultation with physician groups, clinical coders, and others to assure clinical accuracy and utility. Notable improvements in the content and format include: the addition of information relevant to ambulatory and managed care encounters; expanded injury codes; the creation of combination diagnosis/symptom codes to reduce the number of codes needed to fully describe a condition; the addition of a sixth character; incorporation of common 4th and 5th digit subclassifications; laterality; and greater specificity in code assignment. The new structure will allow further expansion than was possible with ICD-9-CM.

There is not yet an anticipated implementation date for the ICD-10-CM. Implementation will be based on the process for adoption of standards under the Health Insurance Portability and Accountability Act of 1996. There will be a two year implementation window once the final notice to implement has been published in the Federal Register.

ICD-9-CM ANATOMICAL ILLUSTRATIONS

A fundamental knowledge and understanding of basic human anatomy and physiology is a prerequisite for accurate diagnosis coding. While a comprehensive treatment of anatomy and physiology is beyond the scope of this text, the large scale, full color anatomical illustrations on the following pages are designed to facilitate the diagnosis coding process for both beginning and experienced coders.

The illustrations provide an anatomical perspective of diagnosis coding by providing a side-by-side view of the major systems of the human body and a corresponding list of the most common diagnoses categories used to support medical, surgical and diagnostic services performed on the illustrated system.

The diagnostic categories listed on the left facing page of each anatomical illustration are three-digit categories and may not be used for coding. These categories are provided as "pointers" to the appropriate section of the ICD-9-CM Volume 1 where the complete listings, including 4th and 5th digits if appropriate, may be found.

ICD-9-CM
ANATOMICAL
ILLUSTRATIONS

PLATE 1. SKIN AND SUBCUTANEOUS TISSUE-MALE

Viral diseases accompanied by exanthem   050-057

Neoplasms
Malignant melanoma of skin   172
Other malignant neoplasm of skin   173
Malignant neoplasm of male breast   175
Kaposi's sarcoma   176
Benign neoplasm of skin   216
Carcinoma in situ of skin   232

Infections of skin and subcutaneous tissue
Carbuncle and furuncle   680
Cellulitis and abscess of finger and toe   681
Other cellulitis and abscess   682
Acute lymphadenitis   683
Impetigo   684
Pilonidal cyst   685
Other local infections of skin and subcutaneous tissue   686

**Other inflammatory conditions of skin
and subcutaneous tissue**
Erythematosquamous dermatosis   690
Atopic dermatitis and related conditions   691
Contact dermatitis and other eczema   692
Dermatitis due to substances taken internally   693
Bullous dermatoses   694
Erythematous conditions   695
Psoriasis and similar disorders   696
Lichen   697
Pruritus and related conditions   698

Other diseases of skin and subcutaneous tissue
Corns and callosities   700
Other hypertrophic and atrophic conditions of skin   701
Diseases of nail   703
Diseases of hair and hair follicles   704
Disorders of sweat glands   705
Diseases of sebaceous glands   706
Chronic ulcer of skin   707
Urticaria   708
Other disorders of skin and subcutaneous tissue   709
Symptoms involving skin and other integumentary tissue   782

Symptoms, signs and ill-defined conditions   780-799

Male Figure
(Anterior View)

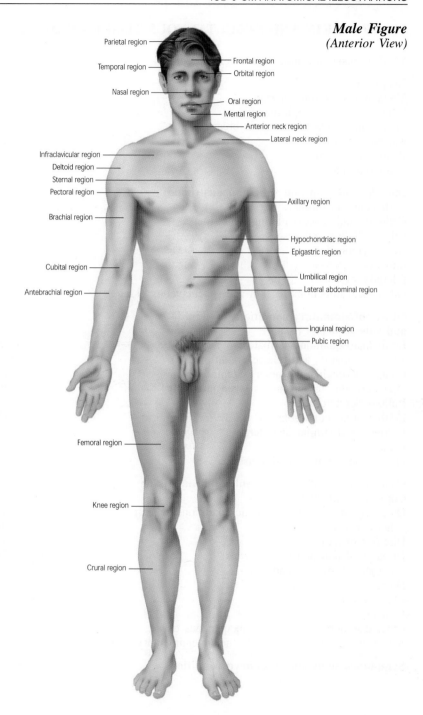

Parietal region

Temporal region

Nasal region

Frontal region

Orbital region

Oral region

Mental region

Anterior neck region

Lateral neck region

Infraclavicular region

Deltoid region

Sternal region

Pectoral region

Brachial region

Axillary region

Hypochondriac region

Epigastric region

Cubital region

Antebrachial region

Umbilical region

Lateral abdominal region

Inguinal region

Pubic region

Femoral region

Knee region

Crural region

©Practice Management Information Corp., Los Angeles, CA

PLATE 2. SKIN AND SUBCUTANEOUS TISSUE - FEMALE

Viral diseases accompanied by exanthem	050-057

Neoplasms

Malignant melanoma of skin	172
Other malignant neoplasm of skin	173
Malignant neoplasm of female breast	174
Kaposi's sarcoma	176
Benign neoplasm of skin	216
Carcinoma in situ of skin	232

Infections of skin and subcutaneous tissue

Carbuncle and furuncle	680
Cellulitis and abscess of finger and toe	681
Other cellulitis and abscess	682
Acute lymphadenitis	683
Impetigo	684
Pilonidal cyst	685
Other local infections of skin and subcutaneous tissue	686

**Other inflammatory conditions of skin
and subcutaneous tissue**

Erythematosquamous dermatosis	690
Atopic dermatitis and related conditions	691
Contact dermatitis and other eczema	692
Dermatitis due to substances taken internally	693
Bullous dermatoses	694
Erythematous conditions	695
Psoriasis and similar disorders	696
Lichen	697
Pruritus and related conditions	698

Other diseases of skin and subcutaneous tissue

Corns and callosities	700
Other hypertrophic and atrophic conditions of skin	701
Other dermatoses	702
Diseases of nail	703
Diseases of hair and hair follicles	704
Disorders of sweat glands	705
Diseases of sebaceous glands	706
Chronic ulcer of skin	707
Urticaria	708
Other disorders of skin and subcutaneous tissue	709
Symptoms involving skin and other integumentary tissue	782

Symptoms, signs and ill-defined conditions	780-799

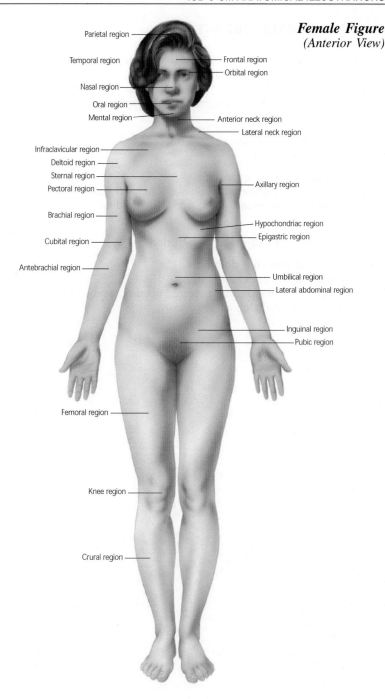

Female Figure
(Anterior View)

Parietal region

Temporal region

Frontal region

Orbital region

Nasal region

Oral region

Mental region

Anterior neck region

Lateral neck region

Infraclavicular region

Deltoid region

Sternal region

Pectoral region

Axillary region

Brachial region

Hypochondriac region

Epigastric region

Cubital region

Antebrachial region

Umbilical region

Lateral abdominal region

Inguinal region

Pubic region

Femoral region

Knee region

Crural region

PLATE 3. FEMALE BREAST

Female Breast

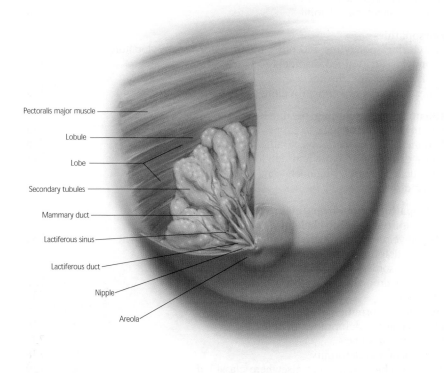

Pectoralis major muscle

Lobule

Lobe

Secondary tubules

Mammary duct

Lactiferous sinus

Lactiferous duct

Nipple

Areola

PLATE 4. MUSCULAR SYSTEM AND CONNECTIVE TISSUE - ANTERIOR VIEW

Muscular System
(Anterior View)

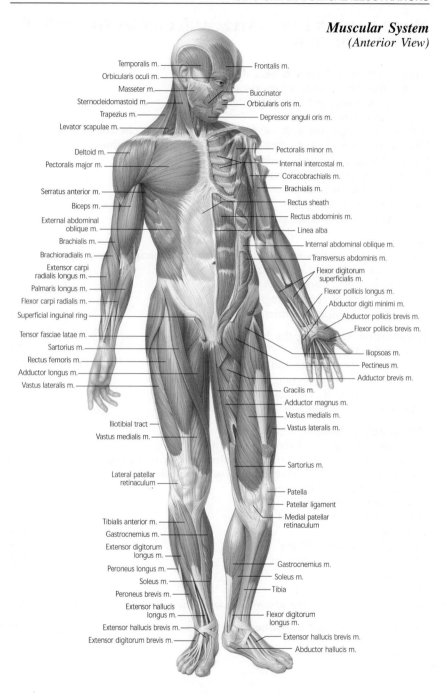

Temporalis m.
Orbicularis oculi m.
Masseter m.
Sternocleidomastoid m.
Trapezius m.
Levator scapulae m.

Frontalis m.
Buccinator
Orbicularis oris m.
Depressor anguli oris m.

Deltoid m.
Pectoralis major m.
Serratus anterior m.
Biceps m.
External abdominal oblique m.
Brachialis m.
Brachioradialis m.
Extensor carpi radialis longus m.
Palmaris longus m.
Flexor carpi radialis m.
Superficial inguinal ring
Tensor fasciae latae m.
Sartorius m.
Rectus femoris m.
Adductor longus m.
Vastus lateralis m.

Pectoralis minor m.
Internal intercostal m.
Coracobrachialis m.
Brachialis m.
Rectus sheath
Rectus abdominis m.
Linea alba
Internal abdominal oblique m.
Transversus abdominis m.
Flexor digitorum superficialis m.
Flexor pollicis longus m.
Abductor digiti minimi m.
Abductor pollicis brevis m.
Flexor pollicis brevis m.
Iliopsoas m.
Pectineus m.
Adductor brevis m.
Gracilis m.
Adductor magnus m.
Vastus medialis m.
Vastus lateralis m.

Iliotibial tract
Vastus medialis m.

Sartorius m.

Lateral patellar retinaculum

Patella
Patellar ligament
Medial patellar retinaculum

Tibialis anterior m.
Gastrocnemius m.
Extensor digitorum longus m.
Peroneus longus m.
Soleus m.
Peroneus brevis m.
Extensor hallucis longus m.
Extensor hallucis brevis m.
Extensor digitorum brevis m.

Gastrocnemius m.
Soleus m.
Tibia
Flexor digitorum longus m.
Extensor hallucis brevis m.
Abductor hallucis m.

PLATE 5. MUSCULAR SYSTEM AND CONNECTIVE TISSUE - POSTERIOR VIEW

Muscular System
(Posterior View)

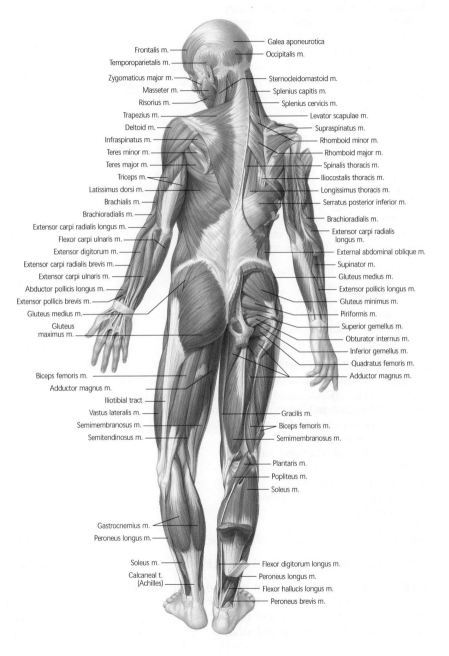

Frontalis m.
Temporoparietalis m.
Zygomaticus major m.
Masseter m.
Risorius m.
Trapezius m.
Deltoid m.
Infraspinatus m.
Teres minor m.
Teres major m.
Triceps m.
Latissimus dorsi m.
Brachialis m.
Brachioradialis m.
Extensor carpi radialis longus m.
Flexor carpi ulnaris m.
Extensor digitorum m.
Extensor carpi radialis brevis m.
Extensor carpi ulnaris m.
Abductor pollicis longus m.
Extensor pollicis brevis m.
Gluteus medius m.
Gluteus maximus m.
Biceps femoris m.
Adductor magnus m.
Iliotibial tract
Vastus lateralis m.
Semimembranosus m.
Semitendinosus m.
Gastrocnemius m.
Peroneus longus m.
Soleus m.
Calcaneal t. (Achilles)

Galea aponeurotica
Occipitalis m.
Sternocleidomastoid m.
Splenius capitis m.
Splenius cervicis m.
Levator scapulae m.
Supraspinatus m.
Rhomboid minor m.
Rhomboid major m.
Spinalis thoracis m.
Iliocostalis thoracis m.
Longissimus thoracis m.
Serratus posterior inferior m.
Brachioradialis m.
Extensor carpi radialis longus m.
External abdominal oblique m.
Supinator m.
Gluteus medius m.
Extensor pollicis longus m.
Gluteus minimus m.
Piriformis m.
Superior gemellus m.
Obturator internus m.
Inferior gemellus m.
Quadratus femoris m.
Adductor magnus m.
Gracilis m.
Biceps femoris m.
Semimembranosus m.
Plantaris m.
Popliteus m.
Soleus m.
Flexor digitorum longus m.
Peroneus longus m.
Flexor hallucis longus m.
Peroneus brevis m.

PLATE 6. MUSCULAR SYSTEM - SHOULDER AND ELBOW

Shoulder and Elbow
(Anterior View)

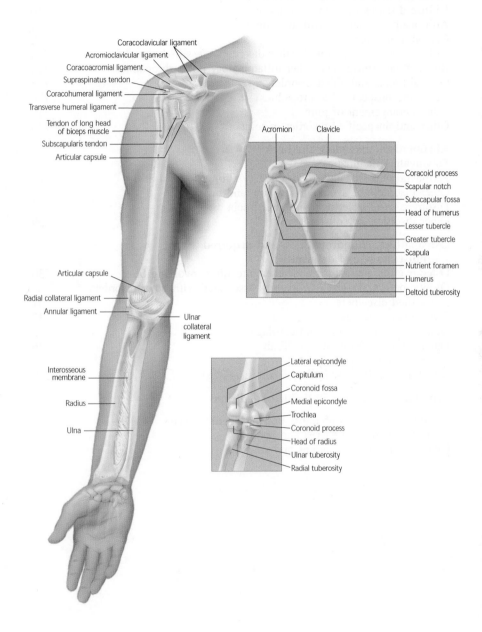

Coracoclavicular ligament
Acromioclavicular ligament
Coracoacromial ligament
Supraspinatus tendon
Coracohumeral ligament
Transverse humeral ligament
Tendon of long head of biceps muscle
Subscapularis tendon
Articular capsule

Acromion
Clavicle

Coracoid process
Scapular notch
Subscapular fossa
Head of humerus
Lesser tubercle
Greater tubercle
Scapula
Nutrient foramen
Humerus
Deltoid tuberosity

Articular capsule
Radial collateral ligament
Annular ligament
Ulnar collateral ligament

Interosseous membrane
Radius
Ulna

Lateral epicondyle
Capitulum
Coronoid fossa
Medial epicondyle
Trochlea
Coronoid process
Head of radius
Ulnar tuberosity
Radial tuberosity

PLATE 7. MUSCULAR SYSTEM - HAND AND WRIST

Hand and Wrist

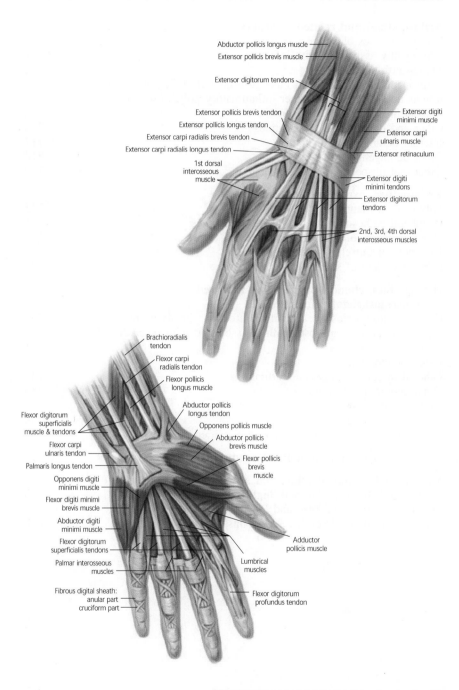

Abductor pollicis longus muscle

Extensor pollicis brevis muscle

Extensor digitorum tendons

Extensor pollicis brevis tendon

Extensor pollicis longus tendon

Extensor carpi radialis brevis tendon

Extensor carpi radialis longus tendon

1st dorsal interosseous muscle

Extensor digiti minimi muscle

Extensor carpi ulnaris muscle

Extensor retinaculum

Extensor digiti minimi tendons

Extensor digitorum tendons

2nd, 3rd, 4th dorsal interosseous muscles

Brachioradialis tendon

Flexor carpi radialis tendon

Flexor pollicis longus muscle

Flexor digitorum superficialis muscle & tendons

Abductor pollicis longus tendon

Opponens pollicis muscle

Abductor pollicis brevis muscle

Flexor pollicis brevis muscle

Flexor carpi ulnaris tendon

Palmaris longus tendon

Opponens digiti minimi muscle

Flexor digiti minimi brevis muscle

Abductor digiti minimi muscle

Flexor digitorum superficialis tendons

Palmar interosseous muscles

Fibrous digital sheath: anular part cruciform part

Adductor pollicis muscle

Lumbrical muscles

Flexor digitorum profundus tendon

PLATE 8. MUSCULOSKELETAL SYSTEM - HIP AND KNEE

Hip and Knee
(Anterior View)

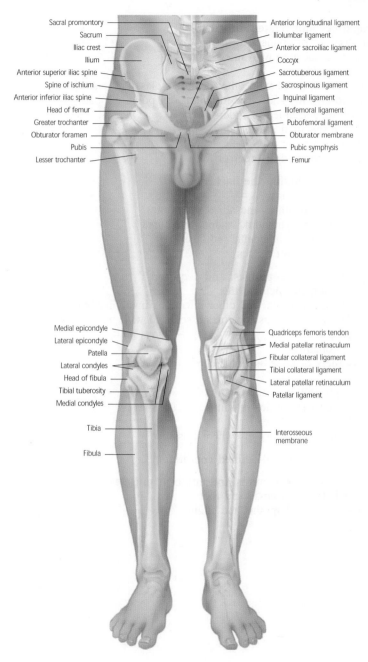

Sacral promontory
Sacrum
Iliac crest
Ilium
Anterior superior iliac spine
Spine of ischium
Anterior inferior iliac spine
Head of femur
Greater trochanter
Obturator foramen
Pubis
Lesser trochanter

Anterior longitudinal ligament
Iliolumbar ligament
Anterior sacroiliac ligament
Coccyx
Sacrotuberous ligament
Sacrospinous ligament
Inguinal ligament
Iliofemoral ligament
Pubofemoral ligament
Obturator membrane
Pubic symphysis
Femur

Medial epicondyle
Lateral epicondyle
Patella
Lateral condyles
Head of fibula
Tibial tuberosity
Medial condyles
Tibia
Fibula

Quadriceps femoris tendon
Medial patellar retinaculum
Fibular collateral ligament
Tibial collateral ligament
Lateral patellar retinaculum
Patellar ligament
Interosseous membrane

PLATE 9. MUSCULOSKELETAL SYSTEM - FOOT AND ANKLE

Foot and Ankle

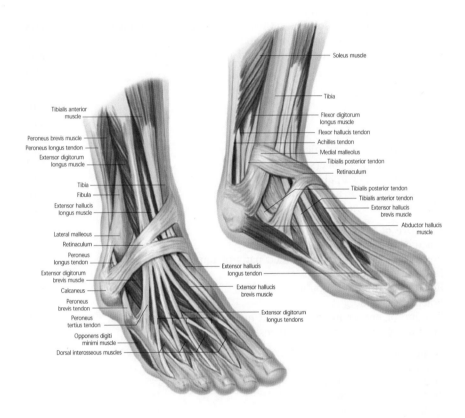

Soleus muscle

Tibia

Flexor digitorum longus muscle

Flexor hallucis tendon

Achilles tendon

Medial malleolus

Tibialis posterior tendon

Retinaculum

Tibialis posterior tendon

Tibialis anterior tendon

Extensor hallucis brevis muscle

Abductor hallucis muscle

Tibialis anterior muscle

Peroneus brevis muscle

Peroneus longus tendon

Extensor digitorum longus muscle

Tibia

Fibula

Extensor hallucis longus muscle

Lateral malleous

Retinaculum

Peroneus longus tendon

Extensor digitorum brevis muscle

Calcaneus

Peroneus brevis tendon

Peroneus tertius tendon

Opponens digiti minimi muscle

Dorsal interosseous muscles

Extensor hallucis longus tendon

Extensor hallucis brevis muscle

Extensor digitorum longus tendons

PLATE 10. SKELETAL SYSTEM - ANTERIOR VIEW

Skeletal System
(Anterior View)

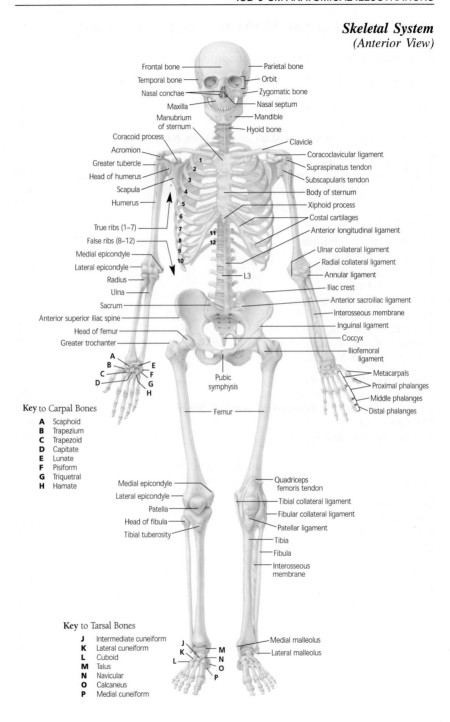

Frontal bone
Parietal bone
Temporal bone
Orbit
Nasal conchae
Zygomatic bone
Maxilla
Nasal septum
Manubrium of sternum
Mandible
Hyoid bone
Coracoid process
Clavicle
Acromion
Coracoclavicular ligament
Greater tubercle
Supraspinatus tendon
Head of humerus
Subscapularis tendon
Scapula
Body of sternum
Humerus
Xiphoid process
Costal cartilages
True ribs (1–7)
Anterior longitudinal ligament
False ribs (8–12)
Medial epicondyle
Ulnar collateral ligament
Lateral epicondyle
Radial collateral ligament
Radius
Annular ligament
Ulna
Iliac crest
Sacrum
Anterior sacroiliac ligament
Anterior superior iliac spine
Interosseous membrane
Head of femur
Inguinal ligament
Greater trochanter
Coccyx
Iliofemoral ligament
Metacarpals
Pubic symphysis
Proximal phalanges
Middle phalanges
Distal phalanges
Femur

L3

Key to Carpal Bones

A	Scaphoid
B	Trapezium
C	Trapezoid
D	Capitate
E	Lunate
F	Pisiform
G	Triquetral
H	Hamate

Medial epicondyle
Quadriceps femoris tendon
Lateral epicondyle
Tibial collateral ligament
Patella
Fibular collateral ligament
Head of fibula
Patellar ligament
Tibial tuberosity
Tibia
Fibula
Interosseous membrane

Key to Tarsal Bones

J	Intermediate cuneiform
K	Lateral cuneiform
L	Cuboid
M	Talus
N	Navicular
O	Calcaneus
P	Medial cuneiform

Medial malleolus
Lateral malleolus

©Scientific Publishing, Ltd., Rolling Meadows, IL

PLATE 11. SKELETAL SYSTEM - POSTERIOR VIEW

Skeletal System
(Posterior View)

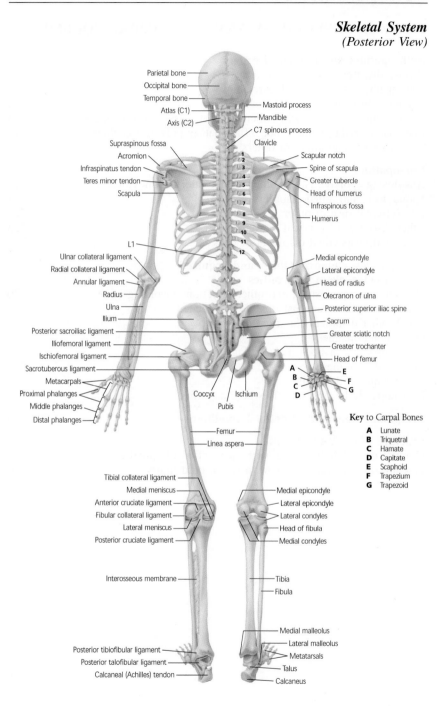

Parietal bone
Occipital bone
Temporal bone
Atlas (C1)
Axis (C2)
Mastoid process
Mandible
C7 spinous process
Clavicle
Supraspinous fossa
Acromion
Scapular notch
Spine of scapula
Infraspinatus tendon
Teres minor tendon
Greater tubercle
Scapula
Head of humerus
Infraspinous fossa
Humerus
1
2
3
4
5
6
7
8
9
10
11
12
L1
Ulnar collateral ligament
Radial collateral ligament
Annular ligament
Radius
Ulna
Ilium
Posterior sacroiliac ligament
Iliofemoral ligament
Ischiofemoral ligament
Sacrotuberous ligament
Metacarpals
Proximal phalanges
Middle phalanges
Distal phalanges
Medial epicondyle
Lateral epicondyle
Head of radius
Olecranon of ulna
Posterior superior iliac spine
Sacrum
Greater sciatic notch
Greater trochanter
Head of femur
A
B
C
D
E
F
G
Coccyx
Ischium
Pubis
Femur
Linea aspera

Key to Carpal Bones
A Lunate
B Triquetral
C Hamate
D Capitate
E Scaphoid
F Trapezium
G Trapezoid

Tibial collateral ligament
Medial meniscus
Anterior cruciate ligament
Fibular collateral ligament
Lateral meniscus
Posterior cruciate ligament
Medial epicondyle
Lateral epicondyle
Lateral condyles
Head of fibula
Medial condyles
Interosseous membrane
Tibia
Fibula
Medial malleolus
Lateral malleolus
Metatarsals
Talus
Calcaneus
Posterior tibiofibular ligament
Posterior talofibular ligament
Calcaneal (Achilles) tendon

©Scientific Publishing, Ltd., Rolling Meadows, IL

PLATE 12. SKELETAL SYSTEM - VERTEBRAL COLUMN

Vertebral Column
(Lateral View)

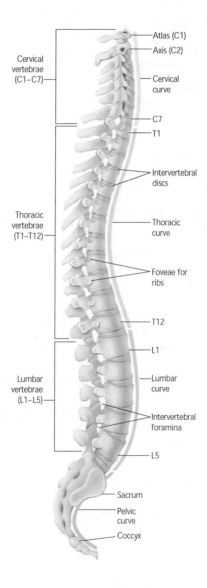

PLATE 13. RESPIRATORY SYSTEM

Neoplasms

Malignant neoplasm of respiratory and intrathoracic organs	160-165
Malignant neoplasm of larynx	161
Malignant neoplasm of trachea, bronchus, and lung	162
Benign neoplasm of respiratory and intrathoracic organs	212
Carcinoma in situ of respiratory system	231

Acute respiratory infections

Acute nasopharyngitis [common cold]	460
Acute sinusitis	461
Acute pharyngitis	462
Acute tonsillitis	463
Acute laryngitis and tracheitis	464
Acute upper respiratory infections of multiple or unspecified sites	465
Acute bronchitis and bronchiolitis	466

Other diseases of upper respiratory tract

Deviated nasal septum	470
Nasal polyps	471
Chronic pharyngitis and nasopharyngitis	472
Chronic sinusitis	473
Chronic disease of tonsils and adenoids	474
Peritonsillar abscess	475
Chronic laryngitis and laryngotracheitis	476
Allergic rhinitis	477

Pneumonia and influenza

Viral pneumonia	480
Pneumococcal pneumonia [Streptococcus pneumoniae pneumonia]	481
Influenza	487

Chronic obstructive pulmonary disease and allied conditions

Chronic bronchitis	491
Emphysema	492
Asthma	493
Bronchiectasis	494
Extrinsic allergic alveolitis	495

Other diseases of respiratory system

Empyema	510
Pleurisy	511
Pneumothorax	512
Abscess of lung and mediastinum	513
Pulmonary congestion and hypostasis	514
Postinflammatory pulmonary fibrosis	515

Respiratory System

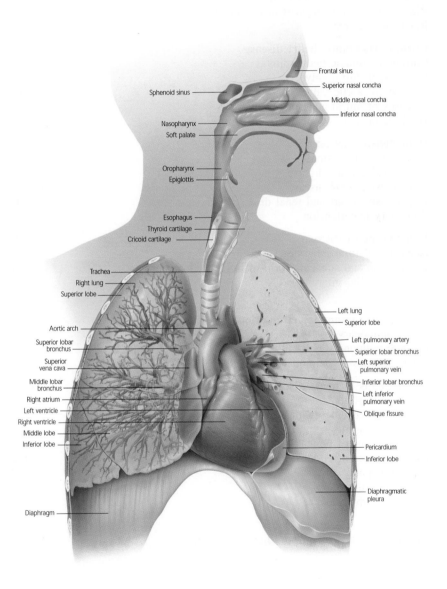

Frontal sinus
Superior nasal concha
Middle nasal concha
Inferior nasal concha
Sphenoid sinus
Nasopharynx
Soft palate
Oropharynx
Epiglottis
Esophagus
Thyroid cartilage
Cricoid cartilage
Trachea
Right lung
Superior lobe
Aortic arch
Superior lobar bronchus
Superior vena cava
Middle lobar bronchus
Right atrium
Left ventricle
Right ventricle
Middle lobe
Inferior lobe
Diaphragm
Left lung
Superior lobe
Left pulmonary artery
Superior lobar bronchus
Left superior pulmonary vein
Inferior lobar bronchus
Left inferior pulmonary vein
Oblique fissure
Pericardium
Inferior lobe
Diaphragmatic pleura

PLATE 14. HEART AND PERICARDIUM

Acute rheumatic fever

Rheumatic fever without mention of heart involvement	390
Rheumatic fever with heart involvement	391
Rheumatic chorea	392

Chronic rheumatic heart disease

Chronic rheumatic pericarditis	393
Diseases of mitral valve	394
Diseases of aortic valve	395
Diseases of mitral and aortic valves	396
Diseases of other endocardial structures	397

Hypertensive disease

Essential hypertension	401
Hypertensive heart disease	402
Hypertensive renal disease	403
Hypertensive heart and renal disease	404
Secondary hypertension	405

Ischemic heart disease

Acute myocardial infarction	410
Other acute and subacute form of ischemic heart disease	411
Old myocardial infarction	412
Angina pectoris	413

Diseases of pulmonary circulation

Acute pulmonary heart disease	415
Chronic pulmonary heart disease	416
Other diseases of pulmonary circulation	417

Other forms of heart disease

Acute pericarditis	420
Acute and subacute endocarditis	421
Acute myocarditis	422
Other diseases of pericardium	423
Other diseases of endocardium	424
Cardiomyopathy	425
Conduction disorders	426
Cardiac dysrhythmias	427
Heart failure	428

Symptoms, signs and ill-defined conditions   780-799

Heart
(External View)

Left common carotid artery
Brachiocephalic artery
Left subclavian artery
Aortic arch
Ligamentum arteriosum
Superior vena cava
Ascending aorta
Left pulmonary artery
Pulmonary trunk
Left auricle
Right coronary artery
Circumflex artery
Right atrium
Great cardiac vein
Right ventricle
Anterior descending (interventricular) artery
Anterior cardiac vein
Left ventricle
Right marginal artery
Small cardiac vein
Apex

Heart
(Internal View)

Superior vena cava
Right pulmonary artery branches
Aorta
Pulmonary trunk
Left pulmonary artery
Left pulmonary veins
Right pulmonary veins
Left atrium
Pulmonary semilunar valve
Aortic semilunar valve
Right atrium
Bicuspid (left AV) valve
Left ventricle
Tricuspid (right AV) valve
Papillary muscle
Interventricular septum
Chordae tendineae
Inferior vena cava
Myocardium
Right ventricle
Trabeculae carneae

PLATE 15. CIRCULATORY SYSTEM

Vascular System

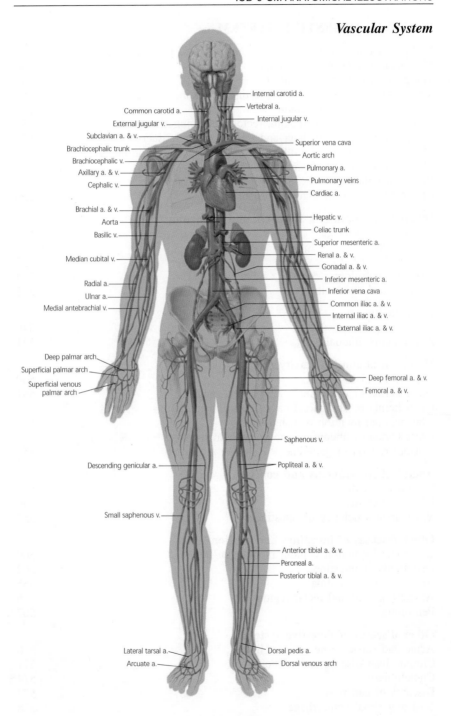

Internal carotid a.
Vertebral a.
Common carotid a.
Internal jugular v.
External jugular v.
Subclavian a. & v.
Superior vena cava
Brachiocephalic trunk
Aortic arch
Brachiocephalic v.
Pulmonary a.
Axillary a. & v.
Pulmonary veins
Cephalic v.
Cardiac a.
Brachial a. & v.
Hepatic v.
Aorta
Celiac trunk
Basilic v.
Superior mesenteric a.
Renal a. & v.
Median cubital v.
Gonadal a. & v.
Inferior mesenteric a.
Radial a.
Inferior vena cava
Ulnar a.
Common iliac a. & v.
Medial antebrachial v.
Internal iliac a. & v.
External iliac a. & v.
Deep palmar arch
Superficial palmar arch
Superficial venous palmar arch
Deep femoral a. & v.
Femoral a. & v.
Saphenous v.
Descending genicular a.
Popliteal a. & v.
Small saphenous v.
Anterior tibial a. & v.
Peroneal a.
Posterior tibial a. & v.
Lateral tarsal a.
Dorsal pedis a.
Arcuate a.
Dorsal venous arch

PLATE 16. DIGESTIVE SYSTEM

Digestive System

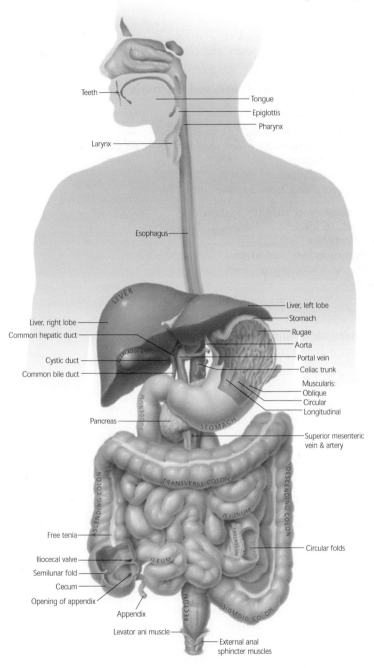

PLATE 17. GENITOURINARY SYSTEM

Urinary System

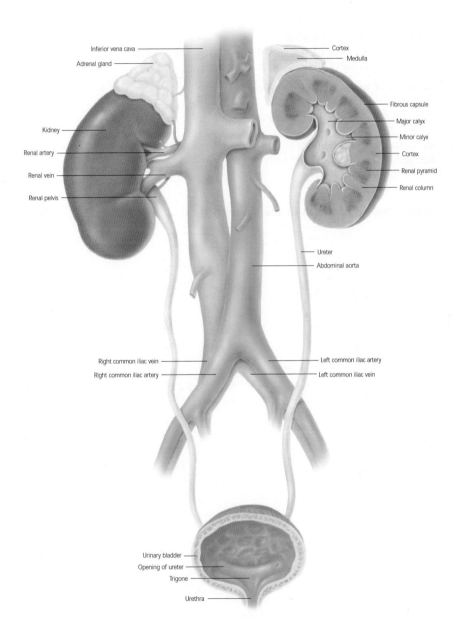

PLATE 18. MALE GENITAL ORGANS

Male Reproductive System

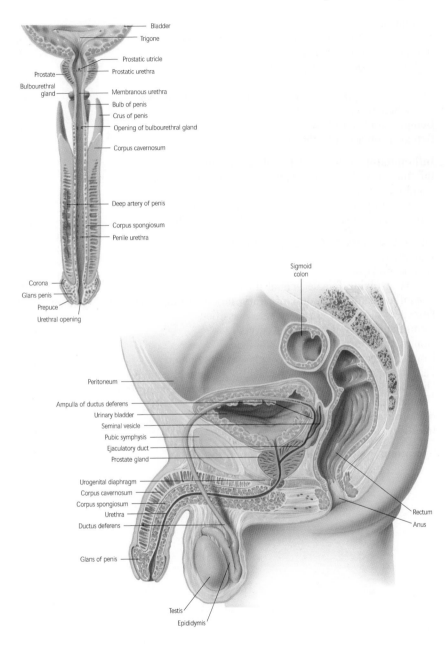

Bladder
Trigone
Prostatic utricle
Prostatic urethra
Prostate
Prostate
Bulbourethral gland
Membranous urethra
Bulb of penis
Crus of penis
Opening of bulbourethral gland
Corpus cavernosum

Deep artery of penis

Corpus spongiosum
Penile urethra

Corona
Glans penis
Prepuce
Urethral opening

Sigmoid colon

Peritoneum

Ampulla of ductus deferens
Urinary bladder
Seminal vesicle
Pubic symphysis
Ejaculatory duct
Prostate gland

Urogenital diaphragm
Corpus cavernosum
Corpus spongiosum
Urethra
Ductus deferens

Rectum
Anus

Glans of penis

Testis
Epididymis

PLATE 19. FEMALE GENITAL ORGANS

Neoplasms

Inflammatory disease of female pelvic organs

Other disorders of female genital tract

Symptoms, signs and ill-defined conditions

Female Reproductive System

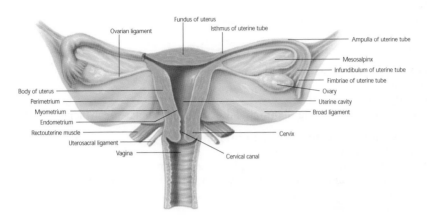

Fundus of uterus
Ovarian ligament
Isthmus of uterine tube
Ampulla of uterine tube
Mesosalpinx
Infundibulum of uterine tube
Fimbriae of uterine tube
Ovary
Body of uterus
Perimetrium
Myometrium
Endometrium
Uterine cavity
Broad ligament
Rectouterine muscle
Uterosacral ligament
Cervix
Vagina
Cervical canal

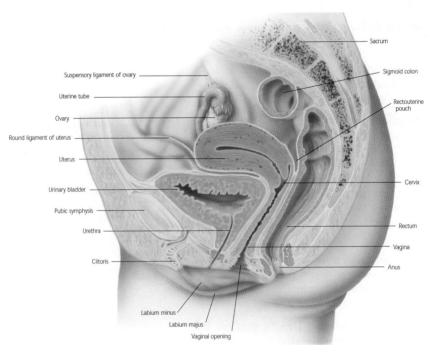

Sacrum
Sigmoid colon
Suspensory ligament of ovary
Uterine tube
Rectouterine pouch
Ovary
Round ligament of uterus
Uterus
Urinary bladder
Pubic symphysis
Cervix
Urethra
Rectum
Clitoris
Vagina
Anus
Labium minus
Labium majus
Vaginal opening

PLATE 20. PREGNANCY, CHILDBIRTH AND THE PUERPERIUM

Female Reproductive System: Pregnancy
(Lateral View)

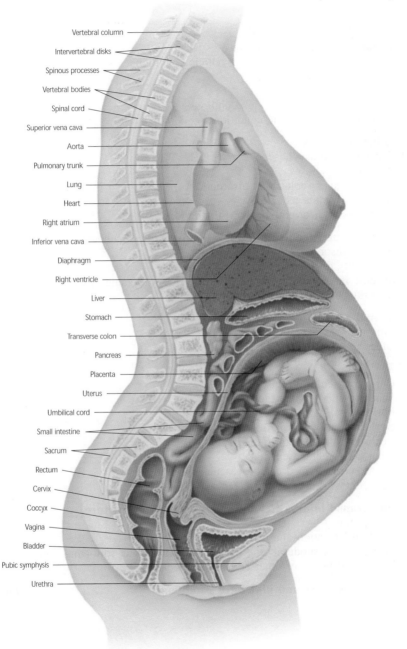

PLATE 21. NERVOUS SYSTEM - BRAIN

Neoplasms

Malignant neoplasm of brain	191

Organic psychotic conditions

Senile and presenile organic psychotic conditions	290
Alcoholic psychoses	291
Drug psychoses	292
Transient organic psychotic conditions	293
Other organic psychotic conditions (conditions)	294

Other psychoses

Schizophrenic psychoses	295
Affective psychoses	296
Paranoid states (delusional disorders)	297
Other nonorganic psychoses	298
Psychoses with origin specific to childhood	299

Neurotic, personality, and other nonpsychotic disorders

Neurotic disorders	300
Personality disorders	301
Specific nonpsychotic mental disorders due to organic brain damage	310
Hyperkinetic syndrome of childhood	314

Mental retardation

Mild mental retardation	317
Other specified mental retardation	318
Unspecified mental retardation	319

Cerebrovascular disease

Subarachnoid hemorrhage	430
Intracerebral hemorrhage	431
Occlusion and stenosis of precerebral arteries	433
Occlusion of cerebral arteries	434
Transient cerebral ischemia	435
Acute but ill-defined cerebrovascular disease	436
Late effects of cerebrovascular disease	438

Intracranial injury, excluding those with skull fracture

Concussion	850
Cerebral laceration and contusion	851
Subarachnoid, subdural, and extradural hemorrhage, following injury	852
Intracranial injury of other and unspecified nature	854

Symptoms, signs and ill-defined conditions 780-799

Brain
(Base View)

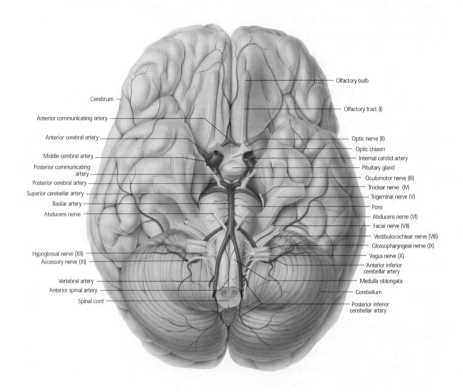

PLATE 22. NERVOUS SYSTEM

Nervous System

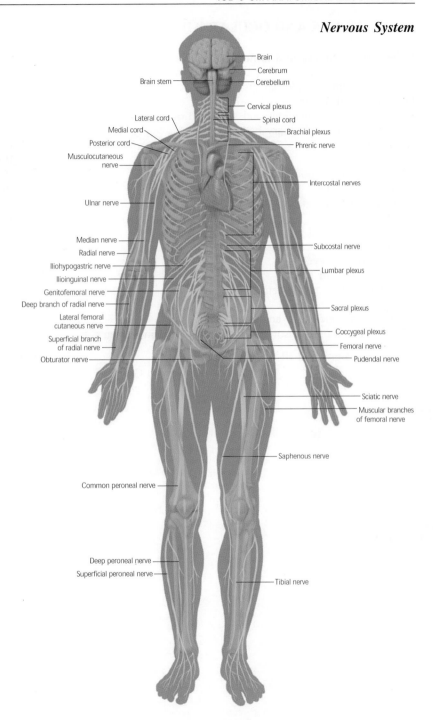

PLATE 23. EYE AND OCULAR ADNEXA

Right Eye
(Horizontal Section)

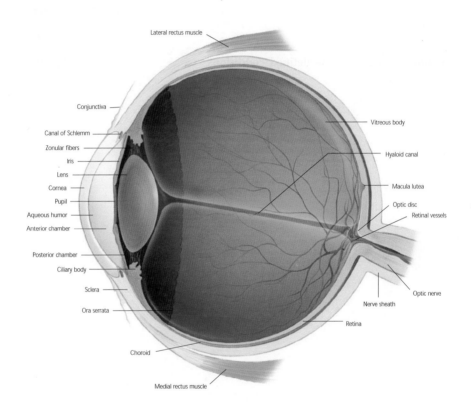

PLATE 24. AUDITORY SYSTEM

The Ear

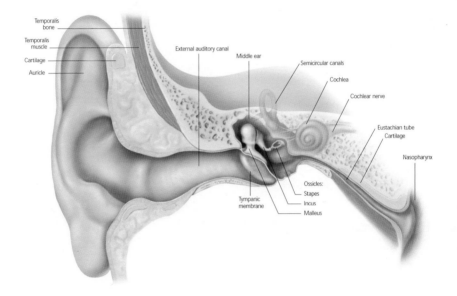

HOW TO FILE A CMS-1500 CLAIM FORM

As with coding systems, historically there have been a variety of insurance claim forms to deal with, the so-called "universal" or "standard" claim form of the American Medical Association, various incarnations of Medicare forms, Blue Shield forms, Medicaid forms, and many, many other forms printed by various insurance carriers. Needless to say, just keeping track of the proper form to use was a major job. Most practices depended on their patients to provide the proper claim form, which the patient usually obtained from their employer.

The American Medical Association recognized the need to simplify and standardize the reporting of physician services under the various types of government programs and third party policies. A task force was established to develop a uniform physician reporting form acceptable to the various government agencies and health insurance carriers. The result of this effort is the Uniform Health Insurance Claim Form, also known as the CMS-1500 form, or Standard Claim Form. As of this writing, the Standard Claim Form is accepted by Medicare, Blue Cross and Blue Shield, the majority of commercial carriers, and most Medicaid plans.

Most of the exceptions to the use of the Standard Claim Form for submitting Medicaid claims occur where computer companies, instead of health insurance carriers, serve as the fiscal intermediary for the Medicaid program. A specific example of this is the Form 401C used to process California Medicaid (Medi-Cal). The Form 401C is designed for what is called optical scanning (machine read) and is very difficult to complete without using a computer.

Note that there are currently two versions of the CMS-1500 insurance claim form which may be required or accepted by insurance carriers. On the following pages you will find examples of both forms with detailed instructions for their completion.

CMS1500 FORM

CMS-1500 CLAIM FORM

The CMS-1500 health insurance claim form answers the needs of many health insurers. It is the basic form prescribed by The Centers for Medicare and Medicaid Services (CMS) formerly known as the Health Care Financing Administration (CMS), for the Medicare and Medicaid programs for claims submitted by physicians and suppliers, except for ambulance services. It has also been adopted by CHAMPUS and has the approval of the AMACouncil on Medical Services.

There are two versions of the CMS-1500 health insurance claim form that may be used to file claims during the first quarter of 2007. The current version (12/90) has been in use since December 1990 and may continue to be used through April 1, 2007. CMS is implementing the new CMS-1500 (08-05) claim form which may be used as of January 2, 2007 and is mandatory for use as of April 2, 2007. However, because CMS frequently delays or extends the implementation dates of various policies, these dates may change.

The major difference between the new CMS-1500 (08-05) form and the prior CMS-1500 (12-90) form is the split provider identifier fields. The split fields will enable NPI reporting in the fields labeled as NPI, and corresponding legacy number reporting in the unlabeled block above each NPI field. In addition, the bar code has been dropped from all versions of the form.

Dual Acceptability Period

There will be a period of time where both versions of the CMS-1500 will be accepted (08-05 and 12-90 versions). From January 2, 2007 through March 30, 2007 providers can use either the current **CMS-1500 (12-90)** version or the revised **CMS-1500 (08-05)** version.

Mandatory Use Date

Only the revised **CMS-1500 (08-05)** is to be used for all claims filed on or after 04/02/2007. All rebilling of claims must use the revised **CMS-1500 (08-05)** from this date forward, even though earlier submissions may have been on the current **CMS-1500 (12-90)**.

Because of the NPI dual usage period, there will be overlap between the use of the old and the new Form CMS-1500. Therefore, you will find information within this chapter that applies to both claim forms. The differences between the two forms will be noted within the body of the text that describes each of the items/boxes/fields of the CMS-1500 health insurance claim form.

On the previous page is a copy of the most current CMS-1500 health insurance claim form. The form is mandatory for all Medicare health insurance claims. Following are field-by-field instructions for completing the CMS-1500 form accurately and completely.

PATIENT INFORMATION

1.   PROGRAM

Enter an "X" in the appropriate box to indicate proper carrier. Do not check all types of coverage that the beneficiary may have.

1A.   INSURED'S IDENTIFICATION NUMBER

Enter the insured's primary identification number including any letters. The number is usually obtained from the patient's or insured's insurance identification card.

Medicare: Enter the Medicare number and suffix.

Medicaid: Enter the Medicaid number from the patient's current Medicaid card.

Commercial: Enter the insured's "member number" or "subscriber number" or "certificate number" from the insurance identification card. Most often this is the insured's social security number.

2.   PATIENT'S NAME

Enter the patient's full name. Do not use nicknames or abbreviated names. The form specifies that the name be entered in last name, first name, middle initial order; however, our experience indicates that listing the name in the more normal order of "first name, middle initial, last name" has no detrimental affect.

3.   DATE OF BIRTH AND SEX

Enter the patient's date of birth in month, day, century and year format, for example 09/01/2003. Enter an "X" in the appropriate box to indicate male or female.

4.   INSURED'S NAME

Enter the full name of the insured, unless the patient is the insured, then enter the word "SAME."

Medicare: If the patient or spouse is age 65 through 69, employed, and covered by an employer health plan, show the insured person's full name.

5.   PATIENT'S ADDRESS

Enter the patient's complete address. Enter the street address on one line followed by the city, and state on the next line, and the zip code and telephone number on the last line.

6.   PATIENT'S RELATIONSHIP TO INSURED

Check the appropriate box.

7.   INSURED'S ADDRESS

Enter insured's street address, city, state and zip code and telephone number. If same as patient's, enter "SAME".

Medicare: Complete this field only if fields 4 and 11 are also completed. If field 4 is blank, this field should also be left blank.

8.   PATIENT STATUS

Enter patient's marital status, employment status, and student status in the appropriate boxes.

9.   OTHER INSURED'S NAME

If the patient is covered by a secondary insurance plan, enter the name of the insured party in this field.

Medicare: Items 9-9d are used only for Medigap purposes and not for supplemental or Medicaid information. *It must be filled out completely and properly for Medigap cross-over to occur.* Only participating physicians who have had Medigap benefits assigned to them by the patient should complete items 9-9d.

Enter the last name, first name, and middle initial of the enrollee in a Medigap policy if it is different from that shown in item 2. Otherwise, use the word SAME. If no Medigap benefits are assigned, leave blank. This field may be used in the future for supplemental insurance plans.

NOTE: Only participating physicians and suppliers are to complete item 9 and its subdivisions and only when the patient wishes to assign his/her benefits under a medigap policy to the participating physician or supplier.

Participating physicians and suppliers enter information required in item 9 and its subdivisions if requested by the patient. Participating physicians/suppliers sign an agreement with Medicare to accept assignment of Medicare benefits for all Medicare patients.Aclaim for which a patient elects to assign his/her benefits under a Medigap policy to a participating physician/supplier is called a mandated Medigap transfer.

Do not list other supplemental coverage in item 9 and its subdivisions at the time a Medicare claim is filed. Other supplemental claims are forwarded automatically to the private insurer if the private insurer contracts with the carrier to send Medicare claim information electronically. If there is no such contract, the beneficiary must file his/her own supplemental claim.

9A.   OTHER INSURED'S POLICY OR GROUP NUMBER

Enter the policy number for the secondary insurance plan.

Medicare: Enter the Medigap policy number, preceded by "MEDIGAP."

9B.   OTHER INSURED'S DATE OF BIRTH

Enter the date of birth in month, day, century and year format (for example, 09/01/2001) and sex of the secondary insured.

Medicare: Enter the Medigap enrollee's date of birth and sex.

9C.   EMPLOYER'S NAME OR SCHOOL NAME

Enter the employer or school name of the secondary insured.

Medicare: If the Medigap carrier has a unique identifier code, sometimes referred to as the "Other Carrier Identification Number" or OCNA, leave field 9c blank and complete 9d.

Leave blank if a Medigap PayerID is entered in item 9d. Otherwise, the claims processing address of the Medigap insurer is shown. Use an abbreviated street address, two letter postal code, and zip code copied from the Medigap insured's Medigap identification card. For example, the address 1257 Anywhere Street, Baltimore, MD 21204 should be listed as "1257 Anywhere St MD 21204."

9D.   INSURANCE PLAN NAME OR PROGRAM NAME

Enter the plan or program name of the secondary insurance.

Medicare: The 9-digit PAYERID number of the Medigap insurer. If no PAYERID number exists, then the Medigap insurance program or plan name is shown. If a participating provider of service or supplier and the patient wants Medicare payment data forwarded to a Medigap insurer under a mandated Medigap transfer, all of the information in items 9, 9a, 9b, and 9d must be complete and accurate.

10.   CONDITION RELATED TO EMPLOYMENT OR ACCIDENT

Check appropriate box(es) if you are treating the patient for either a work related injury or accident related injury. Note that workers' compensation claims are filed with insurance carriers designated by the patient's employer and is not the same carrier as the patient's health insurance carrier. Likewise, accident related claims, such as automobile accidents, are frequently processed by automobile insurance carriers and/or private attorneys.

Medicare: Items 10a thru 10c. "YES" or "NO" must be checked to indicate whether employment, auto liability, or other accident involvement applies to one or more of the services described in item 24. The State postal code must be shown. Any item checked "YES" indicates there may be other insurance primary to Medicare. Primary insurance information must then be shown in item 11.

10D.   RESERVED FOR LOCAL USE

Medicare: This field is now exclusively for Medicaid. Enter the patient's Medicaid number preceded by "MCD."

11.   INSURED'S POLICY GROUP OR FECA NUMBER

Enter the "group number" or "group name" from the insurance identification card if the patient is covered by an employer sponsored health insurance plan.
Medicare: This item must be completed. By completing this item, the physician/supplier acknowledges having made a good faith effort to determine whether Medicare is the primary or secondary payer.

If there is insurance primary to Medicare, enter the insured's policy or group number is entered and then proceed to items 11a - 11c.

NOTE: The appropriate information in item 11c is shown if insurance primary to Medicare is indicated in item 11.

If there is no insurance primary to Medicare, the word "NONE" is used and then proceed to item 12.

If the insured reports a terminating event with regard to insurance which had been primary to Medicare (e.g., insured retired), the word "NONE" is shown and proceed to item 11b.

Insurance Primary to Medicare. Circumstances under which Medicare payment may be secondary to other insurance include:

- Group Health Plan Coverage:

  — Working aged;
  — Disability (large group health plan); and
  — End Stage Renal Disease;

- No Fault and/or Other Liability; and
- Work-Related Illness/Injury:

  — Workers' compensation;
  — Black lung; and
  — Veterans benefits.

NOTE: For a paper claim to be considered for Medicare secondary payer benefits, a copy of the primary payers explanation of benefits (EOB) notice must be forwarded along with the claim form.

11A.   INSURED'S DATE OF BIRTH

Enter the date of birth and sex of the primary insured.

11B.   EMPLOYER'S NAME OR SCHOOL NAME

Enter the employer or school name of the primary insured.

Medicare: If the insured's employment insurance status has changed due to retirement, enter "RETIRED" and the retirement date in month, day, century and year format here.

11C.   INSURANCE PLAN NAME OR PROGRAM NAME

Enter the name of the primary insurance carrier.

Medicare: The 9-digit PAYERID number of the primary insurer. If no PAYERID number exists, then enter the complete primary payer's program or plan name. If the primary payer's EOB does not contain the claims processing address, record the primary payer's claims processing address directly on the EOB.

11D.   IS THERE ANOTHER HEALTH BENEFIT PLAN?

Enter an "X" in the YES box if the patient is covered by any other plan.

Medicare: Leave blank. Not required by Medicare.

12.   RELEASE OF INFORMATION

Either have the patient, or his or her representative sign the health insurance claim form, or attach your own release form to the claim and enter "SEE ATTACHMENT" in this space. If the patient is a minor, the signature must be that of a parent or legal guardian.

Medicare: The patient or authorized representative must sign and enter either a 6-digit date (MM | DD | YY), 8-digit date (MM | DD | CCYY) , or an alphanumeric date (e.g., January 1, 2002) unless the signature is on file.

In lieu of signing the claim, the patient may sign a statement to be retained in the provider, physician, or supplier file. If the patient is physically or mentally unable to sign, a representative may sign on the patient's behalf. In this event, the statement's signature line must indicate the patient's name followed by "by" the representative's name, address, relationship to the patient, and the reason the patient cannot sign. The authorization is effective indefinitely unless patient or the patient's representative revokes this arrangement.

The patient's signature authorizes release of medical information necessary to process the claim. It also authorizes payment of benefits to the provider of service or supplier when the provider of service or supplier accepts assignment on the claim.

Signature by Mark (X). When an illiterate or physically handicapped enrollee signs by mark, a witness must enter his/her name and address next to the mark.

13.   **ASSIGNMENT OF BENEFITS**

The insured's signature in this space directs the insurance carrier to pay any benefits directly to the provider. You may also use a form which combines release of information and assignment of benefits, attached to the health insurance claim form.

Medicare: The signature in this item authorizes payment of mandated Medigap benefits to the participating physician or supplier if required Medigap information is included in item 9 and its subdivisions. The patient or his/her authorized representative signs this item, or the signature must be on file as a separate Medigap authorization. The Medigap assignment on file in the participating provider of service/supplier's office must be insurer specific. It may state that the authorization applies to all occasions of service until it is revoked.

PHYSICIAN INFORMATION

14.   **DATE OF CURRENT (ILLNESS, INJURY OR PREGNANCY)**

Enter, if known, the date (in month, day, century and year format) of onset for illnesses, the date of injury or, for pregnancy, the date of the last menstrual period (LMP). The carriers like to have this information to assist them in determining coverage or exclusions for preexisting conditions; however, in our experience, lack of the information rarely affects processing of a claim.

Medicare: Enter the date of the current illness, date of injury, or date of the last menstrual period.

For chiropractic services, enter the date of the beginning of the course of treatment and enter the x-ray date in field 19.

15.   **DATE(S) OF SAME/SIMILAR ILLNESS OR INJURY**

Enter, if known, the date the patient first came to see you for the condition for which you are submitting the claim. We recommend that you leave this space blank, or, if you do enter the information, do so only on the first claim for the condition.

Medicare: Leave blank.

16.   **DATES PATIENT UNABLE TO WORK IN CURRENT OCCUPATION**

Enter dates in month, day, century and year format only if the patient is entitled to disability benefits, or is being treated for a work related injury.

Medicare: Leave blank.

17.   **NAME OR REFERRING PHYSICIAN OR OTHER SOURCE**

Medicare: Enter the name of the referring or ordering physician if the service or item was ordered or referred by a physician.

The term "physician" refers to:

1. A doctor of medicine or osteopathy legally authorized to practice medicine and surgery by the State in which he/she performs such function or action;

2. A doctor of dental surgery or dental medicine who is legally authorized to practice dentistry by the tate in which he/she performs such functions and who is acting within the scope of his/her license when performing such functions;

3. A doctor of podiatric medicine, but only with respect to functions which he/she is legally authorized to perform as such by the State in which he/she performs them;

4. A doctor of optometry, but only with respect to the provision of items or services which he/she is legally authorized to perform as a doctor of optometry by the State in which he/she performs them; or

5. A chiropractor who is licensed as such by a State (or in a State which does not license chiropractors as such), and is legally authorized to perform the services of a chiropractor in the jurisdiction in which he/she performs such services, and who meets uniform minimum standards, and only with respect to treatment by means of manual manipulation of the spine (to correct a subluxation).

Referring physician - is a physician who requests an item or service for the beneficiary for which payment may be made under the Medicare program.

Ordering physician - is a physician or, when appropriate, a non-physician practitioner who orders non-physician services for the patient. Examples of services that might be ordered include diagnostic laboratory tests, clinical laboratory tests, pharmaceutical services, durable medical equipment, and services incident to that physician's or non-physician practitioner's service.

The ordering/referring requirement became effective January 1, 1992, and is required. All claims for Medicare covered services and items that are the result of a physician's order or referral shall include the ordering/referring physician's name. See Items 17a and 17b below for further guidance on reporting the referring/ordering provider's UPIN and/or NPI. The following services/situations require the submission of the referring/ordering provider information:

- Medicare covered services and items that are the result of a physician's order or referral;
- Parenteral and enteral nutrition;
  Immunosuppressive drug claims;
  Hepatitis B claims;
- Diagnostic laboratory services;
  Diagnostic radiology services;
  Portable x-ray services;
  Consultative services;
  Durable medical equipment;
- When the ordering physician is also the performing physician (as often is the case with in-office clinical laboratory tests);
- When a service is incident to the service of a physician or non-physician practitioner, the name of the physician or non-physician practitioner who performs the initial service and orders the non-physician service must appear in item 17;
- When a physician extender or other limited licensed practitioner refers a patient for consultative service, submit the name of the physician who is supervising the limited licensed practitioner;

17A. Enter the CMS assigned UPIN of the referring/ordering physician listed in item 17. The UPIN may be reported on the CMS-1500 health insurance claim form until May 22, 2007, and MUST be reported if an NPI is not available.

NOTE: FIELD17A and/or FIELD17B is required when a service was ordered or referred by a physician. Effective May 23, 2007, and later, FIELD17A is not to be reported but FIELD17B <u>MUST</u> be reported when a service was ordered or referred by a physician.
When a claim involves multiple referring and/or ordering physicians, a separate CMS-1500 health insurance claim form must be used for each ordering/referring physician. All physicians who order or refer

Medicare beneficiaries or services must report either an NPI or UPIN or both prior to May 23, 2007. After that date, an NPI (but not a UPIN) must be reported even though they may never bill Medicare directly. A physician who has not been assigned a UPIN shall contact the Medicare carrier.

17B.   NPI

CMS-1500 (08-05) - Enter the NPI of the referring/ordering physician listed in item 17 as soon as it is available.

NOTE: FIELD17A and/or FIELD17B is required when a service was ordered or referred by a physician. Effective May 23, 2007, and later, FIELD17A is not to be reported but FIELD17B <u>MUST</u> be reported when a service was ordered or referred by a physician.

18.   HOSPITALIZATION DATES RELATED TO CURRENT SERVICES

Enter dates in month, day, century and year format of admission and/or discharge if
services are rendered as a result of or subsequent to a hospitalization.

19.   RESERVED FOR LOCAL USE

Medicare: The following are acceptable entries for this field:

Enter either a 6-digit (MM | DD | YY) or an 8-digit (MM | DD | CCYY) date patient was last seen and the UPIN (NPI when it becomes effective) of his/her attending physician when a physician providing routine foot care submits claims.

For physical therapy, occupational therapy or speech-language pathology services, effective for claims with dates of service on or after June 6, 2005, the date last seen and the UPIN/NPI of an ordering/referring/attending/certifying physician or non-physician practitioner are not required. If this information is submitted voluntarily, it must be correct or it will cause rejection or denial of the claim. However, when the therapy service is provided incident to the services of a physician or nonphysician practitioner, then incident to policies continue to apply. For example, for identification of the ordering physician who provided the initial service, see Item 17 and 17a, and for the identification of the supervisor, see item 24K of this section.

Enter either a 6-digit (MM | DD | YY) or an 8-digit (MM | DD | CCYY) x-ray date for chiropractor services (if an x-ray, rather than a physical examination was the method used to demonstrate the subluxation). By entering an x-ray date and the initiation date for course of chiropractic treatment in item 14, the chiropractor is certifying that all the relevant information requirements (including level of subluxation) of Pub. 100-02, Medicare Benefit Policy Manual, chapter 15, are on file, along with the appropriate x-ray and all are available for carrier review.

Enter the drug's name and dosage when submitting a claim for Not Otherwise Classified (NOC) drugs.

Enter a concise description of an "unlisted procedure code" or an NOC code if one can be given within the confines of this box. Otherwise an attachment shall be submitted with the claim.

Enter all applicable modifiers when modifier -99 (multiple modifiers) is entered in item 24d. If modifier -99 is entered on multiple line items of a single claim form, all applicable modifiers for each line item containing a -99 modifier should be listed as follows: 1=(mod), where the number 1 represents the line item and "mod" represents all modifiers applicable to the referenced line item.

Enter the statement "Homebound" when an independent laboratory renders an EKG tracing or obtains a specimen from a homebound or institutionalized patient.

Enter the statement, "Patient refuses to assign benefits" when the beneficiary absolutely refuses to assign benefits to a participating provider. In this case, no payment may be made on the claim.

Enter the statement, "Testing for hearing aid" when billing services involving the testing of a hearing aid(s) is used to obtain intentional denials when other payers are involved.

When dental examinations are billed, enter the specific surgery for which the exam is being performed.

Enter the specific name and dosage amount when low osmolar contrast material is billed, but only if HCPCS codes do not cover them.

Enter a 6-digit (MM | DD | YY) or an 8-digit (MM | DD | CCYY) assumed and/or relinquished date for a global surgery claim when providers share post-operative care. Enter demonstration ID number "30" for all national emphysema treatment trial claims. Enter the pin (or NPI when effective) of the physician who is performing a purchased interpretation of a diagnostic test.

Method II suppliers shall enter the most current HCT value for the injection of Aranesp for ESRD beneficiaries on dialysis.

20.   OUTSIDE LABORATORY WORK

If you are billing for laboratory work performed by an outside laboratory, check the "yes" box and enter the your charge for the test(s). If you are billing for laboratory work performed in your own laboratory, check the "no" box or leave blank.

Medicare: This item is completed when billing for diagnostic tests subject to purchase price limitations. The purchase price under charges must be shown if the "yes" block is checked. A "yes" check indicates that an entity other than the entity billing for the service performed the diagnostic test.A"no" check indicates that "no purchased tests are included on the claim." When "yes" is annotated, item 32 must be completed. When billing for purchased diagnostic tests, each test must be submitted on a separate claim form.

21.   DIAGNOSIS OR NATURE OF ILLNESS OR INJURY

Enter up to four (4) ICD-9-CM codes in this space. There is no space for diagnosis
descriptions on this form. The first code listed should clearly define the reason for the current visit or service. An independent lab must enter a diagnosis code only for limited coverage procedures.

Medicare: The patient's diagnosis/condition. All physician and non-physician specialties (i.e., PA, NP, CNS, CRNA) must use an ICD-9-CM code number and code to the highest level of specificity. Enter up to four codes in priority order (primary, secondary condition). An independent laboratory must enter a diagnosis only for limited coverage procedures. All narrative diagnoses for non-physician specialties must be submitted on an attachment.

22.   MEDICAID RESUBMISSION

For Medicaid resubmission claims only, enter the resubmission code and the original reference number.

23.   PRIOR AUTHORIZATION NUMBER

Enter the Quality Improvement Organization (QIO) prior authorization number for those procedures requiring QIO prior approval.

Enter the Investigational Device Exemption (IDE) number when an investigational device is used in an FDA-approved clinical trial. Post Market Approval number should also be placed here when applicable.

For physicians performing care plan oversight services, enter the 6-digit Medicare provider number (or NPI when effective) of the home health agency (HHA) or hospice when CPT code G0181 (HH) or G0182 (Hospice) is billed.

Enter the 10-digit Clinical Laboratory Improvement Act (CLIA) certification number for laboratory services billed by an entity performing CLIA covered procedures.

When a physician provides services to a beneficiary residing in a SNF and the services were rendered to a SNF beneficiary outside of the SNF, the physician shall enter the Medicare facility provider number of the SNF in item 23.

NOTE: Item 23 can contain only one condition. Any additional conditions must be reported on a separate CMS-1500 health insurance claim form.

24.   DATE(S) AND PLACE(S) OF SERVICE

CMS-1500 (08-05) - The six service lines in section 24 have been divided horizontally to accommodate submission of both the NPI and legacy identifier during the NPI transition and to accommodate the submission of supplemental information to support the billed service. The top portion in each of the six service lines is shaded and is the location for reporting supplemental information. It is not intended to allow the billing of 12 service lines. At this time, the shaded area is not used by Medicare. Future guidance will be provided on when and how to use this shaded area for the submission of Medicare claims.

Column A Date(s) of Service

Enter the month, day, century and year (for example, 09/01/2001) that the service or procedure was performed, or supply provided. If using "from" and "to" dates, the number of services should appear in Column F.

Column B Place of Service

Enter the place of service (POS) code using The appropriate place of service code(s) from the following list. Identify the location, using a place of service code, for each item used or service performed. NOTE: When a service is rendered to a hospital inpatient, use the "inpatient hospital" code.

POS   Place of Service Description

11   Office

Location, other than a hospital, SNF, or ICF, where the health professional routinely provides health examinations, diagnosis and treatment of illness or injury on an ambulatory basis.

12   Home

Location, other than a hospital, or other facility, where the patient receives care in a private residence.

21   Inpatient Hospital

A facility, other than psychiatric, which primarily provides diagnostic, therapeutic (both surgical and nonsurgical) and rehabilitation services by or under the supervision of physicians to patients admitted for a variety of medical conditions.

22   Outpatient Hospital

A portion of a hospital which provides diagnostic, therapeutic (both surgical and nonsurgical), and rehabilitation services to sick or injured persons who do not require hospitalization or institutionalization.

23   Emergency Room – Hospital

A portion of a hospital where emergency diagnosis and treatment of illness or injury is provided.

24   Ambulatory Surgical Center

A freestanding facility, other than a physician's office, where surgical and diagnostic services are provided on an ambulatory basis.

25   Birthing Center

A facility, other than a hospital's maternity facilities or a physician's office, which provides a setting for labor, delivery, and immediate post-partum care as well as immediate care of newborn infants.

26   Military Treatment Facility

A medical facility operated by one or more of the Uniformed Services. MTF also refers to certain former U.S. Public Health Service (USPHS) facilities now designated as Uniformed Service Treatment Facilities (USTF).

31   Skilled Nursing Facility

A facility which primarily provides inpatient skilled nursing care and related services to patients who require medical, nursing, or rehabilitative services but does not provide the level of care or treatment available in a hospital.

32   Nursing Facility

A facility which primarily provides to residents skilled nursing care and related services for the rehabilitation of injured, disabled, or sick persons, or, on a regular basis, health-related care services above the level of custodial care to other than mentally retarded individuals.

33   Custodial Care Facility

A facility which provides room, board and other personal assistance services, generally on a long-term basis, and which does not include a medical component.

34   Hospice

A facility, other than a patient's home, in which palliative and supportive care for terminally ill patients and their families are provided.

41   Ambulance – Land

A land vehicle specifically designed, equipped, or staffed for lifesaving and transporting the sick or injured.

42   Ambulance - Air or Water

An air or water vehicle specifically designed, equipped or staffed for lifesaving and transporting the sick or injured.

50   Federally Qualified Health Center

A facility located in a medically underserved area that provides Medicare beneficiaries preventive primary medical care under the general direction of a physician.

51   Inpatient Psychiatric Facility

A facility that provides inpatient psychiatric services for the diagnosis and treatment of mental illness on a 24-hour basis, by or under the supervision of a physician.

52   Psychiatric Facility Partial Hospitalization

A facility for the diagnosis and treatment of mental illness that provides a planned therapeutic program for patients who do not require full-time hospitalization, but who need broader programs than are possible from outpatient visits in a hospital-based or hospital-affiliated facility.

53   Community Mental Health Center

A facility that provides comprehensive mental health services on an ambulatory basis primarily to individuals residing or employed in a defined area.

54   Intermediate Care Facility/Mentally Retarded

A facility which primarily provides health-related care and services above the level of custodial care to mentally retarded individuals, but does not provide the level of care or treatment available in a hospital or skilled nursing facility (SNF).

55   Residential Substance Abuse Treatment Facility

A facility which provides treatment for substance (alcohol and drug) abuse to live-in residents who do not require acute medical care.

Services include individual and group therapy and counseling, family counseling, laboratory tests, drugs and supplies, psychological testing, and room and board.

56   Psychiatric Residential Treatment Center

A facility or distinct part of a facility for psychiatric care which provides a total 24-hour therapeutically planned and professionally staffed group living and learning environment.

60   Mass Immunization Center

A location where providers administer pneumococcal pneumonia and influenza virus vaccinations and submit these services as electronic media claims, paper claims, or using the roster billing method. This generally takes place in a mass immunization setting, such as, a public health center, pharmacy, or mall but may include a physician office setting.

61   Comprehensive Inpatient Rehabilitation Facility

A facility that provides comprehensive rehabilitation services under the supervision of a physician to inpatients with physical disabilities. Services include physical therapy, occupational therapy, speech pathology, social or psychological services, and orthotics and prosthetics services.

62   Comprehensive Outpatient Rehabilitation Facility

A facility that provides comprehensive rehabilitation services under the supervision of a physician to outpatients with physical disabilities. Services include physical therapy, occupational therapy, and speech pathology services.

65   End-Stage Renal Disease Treatment Facility

A facility other than a hospital, which provides dialysis treatment, maintenance, and/or training to patients or care givers on an ambulatory or home-care basis.

71   State or Local Public Health Clinic

A facility maintained by either State or local health departments that provides ambulatory primary medical care under the general direction of a physician.

72   Rural Health Clinic

A certified facility which is located in a rural medically underserved area that provides ambulatory primary medical care under the general direction of a physician.

81   Independent Laboratory

A laboratory certified to perform diagnostic and/or clinical tests independent of an institution or a physician's office.

99   Other Unlisted Facility

Other service facilities not identified above.

If the physician bills for lab services performed in his/her office, the code for "Office" is shown. If the physician bills for a lab test furnished by another physician, who maintains a lab in his/her office, the code for "Other" is shown. If the physician bills for a lab service furnished by an independent lab, the code for "Independent Laboratory" is used. Items 21 and 22 on the Form CMS-1500 must be completed for all laboratory work performed outside a physician's office. If an independent lab bills, the place where the sample was taken is shown. An independent laboratory taking a sample in its laboratory shows "IL" as place of service. If an independent laboratory bills for a test on a sample drawn on a hospital inpatient, it uses the code for "Hospital Inpatient."

Column C Type of Service Code

Leave blank unless otherwise instructed by insurance carriers.

This field is used by Medicare health insurance carriers to record the correct type of service indicator that matched the HCPCS procedure code. This information is provided for reference only. *Do not input these codes on your CMS-1500 claim forms.*

TOS   **Type of Service Description**

0   Whole Blood

1	Medical Care
2	Surgery
3	Consultation
4	Diagnostic Radiology
5	Diagnostic Laboratory
6	Therapeutic Radiology
7	Anesthesia
8	Assistant at Surgery
9	Other Medical Items or Services
A	Used DME
B	High Risk Screening Mammography
C	Low Risk Screening Mammography
D	Ambulance
E	Enteral/Parenteral Nutrients/Supplies
F	Ambulatory Surgical Center
G	Immunosuppressive Drugs
H	Hospice
J	Diabetic Shoes
K	Hearing Items and Services
L	ESRD Supplies
M	Monthly Capitation Payment for Dialysis
N	Kidney Donor
P	Lump Sum Purchase of DME, Prosthetics, Orthotics
Q	Vision Items or Services
R	Rental of DME
S	Surgical Dressings or Other Medical Supplies
T	Outpatient Mental Health Treatment Limitation
U	Occupational Therapy
V	Pneumococcal/Flu Vaccine
W	Physical Therapy

Column D Procedures, Services or Supplies

NOTE: The **CMS-1500 (08-05)** has the ability to capture up to four modifiers.

Procedure Code

Medicare: The procedures, services, or supplies using the Healthcare Common Procedure Coding System (HCPCS). When applicable, show HCPCS modifiers with the HCPCS code.

The specific procedure code must be shown without a narrative description. However, when reporting an "unlisted procedure code" or a NOC code, include a narrative description in item 19 if a coherent description can be given within the confines of that box. Otherwise, an attachment must be submitted with the claim.

Medicaid: Enter the proper procedure code from the most current edition of CPT or other codes as instructed by your MEDICAID carrier.

COMMERCIAL: For all commercial insurance carriers, enter the proper procedure code from the most current edition of the CPT book.

WORKERS' COMP: Use the coding system specified by your State Workers' Compensation Board.

Procedure Description

There is no space available on this form for a procedure description. If you are reporting a procedure or service described as "unlisted" in CPT, you need to include a narrative report with your claim to explain what the unlisted procedure or service was.

Column E Diagnosis Code

The diagnosis code reference number as shown in item 21 to relate the date of service and the procedures performed to the primary diagnosis. Only one reference number per line item. When multiple services are performed, the primary reference number for each service; either a 1, or a 2, or a 3, or a 4 is shown. If a situation arises where two or more diagnoses are required for a procedure code (e.g., pap smears), the provider must reference only one of the diagnoses in item 21.

Column F Charges

Enter the charge for the service, procedure or supply.

Column G Days or Units

Medicare: Enter the number of days or units. This field is most commonly used for multiple visits, units of supplies, anesthesia minutes, or oxygen volume. If only one service is performed, the numeral 1 must be entered.

Some services require that the actual number or quantity billed be clearly indicated on the claim form (e.g., multiple ostomy or urinary supplies, medication dosages, or allergy testing procedures). When multiple services are provided, the actual number provided must be indicated.

For anesthesia, the provider must indicate the elapsed time (minutes) in item 24g. Convert hours into minutes and enter the total minutes required for this procedure.

Suppliers must furnish the units of oxygen contents except for concentrators and initial rental claims for gas and liquid oxygen systems. Rounding of oxygen contents is as follows:

- For stationary gas system rentals, suppliers must indicate oxygen contents in unit multiples of 50 cubic feet in item 24g, rounded to the nearest increment of 50. For example, if 73 cubic feet of oxygen were delivered during the rental month, the unit entry "01" indicating the nearest 50 cubic foot increment is entered in item 24g.
- For stationary liquid systems, units of contents must be specified in multiples of 10 pounds of liquid contents delivered, rounded to the nearest 10 pound increment. For example, if 63 pounds of liquid oxygen were delivered during the applicable rental month billed, the unit entry "06" is entered in item 24g.
- For units of portable contents only (i.e., no stationary gas or liquid system used), round to the nearest five feet or one liquid pound, respectively.

Column H EPSDT Family Plan

Medicaid: Complete if appropriate

All others: Leave blank

Column I EMG

Place an "X" in this column if the service was provided in a hospital emergency
room.

Medicare: **CMS-1500 (12-90)** - Leave blank. Not required by Medicare.

CMS-1500 (08-05) - Enter the ID qualifier 1C in the shaded portion.

Column J COB

Medicare: **CMS-1500 (12-90)** - Leave blank. Not required by Medicare.

CMS-1500 (08-05) - Prior to May 23, 2007, enter the rendering provider's PIN in the shaded portion. In the case of a service provided incident to the service of a physician or non-physician practitioner, when the person who ordered the service is not supervising, enter the PIN of the supervisor in the shaded portion.

Effective May 23, 2007 and later, do not use the shaded portion. Beginning no earlier than October 1, 2006, enter the rendering provider's NPI number in the lower portion. In the case of a service provided incident to the service of a physician or non-physician practitioner, when the person who ordered the service is not supervising, enter the NPI of the supervisor in the lower portion.

Column K Reserved for local use

Medicare: **CMS-1500 (12-90)** – Enter the PIN of the performing provider of service or supplier if the provider is a member of a group practice. When several different providers of service or suppliers within a group are billing on the same Form CMS-1500, show the individual PIN in the corresponding line item. In the case of a service provided incident to the service of a physician or non-physician practitioner, when the person who ordered the service is not supervising, enter the PIN of the supervisor in item 24k.

CMS-1500 (08-05) - There is no Item 24K on this version.

25. **FEDERAL TAX I.D. NUMBER**

Enter the Social Security Number (SSN) or Federal Employer Identification Number (FEIN) and mark an "X" in the appropriate box to indicate which is being used.

26. **PATIENT ACCOUNT NUMBER**

If you use a patient account number system, enter the patient account number in this space. Most Medicare and Medicaid intermediaries, and some commercial carriers, include this information on their Explanation of Benefits, making it easier for you to identify patients for posting of payments.

27.   ACCEPT ASSIGNMENT

The appropriate block must be checked to indicate whether the provider of service or supplier accepts assignment of Medicare benefits. If MEDIGAP is indicated in block 9 and MEDIGAP payment authorization is given in item 13, the provider of service or supplier must also be a Medicare participating provider of service or supplier and must accept assignment of Medicare benefits for all covered charges for all patients.

The following providers of service/suppliers and claims can only be paid on an assignment basis:

- Clinical diagnostic laboratory services
- Physician services to individuals dually entitled to Medicare and Medicaid
- Participating physician/supplier services
- Services of physician assistants, nurse practitioners, clinical nurse specialists, nurse   midwives certified registered nurse anesthetists, clinical psychologists, and clinical   social workers
- Ambulatory surgical center services for covered ASC procedures
- Home dialysis supplies and equipment paid under Method II

28.   TOTAL CHARGE

Enter the total of all charges listed in Section 24 Column F.

29.   AMOUNT PAID

For all private carriers, enter zero or none in this space. This assures that your full charges will be processed for determination of benefits and the resulting payment. Any over payments resulting can be handled between you and your patient.

Medicare: If you are the first provider of service for a Medicare beneficiary at the beginning of a new benefit year, you should collect the deductible and indicate the
payment in this space.

30.   BALANCE DUE

Leave blank.

31.   SIGNATURE OF PHYSICIAN OR SUPPLIER

The physician or supplier, or his or her authorized representative must sign the provider's name and enter the date in month, day, century and year format in this space. For most carriers, impressions such as rubber stamps are acceptable.

Medicare: There is a portion of the statement in this space which refers to information on the back of the health insurance claim form. Medicare carriers are not allowed to process claims which do not have this information printed on the on the back. Keep this is mind if you are having your own health insurance claim forms printed.

32.   NAME AND ADDRESS OF FACILITY WHERE SERVICE WERE RENDERED

If the services were provided at a location other than the provider's office or the patient's home, enter the name and address of the facility in this space.

Medicare: **CMS-1500 (12-90)** – Enter the name and address, and zip code of the facility if the services were furnished in a hospital, clinic, laboratory, or facility other than the patient's home or physician's office. Effective for claims received on or after April 1, 2004, the name, address, and zip code of the service location for all services other than those furnished in place of service home - 12.

Effective for claims received on or after April 1, 2004, on the Form CMS-1500, only one name, address and zip code may be entered in the block. If additional entries are needed, separate claim forms shall be submitted.

Providers of service (namely physicians) shall identify the supplier's name, address, ZIP code and PIN when billing for purchased diagnostic tests. When more than one supplier is used, a separate Form CMS-1500 should be used to bill for each supplier.

For foreign claims, only the enrollee can file for Part B benefits rendered outside of the United States. These claims will not include a valid ZIP code. When a claim is received for these services on a beneficiary submitted

Form CMS-1490S, before the claim is entered in the system, it should be determined if it is a foreign claim. If it is a foreign claim, follow instructions in chapter 1 for disposition of the claim. The carrier processing the foreign claim will have to make necessary accommodations to verify that the claim is not returned as unprocessable due to the lack of a ZIP code.

For durable medical, orthotic, and prosthetic claims, the name address, or PIN of the location where the order was accepted must be entered (DMERC only).

This field is required. When more than one supplier is used, a separate Form CMS-1500 should be used to bill for each supplier.

This item is completed whether the supplier's personnel performs the work at the physician's office or at another location.

If a modifier is billed, indicating the service was rendered in a Health Professional Shortage Area (HPSA) or Physician Scarcity Area (PSA), the physical location where the service was rendered shall be entered if other than home.

If the supplier is a certified mammography screening center, enter the 6-digit FDA approved certification number.

Complete this item for all laboratory work performed outside a physician's office. If an independent laboratory is billing, enter the place where the test was performed, and the PIN.

CMS-1500 (08-05) - Enter the name and address, and ZIP code of the facility if the services were furnished in a hospital, clinic, laboratory, or facility other than the patient's home or physician's office. Effective for claims received on or after April 1, 2004, the name, address, and zip code of the service location for all services other than those furnished in place of service home - 12. Effective for claims received on or after April 1, 2004, on the Form CMS-1500, only one name, address and zip code may be entered in the block. If additional entries are needed, separate claim forms shall be submitted.

Providers of service (namely physicians) shall identify the supplier's name, address, and ZIP code when billing for purchased diagnostic tests. When more than one supplier is used, a separate Form CMS-1500 should be used to bill for each supplier. For foreign claims, only the enrollee can file for Part B benefits rendered outside of the United States. These claims will not include a valid ZIP code. When a claim is received for these services on a beneficiary submitted Form CMS-1490S, before the claim is entered in the system, it should be determined if it is a foreign claim. If it is a foreign claim, follow instructions in chapter 1 for disposition of the claim. The carrier processing the foreign claim will have to make necessary accommodations to verify that the claim is not returned as unprocessable due to the lack of a ZIP code. For durable medical, orthotic, and prosthetic claims, the name and address of the location where the order was accepted must be entered (DMERC only). This field is required. When more than one supplier is used, a separate Form CMS-1500 should be used to bill for each supplier. This item is completed whether the supplier's personnel performs the work at the physician's office or at another location. If a modifier is billed, indicating the service was rendered in a Health Professional Shortage Area (HPSA) or Physician Scarcity Area (PSA), the physical location where the service was rendered shall be entered if other than home.

Complete this item for all laboratory work performed outside a physician's office. If an independent laboratory is billing, enter the place where the test was performed.

32A   **CMS-1500 (12-90)** - There is no ITEM 32A on this version.

CMS-1500 (08-05) - Enter the NPI of the service facility as soon as it is available. The NPI may be reported on the Form CMS-1500 (08-05) as early as October 1, 2006.

32B   **CMS-1500 (12-90)** - There is no ITEM 32A on this version.

CMS-1500 (08-05) - Enter the ID qualifier 1C followed by one blank space and then the PIN of the service facility. Effective May 23, 2007, and later, 32b is not to be reported.

Providers of service (namely physicians) shall identify the supplier's PIN when billing for purchased diagnostic tests.

If the supplier is a certified mammography screening center, enter the 6-digit FDA approved certification number.

For durable medical, orthotic, and prosthetic claims, enter the PIN (of the location where the order was accepted) if the name and address was not provided in item 32 (DMERC only).

33.   PHYSICIAN'S, SUPPLIER'S BILLING NAME

If your health insurance claim forms are not already preprinted with this information, enter the provider number(s), the provider name(s), provider street, city, state, zip code and telephone number.

Medicare: Enter the provider of service/supplier's billing name, address, ZIP code, and telephone number. This is a required field.

Enter the PIN (or NPI when implemented), for the performing provider of service/supplier who is not a member of a group practice.

Enter the group PIN (or NPI when implemented), for the performing provider of service/supplier who is a member of a group practice.

Suppliers billing the DMERC will use the National Supplier Clearinghouse (NSC) number in this item.

Enter the group UPIN, including the 2-digit location identifier, for the performing practitioner/supplier who is a member of a group practice.

33A   CMS-1500 (12-90) - There is no ITEM 33A on this version.

CMS-1500 (08-05) - Effective May 23, 2007, and later, you MUST enter the NPI of the billing provider or group. The NPI may be reported on the Form CMS-1500 (08-05) as early as October 1, 2006. This is a required field.

33B   **CMS-1500 (12-90)** - There is no ITEM 33A on this version.

CMS-1500 (08-05) - Enter the ID qualifier 1C followed by one blank space and then the PIN of the billing provider or group. Effective May 23, 2007, and later, 33b is not to be reported. Suppliers billing the DMERC will use the National Supplier Clearinghouse (NSC) number in this item. Enter the PIN for the performing provider of service/supplier who is not a member of a group practice. Enter the group PIN for the performing provider of service/supplier who is a member of a group practice. Enter the group UPIN, including the 2-digit location identifier, for the performing practitioner/supplier who is a member of a group practice.

CODING & COMPLIANCE GUIDELINES

Keeping track of the various policies, procedures, rules, restrictions, limitations, and reimbursement opportunities involved in reporting CPT codes for medical services and procedures is a difficult task. Changes to only a few codes can have a significant impact on your reimbursement and your audit liability. However, with just under 8,000 CPT codes and almost 3,000 HCPCS Level II codes, it is virtually impossible for anyone to know all the rules for each and every code. In addition the rules for Medicare may be different than those for other health insurance plans, and many of the rules are changed annually.

The guidelines in this section are designed to help you answer important coding and compliance questions about specific CPT codes. Questions like...

- Is this visit for a wound infection one week after surgery covered in the follow-up period?
- Do standard multiple procedure rules apply for this service?
- Do I use modifier -50 to report this bilateral procedure, or list it twice, or report it without modifier -50?
- Will Medicare pay for assistant surgery for this procedure?
- Should I report this add-on procedure separately?

Every day you have to find the answers to dozens of questions like these before you can complete your coding and prepare your health insurance claims.

The CPT codes listed in this section include short and simple descriptions and annotations regarding important coding and compliance issues. Only those CPT codes which have coverage restrictions, and/or special instructions regarding follow-up periods, multiple procedure rules, bilateral procedure rules, assistant surgeons, and add-on codes are included.

STATUS

CMS includes a "status" code in the Medicare Physician's Fee Schedule to help Medicare carriers determine how to process each CPT code. Most CPT codes are covered, subject to various rules, regulations, documentation and limitations. Some CPT codes are designated as "bundled codes" or "restricted coverage" and have special processing rules, and a few others are designated simply as "non-covered service." These CPT codes are specifically identified in the following CPT code listings.

BUNDLED CODE

There are a limited number of CPT codes classified by CMS (formerly known as HCFA) as "bundled codes." There are no RVUs or payment amounts for these CPT codes, and no separate payment is made for these services. When these services are covered, payment for them is included within the payment for the service(s) which includes the service identified by the "bundled" CPT code. These procedures are annotated in the following listings with the phrase "bundled code - no separate payment made." An example of a procedure classified as a bundled code is:

15850 **Remove sutures** ~ bundled code – no separate payment made, multiple procedure concept does not apply, bilateral surgery concept does not apply, assistant surgery concept does not apply

NON-COVERED SERVICE

These procedures are not covered by Medicare and no payment will be made. These procedures are annotated in the following listings with the phrase "non-covered service." An example of a procedure classified as a non-covered service is:

11975 **Insert contraceptive cap** ~ non-covered service, multiple procedure concept does not apply, bilateral surgery concept does not apply, assistant surgery concept does not apply

RESTRICTED COVERAGE

There are a limited number of CPT codes classified by CMS (formerly known as HCFA) as restricted coverage codes. Special coverage instructions apply to these codes and if covered, the service is priced by the Medicare carrier. Generally these services are covered only in unusual circumstances. These procedures are annotated in the following listings with the phrase "restricted coverage - special coverage rules apply." An example of a procedure classified as a restricted coverage procedure is:

15788 **Chemical peel, face, epidermal** ~ restricted coverage - special coverage rules apply, follow-up period is 90 days, standard payment adjustment rules for multiple procedures apply, 150% payment adjustment for bilateral procedures does not apply, assistant surgeon may not be paid

FOLLOW-UP PERIOD

Most surgical procedures are based upon the global surgery concept, wherein all services related to the specific procedure provided within a certain time period are considered to be covered by the initial service. CMS defines three follow-up periods depending upon the complexity of the surgical procedures.

ENDOSCOPIC OR MINOR PROCEDURES

Surgical procedures defined by Medicare as relatively minor surgical or endoscopic procedures have a follow-up period of zero days. These procedures are considered to have no pre- or post-operative work other than that required on the date of the procedure. Any E/M services provided on the same date are generally not reportable unless a documented, separately identifiable service is provided. These procedures are annotated in the following listings with the phrase "endoscopic or minor procedure - E/M services on the same day generally not paid." An example of a procedure classified as a minor surgical procedure with no follow-up days is:

17250   **Chemical cautery, tissue**   ~ endoscopic or minor procedure – E/M services on the same day generally not paid, standard payment adjustment rules for multiple procedures apply, 150% payment adjustment for bilateral procedures does not apply, assistant surgeon may not be paid

MINOR SURGICAL PROCEDURES

Some procedures defined by Medicare as minor surgical procedures include pre-op work on the date of service and post-operative work for a period of up to ten (10) days following the procedure. Any E/M services provided on the same date and for ten (10) days following the procedure are generally not reportable unless a documented, separately identifiable service is provided. These procedures are annotated in the following listings with the phrase "follow-up period is 10 days." An example of a procedure classified as a minor surgical procedure with a 10 day follow-up period is:

27860   **Fixate ankle joint**   ~ follow-up period is 10 days, standard payment adjustment rules for multiple procedures apply, 150% payment adjustment for bilateral procedures does not apply, payment for assistant surgeon subject to documentation of medical necessity

MAJOR SURGICAL PROCEDURES

Surgical procedures as defined by Medicare as major surgical procedures include a one (1) day pre-op period prior to the date of the major surgery and a post-operative period of ninety (90) days following the procedure. Any E/M services provided on the date before, the date of, and for ninety (90) days following the procedure are generally not reportable unless a documented, separately identifiable service is provided. These procedures are annotated in the following listings with the phrase "follow-up period is 90 days." An example of a procedure classified as a major surgical procedure with a 90 day follow-up period is:

50010 **Explore kidney** ~ follow-up period is 90 days, standard payment adjustment rules for multiple procedures apply, 150% payment adjustment for bilateral procedures does not apply, assistant surgeon may be paid

FOLLOW-UP PERIOD INCLUDED IN ANOTHER SERVICE

In addition to services with specifically defined follow-up days, there are some surgical procedures wherein the follow-up services are included in another procedure. These procedures are annotated in the following listings with the phrase "follow-up period is included in another service." An example of a procedure classified as a procedure with follow-up days included in another service is:

11001 **Debride infected skin, add-on** ~ follow-up period included in another service, no payment adjustment rules for multiple procedures apply, 150% payment adjustment for bilateral procedures does not apply, assistant surgeon may not be paid, +add-on code (list separately in addition to primary procedure)

MULTIPLE PROCEDURES - MODIFIER 51

It is common for several surgical procedures to be performed during a single operative session. When multiple procedures are performed during the same operative session, the "major" procedure should be listed first on the health insurance claim form, followed by secondary, additional, or "lessor" procedures. CPT modifier -51 is reported with all procedures listed after the first one. Medicare has several procedure dependent rules regarding payment adjustments for multiple procedures.

NO PAYMENT ADJUSTMENT RULES FOR MULTIPLE PROCEDURES APPLY

If the procedure is reported on the same day as another procedure, the Medicare carrier bases payment on the lower of a) the actual charge or b) the fee schedule amount for the procedure. These procedures are annotated in the following listings with the phrase "no payment adjustment rules for multiple procedures apply." An example of a procedure which is classified as having no payment adjustment rules for multiple procedures is:

15002 **Wound prep, ch/inf, trunk/arm/lg** ~ endoscopies or minor procedure - E/M services on the same day generally not paid, no payment adjustment rules for multiple procedures apply, 150% payment adjustment for bilateral procedures does not apply, payment for assistant surgeon subject to documentation of medical necessity

STANDARD PAYMENT ADJUSTMENT RULES FOR MULTIPLE PROCEDURES APPLY

The "standard" payment adjustment performed by the Medicare carrier is to first rank the procedures by fee schedule amount, and then to apply the appropriate reduction. The reduction formula is 100% for the first procedure and 50% for all other procedures with the exception of "by report" procedures. Following the reduction, payment is based on the lower of a) the actual charge or b) the fee schedule amount reduced by the appropriate percentage. These procedures are annotated in the following listings with the phrase "standard payment adjustment rules for multiple procedures apply." An example of a procedure classified as having standard payment adjustment rules for multiple procedures is:

35483   **Atherectomy, open**   ~ endoscopies or minor procedure - E/M services on the same day generally not paid, <u>standard payment adjustment rules for multiple procedures apply</u>, 150% payment adjustment for bilateral procedures does not apply, assistant surgeon may be paid

SPECIAL RULES FOR MULTIPLE ENDOSCOPIC PROCEDURES

Special rules for multiple endoscopic procedures apply if a procedure is billed with another endoscopy in the same family (i.e., another endoscopy that has the same base procedure). These procedures are annotated in the following listings with the phrase "special rules for multiple endoscopies apply if billed with another endoscopy in the same family." An example of a procedure classified as having special rules for multiple endoscopies is:

29819   **Shoulder arthroscopy/surgery**   ~ follow-up period is 90 days, <u>special rules for multiple endoscopic procedures apply if billed with another endoscopy in the same family</u>, 150% payment adjustment for bilateral procedures applies, assistant surgeon may not be paid

BILATERAL SURGERY - MODIFIER 50

Bilateral surgical procedures are reported by listing the CPT code for the procedure twice on the health insurance claim form. For non-Medicare health insurance claims, CPT modifier -50 is reported with the second CPT code. For Medicare health insurance claims, HCPCS modifier -LT (left) is reported with the first CPT code and HCPCS modifier -RT (right) is reported with the second CPT code (or vice versa). Medicare has several procedure dependent rules regarding payment adjustments for bilateral surgical procedures.

150% PAYMENT ADJUSTMENT FOR BILATERAL PROCEDURES DOES NOT APPLY

Medicare payment is based upon the lower of a) the total actual charge for both sides or b) 100% of the fee schedule amount for a single code. These procedures are annotated in the following listings with the phrase "150% payment adjustment for bilateral procedures does not apply." An example of a procedure where the 150% bilateral payment adjustment does not apply is:

11010   **Debride skin, fracture**   ~ follow-up period is 10 days, standard payment adjustment rules for multiple procedures apply, 150% payment adjustment does not apply - RVUs based on bilateral procedure, assistant surgeon may not be paid

150% PAYMENT ADJUSTMENT RULE FOR BILATERAL PROCEDURES APPLIES

If the code is billed with the bilateral modifier, Medicare payment is based on the lower of a) the total actual charge for both sides or, b) 150% of the fee schedule amount for a single procedure. If the procedure is reported as a bilateral procedure and is also reported with other procedures on the same day (multiple procedure), the Medicare carrier will apply the bilateral procedure adjustment before applying any multiple procedure adjustments.

These procedures are annotated in the following listings with the phrase "150% payment adjustment for bilateral procedures applies > report twice or add -50 modifier." An example of a procedure where the 150% bilateral payment adjustment does apply is:

15820   **Revise lower eyelid**   ~ follow-up period is 90 days, standard payment adjustment rules for multiple procedures apply, 150% payment adjustment for bilateral procedures applies, payment for assistant surgeon subject to documentation of medical necessity

ASSISTANT SURGEON

A routine surgical assist is billed by reporting the CPT code for the surgical procedure with the modifier -80. Most health insurance plans will pay the assistant surgeon a pre-determined percentage of the amount paid to the primary surgeon. Medicare will pay the assistant surgeon 16 percent of the physician fee schedule amount allowed for the primary surgeon.

ASSISTANT SURGEON MAY NOT BE PAID

CMS maintains statistics on the use of assistant surgeons by procedure. For surgical procedures where assistant surgeons are used in less than five percent (5%)of the cases on a national basis, Medicare will not pay for an assistant surgeon. These procedures are annotated in the following listings with the phrase "assistant surgeon may not be paid." An example of a procedure for which CMS will not pay for an assistant surgeon is:

10060   **Drain skin abscess**   ~ follow-up period is 10 days, standard payment adjustment rules for multiple procedures apply, 150% payment adjustment for bilateral procedures does not apply, <u>assistant surgeon may not be paid</u>

PAYMENT FOR ASSISTANT SURGEON SUBJECT TO DOCUMENTATION

Medicare has identified some surgical procedures where the assistant surgeon may be paid if supporting documentation is submitted with the health insurance claim to establish the medical necessity of the assistant surgeon's services. These procedures are annotated in the following listings with the phrase "payment for assistant surgeon subject to documentation of medical necessity."

An example of a procedure for which CMS will pay for an assistant surgeon if medical necessity is documented is:

31510   **Laryngoscopy with biopsy**   ~ endoscopies or minor procedure - E/M services on the same day generally not paid, special rules for multiple endoscopic procedures apply if billed with another endoscopy in the same family, 150% payment adjustment for bilateral procedures does not apply, <u>payment for assistant surgeon subject to documentation of medical necessity</u>

ASSISTANT SURGEON MAY BE PAID

Procedures for which Medicare will routinely pay for the assistant surgeon are annotated in the following listings with the phrase "assistant surgeon may be paid for this procedure." An example of a procedure for which CMS will routinely pay for an assistant surgeon is:

43280   **Laparoscopy, fundoplasty**   ~ follow-up period is 90 days, standard payment adjustment rules for multiple procedures apply, 150% payment adjustment for bilateral procedures does not apply, <u>assistant surgeon may be paid</u>

BILLABLE MEDICAL SUPPLIES

Under the latest CMS guidelines, medical supplies are no longer billable as a separate item. Under resource based practice expense, all billable medical supplies have been incorporated into the practice expense relative values of individual services and procedures.

ADD-ON PROCEDURES

Some surgical procedures defined in CPT are performed only in addition to a primary procedure. These additional or supplementary procedures are designated as "add-on" procedures. "Add-on" procedures are identified in CPT with a + symbol to the immediate left of the CPT code. In addition, the procedure descriptions include phrases such as "add-on," "each additional," or "(List separately in addition to primary procedure)". These procedures are annotated in the following listings with the phrase "+add-on code (list separately in addition to primary procedure)." An example of a primary procedure followed by an add-on procedure is:

11000   **Debride infected skin**   ~ endoscopies or minor procedure - E/M services on the same day generally not paid, standard payment adjustment rules for multiple procedures apply, 150% payment adjustment for bilateral procedures does not apply, assistant surgeon may not be paid

11001   **Debride infected skin, add-on**   ~ follow-up period included in another service, no payment adjustment rules for multiple procedures apply, 150% payment adjustment for bilateral procedures does not apply, assistant surgeon may not be paid, <u>+add-on code (list separately in addition to primary procedure)</u>

To report biopsy of four skin lesions, CPT code 11100 is listed first, and CPT code 11101 is listed three times to report the additional lesions. All CPT add-on codes are exempt from the multiple procedure concept, therefore, do not add modifier -51 when reporting add-on codes.

SURGERY SERVICES
INTEGUMENTARY SYSTEM

Skin, Subcutaneous and Accessory Structures

10021 **FNA w/o image** ~ no payment adjustment rules for multiple procedures apply, 150% payment adjustment for bilateral procedures does not apply, payment for assistant surgeon subject to documentation of medical necessity

10022 **FNA w/image** ~ no payment adjustment rules for multiple procedures apply, 150% payment adjustment for bilateral procedures does not apply, payment for assistant surgeon subject to documentation of medical necessity

10040 **Acne surgery** ~ follow-up period is 10 days, standard payment adjustment rules for multiple procedures apply, 150% payment adjustment for bilateral procedures does not apply, assistant surgeon may not be paid

10060 **Drain skin abscess** ~ follow-up period is 10 days, standard payment adjustment rules for multiple procedures apply, 150% payment adjustment for bilateral procedures does not apply, assistant surgeon may not be paid

10061 **Drain skin abscess** ~ follow-up period is 10 days, standard payment adjustment rules for multiple procedures apply, 150% payment adjustment for bilateral procedures does not apply, assistant surgeon may not be paid

10080 **Drain pilonidal cyst** ~ follow-up period is 10 days, standard payment adjustment rules for multiple procedures apply, 150% payment adjustment for bilateral procedures does not apply, assistant surgeon may not be paid

10081 **Drain pilonidal cyst** ~ follow-up period is 10 days, standard payment adjustment rules for multiple procedures apply, 150% payment adjustment for bilateral procedures does not apply, assistant surgeon may not be paid

10120 **Remove foreign body** ~ follow-up period is 10 days, standard payment adjustment rules for multiple procedures apply, 150% payment adjustment for bilateral procedures does not apply, assistant surgeon may not be paid

10121 **Remove foreign body** ~ follow-up period is 10 days, standard payment adjustment rules for multiple procedures apply, 150% payment adjustment for bilateral procedures does not apply, assistant surgeon may not be paid

10140 **Drain hematoma/fluid** ~ follow-up period is 10 days, standard payment adjustment rules for multiple procedures apply, 150% payment adjustment for bilateral procedures does not apply, assistant surgeon may not be paid

10160   **Puncture drain lesion**   ~ follow-up period is 10 days, standard payment adjustment rules for multiple procedures apply, 150% payment adjustment for bilateral procedures does not apply, assistant surgeon may not be paid

10180   **Complex drain wound**   ~ follow-up period is 10 days, standard payment adjustment rules for multiple procedures apply, 150% payment adjustment for bilateral procedures does not apply, assistant surgeon may not be paid

11000   **Debride infected skin**   ~ endoscopies or minor procedure - E/M services on the same day generally not paid, standard payment adjustment rules for multiple procedures apply, 150% payment adjustment for bilateral procedures does not apply, assistant surgeon may not be paid

11001   **Debride infected skin, add-on**   ~ follow-up period included in another service, no payment adjustment rules for multiple procedures apply, 150% payment adjustment for bilateral procedures does not apply, assistant surgeon may not be paid, +add-on code (list separately in addition to primary procedure)

11004   **Debride genitalia & perineum**   ~ endoscopies or minor procedure - E/M services on the same day generally not paid, standard payment adjustment rules for multiple procedures apply, 150% payment adjustment for bilateral procedures does not apply, assistant surgeon may not be paid

11005   **Debride abdom wall**   ~ endoscopies or minor procedure - E/M services on the same day generally not paid, no payment adjustment rules for multiple procedures apply, 150% payment adjustment for bilateral procedures does not apply, payment for assistant surgeon subject to documentation of medical necessity

11006   **Debride genital/per/abdom wall**   ~ endoscopies or minor procedure - E/M services on the same day generally not paid, standard payment adjustment rules for multiple procedures apply, 150% payment adjustment for bilateral procedures does not apply, assistant surgeon may not be paid

11008   **Remove mesh from abdom wall**   ~ follow-up period included in another service, no payment adjustment rules for multiple procedures apply, 150% payment adjustment for bilateral procedures does not apply, payment for assistant surgeon subject to documentation of medical necessity

11010   **Debride skin, fracture**   ~ follow-up period is 10 days, standard payment adjustment rules for multiple procedures apply, 150% payment adjustment does not apply - RVUs based on bilateral procedure, assistant surgeon may not be paid

11011   **Debride skin/muscle, fracture**   ~ endoscopies or minor procedure - E/M services on the same day generally not paid, standard payment adjustment rules for multiple procedures apply, 150% payment adjustment does not apply - RVUs based on bilateral procedure, assistant surgeon may not be paid

11012 **Debride skin/muscle/bone, fracture** ~ endoscopies or minor procedure - E/M services on the same day generally not paid, standard payment adjustment rules for multiple procedures apply, 150% payment adjustment does not apply - RVUs based on bilateral procedure, assistant surgeon may not be paid

11040 **Debride skin, partial** ~ endoscopies or minor procedure - E/M services on the same day generally not paid, standard payment adjustment rules for multiple procedures apply, 150% payment adjustment for bilateral procedures does not apply, assistant surgeon may not be paid

11041 **Debride skin, full** ~ endoscopies or minor procedure - E/M services on the same day generally not paid, standard payment adjustment rules for multiple procedures apply, 150% payment adjustment for bilateral procedures does not apply, assistant surgeon may not be paid

11042 **Debride skin/tissue** ~ endoscopies or minor procedure - E/M services on the same day generally not paid, standard payment adjustment rules for multiple procedures apply, 150% payment adjustment for bilateral procedures does not apply, assistant surgeon may not be paid

11043 **Debride tissue/muscle** ~ follow-up period is 10 days, standard payment adjustment rules for multiple procedures apply, 150% payment adjustment for bilateral procedures does not apply, assistant surgeon may not be paid

11044 **Debride tissue/muscle/bone** ~ follow-up period is 10 days, standard payment adjustment rules for multiple procedures apply, 150% payment adjustment for bilateral procedures does not apply, assistant surgeon may not be paid

11055 **Trim skin lesion** ~ restricted coverage - special coverage rules apply, endoscopies or minor procedure - E/M services on the same day generally not paid, standard payment adjustment rules for multiple procedures apply, 150% payment adjustment for bilateral procedures does not apply, assistant surgeon may not be paid

11056 **Trim skin lesions, 2 to 4** ~ restricted coverage - special coverage rules apply, endoscopies or minor procedure - E/M services on the same day generally not paid, standard payment adjustment rules for multiple procedures apply, 150% payment adjustment for bilateral procedures does not apply, assistant surgeon may not be paid

11057 **Trim skin lesions, over 4** ~ restricted coverage - special coverage rules apply, endoscopies or minor procedure - E/M services on the same day generally not paid, standard payment adjustment rules for multiple procedures apply, 150% payment adjustment for bilateral procedures does not apply, assistant surgeon may not be paid

11100 **Biopsy skin lesion** ~ endoscopies or minor procedure - E/M services on the same day generally not paid, standard payment adjustment rules for multiple procedures apply, 150% payment adjustment for bilateral procedures does not apply, assistant surgeon may not be paid

---

11101   **Biopsy skin, add-on**   ~ follow-up period included in another service, no payment adjustment rules for multiple procedures apply, 150% payment adjustment for bilateral procedures does not apply, assistant surgeon may not be paid, +add-on code (list separately in addition to primary procedure)

11200   **Remove skin tags**   ~ follow-up period is 10 days, standard payment adjustment rules for multiple procedures apply, 150% payment adjustment for bilateral procedures does not apply, assistant surgeon may not be paid

11201   **Remove skin tags, add-on**   ~ follow-up period included in another service, no payment adjustment rules for multiple procedures apply, 150% payment adjustment for bilateral procedures does not apply, assistant surgeon may not be paid, +add-on code (list separately in addition to primary procedure)

11300   **Shave skin lesion trunk/arm/legs 0.5cm <**
~ endoscopies or minor procedure - E/M services on the same day generally not paid, standard payment adjustment rules for multiple procedures apply, bilateral surgery concept does not apply, payment for assistant surgeon subject to documentation of medical necessity

11301   **Shave skin lesion trunk/arm/legs 0.6-1.0cm**
~ endoscopies or minor procedure - E/M services on the same day generally not paid, standard payment adjustment rules for multiple procedures apply, bilateral surgery concept does not apply, payment for assistant surgeon subject to documentation of medical necessity

11302   **Shave skin lesion trunk/arm/legs 1.1-2.0cm**
~ endoscopies or minor procedure - E/M services on the same day generally not paid, standard payment adjustment rules for multiple procedures apply, bilateral surgery concept does not apply, payment for assistant surgeon subject to documentation of medical necessity

11303   **Shave skin lesion trunk/arm/legs >2.0cm**
~ endoscopies or minor procedure - E/M services on the same day generally not paid, standard payment adjustment rules for multiple procedures apply, bilateral surgery concept does not apply, payment for assistant surgeon subject to documentation of medical necessity

11305   **Shave skin lesion scalp/neck/hand/genital 0.5cm <**
~ endoscopies or minor procedure - E/M services on the same day generally not paid, standard payment adjustment rules for multiple procedures apply, bilateral surgery concept does not apply, payment for assistant surgeon subject to documentation of medical necessity

11306   **Shave skin lesion scalp/neck/hand/genital 0.6-1.0cm**
~ endoscopies or minor procedure - E/M services on the same day generally not paid, standard payment adjustment rules for multiple procedures apply, bilateral surgery concept

does not apply, payment for assistant surgeon subject to documentation of medical necessity

11307 **Shave skin lesion scalp/neck/hand/genital 1.1-2.0cm**
~ endoscopies or minor procedure - E/M services on the same day generally not paid, standard payment adjustment rules for multiple procedures apply, bilateral surgery concept does not apply, payment for assistant surgeon subject to documentation of medical necessity

11308 **Shave skin lesion scalp/neck/hand/genital >2.0cm**
~ endoscopies or minor procedure - E/M services on the same day generally not paid, standard payment adjustment rules for multiple procedures apply, bilateral surgery concept does not apply, payment for assistant surgeon subject to documentation of medical necessity

11310 **Shave skin lesion face/ear/nose/lip 0.5cm <** ~ endoscopies or minor procedure - E/M services on the same day generally not paid, standard payment adjustment rules for multiple procedures apply, bilateral surgery concept does not apply, payment for assistant surgeon subject to documentation of medical necessity

11311 **Shave skin lesion face/ear/nose/lip 0.6-1.0cm**
~ endoscopies or minor procedure - E/M services on the same day generally not paid, standard payment adjustment rules for multiple procedures apply, bilateral surgery concept does not apply, payment for assistant surgeon subject to documentation of medical necessity

11312 **Shave skin lesion face/ear/nose/lip 1.1-2.0cm**
~ endoscopies or minor procedure - E/M services on the same day generally not paid, standard payment adjustment rules for multiple procedures apply, bilateral surgery concept does not apply, payment for assistant surgeon subject to documentation of medical necessity

11313 **Shave skin lesion face/ear/nose/lip >2.0cm**
~ endoscopies or minor procedure - E/M services on the same day generally not paid, standard payment adjustment rules for multiple procedures apply, bilateral surgery concept does not apply, payment for assistant surgeon subject to documentation of medical necessity

11400 **Excise benign lesion trunk/arm/legs 0.5 < cm**
~ follow-up period is 10 days, standard payment adjustment rules for multiple procedures apply, 150% payment adjustment for bilateral procedures does not apply, assistant surgeon may not be paid

11401 **Excise benign lesion trunk/arm/legs 0.6-1 cm**
~ follow-up period is 10 days, standard payment adjustment rules for multiple procedures apply, 150% payment adjustment for bilateral procedures does not apply, assistant surgeon may not be paid

11402 **Excise benign lesion trunk/arm/legs 1.1-2 cm**
~ follow-up period is 10 days, standard payment adjustment rules for multiple procedures apply, 150% payment adjustment for bilateral procedures does not apply, assistant surgeon may not be paid

11403 **Excise benign lesion trunk/arm/legs 2.1-3 cm**
~ follow-up period is 10 days, standard payment adjustment rules for multiple procedures apply, 150% payment adjustment for bilateral procedures does not apply, assistant surgeon may not be paid

11404 **Excise benign lesion trunk/arm/legs 3.1-4 cm**
~ follow-up period is 10 days, standard payment adjustment rules for multiple procedures apply, 150% payment adjustment for bilateral procedures does not apply, assistant surgeon may not be paid

11406 **Excise benign lesion trunk/arm/legs > 4.0 cm**
~ follow-up period is 10 days, standard payment adjustment rules for multiple procedures apply, 150% payment adjustment for bilateral procedures does not apply, assistant surgeon may not be paid

11420 **Excise benign lesion scalp/neck/hand/genital 0.5cm <**
~ follow-up period is 10 days, standard payment adjustment rules for multiple procedures apply, 150% payment adjustment for bilateral procedures does not apply, assistant surgeon may not be paid

11421 **Excise benign lesion scalp/neck/hand/genital 0.6-1.0cm**
~ follow-up period is 10 days, standard payment adjustment rules for multiple procedures apply, 150% payment adjustment for bilateral procedures does not apply, assistant surgeon may not be paid

11422 **Excise benign lesion scalp/neck/hand/genital 1.1-2.0cm**
~ follow-up period is 10 days, standard payment adjustment rules for multiple procedures apply, 150% payment adjustment for bilateral procedures does not apply, assistant surgeon may not be paid

11423 **Excise benign lesion scalp/neck/hand/genital 2.1-3.0cm**
~ follow-up period is 10 days, standard payment adjustment rules for multiple procedures apply, 150% payment adjustment for bilateral procedures does not apply, assistant surgeon may not be paid

11424 **Excise benign lesion scalp/neck/hand/genital 3.1-4.0cm**
~ follow-up period is 10 days, standard payment adjustment rules for multiple procedures apply, 150% payment adjustment for bilateral procedures does not apply, assistant surgeon may not be paid

11426 **Excise benign lesion scalp/neck/hand/genital > 4 cm**

~ follow-up period is 10 days, standard payment adjustment rules for multiple procedures apply, 150% payment adjustment for bilateral procedures does not apply, assistant surgeon may not be paid

11440   Excise benign lesion face/ear/nose/lip 0.5 < cm
~ follow-up period is 10 days, standard payment adjustment rules for multiple procedures apply, 150% payment adjustment for bilateral procedures does not apply, assistant surgeon may not be paid

11441   Excise benign lesion face/ear/nose/lip 0.6-1 cm
~ follow-up period is 10 days, standard payment adjustment rules for multiple procedures apply, 150% payment adjustment for bilateral procedures does not apply, assistant surgeon may not be paid

11442   Excise benign lesion face/ear/nose/lip 1.1-2 cm
~ follow-up period is 10 days, standard payment adjustment rules for multiple procedures apply, 150% payment adjustment for bilateral procedures does not apply, assistant surgeon may not be paid

11443   Excise benign lesion face/ear/nose/lip 2.1-3 cm
~ follow-up period is 10 days, standard payment adjustment rules for multiple procedures apply, 150% payment adjustment for bilateral procedures does not apply, assistant surgeon may not be paid

11444   Excise benign lesion face/ear/nose/lip 3.1-4 cm
~ follow-up period is 10 days, standard payment adjustment rules for multiple procedures apply, 150% payment adjustment for bilateral procedures does not apply, assistant surgeon may not be paid

11446   Excise benign lesion face/ear/nose/lip > 4 cm
~ follow-up period is 10 days, standard payment adjustment rules for multiple procedures apply, 150% payment adjustment for bilateral procedures does not apply, assistant surgeon may not be paid

11450   Excise skin axilla; simple/intermediate
~ follow-up period is 90 days, standard payment adjustment rules for multiple procedures apply, 150% payment adjustment for bilateral procedures does not apply, assistant surgeon may not be paid

11451   Excise skin axilla; complex   ~ follow-up period is 90 days, standard payment adjustment rules for multiple procedures apply, 150% payment adjustment for bilateral procedures does not apply, payment for assistant surgeon subject to documentation of medical necessity

11462   Excise skin inguinal; simple/intermediate ~ follow-up period is 90 days, standard payment adjustment rules for multiple procedures apply, 150% payment adjustment for

---

bilateral procedures does not apply, payment for assistant surgeon subject to documentation of medical necessity

11463   **Excise skin inguinal; complex**   ~ follow-up period is 90 days, standard payment adjustment rules for multiple procedures apply, 150% payment adjustment for bilateral procedures does not apply, payment for assistant surgeon subject to documentation of medical necessity

11470   **Excise skin perianal/umbilical; simple/interm**
~ follow-up period is 90 days, standard payment adjustment rules for multiple procedures apply, 150% payment adjustment for bilateral procedures does not apply, assistant surgeon may not be paid

11471   **Excise skin perianal/umbilical; complex**
~ follow-up period is 90 days, standard payment adjustment rules for multiple procedures apply, 150% payment adjustment for bilateral procedures does not apply, payment for assistant surgeon subject to documentation of medical necessity

11600   **Excise malig lesion trunk/arm/leg 0.5 < cm**
~ follow-up period is 10 days, standard payment adjustment rules for multiple procedures apply, 150% payment adjustment for bilateral procedures does not apply, assistant surgeon may not be paid

11601   **Excise malig lesion trunk/arm/leg 0.6-1 cm**
~ follow-up period is 10 days, standard payment adjustment rules for multiple procedures apply, 150% payment adjustment for bilateral procedures does not apply, assistant surgeon may not be paid

11602   **Excise malig lesion trunk/arm/leg 1.1-2 cm**
~ follow-up period is 10 days, standard payment adjustment rules for multiple procedures apply, 150% payment adjustment for bilateral procedures does not apply, assistant surgeon may not be paid

11603   **Excise malig lesion trunk/arm/leg 2.1-3 cm**
~ follow-up period is 10 days, standard payment adjustment rules for multiple procedures apply, 150% payment adjustment for bilateral procedures does not apply, assistant surgeon may not be paid

11604   **Excise malig lesion trunk/arm/leg 3.1-4 cm**
~ follow-up period is 10 days, standard payment adjustment rules for multiple procedures apply, 150% payment adjustment for bilateral procedures does not apply, assistant surgeon may not be paid

11606   **Excise malig lesion trunk/arm/leg > 4 cm**
~ follow-up period is 10 days, standard payment adjustment rules for multiple procedures apply, 150% payment adjustment for bilateral procedures does not apply, assistant surgeon may not be paid

11620   Excise malig lesion scalp/neck/hand/genital 0.5 <
~ follow-up period is 10 days, standard payment adjustment rules for multiple procedures apply, 150% payment adjustment for bilateral procedures does not apply, assistant surgeon may not be paid

11621   Excise malig lesion scalp/neck/hand/genital 0.6-1
~ follow-up period is 10 days, standard payment adjustment rules for multiple procedures apply, 150% payment adjustment for bilateral procedures does not apply, assistant surgeon may not be paid

11622   Excise malig lesion scalp/neck/hand/genital 1.1-2
~ follow-up period is 10 days, standard payment adjustment rules for multiple procedures apply, 150% payment adjustment for bilateral procedures does not apply, assistant surgeon may not be paid

11623   Excise malig lesion scalp/neck/hand/genital 2.1-3
~ follow-up period is 10 days, standard payment adjustment rules for multiple procedures apply, 150% payment adjustment for bilateral procedures does not apply, assistant surgeon may not be paid

11624   Excise malig lesion scalp/neck/hand/genital 3.1-4
~ follow-up period is 10 days, standard payment adjustment rules for multiple procedures apply, 150% payment adjustment for bilateral procedures does not apply, assistant surgeon may not be paid

11626   Excise malig lesion scalp/neck/hand/genital > 4 cm
~ follow-up period is 10 days, standard payment adjustment rules for multiple procedures apply, 150% payment adjustment for bilateral procedures does not apply, assistant surgeon may not be paid

11640   Excise malig lesion face/ear/nose/lip 0.5 <
~ follow-up period is 10 days, standard payment adjustment rules for multiple procedures apply, 150% payment adjustment for bilateral procedures does not apply, assistant surgeon may not be paid

11641   Excise malig lesion face/ear/nose/lip 0.6-1
~ follow-up period is 10 days, standard payment adjustment rules for multiple procedures apply, 150% payment adjustment for bilateral procedures does not apply, assistant surgeon may not be paid

11642   Excise malig lesion face/ear/nose/lip 1.1-2
~ follow-up period is 10 days, standard payment adjustment rules for multiple procedures apply, 150% payment adjustment for bilateral procedures does not apply, assistant surgeon may not be paid

11643   Excise malig lesion face/ear/nose/lip 2.1-3

~ follow-up period is 10 days, standard payment adjustment rules for multiple procedures apply, 150% payment adjustment for bilateral procedures does not apply, assistant surgeon may not be paid

11644   **Excise malig lesion face/ear/nose/lip 3.1-4**
~ follow-up period is 10 days, standard payment adjustment rules for multiple procedures apply, 150% payment adjustment for bilateral procedures does not apply, assistant surgeon may not be paid

11646   **Excise malig lesion face/ear/nose/lip > 4 cm**
~ follow-up period is 10 days, standard payment adjustment rules for multiple procedures apply, 150% payment adjustment for bilateral procedures does not apply, assistant surgeon may not be paid

Nails

11719   **Trim nail(s)**   ~ restricted coverage - special coverage rules apply, endoscopies or minor procedure - E/M services on the same day generally not paid, standard payment adjustment rules for multiple procedures apply, 150% payment adjustment for bilateral procedures does not apply, assistant surgeon may not be paid

11720   **Debride nail, 1-5**   ~ endoscopies or minor procedure - E/M services on the same day generally not paid, no payment adjustment rules for multiple procedures apply, 150% payment adjustment for bilateral procedures does not apply, assistant surgeon may not be paid

11721   **Debride nail, 6 or more**   ~ endoscopies or minor procedure - E/M services on the same day generally not paid, no payment adjustment rules for multiple procedures apply, 150% payment adjustment for bilateral procedures does not apply, assistant surgeon may not be paid

11730   **Remove nail plate**   ~ endoscopies or minor procedure - E/M services on the same day generally not paid, standard payment adjustment rules for multiple procedures apply, 150% payment adjustment for bilateral procedures does not apply, assistant surgeon may not be paid

11732   **Remove nail plate, add-on**   ~ follow-up period included in another service, no payment adjustment rules for multiple procedures apply, 150% payment adjustment for bilateral procedures does not apply, assistant surgeon may not be paid, +add-on code (list separately in addition to primary procedure)

11740   **Drain blood from under nail**   ~ endoscopies or minor procedure - E/M services on the same day generally not paid, standard payment adjustment rules for multiple procedures apply, 150% payment adjustment for bilateral procedures does not apply, assistant surgeon may not be paid

11750   **Remove nail bed**   ~ follow-up period is 10 days, standard payment adjustment rules for multiple procedures apply, 150% payment adjustment for bilateral procedures does not apply, assistant surgeon may not be paid

11752   **Remove nail bed/finger tip**   ~ follow-up period is 10 days, standard payment adjustment rules for multiple procedures apply, 150% payment adjustment for bilateral procedures does not apply, assistant surgeon may not be paid

11755   **Biopsy nail unit**   ~ endoscopies or minor procedure - E/M services on the same day generally not paid, standard payment adjustment rules for multiple procedures apply, 150% payment adjustment for bilateral procedures does not apply, payment for assistant surgeon subject to documentation of medical necessity

11760   **Repair nail bed**   ~ follow-up period is 10 days, standard payment adjustment rules for multiple procedures apply, 150% payment adjustment for bilateral procedures does not apply, assistant surgeon may not be paid

11762   **Reconstruct nail bed**   ~ follow-up period is 10 days, standard payment adjustment rules for multiple procedures apply, 150% payment adjustment for bilateral procedures does not apply, assistant surgeon may not be paid

11765   **Excise nail fold, toe**   ~ follow-up period is 10 days, standard payment adjustment rules for multiple procedures apply, 150% payment adjustment for bilateral procedures does not apply, assistant surgeon may not be paid

Pilonidal Cyst

11770   **Remove pilonidal lesion**   ~ follow-up period is 10 days, standard payment adjustment rules for multiple procedures apply, 150% payment adjustment for bilateral procedures does not apply, assistant surgeon may not be paid

11771   **Remove pilonidal lesion**   ~ follow-up period is 90 days, standard payment adjustment rules for multiple procedures apply, 150% payment adjustment for bilateral procedures does not apply, assistant surgeon may not be paid

11772   **Remove pilonidal lesion**   ~ follow-up period is 90 days, standard payment adjustment rules for multiple procedures apply, 150% payment adjustment for bilateral procedures does not apply, assistant surgeon may not be paid

Introduction

11900   **Inject into skin lesions**   ~ endoscopies or minor procedure - E/M services on the same day generally not paid, standard payment adjustment rules for multiple procedures apply, 150% payment adjustment for bilateral procedures does not apply, assistant surgeon may not be paid

11901   **Added skin lesions injection**   ~ endoscopies or minor procedure - E/M services on the same day generally not paid, standard payment adjustment rules for multiple procedures apply, 150% payment adjustment for bilateral procedures does not apply, assistant surgeon may not be paid, +add-on code (list separately in addition to primary procedure)

11920   **Correct skin color defects**   ~ restricted coverage - special coverage rules apply, endoscopies or minor procedure - E/M services on the same day generally not paid, standard payment adjustment rules for multiple procedures apply, 150% payment adjustment for bilateral procedures does not apply, payment for assistant surgeon subject to documentation of medical necessity

11921   **Correct skin color defects**   ~ restricted coverage - special coverage rules apply, endoscopies or minor procedure - E/M services on the same day generally not paid, standard payment adjustment rules for multiple procedures apply, 150% payment adjustment for bilateral procedures does not apply, payment for assistant surgeon subject to documentation of medical necessity

11922   **Correct skin color defects**   ~ restricted coverage - special coverage rules apply, follow-up period included in another service, no payment adjustment rules for multiple procedures apply, 150% payment adjustment for bilateral procedures does not apply, payment for assistant surgeon subject to documentation of medical necessity

11950   **Therapy for contour defects**   ~ restricted coverage - special coverage rules apply, endoscopies or minor procedure - E/M services on the same day generally not paid, standard payment adjustment rules for multiple procedures apply, 150% payment adjustment for bilateral procedures does not apply, payment for assistant surgeon subject to documentation of medical necessity

11951   **Therapy for contour defects**   ~ restricted coverage - special coverage rules apply, endoscopies or minor procedure - E/M services on the same day generally not paid, standard payment adjustment rules for multiple procedures apply, 150% payment adjustment for bilateral procedures does not apply, payment for assistant surgeon subject to documentation of medical necessity

11952   **Therapy for contour defects**   ~ restricted coverage - special coverage rules apply, endoscopies or minor procedure - E/M services on the same day generally not paid, standard payment adjustment rules for multiple procedures apply, 150% payment adjustment for bilateral procedures does not apply, payment for assistant surgeon subject to documentation of medical necessity

11954   **Therapy for contour defects**   ~ restricted coverage - special coverage rules apply, endoscopies or minor procedure - E/M services on the same day generally not paid, standard payment adjustment rules for multiple procedures apply, 150% payment adjustment for bilateral procedures does not apply, payment for assistant surgeon subject to documentation of medical necessity

11960   **Insert tissue expander(s)**   ~ follow-up period is 90 days, standard payment adjustment rules for multiple procedures apply, 150% payment adjustment for bilateral procedures does not apply, assistant surgeon may not be paid

11970   **Replace tissue expander**   ~ follow-up period is 90 days, standard payment adjustment rules for multiple procedures apply, 150% payment adjustment for bilateral procedures does not apply, assistant surgeon may not be paid

11971   **Remove tissue expander(s)**   ~ follow-up period is 90 days, standard payment adjustment rules for multiple procedures apply, 150% payment adjustment for bilateral procedures does not apply, payment for assistant surgeon subject to documentation of medical necessity

11975   **Insert contraceptive cap**   ~ non-covered service, multiple procedure concept does not apply, bilateral surgery concept does not apply, assistant surgery concept does not apply

11976   **Remove contraceptive cap**   ~ restricted coverage - special coverage rules apply, endoscopies or minor procedure - E/M services on the same day generally not paid, standard payment adjustment rules for multiple procedures apply, 150% payment adjustment for bilateral procedures does not apply, payment for assistant surgeon subject to documentation of medical necessity

11977   **Remove/reinsert contra cap**   non-covered service, multiple procedure concept does not apply, bilateral surgery concept does not apply, assistant surgery concept does not apply

11980   **Implant hormone pellet(s)**   ~ endoscopies or minor procedure - E/M services on the same day generally not paid, standard payment adjustment rules for multiple procedures apply, 150% payment adjustment for bilateral procedures does not apply, assistant surgeon may not be paid

11981   **Insert drug implant device**   ~ standard payment adjustment rules for multiple procedures apply, 150% payment adjustment for bilateral procedures does not apply, payment for assistant surgeon subject to documentation of medical necessity

11982   **Remove drug implant device**   ~ standard payment adjustment rules for multiple procedures apply, 150% payment adjustment for bilateral procedures does not apply, payment for assistant surgeon subject to documentation of medical necessity

11983   **Remove/insert drug implant**   ~ standard payment adjustment rules for multiple procedures apply, 150% payment adjustment for bilateral procedures does not apply, payment for assistant surgeon subject to documentation of medical necessity

Repair (Closure)

12001   **Repair superficial wound(s)**   ~ follow-up period is 10 days, standard payment adjustment rules for multiple procedures apply, 150% payment adjustment for bilateral procedures does not apply, assistant surgeon may not be paid

12002 **Repair superficial wound(s)** ~ follow-up period is 10 days, standard payment adjustment rules for multiple procedures apply, 150% payment adjustment for bilateral procedures does not apply, assistant surgeon may not be paid

12004 **Repair superficial wound(s)** ~ follow-up period is 10 days, standard payment adjustment rules for multiple procedures apply, 150% payment adjustment for bilateral procedures does not apply, assistant surgeon may not be paid

12005 **Repair superficial wound(s)** ~ follow-up period is 10 days, standard payment adjustment rules for multiple procedures apply, 150% payment adjustment for bilateral procedures does not apply, assistant surgeon may not be paid

12006 **Repair superficial wound(s)** ~ follow-up period is 10 days, standard payment adjustment rules for multiple procedures apply, 150% payment adjustment for bilateral procedures does not apply, assistant surgeon may not be paid

12007 **Repair superficial wound(s)** ~ follow-up period is 10 days, standard payment adjustment rules for multiple procedures apply, 150% payment adjustment for bilateral procedures does not apply, assistant surgeon may not be paid

12011 **Repair superficial wound(s)** ~ follow-up period is 10 days, standard payment adjustment rules for multiple procedures apply, 150% payment adjustment for bilateral procedures does not apply, assistant surgeon may not be paid

12013 **Repair superficial wound(s)** ~ follow-up period is 10 days, standard payment adjustment rules for multiple procedures apply, 150% payment adjustment for bilateral procedures does not apply, assistant surgeon may not be paid

12014 **Repair superficial wound(s)** ~ follow-up period is 10 days, standard payment adjustment rules for multiple procedures apply, 150% payment adjustment for bilateral procedures does not apply, assistant surgeon may not be paid

12015 **Repair superficial wound(s)** ~ follow-up period is 10 days, standard payment adjustment rules for multiple procedures apply, 150% payment adjustment for bilateral procedures does not apply, assistant surgeon may not be paid

12016 **Repair superficial wound(s)** ~ follow-up period is 10 days, standard payment adjustment rules for multiple procedures apply, 150% payment adjustment for bilateral procedures does not apply, assistant surgeon may not be paid

12017 **Repair superficial wound(s)** ~ follow-up period is 10 days, standard payment adjustment rules for multiple procedures apply, 150% payment adjustment for bilateral procedures does not apply, payment for assistant surgeon subject to documentation of medical necessity

12018   **Repair superficial wound(s)**   ~ follow-up period is 10 days, standard payment adjustment rules for multiple procedures apply, 150% payment adjustment for bilateral procedures does not apply, assistant surgeon may be paid

12020   **Closure split wound**   ~ follow-up period is 10 days, standard payment adjustment rules for multiple procedures apply, 150% payment adjustment for bilateral procedures does not apply, assistant surgeon may not be paid

12021   **Closure split wound**   ~ follow-up period is 10 days, standard payment adjustment rules for multiple procedures apply, 150% payment adjustment for bilateral procedures does not apply, assistant surgeon may not be paid

12031   **Layer closure wound(s)**   ~ follow-up period is 10 days, standard payment adjustment rules for multiple procedures apply, 150% payment adjustment for bilateral procedures does not apply, assistant surgeon may not be paid

12032   **Layer closure wound(s)**   ~ follow-up period is 10 days, standard payment adjustment rules for multiple procedures apply, 150% payment adjustment for bilateral procedures does not apply, assistant surgeon may not be paid

12034   **Layer closure wound(s)**   ~ follow-up period is 10 days, standard payment adjustment rules for multiple procedures apply, 150% payment adjustment for bilateral procedures does not apply, assistant surgeon may not be paid

12035   **Layer closure wound(s)**   ~ follow-up period is 10 days, standard payment adjustment rules for multiple procedures apply, 150% payment adjustment for bilateral procedures does not apply, assistant surgeon may not be paid

12036   **Layer closure wound(s)**   ~ follow-up period is 10 days, standard payment adjustment rules for multiple procedures apply, 150% payment adjustment for bilateral procedures does not apply, assistant surgeon may not be paid

12037   **Layer closure wound(s)**   ~ follow-up period is 10 days, standard payment adjustment rules for multiple procedures apply, 150% payment adjustment for bilateral procedures does not apply, payment for assistant surgeon subject to documentation of medical necessity

12041   **Layer closure wound(s)**   ~ follow-up period is 10 days, standard payment adjustment rules for multiple procedures apply, 150% payment adjustment for bilateral procedures does not apply, assistant surgeon may not be paid

12042   **Layer closure wound(s)**   ~ follow-up period is 10 days, standard payment adjustment rules for multiple procedures apply, 150% payment adjustment for bilateral procedures does not apply, assistant surgeon may not be paid

12044   **Layer closure wound(s)**   ~ follow-up period is 10 days, standard payment adjustment rules for multiple procedures apply, 150% payment adjustment for bilateral procedures does not apply, assistant surgeon may not be paid

12045   **Layer closure wound(s)**   ~ follow-up period is 10 days, standard payment adjustment rules for multiple procedures apply, 150% payment adjustment for bilateral procedures does not apply, assistant surgeon may not be paid

12046   **Layer closure wound(s)**   ~ follow-up period is 10 days, standard payment adjustment rules for multiple procedures apply, 150% payment adjustment for bilateral procedures does not apply, payment for assistant surgeon subject to documentation of medical necessity

12047   **Layer closure wound(s)**   ~ follow-up period is 10 days, standard payment adjustment rules for multiple procedures apply, 150% payment adjustment for bilateral procedures does not apply, assistant surgeon may be paid

12051   **Layer closure wound(s)**   ~ follow-up period is 10 days, standard payment adjustment rules for multiple procedures apply, 150% payment adjustment for bilateral procedures does not apply, assistant surgeon may not be paid

12052   **Layer closure wound(s)**   ~ follow-up period is 10 days, standard payment adjustment rules for multiple procedures apply, 150% payment adjustment for bilateral procedures does not apply, assistant surgeon may not be paid

12053   **Layer closure wound(s)**   ~ follow-up period is 10 days, standard payment adjustment rules for multiple procedures apply, 150% payment adjustment for bilateral procedures does not apply, assistant surgeon may not be paid

12054   **Layer closure wound(s)**   ~ follow-up period is 10 days, standard payment adjustment rules for multiple procedures apply, 150% payment adjustment for bilateral procedures does not apply, assistant surgeon may not be paid

12055   **Layer closure wound(s)**   ~ follow-up period is 10 days, standard payment adjustment rules for multiple procedures apply, 150% payment adjustment for bilateral procedures does not apply, assistant surgeon may not be paid

12056   **Layer closure wound(s)**   ~ follow-up period is 10 days, standard payment adjustment rules for multiple procedures apply, 150% payment adjustment for bilateral procedures does not apply, payment for assistant surgeon subject to documentation of medical necessity

12057   **Layer closure wound(s)**   ~ follow-up period is 10 days, standard payment adjustment rules for multiple procedures apply, 150% payment adjustment for bilateral procedures does not apply, assistant surgeon may be paid

13100   **Repair wound or lesion**   ~ follow-up period is 10 days, standard payment adjustment rules for multiple procedures apply, 150% payment adjustment for bilateral procedures does not apply, assistant surgeon may not be paid

13101   **Repair wound or lesion**   ~ follow-up period is 10 days, standard payment adjustment rules for multiple procedures apply, 150% payment adjustment for bilateral procedures does not apply, assistant surgeon may not be paid

13102   **Repair wound/lesion, add-on**   ~ follow-up period included in another service, no payment adjustment rules for multiple procedures apply, 150% payment adjustment for bilateral procedures does not apply, assistant surgeon may not be paid, +add-on code (list separately in addition to primary procedure)

13120   **Repair wound or lesion**   ~ follow-up period is 10 days, standard payment adjustment rules for multiple procedures apply, 150% payment adjustment for bilateral procedures does not apply, assistant surgeon may not be paid

13121   **Repair wound or lesion**   ~ follow-up period is 10 days, standard payment adjustment rules for multiple procedures apply, 150% payment adjustment for bilateral procedures does not apply, assistant surgeon may not be paid

13122   **Repair wound/lesion, add-on**   ~ follow-up period included in another service, no payment adjustment rules for multiple procedures apply, 150% payment adjustment for bilateral procedures does not apply, assistant surgeon may not be paid, +add-on code (list separately in addition to primary procedure)

13131   **Repair wound or lesion**   ~ follow-up period is 10 days, standard payment adjustment rules for multiple procedures apply, 150% payment adjustment for bilateral procedures does not apply, assistant surgeon may not be paid

13132   **Repair wound or lesion**   ~ follow-up period is 10 days, standard payment adjustment rules for multiple procedures apply, 150% payment adjustment for bilateral procedures does not apply, assistant surgeon may not be paid

13133   **Repair wound/lesion, add-on**   ~ follow-up period included in another service, no payment adjustment rules for multiple procedures apply, 150% payment adjustment for bilateral procedures does not apply, assistant surgeon may not be paid, +add-on code (list separately in addition to primary procedure)

13150   **Repair wound or lesion**   ~ follow-up period is 10 days, standard payment adjustment rules for multiple procedures apply, 150% payment adjustment for bilateral procedures does not apply, assistant surgeon may not be paid

13151   **Repair wound or lesion**   ~ follow-up period is 10 days, standard payment adjustment rules for multiple procedures apply, 150% payment adjustment for bilateral procedures does not apply, assistant surgeon may not be paid

13152   **Repair wound or lesion**   ~ follow-up period is 10 days, standard payment adjustment rules for multiple procedures apply, 150% payment adjustment for bilateral procedures does not apply, assistant surgeon may not be paid

13153   **Repair wound/lesion, add-on**   ~ follow-up period included in another service, no payment adjustment rules for multiple procedures apply, 150% payment adjustment for bilateral procedures does not apply, assistant surgeon may not be paid, +add-on code (list separately in addition to primary procedure)

13160   **Late closure wound**   ~ follow-up period is 90 days, standard payment adjustment rules for multiple procedures apply, 150% payment adjustment for bilateral procedures does not apply, assistant surgeon may not be paid

14000   **Skin tissue rearrangement**   ~ follow-up period is 90 days, standard payment adjustment rules for multiple procedures apply, 150% payment adjustment for bilateral procedures does not apply, assistant surgeon may not be paid

14001   **Skin tissue rearrangement**   ~ follow-up period is 90 days, standard payment adjustment rules for multiple procedures apply, 150% payment adjustment for bilateral procedures does not apply, assistant surgeon may not be paid

14020   **Skin tissue rearrangement**   ~ follow-up period is 90 days, standard payment adjustment rules for multiple procedures apply, 150% payment adjustment for bilateral procedures does not apply, assistant surgeon may not be paid

14021   **Skin tissue rearrangement**   ~ follow-up period is 90 days, standard payment adjustment rules for multiple procedures apply, 150% payment adjustment for bilateral procedures does not apply, assistant surgeon may not be paid

14040   **Skin tissue rearrangement**   ~ follow-up period is 90 days, standard payment adjustment rules for multiple procedures apply, 150% payment adjustment for bilateral procedures does not apply, assistant surgeon may not be paid

14041   **Skin tissue rearrangement**   ~ follow-up period is 90 days, standard payment adjustment rules for multiple procedures apply, 150% payment adjustment for bilateral procedures does not apply, assistant surgeon may not be paid

14060   **Skin tissue rearrangement**   ~ follow-up period is 90 days, standard payment adjustment rules for multiple procedures apply, 150% payment adjustment for bilateral procedures does not apply, assistant surgeon may not be paid

14061   **Skin tissue rearrangement**   ~ follow-up period is 90 days, standard payment adjustment rules for multiple procedures apply, 150% payment adjustment for bilateral procedures does not apply, assistant surgeon may not be paid

14300   **Skin tissue rearrangement**   ~ follow-up period is 90 days, standard payment adjustment rules for multiple procedures apply, 150% payment adjustment for bilateral procedures does not apply, assistant surgeon may not be paid

14350   **Skin tissue rearrangement**   ~ follow-up period is 90 days, standard payment adjustment rules for multiple procedures apply, 150% payment adjustment for bilateral procedures does not apply, payment for assistant surgeon subject to documentation of medical necessity

Skin Replacement Surgery and Skin Substitutes

15002   **Wound prep, ch/inf, trunk/arm/lg**   ~ endoscopies or minor procedure - E/M services on the same day generally not paid, no payment adjustment rules for multiple procedures apply, 150% payment adjustment for bilateral procedures does not apply, payment for assistant surgeon subject to documentation of medical necessity

15003   **Wound prep, ch/inf added 100 cm**   ~ follow-up period included in another service, no payment adjustment rules for multiple procedures apply, 150% payment adjustment for bilateral procedures does not apply, payment for assistant surgeon subject to documentation of medical necessity, +add-on code (list separately in addition to primary procedure)

15004   **Wound prepare ch/inf, f/n/hf/g**   ~ endoscopies or minor procedure - E/M services on the same day generally not paid, no payment adjustment rules for multiple procedures apply, 150% payment adjustment for bilateral procedures does not apply, payment for assistant surgeon subject to documentation of medical necessity

15005   **Wound prep, f/n/hf/g, added cm**   ~ follow-up period included in another service, no payment adjustment rules for multiple procedures apply, 150% payment adjustment for bilateral procedures does not apply, payment for assistant surgeon subject to documentation of medical necessity, +add-on code (list separately in addition to primary procedure)

15040   **Harvest cultured skin graft**   ~ endoscopies or minor procedure - E/M services on the same day generally not paid, no payment adjustment rules for multiple procedures apply, 150% payment adjustment for bilateral procedures does not apply, assistant surgeon may not be paid

15050   **Skin pinch graft**   ~ follow-up period is 90 days, standard payment adjustment rules for multiple procedures apply, 150% payment adjustment for bilateral procedures does not apply, assistant surgeon may not be paid

15100   **Skin split graft, trunk/arm/leg**   ~ follow-up period is 90 days, standard payment adjustment rules for multiple procedures apply, 150% payment adjustment for bilateral procedures does not apply, assistant surgeon may not be paid

15101   **Skin split graft t/a/l, add-on**   ~ follow-up period included in another service, no payment adjustment rules for multiple procedures apply, 150% payment adjustment for bilateral procedures does not apply, assistant surgeon may not be paid, +add-on code (list separately in addition to primary procedure)

15110   **Epidermal autograft trunk/arm/leg**   ~ follow-up period is 90 days, standard payment adjustment rules for multiple procedures apply, 150% payment adjustment for bilateral procedures does not apply, assistant surgeon may not be paid

15111   **Epidermal autograft t/a/l, add-on**   ~ follow-up period included in another service, no payment adjustment rules for multiple procedures apply, 150% payment adjustment for bilateral procedures does not apply, assistant surgeon may not be paid, +add-on code (list separately in addition to primary procedure)

15115   **Epidermal a-graft face/neck/hf/g**   ~ follow-up period is 90 days, standard payment adjustment rules for multiple procedures apply, 150% payment adjustment for bilateral procedures does not apply, assistant surgeon may not be paid

15116   **Epidermal a-graft f/n/hf/g added**   ~ follow-up period included in another service, no payment adjustment rules for multiple procedures apply, 150% payment adjustment for bilateral procedures does not apply, assistant surgeon may not be paid, +add-on code (list separately in addition to primary procedure)

15120   **Skin split a-graft face/neck/hands/feet/genitals**~ follow-up period is 90 days, standard payment adjustment rules for multiple procedures apply, 150% payment adjustment for bilateral procedures does not apply, assistant surgeon may not be paid

15121   **Skin split a-graft f/n/hf/g add-on**   ~ follow-up period included in another service, no payment adjustment rules for multiple procedures apply, 150% payment adjustment for bilateral procedures does not apply, assistant surgeon may not be paid, +add-on code (list separately in addition to primary procedure)

15130   **Derm autograft, trunk/arm/leg**   ~ follow-up period is 90 days, standard payment adjustment rules for multiple procedures apply, 150% payment adjustment for bilateral procedures does not apply, assistant surgeon may not be paid

15131   **Derm autograft t/a/l, add-on**   ~ follow-up period included in another service, no payment adjustment rules for multiple procedures apply, 150% payment adjustment for bilateral procedures does not apply, assistant surgeon may not be paid, +add-on code (list separately in addition to primary procedure)

15135   **Derm autograft face/neck/hf/g**   ~ follow-up period is 90 days, standard payment adjustment rules for multiple procedures apply, 150% payment adjustment for bilateral procedures does not apply, assistant surgeon may not be paid

15136   **Derm autograft, f/n/hf/g add-on**   ~ follow-up period included in another service, no payment adjustment rules for multiple procedures apply, 150% payment adjustment for

bilateral procedures does not apply, assistant surgeon may not be paid, +add-on code (list separately in addition to primary procedure)

15150   **Cult epidermal graft t/arm/leg**   ~ follow-up period is 90 days, standard payment adjustment rules for multiple procedures apply, 150% payment adjustment for bilateral procedures does not apply, assistant surgeon may not be paid

15151   **Cult epidermal graft t/a/l added**   ~ follow-up period included in another service, no payment adjustment rules for multiple procedures apply, 150% payment adjustment for bilateral procedures does not apply, assistant surgeon may not be paid, +add-on code (list separately in addition to primary procedure)

15152   **Cult epidermal graft t/a/l +%**   ~ follow-up period included in another service, no payment adjustment rules for multiple procedures apply, 150% payment adjustment for bilateral procedures does not apply, assistant surgeon may not be paid

15155   **Cult epidermal graft, f/n/hf/g**   ~ follow-up period is 90 days, standard payment adjustment rules for multiple procedures apply, 150% payment adjustment for bilateral procedures does not apply, assistant surgeon may not be paid

15156   **Cult epidermal graft f/n/hands/feet/genitals add-on**
~ follow-up period included in another service, no payment adjustment rules for multiple procedures apply, 150% payment adjustment for bilateral procedures does not apply, assistant surgeon may not be paid, +add-on code (list separately in addition to primary procedure)

15157   **Cult epidermal graft f/n/hands/feet/genitals +%**
~ follow-up period included in another service, no payment adjustment rules for multiple procedures apply, 150% payment adjustment for bilateral procedures does not apply, assistant surgeon may not be paid

15170   **Acellular graft trunk/arms/legs**   ~ follow-up period is 90 days, standard payment adjustment rules for multiple procedures apply, 150% payment adjustment for bilateral procedures does not apply, assistant surgeon may not be paid

15171   **Acellular graft t/arm/leg, add-on**   ~ follow-up period included in another service, no payment adjustment rules for multiple procedures apply, 150% payment adjustment for bilateral procedures does not apply, assistant surgeon may not be paid, +add-on code (list separately in addition to primary procedure)

15175   **Acellular graft, f/n/hf/g**   ~ follow-up period is 90 days, standard payment adjustment rules for multiple procedures apply, 150% payment adjustment for bilateral procedures does not apply, assistant surgeon may not be paid

15176   **Acellular graft, f/n/hf/g, add-on**   ~ follow-up period included in another service, no payment adjustment rules for multiple procedures apply, 150% payment adjustment for

bilateral procedures does not apply, assistant surgeon may not be paid, +add-on code (list separately in addition to primary procedure)

15200 **Skin full graft, trunk** ~ follow-up period is 90 days, standard payment adjustment rules for multiple procedures apply, 150% payment adjustment for bilateral procedures does not apply, assistant surgeon may not be paid

15201 **Skin full graft trunk, add-on** ~ follow-up period included in another service, no payment adjustment rules for multiple procedures apply, 150% payment adjustment for bilateral procedures does not apply, payment for assistant surgeon subject to documentation of medical necessity, +add-on code (list separately in addition to primary procedure)

15220 **Skin full graft scalp/arm/leg** ~ follow-up period is 90 days, standard payment adjustment rules for multiple procedures apply, 150% payment adjustment for bilateral procedures does not apply, assistant surgeon may not be paid

15221 **Skin full graft, add-on** ~ follow-up period included in another service, no payment adjustment rules for multiple procedures apply, 150% payment adjustment for bilateral procedures does not apply, assistant surgeon may not be paid, +add-on code (list separately in addition to primary procedure)

15240 **Skin full graft face/genital/hf** ~ follow-up period is 90 days, standard payment adjustment rules for multiple procedures apply, 150% payment adjustment for bilateral procedures does not apply, assistant surgeon may not be paid

15241 **Skin full graft, add-on** ~ follow-up period included in another service, no payment adjustment rules for multiple procedures apply, 150% payment adjustment for bilateral procedures does not apply, assistant surgeon may not be paid, +add-on code (list separately in addition to primary procedure)

15260 **Skin full graft ear/eye/nose & lips** ~ follow-up period is 90 days, standard payment adjustment rules for multiple procedures apply, 150% payment adjustment for bilateral procedures does not apply, assistant surgeon may not be paid

15261 **Skin full graft, add-on** ~ follow-up period included in another service, no payment adjustment rules for multiple procedures apply, 150% payment adjustment for bilateral procedures does not apply, assistant surgeon may not be paid, +add-on code (list separately in addition to primary procedure)

15300 **Apply skin allograft, t/arm/lg** ~ follow-up period is 90 days, standard payment adjustment rules for multiple procedures apply, 150% payment adjustment for bilateral procedures does not apply, assistant surgeon may not be paid

15301 **Apply skin allograft t/a/l added** ~ follow-up period included in another service, no payment adjustment rules for multiple procedures apply, 150% payment adjustment for

bilateral procedures does not apply, assistant surgeon may not be paid, +add-on code (list separately in addition to primary procedure)

15320   **Apply skin allograft f/n/hf/g**   ~ follow-up period is 90 days, standard payment adjustment rules for multiple procedures apply, 150% payment adjustment for bilateral procedures does not apply, assistant surgeon may not be paid

15321   **Apply skin allograft f/n/hands/feet/genitals add**
~ follow-up period included in another service, no payment adjustment rules for multiple procedures apply, 150% payment adjustment for bilateral procedures does not apply, assistant surgeon may not be paid, +add-on code (list separately in addition to primary procedure)

15330   **Apply acellular allograft t/arm/leg**   ~ follow-up period is 90 days, standard payment adjustment rules for multiple procedures apply, 150% payment adjustment for bilateral procedures does not apply, assistant surgeon may not be paid

15331   **Apply acellular graft t/a/l, add-on**   ~ follow-up period included in another service, no payment adjustment rules for multiple procedures apply, 150% payment adjustment for bilateral procedures does not apply, assistant surgeon may not be paid, +add-on code (list separately in addition to primary procedure)

15335   **Apply acellular graft, f/n/hf/g**   ~ follow-up period is 90 days, standard payment adjustment rules for multiple procedures apply, 150% payment adjustment for bilateral procedures does not apply, assistant surgeon may not be paid

15336   **Apply acellular graft f/n/hf/g add**   ~ follow-up period included in another service, no payment adjustment rules for multiple procedures apply, 150% payment adjustment for bilateral procedures does not apply, assistant surgeon may not be paid, +add-on code (list separately in addition to primary procedure)

15340   **Apply cult skin substitute**   ~ follow-up period is 10 days, standard payment adjustment rules for multiple procedures apply, 150% payment adjustment for bilateral procedures does not apply, assistant surgeon may not be paid

15341   **Apply cult skin sub, add-on**   ~ follow-up period included in another service, no payment adjustment rules for multiple procedures apply, 150% payment adjustment for bilateral procedures does not apply, assistant surgeon may not be paid, +add-on code (list separately in addition to primary procedure)

15360   **Apply cult derm sub, t/a/l**   ~ follow-up period is 90 days, standard payment adjustment rules for multiple procedures apply, 150% payment adjustment for bilateral procedures does not apply, assistant surgeon may not be paid

15361   **Apply cult derm sub t/a/l add**   ~ follow-up period included in another service, no payment adjustment rules for multiple procedures apply, 150% payment adjustment for bilateral procedures does not apply, assistant surgeon may not be paid, +add-on code (list separately in addition to primary procedure)

15365   **Apply cult derm sub f/n/hf/g**   ~ follow-up period is 90 days, standard payment adjustment rules for multiple procedures apply, 150% payment adjustment for bilateral procedures does not apply, assistant surgeon may not be paid

15366   **Apply cult derm f/hf/g add**   ~ follow-up period included in another service, no payment adjustment rules for multiple procedures apply, 150% payment adjustment for bilateral procedures does not apply, assistant surgeon may not be paid, +add-on code (list separately in addition to primary procedure)

15400   **Apply skin xenograft, t/a/l**   ~ follow-up period is 90 days, standard payment adjustment rules for multiple procedures apply, 150% payment adjustment for bilateral procedures does not apply, assistant surgeon may not be paid

15401   **Apply skin xenograft t/a/l add**   ~ follow-up period included in another service, no payment adjustment rules for multiple procedures apply, 150% payment adjustment for bilateral procedures does not apply, assistant surgeon may not be paid, +add-on code (list separately in addition to primary procedure)

15420   **Apply skin xenograft, f/n/hf/g**   ~ follow-up period is 90 days, standard payment adjustment rules for multiple procedures apply, 150% payment adjustment for bilateral procedures does not apply, assistant surgeon may not be paid

15421   **Apply skin graft f/n/hf/g add**   ~ follow-up period included in another service, no payment adjustment rules for multiple procedures apply, 150% payment adjustment for bilateral procedures does not apply, assistant surgeon may not be paid

15430   **Apply acellular xenograft**   ~ follow-up period is 90 days, standard payment adjustment rules for multiple procedures apply, 150% payment adjustment for bilateral procedures does not apply, assistant surgeon may not be paid, +add-on code (list separately in addition to primary procedure)

15431   **Apply acellular xenograft add**   ~ follow-up period included in another service, no payment adjustment rules for multiple procedures apply, 150% payment adjustment for bilateral procedures does not apply, payment for assistant surgeon subject to documentation of medical necessity, +add-on code (list separately in addition to primary procedure)

Flaps (Skin and/or Deep Tissues)

15570   **Form skin pedicle flap**   ~ follow-up period is 90 days, standard payment adjustment rules for multiple procedures apply, 150% payment adjustment for bilateral procedures does not apply, assistant surgeon may not be paid

15572   **Form skin pedicle flap**   ~ follow-up period is 90 days, standard payment adjustment rules for multiple procedures apply, 150% payment adjustment for bilateral procedures does not apply, assistant surgeon may not be paid

15574   **Form skin pedicle flap**   ~ follow-up period is 90 days, standard payment adjustment rules for multiple procedures apply, 150% payment adjustment for bilateral procedures does not apply, assistant surgeon may not be paid

15576   **Form skin pedicle flap**   ~ follow-up period is 90 days, standard payment adjustment rules for multiple procedures apply, 150% payment adjustment for bilateral procedures does not apply, assistant surgeon may not be paid

15600   **Skin graft**   ~ follow-up period is 90 days, standard payment adjustment rules for multiple procedures apply, 150% payment adjustment for bilateral procedures does not apply, payment for assistant surgeon subject to documentation of medical necessity

15610   **Skin graft**   ~ follow-up period is 90 days, standard payment adjustment rules for multiple procedures apply, 150% payment adjustment for bilateral procedures does not apply, payment for assistant surgeon subject to documentation of medical necessity

15620   **Skin graft**   ~ follow-up period is 90 days, standard payment adjustment rules for multiple procedures apply, 150% payment adjustment for bilateral procedures does not apply, assistant surgeon may not be paid

15630   **Skin graft**   ~ follow-up period is 90 days, standard payment adjustment rules for multiple procedures apply, 150% payment adjustment for bilateral procedures does not apply, assistant surgeon may not be paid

15650   **Transfer skin pedicle flap**   ~ follow-up period is 90 days, standard payment adjustment rules for multiple procedures apply, 150% payment adjustment for bilateral procedures does not apply, payment for assistant surgeon subject to documentation of medical necessity

15731   **Forehead flap w/vasc pedicle**   ~ follow-up period is 90 days, standard payment adjustment rules for multiple procedures apply, 150% payment adjustment for bilateral procedures does not apply, payment for assistant surgeon subject to documentation of medical necessity

15732   **Muscle-skin graft, head/neck**   ~ follow-up period is 90 days, standard payment adjustment rules for multiple procedures apply, 150% payment adjustment for bilateral procedures does not apply, assistant surgeon may be paid

15734   **Muscle-skin graft, trunk**   ~ follow-up period is 90 days, standard payment adjustment rules for multiple procedures apply, 150% payment adjustment for bilateral procedures does not apply, assistant surgeon may be paid

15736   **Muscle-skin graft, arm**   ~ follow-up period is 90 days, standard payment adjustment rules for multiple procedures apply, 150% payment adjustment for bilateral procedures does not apply, assistant surgeon may not be paid

15738   **Muscle-skin graft, leg**   ~ follow-up period is 90 days, standard payment adjustment rules for multiple procedures apply, 150% payment adjustment for bilateral procedures does not apply, assistant surgeon may be paid

15740   **Island pedicle flap graft**   ~ follow-up period is 90 days, standard payment adjustment rules for multiple procedures apply, 150% payment adjustment for bilateral procedures does not apply, assistant surgeon may not be paid

15750   **Neurovascular pedicle graft**   ~ follow-up period is 90 days, standard payment adjustment rules for multiple procedures apply, 150% payment adjustment for bilateral procedures does not apply, assistant surgeon may be paid

15756   **Free myocutaneous/skin flap microvasc** ~ follow-up period is 90 days, standard payment adjustment rules for multiple procedures apply, 150% payment adjustment for bilateral procedures does not apply, assistant surgeon may be paid

15757   **Free skin flap, microvasc**   ~ follow-up period is 90 days, standard payment adjustment rules for multiple procedures apply, 150% payment adjustment for bilateral procedures does not apply, assistant surgeon may be paid

15758   **Free fascial flap, microvasc**   ~ follow-up period is 90 days, standard payment adjustment rules for multiple procedures apply, 150% payment adjustment for bilateral procedures does not apply, assistant surgeon may be paid

15760   **Composite skin graft**   ~ follow-up period is 90 days, standard payment adjustment rules for multiple procedures apply, 150% payment adjustment for bilateral procedures does not apply, assistant surgeon may not be paid

15770   **Derma-fat-fascia graft**   ~ follow-up period is 90 days, standard payment adjustment rules for multiple procedures apply, 150% payment adjustment for bilateral procedures does not apply, assistant surgeon may be paid

15775   **Hair transplant punch grafts**   ~ restricted coverage - special coverage rules apply, endoscopies or minor procedure - E/M services on the same day generally not paid, standard payment adjustment rules for multiple procedures apply, 150% payment adjustment for bilateral procedures does not apply, payment for assistant surgeon subject to documentation of medical necessity

15776   **Hair transplant punch grafts**   ~ restricted coverage - special coverage rules apply, endoscopies or minor procedure - E/M services on the same day generally not paid, standard payment adjustment rules for multiple procedures apply, 150% payment adjustment for bilateral procedures does not apply, payment for assistant surgeon subject to documentation of medical necessity

15780   **Abrasion treat skin**   ~ follow-up period is 90 days, standard payment adjustment rules for multiple procedures apply, 150% payment adjustment for

bilateral procedures does not apply, payment for assistant surgeon subject to documentation of medical necessity

15781 **Abrasion treat skin** ~ follow-up period is 90 days, standard payment adjustment rules for multiple procedures apply, 150% payment adjustment for bilateral procedures does not apply, assistant surgeon may not be paid

15782 **Abrasion treat skin** ~ follow-up period is 90 days, standard payment adjustment rules for multiple procedures apply, 150% payment adjustment for bilateral procedures does not apply, payment for assistant surgeon subject to documentation of medical necessity

15783 **Abrasion treat skin** ~ follow-up period is 90 days, standard payment adjustment rules for multiple procedures apply, 150% payment adjustment for bilateral procedures does not apply, payment for assistant surgeon subject to documentation of medical necessity

15786 **Abrasion, lesion, single** ~ follow-up period is 10 days, standard payment adjustment rules for multiple procedures apply, 150% payment adjustment for bilateral procedures does not apply, assistant surgeon may not be paid

15787 **Abrasion, lesions, add-on** ~ follow-up period included in another service, no payment adjustment rules for multiple procedures apply, 150% payment adjustment for bilateral procedures does not apply, assistant surgeon may not be paid, +add-on code (list separately in addition to primary procedure)

15788 **Chemical peel, face, epidermal** ~ restricted coverage - special coverage rules apply, follow-up period is 90 days, standard payment adjustment rules for multiple procedures apply, 150% payment adjustment for bilateral procedures does not apply, assistant surgeon may not be paid

15789 **Chemical peel, face, dermal** ~ restricted coverage - special coverage rules apply, follow-up period is 90 days, standard payment adjustment rules for multiple procedures apply, 150% payment adjustment for bilateral procedures does not apply, assistant surgeon may not be paid

15792 **Chemical peel, nonfacial** ~ restricted coverage - special coverage rules apply, follow-up period is 90 days, standard payment adjustment rules for multiple procedures apply, 150% payment adjustment for bilateral procedures does not apply, payment for assistant surgeon subject to documentation of medical necessity

15793 **Chemical peel, nonfacial** ~ follow-up period is 90 days, standard payment adjustment rules for multiple procedures apply, 150% payment adjustment for bilateral procedures does not apply, payment for assistant surgeon subject to documentation of medical necessity

15819   **Plastic surgery, neck**   ~ follow-up period is 90 days, standard payment adjustment rules for multiple procedures apply, 150% payment adjustment for bilateral procedures does not apply, payment for assistant surgeon subject to documentation of medical necessity

15820   **Revise lower eyelid**   ~ follow-up period is 90 days, standard payment adjustment rules for multiple procedures apply, 150% payment adjustment for bilateral procedures applies, payment for assistant surgeon subject to documentation of medical necessity

15821   **Revise lower eyelid**   ~ follow-up period is 90 days, standard payment adjustment rules for multiple procedures apply, 150% payment adjustment for bilateral procedures applies, payment for assistant surgeon subject to documentation of medical necessity

15822   **Revise upper eyelid**   ~ follow-up period is 90 days, standard payment adjustment rules for multiple procedures apply, 150% payment adjustment for bilateral procedures applies, assistant surgeon may not be paid

15823   **Revise upper eyelid**   ~ follow-up period is 90 days, standard payment adjustment rules for multiple procedures apply, 150% payment adjustment for bilateral procedures applies, assistant surgeon may not be paid

15824   **Remove forehead wrinkles**   ~ restricted coverage - special coverage rules apply, endoscopies or minor procedure - E/M services on the same day generally not paid, standard payment adjustment rules for multiple procedures apply, 150% payment adjustment for bilateral procedures applies, payment for assistant surgeon subject to documentation of medical necessity

15825   **Remove neck wrinkles**   ~ restricted coverage - special coverage rules apply, endoscopies or minor procedure - E/M services on the same day generally not paid, standard payment adjustment rules for multiple procedures apply, 150% payment adjustment for bilateral procedures applies, payment for assistant surgeon subject to documentation of medical necessity

15826   **Remove brow wrinkles**   ~ restricted coverage - special coverage rules apply, endoscopies or minor procedure - E/M services on the same day generally not paid, standard payment adjustment rules for multiple procedures apply, 150% payment adjustment for bilateral procedures applies, payment for assistant surgeon subject to documentation of medical necessity

15828   **Remove face wrinkles**   ~ restricted coverage - special coverage rules apply, endoscopies or minor procedure - E/M services on the same day generally not paid, standard payment adjustment rules for multiple procedures apply, 150% payment adjustment for bilateral procedures applies, payment for assistant surgeon subject to documentation of medical necessity

15829   **Remove skin wrinkles**   ~ restricted coverage - special coverage rules
apply, endoscopies or minor procedure - E/M services on the same day generally not paid,
standard payment adjustment rules for multiple procedures apply, 150% payment
adjustment for bilateral procedures applies, payment for assistant surgeon subject to
documentation of medical necessity

15830   **Excise skin abdomen**   ~ restricted coverage - special coverage rules
apply, follow-up period is 90 days, standard payment adjustment rules for multiple
procedures apply, 150% payment adjustment for bilateral procedures does not apply,
assistant surgeon may be paid

15832   **Excise excessive skin tissue**   ~ follow-up period is 90 days, standard
payment adjustment rules for multiple procedures apply, 150% payment adjustment for
bilateral procedures does not apply, assistant surgeon may be paid

15833   **Excise excessive skin tissue**   ~ follow-up period is 90 days, standard
payment adjustment rules for multiple procedures apply, 150% payment adjustment for
bilateral procedures does not apply, payment for assistant surgeon subject to
documentation of medical necessity

15834   **Excise excessive skin tissue**   ~ follow-up period is 90 days, standard
payment adjustment rules for multiple procedures apply, 150% payment adjustment for
bilateral procedures does not apply, payment for assistant surgeon subject to
documentation of medical necessity

15835   **Excise excessive skin tissue**   ~ follow-up period is 90 days, standard
payment adjustment rules for multiple procedures apply, 150% payment adjustment for
bilateral procedures does not apply, payment for assistant surgeon subject to
documentation of medical necessity

15836   **Excise excessive skin tissue**   ~ follow-up period is 90 days, standard
payment adjustment rules for multiple procedures apply, 150% payment adjustment for
bilateral procedures does not apply, payment for assistant surgeon subject to
documentation of medical necessity

15837   **Excise excessive skin tissue**   ~ follow-up period is 90 days, standard
payment adjustment rules for multiple procedures apply, 150% payment adjustment for
bilateral procedures does not apply, payment for assistant surgeon subject to
documentation of medical necessity

15838   **Excise excessive skin tissue**   ~ follow-up period is 90 days, standard
payment adjustment rules for multiple procedures apply, 150% payment adjustment for
bilateral procedures does not apply, payment for assistant surgeon subject to
documentation of medical necessity

15839   **Excise excessive skin tissue**   ~ follow-up period is 90 days, standard
payment adjustment rules for multiple procedures apply, 150% payment adjustment for

bilateral procedures does not apply, payment for assistant surgeon subject to documentation of medical necessity

15840 **Graft for face nerve palsy** ~ follow-up period is 90 days, standard payment adjustment rules for multiple procedures apply, 150% payment adjustment for bilateral procedures does not apply, assistant surgeon may not be paid

15841 **Graft for face nerve palsy** ~ follow-up period is 90 days, standard payment adjustment rules for multiple procedures apply, 150% payment adjustment for bilateral procedures does not apply, assistant surgeon may be paid

15842 **Flap for face nerve palsy** ~ follow-up period is 90 days, standard payment adjustment rules for multiple procedures apply, 150% payment adjustment for bilateral procedures does not apply, assistant surgeon may be paid

15845 **Skin and muscle repair, face** ~ follow-up period is 90 days, standard payment adjustment rules for multiple procedures apply, 150% payment adjustment for bilateral procedures does not apply, assistant surgeon may be paid

15847 **Excise skin abdomen, add-on** ~ medicare carrier determines global period, standard payment adjustment rules for multiple procedures apply, 150% payment adjustment for bilateral procedures does not apply, assistant surgeon may be paid, +add-on code (list separately in addition to primary procedure)

15850 **Remove sutures** ~ bundled code - no separate payment made, multiple procedure concept does not apply, bilateral surgery concept does not apply, assistant surgery concept does not apply

15851 **Remove sutures** ~ endoscopies or minor procedure - E/M services on the same day generally not paid, standard payment adjustment rules for multiple procedures apply, 150% payment adjustment for bilateral procedures does not apply, assistant surgeon may not be paid

15852 **Dressing change not for burn** ~ endoscopies or minor procedure - E/M services on the same day generally not paid, standard payment adjustment rules for multiple procedures apply, 150% payment adjustment for bilateral procedures does not apply, assistant surgeon may not be paid

15860 **Test for blood flow in graft** ~ endoscopies or minor procedure - E/M services on the same day generally not paid, standard payment adjustment rules for multiple procedures apply, 150% payment adjustment for bilateral procedures does not apply, payment for assistant surgeon subject to documentation of medical necessity

15876 **Suction assisted lipectomy** ~ restricted coverage - special coverage rules apply, endoscopies or minor procedure - E/M services on the same day generally not paid, standard payment adjustment rules for multiple procedures apply, 150% payment

adjustment for bilateral procedures does not apply, payment for assistant surgeon subject to documentation of medical necessity

15877   Suction assisted lipectomy   ~ restricted coverage - special coverage rules apply, endoscopies or minor procedure - E/M services on the same day generally not paid, standard payment adjustment rules for multiple procedures apply, 150% payment adjustment for bilateral procedures does not apply, payment for assistant surgeon subject to documentation of medical necessity

15878   Suction assisted lipectomy   ~ restricted coverage - special coverage rules apply, endoscopies or minor procedure - E/M services on the same day generally not paid, standard payment adjustment rules for multiple procedures apply, 150% payment adjustment for bilateral procedures does not apply, payment for assistant surgeon subject to documentation of medical necessity

15879   Suction assisted lipectomy   ~ restricted coverage - special coverage rules apply, endoscopies or minor procedure - E/M services on the same day generally not paid, standard payment adjustment rules for multiple procedures apply, 150% payment adjustment for bilateral procedures does not apply, payment for assistant surgeon subject to documentation of medical necessity

Pressure Ulcers (Decubitus Ulcers)

15920   Remove tail bone ulcer   ~ follow-up period is 90 days, standard payment adjustment rules for multiple procedures apply, 150% payment adjustment for bilateral procedures does not apply, payment for assistant surgeon subject to documentation of medical necessity

15922   Remove tail bone ulcer   ~ follow-up period is 90 days, standard payment adjustment rules for multiple procedures apply, 150% payment adjustment for bilateral procedures does not apply, assistant surgeon may be paid

15931   Remove sacrum pressure sore   ~ follow-up period is 90 days, standard payment adjustment rules for multiple procedures apply, 150% payment adjustment for bilateral procedures does not apply, assistant surgeon may not be paid

15933   Remove sacrum pressure sore   ~ follow-up period is 90 days, standard payment adjustment rules for multiple procedures apply, 150% payment adjustment for bilateral procedures does not apply, payment for assistant surgeon subject to documentation of medical necessity

15934   Remove sacrum pressure sore   ~ follow-up period is 90 days, standard payment adjustment rules for multiple procedures apply, 150% payment adjustment for bilateral procedures does not apply, assistant surgeon may not be paid

15935   **Remove sacrum pressure sore**   ~ follow-up period is 90 days, standard payment adjustment rules for multiple procedures apply, 150% payment adjustment for bilateral procedures does not apply, assistant surgeon may be paid

15936   **Remove sacrum pressure sore**   ~ follow-up period is 90 days, standard payment adjustment rules for multiple procedures apply, 150% payment adjustment for bilateral procedures does not apply, assistant surgeon may not be paid

15937   **Remove sacrum pressure sore**   ~ follow-up period is 90 days, standard payment adjustment rules for multiple procedures apply, 150% payment adjustment for bilateral procedures does not apply, assistant surgeon may be paid

15940   **Remove hip pressure sore**   ~ follow-up period is 90 days, standard payment adjustment rules for multiple procedures apply, 150% payment adjustment for bilateral procedures does not apply, assistant surgeon may not be paid

15941   **Remove hip pressure sore**   ~ follow-up period is 90 days, standard payment adjustment rules for multiple procedures apply, 150% payment adjustment for bilateral procedures does not apply, payment for assistant surgeon subject to documentation of medical necessity

15944   **Remove hip pressure sore**   ~ follow-up period is 90 days, standard payment adjustment rules for multiple procedures apply, 150% payment adjustment for bilateral procedures does not apply, payment for assistant surgeon subject to documentation of medical necessity

15945   **Remove hip pressure sore**   ~ follow-up period is 90 days, standard payment adjustment rules for multiple procedures apply, 150% payment adjustment for bilateral procedures does not apply, payment for assistant surgeon subject to documentation of medical necessity

15946   **Remove hip pressure sore**   ~ follow-up period is 90 days, standard payment adjustment rules for multiple procedures apply, 150% payment adjustment for bilateral procedures does not apply, assistant surgeon may be paid

15950   **Remove thigh pressure sore**   ~ follow-up period is 90 days, standard payment adjustment rules for multiple procedures apply, 150% payment adjustment for bilateral procedures does not apply, assistant surgeon may not be paid

15951   **Remove thigh pressure sore**   ~ follow-up period is 90 days, standard payment adjustment rules for multiple procedures apply, 150% payment adjustment for bilateral procedures does not apply, payment for assistant surgeon subject to documentation of medical necessity

15952   **Remove thigh pressure sore**   ~ follow-up period is 90 days, standard payment adjustment rules for multiple procedures apply, 150% payment adjustment for bilateral procedures does not apply, assistant surgeon may be paid

15953   **Remove thigh pressure sore**   ~ follow-up period is 90 days, standard payment adjustment rules for multiple procedures apply, 150% payment adjustment for bilateral procedures does not apply, assistant surgeon may not be paid

15956   **Remove thigh pressure sore**   ~ follow-up period is 90 days, standard payment adjustment rules for multiple procedures apply, 150% payment adjustment for bilateral procedures does not apply, assistant surgeon may not be paid

15958   **Remove thigh pressure sore**   ~ follow-up period is 90 days, standard payment adjustment rules for multiple procedures apply, 150% payment adjustment for bilateral procedures does not apply, assistant surgeon may be paid

15999   **Remove pressure sore**   ~ medicare carrier determines global period, standard payment adjustment rules for multiple procedures apply, 150% payment adjustment for bilateral procedures does not apply, payment for assistant surgeon subject to documentation of medical necessity

16000   **Initial treat burn(s)**   ~ endoscopies or minor procedure - E/M services on the same day generally not paid, standard payment adjustment rules for multiple procedures apply, 150% payment adjustment for bilateral procedures does not apply, assistant surgeon may not be paid

16020   **Dress/debride p-thick burn, s**   ~ endoscopies or minor procedure - E/M services on the same day generally not paid, standard payment adjustment rules for multiple procedures apply, 150% payment adjustment for bilateral procedures does not apply, assistant surgeon may not be paid

16025   **Dress/debride p-thick burn, m**   ~ endoscopies or minor procedure - E/M services on the same day generally not paid, standard payment adjustment rules for multiple procedures apply, 150% payment adjustment for bilateral procedures does not apply, assistant surgeon may not be paid

16030   **Dress/debride p-thick burn, l**   ~ endoscopies or minor procedure - E/M services on the same day generally not paid, standard payment adjustment rules for multiple procedures apply, 150% payment adjustment for bilateral procedures does not apply, assistant surgeon may not be paid

16035   **Incise burn scab, initial**   ~ follow-up period is 90 days, standard payment adjustment rules for multiple procedures apply, 150% payment adjustment for bilateral procedures does not apply, assistant surgeon may not be paid

16036   **Escharotomy; added incision**   ~ follow-up period included in another service, no payment adjustment rules for multiple procedures apply, 150% payment adjustment for bilateral procedures does not apply, assistant surgeon may not be paid, +add-on code (list separately in addition to primary procedure)

Destruction

17000   **Destroy premalig lesion**   ~ follow-up period is 10 days, standard payment adjustment rules for multiple procedures apply, 150% payment adjustment for bilateral procedures does not apply, assistant surgeon may not be paid

17003   **Destroy premalig les, 2-14**   ~ follow-up period included in another service, no payment adjustment rules for multiple procedures apply, 150% payment adjustment for bilateral procedures does not apply, assistant surgeon may not be paid

17004   **Destroy premalig lesions 15+**   ~ follow-up period is 10 days, no payment adjustment rules for multiple procedures apply, 150% payment adjustment for bilateral procedures does not apply, assistant surgeon may not be paid

17106   **Destroy skin lesions**   ~ follow-up period is 90 days, standard payment adjustment rules for multiple procedures apply, 150% payment adjustment for bilateral procedures does not apply, assistant surgeon may not be paid

17107   **Destroy skin lesions**   ~ follow-up period is 90 days, standard payment adjustment rules for multiple procedures apply, 150% payment adjustment for bilateral procedures does not apply, assistant surgeon may not be paid

17108   **Destroy skin lesions**   ~ follow-up period is 90 days, standard payment adjustment rules for multiple procedures apply, 150% payment adjustment for bilateral procedures does not apply, payment for assistant surgeon subject to documentation of medical necessity

17110   **Destroy b9 lesion, 1-14**   ~ follow-up period is 10 days, standard payment adjustment rules for multiple procedures apply, 150% payment adjustment for bilateral procedures does not apply, assistant surgeon may not be paid

17111   **Destroy lesion, 15 or more**   ~ follow-up period is 10 days, standard payment adjustment rules for multiple procedures apply, 150% payment adjustment for bilateral procedures does not apply, assistant surgeon may not be paid

17250   **Chemical cautery, tissue**   ~ endoscopies or minor procedure - E/M services on the same day generally not paid, standard payment adjustment rules for multiple procedures apply, 150% payment adjustment for bilateral procedures does not apply, assistant surgeon may not be paid

17260   **Destroy skin lesions**   ~ follow-up period is 10 days, standard payment adjustment rules for multiple procedures apply, 150% payment adjustment for bilateral procedures does not apply, assistant surgeon may not be paid

17261   **Destroy skin lesions**   ~ follow-up period is 10 days, standard payment adjustment rules for multiple procedures apply, 150% payment adjustment for bilateral procedures does not apply, assistant surgeon may not be paid

17262   **Destroy skin lesions**   ~ follow-up period is 10 days, standard
payment adjustment rules for multiple procedures apply, 150% payment adjustment for
bilateral procedures does not apply, assistant surgeon may not be paid

17263   **Destroy skin lesions**   ~ follow-up period is 10 days, standard
payment adjustment rules for multiple procedures apply, 150% payment adjustment for
bilateral procedures does not apply, assistant surgeon may not be paid

17264   **Destroy skin lesions**   ~ follow-up period is 10 days, standard
payment adjustment rules for multiple procedures apply, 150% payment adjustment for
bilateral procedures does not apply, assistant surgeon may not be paid

17266   **Destroy skin lesions**   ~ follow-up period is 10 days, standard
payment adjustment rules for multiple procedures apply, 150% payment adjustment for
bilateral procedures does not apply, assistant surgeon may not be paid

17270   **Destroy skin lesions**   ~ follow-up period is 10 days, standard
payment adjustment rules for multiple procedures apply, 150% payment adjustment for
bilateral procedures does not apply, assistant surgeon may not be paid

17271   **Destroy skin lesions**   ~ follow-up period is 10 days, standard
payment adjustment rules for multiple procedures apply, 150% payment adjustment for
bilateral procedures does not apply, assistant surgeon may not be paid

17272   **Destroy skin lesions**   ~ follow-up period is 10 days, standard
payment adjustment rules for multiple procedures apply, 150% payment adjustment for
bilateral procedures does not apply, assistant surgeon may not be paid

17273   **Destroy skin lesions**   ~ follow-up period is 10 days, standard
payment adjustment rules for multiple procedures apply, 150% payment adjustment for
bilateral procedures does not apply, assistant surgeon may not be paid

17274   **Destroy skin lesions**   ~ follow-up period is 10 days, standard
payment adjustment rules for multiple procedures apply, 150% payment adjustment for
bilateral procedures does not apply, assistant surgeon may not be paid

17276   **Destroy skin lesions**   ~ follow-up period is 10 days, standard
payment adjustment rules for multiple procedures apply, 150% payment adjustment for
bilateral procedures does not apply, assistant surgeon may not be paid

17280   **Destroy skin lesions**   ~ follow-up period is 10 days, standard
payment adjustment rules for multiple procedures apply, 150% payment adjustment for
bilateral procedures does not apply, assistant surgeon may not be paid

17281   **Destroy skin lesions**   ~ follow-up period is 10 days, standard
payment adjustment rules for multiple procedures apply, 150% payment adjustment for
bilateral procedures does not apply, assistant surgeon may not be paid

17282   **Destroy skin lesions**   ~ follow-up period is 10 days, standard payment adjustment rules for multiple procedures apply, 150% payment adjustment for bilateral procedures does not apply, assistant surgeon may not be paid

17283   **Destroy skin lesions**   ~ follow-up period is 10 days, standard payment adjustment rules for multiple procedures apply, 150% payment adjustment for bilateral procedures does not apply, assistant surgeon may not be paid

17284   **Destroy skin lesions**   ~ follow-up period is 10 days, standard payment adjustment rules for multiple procedures apply, 150% payment adjustment for bilateral procedures does not apply, assistant surgeon may not be paid

17286   **Destroy skin lesions**   ~ follow-up period is 10 days, standard payment adjustment rules for multiple procedures apply, 150% payment adjustment for bilateral procedures does not apply, assistant surgeon may not be paid

17311   **Mohs, 1 stage, h/n/hf/g**   ~ endoscopies or minor procedure - E/M services on the same day generally not paid, standard payment adjustment rules for multiple procedures apply, 150% payment adjustment for bilateral procedures does not apply, assistant surgeon may not be paid

17312   **Mohs added stage**   ~ follow-up period included in another service, no payment adjustment rules for multiple procedures apply, 150% payment adjustment for bilateral procedures does not apply, assistant surgeon may not be paid, +add-on code (list separately in addition to primary procedure)

17313   **Mohs, 1 stage, t/a/l**   ~ endoscopies or minor procedure - E/M services on the same day generally not paid, standard payment adjustment rules for multiple procedures apply, 150% payment adjustment for bilateral procedures does not apply, assistant surgeon may not be paid

17314   **Mohs, added stage, t/a/l**   ~ follow-up period included in another service, no payment adjustment rules for multiple procedures apply, 150% payment adjustment for bilateral procedures does not apply, assistant surgeon may not be paid, +add-on code (list separately in addition to primary procedure)

17315   **Mohs surg, added block**   ~ follow-up period included in another service, no payment adjustment rules for multiple procedures apply, 150% payment adjustment for bilateral procedures does not apply, assistant surgeon may not be paid, +add-on code (list separately in addition to primary procedure)

17340   **Cryotherapy of skin**   ~ follow-up period is 10 days, standard payment adjustment rules for multiple procedures apply, 150% payment adjustment for bilateral procedures does not apply, assistant surgeon may not be paid

17360   **Skin peel therapy**   ~ follow-up period is 10 days, standard payment adjustment rules for multiple procedures apply, 150% payment adjustment for bilateral procedures does not apply, assistant surgeon may not be paid

17380   **Hair remove by electrolysis**   ~ restricted coverage - special coverage rules apply, endoscopies or minor procedure - E/M services on the same day generally not paid, standard payment adjustment rules for multiple procedures apply, 150% payment adjustment for bilateral procedures does not apply, payment for assistant surgeon subject to documentation of medical necessity

17999   **Skin tissue procedure**   ~ medicare carrier determines global period, standard payment adjustment rules for multiple procedures apply, 150% payment adjustment for bilateral procedures does not apply, payment for assistant surgeon subject to documentation of medical necessity

Breast

19000   **Drain breast lesion**   ~ endoscopies or minor procedure - E/M services on the same day generally not paid, standard payment adjustment rules for multiple procedures apply, 150% payment adjustment for bilateral procedures does not apply, assistant surgeon may not be paid

19001   **Drain breast lesion, add-on**   ~ follow-up period included in another service, no payment adjustment rules for multiple procedures apply, 150% payment adjustment for bilateral procedures does not apply, assistant surgeon may not be paid, +add-on code (list separately in addition to primary procedure)

19020   **Incise breast lesion**   ~ follow-up period is 90 days, standard payment adjustment rules for multiple procedures apply, 150% payment adjustment for bilateral procedures applies, assistant surgeon may not be paid

19030   **Inject for breast x-ray**   ~ endoscopies or minor procedure - E/M services on the same day generally not paid, standard payment adjustment rules for multiple procedures apply, 150% payment adjustment for bilateral procedures applies, assistant surgeon may not be paid

19100   **Biopsy breast percutaneous w/o image**   ~ endoscopies or minor procedure - E/M services on the same day generally not paid, standard payment adjustment rules for multiple procedures apply, 150% payment adjustment for bilateral procedures applies, assistant surgeon may not be paid

19101   **Biopsy breast, open**   ~ follow-up period is 10 days, standard payment adjustment rules for multiple procedures apply, 150% payment adjustment for bilateral procedures applies, assistant surgeon may not be paid

19102   **Biopsy breast percutaneous w/image**   ~ endoscopies or minor procedure - E/M services on the same day generally not paid, standard payment adjustment rules for multiple

procedures apply, 150% payment adjustment for bilateral procedures applies, assistant surgeon may not be paid

19103   **Biopsy breast percutaneous w/device**   ~ endoscopies or minor procedure - E/M services on the same day generally not paid, standard payment adjustment rules for multiple procedures apply, 150% payment adjustment for bilateral procedures applies, assistant surgeon may not be paid

19105   **Cryosurgery ablate fa, each**   ~ endoscopies or minor procedure - E/M services on the same day generally not paid, standard payment adjustment rules for multiple procedures apply, 150% payment adjustment for bilateral procedures applies, assistant surgeon may not be paid

19110   **Nipple exploration**   ~ follow-up period is 90 days, standard payment adjustment rules for multiple procedures apply, 150% payment adjustment for bilateral procedures applies, assistant surgeon may not be paid

19112   **Excise breast duct fistula**   ~ follow-up period is 90 days, standard payment adjustment rules for multiple procedures apply, 150% payment adjustment for bilateral procedures applies, payment for assistant surgeon subject to documentation of medical necessity

19120   **Remove breast lesion**   ~ follow-up period is 90 days, standard payment adjustment rules for multiple procedures apply, 150% payment adjustment for bilateral procedures applies, assistant surgeon may not be paid

19125   **Excise breast lesion**   ~ follow-up period is 90 days, standard payment adjustment rules for multiple procedures apply, 150% payment adjustment for bilateral procedures applies, assistant surgeon may not be paid

19126   **Excise added breast lesion**   ~ follow-up period included in another service, no payment adjustment rules for multiple procedures apply, 150% payment adjustment for bilateral procedures does not apply, assistant surgeon may not be paid, +add-on code (list separately in addition to primary procedure)

19260   **Remove chest wall lesion**   ~ follow-up period is 90 days, standard payment adjustment rules for multiple procedures apply, 150% payment adjustment for bilateral procedures does not apply, assistant surgeon may be paid

19271   **Revise chest wall**   ~ follow-up period is 90 days, standard payment adjustment rules for multiple procedures apply, 150% payment adjustment for bilateral procedures does not apply, assistant surgeon may be paid

19272   **Extensive chest wall surgery**   ~ follow-up period is 90 days, standard payment adjustment rules for multiple procedures apply, 150% payment adjustment for bilateral procedures does not apply, assistant surgeon may be paid

19290   **Place needle wire, breast**   ~ endoscopies or minor procedure - E/M services on the same day generally not paid, standard payment adjustment rules for multiple procedures apply, 150% payment adjustment for bilateral procedures applies, assistant surgeon may not be paid

19291   **Place needle wire, breast**   ~ follow-up period included in another service, no payment adjustment rules for multiple procedures apply, 150% payment adjustment for bilateral procedures does not apply, payment for assistant surgeon subject to documentation of medical necessity

19295   **Place breast clip, percutaneous**   ~ follow-up period included in another service, no payment adjustment rules for multiple procedures apply, 150% payment adjustment for bilateral procedures does not apply, payment for assistant surgeon subject to documentation of medical necessity

19296   **Place po breast cath for radiation**   ~ endoscopies or minor procedure - E/M services on the same day generally not paid, standard payment adjustment rules for multiple procedures apply, 150% payment adjustment for bilateral procedures applies, payment for assistant surgeon subject to documentation of medical necessity

19297   **Place breast cath for radiation**   ~ follow-up period included in another service, no payment adjustment rules for multiple procedures apply, 150% payment adjustment for bilateral procedures does not apply, payment for assistant surgeon subject to documentation of medical necessity

19298   **Place breast radiation tube/caths**   ~ endoscopies or minor procedure - E/M services on the same day generally not paid, standard payment adjustment rules for multiple procedures apply, 150% payment adjustment for bilateral procedures applies, payment for assistant surgeon subject to documentation of medical necessity

19300   **Remove breast tissue**   ~ follow-up period is 90 days, standard payment adjustment rules for multiple procedures apply, 150% payment adjustment for bilateral procedures applies, assistant surgeon may not be paid

19301   **Partial mastectomy**   ~ follow-up period is 90 days, standard payment adjustment rules for multiple procedures apply, 150% payment adjustment for bilateral procedures applies, payment for assistant surgeon subject to documentation of medical necessity

19302   **Part mastectomy w/lymph node remove**   ~ follow-up period is 90 days, standard payment adjustment rules for multiple procedures apply, 150% payment adjustment for bilateral procedures applies, assistant surgeon may be paid

19303   **Mastectomy, simple, complete**   ~ follow-up period is 90 days, standard payment adjustment rules for multiple procedures apply, 150% payment adjustment for bilateral procedures applies, assistant surgeon may be paid

19304   **Mastectomy, subcutaneous**   ~ follow-up period is 90 days, standard payment adjustment rules for multiple procedures apply, 150% payment adjustment for bilateral procedures applies, assistant surgeon may be paid

19305   **Mastectomy, radical**   ~ follow-up period is 90 days, standard payment adjustment rules for multiple procedures apply, 150% payment adjustment for bilateral procedures applies, assistant surgeon may be paid

19306   **Mastectomy, radiation, urban type**   ~ follow-up period is 90 days, standard payment adjustment rules for multiple procedures apply, 150% payment adjustment for bilateral procedures applies, assistant surgeon may be paid

19307   **Mastectomy, mod radiation**   ~ follow-up period is 90 days, standard payment adjustment rules for multiple procedures apply, 150% payment adjustment for bilateral procedures applies, assistant surgeon may be paid

19316   **Suspend breast**   ~ follow-up period is 90 days, standard payment adjustment rules for multiple procedures apply, 150% payment adjustment for bilateral procedures applies, assistant surgeon may be paid

19318   **Reduce large breast**   ~ follow-up period is 90 days, standard payment adjustment rules for multiple procedures apply, 150% payment adjustment for bilateral procedures applies, assistant surgeon may be paid

19324   **Enlarge breast**   ~ follow-up period is 90 days, standard payment adjustment rules for multiple procedures apply, 150% payment adjustment for bilateral procedures applies, payment for assistant surgeon subject to documentation of medical necessity

19325   **Enlarge breast with implant**   ~ follow-up period is 90 days, standard payment adjustment rules for multiple procedures apply, 150% payment adjustment for bilateral procedures applies, payment for assistant surgeon subject to documentation of medical necessity

19328   **Remove breast implant**   ~ follow-up period is 90 days, standard payment adjustment rules for multiple procedures apply, 150% payment adjustment for bilateral procedures applies, assistant surgeon may not be paid

19330   **Remove implant material**   ~ follow-up period is 90 days, standard payment adjustment rules for multiple procedures apply, 150% payment adjustment for bilateral procedures applies, assistant surgeon may not be paid

19340   **Immediate breast prosthesis**   ~ follow-up period included in another service, standard payment adjustment rules for multiple procedures apply, 150% payment adjustment for bilateral procedures applies, assistant surgeon may not be paid

19342 **Delayed breast prosthesis** ~ follow-up period is 90 days, standard payment adjustment rules for multiple procedures apply, 150% payment adjustment for bilateral procedures applies, payment for assistant surgeon subject to documentation of medical necessity

19350 **Breast reconstruct** ~ follow-up period is 90 days, standard payment adjustment rules for multiple procedures apply, 150% payment adjustment for bilateral procedures applies, assistant surgeon may not be paid

19355 **Correct inverted nipple(s)** ~ follow-up period is 90 days, standard payment adjustment rules for multiple procedures apply, 150% payment adjustment for bilateral procedures applies, payment for assistant surgeon subject to documentation of medical necessity

19357 **Breast reconstruct** ~ follow-up period is 90 days, standard payment adjustment rules for multiple procedures apply, 150% payment adjustment for bilateral procedures applies, assistant surgeon may be paid

19361 **Breast reconstruct w/lat flap** ~ follow-up period is 90 days, standard payment adjustment rules for multiple procedures apply, 150% payment adjustment for bilateral procedures applies, assistant surgeon may be paid

19364 **Breast reconstruct** ~ follow-up period is 90 days, standard payment adjustment rules for multiple procedures apply, 150% payment adjustment for bilateral procedures applies, assistant surgeon may be paid

19366 **Breast reconstruct** ~ follow-up period is 90 days, standard payment adjustment rules for multiple procedures apply, 150% payment adjustment for bilateral procedures applies, assistant surgeon may be paid

19367 **Breast reconstruct** ~ follow-up period is 90 days, standard payment adjustment rules for multiple procedures apply, 150% payment adjustment for bilateral procedures applies, assistant surgeon may be paid

19368 **Breast reconstruct** ~ follow-up period is 90 days, standard payment adjustment rules for multiple procedures apply, 150% payment adjustment for bilateral procedures applies, assistant surgeon may be paid

19369 **Breast reconstruct** ~ follow-up period is 90 days, standard payment adjustment rules for multiple procedures apply, 150% payment adjustment for bilateral procedures applies, assistant surgeon may be paid

19370 **Surgery breast capsule** ~ follow-up period is 90 days, standard payment adjustment rules for multiple procedures apply, 150% payment adjustment for bilateral procedures applies, assistant surgeon may not be paid

19371   **Remove breast capsule**   ~ follow-up period is 90 days, standard payment adjustment rules for multiple procedures apply, 150% payment adjustment for bilateral procedures applies, assistant surgeon may not be paid

19380   **Revise breast reconstruct**   ~ follow-up period is 90 days, standard payment adjustment rules for multiple procedures apply, 150% payment adjustment for bilateral procedures applies, assistant surgeon may not be paid

19396   **Design custom breast implant**   ~ endoscopies or minor procedure - E/M services on the same day generally not paid, standard payment adjustment rules for multiple procedures apply, 150% payment adjustment for bilateral procedures applies, payment for assistant surgeon subject to documentation of medical necessity

19499   **Breast surgery procedure**   ~ medicare carrier determines global period, standard payment adjustment rules for multiple procedures apply, 150% payment adjustment for bilateral procedures applies, payment for assistant surgeon subject to documentation of medical necessity

MUSCULOSKELETAL SYSTEM

General

20000   **Incise abscess**   ~ follow-up period is 10 days, standard payment adjustment rules for multiple procedures apply, 150% payment adjustment for bilateral procedures does not apply, assistant surgeon may not be paid

20005   **Incise deep abscess**   ~ follow-up period is 10 days, standard payment adjustment rules for multiple procedures apply, 150% payment adjustment for bilateral procedures does not apply, assistant surgeon may not be paid

Wound exploration

20100   **Explore wound, neck**   ~ follow-up period is 10 days, standard payment adjustment rules for multiple procedures apply, 150% payment adjustment for bilateral procedures applies, assistant surgeon may be paid

20101   **Explore wound, chest**   ~ follow-up period is 10 days, standard payment adjustment rules for multiple procedures apply, 150% payment adjustment for bilateral procedures does not apply, assistant surgeon may not be paid

20102   **Explore wound, abdomen**   ~ follow-up period is 10 days, standard payment adjustment rules for multiple procedures apply, 150% payment adjustment for bilateral procedures does not apply, assistant surgeon may be paid

20103   **Explore wound, extremity**   ~ follow-up period is 10 days, standard payment adjustment rules for multiple procedures apply, 150% payment adjustment for

bilateral procedures does not apply, payment for assistant surgeon subject to documentation of medical necessity

20150 **Excise epiphyseal bar** ~ follow-up period is 90 days, standard payment adjustment rules for multiple procedures apply, 150% payment adjustment for bilateral procedures applies, assistant surgeon may be paid

20200 **Muscle biopsy** ~ endoscopies or minor procedure - E/M services on the same day generally not paid, standard payment adjustment rules for multiple procedures apply, 150% payment adjustment for bilateral procedures does not apply, assistant surgeon may not be paid

20205 **Deep muscle biopsy** ~ endoscopies or minor procedure - E/M services on the same day generally not paid, standard payment adjustment rules for multiple procedures apply, 150% payment adjustment for bilateral procedures does not apply, assistant surgeon may not be paid

20206 **Needle biopsy muscle** ~ endoscopies or minor procedure - E/M services on the same day generally not paid, standard payment adjustment rules for multiple procedures apply, 150% payment adjustment for bilateral procedures does not apply, assistant surgeon may not be paid

20220 **Bone biopsy trocar/needle** ~ endoscopies or minor procedure - E/M services on the same day generally not paid, standard payment adjustment rules for multiple procedures apply, 150% payment adjustment for bilateral procedures does not apply, assistant surgeon may not be paid

20225 **Bone biopsy trocar/needle** ~ endoscopies or minor procedure - E/M services on the same day generally not paid, standard payment adjustment rules for multiple procedures apply, 150% payment adjustment for bilateral procedures does not apply, assistant surgeon may not be paid

20240 **Bone biopsy excisional** ~ follow-up period is 10 days, standard payment adjustment rules for multiple procedures apply, 150% payment adjustment for bilateral procedures does not apply, assistant surgeon may not be paid

20245 **Bone biopsy excisional** ~ follow-up period is 10 days, standard payment adjustment rules for multiple procedures apply, 150% payment adjustment for bilateral procedures does not apply, assistant surgeon may not be paid

20250 **Open bone biopsy** ~ follow-up period is 10 days, standard payment adjustment rules for multiple procedures apply, 150% payment adjustment for bilateral procedures does not apply, assistant surgeon may not be paid

20251 **Open bone biopsy** ~ follow-up period is 10 days, standard payment adjustment rules for multiple procedures apply, 150% payment adjustment for bilateral procedures does not apply, assistant surgeon may be paid

20500   **Injection of sinus tract**   ~ follow-up period is 10 days, standard payment adjustment rules for multiple procedures apply, 150% payment adjustment for bilateral procedures does not apply, assistant surgeon may not be paid

20501   **Inject sinus tract for x-ray**   ~ endoscopies or minor procedure - E/M services on the same day generally not paid, standard payment adjustment rules for multiple procedures apply, 150% payment adjustment for bilateral procedures does not apply, assistant surgeon may not be paid

20520   **Remove foreign body**   ~ follow-up period is 10 days, standard payment adjustment rules for multiple procedures apply, 150% payment adjustment for bilateral procedures does not apply, assistant surgeon may not be paid

20525   **Remove foreign body**   ~ follow-up period is 10 days, standard payment adjustment rules for multiple procedures apply, 150% payment adjustment for bilateral procedures does not apply, assistant surgeon may not be paid

20526   **Therapeutic injection, carp tunnel**   ~ endoscopies or minor procedure - E/M services on the same day generally not paid, standard payment adjustment rules for multiple procedures apply, 150% payment adjustment for bilateral procedures applies, assistant surgeon may not be paid

20550   **Inject tendon sheath/ligament**   ~ endoscopies or minor procedure - E/M services on the same day generally not paid, standard payment adjustment rules for multiple procedures apply, 150% payment adjustment for bilateral procedures does not apply, assistant surgeon may not be paid

20551   **Inject tendon origin/insertion**   ~ endoscopies or minor procedure - E/M services on the same day generally not paid, standard payment adjustment rules for multiple procedures apply, 150% payment adjustment for bilateral procedures does not apply, assistant surgeon may not be paid

20552   **Inject trigger point, 1/2 muscle**   ~ endoscopies or minor procedure - E/M services on the same day generally not paid, standard payment adjustment rules for multiple procedures apply, 150% payment adjustment for bilateral procedures does not apply, assistant surgeon may not be paid

20553   **Inject trigger points, =/> 3**   ~ endoscopies or minor procedure - E/M services on the same day generally not paid, standard payment adjustment rules for multiple procedures apply, 150% payment adjustment for bilateral procedures does not apply, assistant surgeon may not be paid

20600   **Drain/inject, joint/bursa**   ~ endoscopies or minor procedure - E/M services on the same day generally not paid, standard payment adjustment rules for multiple procedures apply, 150% payment adjustment for bilateral procedures applies, assistant surgeon may not be paid

CPT codes and descriptions only copyright American Medical Association

20605   **Drain/inject, joint/bursa**   ~ endoscopies or minor procedure - E/M services on the same day generally not paid, standard payment adjustment rules for multiple procedures apply, 150% payment adjustment for bilateral procedures applies, assistant surgeon may not be paid

20610   **Drain/inject, joint/bursa**   ~ endoscopies or minor procedure - E/M services on the same day generally not paid, standard payment adjustment rules for multiple procedures apply, 150% payment adjustment for bilateral procedures applies, assistant surgeon may not be paid

20612   **Aspirate/inject ganglion cyst**   ~ endoscopies or minor procedure - E/M services on the same day generally not paid, standard payment adjustment rules for multiple procedures apply, 150% payment adjustment for bilateral procedures does not apply, assistant surgeon may not be paid

20615   **Treat bone cyst**   ~ follow-up period is 10 days, standard payment adjustment rules for multiple procedures apply, 150% payment adjustment for bilateral procedures does not apply, assistant surgeon may not be paid

20650   **Insert and remove bone pin**   ~ follow-up period is 10 days, standard payment adjustment rules for multiple procedures apply, 150% payment adjustment for bilateral procedures does not apply, assistant surgeon may not be paid

20660   **Apply, rem fixation device**   ~ endoscopies or minor procedure - E/M services on the same day generally not paid, no payment adjustment rules for multiple procedures apply, 150% payment adjustment for bilateral procedures does not apply, assistant surgeon may not be paid

20661   **Apply head brace**   ~ follow-up period is 90 days, standard payment adjustment rules for multiple procedures apply, 150% payment adjustment for bilateral procedures does not apply, assistant surgeon may not be paid

20662   **Apply pelvis brace**   ~ follow-up period is 90 days, standard payment adjustment rules for multiple procedures apply, 150% payment adjustment for bilateral procedures does not apply, payment for assistant surgeon subject to documentation of medical necessity

20663   **Apply thigh brace**   ~ follow-up period is 90 days, standard payment adjustment rules for multiple procedures apply, 150% payment adjustment for bilateral procedures does not apply, payment for assistant surgeon subject to documentation of medical necessity

20664   **Halo brace application**   ~ follow-up period is 90 days, standard payment adjustment rules for multiple procedures apply, 150% payment adjustment for bilateral procedures does not apply, assistant surgeon may not be paid

20665   **Remove fixation device**   ~ follow-up period is 10 days, standard payment adjustment rules for multiple procedures apply, 150% payment adjustment for bilateral procedures does not apply, payment for assistant surgeon subject to documentation of medical necessity

20670   **Remove support implant**   ~ follow-up period is 10 days, standard payment adjustment rules for multiple procedures apply, 150% payment adjustment for bilateral procedures does not apply, assistant surgeon may not be paid

20680   **Remove support implant**   ~ follow-up period is 90 days, standard payment adjustment rules for multiple procedures apply, 150% payment adjustment for bilateral procedures does not apply, payment for assistant surgeon subject to documentation of medical necessity

20690   **Apply bone fixation device**   ~ follow-up period is 90 days, standard payment adjustment rules for multiple procedures apply, 150% payment adjustment for bilateral procedures applies, assistant surgeon may not be paid

20692   **Apply bone fixation device**   ~ follow-up period is 90 days, standard payment adjustment rules for multiple procedures apply, 150% payment adjustment for bilateral procedures does not apply, assistant surgeon may be paid

20693   **Adjust bone fixation device**   ~ follow-up period is 90 days, standard payment adjustment rules for multiple procedures apply, 150% payment adjustment for bilateral procedures does not apply, assistant surgeon may not be paid

20694   **Remove bone fixation device**   ~ follow-up period is 90 days, standard payment adjustment rules for multiple procedures apply, 150% payment adjustment for bilateral procedures does not apply, assistant surgeon may not be paid

20802   **Replant arm, complete**   ~ follow-up period is 90 days, standard payment adjustment rules for multiple procedures apply, 150% payment adjustment for bilateral procedures applies, assistant surgeon may be paid

20805   **Replant forearm, complete**   ~ follow-up period is 90 days, standard payment adjustment rules for multiple procedures apply, 150% payment adjustment for bilateral procedures applies, assistant surgeon may be paid

20808   **Replant hand, complete**   ~ follow-up period is 90 days, standard payment adjustment rules for multiple procedures apply, 150% payment adjustment for bilateral procedures applies, assistant surgeon may be paid

20816   **Replant digit, complete**   ~ follow-up period is 90 days, standard payment adjustment rules for multiple procedures apply, 150% payment adjustment for bilateral procedures does not apply, assistant surgeon may be paid

20822   **Replant digit, complete**   ~ follow-up period is 90 days, standard payment adjustment rules for multiple procedures apply, 150% payment adjustment for bilateral procedures does not apply, assistant surgeon may be paid

20824   **Replant thumb, complete**   ~ follow-up period is 90 days, standard payment adjustment rules for multiple procedures apply, 150% payment adjustment for bilateral procedures applies, assistant surgeon may be paid

20827   **Replant thumb, complete**   ~ follow-up period is 90 days, standard payment adjustment rules for multiple procedures apply, 150% payment adjustment for bilateral procedures applies, assistant surgeon may be paid

20838   **Replant foot, complete**   ~ follow-up period is 90 days, standard payment adjustment rules for multiple procedures apply, 150% payment adjustment for bilateral procedures applies, assistant surgeon may be paid

20900   **Remove bone for graft**   ~ follow-up period is 90 days, standard payment adjustment rules for multiple procedures apply, 150% payment adjustment for bilateral procedures does not apply, assistant surgeon may be paid

20902   **Remove bone for graft**   ~ follow-up period is 90 days, standard payment adjustment rules for multiple procedures apply, 150% payment adjustment for bilateral procedures does not apply, assistant surgeon may be paid

20910   **Remove cartilage for graft**   ~ follow-up period is 90 days, standard payment adjustment rules for multiple procedures apply, 150% payment adjustment for bilateral procedures does not apply, payment for assistant surgeon subject to documentation of medical necessity

20912   **Remove cartilage for graft**   ~ follow-up period is 90 days, standard payment adjustment rules for multiple procedures apply, 150% payment adjustment for bilateral procedures does not apply, payment for assistant surgeon subject to documentation of medical necessity

20920   **Remove fascia for graft**   ~ follow-up period is 90 days, standard payment adjustment rules for multiple procedures apply, 150% payment adjustment for bilateral procedures does not apply, assistant surgeon may not be paid

20922   **Remove fascia for graft**   ~ follow-up period is 90 days, standard payment adjustment rules for multiple procedures apply, 150% payment adjustment for bilateral procedures does not apply, assistant surgeon may be paid

20924   **Remove tendon for graft**   ~ follow-up period is 90 days, standard payment adjustment rules for multiple procedures apply, 150% payment adjustment for bilateral procedures does not apply, assistant surgeon may be paid

20926   **Remove tissue for graft**   ~ follow-up period is 90 days, no payment adjustment rules for multiple procedures apply, 150% payment adjustment for bilateral procedures does not apply, assistant surgeon may not be paid

20930   **Spinal bone allograft**   ~ bundled code - no separate payment made, multiple procedure concept does not apply, bilateral surgery concept does not apply, assistant surgery concept does not apply

20931   **Spinal bone allograft**   ~ follow-up period included in another service, no payment adjustment rules for multiple procedures apply, 150% payment adjustment for bilateral procedures does not apply, assistant surgeon may not be paid

20936   **Spinal bone autograft**   ~ bundled code - no separate payment made, multiple procedure concept does not apply, bilateral surgery concept does not apply, assistant surgery concept does not apply

20937   **Spinal bone autograft**   ~ follow-up period included in another service, no payment adjustment rules for multiple procedures apply, 150% payment adjustment for bilateral procedures does not apply, assistant surgeon may be paid

20938   **Spinal bone autograft**   ~ follow-up period included in another service, no payment adjustment rules for multiple procedures apply, 150% payment adjustment for bilateral procedures does not apply, assistant surgeon may be paid

20950   **Fluid pressure, muscle**   ~ endoscopies or minor procedure - E/M services on the same day generally not paid, standard payment adjustment rules for multiple procedures apply, 150% payment adjustment for bilateral procedures does not apply, payment for assistant surgeon subject to documentation of medical necessity

20955   **Fibula bone graft, microvasc**   ~ follow-up period is 90 days, standard payment adjustment rules for multiple procedures apply, 150% payment adjustment for bilateral procedures does not apply, assistant surgeon may be paid

20956   **Iliac bone graft, microvasc**   ~ follow-up period is 90 days, standard payment adjustment rules for multiple procedures apply, 150% payment adjustment for bilateral procedures does not apply, assistant surgeon may be paid

20957   **Mt bone graft, microvasc**   ~ follow-up period is 90 days, standard payment adjustment rules for multiple procedures apply, 150% payment adjustment for bilateral procedures does not apply, assistant surgeon may be paid

20962   **Other bone graft, microvasc**   ~ follow-up period is 90 days, standard payment adjustment rules for multiple procedures apply, 150% payment adjustment for bilateral procedures does not apply, assistant surgeon may be paid

20969   **Bone/skin graft, microvasc**   ~ follow-up period is 90 days, standard payment adjustment rules for multiple procedures apply, 150% payment adjustment for bilateral procedures does not apply, assistant surgeon may be paid

20970   **Bone/skin graft, iliac crest**   ~ follow-up period is 90 days, standard payment adjustment rules for multiple procedures apply, 150% payment adjustment for bilateral procedures does not apply, assistant surgeon may be paid

20972   **Bone/skin graft, metatarsal**   ~ follow-up period is 90 days, standard payment adjustment rules for multiple procedures apply, 150% payment adjustment for bilateral procedures does not apply, assistant surgeon may be paid

20973   **Bone/skin graft, great toe**   ~ follow-up period is 90 days, standard payment adjustment rules for multiple procedures apply, 150% payment adjustment for bilateral procedures does not apply, assistant surgeon may be paid

20974   **Electrical bone stimulation**   ~ endoscopies or minor procedure - E/M services on the same day generally not paid, no payment adjustment rules for multiple procedures apply, 150% payment adjustment for bilateral procedures does not apply, assistant surgeon may not be paid

20975   **Electrical bone stimulation**   ~ endoscopies or minor procedure - E/M services on the same day generally not paid, no payment adjustment rules for multiple procedures apply, 150% payment adjustment for bilateral procedures does not apply, assistant surgeon may be paid

20979   **Us bone stimulation**   ~ endoscopies or minor procedure - E/M services on the same day generally not paid, no payment adjustment rules for multiple procedures apply, 150% payment adjustment for bilateral procedures does not apply, assistant surgeon may not be paid

20982   **Ablate, bone tumor(s) percutaneous**   ~ endoscopies or minor procedure - E/M services on the same day generally not paid, standard payment adjustment rules for multiple procedures apply, 150% payment adjustment for bilateral procedures applies, assistant surgeon may be paid

20999   **Musculoskeletal surgery**   ~ medicare carrier determines global period, standard payment adjustment rules for multiple procedures apply, 150% payment adjustment for bilateral procedures does not apply, payment for assistant surgeon subject to documentation of medical necessity

Head

21010   **Incise jaw joint**   ~ follow-up period is 90 days, standard payment adjustment rules for multiple procedures apply, 150% payment adjustment for bilateral procedures applies, payment for assistant surgeon subject to documentation of medical necessity

---

21015   **Resection of facial tumor**   ~ follow-up period is 90 days, standard payment adjustment rules for multiple procedures apply, 150% payment adjustment for bilateral procedures does not apply, assistant surgeon may not be paid

21025   **Excise bone, lower jaw**   ~ follow-up period is 90 days, standard payment adjustment rules for multiple procedures apply, 150% payment adjustment for bilateral procedures does not apply, assistant surgeon may not be paid

21026   **Excise facial bone(s)**   ~ follow-up period is 90 days, standard payment adjustment rules for multiple procedures apply, 150% payment adjustment for bilateral procedures does not apply, assistant surgeon may not be paid

21029   **Contour face bone lesion**   ~ follow-up period is 90 days, standard payment adjustment rules for multiple procedures apply, 150% payment adjustment for bilateral procedures does not apply, payment for assistant surgeon subject to documentation of medical necessity

21030   **Excise max/zygoma b9 tumor**   ~ follow-up period is 90 days, standard payment adjustment rules for multiple procedures apply, 150% payment adjustment for bilateral procedures does not apply, assistant surgeon may not be paid

21031   **Remove exostosis, mandible**   ~ follow-up period is 90 days, standard payment adjustment rules for multiple procedures apply, 150% payment adjustment for bilateral procedures does not apply, assistant surgeon may not be paid

21032   **Remove exostosis, maxilla**   ~ follow-up period is 90 days, standard payment adjustment rules for multiple procedures apply, 150% payment adjustment for bilateral procedures does not apply, assistant surgeon may not be paid

21034   **Excise max/zygoma malig tumor**   ~ follow-up period is 90 days, standard payment adjustment rules for multiple procedures apply, 150% payment adjustment for bilateral procedures does not apply, assistant surgeon may be paid

21040   **Excise mandible lesion**   ~ follow-up period is 90 days, standard payment adjustment rules for multiple procedures apply, 150% payment adjustment for bilateral procedures does not apply, assistant surgeon may not be paid

21044   **Remove jaw bone lesion**   ~ follow-up period is 90 days, standard payment adjustment rules for multiple procedures apply, 150% payment adjustment for bilateral procedures does not apply, assistant surgeon may be paid

21045   **Extensive jaw surgery**   ~ follow-up period is 90 days, standard payment adjustment rules for multiple procedures apply, 150% payment adjustment for bilateral procedures does not apply, assistant surgeon may be paid

21046   **Remove mandible cyst complex**   ~ follow-up period is 90 days, standard payment adjustment rules for multiple procedures apply, 150% payment adjustment for

bilateral procedures does not apply, payment for assistant surgeon subject to documentation of medical necessity

21047   **Excise lower jaw cyst w/repair**   ~ follow-up period is 90 days, standard payment adjustment rules for multiple procedures apply, 150% payment adjustment for bilateral procedures does not apply, assistant surgeon may be paid

21048   **Remove maxilla cyst complex**   ~ follow-up period is 90 days, standard payment adjustment rules for multiple procedures apply, 150% payment adjustment for bilateral procedures does not apply, payment for assistant surgeon subject to documentation of medical necessity

21049   **Excise upper jaw cyst w/repair**   ~ follow-up period is 90 days, standard payment adjustment rules for multiple procedures apply, 150% payment adjustment for bilateral procedures does not apply, assistant surgeon may be paid

21050   **Remove jaw joint**   ~ follow-up period is 90 days, standard payment adjustment rules for multiple procedures apply, 150% payment adjustment for bilateral procedures applies, payment for assistant surgeon subject to documentation of medical necessity

21060   **Remove jaw joint cartilage**   ~ follow-up period is 90 days, standard payment adjustment rules for multiple procedures apply, 150% payment adjustment for bilateral procedures applies, assistant surgeon may be paid

21070   **Remove coronoid process**   ~ follow-up period is 90 days, standard payment adjustment rules for multiple procedures apply, 150% payment adjustment for bilateral procedures applies, payment for assistant surgeon subject to documentation of medical necessity

21076   **Prepare face/oral prosthesis**   ~ follow-up period is 10 days, standard payment adjustment rules for multiple procedures apply, 150% payment adjustment for bilateral procedures does not apply, payment for assistant surgeon subject to documentation of medical necessity

21077   **Prepare face/oral prosthesis**   ~ follow-up period is 90 days, standard payment adjustment rules for multiple procedures apply, 150% payment adjustment for bilateral procedures applies, payment for assistant surgeon subject to documentation of medical necessity

21079   **Prepare face/oral prosthesis**   ~ follow-up period is 90 days, standard payment adjustment rules for multiple procedures apply, 150% payment adjustment for bilateral procedures does not apply, assistant surgeon may not be paid

21080   **Prepare face/oral prosthesis**   ~ follow-up period is 90 days, standard payment adjustment rules for multiple procedures apply, 150% payment adjustment for bilateral procedures does not apply, assistant surgeon may not be paid

21081   **Prepare face/oral prosthesis**   ~ follow-up period is 90 days, standard payment adjustment rules for multiple procedures apply, 150% payment adjustment for bilateral procedures does not apply, payment for assistant surgeon subject to documentation of medical necessity

21082   **Prepare face/oral prosthesis**   ~ follow-up period is 90 days, standard payment adjustment rules for multiple procedures apply, 150% payment adjustment for bilateral procedures does not apply, payment for assistant surgeon subject to documentation of medical necessity

21083   **Prepare face/oral prosthesis**   ~ follow-up period is 90 days, standard payment adjustment rules for multiple procedures apply, 150% payment adjustment for bilateral procedures does not apply, payment for assistant surgeon subject to documentation of medical necessity

21084   **Prepare face/oral prosthesis**   ~ follow-up period is 90 days, standard payment adjustment rules for multiple procedures apply, 150% payment adjustment for bilateral procedures does not apply, payment for assistant surgeon subject to documentation of medical necessity

21085   **Prepare face/oral prosthesis**   ~ follow-up period is 10 days, standard payment adjustment rules for multiple procedures apply, 150% payment adjustment for bilateral procedures does not apply, payment for assistant surgeon subject to documentation of medical necessity

21086   **Prepare face/oral prosthesis**   ~ follow-up period is 90 days, standard payment adjustment rules for multiple procedures apply, 150% payment adjustment for bilateral procedures applies, payment for assistant surgeon subject to documentation of medical necessity

21087   **Prepare face/oral prosthesis**   ~ follow-up period is 90 days, standard payment adjustment rules for multiple procedures apply, 150% payment adjustment for bilateral procedures does not apply, payment for assistant surgeon subject to documentation of medical necessity

21088   **Prepare face/oral prosthesis**   ~ follow-up period is 90 days, no payment adjustment rules for multiple procedures apply, 150% payment adjustment for bilateral procedures does not apply, payment for assistant surgeon subject to documentation of medical necessity

21089   **Prepare face/oral prosthesis**   ~ follow-up period is 90 days, no payment adjustment rules for multiple procedures apply, 150% payment adjustment for bilateral procedures does not apply, assistant surgeon may not be paid

21100   **Maxillofacial fixation**   ~ follow-up period is 90 days, standard payment adjustment rules for multiple procedures apply, 150% payment adjustment for

bilateral procedures does not apply, payment for assistant surgeon subject to documentation of medical necessity

21110   **Interdental fixation**   ~ follow-up period is 90 days, standard payment adjustment rules for multiple procedures apply, 150% payment adjustment for bilateral procedures does not apply, assistant surgeon may not be paid

21116   **Injection, jaw joint x-ray**   ~ endoscopies or minor procedure - E/M services on the same day generally not paid, standard payment adjustment rules for multiple procedures apply, 150% payment adjustment for bilateral procedures does not apply, assistant surgeon may not be paid

21120   **Reconstruct chin**   ~ follow-up period is 90 days, standard payment adjustment rules for multiple procedures apply, 150% payment adjustment for bilateral procedures does not apply, assistant surgeon may not be paid

21121   **Reconstruct chin**   ~ follow-up period is 90 days, standard payment adjustment rules for multiple procedures apply, 150% payment adjustment for bilateral procedures does not apply, assistant surgeon may be paid

21122   **Reconstruct chin**   ~ follow-up period is 90 days, standard payment adjustment rules for multiple procedures apply, 150% payment adjustment for bilateral procedures does not apply, assistant surgeon may be paid

21123   **Reconstruct chin**   ~ follow-up period is 90 days, standard payment adjustment rules for multiple procedures apply, 150% payment adjustment for bilateral procedures does not apply, assistant surgeon may be paid

21125   **Augment lower jaw bone**   ~ follow-up period is 90 days, standard payment adjustment rules for multiple procedures apply, 150% payment adjustment for bilateral procedures does not apply, assistant surgeon may be paid

21127   **Augment lower jaw bone**   ~ follow-up period is 90 days, standard payment adjustment rules for multiple procedures apply, 150% payment adjustment for bilateral procedures does not apply, assistant surgeon may be paid

21137   **Reduce forehead**   ~ follow-up period is 90 days, standard payment adjustment rules for multiple procedures apply, 150% payment adjustment for bilateral procedures does not apply, assistant surgeon may be paid

21138   **Reduce forehead**   ~ follow-up period is 90 days, standard payment adjustment rules for multiple procedures apply, 150% payment adjustment for bilateral procedures does not apply, assistant surgeon may be paid

21139   **Reduce forehead**   ~ follow-up period is 90 days, standard payment adjustment rules for multiple procedures apply, 150% payment adjustment for bilateral procedures does not apply, assistant surgeon may be paid

21141   **Reconstruct midface, lefort**   ~ follow-up period is 90 days, standard payment adjustment rules for multiple procedures apply, 150% payment adjustment for bilateral procedures does not apply, assistant surgeon may be paid

21142   **Reconstruct midface, lefort**   ~ follow-up period is 90 days, standard payment adjustment rules for multiple procedures apply, 150% payment adjustment for bilateral procedures does not apply, assistant surgeon may be paid

21143   **Reconstruct midface, lefort**   ~ follow-up period is 90 days, standard payment adjustment rules for multiple procedures apply, 150% payment adjustment for bilateral procedures does not apply, assistant surgeon may be paid

21145   **Reconstruct midface, lefort**   ~ follow-up period is 90 days, standard payment adjustment rules for multiple procedures apply, 150% payment adjustment for bilateral procedures does not apply, assistant surgeon may be paid

21146   **Reconstruct midface, lefort**   ~ follow-up period is 90 days, standard payment adjustment rules for multiple procedures apply, 150% payment adjustment for bilateral procedures does not apply, assistant surgeon may be paid

21147   **Reconstruct midface, lefort**   ~ follow-up period is 90 days, standard payment adjustment rules for multiple procedures apply, 150% payment adjustment for bilateral procedures does not apply, assistant surgeon may be paid

21150   **Reconstruct midface, lefort**   ~ follow-up period is 90 days, standard payment adjustment rules for multiple procedures apply, 150% payment adjustment for bilateral procedures does not apply, assistant surgeon may be paid

21151   **Reconstruct midface, lefort**   ~ follow-up period is 90 days, standard payment adjustment rules for multiple procedures apply, 150% payment adjustment for bilateral procedures does not apply, assistant surgeon may be paid

21154   **Reconstruct midface, lefort**   ~ follow-up period is 90 days, standard payment adjustment rules for multiple procedures apply, 150% payment adjustment for bilateral procedures does not apply, assistant surgeon may be paid

21155   **Reconstruct midface, lefort**   ~ follow-up period is 90 days, standard payment adjustment rules for multiple procedures apply, 150% payment adjustment for bilateral procedures does not apply, assistant surgeon may be paid

21159   **Reconstruct midface, lefort**   ~ follow-up period is 90 days, standard payment adjustment rules for multiple procedures apply, 150% payment adjustment for bilateral procedures does not apply, assistant surgeon may be paid

21160   **Reconstruct midface, lefort**   ~ follow-up period is 90 days, standard payment adjustment rules for multiple procedures apply, 150% payment adjustment for bilateral procedures does not apply, assistant surgeon may be paid

21172   **Reconstruct orbit/forehead**   ~ follow-up period is 90 days, standard payment adjustment rules for multiple procedures apply, 150% payment adjustment for bilateral procedures does not apply, assistant surgeon may be paid

21175   **Reconstruct orbit/forehead**   ~ follow-up period is 90 days, standard payment adjustment rules for multiple procedures apply, 150% payment adjustment for bilateral procedures does not apply, assistant surgeon may be paid

21179   **Reconstruct entire forehead**   ~ follow-up period is 90 days, standard payment adjustment rules for multiple procedures apply, 150% payment adjustment for bilateral procedures does not apply, assistant surgeon may be paid

21180   **Reconstruct entire forehead**   ~ follow-up period is 90 days, standard payment adjustment rules for multiple procedures apply, 150% payment adjustment for bilateral procedures does not apply, assistant surgeon may be paid

21181   **Contour cranial bone lesion**   ~ follow-up period is 90 days, standard payment adjustment rules for multiple procedures apply, 150% payment adjustment for bilateral procedures does not apply, payment for assistant surgeon subject to documentation of medical necessity

21182   **Reconstruct cranial bone**   ~ follow-up period is 90 days, standard payment adjustment rules for multiple procedures apply, 150% payment adjustment for bilateral procedures does not apply, assistant surgeon may be paid

21183   **Reconstruct cranial bone**   ~ follow-up period is 90 days, standard payment adjustment rules for multiple procedures apply, 150% payment adjustment for bilateral procedures does not apply, assistant surgeon may be paid

21184   **Reconstruct cranial bone**   ~ follow-up period is 90 days, standard payment adjustment rules for multiple procedures apply, 150% payment adjustment for bilateral procedures does not apply, assistant surgeon may be paid

21188   **Reconstruct midface**   ~ follow-up period is 90 days, standard payment adjustment rules for multiple procedures apply, 150% payment adjustment for bilateral procedures does not apply, assistant surgeon may be paid

21193   **Reconstruct lower jaw w/o graft**   ~ follow-up period is 90 days, standard payment adjustment rules for multiple procedures apply, 150% payment adjustment does not apply - RVUs based on bilateral procedure, assistant surgeon may be paid

21194   **Reconstruct lower jaw w/graft**   ~ follow-up period is 90 days, standard payment adjustment rules for multiple procedures apply, 150% payment adjustment does not apply - RVUs based on bilateral procedure, assistant surgeon may be paid

21195 **Reconstruct lower jaw w/o fixation** ~ follow-up period is 90 days, standard payment adjustment rules for multiple procedures apply, 150% payment adjustment does not apply - RVUs based on bilateral procedure, assistant surgeon may be paid

21196 **Reconstruct lower jaw w/fixation** ~ follow-up period is 90 days, standard payment adjustment rules for multiple procedures apply, 150% payment adjustment does not apply - RVUs based on bilateral procedure, assistant surgeon may be paid

21198 **Reconstruct lower jaw segment** ~ follow-up period is 90 days, standard payment adjustment rules for multiple procedures apply, 150% payment adjustment for bilateral procedures does not apply, assistant surgeon may be paid

21199 **Reconstruct lower jaw w/advance** ~ follow-up period is 90 days, standard payment adjustment rules for multiple procedures apply, 150% payment adjustment for bilateral procedures does not apply, assistant surgeon may be paid

21206 **Reconstruct upper jaw bone** ~ follow-up period is 90 days, standard payment adjustment rules for multiple procedures apply, 150% payment adjustment for bilateral procedures does not apply, assistant surgeon may be paid

21208 **Augment facial bones** ~ follow-up period is 90 days, standard payment adjustment rules for multiple procedures apply, 150% payment adjustment for bilateral procedures does not apply, payment for assistant surgeon subject to documentation of medical necessity

21209 **Reduce facial bones** ~ follow-up period is 90 days, standard payment adjustment rules for multiple procedures apply, 150% payment adjustment for bilateral procedures does not apply, assistant surgeon may be paid

21210 **Face bone graft** ~ follow-up period is 90 days, standard payment adjustment rules for multiple procedures apply, 150% payment adjustment for bilateral procedures does not apply, assistant surgeon may not be paid

21215 **Lower jaw bone graft** ~ follow-up period is 90 days, standard payment adjustment rules for multiple procedures apply, 150% payment adjustment for bilateral procedures does not apply, assistant surgeon may not be paid

21230 **Rib cartilage graft** ~ follow-up period is 90 days, standard payment adjustment rules for multiple procedures apply, 150% payment adjustment for bilateral procedures does not apply, payment for assistant surgeon subject to documentation of medical necessity

21235 **Ear cartilage graft** ~ follow-up period is 90 days, standard payment adjustment rules for multiple procedures apply, 150% payment adjustment for bilateral procedures does not apply, assistant surgeon may not be paid

21240   **Reconstruct jaw joint**   ~ follow-up period is 90 days, standard payment adjustment rules for multiple procedures apply, 150% payment adjustment for bilateral procedures applies, assistant surgeon may be paid

21242   **Reconstruct jaw joint**   ~ follow-up period is 90 days, standard payment adjustment rules for multiple procedures apply, 150% payment adjustment for bilateral procedures applies, assistant surgeon may be paid

21243   **Reconstruct jaw joint**   ~ follow-up period is 90 days, standard payment adjustment rules for multiple procedures apply, 150% payment adjustment for bilateral procedures applies, assistant surgeon may be paid

21244   **Reconstruct lower jaw**   ~ follow-up period is 90 days, standard payment adjustment rules for multiple procedures apply, 150% payment adjustment for bilateral procedures does not apply, assistant surgeon may be paid

21245   **Reconstruct jaw**   ~ follow-up period is 90 days, standard payment adjustment rules for multiple procedures apply, 150% payment adjustment for bilateral procedures does not apply, assistant surgeon may be paid

21246   **Reconstruct jaw**   ~ follow-up period is 90 days, standard payment adjustment rules for multiple procedures apply, 150% payment adjustment for bilateral procedures does not apply, assistant surgeon may be paid

21247   **Reconstruct lower jaw bone**   ~ follow-up period is 90 days, standard payment adjustment rules for multiple procedures apply, 150% payment adjustment for bilateral procedures does not apply, assistant surgeon may be paid

21248   **Reconstruct jaw**   ~ follow-up period is 90 days, standard payment adjustment rules for multiple procedures apply, 150% payment adjustment for bilateral procedures does not apply, assistant surgeon may not be paid

21249   **Reconstruct jaw**   ~ follow-up period is 90 days, standard payment adjustment rules for multiple procedures apply, 150% payment adjustment for bilateral procedures does not apply, payment for assistant surgeon subject to documentation of medical necessity

21255   **Reconstruct lower jaw bone**   ~ follow-up period is 90 days, standard payment adjustment rules for multiple procedures apply, 150% payment adjustment for bilateral procedures does not apply, assistant surgeon may be paid

21256   **Reconstruct orbit**   ~ follow-up period is 90 days, standard payment adjustment rules for multiple procedures apply, 150% payment adjustment for bilateral procedures does not apply, assistant surgeon may be paid

21260   **Revise eye sockets**   ~ follow-up period is 90 days, standard payment adjustment rules for multiple procedures apply, 150% payment adjustment for bilateral procedures does not apply, assistant surgeon may be paid

21261   **Revise eye sockets**   ~ follow-up period is 90 days, standard payment adjustment rules for multiple procedures apply, 150% payment adjustment for bilateral procedures does not apply, assistant surgeon may be paid

21263   **Revise eye sockets**   ~ follow-up period is 90 days, standard payment adjustment rules for multiple procedures apply, 150% payment adjustment for bilateral procedures does not apply, assistant surgeon may be paid

21267   **Revise eye sockets**   ~ follow-up period is 90 days, standard payment adjustment rules for multiple procedures apply, 150% payment adjustment for bilateral procedures does not apply, assistant surgeon may be paid

21268   **Revise eye sockets**   ~ follow-up period is 90 days, standard payment adjustment rules for multiple procedures apply, 150% payment adjustment for bilateral procedures does not apply, assistant surgeon may be paid

21270   **Augment cheek bone**   ~ follow-up period is 90 days, standard payment adjustment rules for multiple procedures apply, 150% payment adjustment for bilateral procedures does not apply, assistant surgeon may be paid

21275   **Revise orbitofacial bones**   ~ follow-up period is 90 days, standard payment adjustment rules for multiple procedures apply, 150% payment adjustment for bilateral procedures does not apply, assistant surgeon may be paid

21280   **Revise eyelid**   ~ follow-up period is 90 days, standard payment adjustment rules for multiple procedures apply, 150% payment adjustment for bilateral procedures applies, payment for assistant surgeon subject to documentation of medical necessity

21282   **Revise eyelid**   ~ follow-up period is 90 days, standard payment adjustment rules for multiple procedures apply, 150% payment adjustment for bilateral procedures applies, assistant surgeon may not be paid

21295   **Revise jaw muscle/bone**   ~ follow-up period is 90 days, standard payment adjustment rules for multiple procedures apply, 150% payment adjustment for bilateral procedures does not apply, payment for assistant surgeon subject to documentation of medical necessity

21296   **Revise jaw muscle/bone**   ~ follow-up period is 90 days, standard payment adjustment rules for multiple procedures apply, 150% payment adjustment for bilateral procedures does not apply, payment for assistant surgeon subject to documentation of medical necessity

21299 **Cranio/maxillofacial surgery** ~ medicare carrier determines global period, standard payment adjustment rules for multiple procedures apply, 150% payment adjustment for bilateral procedures does not apply, payment for assistant surgeon subject to documentation of medical necessity

21310 **Treat nose fracture** ~ endoscopies or minor procedure - E/M services on the same day generally not paid, standard payment adjustment rules for multiple procedures apply, 150% payment adjustment for bilateral procedures does not apply, assistant surgeon may not be paid

21315 **Treat nose fracture** ~ follow-up period is 10 days, standard payment adjustment rules for multiple procedures apply, 150% payment adjustment for bilateral procedures does not apply, assistant surgeon may not be paid

21320 **Treat nose fracture** ~ follow-up period is 10 days, standard payment adjustment rules for multiple procedures apply, 150% payment adjustment for bilateral procedures does not apply, assistant surgeon may not be paid

21325 **Treat nose fracture** ~ follow-up period is 90 days, standard payment adjustment rules for multiple procedures apply, 150% payment adjustment for bilateral procedures does not apply, payment for assistant surgeon subject to documentation of medical necessity

21330 **Treat nose fracture** ~ follow-up period is 90 days, standard payment adjustment rules for multiple procedures apply, 150% payment adjustment for bilateral procedures does not apply, payment for assistant surgeon subject to documentation of medical necessity

21335 **Treat nose fracture** ~ follow-up period is 90 days, standard payment adjustment rules for multiple procedures apply, 150% payment adjustment for bilateral procedures does not apply, assistant surgeon may not be paid

21336 **Treat nasal septal fracture** ~ follow-up period is 90 days, standard payment adjustment rules for multiple procedures apply, 150% payment adjustment for bilateral procedures does not apply, payment for assistant surgeon subject to documentation of medical necessity

21337 **Treat nasal septal fracture** ~ follow-up period is 90 days, standard payment adjustment rules for multiple procedures apply, 150% payment adjustment for bilateral procedures does not apply, payment for assistant surgeon subject to documentation of medical necessity

21338 **Treat nasoethmoid fracture** ~ follow-up period is 90 days, standard payment adjustment rules for multiple procedures apply, 150% payment adjustment for bilateral procedures does not apply, payment for assistant surgeon subject to documentation of medical necessity

21339   **Treat nasoethmoid fracture**   ~ follow-up period is 90 days, standard payment adjustment rules for multiple procedures apply, 150% payment adjustment for bilateral procedures does not apply, assistant surgeon may be paid

21340   **Treat nose fracture**   ~ follow-up period is 90 days, standard payment adjustment rules for multiple procedures apply, 150% payment adjustment for bilateral procedures does not apply, payment for assistant surgeon subject to documentation of medical necessity

21343   **Treat sinus fracture**   ~ follow-up period is 90 days, standard payment adjustment rules for multiple procedures apply, 150% payment adjustment for bilateral procedures does not apply, assistant surgeon may be paid

21344   **Treat sinus fracture**   ~ follow-up period is 90 days, standard payment adjustment rules for multiple procedures apply, 150% payment adjustment for bilateral procedures does not apply, assistant surgeon may be paid

21345   **Treat nose/jaw fracture**   ~ follow-up period is 90 days, standard payment adjustment rules for multiple procedures apply, 150% payment adjustment for bilateral procedures does not apply, payment for assistant surgeon subject to documentation of medical necessity

21346   **Treat nose/jaw fracture**   ~ follow-up period is 90 days, standard payment adjustment rules for multiple procedures apply, 150% payment adjustment for bilateral procedures does not apply, assistant surgeon may not be paid

21347   **Treat nose/jaw fracture**   ~ follow-up period is 90 days, standard payment adjustment rules for multiple procedures apply, 150% payment adjustment for bilateral procedures does not apply, assistant surgeon may be paid

21348   **Treat nose/jaw fracture**   ~ follow-up period is 90 days, standard payment adjustment rules for multiple procedures apply, 150% payment adjustment for bilateral procedures does not apply, assistant surgeon may be paid

21355   **Treat cheek bone fracture**   ~ follow-up period is 10 days, standard payment adjustment rules for multiple procedures apply, 150% payment adjustment for bilateral procedures does not apply, payment for assistant surgeon subject to documentation of medical necessity

21356   **Treat cheek bone fracture**   ~ follow-up period is 10 days, standard payment adjustment rules for multiple procedures apply, 150% payment adjustment for bilateral procedures does not apply, payment for assistant surgeon subject to documentation of medical necessity

21360   **Treat cheek bone fracture**   ~ follow-up period is 90 days, standard payment adjustment rules for multiple procedures apply, 150% payment adjustment for bilateral procedures does not apply, assistant surgeon may be paid

21365   **Treat cheek bone fracture**   ~ follow-up period is 90 days, standard payment adjustment rules for multiple procedures apply, 150% payment adjustment for bilateral procedures does not apply, assistant surgeon may be paid

21366   **Treat cheek bone fracture**   ~ follow-up period is 90 days, standard payment adjustment rules for multiple procedures apply, 150% payment adjustment for bilateral procedures does not apply, assistant surgeon may be paid

21385   **Treat eye socket fracture**   ~ follow-up period is 90 days, standard payment adjustment rules for multiple procedures apply, 150% payment adjustment for bilateral procedures does not apply, assistant surgeon may be paid

21386   **Treat eye socket fracture**   ~ follow-up period is 90 days, standard payment adjustment rules for multiple procedures apply, 150% payment adjustment for bilateral procedures does not apply, assistant surgeon may be paid

21387   **Treat eye socket fracture**   ~ follow-up period is 90 days, standard payment adjustment rules for multiple procedures apply, 150% payment adjustment for bilateral procedures does not apply, assistant surgeon may be paid

21390   **Treat eye socket fracture**   ~ follow-up period is 90 days, standard payment adjustment rules for multiple procedures apply, 150% payment adjustment for bilateral procedures does not apply, assistant surgeon may be paid

21395   **Treat eye socket fracture**   ~ follow-up period is 90 days, standard payment adjustment rules for multiple procedures apply, 150% payment adjustment for bilateral procedures does not apply, assistant surgeon may be paid

21400   **Treat eye socket fracture**   ~ follow-up period is 90 days, standard payment adjustment rules for multiple procedures apply, 150% payment adjustment for bilateral procedures does not apply, payment for assistant surgeon subject to documentation of medical necessity

21401   **Treat eye socket fracture**   ~ follow-up period is 90 days, standard payment adjustment rules for multiple procedures apply, 150% payment adjustment for bilateral procedures does not apply, assistant surgeon may be paid

21406   **Treat eye socket fracture**   ~ follow-up period is 90 days, standard payment adjustment rules for multiple procedures apply, 150% payment adjustment for bilateral procedures does not apply, assistant surgeon may be paid

21407   **Treat eye socket fracture**   ~ follow-up period is 90 days, standard payment adjustment rules for multiple procedures apply, 150% payment adjustment for bilateral procedures does not apply, assistant surgeon may be paid

21408   **Treat eye socket fracture**   ~ follow-up period is 90 days, standard payment adjustment rules for multiple procedures apply, 150% payment adjustment for bilateral procedures does not apply, assistant surgeon may be paid

21421   **Treat mouth roof fracture**   ~ follow-up period is 90 days, standard payment adjustment rules for multiple procedures apply, 150% payment adjustment for bilateral procedures does not apply, payment for assistant surgeon subject to documentation of medical necessity

21422   **Treat mouth roof fracture**   ~ follow-up period is 90 days, standard payment adjustment rules for multiple procedures apply, 150% payment adjustment for bilateral procedures does not apply, assistant surgeon may be paid

21423   **Treat mouth roof fracture**   ~ follow-up period is 90 days, standard payment adjustment rules for multiple procedures apply, 150% payment adjustment for bilateral procedures does not apply, assistant surgeon may be paid

21431   **Treat craniofacial fracture**   ~ follow-up period is 90 days, standard payment adjustment rules for multiple procedures apply, 150% payment adjustment for bilateral procedures does not apply, assistant surgeon may be paid

21432   **Treat craniofacial fracture**   ~ follow-up period is 90 days, standard payment adjustment rules for multiple procedures apply, 150% payment adjustment for bilateral procedures does not apply, assistant surgeon may be paid

21433   **Treat craniofacial fracture**   ~ follow-up period is 90 days, standard payment adjustment rules for multiple procedures apply, 150% payment adjustment for bilateral procedures does not apply, assistant surgeon may be paid

21435   **Treat craniofacial fracture**   ~ follow-up period is 90 days, standard payment adjustment rules for multiple procedures apply, 150% payment adjustment for bilateral procedures does not apply, assistant surgeon may be paid

21436   **Treat craniofacial fracture**   ~ follow-up period is 90 days, standard payment adjustment rules for multiple procedures apply, 150% payment adjustment for bilateral procedures does not apply, assistant surgeon may be paid

21440   **Treat dental ridge fracture**   ~ follow-up period is 90 days, standard payment adjustment rules for multiple procedures apply, 150% payment adjustment for bilateral procedures does not apply, payment for assistant surgeon subject to documentation of medical necessity

21445   **Treat dental ridge fracture**   ~ follow-up period is 90 days, standard payment adjustment rules for multiple procedures apply, 150% payment adjustment for bilateral procedures does not apply, assistant surgeon may be paid

21450   **Treat lower jaw fracture**   ~ follow-up period is 90 days, standard payment adjustment rules for multiple procedures apply, 150% payment adjustment for bilateral procedures does not apply, payment for assistant surgeon subject to documentation of medical necessity

21451   **Treat lower jaw fracture**   ~ follow-up period is 90 days, standard payment adjustment rules for multiple procedures apply, 150% payment adjustment for bilateral procedures does not apply, payment for assistant surgeon subject to documentation of medical necessity

21452   **Treat lower jaw fracture**   ~ follow-up period is 90 days, standard payment adjustment rules for multiple procedures apply, 150% payment adjustment for bilateral procedures does not apply, payment for assistant surgeon subject to documentation of medical necessity

21453   **Treat lower jaw fracture**   ~ follow-up period is 90 days, standard payment adjustment rules for multiple procedures apply, 150% payment adjustment for bilateral procedures does not apply, payment for assistant surgeon subject to documentation of medical necessity

21454   **Treat lower jaw fracture**   ~ follow-up period is 90 days, standard payment adjustment rules for multiple procedures apply, 150% payment adjustment for bilateral procedures does not apply, payment for assistant surgeon subject to documentation of medical necessity

21461   **Treat lower jaw fracture**   ~ follow-up period is 90 days, standard payment adjustment rules for multiple procedures apply, 150% payment adjustment for bilateral procedures does not apply, assistant surgeon may be paid

21462   **Treat lower jaw fracture**   ~ follow-up period is 90 days, standard payment adjustment rules for multiple procedures apply, 150% payment adjustment for bilateral procedures does not apply, assistant surgeon may be paid

21465   **Treat lower jaw fracture**   ~ follow-up period is 90 days, standard payment adjustment rules for multiple procedures apply, 150% payment adjustment for bilateral procedures does not apply, assistant surgeon may be paid

21470   **Treat lower jaw fracture**   ~ follow-up period is 90 days, standard payment adjustment rules for multiple procedures apply, 150% payment adjustment for bilateral procedures does not apply, assistant surgeon may be paid

21480   **Reset dislocated jaw**   ~ endoscopies or minor procedure - E/M services on the same day generally not paid, standard payment adjustment rules for multiple procedures apply, 150% payment adjustment for bilateral procedures applies, assistant surgeon may not be paid

21485   **Reset dislocated jaw**   ~ follow-up period is 90 days, standard payment adjustment rules for multiple procedures apply, 150% payment adjustment for bilateral procedures applies, payment for assistant surgeon subject to documentation of medical necessity

21490   **Repair dislocated jaw**   ~ follow-up period is 90 days, standard payment adjustment rules for multiple procedures apply, 150% payment adjustment for bilateral procedures applies, assistant surgeon may be paid

21495   **Treat hyoid bone fracture**   ~ follow-up period is 90 days, standard payment adjustment rules for multiple procedures apply, 150% payment adjustment for bilateral procedures does not apply, assistant surgeon may be paid

21497   **Interdental wiring**   ~ follow-up period is 90 days, standard payment adjustment rules for multiple procedures apply, 150% payment adjustment for bilateral procedures does not apply, payment for assistant surgeon subject to documentation of medical necessity

21499   **Head surgery procedure**   ~ medicare carrier determines global period, standard payment adjustment rules for multiple procedures apply, 150% payment adjustment for bilateral procedures does not apply, payment for assistant surgeon subject to documentation of medical necessity

Neck (Soft Tissues) And Thorax

21501   **Drain neck/chest lesion**   ~ follow-up period is 90 days, standard payment adjustment rules for multiple procedures apply, 150% payment adjustment for bilateral procedures does not apply, assistant surgeon may not be paid

21502   **Drain chest lesion**   ~ follow-up period is 90 days, standard payment adjustment rules for multiple procedures apply, 150% payment adjustment for bilateral procedures does not apply, assistant surgeon may be paid

21510   **Drain bone lesion**   ~ follow-up period is 90 days, standard payment adjustment rules for multiple procedures apply, 150% payment adjustment for bilateral procedures does not apply, payment for assistant surgeon subject to documentation of medical necessity

21550   **Biopsy neck/chest**   ~ follow-up period is 10 days, standard payment adjustment rules for multiple procedures apply, 150% payment adjustment for bilateral procedures does not apply, assistant surgeon may not be paid

21555   **Remove lesion, neck/chest**   ~ follow-up period is 90 days, standard payment adjustment rules for multiple procedures apply, 150% payment adjustment for bilateral procedures does not apply, assistant surgeon may not be paid

21556   **Remove lesion, neck/chest**   ~ follow-up period is 90 days, standard payment adjustment rules for multiple procedures apply, 150% payment adjustment for bilateral procedures does not apply, assistant surgeon may not be paid

21557   **Remove tumor, neck/chest**   ~ follow-up period is 90 days, standard payment adjustment rules for multiple procedures apply, 150% payment adjustment for bilateral procedures does not apply, assistant surgeon may be paid

21600   **Partial remove rib**   ~ follow-up period is 90 days, standard payment adjustment rules for multiple procedures apply, 150% payment adjustment for bilateral procedures does not apply, assistant surgeon may be paid

21610   **Partial remove rib**   ~ follow-up period is 90 days, standard payment adjustment rules for multiple procedures apply, 150% payment adjustment for bilateral procedures does not apply, assistant surgeon may be paid

21615   **Remove rib**   ~ follow-up period is 90 days, standard payment adjustment rules for multiple procedures apply, 150% payment adjustment for bilateral procedures applies, assistant surgeon may be paid

21616   **Remove rib and nerves**   ~ follow-up period is 90 days, standard payment adjustment rules for multiple procedures apply, 150% payment adjustment for bilateral procedures applies, assistant surgeon may be paid

21620   **Partial remove sternum**   ~ follow-up period is 90 days, standard payment adjustment rules for multiple procedures apply, 150% payment adjustment for bilateral procedures does not apply, assistant surgeon may be paid

21627   **Sternal debridement**   ~ follow-up period is 90 days, standard payment adjustment rules for multiple procedures apply, 150% payment adjustment for bilateral procedures does not apply, assistant surgeon may be paid

21630   **Extensive sternum surgery**   ~ follow-up period is 90 days, standard payment adjustment rules for multiple procedures apply, 150% payment adjustment for bilateral procedures does not apply, assistant surgeon may be paid

21632   **Extensive sternum surgery**   ~ follow-up period is 90 days, standard payment adjustment rules for multiple procedures apply, 150% payment adjustment for bilateral procedures does not apply, assistant surgeon may be paid

21685   **Hyoid myotomy & suspension**   ~ follow-up period is 90 days, standard payment adjustment rules for multiple procedures apply, 150% payment adjustment for bilateral procedures does not apply, assistant surgeon may be paid

21700   **Revise neck muscle**   ~ follow-up period is 90 days, standard payment adjustment rules for multiple procedures apply, 150% payment adjustment for bilateral procedures does not apply, assistant surgeon may be paid

21705   **Revise neck muscle/rib** ~ follow-up period is 90 days, standard payment adjustment rules for multiple procedures apply, 150% payment adjustment for bilateral procedures does not apply, assistant surgeon may be paid

21720   **Revise neck muscle** ~ follow-up period is 90 days, standard payment adjustment rules for multiple procedures apply, 150% payment adjustment for bilateral procedures does not apply, assistant surgeon may be paid

21725   **Revise neck muscle** ~ follow-up period is 90 days, standard payment adjustment rules for multiple procedures apply, 150% payment adjustment for bilateral procedures does not apply, assistant surgeon may be paid

21740   **Reconstruct sternum** ~ follow-up period is 90 days, standard payment adjustment rules for multiple procedures apply, 150% payment adjustment for bilateral procedures does not apply, assistant surgeon may be paid

21742   **Repair stern/nuss w/o scope** ~ follow-up period is 90 days, standard payment adjustment rules for multiple procedures apply, 150% payment adjustment for bilateral procedures does not apply, assistant surgeon may be paid

21743   **Repair sternum/nuss w/scope** ~ follow-up period is 90 days, standard payment adjustment rules for multiple procedures apply, 150% payment adjustment for bilateral procedures does not apply, assistant surgeon may be paid

21750   **Repair sternum separation** ~ follow-up period is 90 days, standard payment adjustment rules for multiple procedures apply, 150% payment adjustment for bilateral procedures does not apply, assistant surgeon may be paid

21800   **Treat rib fracture** ~ follow-up period is 90 days, standard payment adjustment rules for multiple procedures apply, 150% payment adjustment for bilateral procedures does not apply, assistant surgeon may not be paid

21805   **Treat rib fracture** ~ follow-up period is 90 days, standard payment adjustment rules for multiple procedures apply, 150% payment adjustment for bilateral procedures does not apply, payment for assistant surgeon subject to documentation of medical necessity

21810   **Treat rib fracture(s)** ~ follow-up period is 90 days, standard payment adjustment rules for multiple procedures apply, 150% payment adjustment for bilateral procedures does not apply, assistant surgeon may be paid

21820   **Treat sternum fracture** ~ follow-up period is 90 days, standard payment adjustment rules for multiple procedures apply, 150% payment adjustment for bilateral procedures does not apply, assistant surgeon may not be paid

21825   **Treat sternum fracture**   ~ follow-up period is 90 days, standard payment adjustment rules for multiple procedures apply, 150% payment adjustment for bilateral procedures does not apply, assistant surgeon may be paid

21899   **Neck/chest surgery procedure**   ~ medicare carrier determines global period, standard payment adjustment rules for multiple procedures apply, 150% payment adjustment for bilateral procedures does not apply, payment for assistant surgeon subject to documentation of medical necessity

Back And Flank

21920   **Biopsy soft tissue of back**   ~ follow-up period is 10 days, standard payment adjustment rules for multiple procedures apply, 150% payment adjustment for bilateral procedures does not apply, assistant surgeon may not be paid

21925   **Biopsy soft tissue of back**   ~ follow-up period is 90 days, standard payment adjustment rules for multiple procedures apply, 150% payment adjustment for bilateral procedures does not apply, assistant surgeon may not be paid

21930   **Remove lesion, back or flank**   ~ follow-up period is 90 days, standard payment adjustment rules for multiple procedures apply, 150% payment adjustment for bilateral procedures does not apply, assistant surgeon may not be paid

21935   **Remove tumor, back**   ~ follow-up period is 90 days, standard payment adjustment rules for multiple procedures apply, 150% payment adjustment for bilateral procedures does not apply, assistant surgeon may not be paid

Spine (Vertebral Column)

22010   **I & D, p-spine, c/t/cervical-thor**   ~ follow-up period is 90 days, standard payment adjustment rules for multiple procedures apply, 150% payment adjustment for bilateral procedures does not apply, payment for assistant surgeon subject to documentation of medical necessity

22015   **I & D, p-spine, l/s/ls**   ~ follow-up period is 90 days, standard payment adjustment rules for multiple procedures apply, 150% payment adjustment for bilateral procedures does not apply, assistant surgeon may not be paid

22100   **Remove part of neck vertebra**   ~ follow-up period is 90 days, standard payment adjustment rules for multiple procedures apply, 150% payment adjustment for bilateral procedures does not apply, assistant surgeon may be paid

22101   **Remove part, thorax vertebra**   ~ follow-up period is 90 days, standard payment adjustment rules for multiple procedures apply, 150% payment adjustment for bilateral procedures does not apply, assistant surgeon may be paid

22102   **Remove part, lumbar vertebra**   ~ follow-up period is 90 days, standard payment adjustment rules for multiple procedures apply, 150% payment adjustment for bilateral procedures does not apply, assistant surgeon may be paid

22103   **Remove extra spine segment**   ~ follow-up period included in another service, no payment adjustment rules for multiple procedures apply, 150% payment adjustment for bilateral procedures does not apply, assistant surgeon may be paid

22110   **Remove part of neck vertebra**   ~ follow-up period is 90 days, standard payment adjustment rules for multiple procedures apply, 150% payment adjustment for bilateral procedures does not apply, assistant surgeon may be paid

22112   **Remove part, thorax vertebra**   ~ follow-up period is 90 days, standard payment adjustment rules for multiple procedures apply, 150% payment adjustment for bilateral procedures does not apply, assistant surgeon may be paid

22114   **Remove part, lumbar vertebra**   ~ follow-up period is 90 days, standard payment adjustment rules for multiple procedures apply, 150% payment adjustment for bilateral procedures does not apply, assistant surgeon may be paid

22116   **Remove extra spine segment**   ~ follow-up period included in another service, no payment adjustment rules for multiple procedures apply, 150% payment adjustment for bilateral procedures does not apply, assistant surgeon may be paid

22210   **Revise neck spine**   ~ follow-up period is 90 days, standard payment adjustment rules for multiple procedures apply, 150% payment adjustment for bilateral procedures does not apply, assistant surgeon may be paid

22212   **Revise thorax spine**   ~ follow-up period is 90 days, standard payment adjustment rules for multiple procedures apply, 150% payment adjustment for bilateral procedures does not apply, assistant surgeon may be paid

22214   **Revise lumbar spine**   ~ follow-up period is 90 days, standard payment adjustment rules for multiple procedures apply, 150% payment adjustment for bilateral procedures does not apply, assistant surgeon may be paid

22216   **Revise, extra spine segment**   ~ follow-up period included in another service, no payment adjustment rules for multiple procedures apply, 150% payment adjustment for bilateral procedures does not apply, assistant surgeon may be paid

22220   **Revise neck spine**   ~ follow-up period is 90 days, standard payment adjustment rules for multiple procedures apply, 150% payment adjustment for bilateral procedures does not apply, assistant surgeon may be paid

22222   **Revise thorax spine**   ~ follow-up period is 90 days, standard payment adjustment rules for multiple procedures apply, 150% payment adjustment for bilateral procedures does not apply, assistant surgeon may be paid

22224 **Revise lumbar spine** ~ follow-up period is 90 days, standard payment adjustment rules for multiple procedures apply, 150% payment adjustment for bilateral procedures does not apply, assistant surgeon may be paid

22226 **Revise, extra spine segment** ~ follow-up period included in another service, no payment adjustment rules for multiple procedures apply, 150% payment adjustment for bilateral procedures does not apply, assistant surgeon may be paid

22305 **Treat spine process fracture** ~ follow-up period is 90 days, standard payment adjustment rules for multiple procedures apply, 150% payment adjustment for bilateral procedures does not apply, assistant surgeon may not be paid

22310 **Treat spine fracture** ~ follow-up period is 90 days, standard payment adjustment rules for multiple procedures apply, 150% payment adjustment for bilateral procedures does not apply, assistant surgeon may not be paid

22315 **Treat spine fracture** ~ follow-up period is 90 days, standard payment adjustment rules for multiple procedures apply, 150% payment adjustment for bilateral procedures does not apply, assistant surgeon may not be paid

22318 **Treat odontoid fracture w/o graft** ~ follow-up period is 90 days, standard payment adjustment rules for multiple procedures apply, 150% payment adjustment for bilateral procedures does not apply, assistant surgeon may be paid

22319 **Treat odontoid fracture w/graft** ~ follow-up period is 90 days, standard payment adjustment rules for multiple procedures apply, 150% payment adjustment for bilateral procedures does not apply, assistant surgeon may be paid

22325 **Treat spine fracture** ~ follow-up period is 90 days, standard payment adjustment rules for multiple procedures apply, 150% payment adjustment for bilateral procedures does not apply, assistant surgeon may be paid

22326 **Treat neck spine fracture** ~ follow-up period is 90 days, standard payment adjustment rules for multiple procedures apply, 150% payment adjustment for bilateral procedures does not apply, assistant surgeon may be paid

22327 **Treat thorax spine fracture** ~ follow-up period is 90 days, standard payment adjustment rules for multiple procedures apply, 150% payment adjustment for bilateral procedures does not apply, assistant surgeon may be paid

22328 **Treat each add spine fracture** ~ follow-up period included in another service, no payment adjustment rules for multiple procedures apply, 150% payment adjustment for bilateral procedures does not apply, assistant surgeon may be paid, +add-on code (list separately in addition to primary procedure)

22505   **Manipulate spine**   ~ follow-up period is 10 days, standard payment adjustment rules for multiple procedures apply, 150% payment adjustment for bilateral procedures does not apply, assistant surgeon may not be paid

22520   **Percutaneous vertebroplasty thor**   ~ follow-up period is 10 days, standard payment adjustment rules for multiple procedures apply, 150% payment adjustment for bilateral procedures does not apply, assistant surgeon may not be paid

22521   **Percutaneous vertebroplasty lumbar**   ~ follow-up period is 10 days, standard payment adjustment rules for multiple procedures apply, 150% payment adjustment for bilateral procedures does not apply, assistant surgeon may not be paid

22522   **Percutaneous vertebroplasty added**   ~ follow-up period included in another service, no payment adjustment rules for multiple procedures apply, 150% payment adjustment for bilateral procedures does not apply, assistant surgeon may not be paid, +add-on code (list separately in addition to primary procedure)

22523   **Percutaneous kyphoplasty, thor**   ~ follow-up period is 10 days, standard payment adjustment rules for multiple procedures apply, 150% payment adjustment for bilateral procedures does not apply, assistant surgeon may not be paid

22524   **Percutaneous kyphoplasty, lumbar**   ~ follow-up period is 10 days, standard payment adjustment rules for multiple procedures apply, 150% payment adjustment for bilateral procedures does not apply, assistant surgeon may not be paid

22525   **Percutaneous kyphoplasty, add-on**   ~ follow-up period included in another service, no payment adjustment rules for multiple procedures apply, 150% payment adjustment for bilateral procedures does not apply, assistant surgeon may not be paid, +add-on code (list separately in addition to primary procedure)

22526   **Idet, single level**   ~ follow-up period is 10 days, standard payment adjustment rules for multiple procedures apply, 150% payment adjustment for bilateral procedures does not apply, assistant surgeon may not be paid

22527   **Idet, 1 or more levels**   ~ follow-up period included in another service, no payment adjustment rules for multiple procedures apply, 150% payment adjustment for bilateral procedures does not apply, assistant surgeon may not be paid

22532   **Lat thorax spine fusion**   ~ follow-up period is 90 days, standard payment adjustment rules for multiple procedures apply, 150% payment adjustment for bilateral procedures does not apply, assistant surgeon may be paid

22533   **Lat lumbar spine fusion**   ~ follow-up period is 90 days, standard payment adjustment rules for multiple procedures apply, 150% payment adjustment for bilateral procedures does not apply, assistant surgeon may be paid

22534   **Lat thor/lumbar, added segment**   ~ follow-up period included in another service, no payment adjustment rules for multiple procedures apply, 150% payment adjustment for

bilateral procedures does not apply, assistant surgeon may be paid, +add-on code (list separately in addition to primary procedure)

22548   **Neck spine fusion**   ~ follow-up period is 90 days, standard payment adjustment rules for multiple procedures apply, 150% payment adjustment for bilateral procedures does not apply, assistant surgeon may be paid

22554   **Neck spine fusion**   ~ follow-up period is 90 days, standard payment adjustment rules for multiple procedures apply, 150% payment adjustment for bilateral procedures does not apply, assistant surgeon may be paid

22556   **Thorax spine fusion**   ~ follow-up period is 90 days, standard payment adjustment rules for multiple procedures apply, 150% payment adjustment for bilateral procedures does not apply, assistant surgeon may be paid

22558   **Lumbar spine fusion**   ~ follow-up period is 90 days, standard payment adjustment rules for multiple procedures apply, 150% payment adjustment for bilateral procedures does not apply, assistant surgeon may be paid

22585   **Additional spinal fusion**   ~ follow-up period included in another service, no payment adjustment rules for multiple procedures apply, 150% payment adjustment for bilateral procedures does not apply, assistant surgeon may be paid, +add-on code (list separately in addition to primary procedure)

22590   **Spine & skull spinal fusion**   ~ follow-up period is 90 days, standard payment adjustment rules for multiple procedures apply, 150% payment adjustment for bilateral procedures does not apply, assistant surgeon may be paid

22595   **Neck spinal fusion**   ~ follow-up period is 90 days, standard payment adjustment rules for multiple procedures apply, 150% payment adjustment for bilateral procedures does not apply, assistant surgeon may be paid

22600   **Neck spine fusion**   ~ follow-up period is 90 days, standard payment adjustment rules for multiple procedures apply, 150% payment adjustment for bilateral procedures does not apply, assistant surgeon may be paid

22610   **Thorax spine fusion**   ~ follow-up period is 90 days, standard payment adjustment rules for multiple procedures apply, 150% payment adjustment for bilateral procedures does not apply, assistant surgeon may be paid

22612   **Lumbar spine fusion**   ~ follow-up period is 90 days, standard payment adjustment rules for multiple procedures apply, 150% payment adjustment for bilateral procedures does not apply, assistant surgeon may be paid

22614   **Spine fuse extra segment**   ~ follow-up period included in another service, no payment adjustment rules for multiple procedures apply, 150% payment adjustment for bilateral procedures does not apply, assistant surgeon may be paid

---

22630   **Lumbar spine fusion**   ~ follow-up period is 90 days, standard payment adjustment rules for multiple procedures apply, 150% payment adjustment for bilateral procedures does not apply, assistant surgeon may be paid

22632   **Spine fuse extra segment**   ~ follow-up period included in another service, no payment adjustment rules for multiple procedures apply, 150% payment adjustment for bilateral procedures does not apply, assistant surgeon may be paid

22800   **Fuse spine**   ~ follow-up period is 90 days, standard payment adjustment rules for multiple procedures apply, 150% payment adjustment for bilateral procedures does not apply, assistant surgeon may be paid

22802   **Fuse spine**   ~ follow-up period is 90 days, standard payment adjustment rules for multiple procedures apply, 150% payment adjustment for bilateral procedures does not apply, assistant surgeon may be paid

22804   **Fuse spine**   ~ follow-up period is 90 days, standard payment adjustment rules for multiple procedures apply, 150% payment adjustment for bilateral procedures does not apply, assistant surgeon may be paid

22808   **Fuse spine**   ~ follow-up period is 90 days, standard payment adjustment rules for multiple procedures apply, 150% payment adjustment for bilateral procedures does not apply, assistant surgeon may be paid

22810   **Fuse spine**   ~ follow-up period is 90 days, standard payment adjustment rules for multiple procedures apply, 150% payment adjustment for bilateral procedures does not apply, assistant surgeon may be paid

22812   **Fuse spine**   ~ follow-up period is 90 days, standard payment adjustment rules for multiple procedures apply, 150% payment adjustment for bilateral procedures does not apply, assistant surgeon may be paid

22818   **Kyphectomy, 1-2 segments**   ~ follow-up period is 90 days, standard payment adjustment rules for multiple procedures apply, 150% payment adjustment for bilateral procedures does not apply, assistant surgeon may be paid

22819   **Kyphectomy, 3 or more**   ~ follow-up period is 90 days, standard payment adjustment rules for multiple procedures apply, 150% payment adjustment for bilateral procedures does not apply, assistant surgeon may be paid

22830   **Explore spinal fusion**   ~ follow-up period is 90 days, standard payment adjustment rules for multiple procedures apply, 150% payment adjustment for bilateral procedures does not apply, assistant surgeon may be paid

22840   **Insert spine fixation device**   ~ follow-up period included in another service, no payment adjustment rules for multiple procedures apply, 150% payment adjustment for bilateral procedures does not apply, assistant surgeon may be paid

22841   **Insert spine fixation device**   ~ bundled code - no separate payment made, multiple procedure concept does not apply, bilateral surgery concept does not apply, assistant surgery concept does not apply

22842   **Insert spine fixation device**   ~ follow-up period included in another service, no payment adjustment rules for multiple procedures apply, 150% payment adjustment for bilateral procedures does not apply, assistant surgeon may be paid

22843   **Insert spine fixation device**   ~ follow-up period included in another service, no payment adjustment rules for multiple procedures apply, 150% payment adjustment for bilateral procedures does not apply, assistant surgeon may be paid

22844   **Insert spine fixation device**   ~ follow-up period included in another service, no payment adjustment rules for multiple procedures apply, 150% payment adjustment for bilateral procedures does not apply, assistant surgeon may be paid

22845   **Insert spine fixation device**   ~ follow-up period included in another service, no payment adjustment rules for multiple procedures apply, 150% payment adjustment for bilateral procedures does not apply, assistant surgeon may be paid

22846   **Insert spine fixation device**   ~ follow-up period included in another service, no payment adjustment rules for multiple procedures apply, 150% payment adjustment for bilateral procedures does not apply, assistant surgeon may be paid

22847   **Insert spine fixation device**   ~ follow-up period included in another service, no payment adjustment rules for multiple procedures apply, 150% payment adjustment for bilateral procedures does not apply, assistant surgeon may be paid

22848   **Insert pelvic fixation device**   ~ follow-up period included in another service, no payment adjustment rules for multiple procedures apply, 150% payment adjustment for bilateral procedures does not apply, assistant surgeon may be paid

22849   **Reinsert spinal fixation**   ~ follow-up period is 90 days, standard payment adjustment rules for multiple procedures apply, 150% payment adjustment for bilateral procedures does not apply, assistant surgeon may be paid

22850   **Remove spine fixation device**   ~ follow-up period is 90 days, standard payment adjustment rules for multiple procedures apply, 150% payment adjustment for bilateral procedures does not apply, assistant surgeon may be paid

22851   **Apply spine prosth device**   ~ follow-up period included in another service, no payment adjustment rules for multiple procedures apply, 150% payment adjustment for bilateral procedures does not apply, assistant surgeon may be paid

22852   **Remove spine fixation device**   ~ follow-up period is 90 days, standard payment adjustment rules for multiple procedures apply, 150% payment adjustment for bilateral procedures does not apply, assistant surgeon may be paid

22855   **Remove spine fixation device**   ~ follow-up period is 90 days, standard payment adjustment rules for multiple procedures apply, 150% payment adjustment for bilateral procedures does not apply, assistant surgeon may be paid

22857   **Lumbar artificial diskectomy**   ~ restricted coverage - special coverage rules apply, follow-up period is 90 days, standard payment adjustment rules for multiple procedures apply, 150% payment adjustment for bilateral procedures does not apply, assistant surgeon may be paid

22862   **Revise lumbar artificial disc**   ~ restricted coverage - special coverage rules apply, follow-up period is 90 days, standard payment adjustment rules for multiple procedures apply, 150% payment adjustment for bilateral procedures does not apply, assistant surgeon may be paid

22865   **Remove lumbar artificial disc**   ~ restricted coverage - special coverage rules apply, follow-up period is 90 days, standard payment adjustment rules for multiple procedures apply, 150% payment adjustment for bilateral procedures does not apply, assistant surgeon may be paid

22899   **Spine surgery procedure**   ~ medicare carrier determines global period, standard payment adjustment rules for multiple procedures apply, 150% payment adjustment for bilateral procedures does not apply, assistant surgeon may be paid

Abdomen

22900   **Remove abdominal wall lesion**   ~ follow-up period is 90 days, standard payment adjustment rules for multiple procedures apply, 150% payment adjustment for bilateral procedures does not apply, assistant surgeon may be paid

22999   **Abdomen surgery procedure**   ~ medicare carrier determines global period, standard payment adjustment rules for multiple procedures apply, 150% payment adjustment for bilateral procedures does not apply, payment for assistant surgeon subject to documentation of medical necessity

Shoulder

23000   **Remove calcium deposits**   ~ follow-up period is 90 days, standard payment adjustment rules for multiple procedures apply, 150% payment adjustment for bilateral procedures does not apply, assistant surgeon may be paid

23020   **Release shoulder joint**   ~ follow-up period is 90 days, standard payment adjustment rules for multiple procedures apply, 150% payment adjustment for bilateral procedures applies, assistant surgeon may be paid

23030   **Drain shoulder lesion**   ~ follow-up period is 10 days, standard payment adjustment rules for multiple procedures apply, 150% payment adjustment for bilateral procedures does not apply, assistant surgeon may not be paid

23031   **Drain shoulder bursa**   ~ follow-up period is 10 days, standard payment adjustment rules for multiple procedures apply, 150% payment adjustment for bilateral procedures applies, assistant surgeon may not be paid

23035   **Drain shoulder bone lesion**   ~ follow-up period is 90 days, standard payment adjustment rules for multiple procedures apply, 150% payment adjustment for bilateral procedures applies, assistant surgeon may be paid

23040   **Exploratory shoulder surgery**   ~ follow-up period is 90 days, standard payment adjustment rules for multiple procedures apply, 150% payment adjustment for bilateral procedures applies, assistant surgeon may be paid

23044   **Exploratory shoulder surgery**   ~ follow-up period is 90 days, standard payment adjustment rules for multiple procedures apply, 150% payment adjustment for bilateral procedures applies, assistant surgeon may not be paid

23065   **Biopsy shoulder tissues**   ~ follow-up period is 10 days, standard payment adjustment rules for multiple procedures apply, 150% payment adjustment for bilateral procedures applies, assistant surgeon may not be paid

23066   **Biopsy shoulder tissues**   ~ follow-up period is 90 days, standard payment adjustment rules for multiple procedures apply, 150% payment adjustment for bilateral procedures applies, assistant surgeon may not be paid

23075   **Remove shoulder lesion**   ~ follow-up period is 10 days, standard payment adjustment rules for multiple procedures apply, 150% payment adjustment for bilateral procedures applies, assistant surgeon may not be paid

23076   **Remove shoulder lesion**   ~ follow-up period is 90 days, standard payment adjustment rules for multiple procedures apply, 150% payment adjustment for bilateral procedures applies, assistant surgeon may not be paid

23077   **Remove tumor of shoulder**   ~ follow-up period is 90 days, standard payment adjustment rules for multiple procedures apply, 150% payment adjustment for bilateral procedures applies, assistant surgeon may be paid

23100   **Biopsy shoulder joint**   ~ follow-up period is 90 days, standard payment adjustment rules for multiple procedures apply, 150% payment adjustment for bilateral procedures applies, assistant surgeon may be paid

23101   **Shoulder joint surgery**   ~ follow-up period is 90 days, standard payment adjustment rules for multiple procedures apply, 150% payment adjustment for bilateral procedures applies, assistant surgeon may not be paid

23105   **Remove shoulder joint lining**   ~ follow-up period is 90 days, standard payment adjustment rules for multiple procedures apply, 150% payment adjustment for bilateral procedures applies, assistant surgeon may be paid

23106   **Incise collarbone joint**   ~ follow-up period is 90 days, standard payment adjustment rules for multiple procedures apply, 150% payment adjustment for bilateral procedures applies, assistant surgeon may not be paid

23107   **Explore treat shoulder joint**   ~ follow-up period is 90 days, standard payment adjustment rules for multiple procedures apply, 150% payment adjustment for bilateral procedures applies, assistant surgeon may be paid

23120   **Partial remove collar bone**   ~ follow-up period is 90 days, standard payment adjustment rules for multiple procedures apply, 150% payment adjustment for bilateral procedures does not apply, assistant surgeon may be paid

23125   **Remove collar bone**   ~ follow-up period is 90 days, standard payment adjustment rules for multiple procedures apply, 150% payment adjustment for bilateral procedures applies, assistant surgeon may be paid

23130   **Remove shoulder bone, part**   ~ follow-up period is 90 days, standard payment adjustment rules for multiple procedures apply, 150% payment adjustment for bilateral procedures applies, assistant surgeon may not be paid

23140   **Remove bone lesion**   ~ follow-up period is 90 days, standard payment adjustment rules for multiple procedures apply, 150% payment adjustment for bilateral procedures applies, assistant surgeon may not be paid

23145   **Remove bone lesion**   ~ follow-up period is 90 days, standard payment adjustment rules for multiple procedures apply, 150% payment adjustment for bilateral procedures applies, assistant surgeon may be paid

23146   **Remove bone lesion**   ~ follow-up period is 90 days, standard payment adjustment rules for multiple procedures apply, 150% payment adjustment for bilateral procedures applies, payment for assistant surgeon subject to documentation of medical necessity

23150   **Remove humerus lesion**   ~ follow-up period is 90 days, standard payment adjustment rules for multiple procedures apply, 150% payment adjustment for bilateral procedures applies, assistant surgeon may be paid

23155   **Remove humerus lesion**   ~ follow-up period is 90 days, standard payment adjustment rules for multiple procedures apply, 150% payment adjustment for bilateral procedures applies, assistant surgeon may be paid

23156   **Remove humerus lesion**   ~ follow-up period is 90 days, standard payment adjustment rules for multiple procedures apply, 150% payment adjustment for bilateral procedures applies, assistant surgeon may be paid

23170   **Remove collar bone lesion**   ~ follow-up period is 90 days, standard payment adjustment rules for multiple procedures apply, 150% payment adjustment for bilateral procedures applies, assistant surgeon may not be paid

23172   **Remove shoulder blade lesion**   ~ follow-up period is 90 days, standard payment adjustment rules for multiple procedures apply, 150% payment adjustment for bilateral procedures applies, assistant surgeon may be paid

23174   **Remove humerus lesion**   ~ follow-up period is 90 days, standard payment adjustment rules for multiple procedures apply, 150% payment adjustment for bilateral procedures applies, assistant surgeon may be paid

23180   **Remove collar bone lesion**   ~ follow-up period is 90 days, standard payment adjustment rules for multiple procedures apply, 150% payment adjustment for bilateral procedures applies, assistant surgeon may not be paid

23182   **Remove shoulder blade lesion**   ~ follow-up period is 90 days, standard payment adjustment rules for multiple procedures apply, 150% payment adjustment for bilateral procedures applies, assistant surgeon may be paid

23184   **Remove humerus lesion**   ~ follow-up period is 90 days, standard payment adjustment rules for multiple procedures apply, 150% payment adjustment for bilateral procedures applies, assistant surgeon may be paid

23190   **Partial remove scapula**   ~ follow-up period is 90 days, standard payment adjustment rules for multiple procedures apply, 150% payment adjustment for bilateral procedures applies, assistant surgeon may be paid

23195   **Remove head of humerus**   ~ follow-up period is 90 days, standard payment adjustment rules for multiple procedures apply, 150% payment adjustment for bilateral procedures applies, assistant surgeon may be paid

23200   **Remove collar bone**   ~ follow-up period is 90 days, standard payment adjustment rules for multiple procedures apply, 150% payment adjustment for bilateral procedures applies, assistant surgeon may be paid

23210   **Remove shoulder blade**   ~ follow-up period is 90 days, standard payment adjustment rules for multiple procedures apply, 150% payment adjustment for bilateral procedures applies, assistant surgeon may be paid

23220   **Partial remove humerus**   ~ follow-up period is 90 days, standard payment adjustment rules for multiple procedures apply, 150% payment adjustment for bilateral procedures applies, assistant surgeon may be paid

23221   **Partial remove humerus**   ~ follow-up period is 90 days, standard payment adjustment rules for multiple procedures apply, 150% payment adjustment for bilateral procedures applies, assistant surgeon may be paid

---

23222   **Partial remove humerus**   ~ follow-up period is 90 days, standard payment adjustment rules for multiple procedures apply, 150% payment adjustment for bilateral procedures applies, assistant surgeon may be paid

23330   **Remove shoulder foreign body**   ~ follow-up period is 10 days, standard payment adjustment rules for multiple procedures apply, 150% payment adjustment for bilateral procedures applies, payment for assistant surgeon subject to documentation of medical necessity

23331   **Remove shoulder foreign body**   ~ follow-up period is 90 days, standard payment adjustment rules for multiple procedures apply, 150% payment adjustment for bilateral procedures applies, payment for assistant surgeon subject to documentation of medical necessity

23332   **Remove shoulder foreign body**   ~ follow-up period is 90 days, standard payment adjustment rules for multiple procedures apply, 150% payment adjustment for bilateral procedures applies, assistant surgeon may be paid

23350   **Inject for shoulder x-ray**   ~ endoscopies or minor procedure - E/M services on the same day generally not paid, standard payment adjustment rules for multiple procedures apply, 150% payment adjustment for bilateral procedures applies, assistant surgeon may not be paid

23395   **Muscle transfer, shoulder/arm**   ~ follow-up period is 90 days, standard payment adjustment rules for multiple procedures apply, 150% payment adjustment for bilateral procedures does not apply, assistant surgeon may be paid

23397   **Muscle transfers**   ~ follow-up period is 90 days, standard payment adjustment rules for multiple procedures apply, 150% payment adjustment for bilateral procedures does not apply, assistant surgeon may be paid

23400   **Fixate shoulder blade**   ~ follow-up period is 90 days, standard payment adjustment rules for multiple procedures apply, 150% payment adjustment for bilateral procedures applies, assistant surgeon may be paid

23405   **Incise tendon & muscle**   ~ follow-up period is 90 days, standard payment adjustment rules for multiple procedures apply, 150% payment adjustment for bilateral procedures does not apply, assistant surgeon may be paid

23406   **Incise tendon(s) & muscle(s)**   ~ follow-up period is 90 days, standard payment adjustment rules for multiple procedures apply, 150% payment adjustment for bilateral procedures does not apply, assistant surgeon may be paid

23410   **Repair rotator cuff, acute**   ~ follow-up period is 90 days, standard payment adjustment rules for multiple procedures apply, 150% payment adjustment for bilateral procedures applies, assistant surgeon may be paid

23412 **Repair rotator cuff, chronic** ~ follow-up period is 90 days, standard payment adjustment rules for multiple procedures apply, 150% payment adjustment for bilateral procedures applies, assistant surgeon may be paid

23415 **Release shoulder ligament** ~ follow-up period is 90 days, standard payment adjustment rules for multiple procedures apply, 150% payment adjustment for bilateral procedures applies, assistant surgeon may not be paid

23420 **Repair shoulder** ~ follow-up period is 90 days, standard payment adjustment rules for multiple procedures apply, 150% payment adjustment for bilateral procedures applies, assistant surgeon may be paid

23430 **Repair biceps tendon** ~ follow-up period is 90 days, standard payment adjustment rules for multiple procedures apply, 150% payment adjustment for bilateral procedures applies, assistant surgeon may be paid

23440 **Remove/transplant tendon** ~ follow-up period is 90 days, standard payment adjustment rules for multiple procedures apply, 150% payment adjustment for bilateral procedures applies, assistant surgeon may be paid

23450 **Repair shoulder capsule** ~ follow-up period is 90 days, standard payment adjustment rules for multiple procedures apply, 150% payment adjustment for bilateral procedures applies, assistant surgeon may be paid

23455 **Repair shoulder capsule** ~ follow-up period is 90 days, standard payment adjustment rules for multiple procedures apply, 150% payment adjustment for bilateral procedures applies, assistant surgeon may be paid

23460 **Repair shoulder capsule** ~ follow-up period is 90 days, standard payment adjustment rules for multiple procedures apply, 150% payment adjustment for bilateral procedures applies, assistant surgeon may be paid

23462 **Repair shoulder capsule** ~ follow-up period is 90 days, standard payment adjustment rules for multiple procedures apply, 150% payment adjustment for bilateral procedures applies, assistant surgeon may be paid

23465 **Repair shoulder capsule** ~ follow-up period is 90 days, standard payment adjustment rules for multiple procedures apply, 150% payment adjustment for bilateral procedures applies, assistant surgeon may be paid

23466 **Repair shoulder capsule** ~ follow-up period is 90 days, standard payment adjustment rules for multiple procedures apply, 150% payment adjustment for bilateral procedures applies, assistant surgeon may be paid

23470 **Reconstruct shoulder joint** ~ follow-up period is 90 days, standard payment adjustment rules for multiple procedures apply, 150% payment adjustment for bilateral procedures applies, assistant surgeon may be paid

23472   **Reconstruct shoulder joint**   ~ follow-up period is 90 days, standard payment adjustment rules for multiple procedures apply, 150% payment adjustment for bilateral procedures applies, assistant surgeon may be paid

23480   **Revise collar bone**   ~ follow-up period is 90 days, standard payment adjustment rules for multiple procedures apply, 150% payment adjustment for bilateral procedures applies, assistant surgeon may not be paid

23485   **Revise collar bone**   ~ follow-up period is 90 days, standard payment adjustment rules for multiple procedures apply, 150% payment adjustment for bilateral procedures applies, assistant surgeon may be paid

23490   **Reinforce clavicle**   ~ follow-up period is 90 days, standard payment adjustment rules for multiple procedures apply, 150% payment adjustment for bilateral procedures applies, assistant surgeon may be paid

23491   **Reinforce shoulder bones**   ~ follow-up period is 90 days, standard payment adjustment rules for multiple procedures apply, 150% payment adjustment for bilateral procedures applies, assistant surgeon may be paid

23500   **Treat clavicle fracture**   ~ follow-up period is 90 days, standard payment adjustment rules for multiple procedures apply, 150% payment adjustment for bilateral procedures applies, assistant surgeon may not be paid

23505   **Treat clavicle fracture**   ~ follow-up period is 90 days, standard payment adjustment rules for multiple procedures apply, 150% payment adjustment for bilateral procedures applies, assistant surgeon may not be paid

23515   **Treat clavicle fracture**   ~ follow-up period is 90 days, standard payment adjustment rules for multiple procedures apply, 150% payment adjustment for bilateral procedures applies, assistant surgeon may be paid

23520   **Treat clavicle dislocation**   ~ follow-up period is 90 days, standard payment adjustment rules for multiple procedures apply, 150% payment adjustment for bilateral procedures applies, payment for assistant surgeon subject to documentation of medical necessity

23525   **Treat clavicle dislocation**   ~ follow-up period is 90 days, standard payment adjustment rules for multiple procedures apply, 150% payment adjustment for bilateral procedures applies, payment for assistant surgeon subject to documentation of medical necessity

23530   **Treat clavicle dislocation**   ~ follow-up period is 90 days, standard payment adjustment rules for multiple procedures apply, 150% payment adjustment for bilateral procedures applies, assistant surgeon may be paid

23532   **Treat clavicle dislocation**   ~ follow-up period is 90 days, standard payment adjustment rules for multiple procedures apply, 150% payment adjustment for bilateral procedures applies, assistant surgeon may be paid

23540   **Treat clavicle dislocation**   ~ follow-up period is 90 days, standard payment adjustment rules for multiple procedures apply, 150% payment adjustment for bilateral procedures applies, assistant surgeon may not be paid

23545   **Treat clavicle dislocation**   ~ follow-up period is 90 days, standard payment adjustment rules for multiple procedures apply, 150% payment adjustment for bilateral procedures applies, payment for assistant surgeon subject to documentation of medical necessity

23550   **Treat clavicle dislocation**   ~ follow-up period is 90 days, standard payment adjustment rules for multiple procedures apply, 150% payment adjustment for bilateral procedures applies, assistant surgeon may be paid

23552   **Treat clavicle dislocation**   ~ follow-up period is 90 days, standard payment adjustment rules for multiple procedures apply, 150% payment adjustment for bilateral procedures applies, assistant surgeon may be paid

23570   **Treat shoulder blade fracture**   ~ follow-up period is 90 days, standard payment adjustment rules for multiple procedures apply, 150% payment adjustment for bilateral procedures applies, assistant surgeon may not be paid

23575   **Treat shoulder blade fracture**   ~ follow-up period is 90 days, standard payment adjustment rules for multiple procedures apply, 150% payment adjustment for bilateral procedures applies, payment for assistant surgeon subject to documentation of medical necessity

23585   **Treat scapula fracture**   ~ follow-up period is 90 days, standard payment adjustment rules for multiple procedures apply, 150% payment adjustment for bilateral procedures applies, assistant surgeon may be paid

23600   **Treat humerus fracture**   ~ follow-up period is 90 days, standard payment adjustment rules for multiple procedures apply, 150% payment adjustment for bilateral procedures applies, assistant surgeon may not be paid

23605   **Treat humerus fracture**   ~ follow-up period is 90 days, standard payment adjustment rules for multiple procedures apply, 150% payment adjustment for bilateral procedures applies, assistant surgeon may not be paid

23615   **Treat humerus fracture**   ~ follow-up period is 90 days, standard payment adjustment rules for multiple procedures apply, 150% payment adjustment for bilateral procedures applies, assistant surgeon may be paid

23616   **Treat humerus fracture**   ~ follow-up period is 90 days, standard payment adjustment rules for multiple procedures apply, 150% payment adjustment for bilateral procedures applies, assistant surgeon may be paid

23620   **Treat humerus fracture**   ~ follow-up period is 90 days, standard payment adjustment rules for multiple procedures apply, 150% payment adjustment for bilateral procedures applies, assistant surgeon may not be paid

23625   **Treat humerus fracture**   ~ follow-up period is 90 days, standard payment adjustment rules for multiple procedures apply, 150% payment adjustment for bilateral procedures applies, assistant surgeon may not be paid

23630   **Treat humerus fracture**   ~ follow-up period is 90 days, standard payment adjustment rules for multiple procedures apply, 150% payment adjustment for bilateral procedures applies, assistant surgeon may be paid

23650   **Treat shoulder dislocation**   ~ follow-up period is 90 days, standard payment adjustment rules for multiple procedures apply, 150% payment adjustment for bilateral procedures applies, assistant surgeon may not be paid

23655   **Treat shoulder dislocation**   ~ follow-up period is 90 days, standard payment adjustment rules for multiple procedures apply, 150% payment adjustment for bilateral procedures applies, assistant surgeon may not be paid

23660   **Treat shoulder dislocation**   ~ follow-up period is 90 days, standard payment adjustment rules for multiple procedures apply, 150% payment adjustment for bilateral procedures applies, assistant surgeon may be paid

23665   **Treat dislocation/fracture**   ~ follow-up period is 90 days, standard payment adjustment rules for multiple procedures apply, 150% payment adjustment for bilateral procedures applies, assistant surgeon may not be paid

23670   **Treat dislocation/fracture**   ~ follow-up period is 90 days, standard payment adjustment rules for multiple procedures apply, 150% payment adjustment for bilateral procedures applies, assistant surgeon may be paid

23675   **Treat dislocation/fracture**   ~ follow-up period is 90 days, standard payment adjustment rules for multiple procedures apply, 150% payment adjustment for bilateral procedures applies, assistant surgeon may not be paid

23680   **Treat dislocation/fracture**   ~ follow-up period is 90 days, standard payment adjustment rules for multiple procedures apply, 150% payment adjustment for bilateral procedures applies, assistant surgeon may be paid

23700   **Fixate shoulder**   ~ follow-up period is 10 days, standard payment adjustment rules for multiple procedures apply, 150% payment adjustment for bilateral procedures does not apply, assistant surgeon may not be paid

23800   **Fuse shoulder joint**   ~ follow-up period is 90 days, standard payment adjustment rules for multiple procedures apply, 150% payment adjustment for bilateral procedures applies, assistant surgeon may be paid

23802   **Fuse shoulder joint**   ~ follow-up period is 90 days, standard payment adjustment rules for multiple procedures apply, 150% payment adjustment for bilateral procedures does not apply, assistant surgeon may be paid

23900   **Amputate arm & girdle**   ~ follow-up period is 90 days, standard payment adjustment rules for multiple procedures apply, 150% payment adjustment for bilateral procedures does not apply, assistant surgeon may be paid

23920   **Amputation at shoulder joint**   ~ follow-up period is 90 days, standard payment adjustment rules for multiple procedures apply, 150% payment adjustment for bilateral procedures does not apply, assistant surgeon may be paid

23921   **Amputation follow-up surgery**   ~ follow-up period is 90 days, standard payment adjustment rules for multiple procedures apply, 150% payment adjustment for bilateral procedures does not apply, assistant surgeon may not be paid

23929   **Shoulder surgery procedure**   ~ medicare carrier determines global period, standard payment adjustment rules for multiple procedures apply, 150% payment adjustment for bilateral procedures does not apply, assistant surgeon may be paid

Humerous (Upper Arm) And Elbow

23930   **Drain arm lesion**   ~ follow-up period is 10 days, standard payment adjustment rules for multiple procedures apply, 150% payment adjustment for bilateral procedures applies, assistant surgeon may not be paid

23931   **Drain arm bursa**   ~ follow-up period is 10 days, standard payment adjustment rules for multiple procedures apply, 150% payment adjustment for bilateral procedures applies, assistant surgeon may not be paid

23935   **Drain arm/elbow bone lesion**   ~ follow-up period is 90 days, standard payment adjustment rules for multiple procedures apply, 150% payment adjustment for bilateral procedures applies, payment for assistant surgeon subject to documentation of medical necessity

24000   **Exploratory elbow surgery**   ~ follow-up period is 90 days, standard payment adjustment rules for multiple procedures apply, 150% payment adjustment for bilateral procedures applies, payment for assistant surgeon subject to documentation of medical necessity

24006   **Release elbow joint**   ~ follow-up period is 90 days, standard payment adjustment rules for multiple procedures apply, 150% payment adjustment for bilateral procedures applies, assistant surgeon may be paid

---

24065   **Biopsy arm/elbow soft tissue**   ~ follow-up period is 10 days, standard payment adjustment rules for multiple procedures apply, 150% payment adjustment for bilateral procedures applies, assistant surgeon may not be paid

24066   **Biopsy arm/elbow soft tissue**   ~ follow-up period is 90 days, standard payment adjustment rules for multiple procedures apply, 150% payment adjustment for bilateral procedures applies, assistant surgeon may not be paid

24075   **Remove arm/elbow lesion**   ~ follow-up period is 90 days, standard payment adjustment rules for multiple procedures apply, 150% payment adjustment for bilateral procedures applies, assistant surgeon may not be paid

24076   **Remove arm/elbow lesion**   ~ follow-up period is 90 days, standard payment adjustment rules for multiple procedures apply, 150% payment adjustment for bilateral procedures applies, assistant surgeon may not be paid

24077   **Remove tumor of arm/elbow**   ~ follow-up period is 90 days, standard payment adjustment rules for multiple procedures apply, 150% payment adjustment for bilateral procedures applies, assistant surgeon may be paid

24100   **Biopsy elbow joint lining**   ~ follow-up period is 90 days, standard payment adjustment rules for multiple procedures apply, 150% payment adjustment for bilateral procedures applies, assistant surgeon may be paid

24101   **Explore/treat elbow joint**   ~ follow-up period is 90 days, standard payment adjustment rules for multiple procedures apply, 150% payment adjustment for bilateral procedures applies, assistant surgeon may be paid

24102   **Remove elbow joint lining**   ~ follow-up period is 90 days, standard payment adjustment rules for multiple procedures apply, 150% payment adjustment for bilateral procedures applies, assistant surgeon may be paid

24105   **Remove elbow bursa**   ~ follow-up period is 90 days, standard payment adjustment rules for multiple procedures apply, 150% payment adjustment for bilateral procedures applies, assistant surgeon may not be paid

24110   **Remove humerus lesion**   ~ follow-up period is 90 days, standard payment adjustment rules for multiple procedures apply, 150% payment adjustment for bilateral procedures applies, assistant surgeon may not be paid

24115   **Remove/graft bone lesion**   ~ follow-up period is 90 days, standard payment adjustment rules for multiple procedures apply, 150% payment adjustment for bilateral procedures applies, assistant surgeon may be paid

24116   **Remove/graft bone lesion**   ~ follow-up period is 90 days, standard payment adjustment rules for multiple procedures apply, 150% payment adjustment for bilateral procedures applies, assistant surgeon may be paid

| 24120 | **Remove elbow lesion** | ~ follow-up period is 90 days, standard payment adjustment rules for multiple procedures apply, 150% payment adjustment for bilateral procedures applies, payment for assistant surgeon subject to documentation of medical necessity |

| 24125 | **Remove/graft bone lesion** | ~ follow-up period is 90 days, standard payment adjustment rules for multiple procedures apply, 150% payment adjustment for bilateral procedures applies, assistant surgeon may be paid |

| 24126 | **Remove/graft bone lesion** | ~ follow-up period is 90 days, standard payment adjustment rules for multiple procedures apply, 150% payment adjustment for bilateral procedures applies, assistant surgeon may be paid |

| 24130 | **Remove head of radius** | ~ follow-up period is 90 days, standard payment adjustment rules for multiple procedures apply, 150% payment adjustment for bilateral procedures applies, assistant surgeon may not be paid |

| 24134 | **Remove arm bone lesion** | ~ follow-up period is 90 days, standard payment adjustment rules for multiple procedures apply, 150% payment adjustment for bilateral procedures applies, assistant surgeon may be paid |

| 24136 | **Remove radius bone lesion** | ~ follow-up period is 90 days, standard payment adjustment rules for multiple procedures apply, 150% payment adjustment for bilateral procedures applies, assistant surgeon may not be paid |

| 24138 | **Remove elbow bone lesion** | ~ follow-up period is 90 days, standard payment adjustment rules for multiple procedures apply, 150% payment adjustment for bilateral procedures applies, assistant surgeon may be paid |

| 24140 | **Partial remove arm bone** | ~ follow-up period is 90 days, standard payment adjustment rules for multiple procedures apply, 150% payment adjustment for bilateral procedures applies, assistant surgeon may be paid |

| 24145 | **Partial remove radius** | ~ follow-up period is 90 days, standard payment adjustment rules for multiple procedures apply, 150% payment adjustment for bilateral procedures applies, assistant surgeon may not be paid |

| 24147 | **Partial remove elbow** | ~ follow-up period is 90 days, standard payment adjustment rules for multiple procedures apply, 150% payment adjustment for bilateral procedures applies, assistant surgeon may not be paid |

| 24149 | **Radical resection of elbow** | ~ follow-up period is 90 days, standard payment adjustment rules for multiple procedures apply, 150% payment adjustment for bilateral procedures applies, assistant surgeon may be paid |

24150 **Extensive humerus surgery** ~ follow-up period is 90 days, standard payment adjustment rules for multiple procedures apply, 150% payment adjustment for bilateral procedures applies, assistant surgeon may be paid

24151 **Extensive humerus surgery** ~ follow-up period is 90 days, standard payment adjustment rules for multiple procedures apply, 150% payment adjustment for bilateral procedures applies, assistant surgeon may be paid

24152 **Extensive radius surgery** ~ follow-up period is 90 days, standard payment adjustment rules for multiple procedures apply, 150% payment adjustment for bilateral procedures applies, assistant surgeon may be paid

24153 **Extensive radius surgery** ~ follow-up period is 90 days, standard payment adjustment rules for multiple procedures apply, 150% payment adjustment for bilateral procedures applies, payment for assistant surgeon subject to documentation of medical necessity

24155 **Remove elbow joint** ~ follow-up period is 90 days, standard payment adjustment rules for multiple procedures apply, 150% payment adjustment for bilateral procedures applies, assistant surgeon may be paid

24160 **Remove elbow joint implant** ~ follow-up period is 90 days, standard payment adjustment rules for multiple procedures apply, 150% payment adjustment for bilateral procedures applies, assistant surgeon may not be paid

24164 **Remove radius head implant** ~ follow-up period is 90 days, standard payment adjustment rules for multiple procedures apply, 150% payment adjustment for bilateral procedures applies, assistant surgeon may not be paid

24200 **Remove arm foreign body** ~ follow-up period is 10 days, standard payment adjustment rules for multiple procedures apply, 150% payment adjustment for bilateral procedures applies, payment for assistant surgeon subject to documentation of medical necessity

24201 **Remove arm foreign body** ~ follow-up period is 90 days, standard payment adjustment rules for multiple procedures apply, 150% payment adjustment for bilateral procedures applies, assistant surgeon may not be paid

24220 **Inject for elbow x-ray** ~ endoscopies or minor procedure - E/M services on the same day generally not paid, standard payment adjustment rules for multiple procedures apply, 150% payment adjustment for bilateral procedures applies, payment for assistant surgeon subject to documentation of medical necessity

24300 **Manipulate elbow w/anesth** ~ follow-up period is 90 days, standard payment adjustment rules for multiple procedures apply, 150% payment adjustment for bilateral procedures applies, assistant surgeon may not be paid

24301   **Muscle/tendon transfer**   ~ follow-up period is 90 days, standard payment adjustment rules for multiple procedures apply, 150% payment adjustment for bilateral procedures does not apply, assistant surgeon may be paid

24305   **Arm tendon lengthening**   ~ follow-up period is 90 days, standard payment adjustment rules for multiple procedures apply, 150% payment adjustment for bilateral procedures does not apply, payment for assistant surgeon subject to documentation of medical necessity

24310   **Revise arm tendon**   ~ follow-up period is 90 days, standard payment adjustment rules for multiple procedures apply, 150% payment adjustment for bilateral procedures does not apply, payment for assistant surgeon subject to documentation of medical necessity

24320   **Repair arm tendon**   ~ follow-up period is 90 days, standard payment adjustment rules for multiple procedures apply, 150% payment adjustment for bilateral procedures does not apply, assistant surgeon may be paid

24330   **Revise arm muscles**   ~ follow-up period is 90 days, standard payment adjustment rules for multiple procedures apply, 150% payment adjustment for bilateral procedures applies, assistant surgeon may be paid

24331   **Revise arm muscles**   ~ follow-up period is 90 days, standard payment adjustment rules for multiple procedures apply, 150% payment adjustment for bilateral procedures applies, assistant surgeon may be paid

24332   **Tenolysis, triceps**   ~ follow-up period is 90 days, standard payment adjustment rules for multiple procedures apply, 150% payment adjustment for bilateral procedures applies, assistant surgeon may not be paid

24340   **Repair biceps tendon**   ~ follow-up period is 90 days, standard payment adjustment rules for multiple procedures apply, 150% payment adjustment for bilateral procedures applies, assistant surgeon may be paid

24341   **Repair arm tendon/muscle**   ~ follow-up period is 90 days, standard payment adjustment rules for multiple procedures apply, 150% payment adjustment for bilateral procedures applies, assistant surgeon may be paid

24342   **Repair ruptured tendon**   ~ follow-up period is 90 days, standard payment adjustment rules for multiple procedures apply, 150% payment adjustment for bilateral procedures applies, assistant surgeon may be paid

24343   **Repair elbow lat ligament w/tissue**   ~ follow-up period is 90 days, standard payment adjustment rules for multiple procedures apply, 150% payment adjustment for bilateral procedures applies, assistant surgeon may be paid

24344   **Reconstruct elbow lat ligament**   ~ follow-up period is 90 days, standard payment adjustment rules for multiple procedures apply, 150% payment adjustment for bilateral procedures applies, assistant surgeon may be paid

24345   **Repair elbow med ligament w/tissue**   ~ follow-up period is 90 days, standard payment adjustment rules for multiple procedures apply, 150% payment adjustment for bilateral procedures applies, assistant surgeon may be paid

24346   **Reconstruct elbow med ligament**   ~ follow-up period is 90 days, standard payment adjustment rules for multiple procedures apply, 150% payment adjustment for bilateral procedures applies, assistant surgeon may be paid

24350   **Repair tennis elbow**   ~ follow-up period is 90 days, standard payment adjustment rules for multiple procedures apply, 150% payment adjustment for bilateral procedures applies, payment for assistant surgeon subject to documentation of medical necessity

24351   **Repair tennis elbow**   ~ follow-up period is 90 days, standard payment adjustment rules for multiple procedures apply, 150% payment adjustment for bilateral procedures applies, payment for assistant surgeon subject to documentation of medical necessity

24352   **Repair tennis elbow**   ~ follow-up period is 90 days, standard payment adjustment rules for multiple procedures apply, 150% payment adjustment for bilateral procedures applies, assistant surgeon may be paid

24354   **Repair tennis elbow**   ~ follow-up period is 90 days, standard payment adjustment rules for multiple procedures apply, 150% payment adjustment for bilateral procedures applies, assistant surgeon may not be paid

24356   **Revise tennis elbow**   ~ follow-up period is 90 days, standard payment adjustment rules for multiple procedures apply, 150% payment adjustment for bilateral procedures applies, payment for assistant surgeon subject to documentation of medical necessity

24360   **Reconstruct elbow joint**   ~ follow-up period is 90 days, standard payment adjustment rules for multiple procedures apply, 150% payment adjustment for bilateral procedures applies, assistant surgeon may be paid

24361   **Reconstruct elbow joint**   ~ follow-up period is 90 days, standard payment adjustment rules for multiple procedures apply, 150% payment adjustment for bilateral procedures applies, assistant surgeon may be paid

24362   **Reconstruct elbow joint**   ~ follow-up period is 90 days, standard payment adjustment rules for multiple procedures apply, 150% payment adjustment for bilateral procedures applies, assistant surgeon may be paid

24363   **Replace elbow joint**   ~ follow-up period is 90 days, standard payment adjustment rules for multiple procedures apply, 150% payment adjustment for bilateral procedures applies, assistant surgeon may be paid

24365   **Reconstruct head of radius**   ~ follow-up period is 90 days, standard payment adjustment rules for multiple procedures apply, 150% payment adjustment for bilateral procedures applies, assistant surgeon may be paid

24366   **Reconstruct head of radius**   ~ follow-up period is 90 days, standard payment adjustment rules for multiple procedures apply, 150% payment adjustment for bilateral procedures applies, assistant surgeon may be paid

24400   **Revise humerus**   ~ follow-up period is 90 days, standard payment adjustment rules for multiple procedures apply, 150% payment adjustment for bilateral procedures applies, assistant surgeon may be paid

24410   **Revise humerus**   ~ follow-up period is 90 days, standard payment adjustment rules for multiple procedures apply, 150% payment adjustment for bilateral procedures applies, assistant surgeon may be paid

24420   **Revise humerus**   ~ follow-up period is 90 days, standard payment adjustment rules for multiple procedures apply, 150% payment adjustment for bilateral procedures applies, assistant surgeon may be paid

24430   **Repair humerus**   ~ follow-up period is 90 days, standard payment adjustment rules for multiple procedures apply, 150% payment adjustment for bilateral procedures applies, assistant surgeon may be paid

24435   **Repair humerus with graft**   ~ follow-up period is 90 days, standard payment adjustment rules for multiple procedures apply, 150% payment adjustment for bilateral procedures applies, assistant surgeon may be paid

24470   **Revise elbow joint**   ~ follow-up period is 90 days, standard payment adjustment rules for multiple procedures apply, 150% payment adjustment for bilateral procedures applies, assistant surgeon may be paid

24495   **Decompress forearm**   ~ follow-up period is 90 days, standard payment adjustment rules for multiple procedures apply, 150% payment adjustment for bilateral procedures applies, payment for assistant surgeon subject to documentation of medical necessity

24498   **Reinforce humerus**   ~ follow-up period is 90 days, standard payment adjustment rules for multiple procedures apply, 150% payment adjustment for bilateral procedures applies, assistant surgeon may be paid

24500 **Treat humerus fracture**   ~ follow-up period is 90 days, standard payment adjustment rules for multiple procedures apply, 150% payment adjustment for bilateral procedures applies, assistant surgeon may not be paid

24505 **Treat humerus fracture**   ~ follow-up period is 90 days, standard payment adjustment rules for multiple procedures apply, 150% payment adjustment for bilateral procedures applies, assistant surgeon may not be paid

24515 **Treat humerus fracture**   ~ follow-up period is 90 days, standard payment adjustment rules for multiple procedures apply, 150% payment adjustment for bilateral procedures applies, assistant surgeon may be paid

24516 **Treat humerus fracture**   ~ follow-up period is 90 days, standard payment adjustment rules for multiple procedures apply, 150% payment adjustment for bilateral procedures applies, assistant surgeon may be paid

24530 **Treat humerus fracture**   ~ follow-up period is 90 days, standard payment adjustment rules for multiple procedures apply, 150% payment adjustment for bilateral procedures applies, assistant surgeon may not be paid

24535 **Treat humerus fracture**   ~ follow-up period is 90 days, standard payment adjustment rules for multiple procedures apply, 150% payment adjustment for bilateral procedures applies, assistant surgeon may not be paid

24538 **Treat humerus fracture**   ~ follow-up period is 90 days, standard payment adjustment rules for multiple procedures apply, 150% payment adjustment for bilateral procedures applies, assistant surgeon may not be paid

24545 **Treat humerus fracture**   ~ follow-up period is 90 days, standard payment adjustment rules for multiple procedures apply, 150% payment adjustment for bilateral procedures applies, assistant surgeon may be paid

24546 **Treat humerus fracture**   ~ follow-up period is 90 days, standard payment adjustment rules for multiple procedures apply, 150% payment adjustment for bilateral procedures applies, assistant surgeon may be paid

24560 **Treat humerus fracture**   ~ follow-up period is 90 days, standard payment adjustment rules for multiple procedures apply, 150% payment adjustment for bilateral procedures applies, assistant surgeon may not be paid

24565 **Treat humerus fracture**   ~ follow-up period is 90 days, standard payment adjustment rules for multiple procedures apply, 150% payment adjustment for bilateral procedures applies, assistant surgeon may not be paid

24566 **Treat humerus fracture**   ~ follow-up period is 90 days, standard payment adjustment rules for multiple procedures apply, 150% payment adjustment for bilateral procedures applies, assistant surgeon may not be paid

24575   **Treat humerus fracture**   ~ follow-up period is 90 days, standard payment adjustment rules for multiple procedures apply, 150% payment adjustment for bilateral procedures applies, assistant surgeon may be paid

24576   **Treat humerus fracture**   ~ follow-up period is 90 days, standard payment adjustment rules for multiple procedures apply, 150% payment adjustment for bilateral procedures applies, assistant surgeon may not be paid

24577   **Treat humerus fracture**   ~ follow-up period is 90 days, standard payment adjustment rules for multiple procedures apply, 150% payment adjustment for bilateral procedures applies, assistant surgeon may not be paid

24579   **Treat humerus fracture**   ~ follow-up period is 90 days, standard payment adjustment rules for multiple procedures apply, 150% payment adjustment for bilateral procedures applies, assistant surgeon may be paid

24582   **Treat humerus fracture**   ~ follow-up period is 90 days, standard payment adjustment rules for multiple procedures apply, 150% payment adjustment for bilateral procedures applies, assistant surgeon may not be paid

24586   **Treat elbow fracture**   ~ follow-up period is 90 days, standard payment adjustment rules for multiple procedures apply, 150% payment adjustment for bilateral procedures applies, assistant surgeon may be paid

24587   **Treat elbow fracture**   ~ follow-up period is 90 days, standard payment adjustment rules for multiple procedures apply, 150% payment adjustment for bilateral procedures applies, assistant surgeon may be paid

24600   **Treat elbow dislocation**   ~ follow-up period is 90 days, standard payment adjustment rules for multiple procedures apply, 150% payment adjustment for bilateral procedures applies, assistant surgeon may not be paid

24605   **Treat elbow dislocation**   ~ follow-up period is 90 days, standard payment adjustment rules for multiple procedures apply, 150% payment adjustment for bilateral procedures applies, assistant surgeon may not be paid

24615   **Treat elbow dislocation**   ~ follow-up period is 90 days, standard payment adjustment rules for multiple procedures apply, 150% payment adjustment for bilateral procedures applies, assistant surgeon may be paid

24620   **Treat elbow fracture**   ~ follow-up period is 90 days, standard payment adjustment rules for multiple procedures apply, 150% payment adjustment for bilateral procedures applies, payment for assistant surgeon subject to documentation of medical necessity

24635   **Treat elbow fracture**   ~ follow-up period is 90 days, standard payment adjustment rules for multiple procedures apply, 150% payment adjustment for bilateral procedures applies, assistant surgeon may be paid

24640   **Treat elbow dislocation**   ~ follow-up period is 10 days, standard payment adjustment rules for multiple procedures apply, 150% payment adjustment for bilateral procedures applies, payment for assistant surgeon subject to documentation of medical necessity

24650   **Treat radius fracture**   ~ follow-up period is 90 days, standard payment adjustment rules for multiple procedures apply, 150% payment adjustment for bilateral procedures applies, assistant surgeon may not be paid

24655   **Treat radius fracture**   ~ follow-up period is 90 days, standard payment adjustment rules for multiple procedures apply, 150% payment adjustment for bilateral procedures applies, assistant surgeon may not be paid

24665   **Treat radius fracture**   ~ follow-up period is 90 days, standard payment adjustment rules for multiple procedures apply, 150% payment adjustment for bilateral procedures applies, assistant surgeon may be paid

24666   **Treat radius fracture**   ~ follow-up period is 90 days, standard payment adjustment rules for multiple procedures apply, 150% payment adjustment for bilateral procedures applies, assistant surgeon may be paid

24670   **Treat ulnar fracture**   ~ follow-up period is 90 days, standard payment adjustment rules for multiple procedures apply, 150% payment adjustment for bilateral procedures applies, assistant surgeon may not be paid

24675   **Treat ulnar fracture**   ~ follow-up period is 90 days, standard payment adjustment rules for multiple procedures apply, 150% payment adjustment for bilateral procedures applies, assistant surgeon may not be paid

24685   **Treat ulnar fracture**   ~ follow-up period is 90 days, standard payment adjustment rules for multiple procedures apply, 150% payment adjustment for bilateral procedures applies, assistant surgeon may be paid

24800   **Fuse elbow joint**   ~ follow-up period is 90 days, standard payment adjustment rules for multiple procedures apply, 150% payment adjustment for bilateral procedures applies, assistant surgeon may be paid

24802   **Fuse/graft of elbow joint**   ~ follow-up period is 90 days, standard payment adjustment rules for multiple procedures apply, 150% payment adjustment for bilateral procedures applies, assistant surgeon may be paid

24900   **Amputate upper arm**   ~ follow-up period is 90 days, standard payment adjustment rules for multiple procedures apply, 150% payment adjustment for bilateral procedures applies, assistant surgeon may be paid

24920   **Amputate upper arm**   ~ follow-up period is 90 days, standard payment adjustment rules for multiple procedures apply, 150% payment adjustment for bilateral procedures applies, assistant surgeon may be paid

24925   **Amputation follow-up surgery**   ~ follow-up period is 90 days, standard payment adjustment rules for multiple procedures apply, 150% payment adjustment for bilateral procedures applies, assistant surgeon may be paid

24930   **Amputation follow-up surgery**   ~ follow-up period is 90 days, standard payment adjustment rules for multiple procedures apply, 150% payment adjustment for bilateral procedures applies, assistant surgeon may be paid

24931   **Amputate upper arm & implant**   ~ follow-up period is 90 days, standard payment adjustment rules for multiple procedures apply, 150% payment adjustment for bilateral procedures applies, assistant surgeon may be paid

24935   **Revise amputation**   ~ follow-up period is 90 days, standard payment adjustment rules for multiple procedures apply, 150% payment adjustment for bilateral procedures applies, payment for assistant surgeon subject to documentation of medical necessity

24940   **Revise upper arm**   ~ follow-up period is 90 days, standard payment adjustment rules for multiple procedures apply, 150% payment adjustment for bilateral procedures applies, assistant surgeon may be paid

24999   **Upper arm/elbow surgery**   ~ medicare carrier determines global period, standard payment adjustment rules for multiple procedures apply, 150% payment adjustment for bilateral procedures applies, payment for assistant surgeon subject to documentation of medical necessity

Forearm and Wrist

25000   **Incise tendon sheath**   ~ follow-up period is 90 days, standard payment adjustment rules for multiple procedures apply, 150% payment adjustment for bilateral procedures applies, assistant surgeon may not be paid

25001   **Incise flexor carpi radialis**   ~ follow-up period is 90 days, standard payment adjustment rules for multiple procedures apply, 150% payment adjustment for bilateral procedures applies, assistant surgeon may not be paid

25020   **Decompress forearm 1 space**   ~ follow-up period is 90 days, standard payment adjustment rules for multiple procedures apply, 150% payment adjustment for bilateral procedures applies, assistant surgeon may not be paid

25023   **Decompress forearm 1 space**   ~ follow-up period is 90 days, standard payment adjustment rules for multiple procedures apply, 150% payment adjustment for bilateral procedures applies, payment for assistant surgeon subject to documentation of medical necessity

25024   **Decompress forearm 2 spaces**   ~ follow-up period is 90 days, standard payment adjustment rules for multiple procedures apply, 150% payment adjustment for bilateral procedures applies, assistant surgeon may not be paid

25025   **Decompress forearm 2 spaces**   ~ follow-up period is 90 days, standard payment adjustment rules for multiple procedures apply, 150% payment adjustment for bilateral procedures applies, payment for assistant surgeon subject to documentation of medical necessity

25028   **Drain forearm lesion**   ~ follow-up period is 90 days, standard payment adjustment rules for multiple procedures apply, 150% payment adjustment for bilateral procedures applies, assistant surgeon may not be paid

25031   **Drain forearm bursa**   ~ follow-up period is 90 days, standard payment adjustment rules for multiple procedures apply, 150% payment adjustment for bilateral procedures applies, payment for assistant surgeon subject to documentation of medical necessity

25035   **Treat forearm bone lesion**   ~ follow-up period is 90 days, standard payment adjustment rules for multiple procedures apply, 150% payment adjustment for bilateral procedures applies, payment for assistant surgeon subject to documentation of medical necessity

25040   **Explore/treat wrist joint**   ~ follow-up period is 90 days, standard payment adjustment rules for multiple procedures apply, 150% payment adjustment for bilateral procedures applies, payment for assistant surgeon subject to documentation of medical necessity

25065   **Biopsy forearm soft tissues**   ~ follow-up period is 10 days, standard payment adjustment rules for multiple procedures apply, 150% payment adjustment for bilateral procedures applies, assistant surgeon may not be paid

25066   **Biopsy forearm soft tissues**   ~ follow-up period is 90 days, standard payment adjustment rules for multiple procedures apply, 150% payment adjustment for bilateral procedures applies, assistant surgeon may not be paid

25075   **Remove forearm lesion subcut**   ~ follow-up period is 90 days, standard payment adjustment rules for multiple procedures apply, 150% payment adjustment for bilateral procedures applies, assistant surgeon may not be paid

25076   **Remove forearm lesion deep**   ~ follow-up period is 90 days, standard payment adjustment rules for multiple procedures apply, 150% payment adjustment for bilateral procedures applies, assistant surgeon may not be paid

25077   **Remove tumor, forearm/wrist**   ~ follow-up period is 90 days, standard payment adjustment rules for multiple procedures apply, 150% payment adjustment for bilateral procedures applies, assistant surgeon may not be paid

25085   **Incise wrist capsule**   ~ follow-up period is 90 days, standard payment adjustment rules for multiple procedures apply, 150% payment adjustment for bilateral procedures applies, assistant surgeon may be paid

25100   **Biopsy wrist joint**   ~ follow-up period is 90 days, standard payment adjustment rules for multiple procedures apply, 150% payment adjustment for bilateral procedures applies, payment for assistant surgeon subject to documentation of medical necessity

25101   **Explore/treat wrist joint**   ~ follow-up period is 90 days, standard payment adjustment rules for multiple procedures apply, 150% payment adjustment for bilateral procedures applies, payment for assistant surgeon subject to documentation of medical necessity

25105   **Remove wrist joint lining**   ~ follow-up period is 90 days, standard payment adjustment rules for multiple procedures apply, 150% payment adjustment for bilateral procedures applies, payment for assistant surgeon subject to documentation of medical necessity

25107   **Remove wrist joint cartilage**   ~ follow-up period is 90 days, standard payment adjustment rules for multiple procedures apply, 150% payment adjustment for bilateral procedures applies, assistant surgeon may be paid

25109   **Excise tendon forearm/wrist**   ~ follow-up period is 90 days, standard payment adjustment rules for multiple procedures apply, 150% payment adjustment for bilateral procedures applies, assistant surgeon may not be paid

25110   **Remove wrist tendon lesion**   ~ follow-up period is 90 days, standard payment adjustment rules for multiple procedures apply, 150% payment adjustment for bilateral procedures applies, assistant surgeon may not be paid

25111   **Remove wrist tendon lesion**   ~ follow-up period is 90 days, standard payment adjustment rules for multiple procedures apply, 150% payment adjustment for bilateral procedures applies, assistant surgeon may not be paid

25112   **Reremove wrist tendon lesion**   ~ follow-up period is 90 days, standard payment adjustment rules for multiple procedures apply, 150% payment adjustment for bilateral procedures applies, assistant surgeon may not be paid

25115 **Remove wrist/forearm lesion** ~ follow-up period is 90 days, standard payment adjustment rules for multiple procedures apply, 150% payment adjustment for bilateral procedures applies, assistant surgeon may not be paid

25116 **Remove wrist/forearm lesion** ~ follow-up period is 90 days, standard payment adjustment rules for multiple procedures apply, 150% payment adjustment for bilateral procedures applies, payment for assistant surgeon subject to documentation of medical necessity

25118 **Excise wrist tendon sheath** ~ follow-up period is 90 days, standard payment adjustment rules for multiple procedures apply, 150% payment adjustment for bilateral procedures applies, assistant surgeon may not be paid

25119 **Partial remove ulna** ~ follow-up period is 90 days, standard payment adjustment rules for multiple procedures apply, 150% payment adjustment for bilateral procedures applies, assistant surgeon may be paid

25120 **Remove forearm lesion** ~ follow-up period is 90 days, standard payment adjustment rules for multiple procedures apply, 150% payment adjustment for bilateral procedures applies, payment for assistant surgeon subject to documentation of medical necessity

25125 **Remove/graft forearm lesion** ~ follow-up period is 90 days, standard payment adjustment rules for multiple procedures apply, 150% payment adjustment for bilateral procedures applies, payment for assistant surgeon subject to documentation of medical necessity

25126 **Remove/graft forearm lesion** ~ follow-up period is 90 days, standard payment adjustment rules for multiple procedures apply, 150% payment adjustment for bilateral procedures applies, assistant surgeon may be paid

25130 **Remove wrist lesion** ~ follow-up period is 90 days, standard payment adjustment rules for multiple procedures apply, 150% payment adjustment for bilateral procedures applies, payment for assistant surgeon subject to documentation of medical necessity

25135 **Remove & graft wrist lesion** ~ follow-up period is 90 days, standard payment adjustment rules for multiple procedures apply, 150% payment adjustment for bilateral procedures applies, assistant surgeon may be paid

25136 **Remove & graft wrist lesion** ~ follow-up period is 90 days, standard payment adjustment rules for multiple procedures apply, 150% payment adjustment for bilateral procedures applies, assistant surgeon may be paid

25145 **Remove forearm bone lesion** ~ follow-up period is 90 days, standard payment adjustment rules for multiple procedures apply, 150% payment adjustment for bilateral procedures applies, assistant surgeon may be paid

25150   **Partial remove ulna**   ~ follow-up period is 90 days, standard payment adjustment rules for multiple procedures apply, 150% payment adjustment for bilateral procedures applies, assistant surgeon may not be paid

25151   **Partial remove radius**   ~ follow-up period is 90 days, standard payment adjustment rules for multiple procedures apply, 150% payment adjustment for bilateral procedures applies, assistant surgeon may be paid

25170   **Extensive forearm surgery**   ~ follow-up period is 90 days, standard payment adjustment rules for multiple procedures apply, 150% payment adjustment for bilateral procedures applies, assistant surgeon may be paid

25210   **Remove wrist bone**   ~ follow-up period is 90 days, standard payment adjustment rules for multiple procedures apply, 150% payment adjustment for bilateral procedures does not apply, payment for assistant surgeon subject to documentation of medical necessity

25215   **Remove wrist bones**   ~ follow-up period is 90 days, standard payment adjustment rules for multiple procedures apply, 150% payment adjustment for bilateral procedures does not apply, assistant surgeon may be paid

25230   **Partial remove radius**   ~ follow-up period is 90 days, standard payment adjustment rules for multiple procedures apply, 150% payment adjustment for bilateral procedures applies, assistant surgeon may not be paid

25240   **Partial remove ulna**   ~ follow-up period is 90 days, standard payment adjustment rules for multiple procedures apply, 150% payment adjustment for bilateral procedures applies, payment for assistant surgeon subject to documentation of medical necessity

25246   **Inject for wrist x-ray**   ~ endoscopies or minor procedure - E/M services on the same day generally not paid, standard payment adjustment rules for multiple procedures apply, 150% payment adjustment for bilateral procedures applies, assistant surgeon may not be paid

25248   **Remove forearm foreign body**   ~ follow-up period is 90 days, standard payment adjustment rules for multiple procedures apply, 150% payment adjustment for bilateral procedures applies, assistant surgeon may not be paid

25250   **Remove wrist prosthesis**   ~ follow-up period is 90 days, standard payment adjustment rules for multiple procedures apply, 150% payment adjustment for bilateral procedures applies, assistant surgeon may be paid

25251   **Remove wrist prosthesis**   ~ follow-up period is 90 days, standard payment adjustment rules for multiple procedures apply, 150% payment adjustment for bilateral procedures does not apply, assistant surgeon may be paid

25259   **Manipulate wrist w/anesthesia**   ~ follow-up period is 90 days, standard payment adjustment rules for multiple procedures apply, 150% payment adjustment for bilateral procedures applies, assistant surgeon may not be paid

25260   **Repair forearm tendon/muscle**   ~ follow-up period is 90 days, standard payment adjustment rules for multiple procedures apply, 150% payment adjustment for bilateral procedures does not apply, assistant surgeon may not be paid

25263   **Repair forearm tendon/muscle**   ~ follow-up period is 90 days, standard payment adjustment rules for multiple procedures apply, 150% payment adjustment for bilateral procedures does not apply, assistant surgeon may be paid

25265   **Repair forearm tendon/muscle**   ~ follow-up period is 90 days, standard payment adjustment rules for multiple procedures apply, 150% payment adjustment for bilateral procedures does not apply, assistant surgeon may be paid

25270   **Repair forearm tendon/muscle**   ~ follow-up period is 90 days, standard payment adjustment rules for multiple procedures apply, 150% payment adjustment for bilateral procedures does not apply, payment for assistant surgeon subject to documentation of medical necessity

25272   **Repair forearm tendon/muscle**   ~ follow-up period is 90 days, standard payment adjustment rules for multiple procedures apply, 150% payment adjustment for bilateral procedures does not apply, payment for assistant surgeon subject to documentation of medical necessity

25274   **Repair forearm tendon/muscle**   ~ follow-up period is 90 days, standard payment adjustment rules for multiple procedures apply, 150% payment adjustment for bilateral procedures does not apply, payment for assistant surgeon subject to documentation of medical necessity

25275   **Repair forearm tendon sheath**   ~ follow-up period is 90 days, standard payment adjustment rules for multiple procedures apply, 150% payment adjustment for bilateral procedures applies, payment for assistant surgeon subject to documentation of medical necessity

25280   **Revise wrist/forearm tendon**   ~ follow-up period is 90 days, standard payment adjustment rules for multiple procedures apply, 150% payment adjustment for bilateral procedures does not apply, payment for assistant surgeon subject to documentation of medical necessity

25290   **Incise wrist/forearm tendon**   ~ follow-up period is 90 days, standard payment adjustment rules for multiple procedures apply, 150% payment adjustment for bilateral procedures does not apply, assistant surgeon may not be paid

25295   **Release wrist/forearm tendon**   ~ follow-up period is 90 days, standard payment adjustment rules for multiple procedures apply, 150% payment adjustment for bilateral procedures does not apply, assistant surgeon may not be paid

25300   **Fuse tendons at wrist**   ~ follow-up period is 90 days, standard payment adjustment rules for multiple procedures apply, 150% payment adjustment for bilateral procedures applies, assistant surgeon may be paid

25301   **Fuse tendons at wrist**   ~ follow-up period is 90 days, standard payment adjustment rules for multiple procedures apply, 150% payment adjustment for bilateral procedures applies, assistant surgeon may be paid

25310   **Transplant forearm tendon**   ~ follow-up period is 90 days, standard payment adjustment rules for multiple procedures apply, 150% payment adjustment for bilateral procedures does not apply, assistant surgeon may be paid

25312   **Transplant forearm tendon**   ~ follow-up period is 90 days, standard payment adjustment rules for multiple procedures apply, 150% payment adjustment for bilateral procedures does not apply, assistant surgeon may be paid

25315   **Revise palsy hand tendon(s)**   ~ follow-up period is 90 days, standard payment adjustment rules for multiple procedures apply, 150% payment adjustment for bilateral procedures applies, assistant surgeon may be paid

25316   **Revise palsy hand tendon(s)**   ~ follow-up period is 90 days, standard payment adjustment rules for multiple procedures apply, 150% payment adjustment for bilateral procedures applies, assistant surgeon may be paid

25320   **Repair/revise wrist joint**   ~ follow-up period is 90 days, standard payment adjustment rules for multiple procedures apply, 150% payment adjustment for bilateral procedures applies, assistant surgeon may be paid

25332   **Revise wrist joint**   ~ follow-up period is 90 days, standard payment adjustment rules for multiple procedures apply, 150% payment adjustment for bilateral procedures applies, assistant surgeon may be paid

25335   **Realignment of hand**   ~ follow-up period is 90 days, standard payment adjustment rules for multiple procedures apply, 150% payment adjustment for bilateral procedures applies, assistant surgeon may be paid

25337   **Reconstruct ulna/radioulnar**   ~ follow-up period is 90 days, standard payment adjustment rules for multiple procedures apply, 150% payment adjustment for bilateral procedures applies, assistant surgeon may not be paid

25350   **Revise radius**   ~ follow-up period is 90 days, standard payment adjustment rules for multiple procedures apply, 150% payment adjustment for bilateral procedures applies, assistant surgeon may be paid

25355 **Revise radius** ~ follow-up period is 90 days, standard payment adjustment rules for multiple procedures apply, 150% payment adjustment for bilateral procedures applies, assistant surgeon may be paid

25360 **Revise ulna** ~ follow-up period is 90 days, standard payment adjustment rules for multiple procedures apply, 150% payment adjustment for bilateral procedures applies, assistant surgeon may be paid

25365 **Revise radius & ulna** ~ follow-up period is 90 days, standard payment adjustment rules for multiple procedures apply, 150% payment adjustment for bilateral procedures applies, assistant surgeon may be paid

25370 **Revise radius or ulna** ~ follow-up period is 90 days, standard payment adjustment rules for multiple procedures apply, 150% payment adjustment for bilateral procedures applies, assistant surgeon may be paid

25375 **Revise radius & ulna** ~ follow-up period is 90 days, standard payment adjustment rules for multiple procedures apply, 150% payment adjustment for bilateral procedures applies, assistant surgeon may be paid

25390 **Shorten radius or ulna** ~ follow-up period is 90 days, standard payment adjustment rules for multiple procedures apply, 150% payment adjustment for bilateral procedures applies, assistant surgeon may be paid

25391 **Lengthen radius or ulna** ~ follow-up period is 90 days, standard payment adjustment rules for multiple procedures apply, 150% payment adjustment for bilateral procedures applies, assistant surgeon may be paid

25392 **Shorten radius & ulna** ~ follow-up period is 90 days, standard payment adjustment rules for multiple procedures apply, 150% payment adjustment for bilateral procedures applies, assistant surgeon may be paid

25393 **Lengthen radius & ulna** ~ follow-up period is 90 days, standard payment adjustment rules for multiple procedures apply, 150% payment adjustment for bilateral procedures applies, assistant surgeon may be paid

25394 **Repair carpal bone, shorten** ~ follow-up period is 90 days, standard payment adjustment rules for multiple procedures apply, 150% payment adjustment for bilateral procedures applies, assistant surgeon may be paid

25400 **Repair radius or ulna** ~ follow-up period is 90 days, standard payment adjustment rules for multiple procedures apply, 150% payment adjustment for bilateral procedures applies, assistant surgeon may be paid

25405 **Repair/graft radius or ulna** ~ follow-up period is 90 days, standard payment adjustment rules for multiple procedures apply, 150% payment adjustment for bilateral procedures applies, assistant surgeon may be paid

25415   **Repair radius & ulna**   ~ follow-up period is 90 days, standard payment adjustment rules for multiple procedures apply, 150% payment adjustment for bilateral procedures applies, assistant surgeon may be paid

25420   **Repair/graft radius & ulna**   ~ follow-up period is 90 days, standard payment adjustment rules for multiple procedures apply, 150% payment adjustment for bilateral procedures applies, assistant surgeon may be paid

25425   **Repair/graft radius or ulna**   ~ follow-up period is 90 days, standard payment adjustment rules for multiple procedures apply, 150% payment adjustment for bilateral procedures applies, assistant surgeon may be paid

25426   **Repair/graft radius & ulna**   ~ follow-up period is 90 days, standard payment adjustment rules for multiple procedures apply, 150% payment adjustment for bilateral procedures applies, assistant surgeon may be paid

25430   **Vasc graft into carpal bone**   ~ follow-up period is 90 days, standard payment adjustment rules for multiple procedures apply, 150% payment adjustment for bilateral procedures applies, assistant surgeon may not be paid

25431   **Repair nonunion carpal bone**   ~ follow-up period is 90 days, standard payment adjustment rules for multiple procedures apply, 150% payment adjustment for bilateral procedures applies, assistant surgeon may be paid

25440   **Repair/graft wrist bone**   ~ follow-up period is 90 days, standard payment adjustment rules for multiple procedures apply, 150% payment adjustment for bilateral procedures applies, assistant surgeon may be paid

25441   **Reconstruct wrist joint**   ~ follow-up period is 90 days, standard payment adjustment rules for multiple procedures apply, 150% payment adjustment for bilateral procedures applies, assistant surgeon may be paid

25442   **Reconstruct wrist joint**   ~ follow-up period is 90 days, standard payment adjustment rules for multiple procedures apply, 150% payment adjustment for bilateral procedures applies, assistant surgeon may be paid

25443   **Reconstruct wrist joint**   ~ follow-up period is 90 days, standard payment adjustment rules for multiple procedures apply, 150% payment adjustment for bilateral procedures applies, assistant surgeon may be paid

25444   **Reconstruct wrist joint**   ~ follow-up period is 90 days, standard payment adjustment rules for multiple procedures apply, 150% payment adjustment for bilateral procedures applies, assistant surgeon may be paid

25445   **Reconstruct wrist joint**   ~ follow-up period is 90 days, standard payment adjustment rules for multiple procedures apply, 150% payment adjustment for bilateral procedures applies, assistant surgeon may not be paid

25446 **Wrist replacement** ~ follow-up period is 90 days, standard payment adjustment rules for multiple procedures apply, 150% payment adjustment for bilateral procedures applies, assistant surgeon may be paid

25447 **Repair wrist joint(s)** ~ follow-up period is 90 days, standard payment adjustment rules for multiple procedures apply, 150% payment adjustment for bilateral procedures applies, assistant surgeon may be paid

25449 **Remove wrist joint implant** ~ follow-up period is 90 days, standard payment adjustment rules for multiple procedures apply, 150% payment adjustment for bilateral procedures applies, assistant surgeon may be paid

25450 **Revise wrist joint** ~ follow-up period is 90 days, standard payment adjustment rules for multiple procedures apply, 150% payment adjustment for bilateral procedures applies, assistant surgeon may not be paid

25455 **Revise wrist joint** ~ follow-up period is 90 days, standard payment adjustment rules for multiple procedures apply, 150% payment adjustment for bilateral procedures applies, assistant surgeon may not be paid

25490 **Reinforce radius** ~ follow-up period is 90 days, standard payment adjustment rules for multiple procedures apply, 150% payment adjustment for bilateral procedures applies, assistant surgeon may be paid

25491 **Reinforce ulna** ~ follow-up period is 90 days, standard payment adjustment rules for multiple procedures apply, 150% payment adjustment for bilateral procedures applies, assistant surgeon may be paid

25492 **Reinforce radius and ulna** ~ follow-up period is 90 days, standard payment adjustment rules for multiple procedures apply, 150% payment adjustment for bilateral procedures applies, assistant surgeon may be paid

25500 **Treat fracture radius** ~ follow-up period is 90 days, standard payment adjustment rules for multiple procedures apply, 150% payment adjustment for bilateral procedures applies, assistant surgeon may not be paid

25505 **Treat fracture radius** ~ follow-up period is 90 days, standard payment adjustment rules for multiple procedures apply, 150% payment adjustment for bilateral procedures applies, assistant surgeon may not be paid

25515 **Treat fracture radius** ~ follow-up period is 90 days, standard payment adjustment rules for multiple procedures apply, 150% payment adjustment for bilateral procedures applies, assistant surgeon may be paid

25520 **Treat fracture radius** ~ follow-up period is 90 days, standard payment adjustment rules for multiple procedures apply, 150% payment adjustment for bilateral procedures applies, assistant surgeon may not be paid

25525   **Treat fracture radius**   ~ follow-up period is 90 days, standard payment adjustment rules for multiple procedures apply, 150% payment adjustment for bilateral procedures applies, assistant surgeon may be paid

25526   **Treat fracture radius**   ~ follow-up period is 90 days, standard payment adjustment rules for multiple procedures apply, 150% payment adjustment for bilateral procedures applies, assistant surgeon may be paid

25530   **Treat fracture ulna**   ~ follow-up period is 90 days, standard payment adjustment rules for multiple procedures apply, 150% payment adjustment for bilateral procedures applies, assistant surgeon may not be paid

25535   **Treat fracture ulna**   ~ follow-up period is 90 days, standard payment adjustment rules for multiple procedures apply, 150% payment adjustment for bilateral procedures applies, assistant surgeon may not be paid

25545   **Treat fracture ulna**   ~ follow-up period is 90 days, standard payment adjustment rules for multiple procedures apply, 150% payment adjustment for bilateral procedures applies, assistant surgeon may be paid

25560   **Treat fracture radius & ulna**   ~ follow-up period is 90 days, standard payment adjustment rules for multiple procedures apply, 150% payment adjustment for bilateral procedures applies, assistant surgeon may not be paid

25565   **Treat fracture radius & ulna**   ~ follow-up period is 90 days, standard payment adjustment rules for multiple procedures apply, 150% payment adjustment for bilateral procedures applies, assistant surgeon may not be paid

25574   **Treat fracture radius & ulna**   ~ follow-up period is 90 days, standard payment adjustment rules for multiple procedures apply, 150% payment adjustment for bilateral procedures applies, assistant surgeon may be paid

25575   **Treat fracture radius/ulna**   ~ follow-up period is 90 days, standard payment adjustment rules for multiple procedures apply, 150% payment adjustment for bilateral procedures applies, assistant surgeon may be paid

25600   **Treat fracture radius/ulna**   ~ follow-up period is 90 days, standard payment adjustment rules for multiple procedures apply, 150% payment adjustment for bilateral procedures applies, assistant surgeon may not be paid

25605   **Treat fracture radius/ulna**   ~ follow-up period is 90 days, standard payment adjustment rules for multiple procedures apply, 150% payment adjustment for bilateral procedures applies, assistant surgeon may not be paid

25606   **Treat fracture distal radial**   ~ follow-up period is 90 days, standard payment adjustment rules for multiple procedures apply, 150% payment adjustment for bilateral procedures applies, assistant surgeon may not be paid

25607   **Treat fracture radiation extra-articular**   ~ follow-up period is 90 days, standard payment adjustment rules for multiple procedures apply, 150% payment adjustment for bilateral procedures applies, assistant surgeon may be paid

25608   **Treat fracture radiation intra-articular**   ~ follow-up period is 90 days, standard payment adjustment rules for multiple procedures apply, 150% payment adjustment for bilateral procedures applies, assistant surgeon may be paid

25609   **Treat fracture radial 3+ fragments**   ~ follow-up period is 90 days, standard payment adjustment rules for multiple procedures apply, 150% payment adjustment for bilateral procedures applies, assistant surgeon may be paid

25622   **Treat wrist bone fracture**   ~ follow-up period is 90 days, standard payment adjustment rules for multiple procedures apply, 150% payment adjustment for bilateral procedures applies, assistant surgeon may not be paid

25624   **Treat wrist bone fracture**   ~ follow-up period is 90 days, standard payment adjustment rules for multiple procedures apply, 150% payment adjustment for bilateral procedures applies, payment for assistant surgeon subject to documentation of medical necessity

25628   **Treat wrist bone fracture**   ~ follow-up period is 90 days, standard payment adjustment rules for multiple procedures apply, 150% payment adjustment for bilateral procedures applies, assistant surgeon may be paid

25630   **Treat wrist bone fracture**   ~ follow-up period is 90 days, standard payment adjustment rules for multiple procedures apply, 150% payment adjustment for bilateral procedures applies, assistant surgeon may not be paid

25635   **Treat wrist bone fracture**   ~ follow-up period is 90 days, standard payment adjustment rules for multiple procedures apply, 150% payment adjustment for bilateral procedures applies, payment for assistant surgeon subject to documentation of medical necessity

25645   **Treat wrist bone fracture**   ~ follow-up period is 90 days, standard payment adjustment rules for multiple procedures apply, 150% payment adjustment for bilateral procedures applies, assistant surgeon may be paid

25650   **Treat wrist bone fracture**   ~ follow-up period is 90 days, standard payment adjustment rules for multiple procedures apply, 150% payment adjustment for bilateral procedures applies, assistant surgeon may not be paid

25651   **Pin ulnar styloid fracture**   ~ follow-up period is 90 days, standard payment adjustment rules for multiple procedures apply, 150% payment adjustment for bilateral procedures applies, payment for assistant surgeon subject to documentation of medical necessity

25652   **Treat fracture ulnar styloid**   ~ follow-up period is 90 days, standard payment adjustment rules for multiple procedures apply, 150% payment adjustment for bilateral procedures applies, assistant surgeon may not be paid

25660   **Treat wrist dislocation**   ~ follow-up period is 90 days, standard payment adjustment rules for multiple procedures apply, 150% payment adjustment for bilateral procedures applies, payment for assistant surgeon subject to documentation of medical necessity

25670   **Treat wrist dislocation**   ~ follow-up period is 90 days, standard payment adjustment rules for multiple procedures apply, 150% payment adjustment for bilateral procedures applies, assistant surgeon may be paid

25671   **Pin radioulnar dislocation**   ~ follow-up period is 90 days, standard payment adjustment rules for multiple procedures apply, 150% payment adjustment for bilateral procedures applies, assistant surgeon may not be paid

25675   **Treat wrist dislocation**   ~ follow-up period is 90 days, standard payment adjustment rules for multiple procedures apply, 150% payment adjustment for bilateral procedures applies, payment for assistant surgeon subject to documentation of medical necessity

25676   **Treat wrist dislocation**   ~ follow-up period is 90 days, standard payment adjustment rules for multiple procedures apply, 150% payment adjustment for bilateral procedures applies, assistant surgeon may be paid

25680   **Treat wrist fracture**   ~ follow-up period is 90 days, standard payment adjustment rules for multiple procedures apply, 150% payment adjustment for bilateral procedures applies, payment for assistant surgeon subject to documentation of medical necessity

25685   **Treat wrist fracture**   ~ follow-up period is 90 days, standard payment adjustment rules for multiple procedures apply, 150% payment adjustment for bilateral procedures applies, assistant surgeon may be paid

25690   **Treat wrist dislocation**   ~ follow-up period is 90 days, standard payment adjustment rules for multiple procedures apply, 150% payment adjustment for bilateral procedures applies, payment for assistant surgeon subject to documentation of medical necessity

25695   **Treat wrist dislocation**   ~ follow-up period is 90 days, standard payment adjustment rules for multiple procedures apply, 150% payment adjustment for bilateral procedures applies, assistant surgeon may be paid

25800   **Fuse wrist joint**   ~ follow-up period is 90 days, standard payment adjustment rules for multiple procedures apply, 150% payment adjustment for bilateral procedures applies, assistant surgeon may be paid

25805   **Fuse/graft of wrist joint**   ~ follow-up period is 90 days, standard payment adjustment rules for multiple procedures apply, 150% payment adjustment for bilateral procedures applies, assistant surgeon may be paid

25810   **Fuse/graft of wrist joint**   ~ follow-up period is 90 days, standard payment adjustment rules for multiple procedures apply, 150% payment adjustment for bilateral procedures applies, assistant surgeon may be paid

25820   **Fuse hand bones**   ~ follow-up period is 90 days, standard payment adjustment rules for multiple procedures apply, 150% payment adjustment for bilateral procedures applies, assistant surgeon may be paid

25825   **Fuse hand bones with graft**   ~ follow-up period is 90 days, standard payment adjustment rules for multiple procedures apply, 150% payment adjustment for bilateral procedures applies, assistant surgeon may be paid

25830   **Fuse radioulnar joint/ulna**   ~ follow-up period is 90 days, standard payment adjustment rules for multiple procedures apply, 150% payment adjustment for bilateral procedures applies, assistant surgeon may be paid

25900   **Amputate forearm**   ~ follow-up period is 90 days, standard payment adjustment rules for multiple procedures apply, 150% payment adjustment for bilateral procedures applies, payment for assistant surgeon subject to documentation of medical necessity

25905   **Amputate forearm**   ~ follow-up period is 90 days, standard payment adjustment rules for multiple procedures apply, 150% payment adjustment for bilateral procedures applies, assistant surgeon may be paid

25907   **Amputation follow-up surgery**   ~ follow-up period is 90 days, standard payment adjustment rules for multiple procedures apply, 150% payment adjustment for bilateral procedures applies, assistant surgeon may be paid

25909   **Amputation follow-up surgery**   ~ follow-up period is 90 days, standard payment adjustment rules for multiple procedures apply, 150% payment adjustment for bilateral procedures applies, assistant surgeon may be paid

25915   **Amputate forearm**   ~ follow-up period is 90 days, standard payment adjustment rules for multiple procedures apply, 150% payment adjustment for bilateral procedures applies, assistant surgeon may be paid

25920   **Amputate hand at wrist**   ~ follow-up period is 90 days, standard payment adjustment rules for multiple procedures apply, 150% payment adjustment for bilateral procedures applies, payment for assistant surgeon subject to documentation of medical necessity

25922   **Amputate hand at wrist**   ~ follow-up period is 90 days, standard payment adjustment rules for multiple procedures apply, 150% payment adjustment for bilateral procedures applies, assistant surgeon may be paid

25924   **Amputation follow-up surgery**   ~ follow-up period is 90 days, standard payment adjustment rules for multiple procedures apply, 150% payment adjustment for bilateral procedures applies, assistant surgeon may be paid

25927   **Amputate hand**   ~ follow-up period is 90 days, standard payment adjustment rules for multiple procedures apply, 150% payment adjustment for bilateral procedures applies, payment for assistant surgeon subject to documentation of medical necessity

25929   **Amputation follow-up surgery**   ~ follow-up period is 90 days, standard payment adjustment rules for multiple procedures apply, 150% payment adjustment for bilateral procedures applies, assistant surgeon may be paid

25931   **Amputation follow-up surgery**   ~ follow-up period is 90 days, standard payment adjustment rules for multiple procedures apply, 150% payment adjustment for bilateral procedures applies, assistant surgeon may not be paid

25999   **Forearm or wrist surgery**   ~ medicare carrier determines global period, standard payment adjustment rules for multiple procedures apply, 150% payment adjustment for bilateral procedures applies, payment for assistant surgeon subject to documentation of medical necessity

Hand and Fingers

26010   **Drain finger abscess**   ~ follow-up period is 10 days, standard payment adjustment rules for multiple procedures apply, 150% payment adjustment for bilateral procedures does not apply, assistant surgeon may not be paid

26011   **Drain finger abscess**   ~ follow-up period is 10 days, standard payment adjustment rules for multiple procedures apply, 150% payment adjustment for bilateral procedures does not apply, assistant surgeon may not be paid

26020   **Drain hand tendon sheath**   ~ follow-up period is 90 days, standard payment adjustment rules for multiple procedures apply, 150% payment adjustment for bilateral procedures does not apply, assistant surgeon may not be paid

26025   **Drain palm bursa**   ~ follow-up period is 90 days, standard payment adjustment rules for multiple procedures apply, 150% payment adjustment for bilateral procedures does not apply, payment for assistant surgeon subject to documentation of medical necessity

26030   **Drain palm bursa(s)**   ~ follow-up period is 90 days, standard payment adjustment rules for multiple procedures apply, 150% payment adjustment for

---

bilateral procedures does not apply, payment for assistant surgeon subject to documentation of medical necessity

26034   **Treat hand bone lesion**   ~ follow-up period is 90 days, standard payment adjustment rules for multiple procedures apply, 150% payment adjustment for bilateral procedures does not apply, assistant surgeon may not be paid

26035   **Decompress fingers/hand**   ~ follow-up period is 90 days, standard payment adjustment rules for multiple procedures apply, 150% payment adjustment for bilateral procedures does not apply, payment for assistant surgeon subject to documentation of medical necessity

26037   **Decompress fingers/hand**   ~ follow-up period is 90 days, standard payment adjustment rules for multiple procedures apply, 150% payment adjustment for bilateral procedures does not apply, payment for assistant surgeon subject to documentation of medical necessity

26040   **Release palm contracture**   ~ follow-up period is 90 days, standard payment adjustment rules for multiple procedures apply, 150% payment adjustment for bilateral procedures applies, assistant surgeon may not be paid

26045   **Release palm contracture**   ~ follow-up period is 90 days, standard payment adjustment rules for multiple procedures apply, 150% payment adjustment for bilateral procedures applies, assistant surgeon may not be paid

26055   **Incise finger tendon sheath**   ~ follow-up period is 90 days, standard payment adjustment rules for multiple procedures apply, 150% payment adjustment for bilateral procedures does not apply, assistant surgeon may not be paid

26060   **Incise finger tendon**   ~ follow-up period is 90 days, standard payment adjustment rules for multiple procedures apply, 150% payment adjustment for bilateral procedures does not apply, payment for assistant surgeon subject to documentation of medical necessity

26070   **Explore/treat hand joint**   ~ follow-up period is 90 days, standard payment adjustment rules for multiple procedures apply, 150% payment adjustment for bilateral procedures applies, assistant surgeon may not be paid

26075   **Explore/treat finger joint**   ~ follow-up period is 90 days, standard payment adjustment rules for multiple procedures apply, 150% payment adjustment for bilateral procedures applies, assistant surgeon may not be paid

26080   **Explore/treat finger joint**   ~ follow-up period is 90 days, standard payment adjustment rules for multiple procedures apply, 150% payment adjustment for bilateral procedures does not apply, assistant surgeon may not be paid

26100   **Biopsy hand joint lining**   ~ follow-up period is 90 days, standard payment adjustment rules for multiple procedures apply, 150% payment adjustment for bilateral procedures applies, payment for assistant surgeon subject to documentation of medical necessity

26105   **Biopsy finger joint lining**   ~ follow-up period is 90 days, standard payment adjustment rules for multiple procedures apply, 150% payment adjustment for bilateral procedures applies, payment for assistant surgeon subject to documentation of medical necessity

26110   **Biopsy finger joint lining**   ~ follow-up period is 90 days, standard payment adjustment rules for multiple procedures apply, 150% payment adjustment for bilateral procedures does not apply, assistant surgeon may not be paid

26115   **Remove hand lesion subcut**   ~ follow-up period is 90 days, standard payment adjustment rules for multiple procedures apply, 150% payment adjustment for bilateral procedures does not apply, assistant surgeon may not be paid

26116   **Remove hand lesion, deep**   ~ follow-up period is 90 days, standard payment adjustment rules for multiple procedures apply, 150% payment adjustment for bilateral procedures does not apply, assistant surgeon may not be paid

26117   **Remove tumor, hand/finger**   ~ follow-up period is 90 days, standard payment adjustment rules for multiple procedures apply, 150% payment adjustment for bilateral procedures does not apply, assistant surgeon may not be paid

26121   **Release palm contracture**   ~ follow-up period is 90 days, standard payment adjustment rules for multiple procedures apply, 150% payment adjustment for bilateral procedures applies, assistant surgeon may not be paid

26123   **Release palm contracture**   ~ follow-up period is 90 days, standard payment adjustment rules for multiple procedures apply, 150% payment adjustment for bilateral procedures applies, assistant surgeon may not be paid

26125   **Release palm contracture**   ~ follow-up period included in another service, no payment adjustment rules for multiple procedures apply, 150% payment adjustment for bilateral procedures does not apply, assistant surgeon may not be paid

26130   **Remove wrist joint lining**   ~ follow-up period is 90 days, standard payment adjustment rules for multiple procedures apply, 150% payment adjustment for bilateral procedures applies, assistant surgeon may not be paid

26135   **Revise finger joint, each**   ~ follow-up period is 90 days, standard payment adjustment rules for multiple procedures apply, 150% payment adjustment for bilateral procedures does not apply, payment for assistant surgeon subject to documentation of medical necessity

26140   **Revise finger joint, each**   ~ follow-up period is 90 days, standard payment adjustment rules for multiple procedures apply, 150% payment adjustment for bilateral procedures does not apply, assistant surgeon may not be paid

26145   **Tendon excise palm/finger**   ~ follow-up period is 90 days, standard payment adjustment rules for multiple procedures apply, 150% payment adjustment for bilateral procedures does not apply, assistant surgeon may not be paid

26160   **Remove tendon sheath lesion**   ~ follow-up period is 90 days, standard payment adjustment rules for multiple procedures apply, 150% payment adjustment for bilateral procedures does not apply, assistant surgeon may not be paid

26170   **Remove palm tendon, each**   ~ follow-up period is 90 days, standard payment adjustment rules for multiple procedures apply, 150% payment adjustment for bilateral procedures does not apply, payment for assistant surgeon subject to documentation of medical necessity

26180   **Remove finger tendon**   ~ follow-up period is 90 days, standard payment adjustment rules for multiple procedures apply, 150% payment adjustment for bilateral procedures does not apply, payment for assistant surgeon subject to documentation of medical necessity

26185   **Remove finger bone**   ~ follow-up period is 90 days, standard payment adjustment rules for multiple procedures apply, 150% payment adjustment for bilateral procedures applies, assistant surgeon may be paid

26200   **Remove hand bone lesion**   ~ follow-up period is 90 days, standard payment adjustment rules for multiple procedures apply, 150% payment adjustment for bilateral procedures does not apply, payment for assistant surgeon subject to documentation of medical necessity

26205   **Remove/graft bone lesion**   ~ follow-up period is 90 days, standard payment adjustment rules for multiple procedures apply, 150% payment adjustment for bilateral procedures does not apply, assistant surgeon may not be paid

26210   **Remove finger lesion**   ~ follow-up period is 90 days, standard payment adjustment rules for multiple procedures apply, 150% payment adjustment for bilateral procedures does not apply, assistant surgeon may not be paid

26215   **Remove/graft finger lesion**   ~ follow-up period is 90 days, standard payment adjustment rules for multiple procedures apply, 150% payment adjustment for bilateral procedures does not apply, assistant surgeon may not be paid

26230   **Partial remove hand bone**   ~ follow-up period is 90 days, standard payment adjustment rules for multiple procedures apply, 150% payment adjustment for bilateral procedures does not apply, payment for assistant surgeon subject to documentation of medical necessity

26235 **Partial remove finger bone** ~ follow-up period is 90 days, standard payment adjustment rules for multiple procedures apply, 150% payment adjustment for bilateral procedures does not apply, payment for assistant surgeon subject to documentation of medical necessity

26236 **Partial remove finger bone** ~ follow-up period is 90 days, standard payment adjustment rules for multiple procedures apply, 150% payment adjustment for bilateral procedures does not apply, assistant surgeon may not be paid

26250 **Extensive hand surgery** ~ follow-up period is 90 days, standard payment adjustment rules for multiple procedures apply, 150% payment adjustment for bilateral procedures does not apply, payment for assistant surgeon subject to documentation of medical necessity

26255 **Extensive hand surgery** ~ follow-up period is 90 days, standard payment adjustment rules for multiple procedures apply, 150% payment adjustment for bilateral procedures does not apply, assistant surgeon may be paid

26260 **Extensive finger surgery** ~ follow-up period is 90 days, standard payment adjustment rules for multiple procedures apply, 150% payment adjustment for bilateral procedures does not apply, assistant surgeon may be paid

26261 **Extensive finger surgery** ~ follow-up period is 90 days, standard payment adjustment rules for multiple procedures apply, 150% payment adjustment for bilateral procedures does not apply, assistant surgeon may be paid

26262 **Partial remove finger** ~ follow-up period is 90 days, standard payment adjustment rules for multiple procedures apply, 150% payment adjustment for bilateral procedures does not apply, assistant surgeon may be paid

26320 **Remove implant from hand** ~ follow-up period is 90 days, standard payment adjustment rules for multiple procedures apply, 150% payment adjustment for bilateral procedures does not apply, assistant surgeon may not be paid

26340 **Manipulate finger w/anesth** ~ follow-up period is 90 days, standard payment adjustment rules for multiple procedures apply, 150% payment adjustment for bilateral procedures applies, assistant surgeon may not be paid

26350 **Repair finger/hand tendon** ~ follow-up period is 90 days, standard payment adjustment rules for multiple procedures apply, 150% payment adjustment for bilateral procedures does not apply, assistant surgeon may not be paid

26352 **Repair/graft hand tendon** ~ follow-up period is 90 days, standard payment adjustment rules for multiple procedures apply, 150% payment adjustment for bilateral procedures does not apply, assistant surgeon may be paid

26356   **Repair finger/hand tendon**   ~ follow-up period is 90 days, standard payment adjustment rules for multiple procedures apply, 150% payment adjustment for bilateral procedures does not apply, assistant surgeon may not be paid

26357   **Repair finger/hand tendon**   ~ follow-up period is 90 days, standard payment adjustment rules for multiple procedures apply, 150% payment adjustment for bilateral procedures does not apply, assistant surgeon may be paid

26358   **Repair/graft hand tendon**   ~ follow-up period is 90 days, standard payment adjustment rules for multiple procedures apply, 150% payment adjustment for bilateral procedures does not apply, assistant surgeon may be paid

26370   **Repair finger/hand tendon**   ~ follow-up period is 90 days, standard payment adjustment rules for multiple procedures apply, 150% payment adjustment for bilateral procedures does not apply, payment for assistant surgeon subject to documentation of medical necessity

26372   **Repair/graft hand tendon**   ~ follow-up period is 90 days, standard payment adjustment rules for multiple procedures apply, 150% payment adjustment for bilateral procedures does not apply, assistant surgeon may be paid

26373   **Repair finger/hand tendon**   ~ follow-up period is 90 days, standard payment adjustment rules for multiple procedures apply, 150% payment adjustment for bilateral procedures does not apply, assistant surgeon may be paid

26390   **Revise hand/finger tendon**   ~ follow-up period is 90 days, standard payment adjustment rules for multiple procedures apply, 150% payment adjustment for bilateral procedures does not apply, assistant surgeon may be paid

26392   **Repair/graft hand tendon**   ~ follow-up period is 90 days, standard payment adjustment rules for multiple procedures apply, 150% payment adjustment for bilateral procedures does not apply, assistant surgeon may be paid

26410   **Repair hand tendon**   ~ follow-up period is 90 days, standard payment adjustment rules for multiple procedures apply, 150% payment adjustment for bilateral procedures does not apply, assistant surgeon may not be paid

26412   **Repair/graft hand tendon**   ~ follow-up period is 90 days, standard payment adjustment rules for multiple procedures apply, 150% payment adjustment for bilateral procedures does not apply, payment for assistant surgeon subject to documentation of medical necessity

26415   **Excise hand/finger tendon**   ~ follow-up period is 90 days, standard payment adjustment rules for multiple procedures apply, 150% payment adjustment for bilateral procedures does not apply, payment for assistant surgeon subject to documentation of medical necessity

26416   **Graft hand or finger tendon**   ~ follow-up period is 90 days, standard payment adjustment rules for multiple procedures apply, 150% payment adjustment for bilateral procedures does not apply, assistant surgeon may not be paid

26418   **Repair finger tendon**   ~ follow-up period is 90 days, standard payment adjustment rules for multiple procedures apply, 150% payment adjustment for bilateral procedures does not apply, assistant surgeon may not be paid

26420   **Repair/graft finger tendon**   ~ follow-up period is 90 days, standard payment adjustment rules for multiple procedures apply, 150% payment adjustment for bilateral procedures does not apply, assistant surgeon may be paid

26426   **Repair finger/hand tendon**   ~ follow-up period is 90 days, standard payment adjustment rules for multiple procedures apply, 150% payment adjustment for bilateral procedures does not apply, assistant surgeon may not be paid

26428   **Repair/graft finger tendon**   ~ follow-up period is 90 days, standard payment adjustment rules for multiple procedures apply, 150% payment adjustment for bilateral procedures does not apply, payment for assistant surgeon subject to documentation of medical necessity

26432   **Repair finger tendon**   ~ follow-up period is 90 days, standard payment adjustment rules for multiple procedures apply, 150% payment adjustment for bilateral procedures does not apply, assistant surgeon may not be paid

26433   **Repair finger tendon**   ~ follow-up period is 90 days, standard payment adjustment rules for multiple procedures apply, 150% payment adjustment for bilateral procedures does not apply, assistant surgeon may not be paid

26434   **Repair/graft finger tendon**   ~ follow-up period is 90 days, standard payment adjustment rules for multiple procedures apply, 150% payment adjustment for bilateral procedures does not apply, assistant surgeon may be paid

26437   **Realignment of tendons**   ~ follow-up period is 90 days, standard payment adjustment rules for multiple procedures apply, 150% payment adjustment for bilateral procedures does not apply, assistant surgeon may not be paid

26440   **Release palm/finger tendon**   ~ follow-up period is 90 days, standard payment adjustment rules for multiple procedures apply, 150% payment adjustment for bilateral procedures does not apply, assistant surgeon may not be paid

26442   **Release palm & finger tendon**   ~ follow-up period is 90 days, standard payment adjustment rules for multiple procedures apply, 150% payment adjustment for bilateral procedures does not apply, assistant surgeon may not be paid

26445 **Release hand/finger tendon** ~ follow-up period is 90 days, standard payment adjustment rules for multiple procedures apply, 150% payment adjustment for bilateral procedures does not apply, assistant surgeon may not be paid

26449 **Release forearm/hand tendon** ~ follow-up period is 90 days, standard payment adjustment rules for multiple procedures apply, 150% payment adjustment for bilateral procedures does not apply, payment for assistant surgeon subject to documentation of medical necessity

26450 **Incise palm tendon** ~ follow-up period is 90 days, standard payment adjustment rules for multiple procedures apply, 150% payment adjustment for bilateral procedures does not apply, payment for assistant surgeon subject to documentation of medical necessity

26455 **Incise finger tendon** ~ follow-up period is 90 days, standard payment adjustment rules for multiple procedures apply, 150% payment adjustment for bilateral procedures does not apply, payment for assistant surgeon subject to documentation of medical necessity

26460 **Incise hand/finger tendon** ~ follow-up period is 90 days, standard payment adjustment rules for multiple procedures apply, 150% payment adjustment for bilateral procedures does not apply, assistant surgeon may not be paid

26471 **Fuse finger tendons** ~ follow-up period is 90 days, standard payment adjustment rules for multiple procedures apply, 150% payment adjustment for bilateral procedures does not apply, payment for assistant surgeon subject to documentation of medical necessity

26474 **Fuse finger tendons** ~ follow-up period is 90 days, standard payment adjustment rules for multiple procedures apply, 150% payment adjustment for bilateral procedures does not apply, assistant surgeon may be paid

26476 **Tendon lengthening** ~ follow-up period is 90 days, standard payment adjustment rules for multiple procedures apply, 150% payment adjustment for bilateral procedures does not apply, assistant surgeon may not be paid

26477 **Tendon shortening** ~ follow-up period is 90 days, standard payment adjustment rules for multiple procedures apply, 150% payment adjustment for bilateral procedures does not apply, assistant surgeon may not be paid

26478 **Lengthening of hand tendon** ~ follow-up period is 90 days, standard payment adjustment rules for multiple procedures apply, 150% payment adjustment for bilateral procedures does not apply, payment for assistant surgeon subject to documentation of medical necessity

26479   **Shortening of hand tendon**   ~ follow-up period is 90 days, standard payment adjustment rules for multiple procedures apply, 150% payment adjustment for bilateral procedures does not apply, assistant surgeon may be paid

26480   **Transplant hand tendon**   ~ follow-up period is 90 days, standard payment adjustment rules for multiple procedures apply, 150% payment adjustment for bilateral procedures does not apply, payment for assistant surgeon subject to documentation of medical necessity

26483   **Transplant/graft hand tendon**   ~ follow-up period is 90 days, standard payment adjustment rules for multiple procedures apply, 150% payment adjustment for bilateral procedures does not apply, assistant surgeon may be paid

26485   **Transplant palm tendon**   ~ follow-up period is 90 days, standard payment adjustment rules for multiple procedures apply, 150% payment adjustment for bilateral procedures does not apply, assistant surgeon may be paid

26489   **Transplant/graft palm tendon**   ~ follow-up period is 90 days, standard payment adjustment rules for multiple procedures apply, 150% payment adjustment for bilateral procedures does not apply, payment for assistant surgeon subject to documentation of medical necessity

26490   **Revise thumb tendon**   ~ follow-up period is 90 days, standard payment adjustment rules for multiple procedures apply, 150% payment adjustment for bilateral procedures does not apply, payment for assistant surgeon subject to documentation of medical necessity

26492   **Tendon transfer with graft**   ~ follow-up period is 90 days, standard payment adjustment rules for multiple procedures apply, 150% payment adjustment for bilateral procedures does not apply, assistant surgeon may be paid

26494   **Hand tendon/muscle transfer**   ~ follow-up period is 90 days, standard payment adjustment rules for multiple procedures apply, 150% payment adjustment for bilateral procedures does not apply, assistant surgeon may be paid

26496   **Revise thumb tendon**   ~ follow-up period is 90 days, standard payment adjustment rules for multiple procedures apply, 150% payment adjustment for bilateral procedures does not apply, payment for assistant surgeon subject to documentation of medical necessity

26497   **Finger tendon transfer**   ~ follow-up period is 90 days, standard payment adjustment rules for multiple procedures apply, 150% payment adjustment for bilateral procedures does not apply, assistant surgeon may be paid

26498   **Finger tendon transfer**   ~ follow-up period is 90 days, standard payment adjustment rules for multiple procedures apply, 150% payment adjustment for bilateral procedures does not apply, assistant surgeon may be paid

26499   **Revise finger**   ~ follow-up period is 90 days, standard payment adjustment rules for multiple procedures apply, 150% payment adjustment for bilateral procedures does not apply, assistant surgeon may be paid

26500   **Hand tendon reconstruct**   ~ follow-up period is 90 days, standard payment adjustment rules for multiple procedures apply, 150% payment adjustment for bilateral procedures does not apply, payment for assistant surgeon subject to documentation of medical necessity

26502   **Hand tendon reconstruct**   ~ follow-up period is 90 days, standard payment adjustment rules for multiple procedures apply, 150% payment adjustment for bilateral procedures does not apply, assistant surgeon may be paid

26508   **Release thumb contracture**   ~ follow-up period is 90 days, standard payment adjustment rules for multiple procedures apply, 150% payment adjustment for bilateral procedures does not apply, payment for assistant surgeon subject to documentation of medical necessity

26510   **Thumb tendon transfer**   ~ follow-up period is 90 days, standard payment adjustment rules for multiple procedures apply, 150% payment adjustment for bilateral procedures does not apply, payment for assistant surgeon subject to documentation of medical necessity

26516   **Fuse knuckle joint**   ~ follow-up period is 90 days, standard payment adjustment rules for multiple procedures apply, 150% payment adjustment for bilateral procedures does not apply, payment for assistant surgeon subject to documentation of medical necessity

26517   **Fuse knuckle joints**   ~ follow-up period is 90 days, standard payment adjustment rules for multiple procedures apply, 150% payment adjustment for bilateral procedures does not apply, assistant surgeon may be paid

26518   **Fuse knuckle joints**   ~ follow-up period is 90 days, standard payment adjustment rules for multiple procedures apply, 150% payment adjustment for bilateral procedures does not apply, assistant surgeon may be paid

26520   **Release knuckle contracture**   ~ follow-up period is 90 days, standard payment adjustment rules for multiple procedures apply, 150% payment adjustment for bilateral procedures does not apply, assistant surgeon may not be paid

26525   **Release finger contracture**   ~ follow-up period is 90 days, standard payment adjustment rules for multiple procedures apply, 150% payment adjustment for bilateral procedures does not apply, assistant surgeon may not be paid

26530   **Revise knuckle joint**   ~ follow-up period is 90 days, standard payment adjustment rules for multiple procedures apply, 150% payment adjustment for bilateral procedures does not apply, assistant surgeon may be paid

26531 **Revise knuckle with implant** ~ follow-up period is 90 days, standard payment adjustment rules for multiple procedures apply, 150% payment adjustment for bilateral procedures does not apply, assistant surgeon may be paid

26535 **Revise finger joint** ~ follow-up period is 90 days, standard payment adjustment rules for multiple procedures apply, 150% payment adjustment for bilateral procedures does not apply, assistant surgeon may not be paid

26536 **Revise/implant finger joint** ~ follow-up period is 90 days, standard payment adjustment rules for multiple procedures apply, 150% payment adjustment for bilateral procedures does not apply, payment for assistant surgeon subject to documentation of medical necessity

26540 **Repair hand joint** ~ follow-up period is 90 days, standard payment adjustment rules for multiple procedures apply, 150% payment adjustment for bilateral procedures does not apply, payment for assistant surgeon subject to documentation of medical necessity

26541 **Repair hand joint with graft** ~ follow-up period is 90 days, standard payment adjustment rules for multiple procedures apply, 150% payment adjustment for bilateral procedures does not apply, assistant surgeon may be paid

26542 **Repair hand joint with graft** ~ follow-up period is 90 days, standard payment adjustment rules for multiple procedures apply, 150% payment adjustment for bilateral procedures does not apply, payment for assistant surgeon subject to documentation of medical necessity

26545 **Reconstruct finger joint** ~ follow-up period is 90 days, standard payment adjustment rules for multiple procedures apply, 150% payment adjustment for bilateral procedures does not apply, payment for assistant surgeon subject to documentation of medical necessity

26546 **Repair nonunion hand** ~ follow-up period is 90 days, standard payment adjustment rules for multiple procedures apply, 150% payment adjustment for bilateral procedures applies, assistant surgeon may be paid

26548 **Reconstruct finger joint** ~ follow-up period is 90 days, standard payment adjustment rules for multiple procedures apply, 150% payment adjustment for bilateral procedures does not apply, payment for assistant surgeon subject to documentation of medical necessity

26550 **Construct thumb replacement** ~ follow-up period is 90 days, standard payment adjustment rules for multiple procedures apply, 150% payment adjustment for bilateral procedures does not apply, assistant surgeon may be paid

26551   **Great toe-hand transfer**   ~ follow-up period is 90 days, standard payment adjustment rules for multiple procedures apply, 150% payment adjustment for bilateral procedures does not apply, assistant surgeon may be paid

26553   **Single transfer, toe-hand**   ~ follow-up period is 90 days, standard payment adjustment rules for multiple procedures apply, 150% payment adjustment for bilateral procedures does not apply, assistant surgeon may be paid

26554   **Double transfer, toe-hand**   ~ follow-up period is 90 days, standard payment adjustment rules for multiple procedures apply, 150% payment adjustment for bilateral procedures does not apply, assistant surgeon may be paid

26555   **Positional change of finger**   ~ follow-up period is 90 days, standard payment adjustment rules for multiple procedures apply, 150% payment adjustment for bilateral procedures does not apply, assistant surgeon may be paid

26556   **Toe joint transfer**   ~ follow-up period is 90 days, standard payment adjustment rules for multiple procedures apply, 150% payment adjustment for bilateral procedures does not apply, assistant surgeon may be paid

26560   **Repair web finger**   ~ follow-up period is 90 days, standard payment adjustment rules for multiple procedures apply, 150% payment adjustment for bilateral procedures does not apply, assistant surgeon may be paid

26561   **Repair web finger**   ~ follow-up period is 90 days, standard payment adjustment rules for multiple procedures apply, 150% payment adjustment for bilateral procedures does not apply, assistant surgeon may be paid

26562   **Repair web finger**   ~ follow-up period is 90 days, standard payment adjustment rules for multiple procedures apply, 150% payment adjustment for bilateral procedures does not apply, assistant surgeon may be paid

26565   **Correct metacarpal flaw**   ~ follow-up period is 90 days, standard payment adjustment rules for multiple procedures apply, 150% payment adjustment for bilateral procedures does not apply, assistant surgeon may be paid

26567   **Correct finger deformity**   ~ follow-up period is 90 days, standard payment adjustment rules for multiple procedures apply, 150% payment adjustment for bilateral procedures does not apply, payment for assistant surgeon subject to documentation of medical necessity

26568   **Lengthen metacarpal/finger**   ~ follow-up period is 90 days, standard payment adjustment rules for multiple procedures apply, 150% payment adjustment for bilateral procedures does not apply, assistant surgeon may be paid

26580 **Repair hand deformity** ~ follow-up period is 90 days, standard payment adjustment rules for multiple procedures apply, 150% payment adjustment for bilateral procedures does not apply, assistant surgeon may be paid

26587 **Reconstruct extra finger** ~ follow-up period is 90 days, standard payment adjustment rules for multiple procedures apply, 150% payment adjustment for bilateral procedures does not apply, assistant surgeon may be paid

26590 **Repair finger deformity** ~ follow-up period is 90 days, standard payment adjustment rules for multiple procedures apply, 150% payment adjustment for bilateral procedures does not apply, assistant surgeon may be paid

26591 **Repair muscles of hand** ~ follow-up period is 90 days, standard payment adjustment rules for multiple procedures apply, 150% payment adjustment for bilateral procedures does not apply, payment for assistant surgeon subject to documentation of medical necessity

26593 **Release muscles of hand** ~ follow-up period is 90 days, standard payment adjustment rules for multiple procedures apply, 150% payment adjustment for bilateral procedures does not apply, assistant surgeon may not be paid

26596 **Excise constricting tissue** ~ follow-up period is 90 days, standard payment adjustment rules for multiple procedures apply, 150% payment adjustment for bilateral procedures does not apply, assistant surgeon may be paid

26600 **Treat metacarpal fracture** ~ follow-up period is 90 days, standard payment adjustment rules for multiple procedures apply, 150% payment adjustment for bilateral procedures does not apply, assistant surgeon may not be paid

26605 **Treat metacarpal fracture** ~ follow-up period is 90 days, standard payment adjustment rules for multiple procedures apply, 150% payment adjustment for bilateral procedures does not apply, assistant surgeon may not be paid

26607 **Treat metacarpal fracture** ~ follow-up period is 90 days, standard payment adjustment rules for multiple procedures apply, 150% payment adjustment for bilateral procedures does not apply, payment for assistant surgeon subject to documentation of medical necessity

26608 **Treat metacarpal fracture** ~ follow-up period is 90 days, standard payment adjustment rules for multiple procedures apply, 150% payment adjustment for bilateral procedures does not apply, payment for assistant surgeon subject to documentation of medical necessity

26615 **Treat metacarpal fracture** ~ follow-up period is 90 days, standard payment adjustment rules for multiple procedures apply, 150% payment adjustment for bilateral procedures does not apply, assistant surgeon may not be paid

26641   **Treat thumb dislocation**   ~ follow-up period is 90 days, standard payment adjustment rules for multiple procedures apply, 150% payment adjustment for bilateral procedures does not apply, payment for assistant surgeon subject to documentation of medical necessity

26645   **Treat thumb fracture**   ~ follow-up period is 90 days, standard payment adjustment rules for multiple procedures apply, 150% payment adjustment for bilateral procedures does not apply, payment for assistant surgeon subject to documentation of medical necessity

26650   **Treat thumb fracture**   ~ follow-up period is 90 days, standard payment adjustment rules for multiple procedures apply, 150% payment adjustment for bilateral procedures does not apply, assistant surgeon may not be paid

26665   **Treat thumb fracture**   ~ follow-up period is 90 days, standard payment adjustment rules for multiple procedures apply, 150% payment adjustment for bilateral procedures does not apply, assistant surgeon may not be paid

26670   **Treat hand dislocation**   ~ follow-up period is 90 days, standard payment adjustment rules for multiple procedures apply, 150% payment adjustment for bilateral procedures does not apply, payment for assistant surgeon subject to documentation of medical necessity

26675   **Treat hand dislocation**   ~ follow-up period is 90 days, standard payment adjustment rules for multiple procedures apply, 150% payment adjustment for bilateral procedures does not apply, payment for assistant surgeon subject to documentation of medical necessity

26676   **Pin hand dislocation**   ~ follow-up period is 90 days, standard payment adjustment rules for multiple procedures apply, 150% payment adjustment for bilateral procedures does not apply, assistant surgeon may not be paid

26685   **Treat hand dislocation**   ~ follow-up period is 90 days, standard payment adjustment rules for multiple procedures apply, 150% payment adjustment for bilateral procedures does not apply, assistant surgeon may not be paid

26686   **Treat hand dislocation**   ~ follow-up period is 90 days, standard payment adjustment rules for multiple procedures apply, 150% payment adjustment for bilateral procedures does not apply, assistant surgeon may be paid

26700   **Treat knuckle dislocation**   ~ follow-up period is 90 days, standard payment adjustment rules for multiple procedures apply, 150% payment adjustment for bilateral procedures does not apply, assistant surgeon may not be paid

26705   **Treat knuckle dislocation**   ~ follow-up period is 90 days, standard payment adjustment rules for multiple procedures apply, 150% payment adjustment for

bilateral procedures does not apply, payment for assistant surgeon subject to documentation of medical necessity

26706   **Pin knuckle dislocation**   ~ follow-up period is 90 days, standard payment adjustment rules for multiple procedures apply, 150% payment adjustment for bilateral procedures does not apply, assistant surgeon may not be paid

26715   **Treat knuckle dislocation**   ~ follow-up period is 90 days, standard payment adjustment rules for multiple procedures apply, 150% payment adjustment for bilateral procedures does not apply, payment for assistant surgeon subject to documentation of medical necessity

26720   **Treat finger fracture, each**   ~ follow-up period is 90 days, standard payment adjustment rules for multiple procedures apply, 150% payment adjustment for bilateral procedures does not apply, assistant surgeon may not be paid

26725   **Treat finger fracture, each**   ~ follow-up period is 90 days, standard payment adjustment rules for multiple procedures apply, 150% payment adjustment for bilateral procedures does not apply, assistant surgeon may not be paid

26727   **Treat finger fracture, each**   ~ follow-up period is 90 days, standard payment adjustment rules for multiple procedures apply, 150% payment adjustment for bilateral procedures does not apply, assistant surgeon may not be paid

26735   **Treat finger fracture, each**   ~ follow-up period is 90 days, standard payment adjustment rules for multiple procedures apply, 150% payment adjustment for bilateral procedures does not apply, assistant surgeon may not be paid

26740   **Treat finger fracture, each**   ~ follow-up period is 90 days, standard payment adjustment rules for multiple procedures apply, 150% payment adjustment for bilateral procedures does not apply, assistant surgeon may not be paid

26742   **Treat finger fracture, each**   ~ follow-up period is 90 days, standard payment adjustment rules for multiple procedures apply, 150% payment adjustment for bilateral procedures does not apply, assistant surgeon may not be paid

26746   **Treat finger fracture, each**   ~ follow-up period is 90 days, standard payment adjustment rules for multiple procedures apply, 150% payment adjustment for bilateral procedures does not apply, assistant surgeon may not be paid

26750   **Treat finger fracture, each**   ~ follow-up period is 90 days, standard payment adjustment rules for multiple procedures apply, 150% payment adjustment for bilateral procedures does not apply, assistant surgeon may not be paid

26755   **Treat finger fracture, each**   ~ follow-up period is 90 days, standard payment adjustment rules for multiple procedures apply, 150% payment adjustment for bilateral procedures does not apply, assistant surgeon may not be paid

26756   **Pin finger fracture, each**   ~ follow-up period is 90 days, standard payment adjustment rules for multiple procedures apply, 150% payment adjustment for bilateral procedures does not apply, payment for assistant surgeon subject to documentation of medical necessity

26765   **Treat finger fracture, each**   ~ follow-up period is 90 days, standard payment adjustment rules for multiple procedures apply, 150% payment adjustment for bilateral procedures does not apply, assistant surgeon may not be paid

26770   **Treat finger dislocation**   ~ follow-up period is 90 days, standard payment adjustment rules for multiple procedures apply, 150% payment adjustment for bilateral procedures does not apply, assistant surgeon may not be paid

26775   **Treat finger dislocation**   ~ follow-up period is 90 days, standard payment adjustment rules for multiple procedures apply, 150% payment adjustment for bilateral procedures does not apply, assistant surgeon may not be paid

26776   **Pin finger dislocation**   ~ follow-up period is 90 days, standard payment adjustment rules for multiple procedures apply, 150% payment adjustment for bilateral procedures does not apply, assistant surgeon may not be paid

26785   **Treat finger dislocation**   ~ follow-up period is 90 days, standard payment adjustment rules for multiple procedures apply, 150% payment adjustment for bilateral procedures does not apply, assistant surgeon may not be paid

26820   **Thumb fuse with graft**   ~ follow-up period is 90 days, standard payment adjustment rules for multiple procedures apply, 150% payment adjustment for bilateral procedures does not apply, assistant surgeon may be paid

26841   **Fuse thumb**   ~ follow-up period is 90 days, standard payment adjustment rules for multiple procedures apply, 150% payment adjustment for bilateral procedures does not apply, payment for assistant surgeon subject to documentation of medical necessity

26842   **Thumb fuse with graft**   ~ follow-up period is 90 days, standard payment adjustment rules for multiple procedures apply, 150% payment adjustment for bilateral procedures does not apply, assistant surgeon may be paid

26843   **Fuse hand joint**   ~ follow-up period is 90 days, standard payment adjustment rules for multiple procedures apply, 150% payment adjustment for bilateral procedures does not apply, assistant surgeon may be paid

26844   **Fuse/graft of hand joint**   ~ follow-up period is 90 days, standard payment adjustment rules for multiple procedures apply, 150% payment adjustment for bilateral procedures does not apply, assistant surgeon may be paid

26850   **Fuse knuckle**   ~ follow-up period is 90 days, standard payment adjustment rules for multiple procedures apply, 150% payment adjustment for

bilateral procedures does not apply, payment for assistant surgeon subject to documentation of medical necessity

26852 **Fuse knuckle with graft**   ~ follow-up period is 90 days, standard payment adjustment rules for multiple procedures apply, 150% payment adjustment for bilateral procedures does not apply, assistant surgeon may be paid

26860 **Fuse finger joint**   ~ follow-up period is 90 days, standard payment adjustment rules for multiple procedures apply, 150% payment adjustment for bilateral procedures does not apply, assistant surgeon may not be paid

26861 **Fuse finger joint, add-on**   ~ follow-up period included in another service, no payment adjustment rules for multiple procedures apply, 150% payment adjustment for bilateral procedures does not apply, assistant surgeon may not be paid, +add-on code (list separately in addition to primary procedure)

26862 **Fuse/graft of finger joint**   ~ follow-up period is 90 days, standard payment adjustment rules for multiple procedures apply, 150% payment adjustment for bilateral procedures does not apply, assistant surgeon may be paid

26863 **Fuse/graft added joint**   ~ follow-up period included in another service, no payment adjustment rules for multiple procedures apply, 150% payment adjustment for bilateral procedures does not apply, assistant surgeon may be paid, +add-on code (list separately in addition to primary procedure)

26910 **Amputate metacarpal bone**   ~ follow-up period is 90 days, standard payment adjustment rules for multiple procedures apply, 150% payment adjustment for bilateral procedures does not apply, assistant surgeon may not be paid

26951 **Amputate finger/thumb**   ~ follow-up period is 90 days, standard payment adjustment rules for multiple procedures apply, 150% payment adjustment for bilateral procedures does not apply, assistant surgeon may not be paid

26952 **Amputate finger/thumb**   ~ follow-up period is 90 days, standard payment adjustment rules for multiple procedures apply, 150% payment adjustment for bilateral procedures does not apply, assistant surgeon may not be paid

26989 **Hand/finger surgery**   ~ medicare carrier determines global period, standard payment adjustment rules for multiple procedures apply, 150% payment adjustment for bilateral procedures does not apply, assistant surgeon may not be paid

Pelvis and Hip Joint

26990 **Drain pelvis lesion**   ~ follow-up period is 90 days, standard payment adjustment rules for multiple procedures apply, 150% payment adjustment for bilateral procedures does not apply, assistant surgeon may not be paid

26991   **Drain pelvis bursa**   ~ follow-up period is 90 days, standard payment adjustment rules for multiple procedures apply, 150% payment adjustment for bilateral procedures does not apply, payment for assistant surgeon subject to documentation of medical necessity

26992   **Drain bone lesion**   ~ follow-up period is 90 days, standard payment adjustment rules for multiple procedures apply, 150% payment adjustment for bilateral procedures does not apply, payment for assistant surgeon subject to documentation of medical necessity

27000   **Incise hip tendon**   ~ follow-up period is 90 days, standard payment adjustment rules for multiple procedures apply, 150% payment adjustment for bilateral procedures applies, assistant surgeon may not be paid

27001   **Incise hip tendon**   ~ follow-up period is 90 days, standard payment adjustment rules for multiple procedures apply, 150% payment adjustment for bilateral procedures applies, assistant surgeon may be paid

27003   **Incise hip tendon**   ~ follow-up period is 90 days, standard payment adjustment rules for multiple procedures apply, 150% payment adjustment for bilateral procedures applies, assistant surgeon may be paid

27005   **Incise hip tendon**   ~ follow-up period is 90 days, standard payment adjustment rules for multiple procedures apply, 150% payment adjustment for bilateral procedures applies, assistant surgeon may be paid

27006   **Incise hip tendons**   ~ follow-up period is 90 days, standard payment adjustment rules for multiple procedures apply, 150% payment adjustment for bilateral procedures applies, assistant surgeon may be paid

27025   **Incise hip/thigh fascia**   ~ follow-up period is 90 days, standard payment adjustment rules for multiple procedures apply, 150% payment adjustment for bilateral procedures applies, payment for assistant surgeon subject to documentation of medical necessity

27030   **Drain hip joint**   ~ follow-up period is 90 days, standard payment adjustment rules for multiple procedures apply, 150% payment adjustment for bilateral procedures applies, assistant surgeon may be paid

27033   **Explore hip joint**   ~ follow-up period is 90 days, standard payment adjustment rules for multiple procedures apply, 150% payment adjustment for bilateral procedures applies, assistant surgeon may be paid

27035   **Denervation of hip joint**   ~ follow-up period is 90 days, standard payment adjustment rules for multiple procedures apply, 150% payment adjustment for bilateral procedures applies, assistant surgeon may be paid

27036 **Excise hip joint/muscle** ~ follow-up period is 90 days, standard payment adjustment rules for multiple procedures apply, 150% payment adjustment for bilateral procedures applies, assistant surgeon may be paid

27040 **Biopsy soft tissues** ~ follow-up period is 10 days, standard payment adjustment rules for multiple procedures apply, 150% payment adjustment for bilateral procedures applies, assistant surgeon may not be paid

27041 **Biopsy soft tissues** ~ follow-up period is 90 days, standard payment adjustment rules for multiple procedures apply, 150% payment adjustment for bilateral procedures applies, assistant surgeon may not be paid

27047 **Remove hip/pelvis lesion** ~ follow-up period is 90 days, standard payment adjustment rules for multiple procedures apply, 150% payment adjustment for bilateral procedures applies, assistant surgeon may not be paid

27048 **Remove hip/pelvis lesion** ~ follow-up period is 90 days, standard payment adjustment rules for multiple procedures apply, 150% payment adjustment for bilateral procedures applies, assistant surgeon may be paid

27049 **Remove tumor, hip/pelvis** ~ follow-up period is 90 days, standard payment adjustment rules for multiple procedures apply, 150% payment adjustment for bilateral procedures applies, assistant surgeon may be paid

27050 **Biopsy sacroiliac joint** ~ follow-up period is 90 days, standard payment adjustment rules for multiple procedures apply, 150% payment adjustment for bilateral procedures applies, payment for assistant surgeon subject to documentation of medical necessity

27052 **Biopsy hip joint** ~ follow-up period is 90 days, standard payment adjustment rules for multiple procedures apply, 150% payment adjustment for bilateral procedures applies, assistant surgeon may be paid

27054 **Remove hip joint lining** ~ follow-up period is 90 days, standard payment adjustment rules for multiple procedures apply, 150% payment adjustment for bilateral procedures applies, assistant surgeon may be paid

27060 **Remove ischial bursa** ~ follow-up period is 90 days, standard payment adjustment rules for multiple procedures apply, 150% payment adjustment for bilateral procedures applies, assistant surgeon may not be paid

27062 **Remove femur lesion/bursa** ~ follow-up period is 90 days, standard payment adjustment rules for multiple procedures apply, 150% payment adjustment for bilateral procedures applies, assistant surgeon may not be paid

27065   **Remove hip bone lesion**   ~ follow-up period is 90 days, standard payment adjustment rules for multiple procedures apply, 150% payment adjustment for bilateral procedures applies, assistant surgeon may be paid

27066   **Remove hip bone lesion**   ~ follow-up period is 90 days, standard payment adjustment rules for multiple procedures apply, 150% payment adjustment for bilateral procedures applies, assistant surgeon may be paid

27067   **Remove/graft hip bone lesion**   ~ follow-up period is 90 days, standard payment adjustment rules for multiple procedures apply, 150% payment adjustment for bilateral procedures applies, assistant surgeon may be paid

27070   **Partial remove hip bone**   ~ follow-up period is 90 days, standard payment adjustment rules for multiple procedures apply, 150% payment adjustment for bilateral procedures applies, assistant surgeon may be paid

27071   **Partial remove hip bone**   ~ follow-up period is 90 days, standard payment adjustment rules for multiple procedures apply, 150% payment adjustment for bilateral procedures applies, assistant surgeon may be paid

27075   **Extensive hip surgery**   ~ follow-up period is 90 days, standard payment adjustment rules for multiple procedures apply, 150% payment adjustment for bilateral procedures does not apply, assistant surgeon may be paid

27076   **Extensive hip surgery**   ~ follow-up period is 90 days, standard payment adjustment rules for multiple procedures apply, 150% payment adjustment for bilateral procedures does not apply, assistant surgeon may be paid

27077   **Extensive hip surgery**   ~ follow-up period is 90 days, standard payment adjustment rules for multiple procedures apply, 150% payment adjustment for bilateral procedures does not apply, assistant surgeon may be paid

27078   **Extensive hip surgery**   ~ follow-up period is 90 days, standard payment adjustment rules for multiple procedures apply, 150% payment adjustment for bilateral procedures does not apply, assistant surgeon may be paid

27079   **Extensive hip surgery**   ~ follow-up period is 90 days, standard payment adjustment rules for multiple procedures apply, 150% payment adjustment for bilateral procedures does not apply, assistant surgeon may be paid

27080   **Remove tail bone**   ~ follow-up period is 90 days, standard payment adjustment rules for multiple procedures apply, 150% payment adjustment for bilateral procedures does not apply, assistant surgeon may be paid

27086   **Remove hip foreign body**   ~ follow-up period is 10 days, standard payment adjustment rules for multiple procedures apply, 150% payment adjustment for

    CPT codes and descriptions only copyright American Medical Association

bilateral procedures applies, payment for assistant surgeon subject to documentation of medical necessity

27087   **Remove hip foreign body**   ~ follow-up period is 90 days, standard payment adjustment rules for multiple procedures apply, 150% payment adjustment for bilateral procedures applies, assistant surgeon may be paid

27090   **Remove hip prosthesis**   ~ follow-up period is 90 days, standard payment adjustment rules for multiple procedures apply, 150% payment adjustment for bilateral procedures applies, assistant surgeon may be paid

27091   **Remove hip prosthesis**   ~ follow-up period is 90 days, standard payment adjustment rules for multiple procedures apply, 150% payment adjustment for bilateral procedures applies, assistant surgeon may be paid

27093   **Inject for hip x-ray**   ~ endoscopies or minor procedure - E/M services on the same day generally not paid, standard payment adjustment rules for multiple procedures apply, 150% payment adjustment for bilateral procedures applies, assistant surgeon may not be paid

27095   **Inject for hip x-ray**   ~ endoscopies or minor procedure - E/M services on the same day generally not paid, standard payment adjustment rules for multiple procedures apply, 150% payment adjustment for bilateral procedures applies, assistant surgeon may not be paid

27096   **Inject sacroiliac joint**   ~ endoscopies or minor procedure - E/M services on the same day generally not paid, standard payment adjustment rules for multiple procedures apply, 150% payment adjustment for bilateral procedures applies, assistant surgeon may not be paid

27097   **Revise hip tendon**   ~ follow-up period is 90 days, standard payment adjustment rules for multiple procedures apply, 150% payment adjustment for bilateral procedures applies, assistant surgeon may be paid

27098   **Transfer tendon to pelvis**   ~ follow-up period is 90 days, standard payment adjustment rules for multiple procedures apply, 150% payment adjustment for bilateral procedures applies, assistant surgeon may be paid

27100   **Transfer of abdominal muscle**   ~ follow-up period is 90 days, standard payment adjustment rules for multiple procedures apply, 150% payment adjustment for bilateral procedures applies, assistant surgeon may be paid

27105   **Transfer of spinal muscle**   ~ follow-up period is 90 days, standard payment adjustment rules for multiple procedures apply, 150% payment adjustment for bilateral procedures applies, assistant surgeon may be paid

27110   **Transfer of iliopsoas muscle**   ~ follow-up period is 90 days, standard payment adjustment rules for multiple procedures apply, 150% payment adjustment for bilateral procedures applies, assistant surgeon may be paid

27111   **Transfer of iliopsoas muscle**   ~ follow-up period is 90 days, standard payment adjustment rules for multiple procedures apply, 150% payment adjustment for bilateral procedures applies, assistant surgeon may be paid

27120   **Reconstruct hip socket**   ~ follow-up period is 90 days, standard payment adjustment rules for multiple procedures apply, 150% payment adjustment for bilateral procedures applies, assistant surgeon may be paid

27122   **Reconstruct hip socket**   ~ follow-up period is 90 days, standard payment adjustment rules for multiple procedures apply, 150% payment adjustment for bilateral procedures applies, assistant surgeon may be paid

27125   **Partial hip replacement**   ~ follow-up period is 90 days, standard payment adjustment rules for multiple procedures apply, 150% payment adjustment for bilateral procedures applies, assistant surgeon may be paid

27130   **Total hip arthroplasty**   ~ follow-up period is 90 days, standard payment adjustment rules for multiple procedures apply, 150% payment adjustment for bilateral procedures applies, assistant surgeon may be paid

27132   **Total hip arthroplasty**   ~ follow-up period is 90 days, standard payment adjustment rules for multiple procedures apply, 150% payment adjustment for bilateral procedures applies, assistant surgeon may be paid

27134   **Revise hip joint replacement**   ~ follow-up period is 90 days, standard payment adjustment rules for multiple procedures apply, 150% payment adjustment for bilateral procedures applies, assistant surgeon may be paid

27137   **Revise hip joint replacement**   ~ follow-up period is 90 days, standard payment adjustment rules for multiple procedures apply, 150% payment adjustment for bilateral procedures applies, assistant surgeon may be paid

27138   **Revise hip joint replacement**   ~ follow-up period is 90 days, standard payment adjustment rules for multiple procedures apply, 150% payment adjustment for bilateral procedures applies, assistant surgeon may be paid

27140   **Transplant femur ridge**   ~ follow-up period is 90 days, standard payment adjustment rules for multiple procedures apply, 150% payment adjustment for bilateral procedures applies, assistant surgeon may be paid

27146   **Incise hip bone**   ~ follow-up period is 90 days, standard payment adjustment rules for multiple procedures apply, 150% payment adjustment for bilateral procedures applies, assistant surgeon may be paid

27147 **Revise hip bone** ~ follow-up period is 90 days, standard payment adjustment rules for multiple procedures apply, 150% payment adjustment for bilateral procedures applies, assistant surgeon may be paid

27151 **Incise hip bones** ~ follow-up period is 90 days, standard payment adjustment rules for multiple procedures apply, 150% payment adjustment for bilateral procedures applies, assistant surgeon may be paid

27156 **Revise hip bones** ~ follow-up period is 90 days, standard payment adjustment rules for multiple procedures apply, 150% payment adjustment for bilateral procedures applies, assistant surgeon may be paid

27158 **Revise pelvis** ~ follow-up period is 90 days, standard payment adjustment rules for multiple procedures apply, 150% payment adjustment does not apply - RVUs based on bilateral procedure, assistant surgeon may be paid

27161 **Incise neck of femur** ~ follow-up period is 90 days, standard payment adjustment rules for multiple procedures apply, 150% payment adjustment for bilateral procedures applies, assistant surgeon may be paid

27165 **Incision/fixate femur** ~ follow-up period is 90 days, standard payment adjustment rules for multiple procedures apply, 150% payment adjustment for bilateral procedures applies, assistant surgeon may be paid

27170 **Repair/graft femur head/neck** ~ follow-up period is 90 days, standard payment adjustment rules for multiple procedures apply, 150% payment adjustment for bilateral procedures applies, assistant surgeon may be paid

27175 **Treat slipped epiphysis** ~ follow-up period is 90 days, standard payment adjustment rules for multiple procedures apply, 150% payment adjustment for bilateral procedures applies, payment for assistant surgeon subject to documentation of medical necessity

27176 **Treat slipped epiphysis** ~ follow-up period is 90 days, standard payment adjustment rules for multiple procedures apply, 150% payment adjustment for bilateral procedures applies, assistant surgeon may be paid

27177 **Treat slipped epiphysis** ~ follow-up period is 90 days, standard payment adjustment rules for multiple procedures apply, 150% payment adjustment for bilateral procedures applies, assistant surgeon may be paid

27178 **Treat slipped epiphysis** ~ follow-up period is 90 days, standard payment adjustment rules for multiple procedures apply, 150% payment adjustment for bilateral procedures applies, assistant surgeon may be paid

27179 **Revise head/neck of femur** ~ follow-up period is 90 days, standard payment adjustment rules for multiple procedures apply, 150% payment adjustment for bilateral procedures applies, assistant surgeon may be paid

27181 **Treat slipped epiphysis** ~ follow-up period is 90 days, standard payment adjustment rules for multiple procedures apply, 150% payment adjustment for bilateral procedures applies, assistant surgeon may be paid

27185 **Revise femur epiphysis** ~ follow-up period is 90 days, standard payment adjustment rules for multiple procedures apply, 150% payment adjustment for bilateral procedures applies, assistant surgeon may not be paid

27187 **Reinforce hip bones** ~ follow-up period is 90 days, standard payment adjustment rules for multiple procedures apply, 150% payment adjustment for bilateral procedures applies, assistant surgeon may be paid

27193 **Treat pelvic ring fracture** ~ follow-up period is 90 days, standard payment adjustment rules for multiple procedures apply, 150% payment adjustment for bilateral procedures applies, assistant surgeon may not be paid

27194 **Treat pelvic ring fracture** ~ follow-up period is 90 days, standard payment adjustment rules for multiple procedures apply, 150% payment adjustment for bilateral procedures does not apply, payment for assistant surgeon subject to documentation of medical necessity

27200 **Treat tail bone fracture** ~ follow-up period is 90 days, standard payment adjustment rules for multiple procedures apply, 150% payment adjustment for bilateral procedures does not apply, assistant surgeon may not be paid

27202 **Treat tail bone fracture** ~ follow-up period is 90 days, standard payment adjustment rules for multiple procedures apply, 150% payment adjustment for bilateral procedures does not apply, assistant surgeon may be paid

27215 **Treat pelvic fracture(s)** ~ follow-up period is 90 days, standard payment adjustment rules for multiple procedures apply, 150% payment adjustment for bilateral procedures does not apply, assistant surgeon may be paid

27216 **Treat pelvic ring fracture** ~ follow-up period is 90 days, standard payment adjustment rules for multiple procedures apply, 150% payment adjustment for bilateral procedures does not apply, assistant surgeon may be paid

27217 **Treat pelvic ring fracture** ~ follow-up period is 90 days, standard payment adjustment rules for multiple procedures apply, 150% payment adjustment for bilateral procedures does not apply, assistant surgeon may be paid

27218   **Treat pelvic ring fracture**   ~ follow-up period is 90 days, standard payment adjustment rules for multiple procedures apply, 150% payment adjustment for bilateral procedures does not apply, assistant surgeon may be paid

27220   **Treat hip socket fracture**   ~ follow-up period is 90 days, standard payment adjustment rules for multiple procedures apply, 150% payment adjustment for bilateral procedures applies, assistant surgeon may not be paid

27222   **Treat hip socket fracture**   ~ follow-up period is 90 days, standard payment adjustment rules for multiple procedures apply, 150% payment adjustment for bilateral procedures applies, assistant surgeon may not be paid

27226   **Treat hip wall fracture**   ~ follow-up period is 90 days, standard payment adjustment rules for multiple procedures apply, 150% payment adjustment for bilateral procedures applies, assistant surgeon may be paid

27227   **Treat hip fracture(s)**   ~ follow-up period is 90 days, standard payment adjustment rules for multiple procedures apply, 150% payment adjustment for bilateral procedures applies, assistant surgeon may be paid

27228   **Treat hip fracture(s)**   ~ follow-up period is 90 days, standard payment adjustment rules for multiple procedures apply, 150% payment adjustment for bilateral procedures applies, assistant surgeon may be paid

27230   **Treat thigh fracture**   ~ follow-up period is 90 days, standard payment adjustment rules for multiple procedures apply, 150% payment adjustment for bilateral procedures applies, assistant surgeon may not be paid

27232   **Treat thigh fracture**   ~ follow-up period is 90 days, standard payment adjustment rules for multiple procedures apply, 150% payment adjustment for bilateral procedures applies, assistant surgeon may not be paid

27235   **Treat thigh fracture**   ~ follow-up period is 90 days, standard payment adjustment rules for multiple procedures apply, 150% payment adjustment for bilateral procedures applies, assistant surgeon may not be paid

27236   **Treat thigh fracture**   ~ follow-up period is 90 days, standard payment adjustment rules for multiple procedures apply, 150% payment adjustment for bilateral procedures applies, assistant surgeon may be paid

27238   **Treat thigh fracture**   ~ follow-up period is 90 days, standard payment adjustment rules for multiple procedures apply, 150% payment adjustment for bilateral procedures applies, assistant surgeon may not be paid

27240   **Treat thigh fracture**   ~ follow-up period is 90 days, standard payment adjustment rules for multiple procedures apply, 150% payment adjustment for bilateral procedures applies, assistant surgeon may not be paid

27244   **Treat thigh fracture**   ~ follow-up period is 90 days, standard payment adjustment rules for multiple procedures apply, 150% payment adjustment for bilateral procedures applies, assistant surgeon may be paid

27245   **Treat thigh fracture**   ~ follow-up period is 90 days, standard payment adjustment rules for multiple procedures apply, 150% payment adjustment for bilateral procedures applies, assistant surgeon may be paid

27246   **Treat thigh fracture**   ~ follow-up period is 90 days, standard payment adjustment rules for multiple procedures apply, 150% payment adjustment for bilateral procedures applies, assistant surgeon may not be paid

27248   **Treat thigh fracture**   ~ follow-up period is 90 days, standard payment adjustment rules for multiple procedures apply, 150% payment adjustment for bilateral procedures applies, assistant surgeon may be paid

27250   **Treat hip dislocation**   ~ follow-up period is 90 days, standard payment adjustment rules for multiple procedures apply, 150% payment adjustment for bilateral procedures applies, assistant surgeon may not be paid

27252   **Treat hip dislocation**   ~ follow-up period is 90 days, standard payment adjustment rules for multiple procedures apply, 150% payment adjustment for bilateral procedures applies, assistant surgeon may not be paid

27253   **Treat hip dislocation**   ~ follow-up period is 90 days, standard payment adjustment rules for multiple procedures apply, 150% payment adjustment for bilateral procedures applies, assistant surgeon may be paid

27254   **Treat hip dislocation**   ~ follow-up period is 90 days, standard payment adjustment rules for multiple procedures apply, 150% payment adjustment for bilateral procedures applies, assistant surgeon may be paid

27256   **Treat hip dislocation**   ~ follow-up period is 10 days, standard payment adjustment rules for multiple procedures apply, 150% payment adjustment for bilateral procedures applies, payment for assistant surgeon subject to documentation of medical necessity

27257   **Treat hip dislocation**   ~ follow-up period is 10 days, standard payment adjustment rules for multiple procedures apply, 150% payment adjustment for bilateral procedures applies, payment for assistant surgeon subject to documentation of medical necessity

27258   **Treat hip dislocation**   ~ follow-up period is 90 days, standard payment adjustment rules for multiple procedures apply, 150% payment adjustment for bilateral procedures applies, assistant surgeon may be paid

     CPT codes and descriptions only copyright American Medical Association

27259   **Treat hip dislocation**   ~ follow-up period is 90 days, standard payment adjustment rules for multiple procedures apply, 150% payment adjustment for bilateral procedures applies, assistant surgeon may be paid

27265   **Treat hip dislocation**   ~ follow-up period is 90 days, standard payment adjustment rules for multiple procedures apply, 150% payment adjustment for bilateral procedures applies, assistant surgeon may not be paid

27266   **Treat hip dislocation**   ~ follow-up period is 90 days, standard payment adjustment rules for multiple procedures apply, 150% payment adjustment for bilateral procedures applies, assistant surgeon may not be paid

27275   **Manipulate hip joint**   ~ follow-up period is 10 days, standard payment adjustment rules for multiple procedures apply, 150% payment adjustment for bilateral procedures does not apply, assistant surgeon may not be paid

27280   **Fuse sacroiliac joint**   ~ follow-up period is 90 days, standard payment adjustment rules for multiple procedures apply, 150% payment adjustment for bilateral procedures applies, assistant surgeon may be paid

27282   **Fuse pubic bones**   ~ follow-up period is 90 days, standard payment adjustment rules for multiple procedures apply, 150% payment adjustment for bilateral procedures does not apply, assistant surgeon may be paid

27284   **Fuse hip joint**   ~ follow-up period is 90 days, standard payment adjustment rules for multiple procedures apply, 150% payment adjustment for bilateral procedures applies, assistant surgeon may be paid

27286   **Fuse hip joint**   ~ follow-up period is 90 days, standard payment adjustment rules for multiple procedures apply, 150% payment adjustment for bilateral procedures applies, assistant surgeon may be paid

27290   **Amputate leg at hip**   ~ follow-up period is 90 days, standard payment adjustment rules for multiple procedures apply, 150% payment adjustment for bilateral procedures does not apply, assistant surgeon may be paid

27295   **Amputate leg at hip**   ~ follow-up period is 90 days, standard payment adjustment rules for multiple procedures apply, 150% payment adjustment for bilateral procedures does not apply, assistant surgeon may be paid

27299   **Pelvis/hip joint surgery**   ~ medicare carrier determines global period, standard payment adjustment rules for multiple procedures apply, 150% payment adjustment for bilateral procedures applies, assistant surgeon may be paid

27301   **Drain thigh/knee lesion**   ~ follow-up period is 90 days, standard payment adjustment rules for multiple procedures apply, 150% payment adjustment for bilateral procedures applies, assistant surgeon may not be paid

27303   **Drain bone lesion**   ~ follow-up period is 90 days, standard payment adjustment rules for multiple procedures apply, 150% payment adjustment for bilateral procedures applies, assistant surgeon may be paid

Femur (Thigh Region) and Knee Joint

27305   **Incise thigh tendon & fascia**   ~ follow-up period is 90 days, standard payment adjustment rules for multiple procedures apply, 150% payment adjustment for bilateral procedures applies, assistant surgeon may be paid

27306   **Incise thigh tendon**   ~ follow-up period is 90 days, standard payment adjustment rules for multiple procedures apply, 150% payment adjustment for bilateral procedures applies, assistant surgeon may be paid

27307   **Incise thigh tendons**   ~ follow-up period is 90 days, standard payment adjustment rules for multiple procedures apply, 150% payment adjustment for bilateral procedures applies, payment for assistant surgeon subject to documentation of medical necessity

27310   **Explore knee joint**   ~ follow-up period is 90 days, standard payment adjustment rules for multiple procedures apply, 150% payment adjustment for bilateral procedures applies, assistant surgeon may be paid

27323   **Biopsy thigh soft tissues**   ~ follow-up period is 10 days, standard payment adjustment rules for multiple procedures apply, 150% payment adjustment for bilateral procedures applies, assistant surgeon may not be paid

27324   **Biopsy thigh soft tissues**   ~ follow-up period is 90 days, standard payment adjustment rules for multiple procedures apply, 150% payment adjustment for bilateral procedures applies, assistant surgeon may not be paid

27325   **Neurectomy, hamstring**   ~ follow-up period is 90 days, standard payment adjustment rules for multiple procedures apply, 150% payment adjustment for bilateral procedures applies, assistant surgeon may be paid

27326   **Neurectomy, popliteal**   ~ follow-up period is 90 days, standard payment adjustment rules for multiple procedures apply, 150% payment adjustment for bilateral procedures applies, assistant surgeon may be paid

27327   **Remove thigh lesion**   ~ follow-up period is 90 days, standard payment adjustment rules for multiple procedures apply, 150% payment adjustment for bilateral procedures applies, assistant surgeon may not be paid

27328   **Remove thigh lesion**   ~ follow-up period is 90 days, standard payment adjustment rules for multiple procedures apply, 150% payment adjustment for bilateral procedures applies, assistant surgeon may not be paid

27329   **Remove tumor, thigh/knee**   ~ follow-up period is 90 days, standard payment adjustment rules for multiple procedures apply, 150% payment adjustment for bilateral procedures applies, assistant surgeon may be paid

27330   **Biopsy knee joint lining**   ~ follow-up period is 90 days, standard payment adjustment rules for multiple procedures apply, 150% payment adjustment for bilateral procedures applies, assistant surgeon may not be paid

27331   **Explore/treat knee joint**   ~ follow-up period is 90 days, standard payment adjustment rules for multiple procedures apply, 150% payment adjustment for bilateral procedures applies, assistant surgeon may be paid

27332   **Remove knee cartilage**   ~ follow-up period is 90 days, standard payment adjustment rules for multiple procedures apply, 150% payment adjustment for bilateral procedures applies, assistant surgeon may be paid

27333   **Remove knee cartilage**   ~ follow-up period is 90 days, standard payment adjustment rules for multiple procedures apply, 150% payment adjustment for bilateral procedures applies, assistant surgeon may be paid

27334   **Remove knee joint lining**   ~ follow-up period is 90 days, standard payment adjustment rules for multiple procedures apply, 150% payment adjustment for bilateral procedures applies, assistant surgeon may be paid

27335   **Remove knee joint lining**   ~ follow-up period is 90 days, standard payment adjustment rules for multiple procedures apply, 150% payment adjustment for bilateral procedures applies, assistant surgeon may be paid

27340   **Remove kneecap bursa**   ~ follow-up period is 90 days, standard payment adjustment rules for multiple procedures apply, 150% payment adjustment for bilateral procedures applies, assistant surgeon may not be paid

27345   **Remove knee cyst**   ~ follow-up period is 90 days, standard payment adjustment rules for multiple procedures apply, 150% payment adjustment for bilateral procedures applies, assistant surgeon may be paid

27347   **Remove knee cyst**   ~ follow-up period is 90 days, standard payment adjustment rules for multiple procedures apply, 150% payment adjustment for bilateral procedures applies, assistant surgeon may be paid

27350   **Remove kneecap**   ~ follow-up period is 90 days, standard payment adjustment rules for multiple procedures apply, 150% payment adjustment for bilateral procedures applies, assistant surgeon may be paid

27355   **Remove femur lesion**   ~ follow-up period is 90 days, standard payment adjustment rules for multiple procedures apply, 150% payment adjustment for bilateral procedures applies, assistant surgeon may be paid

27356   **Remove femur lesion/graft**   ~ follow-up period is 90 days, standard payment adjustment rules for multiple procedures apply, 150% payment adjustment for bilateral procedures applies, assistant surgeon may be paid

27357   **Remove femur lesion/graft**   ~ follow-up period is 90 days, standard payment adjustment rules for multiple procedures apply, 150% payment adjustment for bilateral procedures applies, assistant surgeon may be paid

27358   **Remove femur lesion/fixation**   ~ follow-up period included in another service, no payment adjustment rules for multiple procedures apply, 150% payment adjustment for bilateral procedures does not apply, assistant surgeon may be paid

27360   **Partial remove leg bone(s)**   ~ follow-up period is 90 days, standard payment adjustment rules for multiple procedures apply, 150% payment adjustment for bilateral procedures applies, assistant surgeon may be paid

27365   **Extensive leg surgery**   ~ follow-up period is 90 days, standard payment adjustment rules for multiple procedures apply, 150% payment adjustment for bilateral procedures applies, assistant surgeon may be paid

27370   **Inject for knee x-ray**   ~ endoscopies or minor procedure - E/M services on the same day generally not paid, standard payment adjustment rules for multiple procedures apply, 150% payment adjustment for bilateral procedures applies, assistant surgeon may not be paid

27372   **Remove foreign body**   ~ follow-up period is 90 days, standard payment adjustment rules for multiple procedures apply, 150% payment adjustment for bilateral procedures applies, payment for assistant surgeon subject to documentation of medical necessity

27380   **Repair kneecap tendon**   ~ follow-up period is 90 days, standard payment adjustment rules for multiple procedures apply, 150% payment adjustment for bilateral procedures applies, assistant surgeon may be paid

27381   **Repair/graft kneecap tendon**   ~ follow-up period is 90 days, standard payment adjustment rules for multiple procedures apply, 150% payment adjustment for bilateral procedures applies, assistant surgeon may be paid

27385   **Repair thigh muscle**   ~ follow-up period is 90 days, standard payment adjustment rules for multiple procedures apply, 150% payment adjustment for bilateral procedures applies, assistant surgeon may be paid

27386   **Repair/graft of thigh muscle**   ~ follow-up period is 90 days, standard payment adjustment rules for multiple procedures apply, 150% payment adjustment for bilateral procedures applies, assistant surgeon may be paid

27390   **Incise thigh tendon**   ~ follow-up period is 90 days, standard payment adjustment rules for multiple procedures apply, 150% payment adjustment for bilateral procedures does not apply, assistant surgeon may be paid

27391   **Incise thigh tendons**   ~ follow-up period is 90 days, standard payment adjustment rules for multiple procedures apply, 150% payment adjustment for bilateral procedures does not apply, payment for assistant surgeon subject to documentation of medical necessity

27392   **Incise thigh tendons**   ~ follow-up period is 90 days, standard payment adjustment rules for multiple procedures apply, 150% payment adjustment does not apply - RVUs based on bilateral procedure, assistant surgeon may be paid

27393   **Lengthening of thigh tendon**   ~ follow-up period is 90 days, standard payment adjustment rules for multiple procedures apply, 150% payment adjustment for bilateral procedures does not apply, assistant surgeon may be paid

27394   **Lengthening of thigh tendons**   ~ follow-up period is 90 days, standard payment adjustment rules for multiple procedures apply, 150% payment adjustment for bilateral procedures does not apply, assistant surgeon may be paid

27395   **Lengthening of thigh tendons**   ~ follow-up period is 90 days, standard payment adjustment rules for multiple procedures apply, 150% payment adjustment does not apply - RVUs based on bilateral procedure, assistant surgeon may be paid

27396   **Transplant of thigh tendon**   ~ follow-up period is 90 days, standard payment adjustment rules for multiple procedures apply, 150% payment adjustment for bilateral procedures does not apply, assistant surgeon may be paid

27397   **Transplant thigh tendons**   ~ follow-up period is 90 days, standard payment adjustment rules for multiple procedures apply, 150% payment adjustment for bilateral procedures does not apply, assistant surgeon may be paid

27400   **Revise thigh muscles/tendons**   ~ follow-up period is 90 days, standard payment adjustment rules for multiple procedures apply, 150% payment adjustment for bilateral procedures applies, assistant surgeon may be paid

27403   **Repair knee cartilage**   ~ follow-up period is 90 days, standard payment adjustment rules for multiple procedures apply, 150% payment adjustment for bilateral procedures applies, assistant surgeon may be paid

27405   **Repair knee ligament**   ~ follow-up period is 90 days, standard payment adjustment rules for multiple procedures apply, 150% payment adjustment for bilateral procedures applies, assistant surgeon may be paid

27407 **Repair knee ligament** ~ follow-up period is 90 days, standard payment adjustment rules for multiple procedures apply, 150% payment adjustment for bilateral procedures applies, assistant surgeon may be paid

27409 **Repair knee ligaments** ~ follow-up period is 90 days, standard payment adjustment rules for multiple procedures apply, 150% payment adjustment for bilateral procedures applies, assistant surgeon may be paid

27412 **Autochondrocyte implant knee** ~ follow-up period is 90 days, standard payment adjustment rules for multiple procedures apply, 150% payment adjustment for bilateral procedures applies, assistant surgeon may be paid

27415 **Osteochondral knee allograft** ~ follow-up period is 90 days, standard payment adjustment rules for multiple procedures apply, 150% payment adjustment for bilateral procedures applies, assistant surgeon may be paid

27418 **Repair degenerated kneecap** ~ follow-up period is 90 days, standard payment adjustment rules for multiple procedures apply, 150% payment adjustment for bilateral procedures applies, assistant surgeon may be paid

27420 **Revise unstable kneecap** ~ follow-up period is 90 days, standard payment adjustment rules for multiple procedures apply, 150% payment adjustment for bilateral procedures applies, assistant surgeon may be paid

27422 **Revise unstable kneecap** ~ follow-up period is 90 days, standard payment adjustment rules for multiple procedures apply, 150% payment adjustment for bilateral procedures applies, assistant surgeon may be paid

27424 **Revision/remove kneecap** ~ follow-up period is 90 days, standard payment adjustment rules for multiple procedures apply, 150% payment adjustment for bilateral procedures applies, assistant surgeon may be paid

27425 **Lat retinacular release open** ~ follow-up period is 90 days, standard payment adjustment rules for multiple procedures apply, 150% payment adjustment for bilateral procedures applies, assistant surgeon may not be paid

27427 **Reconstruct knee** ~ follow-up period is 90 days, standard payment adjustment rules for multiple procedures apply, 150% payment adjustment for bilateral procedures applies, assistant surgeon may be paid

27428 **Reconstruct knee** ~ follow-up period is 90 days, standard payment adjustment rules for multiple procedures apply, 150% payment adjustment for bilateral procedures applies, assistant surgeon may be paid

27429 **Reconstruct knee** ~ follow-up period is 90 days, standard payment adjustment rules for multiple procedures apply, 150% payment adjustment for bilateral procedures applies, assistant surgeon may be paid

27430   **Revise thigh muscles**   ~ follow-up period is 90 days, standard payment adjustment rules for multiple procedures apply, 150% payment adjustment for bilateral procedures applies, assistant surgeon may be paid

27435   **Incise knee joint**   ~ follow-up period is 90 days, standard payment adjustment rules for multiple procedures apply, 150% payment adjustment for bilateral procedures applies, assistant surgeon may be paid

27437   **Revise kneecap**   ~ follow-up period is 90 days, standard payment adjustment rules for multiple procedures apply, 150% payment adjustment for bilateral procedures applies, assistant surgeon may not be paid

27438   **Revise kneecap with implant**   ~ follow-up period is 90 days, standard payment adjustment rules for multiple procedures apply, 150% payment adjustment for bilateral procedures applies, assistant surgeon may be paid

27440   **Revise knee joint**   ~ follow-up period is 90 days, standard payment adjustment rules for multiple procedures apply, 150% payment adjustment for bilateral procedures applies, assistant surgeon may be paid

27441   **Revise knee joint**   ~ follow-up period is 90 days, standard payment adjustment rules for multiple procedures apply, 150% payment adjustment for bilateral procedures applies, assistant surgeon may be paid

27442   **Revise knee joint**   ~ follow-up period is 90 days, standard payment adjustment rules for multiple procedures apply, 150% payment adjustment for bilateral procedures applies, assistant surgeon may be paid

27443   **Revise knee joint**   ~ follow-up period is 90 days, standard payment adjustment rules for multiple procedures apply, 150% payment adjustment for bilateral procedures applies, assistant surgeon may be paid

27445   **Revise knee joint**   ~ follow-up period is 90 days, standard payment adjustment rules for multiple procedures apply, 150% payment adjustment for bilateral procedures applies, assistant surgeon may be paid

27446   **Revise knee joint**   ~ follow-up period is 90 days, standard payment adjustment rules for multiple procedures apply, 150% payment adjustment for bilateral procedures applies, assistant surgeon may be paid

27447   **Total knee arthroplasty**   ~ follow-up period is 90 days, standard payment adjustment rules for multiple procedures apply, 150% payment adjustment for bilateral procedures applies, assistant surgeon may be paid

27448   **Incise thigh**   ~ follow-up period is 90 days, standard payment adjustment rules for multiple procedures apply, 150% payment adjustment for bilateral procedures applies, assistant surgeon may be paid

27450   **Incise thigh**   ~ follow-up period is 90 days, standard payment adjustment rules for multiple procedures apply, 150% payment adjustment for bilateral procedures applies, assistant surgeon may be paid

27454   **Realignment of thigh bone**   ~ follow-up period is 90 days, standard payment adjustment rules for multiple procedures apply, 150% payment adjustment for bilateral procedures applies, assistant surgeon may be paid

27455   **Realignment of knee**   ~ follow-up period is 90 days, standard payment adjustment rules for multiple procedures apply, 150% payment adjustment for bilateral procedures applies, assistant surgeon may be paid

27457   **Realignment of knee**   ~ follow-up period is 90 days, standard payment adjustment rules for multiple procedures apply, 150% payment adjustment for bilateral procedures applies, assistant surgeon may be paid

27465   **Shortening of thigh bone**   ~ follow-up period is 90 days, standard payment adjustment rules for multiple procedures apply, 150% payment adjustment for bilateral procedures applies, assistant surgeon may be paid

27466   **Lengthening of thigh bone**   ~ follow-up period is 90 days, standard payment adjustment rules for multiple procedures apply, 150% payment adjustment for bilateral procedures applies, assistant surgeon may be paid

27468   **Shorten/lengthen thighs**   ~ follow-up period is 90 days, standard payment adjustment rules for multiple procedures apply, 150% payment adjustment for bilateral procedures applies, assistant surgeon may be paid

27470   **Repair thigh**   ~ follow-up period is 90 days, standard payment adjustment rules for multiple procedures apply, 150% payment adjustment for bilateral procedures applies, assistant surgeon may be paid

27472   **Repair/graft of thigh**   ~ follow-up period is 90 days, standard payment adjustment rules for multiple procedures apply, 150% payment adjustment for bilateral procedures applies, assistant surgeon may be paid

27475   **Surgery to stop leg growth**   ~ follow-up period is 90 days, standard payment adjustment rules for multiple procedures apply, 150% payment adjustment for bilateral procedures applies, assistant surgeon may not be paid

27477   **Surgery to stop leg growth**   ~ follow-up period is 90 days, standard payment adjustment rules for multiple procedures apply, 150% payment adjustment for bilateral procedures applies, assistant surgeon may not be paid

27479   **Surgery to stop leg growth**   ~ follow-up period is 90 days, standard payment adjustment rules for multiple procedures apply, 150% payment adjustment for bilateral procedures applies, assistant surgeon may be paid

27485   **Surgery to stop leg growth**   ~ follow-up period is 90 days, standard payment adjustment rules for multiple procedures apply, 150% payment adjustment for bilateral procedures applies, assistant surgeon may not be paid

27486   **Revise/replace knee joint**   ~ follow-up period is 90 days, standard payment adjustment rules for multiple procedures apply, 150% payment adjustment for bilateral procedures applies, assistant surgeon may be paid

27487   **Revise/replace knee joint**   ~ follow-up period is 90 days, standard payment adjustment rules for multiple procedures apply, 150% payment adjustment for bilateral procedures applies, assistant surgeon may be paid

27488   **Remove knee prosthesis**   ~ follow-up period is 90 days, standard payment adjustment rules for multiple procedures apply, 150% payment adjustment for bilateral procedures applies, assistant surgeon may be paid

27495   **Reinforce thigh**   ~ follow-up period is 90 days, standard payment adjustment rules for multiple procedures apply, 150% payment adjustment for bilateral procedures applies, assistant surgeon may be paid

27496   **Decompress thigh/knee**   ~ follow-up period is 90 days, standard payment adjustment rules for multiple procedures apply, 150% payment adjustment for bilateral procedures applies, assistant surgeon may not be paid

27497   **Decompress thigh/knee**   ~ follow-up period is 90 days, standard payment adjustment rules for multiple procedures apply, 150% payment adjustment for bilateral procedures applies, payment for assistant surgeon subject to documentation of medical necessity

27498   **Decompress thigh/knee**   ~ follow-up period is 90 days, standard payment adjustment rules for multiple procedures apply, 150% payment adjustment for bilateral procedures applies, assistant surgeon may be paid

27499   **Decompress thigh/knee**   ~ follow-up period is 90 days, standard payment adjustment rules for multiple procedures apply, 150% payment adjustment for bilateral procedures applies, assistant surgeon may be paid

27500   **Treat thigh fracture**   ~ follow-up period is 90 days, standard payment adjustment rules for multiple procedures apply, 150% payment adjustment for bilateral procedures applies, assistant surgeon may not be paid

27501   **Treat thigh fracture**   ~ follow-up period is 90 days, standard payment adjustment rules for multiple procedures apply, 150% payment adjustment for bilateral procedures applies, payment for assistant surgeon subject to documentation of medical necessity

27502   **Treat thigh fracture**   ~ follow-up period is 90 days, standard payment adjustment rules for multiple procedures apply, 150% payment adjustment for bilateral procedures applies, assistant surgeon may not be paid

27503   **Treat thigh fracture**   ~ follow-up period is 90 days, standard payment adjustment rules for multiple procedures apply, 150% payment adjustment for bilateral procedures applies, payment for assistant surgeon subject to documentation of medical necessity

27506   **Treat thigh fracture**   ~ follow-up period is 90 days, standard payment adjustment rules for multiple procedures apply, 150% payment adjustment for bilateral procedures applies, assistant surgeon may be paid

27507   **Treat thigh fracture**   ~ follow-up period is 90 days, standard payment adjustment rules for multiple procedures apply, 150% payment adjustment for bilateral procedures applies, assistant surgeon may be paid

27508   **Treat thigh fracture**   ~ follow-up period is 90 days, standard payment adjustment rules for multiple procedures apply, 150% payment adjustment for bilateral procedures applies, assistant surgeon may not be paid

27509   **Treat thigh fracture**   ~ follow-up period is 90 days, standard payment adjustment rules for multiple procedures apply, 150% payment adjustment for bilateral procedures applies, payment for assistant surgeon subject to documentation of medical necessity

27510   **Treat thigh fracture**   ~ follow-up period is 90 days, standard payment adjustment rules for multiple procedures apply, 150% payment adjustment for bilateral procedures applies, assistant surgeon may not be paid

27511   **Treat thigh fracture**   ~ follow-up period is 90 days, standard payment adjustment rules for multiple procedures apply, 150% payment adjustment for bilateral procedures applies, assistant surgeon may be paid

27513   **Treat thigh fracture**   ~ follow-up period is 90 days, standard payment adjustment rules for multiple procedures apply, 150% payment adjustment for bilateral procedures applies, assistant surgeon may be paid

27514   **Treat thigh fracture**   ~ follow-up period is 90 days, standard payment adjustment rules for multiple procedures apply, 150% payment adjustment for bilateral procedures applies, assistant surgeon may be paid

27516   **Treat thigh fracture growth plate**   ~ follow-up period is 90 days, standard payment adjustment rules for multiple procedures apply, 150% payment adjustment for bilateral procedures applies, assistant surgeon may not be paid

27517 **Treat thigh fracture growth plate** ~ follow-up period is 90 days, standard payment adjustment rules for multiple procedures apply, 150% payment adjustment for bilateral procedures applies, payment for assistant surgeon subject to documentation of medical necessity

27519 **Treat thigh fracture growth plate** ~ follow-up period is 90 days, standard payment adjustment rules for multiple procedures apply, 150% payment adjustment for bilateral procedures applies, assistant surgeon may be paid

27520 **Treat kneecap fracture** ~ follow-up period is 90 days, standard payment adjustment rules for multiple procedures apply, 150% payment adjustment for bilateral procedures applies, assistant surgeon may not be paid

27524 **Treat kneecap fracture** ~ follow-up period is 90 days, standard payment adjustment rules for multiple procedures apply, 150% payment adjustment for bilateral procedures applies, assistant surgeon may be paid

27530 **Treat knee fracture** ~ follow-up period is 90 days, standard payment adjustment rules for multiple procedures apply, 150% payment adjustment for bilateral procedures applies, assistant surgeon may not be paid

27532 **Treat knee fracture** ~ follow-up period is 90 days, standard payment adjustment rules for multiple procedures apply, 150% payment adjustment for bilateral procedures applies, assistant surgeon may not be paid

27535 **Treat knee fracture** ~ follow-up period is 90 days, standard payment adjustment rules for multiple procedures apply, 150% payment adjustment for bilateral procedures applies, assistant surgeon may be paid

27536 **Treat knee fracture** ~ follow-up period is 90 days, standard payment adjustment rules for multiple procedures apply, 150% payment adjustment for bilateral procedures applies, assistant surgeon may be paid

27538 **Treat knee fracture(s)** ~ follow-up period is 90 days, standard payment adjustment rules for multiple procedures apply, 150% payment adjustment for bilateral procedures applies, payment for assistant surgeon subject to documentation of medical necessity

27540 **Treat knee fracture** ~ follow-up period is 90 days, standard payment adjustment rules for multiple procedures apply, 150% payment adjustment for bilateral procedures applies, assistant surgeon may be paid

27550 **Treat knee dislocation** ~ follow-up period is 90 days, standard payment adjustment rules for multiple procedures apply, 150% payment adjustment for bilateral procedures applies, payment for assistant surgeon subject to documentation of medical necessity

27552 **Treat knee dislocation** ~ follow-up period is 90 days, standard payment adjustment rules for multiple procedures apply, 150% payment adjustment for bilateral procedures applies, payment for assistant surgeon subject to documentation of medical necessity

27556 **Treat knee dislocation** ~ follow-up period is 90 days, standard payment adjustment rules for multiple procedures apply, 150% payment adjustment for bilateral procedures applies, assistant surgeon may be paid

27557 **Treat knee dislocation** ~ follow-up period is 90 days, standard payment adjustment rules for multiple procedures apply, 150% payment adjustment for bilateral procedures applies, assistant surgeon may be paid

27558 **Treat knee dislocation** ~ follow-up period is 90 days, standard payment adjustment rules for multiple procedures apply, 150% payment adjustment for bilateral procedures applies, assistant surgeon may be paid

27560 **Treat kneecap dislocation** ~ follow-up period is 90 days, standard payment adjustment rules for multiple procedures apply, 150% payment adjustment for bilateral procedures applies, assistant surgeon may not be paid

27562 **Treat kneecap dislocation** ~ follow-up period is 90 days, standard payment adjustment rules for multiple procedures apply, 150% payment adjustment for bilateral procedures applies, payment for assistant surgeon subject to documentation of medical necessity

27566 **Treat kneecap dislocation** ~ follow-up period is 90 days, standard payment adjustment rules for multiple procedures apply, 150% payment adjustment for bilateral procedures applies, assistant surgeon may be paid

27570 **Fixate knee joint** ~ follow-up period is 10 days, standard payment adjustment rules for multiple procedures apply, 150% payment adjustment for bilateral procedures does not apply, assistant surgeon may not be paid

27580 **Fuse knee** ~ follow-up period is 90 days, standard payment adjustment rules for multiple procedures apply, 150% payment adjustment for bilateral procedures applies, assistant surgeon may be paid

27590 **Amputate leg at thigh** ~ follow-up period is 90 days, standard payment adjustment rules for multiple procedures apply, 150% payment adjustment for bilateral procedures applies, assistant surgeon may be paid

27591 **Amputate leg at thigh** ~ follow-up period is 90 days, standard payment adjustment rules for multiple procedures apply, 150% payment adjustment for bilateral procedures applies, assistant surgeon may be paid

27592 **Amputate leg at thigh** ~ follow-up period is 90 days, standard payment adjustment rules for multiple procedures apply, 150% payment adjustment for bilateral procedures applies, assistant surgeon may be paid

27594 **Amputation follow-up surgery** ~ follow-up period is 90 days, standard payment adjustment rules for multiple procedures apply, 150% payment adjustment for bilateral procedures applies, assistant surgeon may not be paid

27596 **Amputation follow-up surgery** ~ follow-up period is 90 days, standard payment adjustment rules for multiple procedures apply, 150% payment adjustment for bilateral procedures applies, assistant surgeon may not be paid

27598 **Amputate lower leg at knee** ~ follow-up period is 90 days, standard payment adjustment rules for multiple procedures apply, 150% payment adjustment for bilateral procedures applies, assistant surgeon may be paid

27599 **Leg surgery procedure** ~ medicare carrier determines global period, standard payment adjustment rules for multiple procedures apply, 150% payment adjustment for bilateral procedures applies, assistant surgeon may be paid

Leg (Tibia and Fibula) and Ankle Joint

27600 **Decompress lower leg** ~ follow-up period is 90 days, standard payment adjustment rules for multiple procedures apply, 150% payment adjustment for bilateral procedures applies, assistant surgeon may not be paid

27601 **Decompress lower leg** ~ follow-up period is 90 days, standard payment adjustment rules for multiple procedures apply, 150% payment adjustment for bilateral procedures applies, assistant surgeon may not be paid

27602 **Decompress lower leg** ~ follow-up period is 90 days, standard payment adjustment rules for multiple procedures apply, 150% payment adjustment for bilateral procedures applies, assistant surgeon may be paid

27603 **Drain lower leg lesion** ~ follow-up period is 90 days, standard payment adjustment rules for multiple procedures apply, 150% payment adjustment for bilateral procedures applies, assistant surgeon may not be paid

27604 **Drain lower leg bursa** ~ follow-up period is 90 days, standard payment adjustment rules for multiple procedures apply, 150% payment adjustment for bilateral procedures applies, payment for assistant surgeon subject to documentation of medical necessity

27605 **Incise achilles tendon** ~ follow-up period is 10 days, standard payment adjustment rules for multiple procedures apply, 150% payment adjustment for bilateral procedures applies, payment for assistant surgeon subject to documentation of medical necessity

27606   **Incise achilles tendon**   ~ follow-up period is 10 days, standard payment adjustment rules for multiple procedures apply, 150% payment adjustment for bilateral procedures applies, assistant surgeon may not be paid

27607   **Treat lower leg bone lesion**   ~ follow-up period is 90 days, standard payment adjustment rules for multiple procedures apply, 150% payment adjustment for bilateral procedures applies, assistant surgeon may not be paid

27610   **Explore/treat ankle joint**   ~ follow-up period is 90 days, standard payment adjustment rules for multiple procedures apply, 150% payment adjustment for bilateral procedures applies, assistant surgeon may not be paid

27612   **Explore ankle joint**   ~ follow-up period is 90 days, standard payment adjustment rules for multiple procedures apply, 150% payment adjustment for bilateral procedures applies, assistant surgeon may be paid

27613   **Biopsy lower leg soft tissue**   ~ follow-up period is 10 days, standard payment adjustment rules for multiple procedures apply, 150% payment adjustment for bilateral procedures applies, assistant surgeon may not be paid

27614   **Biopsy lower leg soft tissue**   ~ follow-up period is 90 days, standard payment adjustment rules for multiple procedures apply, 150% payment adjustment for bilateral procedures applies, assistant surgeon may not be paid

27615   **Remove tumor, lower leg**   ~ follow-up period is 90 days, standard payment adjustment rules for multiple procedures apply, 150% payment adjustment for bilateral procedures applies, payment for assistant surgeon subject to documentation of medical necessity

27618   **Remove lower leg lesion**   ~ follow-up period is 90 days, standard payment adjustment rules for multiple procedures apply, 150% payment adjustment for bilateral procedures applies, assistant surgeon may not be paid

27619   **Remove lower leg lesion**   ~ follow-up period is 90 days, standard payment adjustment rules for multiple procedures apply, 150% payment adjustment for bilateral procedures applies, assistant surgeon may not be paid

27620   **Explore/treat ankle joint**   ~ follow-up period is 90 days, standard payment adjustment rules for multiple procedures apply, 150% payment adjustment for bilateral procedures applies, assistant surgeon may be paid

27625   **Remove ankle joint lining**   ~ follow-up period is 90 days, standard payment adjustment rules for multiple procedures apply, 150% payment adjustment for bilateral procedures applies, assistant surgeon may be paid

27626   **Remove ankle joint lining**   ~ follow-up period is 90 days, standard payment adjustment rules for multiple procedures apply, 150% payment adjustment for bilateral procedures applies, assistant surgeon may be paid

27630   **Remove tendon lesion**   ~ follow-up period is 90 days, standard payment adjustment rules for multiple procedures apply, 150% payment adjustment for bilateral procedures applies, assistant surgeon may not be paid

27635   **Remove lower leg bone lesion**   ~ follow-up period is 90 days, standard payment adjustment rules for multiple procedures apply, 150% payment adjustment for bilateral procedures applies, assistant surgeon may not be paid

27637   **Remove/graft leg bone lesion**   ~ follow-up period is 90 days, standard payment adjustment rules for multiple procedures apply, 150% payment adjustment for bilateral procedures applies, assistant surgeon may be paid

27638   **Remove/graft leg bone lesion**   ~ follow-up period is 90 days, standard payment adjustment rules for multiple procedures apply, 150% payment adjustment for bilateral procedures applies, assistant surgeon may be paid

27640   **Partial remove tibia**   ~ follow-up period is 90 days, standard payment adjustment rules for multiple procedures apply, 150% payment adjustment for bilateral procedures applies, assistant surgeon may not be paid

27641   **Partial remove fibula**   ~ follow-up period is 90 days, standard payment adjustment rules for multiple procedures apply, 150% payment adjustment for bilateral procedures applies, assistant surgeon may not be paid

27645   **Extensive lower leg surgery**   ~ follow-up period is 90 days, standard payment adjustment rules for multiple procedures apply, 150% payment adjustment for bilateral procedures applies, assistant surgeon may be paid

27646   **Extensive lower leg surgery**   ~ follow-up period is 90 days, standard payment adjustment rules for multiple procedures apply, 150% payment adjustment for bilateral procedures applies, assistant surgeon may be paid

27647   **Extensive ankle/heel surgery**   ~ follow-up period is 90 days, standard payment adjustment rules for multiple procedures apply, 150% payment adjustment for bilateral procedures applies, assistant surgeon may be paid

27648   **Inject for ankle x-ray**   ~ endoscopies or minor procedure - E/M services on the same day generally not paid, standard payment adjustment rules for multiple procedures apply, 150% payment adjustment for bilateral procedures applies, payment for assistant surgeon subject to documentation of medical necessity

27650   **Repair achilles tendon**   ~ follow-up period is 90 days, standard payment adjustment rules for multiple procedures apply, 150% payment adjustment for bilateral procedures applies, assistant surgeon may be paid

27652   **Repair/graft achilles tendon**   ~ follow-up period is 90 days, standard payment adjustment rules for multiple procedures apply, 150% payment adjustment for bilateral procedures applies, assistant surgeon may not be paid

27654   **Repair achilles tendon**   ~ follow-up period is 90 days, standard payment adjustment rules for multiple procedures apply, 150% payment adjustment for bilateral procedures applies, assistant surgeon may be paid

27656   **Repair leg fascia defect**   ~ follow-up period is 90 days, standard payment adjustment rules for multiple procedures apply, 150% payment adjustment for bilateral procedures applies, assistant surgeon may be paid

27658   **Repair leg tendon, each**   ~ follow-up period is 90 days, standard payment adjustment rules for multiple procedures apply, 150% payment adjustment for bilateral procedures does not apply, assistant surgeon may be paid

27659   **Repair leg tendon, each**   ~ follow-up period is 90 days, standard payment adjustment rules for multiple procedures apply, 150% payment adjustment for bilateral procedures does not apply, assistant surgeon may be paid

27664   **Repair leg tendon, each**   ~ follow-up period is 90 days, standard payment adjustment rules for multiple procedures apply, 150% payment adjustment for bilateral procedures does not apply, payment for assistant surgeon subject to documentation of medical necessity

27665   **Repair leg tendon, each**   ~ follow-up period is 90 days, standard payment adjustment rules for multiple procedures apply, 150% payment adjustment for bilateral procedures does not apply, assistant surgeon may be paid

27675   **Repair lower leg tendons**   ~ follow-up period is 90 days, standard payment adjustment rules for multiple procedures apply, 150% payment adjustment for bilateral procedures applies, assistant surgeon may be paid

27676   **Repair lower leg tendons**   ~ follow-up period is 90 days, standard payment adjustment rules for multiple procedures apply, 150% payment adjustment for bilateral procedures applies, assistant surgeon may be paid

27680   **Release lower leg tendon**   ~ follow-up period is 90 days, standard payment adjustment rules for multiple procedures apply, 150% payment adjustment for bilateral procedures does not apply, assistant surgeon may not be paid

27681   **Release lower leg tendons**   ~ follow-up period is 90 days, standard payment adjustment rules for multiple procedures apply, 150% payment adjustment for bilateral procedures does not apply, assistant surgeon may not be paid

27685   **Revise lower leg tendon**   ~ follow-up period is 90 days, standard payment adjustment rules for multiple procedures apply, 150% payment adjustment for bilateral procedures does not apply, assistant surgeon may be paid

27686   **Revise lower leg tendons**   ~ follow-up period is 90 days, standard payment adjustment rules for multiple procedures apply, 150% payment adjustment for bilateral procedures does not apply, assistant surgeon may not be paid

27687   **Revise calf tendon**   ~ follow-up period is 90 days, standard payment adjustment rules for multiple procedures apply, 150% payment adjustment for bilateral procedures applies, assistant surgeon may be paid

27690   **Revise lower leg tendon**   ~ follow-up period is 90 days, standard payment adjustment rules for multiple procedures apply, 150% payment adjustment for bilateral procedures applies, assistant surgeon may be paid

27691   **Revise lower leg tendon**   ~ follow-up period is 90 days, standard payment adjustment rules for multiple procedures apply, 150% payment adjustment for bilateral procedures applies, assistant surgeon may be paid

27692   **Revise additional leg tendon**   ~ follow-up period included in another service, no payment adjustment rules for multiple procedures apply, 150% payment adjustment for bilateral procedures does not apply, assistant surgeon may be paid, +add-on code (list separately in addition to primary procedure)

27695   **Repair ankle ligament**   ~ follow-up period is 90 days, standard payment adjustment rules for multiple procedures apply, 150% payment adjustment for bilateral procedures applies, assistant surgeon may not be paid

27696   **Repair ankle ligaments**   ~ follow-up period is 90 days, standard payment adjustment rules for multiple procedures apply, 150% payment adjustment for bilateral procedures applies, assistant surgeon may not be paid

27698   **Repair ankle ligament**   ~ follow-up period is 90 days, standard payment adjustment rules for multiple procedures apply, 150% payment adjustment for bilateral procedures applies, assistant surgeon may be paid

27700   **Revise ankle joint**   ~ follow-up period is 90 days, standard payment adjustment rules for multiple procedures apply, 150% payment adjustment for bilateral procedures applies, assistant surgeon may be paid

27702   **Reconstruct ankle joint**   ~ follow-up period is 90 days, standard payment adjustment rules for multiple procedures apply, 150% payment adjustment for bilateral procedures applies, assistant surgeon may be paid

27703   **Reconstruct ankle joint**   ~ follow-up period is 90 days, standard payment adjustment rules for multiple procedures apply, 150% payment adjustment for bilateral procedures applies, assistant surgeon may be paid

27704   **Remove ankle implant**   ~ follow-up period is 90 days, standard payment adjustment rules for multiple procedures apply, 150% payment adjustment for bilateral procedures applies, assistant surgeon may not be paid

27705   **Incise tibia**   ~ follow-up period is 90 days, standard payment adjustment rules for multiple procedures apply, 150% payment adjustment for bilateral procedures applies, assistant surgeon may be paid

27707   **Incise fibula**   ~ follow-up period is 90 days, standard payment adjustment rules for multiple procedures apply, 150% payment adjustment for bilateral procedures applies, assistant surgeon may not be paid

27709   **Incise tibia & fibula**   ~ follow-up period is 90 days, standard payment adjustment rules for multiple procedures apply, 150% payment adjustment for bilateral procedures applies, assistant surgeon may be paid

27712   **Realignment of lower leg**   ~ follow-up period is 90 days, standard payment adjustment rules for multiple procedures apply, 150% payment adjustment for bilateral procedures applies, assistant surgeon may be paid

27715   **Revise lower leg**   ~ follow-up period is 90 days, standard payment adjustment rules for multiple procedures apply, 150% payment adjustment for bilateral procedures applies, assistant surgeon may be paid

27720   **Repair tibia**   ~ follow-up period is 90 days, standard payment adjustment rules for multiple procedures apply, 150% payment adjustment for bilateral procedures applies, assistant surgeon may be paid

27722   **Repair/graft of tibia**   ~ follow-up period is 90 days, standard payment adjustment rules for multiple procedures apply, 150% payment adjustment for bilateral procedures applies, assistant surgeon may be paid

27724   **Repair/graft of tibia**   ~ follow-up period is 90 days, standard payment adjustment rules for multiple procedures apply, 150% payment adjustment for bilateral procedures applies, assistant surgeon may be paid

27725   **Repair lower leg**   ~ follow-up period is 90 days, standard payment adjustment rules for multiple procedures apply, 150% payment adjustment for bilateral procedures applies, assistant surgeon may be paid

27727   **Repair lower leg**   ~ follow-up period is 90 days, standard payment adjustment rules for multiple procedures apply, 150% payment adjustment for bilateral procedures applies, assistant surgeon may be paid

27730   **Repair tibia epiphysis**   ~ follow-up period is 90 days, standard payment adjustment rules for multiple procedures apply, 150% payment adjustment for bilateral procedures applies, assistant surgeon may not be paid

27732   **Repair fibula epiphysis**   ~ follow-up period is 90 days, standard payment adjustment rules for multiple procedures apply, 150% payment adjustment for bilateral procedures applies, assistant surgeon may not be paid

27734   **Repair lower leg epiphyses**   ~ follow-up period is 90 days, standard payment adjustment rules for multiple procedures apply, 150% payment adjustment for bilateral procedures applies, assistant surgeon may not be paid

27740   **Repair leg epiphyses**   ~ follow-up period is 90 days, standard payment adjustment rules for multiple procedures apply, 150% payment adjustment for bilateral procedures applies, assistant surgeon may be paid

27742   **Repair leg epiphyses**   ~ follow-up period is 90 days, standard payment adjustment rules for multiple procedures apply, 150% payment adjustment for bilateral procedures applies, assistant surgeon may be paid

27745   **Reinforce tibia**   ~ follow-up period is 90 days, standard payment adjustment rules for multiple procedures apply, 150% payment adjustment for bilateral procedures applies, assistant surgeon may be paid

27750   **Treat tibia fracture**   ~ follow-up period is 90 days, standard payment adjustment rules for multiple procedures apply, 150% payment adjustment for bilateral procedures applies, assistant surgeon may not be paid

27752   **Treat tibia fracture**   ~ follow-up period is 90 days, standard payment adjustment rules for multiple procedures apply, 150% payment adjustment for bilateral procedures applies, assistant surgeon may not be paid

27756   **Treat tibia fracture**   ~ follow-up period is 90 days, standard payment adjustment rules for multiple procedures apply, 150% payment adjustment for bilateral procedures applies, assistant surgeon may be paid

27758   **Treat tibia fracture**   ~ follow-up period is 90 days, standard payment adjustment rules for multiple procedures apply, 150% payment adjustment for bilateral procedures applies, assistant surgeon may be paid

27759   **Treat tibia fracture**   ~ follow-up period is 90 days, standard payment adjustment rules for multiple procedures apply, 150% payment adjustment for bilateral procedures applies, assistant surgeon may be paid

27760   **Treat ankle fracture**   ~ follow-up period is 90 days, standard payment adjustment rules for multiple procedures apply, 150% payment adjustment for bilateral procedures applies, assistant surgeon may not be paid

27762   **Treat ankle fracture**   ~ follow-up period is 90 days, standard payment adjustment rules for multiple procedures apply, 150% payment adjustment for bilateral procedures applies, assistant surgeon may not be paid

27766   **Treat ankle fracture**   ~ follow-up period is 90 days, standard payment adjustment rules for multiple procedures apply, 150% payment adjustment for bilateral procedures applies, assistant surgeon may not be paid

27780   **Treat fibula fracture**   ~ follow-up period is 90 days, standard payment adjustment rules for multiple procedures apply, 150% payment adjustment for bilateral procedures applies, assistant surgeon may not be paid

27781   **Treat fibula fracture**   ~ follow-up period is 90 days, standard payment adjustment rules for multiple procedures apply, 150% payment adjustment for bilateral procedures applies, assistant surgeon may not be paid

27784   **Treat fibula fracture**   ~ follow-up period is 90 days, standard payment adjustment rules for multiple procedures apply, 150% payment adjustment for bilateral procedures applies, assistant surgeon may not be paid

27786   **Treat ankle fracture**   ~ follow-up period is 90 days, standard payment adjustment rules for multiple procedures apply, 150% payment adjustment for bilateral procedures applies, assistant surgeon may not be paid

27788   **Treat ankle fracture**   ~ follow-up period is 90 days, standard payment adjustment rules for multiple procedures apply, 150% payment adjustment for bilateral procedures applies, assistant surgeon may not be paid

27792   **Treat ankle fracture**   ~ follow-up period is 90 days, standard payment adjustment rules for multiple procedures apply, 150% payment adjustment for bilateral procedures applies, assistant surgeon may not be paid

27808   **Treat ankle fracture**   ~ follow-up period is 90 days, standard payment adjustment rules for multiple procedures apply, 150% payment adjustment for bilateral procedures applies, assistant surgeon may not be paid

27810   **Treat ankle fracture**   ~ follow-up period is 90 days, standard payment adjustment rules for multiple procedures apply, 150% payment adjustment for bilateral procedures applies, assistant surgeon may not be paid

27814   **Treat ankle fracture**   ~ follow-up period is 90 days, standard payment adjustment rules for multiple procedures apply, 150% payment adjustment for bilateral procedures applies, assistant surgeon may be paid

27816 **Treat ankle fracture** ~ follow-up period is 90 days, standard payment adjustment rules for multiple procedures apply, 150% payment adjustment for bilateral procedures applies, assistant surgeon may not be paid

27818 **Treat ankle fracture** ~ follow-up period is 90 days, standard payment adjustment rules for multiple procedures apply, 150% payment adjustment for bilateral procedures applies, assistant surgeon may not be paid

27822 **Treat ankle fracture** ~ follow-up period is 90 days, standard payment adjustment rules for multiple procedures apply, 150% payment adjustment for bilateral procedures applies, assistant surgeon may be paid

27823 **Treat ankle fracture** ~ follow-up period is 90 days, standard payment adjustment rules for multiple procedures apply, 150% payment adjustment for bilateral procedures applies, assistant surgeon may be paid

27824 **Treat lower leg fracture** ~ follow-up period is 90 days, standard payment adjustment rules for multiple procedures apply, 150% payment adjustment for bilateral procedures applies, assistant surgeon may not be paid

27825 **Treat lower leg fracture** ~ follow-up period is 90 days, standard payment adjustment rules for multiple procedures apply, 150% payment adjustment for bilateral procedures applies, payment for assistant surgeon subject to documentation of medical necessity

27826 **Treat lower leg fracture** ~ follow-up period is 90 days, standard payment adjustment rules for multiple procedures apply, 150% payment adjustment for bilateral procedures applies, assistant surgeon may be paid

27827 **Treat lower leg fracture** ~ follow-up period is 90 days, standard payment adjustment rules for multiple procedures apply, 150% payment adjustment for bilateral procedures applies, assistant surgeon may be paid

27828 **Treat lower leg fracture** ~ follow-up period is 90 days, standard payment adjustment rules for multiple procedures apply, 150% payment adjustment for bilateral procedures applies, assistant surgeon may be paid

27829 **Treat lower leg joint** ~ follow-up period is 90 days, standard payment adjustment rules for multiple procedures apply, 150% payment adjustment for bilateral procedures applies, assistant surgeon may be paid

27830 **Treat lower leg dislocation** ~ follow-up period is 90 days, standard payment adjustment rules for multiple procedures apply, 150% payment adjustment for bilateral procedures applies, payment for assistant surgeon subject to documentation of medical necessity

27831   **Treat lower leg dislocation**   ~ follow-up period is 90 days, standard payment adjustment rules for multiple procedures apply, 150% payment adjustment for bilateral procedures applies, payment for assistant surgeon subject to documentation of medical necessity

27832   **Treat lower leg dislocation**   ~ follow-up period is 90 days, standard payment adjustment rules for multiple procedures apply, 150% payment adjustment for bilateral procedures applies, assistant surgeon may be paid

27840   **Treat ankle dislocation**   ~ follow-up period is 90 days, standard payment adjustment rules for multiple procedures apply, 150% payment adjustment for bilateral procedures applies, assistant surgeon may not be paid

27842   **Treat ankle dislocation**   ~ follow-up period is 90 days, standard payment adjustment rules for multiple procedures apply, 150% payment adjustment for bilateral procedures applies, assistant surgeon may not be paid

27846   **Treat ankle dislocation**   ~ follow-up period is 90 days, standard payment adjustment rules for multiple procedures apply, 150% payment adjustment for bilateral procedures applies, assistant surgeon may be paid

27848   **Treat ankle dislocation**   ~ follow-up period is 90 days, standard payment adjustment rules for multiple procedures apply, 150% payment adjustment for bilateral procedures applies, assistant surgeon may be paid

27860   **Fixate ankle joint**   ~ follow-up period is 10 days, standard payment adjustment rules for multiple procedures apply, 150% payment adjustment for bilateral procedures does not apply, payment for assistant surgeon subject to documentation of medical necessity

27870   **Fuse ankle joint, open**   ~ follow-up period is 90 days, standard payment adjustment rules for multiple procedures apply, 150% payment adjustment for bilateral procedures applies, assistant surgeon may be paid

27871   **Fuse tibiofibular joint**   ~ follow-up period is 90 days, standard payment adjustment rules for multiple procedures apply, 150% payment adjustment for bilateral procedures applies, assistant surgeon may be paid

27880   **Amputate lower leg**   ~ follow-up period is 90 days, standard payment adjustment rules for multiple procedures apply, 150% payment adjustment for bilateral procedures applies, assistant surgeon may be paid

27881   **Amputate lower leg**   ~ follow-up period is 90 days, standard payment adjustment rules for multiple procedures apply, 150% payment adjustment for bilateral procedures applies, assistant surgeon may be paid

27882   **Amputate lower leg**   ~ follow-up period is 90 days, standard payment adjustment rules for multiple procedures apply, 150% payment adjustment for bilateral procedures applies, payment for assistant surgeon subject to documentation of medical necessity

27884   **Amputation follow-up surgery**   ~ follow-up period is 90 days, standard payment adjustment rules for multiple procedures apply, 150% payment adjustment for bilateral procedures applies, assistant surgeon may not be paid

27886   **Amputation follow-up surgery**   ~ follow-up period is 90 days, standard payment adjustment rules for multiple procedures apply, 150% payment adjustment for bilateral procedures applies, assistant surgeon may not be paid

27888   **Amputate foot at ankle**   ~ follow-up period is 90 days, standard payment adjustment rules for multiple procedures apply, 150% payment adjustment for bilateral procedures applies, assistant surgeon may be paid

27889   **Amputate foot at ankle**   ~ follow-up period is 90 days, standard payment adjustment rules for multiple procedures apply, 150% payment adjustment for bilateral procedures applies, assistant surgeon may not be paid

27892   **Decompress leg**   ~ follow-up period is 90 days, standard payment adjustment rules for multiple procedures apply, 150% payment adjustment for bilateral procedures applies, payment for assistant surgeon subject to documentation of medical necessity

27893   **Decompress leg**   ~ follow-up period is 90 days, standard payment adjustment rules for multiple procedures apply, 150% payment adjustment for bilateral procedures applies, payment for assistant surgeon subject to documentation of medical necessity

27894   **Decompress leg**   ~ follow-up period is 90 days, standard payment adjustment rules for multiple procedures apply, 150% payment adjustment for bilateral procedures applies, assistant surgeon may be paid

27899   **Leg/ankle surgery procedure**   ~ medicare carrier determines global period, standard payment adjustment rules for multiple procedures apply, 150% payment adjustment for bilateral procedures applies, payment for assistant surgeon subject to documentation of medical necessity

Foot and Toes

28001   **Drain bursa of foot**   ~ follow-up period is 10 days, standard payment adjustment rules for multiple procedures apply, 150% payment adjustment for bilateral procedures does not apply, assistant surgeon may not be paid

28002   **Treat foot infection**   ~ follow-up period is 10 days, standard payment adjustment rules for multiple procedures apply, 150% payment adjustment for bilateral procedures does not apply, assistant surgeon may not be paid

28003   **Treat foot infection**   ~ follow-up period is 90 days, standard payment adjustment rules for multiple procedures apply, 150% payment adjustment for bilateral procedures does not apply, assistant surgeon may not be paid

28005   **Treat foot bone lesion**   ~ follow-up period is 90 days, standard payment adjustment rules for multiple procedures apply, 150% payment adjustment for bilateral procedures does not apply, assistant surgeon may not be paid

28008   **Incise foot fascia**   ~ follow-up period is 90 days, standard payment adjustment rules for multiple procedures apply, 150% payment adjustment for bilateral procedures applies, assistant surgeon may not be paid

28010   **Incise toe tendon**   ~ follow-up period is 90 days, standard payment adjustment rules for multiple procedures apply, 150% payment adjustment for bilateral procedures does not apply, assistant surgeon may not be paid

28011   **Incise toe tendons**   ~ follow-up period is 90 days, standard payment adjustment rules for multiple procedures apply, 150% payment adjustment for bilateral procedures does not apply, assistant surgeon may not be paid

28020   **Explore foot joint**   ~ follow-up period is 90 days, standard payment adjustment rules for multiple procedures apply, 150% payment adjustment for bilateral procedures does not apply, assistant surgeon may not be paid

28022   **Explore foot joint**   ~ follow-up period is 90 days, standard payment adjustment rules for multiple procedures apply, 150% payment adjustment for bilateral procedures does not apply, assistant surgeon may not be paid

28024   **Explore toe joint**   ~ follow-up period is 90 days, standard payment adjustment rules for multiple procedures apply, 150% payment adjustment for bilateral procedures does not apply, assistant surgeon may not be paid

28035   **Decompress tibia nerve**   ~ follow-up period is 90 days, standard payment adjustment rules for multiple procedures apply, 150% payment adjustment for bilateral procedures does not apply, assistant surgeon may not be paid

28043   **Excise foot lesion**   ~ follow-up period is 90 days, standard payment adjustment rules for multiple procedures apply, 150% payment adjustment for bilateral procedures applies, assistant surgeon may not be paid

28045   **Excise foot lesion**   ~ follow-up period is 90 days, standard payment adjustment rules for multiple procedures apply, 150% payment adjustment for

bilateral procedures applies, payment for assistant surgeon subject to documentation of medical necessity

28046   **Resection of tumor, foot**   ~ follow-up period is 90 days, standard payment adjustment rules for multiple procedures apply, 150% payment adjustment for bilateral procedures applies, assistant surgeon may not be paid

28050   **Biopsy foot joint lining**   ~ follow-up period is 90 days, standard payment adjustment rules for multiple procedures apply, 150% payment adjustment for bilateral procedures applies, assistant surgeon may not be paid

28052   **Biopsy foot joint lining**   ~ follow-up period is 90 days, standard payment adjustment rules for multiple procedures apply, 150% payment adjustment for bilateral procedures applies, assistant surgeon may not be paid

28054   **Biopsy toe joint lining**   ~ follow-up period is 90 days, standard payment adjustment rules for multiple procedures apply, 150% payment adjustment for bilateral procedures applies, payment for assistant surgeon subject to documentation of medical necessity

28055   **Neurectomy, foot**   ~ follow-up period is 90 days, standard payment adjustment rules for multiple procedures apply, 150% payment adjustment for bilateral procedures does not apply, payment for assistant surgeon subject to documentation of medical necessity

28060   **Partial remove foot fascia**   ~ follow-up period is 90 days, standard payment adjustment rules for multiple procedures apply, 150% payment adjustment for bilateral procedures applies, assistant surgeon may not be paid

28062   **Remove foot fascia**   ~ follow-up period is 90 days, standard payment adjustment rules for multiple procedures apply, 150% payment adjustment for bilateral procedures does not apply, assistant surgeon may not be paid

28070   **Remove foot joint lining**   ~ follow-up period is 90 days, standard payment adjustment rules for multiple procedures apply, 150% payment adjustment for bilateral procedures does not apply, assistant surgeon may not be paid

28072   **Remove foot joint lining**   ~ follow-up period is 90 days, standard payment adjustment rules for multiple procedures apply, 150% payment adjustment for bilateral procedures does not apply, assistant surgeon may not be paid

28080   **Remove foot lesion**   ~ follow-up period is 90 days, standard payment adjustment rules for multiple procedures apply, 150% payment adjustment for bilateral procedures does not apply, payment for assistant surgeon subject to documentation of medical necessity

28086   **Excise foot tendon sheath**   ~ follow-up period is 90 days, standard payment adjustment rules for multiple procedures apply, 150% payment adjustment for bilateral procedures applies, assistant surgeon may be paid

28088   **Excise foot tendon sheath**   ~ follow-up period is 90 days, standard payment adjustment rules for multiple procedures apply, 150% payment adjustment for bilateral procedures applies, payment for assistant surgeon subject to documentation of medical necessity

28090   **Remove foot lesion**   ~ follow-up period is 90 days, standard payment adjustment rules for multiple procedures apply, 150% payment adjustment for bilateral procedures applies, assistant surgeon may not be paid

28092   **Remove toe lesions**   ~ follow-up period is 90 days, standard payment adjustment rules for multiple procedures apply, 150% payment adjustment for bilateral procedures does not apply, assistant surgeon may not be paid

28100   **Remove ankle/heel lesion**   ~ follow-up period is 90 days, standard payment adjustment rules for multiple procedures apply, 150% payment adjustment for bilateral procedures applies, assistant surgeon may be paid

28102   **Remove/graft foot lesion**   ~ follow-up period is 90 days, standard payment adjustment rules for multiple procedures apply, 150% payment adjustment for bilateral procedures applies, assistant surgeon may be paid

28103   **Remove/graft foot lesion**   ~ follow-up period is 90 days, standard payment adjustment rules for multiple procedures apply, 150% payment adjustment for bilateral procedures applies, assistant surgeon may be paid

28104   **Remove foot lesion**   ~ follow-up period is 90 days, standard payment adjustment rules for multiple procedures apply, 150% payment adjustment for bilateral procedures does not apply, assistant surgeon may be paid

28106   **Remove/graft foot lesion**   ~ follow-up period is 90 days, standard payment adjustment rules for multiple procedures apply, 150% payment adjustment for bilateral procedures does not apply, assistant surgeon may be paid

28107   **Remove/graft foot lesion**   ~ follow-up period is 90 days, standard payment adjustment rules for multiple procedures apply, 150% payment adjustment for bilateral procedures does not apply, assistant surgeon may be paid

28108   **Remove toe lesions**   ~ follow-up period is 90 days, standard payment adjustment rules for multiple procedures apply, 150% payment adjustment for bilateral procedures does not apply, assistant surgeon may not be paid

28110   **Partial remove metatarsal**   ~ follow-up period is 90 days, standard payment adjustment rules for multiple procedures apply, 150% payment adjustment for bilateral procedures applies, assistant surgeon may not be paid

28111   **Partial remove metatarsal**   ~ follow-up period is 90 days, standard payment adjustment rules for multiple procedures apply, 150% payment adjustment for bilateral procedures applies, assistant surgeon may not be paid

28112   **Partial remove metatarsal**   ~ follow-up period is 90 days, standard payment adjustment rules for multiple procedures apply, 150% payment adjustment for bilateral procedures applies, assistant surgeon may not be paid

28113   **Partial remove metatarsal**   ~ follow-up period is 90 days, standard payment adjustment rules for multiple procedures apply, 150% payment adjustment for bilateral procedures applies, payment for assistant surgeon subject to documentation of medical necessity

28114   **Remove metatarsal heads**   ~ follow-up period is 90 days, standard payment adjustment rules for multiple procedures apply, 150% payment adjustment for bilateral procedures applies, assistant surgeon may be paid

28116   **Revise foot**   ~ follow-up period is 90 days, standard payment adjustment rules for multiple procedures apply, 150% payment adjustment for bilateral procedures applies, assistant surgeon may not be paid

28118   **Remove heel bone**   ~ follow-up period is 90 days, standard payment adjustment rules for multiple procedures apply, 150% payment adjustment for bilateral procedures applies, assistant surgeon may be paid

28119   **Remove heel spur**   ~ follow-up period is 90 days, standard payment adjustment rules for multiple procedures apply, 150% payment adjustment for bilateral procedures applies, assistant surgeon may not be paid

28120   **Partial remove ankle/heel**   ~ follow-up period is 90 days, standard payment adjustment rules for multiple procedures apply, 150% payment adjustment for bilateral procedures applies, assistant surgeon may not be paid

28122   **Partial remove foot bone**   ~ follow-up period is 90 days, standard payment adjustment rules for multiple procedures apply, 150% payment adjustment for bilateral procedures applies, assistant surgeon may be paid

28124   **Partial remove toe**   ~ follow-up period is 90 days, standard payment adjustment rules for multiple procedures apply, 150% payment adjustment for bilateral procedures applies, assistant surgeon may not be paid

28126   **Partial remove toe**   ~ follow-up period is 90 days, standard payment adjustment rules for multiple procedures apply, 150% payment adjustment for bilateral procedures does not apply, assistant surgeon may not be paid

28130   **Remove ankle bone**   ~ follow-up period is 90 days, standard payment adjustment rules for multiple procedures apply, 150% payment adjustment for bilateral procedures applies, assistant surgeon may be paid

28140   **Remove metatarsal**   ~ follow-up period is 90 days, standard payment adjustment rules for multiple procedures apply, 150% payment adjustment for bilateral procedures does not apply, assistant surgeon may not be paid

28150   **Remove toe**   ~ follow-up period is 90 days, standard payment adjustment rules for multiple procedures apply, 150% payment adjustment for bilateral procedures does not apply, assistant surgeon may not be paid

28153   **Partial remove toe**   ~ follow-up period is 90 days, standard payment adjustment rules for multiple procedures apply, 150% payment adjustment for bilateral procedures does not apply, assistant surgeon may not be paid

28160   **Partial remove toe**   ~ follow-up period is 90 days, standard payment adjustment rules for multiple procedures apply, 150% payment adjustment for bilateral procedures does not apply, assistant surgeon may not be paid

28171   **Extensive foot surgery**   ~ follow-up period is 90 days, standard payment adjustment rules for multiple procedures apply, 150% payment adjustment for bilateral procedures does not apply, assistant surgeon may be paid

28173   **Extensive foot surgery**   ~ follow-up period is 90 days, standard payment adjustment rules for multiple procedures apply, 150% payment adjustment for bilateral procedures does not apply, assistant surgeon may not be paid

28175   **Extensive foot surgery**   ~ follow-up period is 90 days, standard payment adjustment rules for multiple procedures apply, 150% payment adjustment for bilateral procedures does not apply, assistant surgeon may not be paid

28190   **Remove foot foreign body**   ~ follow-up period is 10 days, standard payment adjustment rules for multiple procedures apply, 150% payment adjustment for bilateral procedures applies, assistant surgeon may not be paid

28192   **Remove foot foreign body**   ~ follow-up period is 90 days, standard payment adjustment rules for multiple procedures apply, 150% payment adjustment for bilateral procedures applies, assistant surgeon may not be paid

28193   **Remove foot foreign body**   ~ follow-up period is 90 days, standard payment adjustment rules for multiple procedures apply, 150% payment adjustment for bilateral procedures applies, assistant surgeon may not be paid

28200   **Repair foot tendon**   ~ follow-up period is 90 days, standard payment adjustment rules for multiple procedures apply, 150% payment adjustment for bilateral procedures does not apply, assistant surgeon may not be paid

28202   **Repair/graft of foot tendon**   ~ follow-up period is 90 days, standard payment adjustment rules for multiple procedures apply, 150% payment adjustment for bilateral procedures does not apply, assistant surgeon may be paid

28208   **Repair foot tendon**   ~ follow-up period is 90 days, standard payment adjustment rules for multiple procedures apply, 150% payment adjustment for bilateral procedures does not apply, assistant surgeon may not be paid

28210   **Repair/graft of foot tendon**   ~ follow-up period is 90 days, standard payment adjustment rules for multiple procedures apply, 150% payment adjustment for bilateral procedures does not apply, assistant surgeon may be paid

28220   **Release foot tendon**   ~ follow-up period is 90 days, standard payment adjustment rules for multiple procedures apply, 150% payment adjustment for bilateral procedures does not apply, assistant surgeon may not be paid

28222   **Release foot tendons**   ~ follow-up period is 90 days, standard payment adjustment rules for multiple procedures apply, 150% payment adjustment for bilateral procedures does not apply, assistant surgeon may not be paid

28225   **Release foot tendon**   ~ follow-up period is 90 days, standard payment adjustment rules for multiple procedures apply, 150% payment adjustment for bilateral procedures does not apply, assistant surgeon may not be paid

28226   **Release foot tendons**   ~ follow-up period is 90 days, standard payment adjustment rules for multiple procedures apply, 150% payment adjustment for bilateral procedures does not apply, assistant surgeon may not be paid

28230   **Incise foot tendon(s)**   ~ follow-up period is 90 days, standard payment adjustment rules for multiple procedures apply, 150% payment adjustment for bilateral procedures does not apply, assistant surgeon may not be paid

28232   **Incise toe tendon**   ~ follow-up period is 90 days, standard payment adjustment rules for multiple procedures apply, 150% payment adjustment for bilateral procedures does not apply, assistant surgeon may not be paid

28234   **Incise foot tendon**   ~ follow-up period is 90 days, standard payment adjustment rules for multiple procedures apply, 150% payment adjustment for bilateral procedures does not apply, assistant surgeon may not be paid

28238   **Revise foot tendon**   ~ follow-up period is 90 days, standard payment adjustment rules for multiple procedures apply, 150% payment adjustment for bilateral procedures applies, assistant surgeon may be paid

28240 **Release big toe** ~ follow-up period is 90 days, standard payment adjustment rules for multiple procedures apply, 150% payment adjustment for bilateral procedures applies, assistant surgeon may not be paid

28250 **Revise foot fascia** ~ follow-up period is 90 days, standard payment adjustment rules for multiple procedures apply, 150% payment adjustment for bilateral procedures applies, assistant surgeon may be paid

28260 **Release midfoot joint** ~ follow-up period is 90 days, standard payment adjustment rules for multiple procedures apply, 150% payment adjustment for bilateral procedures applies, assistant surgeon may be paid

28261 **Revise foot tendon** ~ follow-up period is 90 days, standard payment adjustment rules for multiple procedures apply, 150% payment adjustment for bilateral procedures applies, payment for assistant surgeon subject to documentation of medical necessity

28262 **Revise foot and ankle** ~ follow-up period is 90 days, standard payment adjustment rules for multiple procedures apply, 150% payment adjustment for bilateral procedures applies, assistant surgeon may be paid

28264 **Release midfoot joint** ~ follow-up period is 90 days, standard payment adjustment rules for multiple procedures apply, 150% payment adjustment for bilateral procedures applies, assistant surgeon may be paid

28270 **Release foot contracture** ~ follow-up period is 90 days, standard payment adjustment rules for multiple procedures apply, 150% payment adjustment for bilateral procedures applies, assistant surgeon may not be paid

28272 **Release toe joint, each** ~ follow-up period is 90 days, standard payment adjustment rules for multiple procedures apply, 150% payment adjustment for bilateral procedures applies, assistant surgeon may not be paid

28280 **Fuse toes** ~ follow-up period is 90 days, standard payment adjustment rules for multiple procedures apply, 150% payment adjustment for bilateral procedures applies, payment for assistant surgeon subject to documentation of medical necessity

28285 **Repair hammertoe** ~ follow-up period is 90 days, standard payment adjustment rules for multiple procedures apply, 150% payment adjustment for bilateral procedures applies, assistant surgeon may not be paid

28286 **Repair hammertoe** ~ follow-up period is 90 days, standard payment adjustment rules for multiple procedures apply, 150% payment adjustment for bilateral procedures does not apply, assistant surgeon may not be paid

28288 **Partial remove foot bone** ~ follow-up period is 90 days, standard payment adjustment rules for multiple procedures apply, 150% payment adjustment for bilateral procedures does not apply, assistant surgeon may not be paid

28289 **Repair hallux rigidus** ~ follow-up period is 90 days, standard payment adjustment rules for multiple procedures apply, 150% payment adjustment for bilateral procedures applies, assistant surgeon may be paid

28290 **Correct bunion** ~ follow-up period is 90 days, standard payment adjustment rules for multiple procedures apply, 150% payment adjustment for bilateral procedures applies, assistant surgeon may not be paid

28292 **Correct bunion** ~ follow-up period is 90 days, standard payment adjustment rules for multiple procedures apply, 150% payment adjustment for bilateral procedures applies, assistant surgeon may be paid

28293 **Correct bunion** ~ follow-up period is 90 days, standard payment adjustment rules for multiple procedures apply, 150% payment adjustment for bilateral procedures applies, assistant surgeon may be paid

28294 **Correct bunion** ~ follow-up period is 90 days, standard payment adjustment rules for multiple procedures apply, 150% payment adjustment for bilateral procedures applies, assistant surgeon may be paid

28296 **Correct bunion** ~ follow-up period is 90 days, standard payment adjustment rules for multiple procedures apply, 150% payment adjustment for bilateral procedures applies, assistant surgeon may be paid

28297 **Correct bunion** ~ follow-up period is 90 days, standard payment adjustment rules for multiple procedures apply, 150% payment adjustment for bilateral procedures applies, assistant surgeon may be paid

28298 **Correct bunion** ~ follow-up period is 90 days, standard payment adjustment rules for multiple procedures apply, 150% payment adjustment for bilateral procedures applies, assistant surgeon may be paid

28299 **Correct bunion** ~ follow-up period is 90 days, standard payment adjustment rules for multiple procedures apply, 150% payment adjustment for bilateral procedures applies, assistant surgeon may be paid

28300 **Incise heel bone** ~ follow-up period is 90 days, standard payment adjustment rules for multiple procedures apply, 150% payment adjustment for bilateral procedures applies, assistant surgeon may be paid

28302 **Incise ankle bone** ~ follow-up period is 90 days, standard payment adjustment rules for multiple procedures apply, 150% payment adjustment for bilateral procedures applies, assistant surgeon may be paid

28304   **Incise midfoot bones**   ~ follow-up period is 90 days, standard payment adjustment rules for multiple procedures apply, 150% payment adjustment for bilateral procedures applies, assistant surgeon may be paid

28305   **Incise/graft midfoot bones**   ~ follow-up period is 90 days, standard payment adjustment rules for multiple procedures apply, 150% payment adjustment for bilateral procedures applies, assistant surgeon may be paid

28306   **Incise metatarsal**   ~ follow-up period is 90 days, standard payment adjustment rules for multiple procedures apply, 150% payment adjustment for bilateral procedures applies, assistant surgeon may be paid

28307   **Incise metatarsal**   ~ follow-up period is 90 days, standard payment adjustment rules for multiple procedures apply, 150% payment adjustment for bilateral procedures applies, payment for assistant surgeon subject to documentation of medical necessity

28308   **Incise metatarsal**   ~ follow-up period is 90 days, standard payment adjustment rules for multiple procedures apply, 150% payment adjustment for bilateral procedures applies, assistant surgeon may be paid

28309   **Incise metatarsals**   ~ follow-up period is 90 days, standard payment adjustment rules for multiple procedures apply, 150% payment adjustment for bilateral procedures applies, payment for assistant surgeon subject to documentation of medical necessity

28310   **Revise big toe**   ~ follow-up period is 90 days, standard payment adjustment rules for multiple procedures apply, 150% payment adjustment for bilateral procedures does not apply, assistant surgeon may not be paid

28312   **Revise toe**   ~ follow-up period is 90 days, standard payment adjustment rules for multiple procedures apply, 150% payment adjustment for bilateral procedures does not apply, assistant surgeon may not be paid

28313   **Repair deformity of toe**   ~ follow-up period is 90 days, standard payment adjustment rules for multiple procedures apply, 150% payment adjustment for bilateral procedures does not apply, assistant surgeon may not be paid

28315   **Remove sesamoid bone**   ~ follow-up period is 90 days, standard payment adjustment rules for multiple procedures apply, 150% payment adjustment for bilateral procedures applies, assistant surgeon may not be paid

28320   **Repair foot bones**   ~ follow-up period is 90 days, standard payment adjustment rules for multiple procedures apply, 150% payment adjustment for bilateral procedures does not apply, assistant surgeon may be paid

28322   **Repair metatarsals**   ~ follow-up period is 90 days, standard payment adjustment rules for multiple procedures apply, 150% payment adjustment for bilateral procedures does not apply, assistant surgeon may be paid

28340   **Resect enlarged toe tissue**   ~ follow-up period is 90 days, standard payment adjustment rules for multiple procedures apply, 150% payment adjustment for bilateral procedures does not apply, assistant surgeon may not be paid

28341   **Resect enlarged toe**   ~ follow-up period is 90 days, standard payment adjustment rules for multiple procedures apply, 150% payment adjustment for bilateral procedures does not apply, assistant surgeon may not be paid

28344   **Repair extra toe(s)**   ~ follow-up period is 90 days, standard payment adjustment rules for multiple procedures apply, 150% payment adjustment for bilateral procedures does not apply, assistant surgeon may not be paid

28345   **Repair webbed toe(s)**   ~ follow-up period is 90 days, standard payment adjustment rules for multiple procedures apply, 150% payment adjustment for bilateral procedures does not apply, payment for assistant surgeon subject to documentation of medical necessity

28360   **Reconstruct cleft foot**   ~ follow-up period is 90 days, standard payment adjustment rules for multiple procedures apply, 150% payment adjustment for bilateral procedures does not apply, assistant surgeon may be paid

28400   **Treat heel fracture**   ~ follow-up period is 90 days, standard payment adjustment rules for multiple procedures apply, 150% payment adjustment for bilateral procedures applies, assistant surgeon may not be paid

28405   **Treat heel fracture**   ~ follow-up period is 90 days, standard payment adjustment rules for multiple procedures apply, 150% payment adjustment for bilateral procedures applies, payment for assistant surgeon subject to documentation of medical necessity

28406   **Treat heel fracture**   ~ follow-up period is 90 days, standard payment adjustment rules for multiple procedures apply, 150% payment adjustment for bilateral procedures applies, payment for assistant surgeon subject to documentation of medical necessity

28415   **Treat heel fracture**   ~ follow-up period is 90 days, standard payment adjustment rules for multiple procedures apply, 150% payment adjustment for bilateral procedures applies, assistant surgeon may be paid

28420   **Treat/graft heel fracture**   ~ follow-up period is 90 days, standard payment adjustment rules for multiple procedures apply, 150% payment adjustment for bilateral procedures applies, assistant surgeon may be paid

28430   **Treat ankle fracture**   ~ follow-up period is 90 days, standard payment adjustment rules for multiple procedures apply, 150% payment adjustment for bilateral procedures applies, assistant surgeon may not be paid

28435   **Treat ankle fracture**   ~ follow-up period is 90 days, standard payment adjustment rules for multiple procedures apply, 150% payment adjustment for bilateral procedures applies, payment for assistant surgeon subject to documentation of medical necessity

28436   **Treat ankle fracture**   ~ follow-up period is 90 days, standard payment adjustment rules for multiple procedures apply, 150% payment adjustment for bilateral procedures applies, assistant surgeon may not be paid

28445   **Treat ankle fracture**   ~ follow-up period is 90 days, standard payment adjustment rules for multiple procedures apply, 150% payment adjustment for bilateral procedures applies, assistant surgeon may be paid

28450   **Treat midfoot fracture, each**   ~ follow-up period is 90 days, standard payment adjustment rules for multiple procedures apply, 150% payment adjustment for bilateral procedures does not apply, assistant surgeon may not be paid

28455   **Treat midfoot fracture, each**   ~ follow-up period is 90 days, standard payment adjustment rules for multiple procedures apply, 150% payment adjustment for bilateral procedures does not apply, payment for assistant surgeon subject to documentation of medical necessity

28456   **Treat midfoot fracture**   ~ follow-up period is 90 days, standard payment adjustment rules for multiple procedures apply, 150% payment adjustment for bilateral procedures does not apply, assistant surgeon may not be paid

28465   **Treat midfoot fracture, each**   ~ follow-up period is 90 days, standard payment adjustment rules for multiple procedures apply, 150% payment adjustment for bilateral procedures does not apply, assistant surgeon may not be paid

28470   **Treat metatarsal fracture**   ~ follow-up period is 90 days, standard payment adjustment rules for multiple procedures apply, 150% payment adjustment for bilateral procedures does not apply, assistant surgeon may not be paid

28475   **Treat metatarsal fracture**   ~ follow-up period is 90 days, standard payment adjustment rules for multiple procedures apply, 150% payment adjustment for bilateral procedures does not apply, assistant surgeon may not be paid

28476   **Treat metatarsal fracture**   ~ follow-up period is 90 days, standard payment adjustment rules for multiple procedures apply, 150% payment adjustment for bilateral procedures does not apply, payment for assistant surgeon subject to documentation of medical necessity

28485   **Treat metatarsal fracture**   ~ follow-up period is 90 days, standard payment adjustment rules for multiple procedures apply, 150% payment adjustment for bilateral procedures does not apply, assistant surgeon may not be paid

28490   **Treat big toe fracture**   ~ follow-up period is 90 days, standard payment adjustment rules for multiple procedures apply, 150% payment adjustment for bilateral procedures does not apply, assistant surgeon may not be paid

28495   **Treat big toe fracture**   ~ follow-up period is 90 days, standard payment adjustment rules for multiple procedures apply, 150% payment adjustment for bilateral procedures does not apply, assistant surgeon may not be paid

28496   **Treat big toe fracture**   ~ follow-up period is 90 days, standard payment adjustment rules for multiple procedures apply, 150% payment adjustment for bilateral procedures does not apply, assistant surgeon may not be paid

28505   **Treat big toe fracture**   ~ follow-up period is 90 days, standard payment adjustment rules for multiple procedures apply, 150% payment adjustment for bilateral procedures does not apply, assistant surgeon may not be paid

28510   **Treat toe fracture**   ~ follow-up period is 90 days, standard payment adjustment rules for multiple procedures apply, 150% payment adjustment for bilateral procedures does not apply, assistant surgeon may not be paid

28515   **Treat toe fracture**   ~ follow-up period is 90 days, standard payment adjustment rules for multiple procedures apply, 150% payment adjustment for bilateral procedures does not apply, assistant surgeon may not be paid

28525   **Treat toe fracture**   ~ follow-up period is 90 days, standard payment adjustment rules for multiple procedures apply, 150% payment adjustment for bilateral procedures does not apply, payment for assistant surgeon subject to documentation of medical necessity

28530   **Treat sesamoid bone fracture**   ~ follow-up period is 90 days, standard payment adjustment rules for multiple procedures apply, 150% payment adjustment for bilateral procedures does not apply, payment for assistant surgeon subject to documentation of medical necessity

28531   **Treat sesamoid bone fracture**   ~ follow-up period is 90 days, standard payment adjustment rules for multiple procedures apply, 150% payment adjustment for bilateral procedures does not apply, assistant surgeon may not be paid

28540   **Treat foot dislocation**   ~ follow-up period is 90 days, standard payment adjustment rules for multiple procedures apply, 150% payment adjustment for bilateral procedures does not apply, payment for assistant surgeon subject to documentation of medical necessity

---

28545   **Treat foot dislocation**   ~ follow-up period is 90 days, standard payment adjustment rules for multiple procedures apply, 150% payment adjustment for bilateral procedures does not apply, payment for assistant surgeon subject to documentation of medical necessity

28546   **Treat foot dislocation**   ~ follow-up period is 90 days, standard payment adjustment rules for multiple procedures apply, 150% payment adjustment for bilateral procedures does not apply, payment for assistant surgeon subject to documentation of medical necessity

28555   **Repair foot dislocation**   ~ follow-up period is 90 days, standard payment adjustment rules for multiple procedures apply, 150% payment adjustment for bilateral procedures does not apply, assistant surgeon may be paid

28570   **Treat foot dislocation**   ~ follow-up period is 90 days, standard payment adjustment rules for multiple procedures apply, 150% payment adjustment for bilateral procedures does not apply, payment for assistant surgeon subject to documentation of medical necessity

28575   **Treat foot dislocation**   ~ follow-up period is 90 days, standard payment adjustment rules for multiple procedures apply, 150% payment adjustment for bilateral procedures does not apply, payment for assistant surgeon subject to documentation of medical necessity

28576   **Treat foot dislocation**   ~ follow-up period is 90 days, standard payment adjustment rules for multiple procedures apply, 150% payment adjustment for bilateral procedures does not apply, payment for assistant surgeon subject to documentation of medical necessity

28585   **Repair foot dislocation**   ~ follow-up period is 90 days, standard payment adjustment rules for multiple procedures apply, 150% payment adjustment for bilateral procedures does not apply, assistant surgeon may be paid

28600   **Treat foot dislocation**   ~ follow-up period is 90 days, standard payment adjustment rules for multiple procedures apply, 150% payment adjustment for bilateral procedures does not apply, payment for assistant surgeon subject to documentation of medical necessity

28605   **Treat foot dislocation**   ~ follow-up period is 90 days, standard payment adjustment rules for multiple procedures apply, 150% payment adjustment for bilateral procedures does not apply, payment for assistant surgeon subject to documentation of medical necessity

28606   **Treat foot dislocation**   ~ follow-up period is 90 days, standard payment adjustment rules for multiple procedures apply, 150% payment adjustment for bilateral procedures does not apply, assistant surgeon may not be paid

28615   **Repair foot dislocation**   ~ follow-up period is 90 days, standard payment adjustment rules for multiple procedures apply, 150% payment adjustment for bilateral procedures does not apply, assistant surgeon may be paid

28630   **Treat toe dislocation**   ~ follow-up period is 10 days, standard payment adjustment rules for multiple procedures apply, 150% payment adjustment for bilateral procedures does not apply, payment for assistant surgeon subject to documentation of medical necessity

28635   **Treat toe dislocation**   ~ follow-up period is 10 days, standard payment adjustment rules for multiple procedures apply, 150% payment adjustment for bilateral procedures does not apply, payment for assistant surgeon subject to documentation of medical necessity

28636   **Treat toe dislocation**   ~ follow-up period is 10 days, standard payment adjustment rules for multiple procedures apply, 150% payment adjustment for bilateral procedures does not apply, assistant surgeon may not be paid

28645   **Repair toe dislocation**   ~ follow-up period is 90 days, standard payment adjustment rules for multiple procedures apply, 150% payment adjustment for bilateral procedures does not apply, assistant surgeon may not be paid

28660   **Treat toe dislocation**   ~ follow-up period is 10 days, standard payment adjustment rules for multiple procedures apply, 150% payment adjustment for bilateral procedures does not apply, assistant surgeon may not be paid

28665   **Treat toe dislocation**   ~ follow-up period is 10 days, standard payment adjustment rules for multiple procedures apply, 150% payment adjustment for bilateral procedures does not apply, payment for assistant surgeon subject to documentation of medical necessity

28666   **Treat toe dislocation**   ~ follow-up period is 10 days, standard payment adjustment rules for multiple procedures apply, 150% payment adjustment for bilateral procedures does not apply, assistant surgeon may not be paid

28675   **Repair toe dislocation**   ~ follow-up period is 90 days, standard payment adjustment rules for multiple procedures apply, 150% payment adjustment for bilateral procedures does not apply, assistant surgeon may not be paid

28705   **Fuse foot bones**   ~ follow-up period is 90 days, standard payment adjustment rules for multiple procedures apply, 150% payment adjustment for bilateral procedures does not apply, assistant surgeon may be paid

28715   **Fuse foot bones**   ~ follow-up period is 90 days, standard payment adjustment rules for multiple procedures apply, 150% payment adjustment for bilateral procedures does not apply, assistant surgeon may be paid

28725   **Fuse foot bones**   ~ follow-up period is 90 days, standard payment adjustment rules for multiple procedures apply, 150% payment adjustment for bilateral procedures does not apply, assistant surgeon may be paid

28730   **Fuse foot bones**   ~ follow-up period is 90 days, standard payment adjustment rules for multiple procedures apply, 150% payment adjustment for bilateral procedures does not apply, assistant surgeon may be paid

28735   **Fuse foot bones**   ~ follow-up period is 90 days, standard payment adjustment rules for multiple procedures apply, 150% payment adjustment for bilateral procedures does not apply, assistant surgeon may be paid

28737   **Revise foot bones**   ~ follow-up period is 90 days, standard payment adjustment rules for multiple procedures apply, 150% payment adjustment for bilateral procedures does not apply, assistant surgeon may be paid

28740   **Fuse foot bones**   ~ follow-up period is 90 days, standard payment adjustment rules for multiple procedures apply, 150% payment adjustment for bilateral procedures does not apply, assistant surgeon may be paid

28750   **Fuse big toe joint**   ~ follow-up period is 90 days, standard payment adjustment rules for multiple procedures apply, 150% payment adjustment for bilateral procedures applies, payment for assistant surgeon subject to documentation of medical necessity

28755   **Fuse big toe joint**   ~ follow-up period is 90 days, standard payment adjustment rules for multiple procedures apply, 150% payment adjustment for bilateral procedures applies, assistant surgeon may not be paid

28760   **Fuse big toe joint**   ~ follow-up period is 90 days, standard payment adjustment rules for multiple procedures apply, 150% payment adjustment for bilateral procedures applies, assistant surgeon may be paid

28800   **Amputate midfoot**   ~ follow-up period is 90 days, standard payment adjustment rules for multiple procedures apply, 150% payment adjustment for bilateral procedures applies, assistant surgeon may be paid

28805   **Amputation thru metatarsal**   ~ follow-up period is 90 days, standard payment adjustment rules for multiple procedures apply, 150% payment adjustment for bilateral procedures applies, payment for assistant surgeon subject to documentation of medical necessity

28810   **Amputation toe & metatarsal**   ~ follow-up period is 90 days, standard payment adjustment rules for multiple procedures apply, 150% payment adjustment for bilateral procedures does not apply, payment for assistant surgeon subject to documentation of medical necessity

28820   **Amputate toe**   ~ follow-up period is 90 days, standard payment adjustment rules for multiple procedures apply, 150% payment adjustment for bilateral procedures does not apply, assistant surgeon may not be paid

28825   **Partial amputate toe**   ~ follow-up period is 90 days, standard payment adjustment rules for multiple procedures apply, 150% payment adjustment for bilateral procedures does not apply, assistant surgeon may not be paid

28890   **High energy eswt, plantar f**   ~ follow-up period is 90 days, standard payment adjustment rules for multiple procedures apply, 150% payment adjustment for bilateral procedures applies, assistant surgeon may be paid

28899   **Foot/toes surgery procedure**   ~ medicare carrier determines global period, standard payment adjustment rules for multiple procedures apply, 150% payment adjustment for bilateral procedures does not apply, payment for assistant surgeon subject to documentation of medical necessity

Application of Casts And Strapping

29000   **Apply body cast**   ~ endoscopies or minor procedure - E/M services on the same day generally not paid, standard payment adjustment rules for multiple procedures apply, 150% payment adjustment for bilateral procedures does not apply, payment for assistant surgeon subject to documentation of medical necessity

29010   **Apply body cast**   ~ endoscopies or minor procedure - E/M services on the same day generally not paid, standard payment adjustment rules for multiple procedures apply, 150% payment adjustment for bilateral procedures does not apply, payment for assistant surgeon subject to documentation of medical necessity

29015   **Apply body cast**   ~ endoscopies or minor procedure - E/M services on the same day generally not paid, standard payment adjustment rules for multiple procedures apply, 150% payment adjustment for bilateral procedures does not apply, payment for assistant surgeon subject to documentation of medical necessity

29020   **Apply body cast**   ~ endoscopies or minor procedure - E/M services on the same day generally not paid, standard payment adjustment rules for multiple procedures apply, 150% payment adjustment for bilateral procedures does not apply, payment for assistant surgeon subject to documentation of medical necessity

29025   **Apply body cast**   ~ endoscopies or minor procedure - E/M services on the same day generally not paid, standard payment adjustment rules for multiple procedures apply, 150% payment adjustment for bilateral procedures does not apply, payment for assistant surgeon subject to documentation of medical necessity

29035   **Apply body cast**   ~ endoscopies or minor procedure - E/M services on the same day generally not paid, standard payment adjustment rules for multiple

procedures apply, 150% payment adjustment for bilateral procedures does not apply, payment for assistant surgeon subject to documentation of medical necessity

29040 **Apply body cast** ~ endoscopies or minor procedure - E/M services on the same day generally not paid, standard payment adjustment rules for multiple procedures apply, 150% payment adjustment for bilateral procedures does not apply, payment for assistant surgeon subject to documentation of medical necessity

29044 **Apply body cast** ~ endoscopies or minor procedure - E/M services on the same day generally not paid, standard payment adjustment rules for multiple procedures apply, 150% payment adjustment for bilateral procedures does not apply, payment for assistant surgeon subject to documentation of medical necessity

29046 **Apply body cast** ~ endoscopies or minor procedure - E/M services on the same day generally not paid, standard payment adjustment rules for multiple procedures apply, 150% payment adjustment for bilateral procedures does not apply, payment for assistant surgeon subject to documentation of medical necessity

29049 **Apply figure eight** ~ endoscopies or minor procedure - E/M services on the same day generally not paid, standard payment adjustment rules for multiple procedures apply, 150% payment adjustment for bilateral procedures does not apply, payment for assistant surgeon subject to documentation of medical necessity

29055 **Apply shoulder cast** ~ endoscopies or minor procedure - E/M services on the same day generally not paid, standard payment adjustment rules for multiple procedures apply, 150% payment adjustment for bilateral procedures does not apply, payment for assistant surgeon subject to documentation of medical necessity

29058 **Apply shoulder cast** ~ endoscopies or minor procedure - E/M services on the same day generally not paid, standard payment adjustment rules for multiple procedures apply, 150% payment adjustment for bilateral procedures does not apply, payment for assistant surgeon subject to documentation of medical necessity

29065 **Apply long arm cast** ~ endoscopies or minor procedure - E/M services on the same day generally not paid, standard payment adjustment rules for multiple procedures apply, 150% payment adjustment for bilateral procedures applies, assistant surgeon may not be paid

29075 **Apply forearm cast** ~ endoscopies or minor procedure - E/M services on the same day generally not paid, standard payment adjustment rules for multiple procedures apply, 150% payment adjustment for bilateral procedures applies, assistant surgeon may not be paid

29085 **Apply hand/wrist cast** ~ endoscopies or minor procedure - E/M services on the same day generally not paid, standard payment adjustment rules for multiple procedures apply, 150% payment adjustment for bilateral procedures applies, assistant surgeon may not be paid

29086 **Apply finger cast** ~ endoscopies or minor procedure - E/M services on the same day generally not paid, standard payment adjustment rules for multiple procedures apply, 150% payment adjustment for bilateral procedures applies, assistant surgeon may not be paid

29105 **Apply long arm splint** ~ endoscopies or minor procedure - E/M services on the same day generally not paid, standard payment adjustment rules for multiple procedures apply, 150% payment adjustment for bilateral procedures applies, assistant surgeon may not be paid

29125 **Apply forearm splint** ~ endoscopies or minor procedure - E/M services on the same day generally not paid, standard payment adjustment rules for multiple procedures apply, 150% payment adjustment for bilateral procedures applies, assistant surgeon may not be paid

29126 **Apply forearm splint** ~ endoscopies or minor procedure - E/M services on the same day generally not paid, standard payment adjustment rules for multiple procedures apply, 150% payment adjustment for bilateral procedures applies, assistant surgeon may not be paid

29130 **Apply finger splint** ~ endoscopies or minor procedure - E/M services on the same day generally not paid, standard payment adjustment rules for multiple procedures apply, 150% payment adjustment for bilateral procedures applies, assistant surgeon may not be paid

29131 **Apply finger splint** ~ endoscopies or minor procedure - E/M services on the same day generally not paid, standard payment adjustment rules for multiple procedures apply, 150% payment adjustment for bilateral procedures applies, assistant surgeon may not be paid

29200 **Strap chest** ~ endoscopies or minor procedure - E/M services on the same day generally not paid, standard payment adjustment rules for multiple procedures apply, 150% payment adjustment for bilateral procedures does not apply, assistant surgeon may not be paid

29220 **Strap low back** ~ endoscopies or minor procedure - E/M services on the same day generally not paid, standard payment adjustment rules for multiple procedures apply, 150% payment adjustment for bilateral procedures does not apply, assistant surgeon may not be paid

29240 **Strap shoulder** ~ endoscopies or minor procedure - E/M services on the same day generally not paid, standard payment adjustment rules for multiple procedures apply, 150% payment adjustment for bilateral procedures does not apply, assistant surgeon may not be paid

29260 **Strap elbow or wrist** ~ endoscopies or minor procedure - E/M services on the same day generally not paid, standard payment adjustment rules for multiple

procedures apply, 150% payment adjustment for bilateral procedures applies, assistant surgeon may not be paid

29280   **Strap hand or finger**   ~ endoscopies or minor procedure - E/M services on the same day generally not paid, standard payment adjustment rules for multiple procedures apply, 150% payment adjustment for bilateral procedures applies, assistant surgeon may not be paid

29305   **Apply hip cast**   ~ endoscopies or minor procedure - E/M services on the same day generally not paid, standard payment adjustment rules for multiple procedures apply, 150% payment adjustment for bilateral procedures does not apply, payment for assistant surgeon subject to documentation of medical necessity

29325   **Apply hip casts**   ~ endoscopies or minor procedure - E/M services on the same day generally not paid, standard payment adjustment rules for multiple procedures apply, 150% payment adjustment for bilateral procedures does not apply, payment for assistant surgeon subject to documentation of medical necessity

29345   **Apply long leg cast**   ~ endoscopies or minor procedure - E/M services on the same day generally not paid, standard payment adjustment rules for multiple procedures apply, 150% payment adjustment for bilateral procedures applies, assistant surgeon may not be paid

29355   **Apply long leg cast**   ~ endoscopies or minor procedure - E/M services on the same day generally not paid, standard payment adjustment rules for multiple procedures apply, 150% payment adjustment for bilateral procedures applies, assistant surgeon may not be paid

29358   **Apply long leg cast brace**   ~ endoscopies or minor procedure - E/M services on the same day generally not paid, standard payment adjustment rules for multiple procedures apply, 150% payment adjustment for bilateral procedures applies, assistant surgeon may not be paid

29365   **Apply long leg cast**   ~ endoscopies or minor procedure - E/M services on the same day generally not paid, standard payment adjustment rules for multiple procedures apply, 150% payment adjustment for bilateral procedures applies, assistant surgeon may not be paid

29405   **Apply short leg cast**   ~ endoscopies or minor procedure - E/M services on the same day generally not paid, standard payment adjustment rules for multiple procedures apply, 150% payment adjustment for bilateral procedures applies, assistant surgeon may not be paid

29425   **Apply short leg cast**   ~ endoscopies or minor procedure - E/M services on the same day generally not paid, standard payment adjustment rules for multiple procedures apply, 150% payment adjustment for bilateral procedures applies, assistant surgeon may not be paid

29435   **Apply short leg cast**   ~ endoscopies or minor procedure - E/M services on the same day generally not paid, standard payment adjustment rules for multiple procedures apply, 150% payment adjustment for bilateral procedures applies, assistant surgeon may not be paid

29440   **Addition of walker to cast**   ~ endoscopies or minor procedure - E/M services on the same day generally not paid, standard payment adjustment rules for multiple procedures apply, 150% payment adjustment for bilateral procedures applies, assistant surgeon may not be paid

29445   **Apply rigid leg cast**   ~ endoscopies or minor procedure - E/M services on the same day generally not paid, standard payment adjustment rules for multiple procedures apply, 150% payment adjustment for bilateral procedures applies, assistant surgeon may not be paid

29450   **Apply leg cast**   ~ endoscopies or minor procedure - E/M services on the same day generally not paid, standard payment adjustment rules for multiple procedures apply, 150% payment adjustment for bilateral procedures applies, assistant surgeon may not be paid

29505   **Application, long leg splint**   ~ endoscopies or minor procedure - E/M services on the same day generally not paid, standard payment adjustment rules for multiple procedures apply, 150% payment adjustment for bilateral procedures applies, assistant surgeon may not be paid

29515   **Application lower leg splint**   ~ endoscopies or minor procedure - E/M services on the same day generally not paid, standard payment adjustment rules for multiple procedures apply, 150% payment adjustment for bilateral procedures applies, assistant surgeon may not be paid

29520   **Strap hip**   ~ endoscopies or minor procedure - E/M services on the same day generally not paid, standard payment adjustment rules for multiple procedures apply, 150% payment adjustment for bilateral procedures does not apply, payment for assistant surgeon subject to documentation of medical necessity

29530   **Strap knee**   ~ endoscopies or minor procedure - E/M services on the same day generally not paid, standard payment adjustment rules for multiple procedures apply, 150% payment adjustment for bilateral procedures does not apply, assistant surgeon may not be paid

29540   **Strap ankle and/or ft**   ~ endoscopies or minor procedure - E/M services on the same day generally not paid, standard payment adjustment rules for multiple procedures apply, 150% payment adjustment for bilateral procedures does not apply, assistant surgeon may not be paid

29550   **Strap toes**   ~ endoscopies or minor procedure - E/M services on the same day generally not paid, standard payment adjustment rules for multiple

---

procedures apply, 150% payment adjustment for bilateral procedures does not apply, assistant surgeon may not be paid

29580 **Apply paste boot** ~ endoscopies or minor procedure - E/M services on the same day generally not paid, standard payment adjustment rules for multiple procedures apply, 150% payment adjustment for bilateral procedures applies, assistant surgeon may not be paid

29590 **Apply foot splint** ~ endoscopies or minor procedure - E/M services on the same day generally not paid, standard payment adjustment rules for multiple procedures apply, 150% payment adjustment for bilateral procedures does not apply, assistant surgeon may not be paid

29700 **Remove/revise cast** ~ endoscopies or minor procedure - E/M services on the same day generally not paid, standard payment adjustment rules for multiple procedures apply, 150% payment adjustment for bilateral procedures does not apply, assistant surgeon may not be paid

29705 **Remove/revise cast** ~ endoscopies or minor procedure - E/M services on the same day generally not paid, standard payment adjustment rules for multiple procedures apply, 150% payment adjustment for bilateral procedures applies, assistant surgeon may not be paid

29710 **Remove/revise cast** ~ endoscopies or minor procedure - E/M services on the same day generally not paid, standard payment adjustment rules for multiple procedures apply, 150% payment adjustment for bilateral procedures applies, payment for assistant surgeon subject to documentation of medical necessity

29715 **Remove/revise cast** ~ endoscopies or minor procedure - E/M services on the same day generally not paid, standard payment adjustment rules for multiple procedures apply, 150% payment adjustment for bilateral procedures does not apply, payment for assistant surgeon subject to documentation of medical necessity

29720 **Repair body cast** ~ endoscopies or minor procedure - E/M services on the same day generally not paid, standard payment adjustment rules for multiple procedures apply, 150% payment adjustment for bilateral procedures does not apply, assistant surgeon may not be paid

29730 **Windowing of cast** ~ endoscopies or minor procedure - E/M services on the same day generally not paid, standard payment adjustment rules for multiple procedures apply, 150% payment adjustment for bilateral procedures does not apply, assistant surgeon may not be paid

29740 **Wedging of cast** ~ endoscopies or minor procedure - E/M services on the same day generally not paid, standard payment adjustment rules for multiple procedures apply, 150% payment adjustment for bilateral procedures does not apply, assistant surgeon may not be paid

29750 **Wedging of clubfoot cast** ~ endoscopies or minor procedure - E/M services on the same day generally not paid, standard payment adjustment rules for multiple procedures apply, 150% payment adjustment for bilateral procedures applies, payment for assistant surgeon subject to documentation of medical necessity

29799 **Casting/strapping procedure** ~ medicare carrier determines global period, standard payment adjustment rules for multiple procedures apply, 150% payment adjustment for bilateral procedures does not apply, payment for assistant surgeon subject to documentation of medical necessity

29800 **Jaw arthroscopy/surgery** ~ follow-up period is 90 days, standard payment adjustment rules for multiple procedures apply, 150% payment adjustment for bilateral procedures applies, payment for assistant surgeon subject to documentation of medical necessity

29804 **Jaw arthroscopy/surgery** ~ follow-up period is 90 days, standard payment adjustment rules for multiple procedures apply, 150% payment adjustment for bilateral procedures applies, assistant surgeon may be paid

29805 **Shoulder arthroscopy, dx** ~ follow-up period is 90 days, standard payment adjustment rules for multiple procedures apply, 150% payment adjustment for bilateral procedures applies, assistant surgeon may not be paid

29806 **Shoulder arthroscopy/surgery** ~ follow-up period is 90 days, special rules for multiple endoscopic procedures apply if billed with another endoscopy in the same family, 150% payment adjustment for bilateral procedures applies, assistant surgeon may not be paid

29807 **Shoulder arthroscopy/surgery** ~ follow-up period is 90 days, special rules for multiple endoscopic procedures apply if billed with another endoscopy in the same family, 150% payment adjustment for bilateral procedures applies, assistant surgeon may not be paid

29819 **Shoulder arthroscopy/surgery** ~ follow-up period is 90 days, special rules for multiple endoscopic procedures apply if billed with another endoscopy in the same family, 150% payment adjustment for bilateral procedures applies, assistant surgeon may not be paid

29820 **Shoulder arthroscopy/surgery** ~ follow-up period is 90 days, special rules for multiple endoscopic procedures apply if billed with another endoscopy in the same family, 150% payment adjustment for bilateral procedures applies, assistant surgeon may be paid

29821 **Shoulder arthroscopy/surgery** ~ follow-up period is 90 days, special rules for multiple endoscopic procedures apply if billed with another endoscopy in the same family, 150% payment adjustment for bilateral procedures applies, assistant surgeon may be paid

29822   **Shoulder arthroscopy/surgery**   ~ follow-up period is 90 days, special rules for multiple endoscopic procedures apply if billed with another endoscopy in the same family, 150% payment adjustment for bilateral procedures applies, assistant surgeon may be paid

29823   **Shoulder arthroscopy/surgery**   ~ follow-up period is 90 days, special rules for multiple endoscopic procedures apply if billed with another endoscopy in the same family, 150% payment adjustment for bilateral procedures applies, assistant surgeon may be paid

29824   **Shoulder arthroscopy/surgery**   ~ follow-up period is 90 days, special rules for multiple endoscopic procedures apply if billed with another endoscopy in the same family, 150% payment adjustment for bilateral procedures applies, assistant surgeon may be paid

29825   **Shoulder arthroscopy/surgery**   ~ follow-up period is 90 days, special rules for multiple endoscopic procedures apply if billed with another endoscopy in the same family, 150% payment adjustment for bilateral procedures applies, assistant surgeon may be paid

29826   **Shoulder arthroscopy/surgery**   ~ follow-up period is 90 days, special rules for multiple endoscopic procedures apply if billed with another endoscopy in the same family, 150% payment adjustment for bilateral procedures applies, assistant surgeon may be paid

29827   **Arthroscopy rotator cuff repair**   ~ follow-up period is 90 days, standard payment adjustment rules for multiple procedures apply, 150% payment adjustment for bilateral procedures applies, assistant surgeon may be paid

29830   **Elbow arthroscopy**   ~ follow-up period is 90 days, standard payment adjustment rules for multiple procedures apply, 150% payment adjustment for bilateral procedures applies, assistant surgeon may not be paid

29834   **Elbow arthroscopy/surgery**   ~ follow-up period is 90 days, special rules for multiple endoscopic procedures apply if billed with another endoscopy in the same family, 150% payment adjustment for bilateral procedures applies, assistant surgeon may be paid

29835   **Elbow arthroscopy/surgery**   ~ follow-up period is 90 days, special rules for multiple endoscopic procedures apply if billed with another endoscopy in the same family, 150% payment adjustment for bilateral procedures applies, assistant surgeon may be paid

29836   **Elbow arthroscopy/surgery**   ~ follow-up period is 90 days, special rules for multiple endoscopic procedures apply if billed with another endoscopy in the same family, 150% payment adjustment for bilateral procedures applies, assistant surgeon may be paid

29837   **Elbow arthroscopy/surgery**   ~ follow-up period is 90 days, special rules for multiple endoscopic procedures apply if billed with another endoscopy in the same family, 150% payment adjustment for bilateral procedures applies, assistant surgeon may be paid

29838   **Elbow arthroscopy/surgery**   ~ follow-up period is 90 days, special rules for multiple endoscopic procedures apply if billed with another endoscopy in the same family,

150% payment adjustment for bilateral procedures applies, payment for assistant surgeon subject to documentation of medical necessity

29840   **Wrist arthroscopy**   ~ follow-up period is 90 days, standard payment adjustment rules for multiple procedures apply, 150% payment adjustment for bilateral procedures applies, payment for assistant surgeon subject to documentation of medical necessity

29843   **Wrist arthroscopy/surgery**   ~ follow-up period is 90 days, special rules for multiple endoscopic procedures apply if billed with another endoscopy in the same family, 150% payment adjustment for bilateral procedures applies, assistant surgeon may be paid

29844   **Wrist arthroscopy/surgery**   ~ follow-up period is 90 days, special rules for multiple endoscopic procedures apply if billed with another endoscopy in the same family, 150% payment adjustment for bilateral procedures applies, assistant surgeon may be paid

29845   **Wrist arthroscopy/surgery**   ~ follow-up period is 90 days, special rules for multiple endoscopic procedures apply if billed with another endoscopy in the same family, 150% payment adjustment for bilateral procedures applies, assistant surgeon may be paid

29846   **Wrist arthroscopy/surgery**   ~ follow-up period is 90 days, special rules for multiple endoscopic procedures apply if billed with another endoscopy in the same family, 150% payment adjustment for bilateral procedures applies, payment for assistant surgeon subject to documentation of medical necessity

29847   **Wrist arthroscopy/surgery**   ~ follow-up period is 90 days, special rules for multiple endoscopic procedures apply if billed with another endoscopy in the same family, 150% payment adjustment for bilateral procedures applies, assistant surgeon may be paid

29848   **Wrist endoscopy/surgery**   ~ follow-up period is 90 days, standard payment adjustment rules for multiple procedures apply, 150% payment adjustment for bilateral procedures applies, assistant surgeon may not be paid

29850   **Knee arthroscopy/surgery**   ~ follow-up period is 90 days, standard payment adjustment rules for multiple procedures apply, 150% payment adjustment for bilateral procedures applies, payment for assistant surgeon subject to documentation of medical necessity

29851   **Knee arthroscopy/surgery**   ~ follow-up period is 90 days, standard payment adjustment rules for multiple procedures apply, 150% payment adjustment for bilateral procedures applies, assistant surgeon may be paid

29855   **Tibial arthroscopy/surgery**   ~ follow-up period is 90 days, standard payment adjustment rules for multiple procedures apply, 150% payment adjustment for bilateral procedures applies, assistant surgeon may be paid

29856   **Tibial arthroscopy/surgery**   ~ follow-up period is 90 days, standard payment adjustment rules for multiple procedures apply, 150% payment adjustment for bilateral procedures applies, assistant surgeon may be paid

29860   **Hip arthroscopy, dx**   ~ follow-up period is 90 days, standard payment adjustment rules for multiple procedures apply, 150% payment adjustment for bilateral procedures applies, assistant surgeon may be paid

29861   **Hip arthroscopy/surgery**   ~ follow-up period is 90 days, special rules for multiple endoscopic procedures apply if billed with another endoscopy in the same family, 150% payment adjustment for bilateral procedures applies, assistant surgeon may be paid

29862   **Hip arthroscopy/surgery**   ~ follow-up period is 90 days, special rules for multiple endoscopic procedures apply if billed with another endoscopy in the same family, 150% payment adjustment for bilateral procedures applies, assistant surgeon may be paid

29863   **Hip arthroscopy/surgery**   ~ follow-up period is 90 days, special rules for multiple endoscopic procedures apply if billed with another endoscopy in the same family, 150% payment adjustment for bilateral procedures applies, assistant surgeon may be paid

29866   **Autograft implant, knee w/scope**   ~ follow-up period is 90 days, standard payment adjustment rules for multiple procedures apply, 150% payment adjustment for bilateral procedures applies, payment for assistant surgeon subject to documentation of medical necessity

29867   **Allograft implant, knee w/scope**   ~ follow-up period is 90 days, standard payment adjustment rules for multiple procedures apply, 150% payment adjustment for bilateral procedures applies, payment for assistant surgeon subject to documentation of medical necessity

29868   **Meniscal transplant, knee w/scope**   ~ follow-up period is 90 days, standard payment adjustment rules for multiple procedures apply, 150% payment adjustment for bilateral procedures applies, payment for assistant surgeon subject to documentation of medical necessity

29870   **Knee arthroscopy, dx**   ~ follow-up period is 90 days, standard payment adjustment rules for multiple procedures apply, 150% payment adjustment for bilateral procedures applies, assistant surgeon may not be paid

29871   **Knee arthroscopy/drainage**   ~ follow-up period is 90 days, special rules for multiple endoscopic procedures apply if billed with another endoscopy in the same family, 150% payment adjustment for bilateral procedures applies, assistant surgeon may not be paid

29873   **Knee arthroscopy/surgery**   ~ follow-up period is 90 days, special rules for multiple endoscopic procedures apply if billed with another endoscopy in the same family,

150% payment adjustment for bilateral procedures applies, assistant surgeon may not be paid

29874 **Knee arthroscopy/surgery** ~ follow-up period is 90 days, special rules for multiple endoscopic procedures apply if billed with another endoscopy in the same family, 150% payment adjustment for bilateral procedures applies, payment for assistant surgeon subject to documentation of medical necessity

29875 **Knee arthroscopy/surgery** ~ follow-up period is 90 days, special rules for multiple endoscopic procedures apply if billed with another endoscopy in the same family, 150% payment adjustment for bilateral procedures applies, payment for assistant surgeon subject to documentation of medical necessity

29876 **Knee arthroscopy/surgery** ~ follow-up period is 90 days, special rules for multiple endoscopic procedures apply if billed with another endoscopy in the same family, 150% payment adjustment for bilateral procedures applies, assistant surgeon may not be paid

29877 **Knee arthroscopy/surgery** ~ follow-up period is 90 days, special rules for multiple endoscopic procedures apply if billed with another endoscopy in the same family, 150% payment adjustment for bilateral procedures applies, payment for assistant surgeon subject to documentation of medical necessity

29879 **Knee arthroscopy/surgery** ~ follow-up period is 90 days, special rules for multiple endoscopic procedures apply if billed with another endoscopy in the same family, 150% payment adjustment for bilateral procedures applies, payment for assistant surgeon subject to documentation of medical necessity

29880 **Knee arthroscopy/surgery** ~ follow-up period is 90 days, special rules for multiple endoscopic procedures apply if billed with another endoscopy in the same family, 150% payment adjustment for bilateral procedures applies, payment for assistant surgeon subject to documentation of medical necessity

29881 **Knee arthroscopy/surgery** ~ follow-up period is 90 days, special rules for multiple endoscopic procedures apply if billed with another endoscopy in the same family, 150% payment adjustment for bilateral procedures applies, payment for assistant surgeon subject to documentation of medical necessity

29882 **Knee arthroscopy/surgery** ~ follow-up period is 90 days, special rules for multiple endoscopic procedures apply if billed with another endoscopy in the same family, 150% payment adjustment for bilateral procedures applies, assistant surgeon may not be paid

29883 **Knee arthroscopy/surgery** ~ follow-up period is 90 days, special rules for multiple endoscopic procedures apply if billed with another endoscopy in the same family, 150% payment adjustment for bilateral procedures applies, payment for assistant surgeon subject to documentation of medical necessity

29884   **Knee arthroscopy/surgery**   ~ follow-up period is 90 days, special rules for multiple endoscopic procedures apply if billed with another endoscopy in the same family, 150% payment adjustment for bilateral procedures applies, assistant surgeon may be paid

29885   **Knee arthroscopy/surgery**   ~ follow-up period is 90 days, special rules for multiple endoscopic procedures apply if billed with another endoscopy in the same family, 150% payment adjustment for bilateral procedures applies, assistant surgeon may be paid

29886   **Knee arthroscopy/surgery**   ~ follow-up period is 90 days, special rules for multiple endoscopic procedures apply if billed with another endoscopy in the same family, 150% payment adjustment for bilateral procedures applies, assistant surgeon may not be paid

29887   **Knee arthroscopy/surgery**   ~ follow-up period is 90 days, special rules for multiple endoscopic procedures apply if billed with another endoscopy in the same family, 150% payment adjustment for bilateral procedures applies, assistant surgeon may be paid

29888   **Knee arthroscopy/surgery**   ~ follow-up period is 90 days, standard payment adjustment rules for multiple procedures apply, 150% payment adjustment for bilateral procedures applies, assistant surgeon may be paid

29889   **Knee arthroscopy/surgery**   ~ follow-up period is 90 days, standard payment adjustment rules for multiple procedures apply, 150% payment adjustment for bilateral procedures applies, assistant surgeon may be paid

29891   **Ankle arthroscopy/surgery**   ~ follow-up period is 90 days, standard payment adjustment rules for multiple procedures apply, 150% payment adjustment for bilateral procedures applies, assistant surgeon may be paid

29892   **Ankle arthroscopy/surgery**   ~ follow-up period is 90 days, standard payment adjustment rules for multiple procedures apply, 150% payment adjustment for bilateral procedures applies, assistant surgeon may be paid

29893   **Scope, plantar fasciotomy**   ~ follow-up period is 90 days, standard payment adjustment rules for multiple procedures apply, 150% payment adjustment for bilateral procedures applies, assistant surgeon may be paid

29894   **Ankle arthroscopy/surgery**   ~ follow-up period is 90 days, standard payment adjustment rules for multiple procedures apply, 150% payment adjustment for bilateral procedures applies, assistant surgeon may be paid

29895   **Ankle arthroscopy/surgery**   ~ follow-up period is 90 days, standard payment adjustment rules for multiple procedures apply, 150% payment adjustment for bilateral procedures applies, assistant surgeon may be paid

29897   **Ankle arthroscopy/surgery**   ~ follow-up period is 90 days, standard payment adjustment rules for multiple procedures apply, 150% payment adjustment for bilateral procedures applies, assistant surgeon may be paid

29898   **Ankle arthroscopy/surgery**   ~ follow-up period is 90 days, standard payment adjustment rules for multiple procedures apply, 150% payment adjustment for bilateral procedures applies, assistant surgeon may be paid

29899   **Ankle arthroscopy/surgery**   ~ follow-up period is 90 days, standard payment adjustment rules for multiple procedures apply, 150% payment adjustment for bilateral procedures applies, assistant surgeon may be paid

29900   **Mcp joint arthroscopy, dx**   ~ follow-up period is 90 days, standard payment adjustment rules for multiple procedures apply, 150% payment adjustment for bilateral procedures applies, payment for assistant surgeon subject to documentation of medical necessity

29901   **Mcp joint arthroscopy, surg**   ~ follow-up period is 90 days, standard payment adjustment rules for multiple procedures apply, 150% payment adjustment for bilateral procedures applies, payment for assistant surgeon subject to documentation of medical necessity

29902   **Mcp joint arthroscopy, surg**   ~ follow-up period is 90 days, standard payment adjustment rules for multiple procedures apply, 150% payment adjustment for bilateral procedures applies, payment for assistant surgeon subject to documentation of medical necessity

29999   **Arthroscopy of joint**   ~ medicare carrier determines global period, standard payment adjustment rules for multiple procedures apply, 150% payment adjustment for bilateral procedures applies, payment for assistant surgeon subject to documentation of medical necessity

RESPIRATORY SYSTEM

Nose

30000   **Drain nose lesion**   ~ follow-up period is 10 days, standard payment adjustment rules for multiple procedures apply, 150% payment adjustment for bilateral procedures does not apply, payment for assistant surgeon subject to documentation of medical necessity

30020   **Drain nose lesion**   ~ follow-up period is 10 days, standard payment adjustment rules for multiple procedures apply, 150% payment adjustment for bilateral procedures does not apply, assistant surgeon may not be paid

30100   **Intranasal biopsy**   ~ endoscopies or minor procedure - E/M services on the same day generally not paid, standard payment adjustment rules for multiple procedures apply, 150% payment adjustment for bilateral procedures does not apply, assistant surgeon may not be paid

30110   **Remove nose polyp(s)**   ~ follow-up period is 10 days, standard payment adjustment rules for multiple procedures apply, 150% payment adjustment for bilateral procedures applies, assistant surgeon may not be paid

30115   **Remove nose polyp(s)**   ~ follow-up period is 90 days, standard payment adjustment rules for multiple procedures apply, 150% payment adjustment for bilateral procedures applies, assistant surgeon may not be paid

30117   **Remove intranasal lesion**   ~ follow-up period is 90 days, standard payment adjustment rules for multiple procedures apply, 150% payment adjustment for bilateral procedures does not apply, assistant surgeon may not be paid

30118   **Remove intranasal lesion**   ~ follow-up period is 90 days, standard payment adjustment rules for multiple procedures apply, 150% payment adjustment for bilateral procedures does not apply, assistant surgeon may be paid

30120   **Revise nose**   ~ follow-up period is 90 days, standard payment adjustment rules for multiple procedures apply, 150% payment adjustment for bilateral procedures does not apply, assistant surgeon may not be paid

30124   **Remove nose lesion**   ~ follow-up period is 90 days, standard payment adjustment rules for multiple procedures apply, 150% payment adjustment for bilateral procedures does not apply, assistant surgeon may not be paid

30125   **Remove nose lesion**   ~ follow-up period is 90 days, standard payment adjustment rules for multiple procedures apply, 150% payment adjustment for bilateral procedures does not apply, assistant surgeon may be paid

30130   **Excise inferior turbinate**   ~ follow-up period is 90 days, standard payment adjustment rules for multiple procedures apply, 150% payment adjustment for bilateral procedures applies, assistant surgeon may not be paid

30140   **Resect inferior turbinate**   ~ follow-up period is 90 days, standard payment adjustment rules for multiple procedures apply, 150% payment adjustment for bilateral procedures applies, assistant surgeon may not be paid

30150   **Partial remove nose**   ~ follow-up period is 90 days, standard payment adjustment rules for multiple procedures apply, 150% payment adjustment for bilateral procedures does not apply, assistant surgeon may not be paid

30160   **Remove nose**   ~ follow-up period is 90 days, standard payment adjustment rules for multiple procedures apply, 150% payment adjustment for bilateral procedures does not apply, assistant surgeon may be paid

30200   **Injection treat nose**   ~ endoscopies or minor procedure - E/M services on the same day generally not paid, standard payment adjustment rules for multiple procedures apply, 150% payment adjustment for bilateral procedures does not apply, assistant surgeon may not be paid

30210   **Nasal sinus therapy**   ~ follow-up period is 10 days, standard payment adjustment rules for multiple procedures apply, 150% payment adjustment for bilateral procedures does not apply, assistant surgeon may not be paid

30220   **Insert nasal septal button**   ~ follow-up period is 10 days, standard payment adjustment rules for multiple procedures apply, 150% payment adjustment for bilateral procedures does not apply, assistant surgeon may not be paid

30300   **Remove nasal foreign body**   ~ follow-up period is 10 days, standard payment adjustment rules for multiple procedures apply, 150% payment adjustment for bilateral procedures does not apply, assistant surgeon may not be paid

30310   **Remove nasal foreign body**   ~ follow-up period is 10 days, standard payment adjustment rules for multiple procedures apply, 150% payment adjustment for bilateral procedures does not apply, payment for assistant surgeon subject to documentation of medical necessity

30320   **Remove nasal foreign body**   ~ follow-up period is 90 days, standard payment adjustment rules for multiple procedures apply, 150% payment adjustment for bilateral procedures does not apply, payment for assistant surgeon subject to documentation of medical necessity

30400   **Reconstruct nose**   ~ restricted coverage - special coverage rules apply, follow-up period is 90 days, standard payment adjustment rules for multiple procedures apply, 150% payment adjustment for bilateral procedures does not apply, payment for assistant surgeon subject to documentation of medical necessity

30410   **Reconstruct nose**   ~ restricted coverage - special coverage rules apply, follow-up period is 90 days, standard payment adjustment rules for multiple procedures apply, 150% payment adjustment for bilateral procedures does not apply, assistant surgeon may be paid

30420   **Reconstruct nose**   ~ restricted coverage - special coverage rules apply, follow-up period is 90 days, standard payment adjustment rules for multiple procedures apply, 150% payment adjustment for bilateral procedures does not apply, assistant surgeon may not be paid

---

30430   **Revise nose**   ~ restricted coverage - special coverage rules apply, follow-up period is 90 days, standard payment adjustment rules for multiple procedures apply, 150% payment adjustment for bilateral procedures does not apply, assistant surgeon may be paid

30435   **Revise nose**   ~ restricted coverage - special coverage rules apply, follow-up period is 90 days, standard payment adjustment rules for multiple procedures apply, 150% payment adjustment for bilateral procedures does not apply, assistant surgeon may be paid

30450   **Revise nose**   ~ restricted coverage - special coverage rules apply, follow-up period is 90 days, standard payment adjustment rules for multiple procedures apply, 150% payment adjustment for bilateral procedures does not apply, assistant surgeon may be paid

30460   **Revise nose**   ~ follow-up period is 90 days, standard payment adjustment rules for multiple procedures apply, 150% payment adjustment for bilateral procedures does not apply, assistant surgeon may be paid

30462   **Revise nose**   ~ follow-up period is 90 days, standard payment adjustment rules for multiple procedures apply, 150% payment adjustment for bilateral procedures does not apply, assistant surgeon may be paid

30465   **Repair nasal stenosis**   ~ follow-up period is 90 days, standard payment adjustment rules for multiple procedures apply, 150% payment adjustment for bilateral procedures does not apply, payment for assistant surgeon subject to documentation of medical necessity

30520   **Repair nasal septum**   ~ follow-up period is 90 days, standard payment adjustment rules for multiple procedures apply, 150% payment adjustment for bilateral procedures does not apply, assistant surgeon may not be paid

30540   **Repair nasal defect**   ~ follow-up period is 90 days, standard payment adjustment rules for multiple procedures apply, 150% payment adjustment for bilateral procedures does not apply, assistant surgeon may be paid

30545   **Repair nasal defect**   ~ follow-up period is 90 days, standard payment adjustment rules for multiple procedures apply, 150% payment adjustment for bilateral procedures does not apply, assistant surgeon may be paid

30560   **Release nasal adhesions**   ~ follow-up period is 10 days, standard payment adjustment rules for multiple procedures apply, 150% payment adjustment for bilateral procedures does not apply, assistant surgeon may not be paid

30580   **Repair upper jaw fistula**   ~ follow-up period is 90 days, standard payment adjustment rules for multiple procedures apply, 150% payment adjustment for bilateral procedures does not apply, assistant surgeon may not be paid

30600   **Repair mouth/nose fistula**   ~ follow-up period is 90 days, standard payment adjustment rules for multiple procedures apply, 150% payment adjustment for bilateral procedures does not apply, payment for assistant surgeon subject to documentation of medical necessity

30620   **Intranasal reconstruct**   ~ follow-up period is 90 days, standard payment adjustment rules for multiple procedures apply, 150% payment adjustment for bilateral procedures does not apply, assistant surgeon may not be paid

30630   **Repair nasal septum defect**   ~ follow-up period is 90 days, standard payment adjustment rules for multiple procedures apply, 150% payment adjustment for bilateral procedures does not apply, payment for assistant surgeon subject to documentation of medical necessity

30801   **Ablate inf turbinate, superficial**   ~ follow-up period is 10 days, standard payment adjustment rules for multiple procedures apply, 150% payment adjustment does not apply - RVUs based on bilateral procedure, assistant surgeon may not be paid

30802   **Cauterization, inner nose**   ~ follow-up period is 10 days, standard payment adjustment rules for multiple procedures apply, 150% payment adjustment does not apply - RVUs based on bilateral procedure, assistant surgeon may not be paid

30901   **Control nosebleed**   ~ endoscopies or minor procedure - E/M services on the same day generally not paid, standard payment adjustment rules for multiple procedures apply, 150% payment adjustment for bilateral procedures applies, assistant surgeon may not be paid

30903   **Control nosebleed**   ~ endoscopies or minor procedure - E/M services on the same day generally not paid, standard payment adjustment rules for multiple procedures apply, 150% payment adjustment for bilateral procedures applies, assistant surgeon may not be paid

30905   **Control nosebleed**   ~ endoscopies or minor procedure - E/M services on the same day generally not paid, standard payment adjustment rules for multiple procedures apply, 150% payment adjustment does not apply - RVUs based on bilateral procedure, assistant surgeon may not be paid

30906   **Repeat control nosebleed**   ~ endoscopies or minor procedure - E/M services on the same day generally not paid, standard payment adjustment rules for multiple procedures apply, 150% payment adjustment does not apply - RVUs based on bilateral procedure, assistant surgeon may not be paid

30915   **Ligate nasal sinus artery**   ~ follow-up period is 90 days, standard payment adjustment rules for multiple procedures apply, 150% payment adjustment for bilateral procedures does not apply, assistant surgeon may not be paid

30920   **Ligate upper jaw artery**   ~ follow-up period is 90 days, standard payment adjustment rules for multiple procedures apply, 150% payment adjustment for bilateral procedures does not apply, assistant surgeon may not be paid

30930   **Therapeutic fracture, nasal inf turbinate**   ~ follow-up period is 10 days, standard payment adjustment rules for multiple procedures apply, 150% payment adjustment for bilateral procedures applies, assistant surgeon may not be paid

30999   **Nasal surgery procedure**   ~ medicare carrier determines global period, standard payment adjustment rules for multiple procedures apply, 150% payment adjustment for bilateral procedures does not apply, payment for assistant surgeon subject to documentation of medical necessity

Accessory Sinuses

31000   **Irrigation, maxillary sinus**   ~ follow-up period is 10 days, standard payment adjustment rules for multiple procedures apply, 150% payment adjustment for bilateral procedures applies, assistant surgeon may not be paid

31002   **Irrigation, sphenoid sinus**   ~ follow-up period is 10 days, standard payment adjustment rules for multiple procedures apply, 150% payment adjustment for bilateral procedures applies, payment for assistant surgeon subject to documentation of medical necessity

31020   **Explore maxillary sinus**   ~ follow-up period is 90 days, standard payment adjustment rules for multiple procedures apply, 150% payment adjustment for bilateral procedures applies, assistant surgeon may not be paid

31030   **Explore maxillary sinus**   ~ follow-up period is 90 days, standard payment adjustment rules for multiple procedures apply, 150% payment adjustment for bilateral procedures applies, assistant surgeon may not be paid

31032   **Explore sinus, remove polyps**   ~ follow-up period is 90 days, standard payment adjustment rules for multiple procedures apply, 150% payment adjustment for bilateral procedures applies, assistant surgeon may not be paid

31040   **Explore behind upper jaw**   ~ follow-up period is 90 days, standard payment adjustment rules for multiple procedures apply, 150% payment adjustment for bilateral procedures does not apply, assistant surgeon may not be paid

31050   **Explore sphenoid sinus**   ~ follow-up period is 90 days, standard payment adjustment rules for multiple procedures apply, 150% payment adjustment for bilateral procedures applies, assistant surgeon may not be paid

31051   **Sphenoid sinus surgery**   ~ follow-up period is 90 days, standard payment adjustment rules for multiple procedures apply, 150% payment adjustment for bilateral procedures applies, assistant surgeon may not be paid

31070   **Explore frontal sinus**   ~ follow-up period is 90 days, standard payment adjustment rules for multiple procedures apply, 150% payment adjustment for bilateral procedures applies, assistant surgeon may not be paid

31075   **Explore frontal sinus**   ~ follow-up period is 90 days, standard payment adjustment rules for multiple procedures apply, 150% payment adjustment for bilateral procedures applies, assistant surgeon may be paid

31080   **Remove frontal sinus**   ~ follow-up period is 90 days, standard payment adjustment rules for multiple procedures apply, 150% payment adjustment for bilateral procedures applies, assistant surgeon may be paid

31081   **Remove frontal sinus**   ~ follow-up period is 90 days, standard payment adjustment rules for multiple procedures apply, 150% payment adjustment for bilateral procedures applies, assistant surgeon may be paid

31084   **Remove frontal sinus**   ~ follow-up period is 90 days, standard payment adjustment rules for multiple procedures apply, 150% payment adjustment for bilateral procedures applies, assistant surgeon may be paid

31085   **Remove frontal sinus**   ~ follow-up period is 90 days, standard payment adjustment rules for multiple procedures apply, 150% payment adjustment for bilateral procedures applies, assistant surgeon may be paid

31086   **Remove frontal sinus**   ~ follow-up period is 90 days, standard payment adjustment rules for multiple procedures apply, 150% payment adjustment for bilateral procedures applies, assistant surgeon may be paid

31087   **Remove frontal sinus**   ~ follow-up period is 90 days, standard payment adjustment rules for multiple procedures apply, 150% payment adjustment for bilateral procedures applies, assistant surgeon may be paid

31090   **Explore sinuses**   ~ follow-up period is 90 days, standard payment adjustment rules for multiple procedures apply, 150% payment adjustment for bilateral procedures applies, assistant surgeon may not be paid

31200   **Remove ethmoid sinus**   ~ follow-up period is 90 days, standard payment adjustment rules for multiple procedures apply, 150% payment adjustment for bilateral procedures applies, assistant surgeon may not be paid

31201   **Remove ethmoid sinus**   ~ follow-up period is 90 days, standard payment adjustment rules for multiple procedures apply, 150% payment adjustment for bilateral procedures applies, assistant surgeon may not be paid

31205   **Remove ethmoid sinus**   ~ follow-up period is 90 days, standard payment adjustment rules for multiple procedures apply, 150% payment adjustment for bilateral procedures applies, assistant surgeon may be paid

31225   **Remove upper jaw**   ~ follow-up period is 90 days, standard payment adjustment rules for multiple procedures apply, 150% payment adjustment for bilateral procedures applies, assistant surgeon may be paid

31230   **Remove upper jaw**   ~ follow-up period is 90 days, standard payment adjustment rules for multiple procedures apply, 150% payment adjustment for bilateral procedures applies, assistant surgeon may be paid

31231   **Nasal endoscopy, dx**   ~ endoscopies or minor procedure - E/M services on the same day generally not paid, standard payment adjustment rules for multiple procedures apply, 150% payment adjustment does not apply - RVUs based on bilateral procedure, assistant surgeon may not be paid

31233   **Nasal/sinus endoscopy, dx**   ~ endoscopies or minor procedure - E/M services on the same day generally not paid, standard payment adjustment rules for multiple procedures apply, 150% payment adjustment for bilateral procedures applies, assistant surgeon may not be paid

31235   **Nasal/sinus endoscopy, dx**   ~ endoscopies or minor procedure - E/M services on the same day generally not paid, standard payment adjustment rules for multiple procedures apply, 150% payment adjustment for bilateral procedures applies, assistant surgeon may not be paid

31237   **Nasal/sinus endoscopy, surg**   ~ endoscopies or minor procedure - E/M services on the same day generally not paid, standard payment adjustment rules for multiple procedures apply, 150% payment adjustment for bilateral procedures applies, assistant surgeon may not be paid

31238   **Nasal/sinus endoscopy, surg**   ~ endoscopies or minor procedure - E/M services on the same day generally not paid, standard payment adjustment rules for multiple procedures apply, 150% payment adjustment for bilateral procedures applies, payment for assistant surgeon subject to documentation of medical necessity

31239   **Nasal/sinus endoscopy, surg**   ~ follow-up period is 10 days, standard payment adjustment rules for multiple procedures apply, 150% payment adjustment for bilateral procedures applies, payment for assistant surgeon subject to documentation of medical necessity

31240   **Nasal/sinus endoscopy, surg**   ~ endoscopies or minor procedure - E/M services on the same day generally not paid, standard payment adjustment rules for multiple procedures apply, 150% payment adjustment for bilateral procedures applies, payment for assistant surgeon subject to documentation of medical necessity

31254   **Revise ethmoid sinus**   ~ endoscopies or minor procedure - E/M services on the same day generally not paid, standard payment adjustment rules for multiple procedures apply, 150% payment adjustment for bilateral procedures applies, assistant surgeon may not be paid

31255 **Remove ethmoid sinus**   ~ endoscopies or minor procedure - E/M services on the same day generally not paid, standard payment adjustment rules for multiple procedures apply, 150% payment adjustment for bilateral procedures applies, assistant surgeon may not be paid

31256 **Explore maxillary sinus**   ~ endoscopies or minor procedure - E/M services on the same day generally not paid, standard payment adjustment rules for multiple procedures apply, 150% payment adjustment for bilateral procedures applies, assistant surgeon may not be paid

31267 **Endoscopy, maxillary sinus**   ~ endoscopies or minor procedure - E/M services on the same day generally not paid, standard payment adjustment rules for multiple procedures apply, 150% payment adjustment for bilateral procedures applies, assistant surgeon may not be paid

31276 **Sinus endoscopy, surgical**   ~ endoscopies or minor procedure - E/M services on the same day generally not paid, standard payment adjustment rules for multiple procedures apply, 150% payment adjustment for bilateral procedures applies, assistant surgeon may not be paid

31287 **Nasal/sinus endoscopy, surg**   ~ endoscopies or minor procedure - E/M services on the same day generally not paid, standard payment adjustment rules for multiple procedures apply, 150% payment adjustment for bilateral procedures applies, payment for assistant surgeon subject to documentation of medical necessity

31288 **Nasal/sinus endoscopy, surg**   ~ endoscopies or minor procedure - E/M services on the same day generally not paid, standard payment adjustment rules for multiple procedures apply, 150% payment adjustment for bilateral procedures applies, payment for assistant surgeon subject to documentation of medical necessity

31290 **Nasal/sinus endoscopy, surg**   ~ follow-up period is 10 days, standard payment adjustment rules for multiple procedures apply, 150% payment adjustment for bilateral procedures applies, payment for assistant surgeon subject to documentation of medical necessity

31291 **Nasal/sinus endoscopy, surg**   ~ follow-up period is 10 days, standard payment adjustment rules for multiple procedures apply, 150% payment adjustment for bilateral procedures applies, payment for assistant surgeon subject to documentation of medical necessity

31292 **Nasal/sinus endoscopy, surg**   ~ follow-up period is 10 days, standard payment adjustment rules for multiple procedures apply, 150% payment adjustment for bilateral procedures applies, payment for assistant surgeon subject to documentation of medical necessity

31293 **Nasal/sinus endoscopy, surg**   ~ follow-up period is 10 days, standard payment adjustment rules for multiple procedures apply, 150% payment adjustment for

bilateral procedures applies, payment for assistant surgeon subject to documentation of medical necessity

31294 **Nasal/sinus endoscopy, surg** ~ follow-up period is 10 days, standard payment adjustment rules for multiple procedures apply, 150% payment adjustment for bilateral procedures applies, payment for assistant surgeon subject to documentation of medical necessity

31299 **Sinus surgery procedure** ~ medicare carrier determines global period, standard payment adjustment rules for multiple procedures apply, 150% payment adjustment for bilateral procedures does not apply, payment for assistant surgeon subject to documentation of medical necessity

31300 **Remove larynx lesion** ~ follow-up period is 90 days, standard payment adjustment rules for multiple procedures apply, 150% payment adjustment for bilateral procedures does not apply, assistant surgeon may be paid

31320 **Diagnostic incise larynx** ~ follow-up period is 90 days, standard payment adjustment rules for multiple procedures apply, 150% payment adjustment for bilateral procedures does not apply, payment for assistant surgeon subject to documentation of medical necessity

31360 **Remove larynx** ~ follow-up period is 90 days, standard payment adjustment rules for multiple procedures apply, 150% payment adjustment for bilateral procedures does not apply, assistant surgeon may be paid

31365 **Remove larynx** ~ follow-up period is 90 days, standard payment adjustment rules for multiple procedures apply, 150% payment adjustment for bilateral procedures does not apply, assistant surgeon may be paid

31367 **Partial remove larynx** ~ follow-up period is 90 days, standard payment adjustment rules for multiple procedures apply, 150% payment adjustment for bilateral procedures does not apply, assistant surgeon may be paid

31368 **Partial remove larynx** ~ follow-up period is 90 days, standard payment adjustment rules for multiple procedures apply, 150% payment adjustment for bilateral procedures does not apply, assistant surgeon may be paid

31370 **Partial remove larynx** ~ follow-up period is 90 days, standard payment adjustment rules for multiple procedures apply, 150% payment adjustment for bilateral procedures does not apply, assistant surgeon may be paid

31375 **Partial remove larynx** ~ follow-up period is 90 days, standard payment adjustment rules for multiple procedures apply, 150% payment adjustment for bilateral procedures does not apply, assistant surgeon may be paid

31380   **Partial remove larynx**   ~ follow-up period is 90 days, standard payment adjustment rules for multiple procedures apply, 150% payment adjustment for bilateral procedures does not apply, assistant surgeon may be paid

31382   **Partial remove larynx**   ~ follow-up period is 90 days, standard payment adjustment rules for multiple procedures apply, 150% payment adjustment for bilateral procedures does not apply, assistant surgeon may be paid

31390   **Remove larynx & pharynx**   ~ follow-up period is 90 days, standard payment adjustment rules for multiple procedures apply, 150% payment adjustment for bilateral procedures does not apply, assistant surgeon may be paid

31395   **Reconstruct larynx & pharynx**   ~ follow-up period is 90 days, standard payment adjustment rules for multiple procedures apply, 150% payment adjustment for bilateral procedures does not apply, assistant surgeon may be paid

31400   **Revise larynx**   ~ follow-up period is 90 days, standard payment adjustment rules for multiple procedures apply, 150% payment adjustment for bilateral procedures does not apply, assistant surgeon may be paid

31420   **Remove epiglottis**   ~ follow-up period is 90 days, standard payment adjustment rules for multiple procedures apply, 150% payment adjustment for bilateral procedures does not apply, assistant surgeon may be paid

31500   **Insert emergency airway**   ~ endoscopies or minor procedure - E/M services on the same day generally not paid, no payment adjustment rules for multiple procedures apply, 150% payment adjustment for bilateral procedures does not apply, assistant surgeon may not be paid

31502   **Change of windpipe airway**   ~ endoscopies or minor procedure - E/M services on the same day generally not paid, standard payment adjustment rules for multiple procedures apply, 150% payment adjustment for bilateral procedures does not apply, assistant surgeon may not be paid

31505   **Diagnostic laryngoscopy**   ~ endoscopies or minor procedure - E/M services on the same day generally not paid, standard payment adjustment rules for multiple procedures apply, 150% payment adjustment for bilateral procedures does not apply, assistant surgeon may not be paid

31510   **Laryngoscopy with biopsy**   ~ endoscopies or minor procedure - E/M services on the same day generally not paid, special rules for multiple endoscopic procedures apply if billed with another endoscopy in the same family, 150% payment adjustment for bilateral procedures does not apply, payment for assistant surgeon subject to documentation of medical necessity

31511   **Remove foreign body larynx**   ~ endoscopies or minor procedure - E/M services on the same day generally not paid, special rules for multiple endoscopic

procedures apply if billed with another endoscopy in the same family, 150% payment adjustment for bilateral procedures does not apply, assistant surgeon may not be paid

31512 **Remove larynx lesion**   ~ endoscopies or minor procedure - E/M services on the same day generally not paid, special rules for multiple endoscopic procedures apply if billed with another endoscopy in the same family, 150% payment adjustment for bilateral procedures does not apply, payment for assistant surgeon subject to documentation of medical necessity

31513 **Inject into vocal cord**   ~ endoscopies or minor procedure - E/M services on the same day generally not paid, special rules for multiple endoscopic procedures apply if billed with another endoscopy in the same family, 150% payment adjustment for bilateral procedures does not apply, payment for assistant surgeon subject to documentation of medical necessity

31515 **Laryngoscopy for aspiration** ~ endoscopies or minor procedure - E/M services on the same day generally not paid, standard payment adjustment rules for multiple procedures apply, 150% payment adjustment for bilateral procedures does not apply, assistant surgeon may not be paid

31520 **Dx laryngoscopy, newborn** ~ endoscopies or minor procedure - E/M services on the same day generally not paid, standard payment adjustment rules for multiple procedures apply, 150% payment adjustment for bilateral procedures does not apply, payment for assistant surgeon subject to documentation of medical necessity

31525 **Dx laryngoscopy excl newborn** ~ endoscopies or minor procedure - E/M services on the same day generally not paid, standard payment adjustment rules for multiple procedures apply, 150% payment adjustment for bilateral procedures does not apply, assistant surgeon may not be paid

31526 **Dx laryngoscopy w/operating scope** ~ endoscopies or minor procedure - E/M services on the same day generally not paid, standard payment adjustment rules for multiple procedures apply, 150% payment adjustment for bilateral procedures does not apply, assistant surgeon may not be paid

31527 **Laryngoscopy for treatment** ~ endoscopies or minor procedure - E/M services on the same day generally not paid, special rules for multiple endoscopic procedures apply if billed with another endoscopy in the same family, 150% payment adjustment for bilateral procedures does not apply, payment for assistant surgeon subject to documentation of medical necessity

31528 **Laryngoscopy and dilate**   ~ endoscopies or minor procedure - E/M services on the same day generally not paid, special rules for multiple endoscopic procedures apply if billed with another endoscopy in the same family, 150% payment adjustment for bilateral procedures does not apply, payment for assistant surgeon subject to documentation of medical necessity

31529   **Laryngoscopy and dilate**   ~ endoscopies or minor procedure - E/M services on the same day generally not paid, special rules for multiple endoscopic procedures apply if billed with another endoscopy in the same family, 150% payment adjustment for bilateral procedures does not apply, payment for assistant surgeon subject to documentation of medical necessity

31530   **Laryngoscopy w/foreign body remove**   ~ endoscopies or minor procedure - E/M services on the same day generally not paid, special rules for multiple endoscopic procedures apply if billed with another endoscopy in the same family, 150% payment adjustment for bilateral procedures does not apply, assistant surgeon may not be paid

31531   **Laryngoscopy w/foreign body & op scope** ~ endoscopies or minor procedure - E/M services on the same day generally not paid, special rules for multiple endoscopic procedures apply if billed with another endoscopy in the same family, 150% payment adjustment for bilateral procedures does not apply, payment for assistant surgeon subject to documentation of medical necessity

31535   **Laryngoscopy w/biopsy**   ~ endoscopies or minor procedure - E/M services on the same day generally not paid, special rules for multiple endoscopic procedures apply if billed with another endoscopy in the same family, 150% payment adjustment for bilateral procedures does not apply, assistant surgeon may not be paid

31536   **Laryngoscopy w/biopsy & op scope**   ~ endoscopies or minor procedure - E/M services on the same day generally not paid, special rules for multiple endoscopic procedures apply if billed with another endoscopy in the same family, 150% payment adjustment for bilateral procedures does not apply, assistant surgeon may not be paid

31540   **Laryngoscopy w/excise of tumor**   ~ endoscopies or minor procedure - E/M services on the same day generally not paid, special rules for multiple endoscopic procedures apply if billed with another endoscopy in the same family, 150% payment adjustment for bilateral procedures does not apply, assistant surgeon may not be paid

31541   **Laryngoscopy w/tumor excise + scope**   ~ endoscopies or minor procedure - E/M services on the same day generally not paid, special rules for multiple endoscopic procedures apply if billed with another endoscopy in the same family, 150% payment adjustment for bilateral procedures does not apply, assistant surgeon may not be paid

31545   **Remove vc lesion w/scope**   ~ endoscopies or minor procedure - E/M services on the same day generally not paid, special rules for multiple endoscopic procedures apply if billed with another endoscopy in the same family, 150% payment adjustment for bilateral procedures does not apply, assistant surgeon may not be paid

31546   **Remove vc lesion scope/graft**   ~ endoscopies or minor procedure - E/M services on the same day generally not paid, special rules for multiple endoscopic procedures apply if billed with another endoscopy in the same family, 150% payment adjustment for bilateral procedures does not apply, assistant surgeon may not be paid

---

31560 **Laryngoscope w/arytenoidectomy** ~ endoscopies or minor procedure - E/M services on the same day generally not paid, special rules for multiple endoscopic procedures apply if billed with another endoscopy in the same family, 150% payment adjustment for bilateral procedures does not apply, payment for assistant surgeon subject to documentation of medical necessity

31561 **Laryngoscopy, remove cart + scope** ~ endoscopies or minor procedure - E/M services on the same day generally not paid, special rules for multiple endoscopic procedures apply if billed with another endoscopy in the same family, 150% payment adjustment for bilateral procedures does not apply, payment for assistant surgeon subject to documentation of medical necessity

31570 **Laryngoscope w/vc inject** ~ endoscopies or minor procedure - E/M services on the same day generally not paid, special rules for multiple endoscopic procedures apply if billed with another endoscopy in the same family, 150% payment adjustment for bilateral procedures does not apply, assistant surgeon may not be paid

31571 **Laryngoscopy w/vc inject + scope** ~ endoscopies or minor procedure - E/M services on the same day generally not paid, special rules for multiple endoscopic procedures apply if billed with another endoscopy in the same family, 150% payment adjustment for bilateral procedures does not apply, assistant surgeon may not be paid

31575 **Diagnostic laryngoscopy** ~ endoscopies or minor procedure - E/M services on the same day generally not paid, standard payment adjustment rules for multiple procedures apply, 150% payment adjustment for bilateral procedures does not apply, assistant surgeon may not be paid

31576 **Laryngoscopy with biopsy** ~ endoscopies or minor procedure - E/M services on the same day generally not paid, special rules for multiple endoscopic procedures apply if billed with another endoscopy in the same family, 150% payment adjustment for bilateral procedures does not apply, assistant surgeon may not be paid

31577 **Remove foreign body larynx** ~ endoscopies or minor procedure - E/M services on the same day generally not paid, special rules for multiple endoscopic procedures apply if billed with another endoscopy in the same family, 150% payment adjustment for bilateral procedures does not apply, payment for assistant surgeon subject to documentation of medical necessity

31578 **Remove larynx lesion** ~ endoscopies or minor procedure - E/M services on the same day generally not paid, special rules for multiple endoscopic procedures apply if billed with another endoscopy in the same family, 150% payment adjustment for bilateral procedures does not apply, payment for assistant surgeon subject to documentation of medical necessity

31579 **Diagnostic laryngoscopy** ~ endoscopies or minor procedure - E/M services on the same day generally not paid, special rules for multiple endoscopic

procedures apply if billed with another endoscopy in the same family, 150% payment adjustment for bilateral procedures does not apply, assistant surgeon may not be paid

31580 **Revise larynx** ~ follow-up period is 90 days, standard payment adjustment rules for multiple procedures apply, 150% payment adjustment for bilateral procedures does not apply, assistant surgeon may be paid

31582 **Revise larynx** ~ follow-up period is 90 days, standard payment adjustment rules for multiple procedures apply, 150% payment adjustment for bilateral procedures does not apply, assistant surgeon may not be paid

31584 **Treat larynx fracture** ~ follow-up period is 90 days, standard payment adjustment rules for multiple procedures apply, 150% payment adjustment for bilateral procedures does not apply, assistant surgeon may be paid

31587 **Revise larynx** ~ follow-up period is 90 days, standard payment adjustment rules for multiple procedures apply, 150% payment adjustment for bilateral procedures does not apply, assistant surgeon may be paid

31588 **Revise larynx** ~ follow-up period is 90 days, standard payment adjustment rules for multiple procedures apply, 150% payment adjustment for bilateral procedures does not apply, assistant surgeon may be paid

31590 **Reinnervate larynx** ~ follow-up period is 90 days, standard payment adjustment rules for multiple procedures apply, 150% payment adjustment for bilateral procedures does not apply, assistant surgeon may be paid

31595 **Larynx nerve surgery** ~ follow-up period is 90 days, standard payment adjustment rules for multiple procedures apply, 150% payment adjustment for bilateral procedures does not apply, assistant surgeon may be paid

31599 **Larynx surgery procedure** ~ medicare carrier determines global period, standard payment adjustment rules for multiple procedures apply, 150% payment adjustment for bilateral procedures does not apply, payment for assistant surgeon subject to documentation of medical necessity

Trachea and Bronchi

31600 **Incise windpipe** ~ endoscopies or minor procedure - E/M services on the same day generally not paid, standard payment adjustment rules for multiple procedures apply, 150% payment adjustment for bilateral procedures does not apply, assistant surgeon may not be paid

31601 **Incise windpipe** ~ endoscopies or minor procedure - E/M services on the same day generally not paid, standard payment adjustment rules for multiple procedures apply, 150% payment adjustment for bilateral procedures does not apply, assistant surgeon may be paid

31603   **Incise windpipe**   ~ endoscopies or minor procedure - E/M services on the same day generally not paid, standard payment adjustment rules for multiple procedures apply, 150% payment adjustment for bilateral procedures does not apply, assistant surgeon may not be paid

31605   **Incise windpipe**   ~ endoscopies or minor procedure - E/M services on the same day generally not paid, standard payment adjustment rules for multiple procedures apply, 150% payment adjustment for bilateral procedures does not apply, assistant surgeon may not be paid

31610   **Incise windpipe**   ~ follow-up period is 90 days, standard payment adjustment rules for multiple procedures apply, 150% payment adjustment for bilateral procedures does not apply, assistant surgeon may not be paid

31611   **Surgery/speech prosthesis**   ~ follow-up period is 90 days, standard payment adjustment rules for multiple procedures apply, 150% payment adjustment for bilateral procedures does not apply, assistant surgeon may be paid

31612   **Puncture/clear windpipe**   ~ endoscopies or minor procedure - E/M services on the same day generally not paid, standard payment adjustment rules for multiple procedures apply, 150% payment adjustment for bilateral procedures does not apply, payment for assistant surgeon subject to documentation of medical necessity

31613   **Repair windpipe opening**   ~ follow-up period is 90 days, standard payment adjustment rules for multiple procedures apply, 150% payment adjustment for bilateral procedures does not apply, assistant surgeon may not be paid

31614   **Repair windpipe opening**   ~ follow-up period is 90 days, standard payment adjustment rules for multiple procedures apply, 150% payment adjustment for bilateral procedures does not apply, assistant surgeon may not be paid

31615   **Visualization of windpipe**   ~ endoscopies or minor procedure - E/M services on the same day generally not paid, standard payment adjustment rules for multiple procedures apply, 150% payment adjustment for bilateral procedures does not apply, assistant surgeon may not be paid

31620   **Endobronchial us, add-on**   ~ follow-up period included in another service, no payment adjustment rules for multiple procedures apply, 150% payment adjustment for bilateral procedures does not apply, assistant surgeon may not be paid, +add-on code (list separately in addition to primary procedure)

31622   **Dx bronchoscope/wash**   ~ endoscopies or minor procedure - E/M services on the same day generally not paid, standard payment adjustment rules for multiple procedures apply, 150% payment adjustment for bilateral procedures does not apply, assistant surgeon may not be paid

31623 **Dx bronchoscope/brush** ~ endoscopies or minor procedure - E/M services on the same day generally not paid, special rules for multiple endoscopic procedures apply if billed with another endoscopy in the same family, 150% payment adjustment for bilateral procedures does not apply, assistant surgeon may not be paid

31624 **Dx bronchoscope/lavage** ~ endoscopies or minor procedure - E/M services on the same day generally not paid, special rules for multiple endoscopic procedures apply if billed with another endoscopy in the same family, 150% payment adjustment for bilateral procedures does not apply, assistant surgeon may not be paid

31625 **Bronchoscopy w/biopsy(s)** ~ endoscopies or minor procedure - E/M services on the same day generally not paid, special rules for multiple endoscopic procedures apply if billed with another endoscopy in the same family, 150% payment adjustment for bilateral procedures does not apply, assistant surgeon may not be paid

31628 **Bronchoscopy/lung biopsy, each** ~ endoscopies or minor procedure - E/M services on the same day generally not paid, special rules for multiple endoscopic procedures apply if billed with another endoscopy in the same family, 150% payment adjustment for bilateral procedures does not apply, assistant surgeon may not be paid

31629 **Bronchoscopy/needle biopsy, each** ~ endoscopies or minor procedure - E/M services on the same day generally not paid, special rules for multiple endoscopic procedures apply if billed with another endoscopy in the same family, 150% payment adjustment for bilateral procedures does not apply, assistant surgeon may not be paid

31630 **Bronchoscopy dilate/fracture repair** ~ endoscopies or minor procedure - E/M services on the same day generally not paid, special rules for multiple endoscopic procedures apply if billed with another endoscopy in the same family, 150% payment adjustment for bilateral procedures does not apply, assistant surgeon may not be paid

31631 **Bronchoscopy, dilate w/stent** ~ endoscopies or minor procedure - E/M services on the same day generally not paid, special rules for multiple endoscopic procedures apply if billed with another endoscopy in the same family, 150% payment adjustment for bilateral procedures does not apply, assistant surgeon may not be paid

31632 **Bronchoscopy/lung biopsy, added** ~ follow-up period included in another service, no payment adjustment rules for multiple procedures apply, 150% payment adjustment for bilateral procedures does not apply, assistant surgeon may not be paid, +add-on code (list separately in addition to primary procedure)

31633 **Bronchoscopy/needle biopsy added** ~ follow-up period included in another service, no payment adjustment rules for multiple procedures apply, 150% payment adjustment for bilateral procedures does not apply, assistant surgeon may not be paid, +add-on code (list separately in addition to primary procedure)

31635 **Bronchoscopy w/foreign body remove** ~ endoscopies or minor procedure - E/M services on the same day generally not paid, special rules for multiple endoscopic

procedures apply if billed with another endoscopy in the same family, 150% payment adjustment for bilateral procedures does not apply, assistant surgeon may not be paid

31636 **Bronchoscopy, bronchial stents** ~ endoscopies or minor procedure - E/M services on the same day generally not paid, special rules for multiple endoscopic procedures apply if billed with another endoscopy in the same family, 150% payment adjustment for bilateral procedures does not apply, assistant surgeon may not be paid

31637 **Bronchoscopy, stent, add-on** ~ follow-up period included in another service, no payment adjustment rules for multiple procedures apply, 150% payment adjustment for bilateral procedures does not apply, assistant surgeon may not be paid, +add-on code (list separately in addition to primary procedure)

31638 **Bronchoscopy, revise stent** ~ endoscopies or minor procedure - E/M services on the same day generally not paid, special rules for multiple endoscopic procedures apply if billed with another endoscopy in the same family, 150% payment adjustment for bilateral procedures does not apply, assistant surgeon may not be paid

31640 **Bronchoscopy w/tumor excise** ~ endoscopies or minor procedure - E/M services on the same day generally not paid, special rules for multiple endoscopic procedures apply if billed with another endoscopy in the same family, 150% payment adjustment for bilateral procedures does not apply, assistant surgeon may not be paid

31641 **Bronchoscopy, treat blockage** ~ endoscopies or minor procedure - E/M services on the same day generally not paid, special rules for multiple endoscopic procedures apply if billed with another endoscopy in the same family, 150% payment adjustment for bilateral procedures does not apply, assistant surgeon may not be paid

31643 **Diag bronchoscope/catheter** ~ endoscopies or minor procedure - E/M services on the same day generally not paid, standard payment adjustment rules for multiple procedures apply, 150% payment adjustment for bilateral procedures does not apply, assistant surgeon may not be paid

31645 **Bronchoscopy, clear airways** ~ endoscopies or minor procedure - E/M services on the same day generally not paid, special rules for multiple endoscopic procedures apply if billed with another endoscopy in the same family, 150% payment adjustment for bilateral procedures does not apply, assistant surgeon may not be paid

31646 **Bronchoscopy, reclear airway** ~ endoscopies or minor procedure - E/M services on the same day generally not paid, standard payment adjustment rules for multiple procedures apply, 150% payment adjustment for bilateral procedures does not apply, assistant surgeon may not be paid

31656 **Bronchoscopy, inject for x-ray** ~ endoscopies or minor procedure - E/M services on the same day generally not paid, standard payment adjustment rules for multiple procedures apply, 150% payment adjustment for bilateral procedures does not apply, payment for assistant surgeon subject to documentation of medical necessity

31715   **Inject for bronchus x-ray**   ~ endoscopies or minor procedure - E/M services on the same day generally not paid, standard payment adjustment rules for multiple procedures apply, 150% payment adjustment for bilateral procedures applies, payment for assistant surgeon subject to documentation of medical necessity

31717   **Bronchial brush biopsy**   ~ endoscopies or minor procedure - E/M services on the same day generally not paid, standard payment adjustment rules for multiple procedures apply, 150% payment adjustment for bilateral procedures does not apply, assistant surgeon may not be paid

31720   **Clear airways**   ~ endoscopies or minor procedure - E/M services on the same day generally not paid, standard payment adjustment rules for multiple procedures apply, 150% payment adjustment for bilateral procedures does not apply, assistant surgeon may not be paid

31725   **Clear airways**   ~ endoscopies or minor procedure - E/M services on the same day generally not paid, standard payment adjustment rules for multiple procedures apply, 150% payment adjustment for bilateral procedures does not apply, assistant surgeon may not be paid

31730   **Introduce windpipe wire/tube**   ~ endoscopies or minor procedure - E/M services on the same day generally not paid, standard payment adjustment rules for multiple procedures apply, 150% payment adjustment for bilateral procedures does not apply, assistant surgeon may not be paid

31750   **Repair windpipe**   ~ follow-up period is 90 days, standard payment adjustment rules for multiple procedures apply, 150% payment adjustment for bilateral procedures does not apply, assistant surgeon may be paid

31755   **Repair windpipe**   ~ follow-up period is 90 days, standard payment adjustment rules for multiple procedures apply, 150% payment adjustment for bilateral procedures does not apply, assistant surgeon may be paid

31760   **Repair windpipe**   ~ follow-up period is 90 days, standard payment adjustment rules for multiple procedures apply, 150% payment adjustment for bilateral procedures does not apply, assistant surgeon may be paid

31766   **Reconstruct windpipe**   ~ follow-up period is 90 days, standard payment adjustment rules for multiple procedures apply, 150% payment adjustment for bilateral procedures does not apply, assistant surgeon may be paid

31770   **Repair/graft of bronchus**   ~ follow-up period is 90 days, standard payment adjustment rules for multiple procedures apply, 150% payment adjustment for bilateral procedures does not apply, assistant surgeon may be paid

31775 **Reconstruct bronchus** ~ follow-up period is 90 days, standard payment adjustment rules for multiple procedures apply, 150% payment adjustment for bilateral procedures does not apply, assistant surgeon may be paid

31780 **Reconstruct windpipe** ~ follow-up period is 90 days, standard payment adjustment rules for multiple procedures apply, 150% payment adjustment for bilateral procedures does not apply, assistant surgeon may be paid

31781 **Reconstruct windpipe** ~ follow-up period is 90 days, standard payment adjustment rules for multiple procedures apply, 150% payment adjustment for bilateral procedures does not apply, assistant surgeon may be paid

31785 **Remove windpipe lesion** ~ follow-up period is 90 days, standard payment adjustment rules for multiple procedures apply, 150% payment adjustment for bilateral procedures does not apply, assistant surgeon may be paid

31786 **Remove windpipe lesion** ~ follow-up period is 90 days, standard payment adjustment rules for multiple procedures apply, 150% payment adjustment for bilateral procedures does not apply, assistant surgeon may be paid

31800 **Repair windpipe injury** ~ follow-up period is 90 days, standard payment adjustment rules for multiple procedures apply, 150% payment adjustment for bilateral procedures does not apply, payment for assistant surgeon subject to documentation of medical necessity

31805 **Repair windpipe injury** ~ follow-up period is 90 days, standard payment adjustment rules for multiple procedures apply, 150% payment adjustment for bilateral procedures does not apply, assistant surgeon may be paid

31820 **Closure windpipe lesion** ~ follow-up period is 90 days, standard payment adjustment rules for multiple procedures apply, 150% payment adjustment for bilateral procedures does not apply, payment for assistant surgeon subject to documentation of medical necessity

31825 **Repair windpipe defect** ~ follow-up period is 90 days, standard payment adjustment rules for multiple procedures apply, 150% payment adjustment for bilateral procedures does not apply, payment for assistant surgeon subject to documentation of medical necessity

31830 **Revise windpipe scar** ~ follow-up period is 90 days, standard payment adjustment rules for multiple procedures apply, 150% payment adjustment for bilateral procedures does not apply, payment for assistant surgeon subject to documentation of medical necessity

31899 **Airways surgical procedure** ~ medicare carrier determines global period, standard payment adjustment rules for multiple procedures apply, 150% payment

adjustment for bilateral procedures does not apply, payment for assistant surgeon subject to documentation of medical necessity

Lungs and Pleura

32000   **Drain chest**   ~ endoscopies or minor procedure - E/M services on the same day generally not paid, no payment adjustment rules for multiple procedures apply, 150% payment adjustment for bilateral procedures applies, assistant surgeon may not be paid

32002   **Treat collapsed lung**   ~ endoscopies or minor procedure - E/M services on the same day generally not paid, no payment adjustment rules for multiple procedures apply, 150% payment adjustment for bilateral procedures applies, assistant surgeon may not be paid

32005   **Treat lung lining chemically**   ~ endoscopies or minor procedure - E/M services on the same day generally not paid, standard payment adjustment rules for multiple procedures apply, 150% payment adjustment for bilateral procedures does not apply, assistant surgeon may not be paid

32019   **Insert pleural catheter**   ~ endoscopies or minor procedure - E/M services on the same day generally not paid, no payment adjustment rules for multiple procedures apply, 150% payment adjustment for bilateral procedures does not apply, assistant surgeon may not be paid

32020   **Insert chest tube**   ~ endoscopies or minor procedure - E/M services on the same day generally not paid, no payment adjustment rules for multiple procedures apply, 150% payment adjustment for bilateral procedures applies, assistant surgeon may not be paid

32035   **Explore chest**   ~ follow-up period is 90 days, standard payment adjustment rules for multiple procedures apply, 150% payment adjustment for bilateral procedures does not apply, assistant surgeon may be paid

32036   **Explore chest**   ~ follow-up period is 90 days, standard payment adjustment rules for multiple procedures apply, 150% payment adjustment for bilateral procedures does not apply, assistant surgeon may be paid

32095   **Biopsy through chest wall**   ~ follow-up period is 90 days, standard payment adjustment rules for multiple procedures apply, 150% payment adjustment for bilateral procedures does not apply, assistant surgeon may be paid

32100   **Explore/biopsy chest**   ~ follow-up period is 90 days, standard payment adjustment rules for multiple procedures apply, 150% payment adjustment for bilateral procedures does not apply, assistant surgeon may be paid

32110 **Explore/repair chest** ~ follow-up period is 90 days, standard payment adjustment rules for multiple procedures apply, 150% payment adjustment for bilateral procedures does not apply, assistant surgeon may be paid

32120 **Re-explore chest** ~ follow-up period is 90 days, standard payment adjustment rules for multiple procedures apply, 150% payment adjustment for bilateral procedures does not apply, assistant surgeon may be paid

32124 **Explore chest free adhesions** ~ follow-up period is 90 days, standard payment adjustment rules for multiple procedures apply, 150% payment adjustment for bilateral procedures does not apply, assistant surgeon may be paid

32140 **Remove lung lesion(s)** ~ follow-up period is 90 days, standard payment adjustment rules for multiple procedures apply, 150% payment adjustment for bilateral procedures does not apply, assistant surgeon may be paid

32141 **Remove/treat lung lesions** ~ follow-up period is 90 days, standard payment adjustment rules for multiple procedures apply, 150% payment adjustment for bilateral procedures does not apply, assistant surgeon may be paid

32150 **Remove lung lesion(s)** ~ follow-up period is 90 days, standard payment adjustment rules for multiple procedures apply, 150% payment adjustment for bilateral procedures does not apply, assistant surgeon may be paid

32151 **Remove lung foreign body** ~ follow-up period is 90 days, standard payment adjustment rules for multiple procedures apply, 150% payment adjustment for bilateral procedures does not apply, assistant surgeon may be paid

32160 **Open chest heart massage** ~ follow-up period is 90 days, standard payment adjustment rules for multiple procedures apply, 150% payment adjustment for bilateral procedures does not apply, assistant surgeon may be paid

32200 **Drain, open, lung lesion** ~ follow-up period is 90 days, standard payment adjustment rules for multiple procedures apply, 150% payment adjustment for bilateral procedures does not apply, assistant surgeon may be paid

32201 **Drain, percutaneous, lung lesion** ~ endoscopies or minor procedure - E/M services on the same day generally not paid, standard payment adjustment rules for multiple procedures apply, 150% payment adjustment for bilateral procedures does not apply, assistant surgeon may be paid

32215 **Treat chest lining** ~ follow-up period is 90 days, standard payment adjustment rules for multiple procedures apply, 150% payment adjustment for bilateral procedures does not apply, assistant surgeon may be paid

32220   **Release lung**   ~ follow-up period is 90 days, standard payment adjustment rules for multiple procedures apply, 150% payment adjustment for bilateral procedures does not apply, assistant surgeon may be paid

32225   **Partial release lung**   ~ follow-up period is 90 days, standard payment adjustment rules for multiple procedures apply, 150% payment adjustment for bilateral procedures does not apply, assistant surgeon may be paid

32310   **Remove chest lining**   ~ follow-up period is 90 days, standard payment adjustment rules for multiple procedures apply, 150% payment adjustment for bilateral procedures does not apply, assistant surgeon may be paid

32320   **Free/remove chest lining**   ~ follow-up period is 90 days, standard payment adjustment rules for multiple procedures apply, 150% payment adjustment for bilateral procedures does not apply, assistant surgeon may be paid

32400   **Needle biopsy chest lining**   ~ endoscopies or minor procedure - E/M services on the same day generally not paid, standard payment adjustment rules for multiple procedures apply, 150% payment adjustment for bilateral procedures does not apply, assistant surgeon may not be paid

32402   **Open biopsy chest lining**   ~ follow-up period is 90 days, standard payment adjustment rules for multiple procedures apply, 150% payment adjustment for bilateral procedures does not apply, assistant surgeon may be paid

32405   **Biopsy lung or mediastinum**   ~ endoscopies or minor procedure - E/M services on the same day generally not paid, standard payment adjustment rules for multiple procedures apply, 150% payment adjustment for bilateral procedures does not apply, assistant surgeon may not be paid

32420   **Puncture/clear lung**   ~ endoscopies or minor procedure - E/M services on the same day generally not paid, standard payment adjustment rules for multiple procedures apply, 150% payment adjustment for bilateral procedures does not apply, assistant surgeon may be paid

32440   **Remove lung**   ~ follow-up period is 90 days, standard payment adjustment rules for multiple procedures apply, 150% payment adjustment for bilateral procedures does not apply, assistant surgeon may be paid

32442   **Sleeve pneumonectomy**   ~ follow-up period is 90 days, standard payment adjustment rules for multiple procedures apply, 150% payment adjustment for bilateral procedures does not apply, assistant surgeon may be paid

32445   **Remove lung**   ~ follow-up period is 90 days, standard payment adjustment rules for multiple procedures apply, 150% payment adjustment for bilateral procedures does not apply, assistant surgeon may be paid

32480   **Partial remove lung**   ~ follow-up period is 90 days, standard payment adjustment rules for multiple procedures apply, 150% payment adjustment for bilateral procedures does not apply, assistant surgeon may be paid

32482   **Bilobectomy**   ~ follow-up period is 90 days, standard payment adjustment rules for multiple procedures apply, 150% payment adjustment for bilateral procedures does not apply, assistant surgeon may be paid

32484   **Segmentectomy**   ~ follow-up period is 90 days, standard payment adjustment rules for multiple procedures apply, 150% payment adjustment for bilateral procedures does not apply, assistant surgeon may be paid

32486   **Sleeve lobectomy**   ~ follow-up period is 90 days, standard payment adjustment rules for multiple procedures apply, 150% payment adjustment for bilateral procedures does not apply, assistant surgeon may be paid

32488   **Completion pneumonectomy**   ~ follow-up period is 90 days, standard payment adjustment rules for multiple procedures apply, 150% payment adjustment for bilateral procedures does not apply, assistant surgeon may be paid

32491   **Lung volume reduction**   ~ restricted coverage - special coverage rules apply, follow-up period is 90 days, standard payment adjustment rules for multiple procedures apply, 150% payment adjustment for bilateral procedures applies, assistant surgeon may be paid

32500   **Partial remove lung**   ~ follow-up period is 90 days, standard payment adjustment rules for multiple procedures apply, 150% payment adjustment for bilateral procedures does not apply, assistant surgeon may be paid

32501   **Repair bronchus, add-on**   ~ follow-up period included in another service, no payment adjustment rules for multiple procedures apply, 150% payment adjustment for bilateral procedures does not apply, assistant surgeon may be paid, +add-on code (list separately in addition to primary procedure)

32503   **Resect apical lung tumor**   ~ follow-up period is 90 days, standard payment adjustment rules for multiple procedures apply, 150% payment adjustment for bilateral procedures does not apply, assistant surgeon may be paid

32504   **Resect apical lung tumor/chest**   ~ follow-up period is 90 days, standard payment adjustment rules for multiple procedures apply, 150% payment adjustment for bilateral procedures does not apply, assistant surgeon may be paid

32540   **Remove lung lesion**   ~ follow-up period is 90 days, standard payment adjustment rules for multiple procedures apply, 150% payment adjustment for bilateral procedures does not apply, assistant surgeon may be paid

32601   **Thoracoscopy, diagnostic**   ~ endoscopies or minor procedure - E/M services on the same day generally not paid, standard payment adjustment rules for multiple procedures apply, 150% payment adjustment for bilateral procedures does not apply, payment for assistant surgeon subject to documentation of medical necessity

32602   **Thoracoscopy, diagnostic**   ~ endoscopies or minor procedure - E/M services on the same day generally not paid, standard payment adjustment rules for multiple procedures apply, 150% payment adjustment for bilateral procedures does not apply, payment for assistant surgeon subject to documentation of medical necessity

32603   **Thoracoscopy, diagnostic**   ~ endoscopies or minor procedure - E/M services on the same day generally not paid, standard payment adjustment rules for multiple procedures apply, 150% payment adjustment for bilateral procedures does not apply, payment for assistant surgeon subject to documentation of medical necessity

32604   **Thoracoscopy, diagnostic**   ~ endoscopies or minor procedure - E/M services on the same day generally not paid, standard payment adjustment rules for multiple procedures apply, 150% payment adjustment for bilateral procedures does not apply, payment for assistant surgeon subject to documentation of medical necessity

32605   **Thoracoscopy, diagnostic**   ~ endoscopies or minor procedure - E/M services on the same day generally not paid, standard payment adjustment rules for multiple procedures apply, 150% payment adjustment for bilateral procedures does not apply, payment for assistant surgeon subject to documentation of medical necessity

32606   **Thoracoscopy, diagnostic**   ~ endoscopies or minor procedure - E/M services on the same day generally not paid, standard payment adjustment rules for multiple procedures apply, 150% payment adjustment for bilateral procedures does not apply, payment for assistant surgeon subject to documentation of medical necessity

32650   **Thoracoscopy, surgical**   ~ follow-up period is 90 days, standard payment adjustment rules for multiple procedures apply, 150% payment adjustment for bilateral procedures does not apply, assistant surgeon may be paid

32651   **Thoracoscopy, surgical**   ~ follow-up period is 90 days, standard payment adjustment rules for multiple procedures apply, 150% payment adjustment for bilateral procedures does not apply, assistant surgeon may be paid

32652   **Thoracoscopy, surgical**   ~ follow-up period is 90 days, standard payment adjustment rules for multiple procedures apply, 150% payment adjustment for bilateral procedures does not apply, assistant surgeon may be paid

32653   **Thoracoscopy, surgical**   ~ follow-up period is 90 days, standard payment adjustment rules for multiple procedures apply, 150% payment adjustment for bilateral procedures does not apply, assistant surgeon may be paid

32654   **Thoracoscopy, surgical** ~ follow-up period is 90 days, standard payment adjustment rules for multiple procedures apply, 150% payment adjustment for bilateral procedures does not apply, assistant surgeon may be paid

32655   **Thoracoscopy, surgical** ~ follow-up period is 90 days, standard payment adjustment rules for multiple procedures apply, 150% payment adjustment for bilateral procedures does not apply, assistant surgeon may be paid

32656   **Thoracoscopy, surgical** ~ follow-up period is 90 days, standard payment adjustment rules for multiple procedures apply, 150% payment adjustment for bilateral procedures does not apply, assistant surgeon may be paid

32657   **Thoracoscopy, surgical** ~ follow-up period is 90 days, standard payment adjustment rules for multiple procedures apply, 150% payment adjustment for bilateral procedures does not apply, assistant surgeon may be paid

32658   **Thoracoscopy, surgical** ~ follow-up period is 90 days, standard payment adjustment rules for multiple procedures apply, 150% payment adjustment for bilateral procedures does not apply, assistant surgeon may be paid

32659   **Thoracoscopy, surgical** ~ follow-up period is 90 days, standard payment adjustment rules for multiple procedures apply, 150% payment adjustment for bilateral procedures does not apply, assistant surgeon may be paid

32660   **Thoracoscopy, surgical** ~ follow-up period is 90 days, standard payment adjustment rules for multiple procedures apply, 150% payment adjustment for bilateral procedures does not apply, assistant surgeon may be paid

32661   **Thoracoscopy, surgical** ~ follow-up period is 90 days, standard payment adjustment rules for multiple procedures apply, 150% payment adjustment for bilateral procedures does not apply, assistant surgeon may be paid

32662   **Thoracoscopy, surgical** ~ follow-up period is 90 days, standard payment adjustment rules for multiple procedures apply, 150% payment adjustment for bilateral procedures does not apply, assistant surgeon may be paid

32663   **Thoracoscopy, surgical** ~ follow-up period is 90 days, standard payment adjustment rules for multiple procedures apply, 150% payment adjustment for bilateral procedures does not apply, assistant surgeon may be paid

32664   **Thoracoscopy, surgical** ~ follow-up period is 90 days, standard payment adjustment rules for multiple procedures apply, 150% payment adjustment for bilateral procedures applies, assistant surgeon may be paid

32665   **Thoracoscopy, surgical** ~ follow-up period is 90 days, standard payment adjustment rules for multiple procedures apply, 150% payment adjustment for bilateral procedures does not apply, assistant surgeon may be paid

32800 **Repair lung hernia**   ~ follow-up period is 90 days, standard payment adjustment rules for multiple procedures apply, 150% payment adjustment for bilateral procedures does not apply, assistant surgeon may be paid

32810 **Close chest after drainage**   ~ follow-up period is 90 days, standard payment adjustment rules for multiple procedures apply, 150% payment adjustment for bilateral procedures does not apply, assistant surgeon may be paid

32815 **Close bronchial fistula**   ~ follow-up period is 90 days, standard payment adjustment rules for multiple procedures apply, 150% payment adjustment for bilateral procedures does not apply, assistant surgeon may be paid

32820 **Reconstruct injured chest**   ~ follow-up period is 90 days, standard payment adjustment rules for multiple procedures apply, 150% payment adjustment for bilateral procedures does not apply, assistant surgeon may be paid

32850 **Donor pneumonectomy**   ~ multiple procedure concept does not apply, bilateral surgery concept does not apply, assistant surgery concept does not apply

32851 **Lung transplant, single**   ~ follow-up period is 90 days, standard payment adjustment rules for multiple procedures apply, 150% payment adjustment for bilateral procedures does not apply, assistant surgeon may be paid

32852 **Lung transplant with bypass**   ~ follow-up period is 90 days, standard payment adjustment rules for multiple procedures apply, 150% payment adjustment for bilateral procedures does not apply, assistant surgeon may be paid

32853 **Lung transplant, double**   ~ follow-up period is 90 days, standard payment adjustment rules for multiple procedures apply, 150% payment adjustment does not apply - RVUs based on bilateral procedure, assistant surgeon may be paid

32854 **Lung transplant with bypass**   ~ follow-up period is 90 days, standard payment adjustment rules for multiple procedures apply, 150% payment adjustment does not apply - RVUs based on bilateral procedure, assistant surgeon may be paid

32855 **Prepare donor lung, single**   ~ standard payment adjustment rules for multiple procedures apply, 150% payment adjustment for bilateral procedures does not apply, assistant surgeon may be paid

32856 **Prepare donor lung, double**   ~ standard payment adjustment rules for multiple procedures apply, 150% payment adjustment for bilateral procedures does not apply, assistant surgeon may be paid

32900 **Remove rib(s)**   ~ follow-up period is 90 days, standard payment adjustment rules for multiple procedures apply, 150% payment adjustment for bilateral procedures does not apply, assistant surgeon may be paid

32905   **Revise & repair chest wall**   ~ follow-up period is 90 days, standard payment adjustment rules for multiple procedures apply, 150% payment adjustment for bilateral procedures does not apply, assistant surgeon may be paid

32906   **Revise & repair chest wall**   ~ follow-up period is 90 days, standard payment adjustment rules for multiple procedures apply, 150% payment adjustment for bilateral procedures does not apply, assistant surgeon may be paid

32940   **Revise lung**   ~ follow-up period is 90 days, standard payment adjustment rules for multiple procedures apply, 150% payment adjustment for bilateral procedures does not apply, assistant surgeon may be paid

32960   **Therapeutic pneumothorax**   ~ endoscopies or minor procedure - E/M services on the same day generally not paid, standard payment adjustment rules for multiple procedures apply, 150% payment adjustment for bilateral procedures does not apply, assistant surgeon may not be paid

32997   **Total lung lavage**   ~ endoscopies or minor procedure - E/M services on the same day generally not paid, standard payment adjustment rules for multiple procedures apply, 150% payment adjustment for bilateral procedures does not apply, assistant surgeon may not be paid

32998   **Percutaneous rf ablate tx, pulmonary tumor** ~ endoscopies or minor procedure - E/M services on the same day generally not paid, standard payment adjustment rules for multiple procedures apply, 150% payment adjustment for bilateral procedures does not apply, assistant surgeon may be paid

32999   **Chest surgery procedure**   ~ medicare carrier determines global period, standard payment adjustment rules for multiple procedures apply, 150% payment adjustment for bilateral procedures does not apply, assistant surgeon may be paid

CARDIOVASCULAR SYSTEM

Heart and Pericardium

33010   **Drain heart sac**   ~ endoscopies or minor procedure - E/M services on the same day generally not paid, standard payment adjustment rules for multiple procedures apply, 150% payment adjustment for bilateral procedures does not apply, assistant surgeon may not be paid

33011   **Repeat drain heart sac**   ~ endoscopies or minor procedure - E/M services on the same day generally not paid, standard payment adjustment rules for multiple procedures apply, 150% payment adjustment for bilateral procedures does not apply, payment for assistant surgeon subject to documentation of medical necessity

33015   **Incise heart sac**   ~ follow-up period is 90 days, standard payment adjustment rules for multiple procedures apply, 150% payment adjustment for bilateral procedures does not apply, assistant surgeon may not be paid

33020   **Incise heart sac**   ~ follow-up period is 90 days, standard payment adjustment rules for multiple procedures apply, 150% payment adjustment for bilateral procedures does not apply, assistant surgeon may be paid

33025   **Incise heart sac**   ~ follow-up period is 90 days, standard payment adjustment rules for multiple procedures apply, 150% payment adjustment for bilateral procedures does not apply, assistant surgeon may be paid

33030   **Partial remove heart sac**   ~ follow-up period is 90 days, standard payment adjustment rules for multiple procedures apply, 150% payment adjustment for bilateral procedures does not apply, assistant surgeon may be paid

33031   **Partial remove heart sac**   ~ follow-up period is 90 days, standard payment adjustment rules for multiple procedures apply, 150% payment adjustment for bilateral procedures does not apply, assistant surgeon may be paid

33050   **Remove heart sac lesion**   ~ follow-up period is 90 days, standard payment adjustment rules for multiple procedures apply, 150% payment adjustment for bilateral procedures does not apply, assistant surgeon may be paid

33120   **Remove heart lesion**   ~ follow-up period is 90 days, standard payment adjustment rules for multiple procedures apply, 150% payment adjustment for bilateral procedures does not apply, assistant surgeon may be paid

33130   **Remove heart lesion**   ~ follow-up period is 90 days, standard payment adjustment rules for multiple procedures apply, 150% payment adjustment for bilateral procedures does not apply, assistant surgeon may be paid

33140   **Heart revascularize (tmr)**   ~ follow-up period is 90 days, standard payment adjustment rules for multiple procedures apply, 150% payment adjustment for bilateral procedures does not apply, assistant surgeon may be paid

33141   **Heart tmr w/other procedure**   ~ follow-up period included in another service, no payment adjustment rules for multiple procedures apply, 150% payment adjustment for bilateral procedures does not apply, assistant surgeon may be paid

33202   **Insert epicardial electrode, open**   ~ follow-up period is 90 days, standard payment adjustment rules for multiple procedures apply, 150% payment adjustment for bilateral procedures does not apply, assistant surgeon may not be paid

33203   **Insert epicardial electrode, endo**   ~ follow-up period is 90 days, standard payment adjustment rules for multiple procedures apply, 150% payment adjustment for bilateral procedures does not apply, assistant surgeon may not be paid

---

33206   **Insert heart pacemaker**   ~ follow-up period is 90 days, standard payment adjustment rules for multiple procedures apply, 150% payment adjustment for bilateral procedures does not apply, assistant surgeon may not be paid

33207   **Insert heart pacemaker**   ~ follow-up period is 90 days, standard payment adjustment rules for multiple procedures apply, 150% payment adjustment for bilateral procedures does not apply, assistant surgeon may not be paid

33208   **Insert heart pacemaker**   ~ follow-up period is 90 days, standard payment adjustment rules for multiple procedures apply, 150% payment adjustment for bilateral procedures does not apply, assistant surgeon may not be paid

33210   **Insert heart electrode**   ~ endoscopies or minor procedure - E/M services on the same day generally not paid, standard payment adjustment rules for multiple procedures apply, 150% payment adjustment for bilateral procedures does not apply, assistant surgeon may not be paid

33211   **Insert heart electrode**   ~ endoscopies or minor procedure - E/M services on the same day generally not paid, standard payment adjustment rules for multiple procedures apply, 150% payment adjustment for bilateral procedures does not apply, assistant surgeon may not be paid

33212   **Insert pulse generator**   ~ follow-up period is 90 days, standard payment adjustment rules for multiple procedures apply, 150% payment adjustment for bilateral procedures does not apply, assistant surgeon may not be paid

33213   **Insert pulse generator**   ~ follow-up period is 90 days, standard payment adjustment rules for multiple procedures apply, 150% payment adjustment for bilateral procedures does not apply, assistant surgeon may not be paid

33214   **Upgrade of pacemaker system**   ~ follow-up period is 90 days, standard payment adjustment rules for multiple procedures apply, 150% payment adjustment for bilateral procedures does not apply, payment for assistant surgeon subject to documentation of medical necessity

33215   **Reposition pacing-defib lead**   ~ follow-up period is 90 days, standard payment adjustment rules for multiple procedures apply, 150% payment adjustment for bilateral procedures does not apply, assistant surgeon may not be paid

33216   **Insert lead pace-defib, one**   ~ follow-up period is 90 days, standard payment adjustment rules for multiple procedures apply, 150% payment adjustment for bilateral procedures does not apply, assistant surgeon may not be paid

33217   **Insert lead pace-defib, dual**   ~ follow-up period is 90 days, standard payment adjustment rules for multiple procedures apply, 150% payment adjustment for bilateral procedures does not apply, assistant surgeon may not be paid

33218   **Repair lead pace-defib, one**   ~ follow-up period is 90 days, standard payment adjustment rules for multiple procedures apply, 150% payment adjustment for bilateral procedures does not apply, assistant surgeon may not be paid

33220   **Repair lead pace-defib, dual**   ~ follow-up period is 90 days, standard payment adjustment rules for multiple procedures apply, 150% payment adjustment for bilateral procedures does not apply, assistant surgeon may not be paid

33222   **Revise pocket, pacemaker**   ~ follow-up period is 90 days, standard payment adjustment rules for multiple procedures apply, 150% payment adjustment for bilateral procedures does not apply, assistant surgeon may not be paid

33223   **Revise pocket, pacing-defib**   ~ follow-up period is 90 days, standard payment adjustment rules for multiple procedures apply, 150% payment adjustment for bilateral procedures does not apply, payment for assistant surgeon subject to documentation of medical necessity

33224   **Insert pacing lead & connect**   ~ endoscopies or minor procedure - E/M services on the same day generally not paid, standard payment adjustment rules for multiple procedures apply, 150% payment adjustment for bilateral procedures does not apply, assistant surgeon may not be paid

33225   **Left ventricle pacing lead, add-on**   ~ follow-up period included in another service, no payment adjustment rules for multiple procedures apply, 150% payment adjustment for bilateral procedures does not apply, assistant surgeon may not be paid, +add-on code (list separately in addition to primary procedure)

33226   **Reposition left ventricle lead**   ~ endoscopies or minor procedure - E/M services on the same day generally not paid, standard payment adjustment rules for multiple procedures apply, 150% payment adjustment for bilateral procedures does not apply, assistant surgeon may not be paid

33233   **Remove pacemaker system**   ~ follow-up period is 90 days, standard payment adjustment rules for multiple procedures apply, 150% payment adjustment for bilateral procedures does not apply, assistant surgeon may not be paid

33234   **Remove pacemaker system**   ~ follow-up period is 90 days, standard payment adjustment rules for multiple procedures apply, 150% payment adjustment for bilateral procedures does not apply, assistant surgeon may not be paid

33235   **Remove pacemaker electrode**   ~ follow-up period is 90 days, standard payment adjustment rules for multiple procedures apply, 150% payment adjustment for bilateral procedures does not apply, assistant surgeon may not be paid

33236   **Remove electrode/thoracotomy**   ~ follow-up period is 90 days, standard payment adjustment rules for multiple procedures apply, 150% payment adjustment for

bilateral procedures does not apply, payment for assistant surgeon subject to documentation of medical necessity

33237 **Remove electrode/thoracotomy** ~ follow-up period is 90 days, standard payment adjustment rules for multiple procedures apply, 150% payment adjustment for bilateral procedures does not apply, payment for assistant surgeon subject to documentation of medical necessity

33238 **Remove electrode/thoracotomy** ~ follow-up period is 90 days, standard payment adjustment rules for multiple procedures apply, 150% payment adjustment for bilateral procedures does not apply, payment for assistant surgeon subject to documentation of medical necessity

33240 **Insert pulse generator** ~ follow-up period is 90 days, standard payment adjustment rules for multiple procedures apply, 150% payment adjustment for bilateral procedures does not apply, assistant surgeon may not be paid

33241 **Remove pulse generator** ~ follow-up period is 90 days, standard payment adjustment rules for multiple procedures apply, 150% payment adjustment for bilateral procedures does not apply, payment for assistant surgeon subject to documentation of medical necessity

33243 **Remove electrode/thoracotomy** ~ follow-up period is 90 days, standard payment adjustment rules for multiple procedures apply, 150% payment adjustment for bilateral procedures does not apply, assistant surgeon may be paid

33244 **Remove electrode, transvenous** ~ follow-up period is 90 days, standard payment adjustment rules for multiple procedures apply, 150% payment adjustment for bilateral procedures does not apply, assistant surgeon may not be paid

33249 **Electrode/insert pace-defib** ~ follow-up period is 90 days, standard payment adjustment rules for multiple procedures apply, 150% payment adjustment for bilateral procedures does not apply, assistant surgeon may not be paid

33250 **Ablate heart dysrhythm focus** ~ follow-up period is 90 days, standard payment adjustment rules for multiple procedures apply, 150% payment adjustment for bilateral procedures does not apply, assistant surgeon may be paid

33251 **Ablate heart dysrhythm focus** ~ follow-up period is 90 days, standard payment adjustment rules for multiple procedures apply, 150% payment adjustment for bilateral procedures does not apply, assistant surgeon may be paid

33254 **Ablate atria, limited** ~ follow-up period is 90 days, standard payment adjustment rules for multiple procedures apply, 150% payment adjustment for bilateral procedures does not apply, assistant surgeon may be paid

33255   **Ablate atria w/o bypass, ext**   ~ follow-up period is 90 days, standard payment adjustment rules for multiple procedures apply, 150% payment adjustment for bilateral procedures does not apply, assistant surgeon may be paid

33256   **Ablate atria w/bypass, extensive**   ~ follow-up period is 90 days, standard payment adjustment rules for multiple procedures apply, 150% payment adjustment for bilateral procedures does not apply, assistant surgeon may be paid

33261   **Ablate heart dysrhythm focus**   ~ follow-up period is 90 days, standard payment adjustment rules for multiple procedures apply, 150% payment adjustment for bilateral procedures does not apply, assistant surgeon may be paid

33265   **Ablate atria w/bypass, endo**   ~ follow-up period is 90 days, standard payment adjustment rules for multiple procedures apply, 150% payment adjustment for bilateral procedures does not apply, assistant surgeon may be paid

33266   **Ablate atria w/o bypass endo**   ~ follow-up period is 90 days, standard payment adjustment rules for multiple procedures apply, 150% payment adjustment for bilateral procedures does not apply, assistant surgeon may be paid

33282   **Implant pat-active heart record**   ~ follow-up period is 90 days, standard payment adjustment rules for multiple procedures apply, 150% payment adjustment for bilateral procedures does not apply, assistant surgeon may not be paid

33284   **Remove pat-active heart record**   ~ follow-up period is 90 days, standard payment adjustment rules for multiple procedures apply, 150% payment adjustment for bilateral procedures does not apply, assistant surgeon may not be paid

33300   **Repair heart wound**   ~ follow-up period is 90 days, standard payment adjustment rules for multiple procedures apply, 150% payment adjustment for bilateral procedures does not apply, assistant surgeon may be paid

33305   **Repair heart wound**   ~ follow-up period is 90 days, standard payment adjustment rules for multiple procedures apply, 150% payment adjustment for bilateral procedures does not apply, assistant surgeon may be paid

33310   **Exploratory heart surgery**   ~ follow-up period is 90 days, standard payment adjustment rules for multiple procedures apply, 150% payment adjustment for bilateral procedures does not apply, assistant surgeon may be paid

33315   **Exploratory heart surgery**   ~ follow-up period is 90 days, standard payment adjustment rules for multiple procedures apply, 150% payment adjustment for bilateral procedures does not apply, assistant surgeon may be paid

33320   **Repair major blood vessel(s)**   ~ follow-up period is 90 days, standard payment adjustment rules for multiple procedures apply, 150% payment adjustment for bilateral procedures does not apply, assistant surgeon may be paid

33321   **Repair major vessel**   ~ follow-up period is 90 days, standard payment adjustment rules for multiple procedures apply, 150% payment adjustment for bilateral procedures does not apply, assistant surgeon may be paid

33322   **Repair major blood vessel(s)**   ~ follow-up period is 90 days, standard payment adjustment rules for multiple procedures apply, 150% payment adjustment for bilateral procedures does not apply, assistant surgeon may be paid

33330   **Insert major vessel graft**   ~ follow-up period is 90 days, standard payment adjustment rules for multiple procedures apply, 150% payment adjustment for bilateral procedures does not apply, assistant surgeon may be paid

33332   **Insert major vessel graft**   ~ follow-up period is 90 days, standard payment adjustment rules for multiple procedures apply, 150% payment adjustment for bilateral procedures does not apply, assistant surgeon may be paid

33335   **Insert major vessel graft**   ~ follow-up period is 90 days, standard payment adjustment rules for multiple procedures apply, 150% payment adjustment for bilateral procedures does not apply, assistant surgeon may be paid

33400   **Repair aortic valve**   ~ follow-up period is 90 days, standard payment adjustment rules for multiple procedures apply, 150% payment adjustment for bilateral procedures does not apply, assistant surgeon may be paid

33401   **Valvuloplasty, open**   ~ follow-up period is 90 days, standard payment adjustment rules for multiple procedures apply, 150% payment adjustment for bilateral procedures does not apply, assistant surgeon may be paid

33403   **Valvuloplasty, w/cp bypass**   ~ follow-up period is 90 days, standard payment adjustment rules for multiple procedures apply, 150% payment adjustment for bilateral procedures does not apply, assistant surgeon may be paid

33404   **Prepare heart-aorta conduit**   ~ follow-up period is 90 days, standard payment adjustment rules for multiple procedures apply, 150% payment adjustment for bilateral procedures does not apply, assistant surgeon may be paid

33405   **Replace aortic valve**   ~ follow-up period is 90 days, standard payment adjustment rules for multiple procedures apply, 150% payment adjustment for bilateral procedures does not apply, assistant surgeon may be paid

33406   **Replace aortic valve**   ~ follow-up period is 90 days, standard payment adjustment rules for multiple procedures apply, 150% payment adjustment for bilateral procedures does not apply, assistant surgeon may be paid

33410   **Replace aortic valve**   ~ follow-up period is 90 days, standard payment adjustment rules for multiple procedures apply, 150% payment adjustment for bilateral procedures does not apply, assistant surgeon may be paid

33411   **Replace aortic valve**   ~ follow-up period is 90 days, standard payment adjustment rules for multiple procedures apply, 150% payment adjustment for bilateral procedures does not apply, assistant surgeon may be paid

33412   **Replace aortic valve**   ~ follow-up period is 90 days, standard payment adjustment rules for multiple procedures apply, 150% payment adjustment for bilateral procedures does not apply, assistant surgeon may be paid

33413   **Replace aortic valve**   ~ follow-up period is 90 days, standard payment adjustment rules for multiple procedures apply, 150% payment adjustment for bilateral procedures does not apply, assistant surgeon may be paid

33414   **Repair aortic valve**   ~ follow-up period is 90 days, standard payment adjustment rules for multiple procedures apply, 150% payment adjustment for bilateral procedures does not apply, assistant surgeon may be paid

33415   **Revise subvalvular tissue**   ~ follow-up period is 90 days, standard payment adjustment rules for multiple procedures apply, 150% payment adjustment for bilateral procedures does not apply, assistant surgeon may be paid

33416   **Revise ventricle muscle**   ~ follow-up period is 90 days, standard payment adjustment rules for multiple procedures apply, 150% payment adjustment for bilateral procedures does not apply, assistant surgeon may be paid

33417   **Repair aortic valve**   ~ follow-up period is 90 days, standard payment adjustment rules for multiple procedures apply, 150% payment adjustment for bilateral procedures does not apply, assistant surgeon may be paid

33420   **Revise mitral valve**   ~ follow-up period is 90 days, standard payment adjustment rules for multiple procedures apply, 150% payment adjustment for bilateral procedures does not apply, assistant surgeon may not be paid

33422   **Revise mitral valve**   ~ follow-up period is 90 days, standard payment adjustment rules for multiple procedures apply, 150% payment adjustment for bilateral procedures does not apply, assistant surgeon may be paid

33425   **Repair mitral valve**   ~ follow-up period is 90 days, standard payment adjustment rules for multiple procedures apply, 150% payment adjustment for bilateral procedures does not apply, assistant surgeon may be paid

33426   **Repair mitral valve**   ~ follow-up period is 90 days, standard payment adjustment rules for multiple procedures apply, 150% payment adjustment for bilateral procedures does not apply, assistant surgeon may be paid

33427   **Repair mitral valve**   ~ follow-up period is 90 days, standard payment adjustment rules for multiple procedures apply, 150% payment adjustment for bilateral procedures does not apply, assistant surgeon may be paid

33430   **Replace mitral valve**   ~ follow-up period is 90 days, standard payment adjustment rules for multiple procedures apply, 150% payment adjustment for bilateral procedures does not apply, assistant surgeon may be paid

33460   **Revise tricuspid valve**   ~ follow-up period is 90 days, standard payment adjustment rules for multiple procedures apply, 150% payment adjustment for bilateral procedures does not apply, assistant surgeon may be paid

33463   **Valvuloplasty, tricuspid**   ~ follow-up period is 90 days, standard payment adjustment rules for multiple procedures apply, 150% payment adjustment for bilateral procedures does not apply, assistant surgeon may be paid

33464   **Valvuloplasty, tricuspid**   ~ follow-up period is 90 days, standard payment adjustment rules for multiple procedures apply, 150% payment adjustment for bilateral procedures does not apply, assistant surgeon may be paid

33465   **Replace tricuspid valve**   ~ follow-up period is 90 days, standard payment adjustment rules for multiple procedures apply, 150% payment adjustment for bilateral procedures does not apply, assistant surgeon may be paid

33468   **Revise tricuspid valve**   ~ follow-up period is 90 days, standard payment adjustment rules for multiple procedures apply, 150% payment adjustment for bilateral procedures does not apply, assistant surgeon may be paid

33470   **Revise pulmonary valve**   ~ follow-up period is 90 days, standard payment adjustment rules for multiple procedures apply, 150% payment adjustment for bilateral procedures does not apply, assistant surgeon may be paid

33471   **Valvotomy, pulmonary valve**   ~ follow-up period is 90 days, standard payment adjustment rules for multiple procedures apply, 150% payment adjustment for bilateral procedures does not apply, assistant surgeon may be paid

33472   **Revise pulmonary valve**   ~ follow-up period is 90 days, standard payment adjustment rules for multiple procedures apply, 150% payment adjustment for bilateral procedures does not apply, assistant surgeon may be paid

33474   **Revise pulmonary valve**   ~ follow-up period is 90 days, standard payment adjustment rules for multiple procedures apply, 150% payment adjustment for bilateral procedures does not apply, assistant surgeon may be paid

33475   **Replacement, pulmonary valve**   ~ follow-up period is 90 days, standard payment adjustment rules for multiple procedures apply, 150% payment adjustment for bilateral procedures does not apply, assistant surgeon may be paid

33476   **Revise heart chamber**   ~ follow-up period is 90 days, standard payment adjustment rules for multiple procedures apply, 150% payment adjustment for bilateral procedures does not apply, assistant surgeon may be paid

33478   **Revise heart chamber**   ~ follow-up period is 90 days, standard payment adjustment rules for multiple procedures apply, 150% payment adjustment for bilateral procedures does not apply, assistant surgeon may be paid

33496   **Repair, prosth valve clot**   ~ follow-up period is 90 days, standard payment adjustment rules for multiple procedures apply, 150% payment adjustment for bilateral procedures does not apply, assistant surgeon may be paid

33500   **Repair heart vessel fistula**   ~ follow-up period is 90 days, standard payment adjustment rules for multiple procedures apply, 150% payment adjustment for bilateral procedures does not apply, assistant surgeon may be paid

33501   **Repair heart vessel fistula**   ~ follow-up period is 90 days, standard payment adjustment rules for multiple procedures apply, 150% payment adjustment for bilateral procedures does not apply, assistant surgeon may be paid

33502   **Coronary artery correct**   ~ follow-up period is 90 days, standard payment adjustment rules for multiple procedures apply, 150% payment adjustment for bilateral procedures does not apply, assistant surgeon may be paid

33503   **Coronary artery graft**   ~ follow-up period is 90 days, standard payment adjustment rules for multiple procedures apply, 150% payment adjustment for bilateral procedures does not apply, payment for assistant surgeon subject to documentation of medical necessity

33504   **Coronary artery graft**   ~ follow-up period is 90 days, standard payment adjustment rules for multiple procedures apply, 150% payment adjustment for bilateral procedures does not apply, assistant surgeon may be paid

33505   **Repair artery w/tunnel**   ~ follow-up period is 90 days, standard payment adjustment rules for multiple procedures apply, 150% payment adjustment for bilateral procedures does not apply, assistant surgeon may be paid

33506   **Repair artery, translocation**   ~ follow-up period is 90 days, standard payment adjustment rules for multiple procedures apply, 150% payment adjustment for bilateral procedures does not apply, assistant surgeon may be paid

33507   **Repair artery, intramural**   ~ follow-up period is 90 days, standard payment adjustment rules for multiple procedures apply, 150% payment adjustment for bilateral procedures does not apply, assistant surgeon may be paid

33508   **Endoscopic vein harvest**   ~ follow-up period included in another service, no payment adjustment rules for multiple procedures apply, 150% payment adjustment for bilateral procedures does not apply, assistant surgeon may be paid

33510   **CABG, vein, single**   ~ follow-up period is 90 days, standard payment adjustment rules for multiple procedures apply, 150% payment adjustment for bilateral procedures does not apply, assistant surgeon may be paid

33511   **CABG, vein, two**   ~ follow-up period is 90 days, standard payment adjustment rules for multiple procedures apply, 150% payment adjustment for bilateral procedures does not apply, assistant surgeon may be paid

33512   **CABG, vein, three**   ~ follow-up period is 90 days, standard payment adjustment rules for multiple procedures apply, 150% payment adjustment for bilateral procedures does not apply, assistant surgeon may be paid

33513   **CABG, vein, four**   ~ follow-up period is 90 days, standard payment adjustment rules for multiple procedures apply, 150% payment adjustment for bilateral procedures does not apply, assistant surgeon may be paid

33514   **CABG, vein, five**   ~ follow-up period is 90 days, standard payment adjustment rules for multiple procedures apply, 150% payment adjustment for bilateral procedures does not apply, assistant surgeon may be paid

33516   **CABG, vein, six or more**   ~ follow-up period is 90 days, standard payment adjustment rules for multiple procedures apply, 150% payment adjustment for bilateral procedures does not apply, assistant surgeon may be paid

33517   **CABG, artery-vein, single**   ~ follow-up period included in another service, no payment adjustment rules for multiple procedures apply, 150% payment adjustment for bilateral procedures does not apply, assistant surgeon may be paid

33518   **CABG, artery-vein, two**   ~ follow-up period included in another service, no payment adjustment rules for multiple procedures apply, 150% payment adjustment for bilateral procedures does not apply, assistant surgeon may be paid

33519   **CABG, artery-vein, three**   ~ follow-up period included in another service, no payment adjustment rules for multiple procedures apply, 150% payment adjustment for bilateral procedures does not apply, assistant surgeon may be paid

33521   **CABG, artery-vein, four**   ~ follow-up period included in another service, no payment adjustment rules for multiple procedures apply, 150% payment adjustment for bilateral procedures does not apply, assistant surgeon may be paid

33522   **CABG, artery-vein, five**   ~ follow-up period included in another service, no payment adjustment rules for multiple procedures apply, 150% payment adjustment for bilateral procedures does not apply, assistant surgeon may be paid

33523   **CABG, art-vein, six or more**   ~ follow-up period included in another service, no payment adjustment rules for multiple procedures apply, 150% payment adjustment for bilateral procedures does not apply, assistant surgeon may be paid

33530   **CABG, reoperate**   ~ follow-up period included in another service, no payment adjustment rules for multiple procedures apply, 150% payment adjustment for bilateral procedures does not apply, assistant surgeon may be paid

33533   **CABG, arterial, single**   ~ follow-up period is 90 days, standard payment adjustment rules for multiple procedures apply, 150% payment adjustment for bilateral procedures does not apply, assistant surgeon may be paid

33534   **CABG, arterial, two**   ~ follow-up period is 90 days, standard payment adjustment rules for multiple procedures apply, 150% payment adjustment for bilateral procedures does not apply, assistant surgeon may be paid

33535   **CABG, arterial, three**   ~ follow-up period is 90 days, standard payment adjustment rules for multiple procedures apply, 150% payment adjustment for bilateral procedures does not apply, assistant surgeon may be paid

33536   **CABG, arterial, four or more**   ~ follow-up period is 90 days, standard payment adjustment rules for multiple procedures apply, 150% payment adjustment for bilateral procedures does not apply, assistant surgeon may be paid

33542   **Remove heart lesion**   ~ follow-up period is 90 days, standard payment adjustment rules for multiple procedures apply, 150% payment adjustment for bilateral procedures does not apply, assistant surgeon may be paid

33545   **Repair heart damage**   ~ follow-up period is 90 days, standard payment adjustment rules for multiple procedures apply, 150% payment adjustment for bilateral procedures does not apply, assistant surgeon may be paid

33548   **Restore/remodel, ventricle**   ~ follow-up period is 90 days, standard payment adjustment rules for multiple procedures apply, 150% payment adjustment for bilateral procedures does not apply, assistant surgeon may be paid

33572   **Open coronary endarterectomy**   ~ follow-up period included in another service, no payment adjustment rules for multiple procedures apply, 150% payment adjustment for bilateral procedures does not apply, assistant surgeon may be paid

33600   **Closure valve**   ~ follow-up period is 90 days, standard payment adjustment rules for multiple procedures apply, 150% payment adjustment for bilateral procedures does not apply, assistant surgeon may be paid

33602   **Closure valve**   ~ follow-up period is 90 days, standard payment adjustment rules for multiple procedures apply, 150% payment adjustment for bilateral procedures does not apply, assistant surgeon may be paid

33606   **Anastomosis/artery-aorta**   ~ follow-up period is 90 days, standard payment adjustment rules for multiple procedures apply, 150% payment adjustment for bilateral procedures does not apply, assistant surgeon may be paid

33608   **Repair anomaly w/conduit**   ~ follow-up period is 90 days, standard payment adjustment rules for multiple procedures apply, 150% payment adjustment for bilateral procedures does not apply, assistant surgeon may be paid

33610   **Repair by enlargement**   ~ follow-up period is 90 days, standard payment adjustment rules for multiple procedures apply, 150% payment adjustment for bilateral procedures does not apply, assistant surgeon may be paid

33611   **Repair double ventricle**   ~ follow-up period is 90 days, standard payment adjustment rules for multiple procedures apply, 150% payment adjustment for bilateral procedures does not apply, assistant surgeon may be paid

33612   **Repair double ventricle**   ~ follow-up period is 90 days, standard payment adjustment rules for multiple procedures apply, 150% payment adjustment for bilateral procedures does not apply, assistant surgeon may be paid

33615   **Repair, modified fontan**   ~ follow-up period is 90 days, standard payment adjustment rules for multiple procedures apply, 150% payment adjustment for bilateral procedures does not apply, assistant surgeon may be paid

33617   **Repair single ventricle**   ~ follow-up period is 90 days, standard payment adjustment rules for multiple procedures apply, 150% payment adjustment for bilateral procedures does not apply, assistant surgeon may be paid

33619   **Repair single ventricle**   ~ follow-up period is 90 days, standard payment adjustment rules for multiple procedures apply, 150% payment adjustment for bilateral procedures does not apply, assistant surgeon may be paid

33641   **Repair heart septum defect**   ~ follow-up period is 90 days, standard payment adjustment rules for multiple procedures apply, 150% payment adjustment for bilateral procedures does not apply, assistant surgeon may be paid

33645   **Revise heart veins**   ~ follow-up period is 90 days, standard payment adjustment rules for multiple procedures apply, 150% payment adjustment for bilateral procedures does not apply, assistant surgeon may be paid

33647   **Repair heart septum defects**   ~ follow-up period is 90 days, standard payment adjustment rules for multiple procedures apply, 150% payment adjustment for bilateral procedures does not apply, assistant surgeon may be paid

33660   **Repair heart defects**   ~ follow-up period is 90 days, standard payment adjustment rules for multiple procedures apply, 150% payment adjustment for bilateral procedures does not apply, assistant surgeon may be paid

33665   **Repair heart defects**   ~ follow-up period is 90 days, standard payment adjustment rules for multiple procedures apply, 150% payment adjustment for bilateral procedures does not apply, assistant surgeon may be paid

33670   **Repair heart chambers**   ~ follow-up period is 90 days, standard payment adjustment rules for multiple procedures apply, 150% payment adjustment for bilateral procedures does not apply, assistant surgeon may be paid

33675   **Close multiple vsd**   ~ follow-up period is 90 days, standard payment adjustment rules for multiple procedures apply, 150% payment adjustment for bilateral procedures does not apply, assistant surgeon may be paid

33676   **Close multiple vsd w/resection**   ~ follow-up period is 90 days, standard payment adjustment rules for multiple procedures apply, 150% payment adjustment for bilateral procedures does not apply, assistant surgeon may be paid

33677   **Close multiple vsd w/rem pulmonary band** ~ follow-up period is 90 days, standard payment adjustment rules for multiple procedures apply, 150% payment adjustment for bilateral procedures does not apply, assistant surgeon may be paid

33681   **Repair heart septum defect**   ~ follow-up period is 90 days, standard payment adjustment rules for multiple procedures apply, 150% payment adjustment for bilateral procedures does not apply, assistant surgeon may be paid

33684   **Repair heart septum defect**   ~ follow-up period is 90 days, standard payment adjustment rules for multiple procedures apply, 150% payment adjustment for bilateral procedures does not apply, assistant surgeon may be paid

33688   **Repair heart septum defect**   ~ follow-up period is 90 days, standard payment adjustment rules for multiple procedures apply, 150% payment adjustment for bilateral procedures does not apply, assistant surgeon may be paid

33690   **Reinforce pulmonary artery**   ~ follow-up period is 90 days, standard payment adjustment rules for multiple procedures apply, 150% payment adjustment for bilateral procedures does not apply, assistant surgeon may be paid

33692   **Repair heart defects**   ~ follow-up period is 90 days, standard payment adjustment rules for multiple procedures apply, 150% payment adjustment for bilateral procedures does not apply, assistant surgeon may be paid

33694   **Repair heart defects**   ~ follow-up period is 90 days, standard payment adjustment rules for multiple procedures apply, 150% payment adjustment for bilateral procedures does not apply, assistant surgeon may be paid

33697   **Repair heart defects**   ~ follow-up period is 90 days, standard payment adjustment rules for multiple procedures apply, 150% payment adjustment for bilateral procedures does not apply, assistant surgeon may be paid

33702   **Repair heart defects**   ~ follow-up period is 90 days, standard payment adjustment rules for multiple procedures apply, 150% payment adjustment for bilateral procedures does not apply, assistant surgeon may be paid

33710   **Repair heart defects**   ~ follow-up period is 90 days, standard
payment adjustment rules for multiple procedures apply, 150% payment adjustment for
bilateral procedures does not apply, assistant surgeon may be paid

33720   **Repair heart defect**   ~ follow-up period is 90 days, standard
payment adjustment rules for multiple procedures apply, 150% payment adjustment for
bilateral procedures does not apply, assistant surgeon may be paid

33722   **Repair heart defect**   ~ follow-up period is 90 days, standard
payment adjustment rules for multiple procedures apply, 150% payment adjustment for
bilateral procedures does not apply, assistant surgeon may be paid

33724   **Repair venous anomaly**   ~ follow-up period is 90 days, standard
payment adjustment rules for multiple procedures apply, 150% payment adjustment for
bilateral procedures does not apply, assistant surgeon may be paid

33726   **Repair pulmonary venous stenosis**   ~ follow-up period is 90 days, standard
payment adjustment rules for multiple procedures apply, 150% payment adjustment for
bilateral procedures does not apply, assistant surgeon may be paid

33730   **Repair heart-vein defect(s)**   ~ follow-up period is 90 days, standard
payment adjustment rules for multiple procedures apply, 150% payment adjustment for
bilateral procedures does not apply, assistant surgeon may be paid

33732   **Repair heart-vein defect**   ~ follow-up period is 90 days, standard
payment adjustment rules for multiple procedures apply, 150% payment adjustment for
bilateral procedures does not apply, assistant surgeon may be paid

33735   **Revise heart chamber**   ~ follow-up period is 90 days, standard
payment adjustment rules for multiple procedures apply, 150% payment adjustment for
bilateral procedures does not apply, assistant surgeon may be paid

33736   **Revise heart chamber**   ~ follow-up period is 90 days, standard
payment adjustment rules for multiple procedures apply, 150% payment adjustment for
bilateral procedures does not apply, assistant surgeon may be paid

33737   **Revise heart chamber**   ~ follow-up period is 90 days, standard
payment adjustment rules for multiple procedures apply, 150% payment adjustment for
bilateral procedures does not apply, assistant surgeon may be paid

33750   **Major vessel shunt**   ~ follow-up period is 90 days, standard
payment adjustment rules for multiple procedures apply, 150% payment adjustment for
bilateral procedures does not apply, assistant surgeon may be paid

33755   **Major vessel shunt**   ~ follow-up period is 90 days, standard
payment adjustment rules for multiple procedures apply, 150% payment adjustment for
bilateral procedures does not apply, assistant surgeon may be paid

33762 **Major vessel shunt** ~ follow-up period is 90 days, standard payment adjustment rules for multiple procedures apply, 150% payment adjustment for bilateral procedures does not apply, assistant surgeon may be paid

33764 **Major vessel shunt & graft** ~ follow-up period is 90 days, standard payment adjustment rules for multiple procedures apply, 150% payment adjustment for bilateral procedures does not apply, assistant surgeon may be paid

33766 **Major vessel shunt** ~ follow-up period is 90 days, standard payment adjustment rules for multiple procedures apply, 150% payment adjustment for bilateral procedures does not apply, assistant surgeon may be paid

33767 **Major vessel shunt** ~ follow-up period is 90 days, standard payment adjustment rules for multiple procedures apply, 150% payment adjustment for bilateral procedures does not apply, assistant surgeon may be paid

33768 **Cavopulmonary shunting** ~ follow-up period included in another service, no payment adjustment rules for multiple procedures apply, 150% payment adjustment for bilateral procedures does not apply, assistant surgeon may be paid

33770 **Repair great vessels defect** ~ follow-up period is 90 days, standard payment adjustment rules for multiple procedures apply, 150% payment adjustment for bilateral procedures does not apply, assistant surgeon may be paid

33771 **Repair great vessels defect** ~ follow-up period is 90 days, standard payment adjustment rules for multiple procedures apply, 150% payment adjustment for bilateral procedures does not apply, assistant surgeon may be paid

33774 **Repair great vessels defect** ~ follow-up period is 90 days, standard payment adjustment rules for multiple procedures apply, 150% payment adjustment for bilateral procedures does not apply, assistant surgeon may be paid

33775 **Repair great vessels defect** ~ follow-up period is 90 days, standard payment adjustment rules for multiple procedures apply, 150% payment adjustment for bilateral procedures does not apply, assistant surgeon may be paid

33776 **Repair great vessels defect** ~ follow-up period is 90 days, standard payment adjustment rules for multiple procedures apply, 150% payment adjustment for bilateral procedures does not apply, assistant surgeon may be paid

33777 **Repair great vessels defect** ~ follow-up period is 90 days, standard payment adjustment rules for multiple procedures apply, 150% payment adjustment for bilateral procedures does not apply, assistant surgeon may be paid

33778 **Repair great vessels defect** ~ follow-up period is 90 days, standard payment adjustment rules for multiple procedures apply, 150% payment adjustment for bilateral procedures does not apply, assistant surgeon may be paid

33779   **Repair great vessels defect**   ~ follow-up period is 90 days, standard payment adjustment rules for multiple procedures apply, 150% payment adjustment for bilateral procedures does not apply, assistant surgeon may be paid

33780   **Repair great vessels defect**   ~ follow-up period is 90 days, standard payment adjustment rules for multiple procedures apply, 150% payment adjustment for bilateral procedures does not apply, assistant surgeon may be paid

33781   **Repair great vessels defect**   ~ follow-up period is 90 days, standard payment adjustment rules for multiple procedures apply, 150% payment adjustment for bilateral procedures does not apply, assistant surgeon may be paid

33786   **Repair arterial trunk**   ~ follow-up period is 90 days, standard payment adjustment rules for multiple procedures apply, 150% payment adjustment for bilateral procedures does not apply, assistant surgeon may be paid

33788   **Revise pulmonary artery**   ~ follow-up period is 90 days, standard payment adjustment rules for multiple procedures apply, 150% payment adjustment for bilateral procedures does not apply, assistant surgeon may be paid

33800   **Aortic suspension**   ~ follow-up period is 90 days, standard payment adjustment rules for multiple procedures apply, 150% payment adjustment for bilateral procedures does not apply, assistant surgeon may be paid

33802   **Repair vessel defect**   ~ follow-up period is 90 days, standard payment adjustment rules for multiple procedures apply, 150% payment adjustment for bilateral procedures does not apply, assistant surgeon may be paid

33803   **Repair vessel defect**   ~ follow-up period is 90 days, standard payment adjustment rules for multiple procedures apply, 150% payment adjustment for bilateral procedures does not apply, assistant surgeon may be paid

33813   **Repair septal defect**   ~ follow-up period is 90 days, standard payment adjustment rules for multiple procedures apply, 150% payment adjustment for bilateral procedures does not apply, assistant surgeon may be paid

33814   **Repair septal defect**   ~ follow-up period is 90 days, standard payment adjustment rules for multiple procedures apply, 150% payment adjustment for bilateral procedures does not apply, assistant surgeon may be paid

33820   **Revise major vessel**   ~ follow-up period is 90 days, standard payment adjustment rules for multiple procedures apply, 150% payment adjustment for bilateral procedures does not apply, assistant surgeon may be paid

33822   **Revise major vessel**   ~ follow-up period is 90 days, standard payment adjustment rules for multiple procedures apply, 150% payment adjustment for bilateral procedures does not apply, assistant surgeon may be paid

33824   **Revise major vessel**   ~ follow-up period is 90 days, standard payment adjustment rules for multiple procedures apply, 150% payment adjustment for bilateral procedures does not apply, assistant surgeon may be paid

33840   **Remove aorta constriction**   ~ follow-up period is 90 days, standard payment adjustment rules for multiple procedures apply, 150% payment adjustment for bilateral procedures does not apply, assistant surgeon may be paid

33845   **Remove aorta constriction**   ~ follow-up period is 90 days, standard payment adjustment rules for multiple procedures apply, 150% payment adjustment for bilateral procedures does not apply, assistant surgeon may be paid

33851   **Remove aorta constriction**   ~ follow-up period is 90 days, standard payment adjustment rules for multiple procedures apply, 150% payment adjustment for bilateral procedures does not apply, assistant surgeon may be paid

33852   **Repair septal defect**   ~ follow-up period is 90 days, standard payment adjustment rules for multiple procedures apply, 150% payment adjustment for bilateral procedures does not apply, assistant surgeon may be paid

33853   **Repair septal defect**   ~ follow-up period is 90 days, standard payment adjustment rules for multiple procedures apply, 150% payment adjustment for bilateral procedures does not apply, assistant surgeon may be paid

33860   **Ascending aortic graft**   ~ follow-up period is 90 days, standard payment adjustment rules for multiple procedures apply, 150% payment adjustment for bilateral procedures does not apply, assistant surgeon may be paid

33861   **Ascending aortic graft**   ~ follow-up period is 90 days, standard payment adjustment rules for multiple procedures apply, 150% payment adjustment for bilateral procedures does not apply, assistant surgeon may be paid

33863   **Ascending aortic graft**   ~ follow-up period is 90 days, standard payment adjustment rules for multiple procedures apply, 150% payment adjustment for bilateral procedures does not apply, assistant surgeon may be paid

33870   **Transverse aortic arch graft**   ~ follow-up period is 90 days, standard payment adjustment rules for multiple procedures apply, 150% payment adjustment for bilateral procedures does not apply, assistant surgeon may be paid

33875   **Thoracic aortic graft**   ~ follow-up period is 90 days, standard payment adjustment rules for multiple procedures apply, 150% payment adjustment for bilateral procedures does not apply, assistant surgeon may be paid

33877   **Thoracoabdominal graft**   ~ follow-up period is 90 days, standard payment adjustment rules for multiple procedures apply, 150% payment adjustment for bilateral procedures does not apply, assistant surgeon may be paid

33880   **Endovascular taa repair including subclavian** ~ follow-up period is 90 days, standard payment adjustment rules for multiple procedures apply, 150% payment adjustment does not apply - RVUs based on bilateral procedure, assistant surgeon may be paid

33881   **Endovascular taa repair w/o subclavian** ~ follow-up period is 90 days, standard payment adjustment rules for multiple procedures apply, 150% payment adjustment does not apply - RVUs based on bilateral procedure, assistant surgeon may be paid

33883   **Insert endovascular prosth, taa** ~ follow-up period is 90 days, standard payment adjustment rules for multiple procedures apply, 150% payment adjustment for bilateral procedures does not apply, assistant surgeon may be paid

33884   **Endovascular prosth, taa, add-on** ~ follow-up period included in another service, no payment adjustment rules for multiple procedures apply, 150% payment adjustment for bilateral procedures does not apply, assistant surgeon may be paid, +add-on code (list separately in addition to primary procedure)

33886   **Endovascular prosth, delayed** ~ follow-up period is 90 days, standard payment adjustment rules for multiple procedures apply, 150% payment adjustment for bilateral procedures does not apply, assistant surgeon may be paid

33889   **Artery transpose/endovascular taa** ~ endoscopies or minor procedure - E/M services on the same day generally not paid, standard payment adjustment rules for multiple procedures apply, 150% payment adjustment for bilateral procedures applies, assistant surgeon may be paid

33891   **Car-car bp graft/endovascular taa** ~ endoscopies or minor procedure - E/M services on the same day generally not paid, standard payment adjustment rules for multiple procedures apply, 150% payment adjustment for bilateral procedures applies, assistant surgeon may be paid

33910   **Remove lung artery emboli** ~ follow-up period is 90 days, standard payment adjustment rules for multiple procedures apply, 150% payment adjustment for bilateral procedures does not apply, assistant surgeon may be paid

33915   **Remove lung artery emboli** ~ follow-up period is 90 days, standard payment adjustment rules for multiple procedures apply, 150% payment adjustment for bilateral procedures does not apply, assistant surgeon may be paid

33916   **Surgery great vessel** ~ follow-up period is 90 days, standard payment adjustment rules for multiple procedures apply, 150% payment adjustment for bilateral procedures does not apply, assistant surgeon may be paid

33917   **Repair pulmonary artery** ~ follow-up period is 90 days, standard payment adjustment rules for multiple procedures apply, 150% payment adjustment for bilateral procedures does not apply, assistant surgeon may be paid

33920 **Repair pulmonary atresia** ~ follow-up period is 90 days, standard payment adjustment rules for multiple procedures apply, 150% payment adjustment for bilateral procedures does not apply, assistant surgeon may be paid

33922 **Transect pulmonary artery** ~ follow-up period is 90 days, standard payment adjustment rules for multiple procedures apply, 150% payment adjustment for bilateral procedures does not apply, assistant surgeon may be paid

33924 **Remove pulmonary shunt** ~ follow-up period included in another service, no payment adjustment rules for multiple procedures apply, 150% payment adjustment for bilateral procedures does not apply, assistant surgeon may be paid

33925 **Repair pulmonary art unifocal w/o cpb** ~ follow-up period is 90 days, standard payment adjustment rules for multiple procedures apply, 150% payment adjustment for bilateral procedures does not apply, assistant surgeon may be paid

33926 **Repair pulmonary art, unifocal w/cpb** ~ follow-up period is 90 days, standard payment adjustment rules for multiple procedures apply, 150% payment adjustment for bilateral procedures does not apply, assistant surgeon may be paid

33930 **Remove donor heart/lung** ~ multiple procedure concept does not apply, bilateral surgery concept does not apply, assistant surgery concept does not apply

33933 **Prepare donor heart/lung** ~ standard payment adjustment rules for multiple procedures apply, 150% payment adjustment for bilateral procedures does not apply, assistant surgeon may be paid

33935 **Transplant heart/lung** ~ restricted coverage - special coverage rules apply, follow-up period is 90 days, standard payment adjustment rules for multiple procedures apply, 150% payment adjustment for bilateral procedures does not apply, assistant surgeon may be paid

33940 **Remove donor heart** ~ multiple procedure concept does not apply, bilateral surgery concept does not apply, assistant surgery concept does not apply

33944 **Prepare donor heart,** ~ standard payment adjustment rules for multiple procedures apply, 150% payment adjustment for bilateral procedures does not apply, assistant surgeon may be paid

33945 **Transplant heart** ~ restricted coverage - special coverage rules apply, follow-up period is 90 days, standard payment adjustment rules for multiple procedures apply, 150% payment adjustment for bilateral procedures does not apply, assistant surgeon may be paid

33960 **External circulation assist** ~ endoscopies or minor procedure - E/M services on the same day generally not paid, no payment adjustment rules for multiple

---

procedures apply, 150% payment adjustment for bilateral procedures does not apply, assistant surgeon may be paid

33961   **External circulation assist**   ~ follow-up period included in another service, no payment adjustment rules for multiple procedures apply, 150% payment adjustment for bilateral procedures does not apply, assistant surgeon may be paid

33967   **Insert ia percutaneous device**   ~ endoscopies or minor procedure - E/M services on the same day generally not paid, standard payment adjustment rules for multiple procedures apply, 150% payment adjustment for bilateral procedures does not apply, payment for assistant surgeon subject to documentation of medical necessity

33968   **Remove aortic assist device**   ~ endoscopies or minor procedure - E/M services on the same day generally not paid, no payment adjustment rules for multiple procedures apply, 150% payment adjustment for bilateral procedures does not apply, assistant surgeon may not be paid

33970   **Aortic circulation assist**   ~ endoscopies or minor procedure - E/M services on the same day generally not paid, standard payment adjustment rules for multiple procedures apply, 150% payment adjustment for bilateral procedures does not apply, assistant surgeon may be paid

33971   **Aortic circulation assist**   ~ follow-up period is 90 days, standard payment adjustment rules for multiple procedures apply, 150% payment adjustment for bilateral procedures does not apply, assistant surgeon may not be paid

33973   **Insert balloon device**   ~ endoscopies or minor procedure - E/M services on the same day generally not paid, standard payment adjustment rules for multiple procedures apply, 150% payment adjustment for bilateral procedures does not apply, assistant surgeon may be paid

33974   **Remove intra-aortic balloon**   ~ follow-up period is 90 days, standard payment adjustment rules for multiple procedures apply, 150% payment adjustment for bilateral procedures does not apply, assistant surgeon may not be paid

33975   **Implant ventricular device**   ~ standard payment adjustment rules for multiple procedures apply, 150% payment adjustment for bilateral procedures does not apply, assistant surgeon may be paid

33976   **Implant ventricular device**   ~ standard payment adjustment rules for multiple procedures apply, 150% payment adjustment does not apply - RVUs based on bilateral procedure, assistant surgeon may be paid

33977   **Remove ventricular device**   ~ follow-up period is 90 days, standard payment adjustment rules for multiple procedures apply, 150% payment adjustment for bilateral procedures does not apply, assistant surgeon may be paid

33978   **Remove ventricular device**   ~ follow-up period is 90 days, standard payment adjustment rules for multiple procedures apply, 150% payment adjustment does not apply - RVUs based on bilateral procedure, assistant surgeon may be paid

33979   **Insert intracorporeal device**   ~ standard payment adjustment rules for multiple procedures apply, 150% payment adjustment for bilateral procedures does not apply, assistant surgeon may be paid

33980   **Remove intracorporeal device**   ~ follow-up period is 90 days, standard payment adjustment rules for multiple procedures apply, 150% payment adjustment for bilateral procedures does not apply, assistant surgeon may be paid

33999   **Cardiac surgery procedure**   ~ medicare carrier determines global period, standard payment adjustment rules for multiple procedures apply, 150% payment adjustment for bilateral procedures does not apply, assistant surgeon may be paid

Arteries and Veins

34001   **Remove artery clot**   ~ follow-up period is 90 days, standard payment adjustment rules for multiple procedures apply, 150% payment adjustment for bilateral procedures applies, assistant surgeon may be paid

34051   **Remove artery clot**   ~ follow-up period is 90 days, standard payment adjustment rules for multiple procedures apply, 150% payment adjustment for bilateral procedures applies, assistant surgeon may be paid

34101   **Remove artery clot**   ~ follow-up period is 90 days, standard payment adjustment rules for multiple procedures apply, 150% payment adjustment for bilateral procedures applies, assistant surgeon may be paid

34111   **Remove arm artery clot**   ~ follow-up period is 90 days, standard payment adjustment rules for multiple procedures apply, 150% payment adjustment for bilateral procedures applies, assistant surgeon may be paid

34151   **Remove artery clot**   ~ follow-up period is 90 days, standard payment adjustment rules for multiple procedures apply, 150% payment adjustment for bilateral procedures applies, assistant surgeon may be paid

34201   **Remove artery clot**   ~ follow-up period is 90 days, standard payment adjustment rules for multiple procedures apply, 150% payment adjustment for bilateral procedures applies, assistant surgeon may be paid

34203   **Remove leg artery clot**   ~ follow-up period is 90 days, standard payment adjustment rules for multiple procedures apply, 150% payment adjustment for bilateral procedures applies, assistant surgeon may be paid

34401   **Remove vein clot**   ~ follow-up period is 90 days, standard payment adjustment rules for multiple procedures apply, 150% payment adjustment for bilateral procedures applies, assistant surgeon may be paid

34421   **Remove vein clot**   ~ follow-up period is 90 days, standard payment adjustment rules for multiple procedures apply, 150% payment adjustment for bilateral procedures applies, assistant surgeon may be paid

34451   **Remove vein clot**   ~ follow-up period is 90 days, standard payment adjustment rules for multiple procedures apply, 150% payment adjustment for bilateral procedures applies, assistant surgeon may be paid

34471   **Remove vein clot**   ~ follow-up period is 90 days, standard payment adjustment rules for multiple procedures apply, 150% payment adjustment for bilateral procedures applies, assistant surgeon may not be paid

34490   **Remove vein clot**   ~ follow-up period is 90 days, standard payment adjustment rules for multiple procedures apply, 150% payment adjustment for bilateral procedures applies, assistant surgeon may not be paid

34501   **Repair valve, femoral vein**   ~ follow-up period is 90 days, standard payment adjustment rules for multiple procedures apply, 150% payment adjustment for bilateral procedures applies, assistant surgeon may be paid

34502   **Reconstruct vena cava**   ~ follow-up period is 90 days, standard payment adjustment rules for multiple procedures apply, 150% payment adjustment for bilateral procedures does not apply, assistant surgeon may be paid

34510   **Transpose vein valve**   ~ follow-up period is 90 days, standard payment adjustment rules for multiple procedures apply, 150% payment adjustment for bilateral procedures applies, assistant surgeon may be paid

34520   **Cross-over vein graft**   ~ follow-up period is 90 days, standard payment adjustment rules for multiple procedures apply, 150% payment adjustment for bilateral procedures applies, assistant surgeon may be paid

34530   **Leg vein fusion**   ~ follow-up period is 90 days, standard payment adjustment rules for multiple procedures apply, 150% payment adjustment for bilateral procedures applies, assistant surgeon may be paid

34800   **Endovascular aaa repair w/sm tube**   ~ follow-up period is 90 days, standard payment adjustment rules for multiple procedures apply, 150% payment adjustment for bilateral procedures does not apply, assistant surgeon may be paid

34802   **Endovascular aaa repair w/2-p part**   ~ follow-up period is 90 days, standard payment adjustment rules for multiple procedures apply, 150% payment adjustment for bilateral procedures does not apply, assistant surgeon may be paid

34803   **Endovascular aaa repair w/3-p part**   ~ follow-up period is 90 days, standard payment adjustment rules for multiple procedures apply, 150% payment adjustment does not apply - RVUs based on bilateral procedure, assistant surgeon may be paid

34804   **Endovascular aaa repair w/1-p part**   ~ follow-up period is 90 days, standard payment adjustment rules for multiple procedures apply, 150% payment adjustment for bilateral procedures does not apply, assistant surgeon may be paid

34805   **Endovascular aaa repair w/long tube**   ~ follow-up period is 90 days, standard payment adjustment rules for multiple procedures apply, 150% payment adjustment for bilateral procedures does not apply, assistant surgeon may be paid

34808   **Endovascular iliac a device add on**   ~ follow-up period included in another service, no payment adjustment rules for multiple procedures apply, 150% payment adjustment for bilateral procedures does not apply, assistant surgeon may be paid, +add-on code (list separately in addition to primary procedure)

34812   **Expose for endoprosthesis, femoral**   ~ endoscopies or minor procedure - E/M services on the same day generally not paid, standard payment adjustment rules for multiple procedures apply, 150% payment adjustment for bilateral procedures applies, assistant surgeon may be paid

34813   **Femoral endovascular graft, add-on**   ~ follow-up period included in another service, no payment adjustment rules for multiple procedures apply, 150% payment adjustment for bilateral procedures does not apply, assistant surgeon may be paid, +add-on code (list separately in addition to primary procedure)

34820   **Expose for endoprosthesis, iliac**   ~ endoscopies or minor procedure - E/M services on the same day generally not paid, standard payment adjustment rules for multiple procedures apply, 150% payment adjustment for bilateral procedures applies, assistant surgeon may be paid

34825   **Endovascular extend prosth, init**   ~ follow-up period is 90 days, standard payment adjustment rules for multiple procedures apply, 150% payment adjustment for bilateral procedures does not apply, assistant surgeon may be paid

34826   **Endovascular extensive prosth, added**   ~ follow-up period included in another service, no payment adjustment rules for multiple procedures apply, 150% payment adjustment for bilateral procedures does not apply, assistant surgeon may be paid, +add-on code (list separately in addition to primary procedure)

34830   **Open aortic tube prosth repair**   ~ follow-up period is 90 days, standard payment adjustment rules for multiple procedures apply, 150% payment adjustment for bilateral procedures does not apply, payment for assistant surgeon subject to documentation of medical necessity

34831   **Open aortoiliac prosth repair**   ~ follow-up period is 90 days, standard payment adjustment rules for multiple procedures apply, 150% payment adjustment for bilateral procedures does not apply, payment for assistant surgeon subject to documentation of medical necessity

34832   **Open aortofemoral prosth repair**   ~ follow-up period is 90 days, standard payment adjustment rules for multiple procedures apply, 150% payment adjustment for bilateral procedures does not apply, payment for assistant surgeon subject to documentation of medical necessity

34833   **Expose for endoprosthesis, iliac**   ~ endoscopies or minor procedure - E/M services on the same day generally not paid, standard payment adjustment rules for multiple procedures apply, 150% payment adjustment for bilateral procedures applies, assistant surgeon may be paid

34834   **Expose, endoprosthesis, brachial**   ~ endoscopies or minor procedure - E/M services on the same day generally not paid, standard payment adjustment rules for multiple procedures apply, 150% payment adjustment for bilateral procedures applies, assistant surgeon may be paid

34900   **Endovascular iliac repair w/graft**   ~ follow-up period is 90 days, standard payment adjustment rules for multiple procedures apply, 150% payment adjustment for bilateral procedures applies, assistant surgeon may be paid

35001   **Repair defect artery**   ~ follow-up period is 90 days, standard payment adjustment rules for multiple procedures apply, 150% payment adjustment for bilateral procedures applies, assistant surgeon may be paid

35002   **Repair artery rupture, neck**   ~ follow-up period is 90 days, standard payment adjustment rules for multiple procedures apply, 150% payment adjustment for bilateral procedures applies, assistant surgeon may be paid

35005   **Repair defect artery**   ~ follow-up period is 90 days, standard payment adjustment rules for multiple procedures apply, 150% payment adjustment for bilateral procedures applies, assistant surgeon may be paid

35011   **Repair defect artery**   ~ follow-up period is 90 days, standard payment adjustment rules for multiple procedures apply, 150% payment adjustment for bilateral procedures applies, assistant surgeon may be paid

35013   **Repair artery rupture, arm**   ~ follow-up period is 90 days, standard payment adjustment rules for multiple procedures apply, 150% payment adjustment for bilateral procedures applies, assistant surgeon may be paid

35021   **Repair defect artery**   ~ follow-up period is 90 days, standard payment adjustment rules for multiple procedures apply, 150% payment adjustment for bilateral procedures applies, assistant surgeon may be paid

35022   **Repair artery rupture, chest**   ~ follow-up period is 90 days, standard payment adjustment rules for multiple procedures apply, 150% payment adjustment for bilateral procedures applies, assistant surgeon may be paid

35045   **Repair defect arm artery**   ~ follow-up period is 90 days, standard payment adjustment rules for multiple procedures apply, 150% payment adjustment for bilateral procedures applies, assistant surgeon may be paid

35081   **Repair defect artery**   ~ follow-up period is 90 days, standard payment adjustment rules for multiple procedures apply, 150% payment adjustment for bilateral procedures does not apply, assistant surgeon may be paid

35082   **Repair artery rupture, aorta**   ~ follow-up period is 90 days, standard payment adjustment rules for multiple procedures apply, 150% payment adjustment for bilateral procedures does not apply, assistant surgeon may be paid

35091   **Repair defect artery**   ~ follow-up period is 90 days, standard payment adjustment rules for multiple procedures apply, 150% payment adjustment for bilateral procedures applies, assistant surgeon may be paid

35092   **Repair artery rupture, aorta**   ~ follow-up period is 90 days, standard payment adjustment rules for multiple procedures apply, 150% payment adjustment for bilateral procedures applies, assistant surgeon may be paid

35102   **Repair defect artery**   ~ follow-up period is 90 days, standard payment adjustment rules for multiple procedures apply, 150% payment adjustment for bilateral procedures applies, assistant surgeon may be paid

35103   **Repair artery rupture, groin**   ~ follow-up period is 90 days, standard payment adjustment rules for multiple procedures apply, 150% payment adjustment for bilateral procedures applies, assistant surgeon may be paid

35111   **Repair defect artery**   ~ follow-up period is 90 days, standard payment adjustment rules for multiple procedures apply, 150% payment adjustment for bilateral procedures applies, assistant surgeon may be paid

35112   **Repair artery rupture, spleen**   ~ follow-up period is 90 days, standard payment adjustment rules for multiple procedures apply, 150% payment adjustment for bilateral procedures applies, assistant surgeon may be paid

35121   **Repair defect artery**   ~ follow-up period is 90 days, standard payment adjustment rules for multiple procedures apply, 150% payment adjustment for bilateral procedures applies, assistant surgeon may be paid

35122   **Repair artery rupture, belly**   ~ follow-up period is 90 days, standard payment adjustment rules for multiple procedures apply, 150% payment adjustment for bilateral procedures applies, assistant surgeon may be paid

35131   **Repair defect artery**   ~ follow-up period is 90 days, standard payment adjustment rules for multiple procedures apply, 150% payment adjustment for bilateral procedures applies, assistant surgeon may be paid

35132   **Repair artery rupture, groin**   ~ follow-up period is 90 days, standard payment adjustment rules for multiple procedures apply, 150% payment adjustment for bilateral procedures applies, assistant surgeon may be paid

35141   **Repair defect artery**   ~ follow-up period is 90 days, standard payment adjustment rules for multiple procedures apply, 150% payment adjustment for bilateral procedures applies, assistant surgeon may be paid

35142   **Repair artery rupture, thigh**   ~ follow-up period is 90 days, standard payment adjustment rules for multiple procedures apply, 150% payment adjustment for bilateral procedures applies, assistant surgeon may be paid

35151   **Repair defect artery**   ~ follow-up period is 90 days, standard payment adjustment rules for multiple procedures apply, 150% payment adjustment for bilateral procedures applies, assistant surgeon may be paid

35152   **Repair artery rupture, knee**   ~ follow-up period is 90 days, standard payment adjustment rules for multiple procedures apply, 150% payment adjustment for bilateral procedures applies, assistant surgeon may be paid

35180   **Repair blood vessel lesion**   ~ follow-up period is 90 days, standard payment adjustment rules for multiple procedures apply, 150% payment adjustment for bilateral procedures does not apply, assistant surgeon may be paid

35182   **Repair blood vessel lesion**   ~ follow-up period is 90 days, standard payment adjustment rules for multiple procedures apply, 150% payment adjustment for bilateral procedures does not apply, assistant surgeon may be paid

35184   **Repair blood vessel lesion**   ~ follow-up period is 90 days, standard payment adjustment rules for multiple procedures apply, 150% payment adjustment for bilateral procedures does not apply, assistant surgeon may be paid

35188   **Repair blood vessel lesion**   ~ follow-up period is 90 days, standard payment adjustment rules for multiple procedures apply, 150% payment adjustment for bilateral procedures does not apply, assistant surgeon may be paid

35189   **Repair blood vessel lesion**   ~ follow-up period is 90 days, standard payment adjustment rules for multiple procedures apply, 150% payment adjustment for bilateral procedures does not apply, assistant surgeon may be paid

35190   **Repair blood vessel lesion**   ~ follow-up period is 90 days, standard payment adjustment rules for multiple procedures apply, 150% payment adjustment for bilateral procedures does not apply, assistant surgeon may be paid

35201   **Repair blood vessel lesion**   ~ follow-up period is 90 days, standard payment adjustment rules for multiple procedures apply, 150% payment adjustment for bilateral procedures applies, assistant surgeon may be paid

35206   **Repair blood vessel lesion**   ~ follow-up period is 90 days, standard payment adjustment rules for multiple procedures apply, 150% payment adjustment for bilateral procedures applies, assistant surgeon may be paid

35207   **Repair blood vessel lesion**   ~ follow-up period is 90 days, standard payment adjustment rules for multiple procedures apply, 150% payment adjustment for bilateral procedures applies, assistant surgeon may not be paid

35211   **Repair blood vessel lesion**   ~ follow-up period is 90 days, standard payment adjustment rules for multiple procedures apply, 150% payment adjustment for bilateral procedures applies, assistant surgeon may be paid

35216   **Repair blood vessel lesion**   ~ follow-up period is 90 days, standard payment adjustment rules for multiple procedures apply, 150% payment adjustment for bilateral procedures applies, assistant surgeon may be paid

35221   **Repair blood vessel lesion**   ~ follow-up period is 90 days, standard payment adjustment rules for multiple procedures apply, 150% payment adjustment for bilateral procedures applies, assistant surgeon may be paid

35226   **Repair blood vessel lesion**   ~ follow-up period is 90 days, standard payment adjustment rules for multiple procedures apply, 150% payment adjustment for bilateral procedures applies, assistant surgeon may be paid

35231   **Repair blood vessel lesion**   ~ follow-up period is 90 days, standard payment adjustment rules for multiple procedures apply, 150% payment adjustment for bilateral procedures applies, assistant surgeon may be paid

35236   **Repair blood vessel lesion**   ~ follow-up period is 90 days, standard payment adjustment rules for multiple procedures apply, 150% payment adjustment for bilateral procedures applies, assistant surgeon may be paid

35241   **Repair blood vessel lesion**   ~ follow-up period is 90 days, standard payment adjustment rules for multiple procedures apply, 150% payment adjustment for bilateral procedures applies, assistant surgeon may be paid

35246   **Repair blood vessel lesion**   ~ follow-up period is 90 days, standard payment adjustment rules for multiple procedures apply, 150% payment adjustment for bilateral procedures applies, assistant surgeon may be paid

35251   **Repair blood vessel lesion**   ~ follow-up period is 90 days, standard payment adjustment rules for multiple procedures apply, 150% payment adjustment for bilateral procedures applies, assistant surgeon may be paid

35256   **Repair blood vessel lesion**   ~ follow-up period is 90 days, standard payment adjustment rules for multiple procedures apply, 150% payment adjustment for bilateral procedures applies, assistant surgeon may be paid

35261   **Repair blood vessel lesion**   ~ follow-up period is 90 days, standard payment adjustment rules for multiple procedures apply, 150% payment adjustment for bilateral procedures applies, assistant surgeon may be paid

35266   **Repair blood vessel lesion**   ~ follow-up period is 90 days, standard payment adjustment rules for multiple procedures apply, 150% payment adjustment for bilateral procedures applies, assistant surgeon may be paid

35271   **Repair blood vessel lesion**   ~ follow-up period is 90 days, standard payment adjustment rules for multiple procedures apply, 150% payment adjustment for bilateral procedures applies, assistant surgeon may be paid

35276   **Repair blood vessel lesion**   ~ follow-up period is 90 days, standard payment adjustment rules for multiple procedures apply, 150% payment adjustment for bilateral procedures applies, assistant surgeon may be paid

35281   **Repair blood vessel lesion**   ~ follow-up period is 90 days, standard payment adjustment rules for multiple procedures apply, 150% payment adjustment for bilateral procedures applies, assistant surgeon may be paid

35286   **Repair blood vessel lesion**   ~ follow-up period is 90 days, standard payment adjustment rules for multiple procedures apply, 150% payment adjustment for bilateral procedures applies, assistant surgeon may be paid

35301   **Rechannel artery**   ~ follow-up period is 90 days, standard payment adjustment rules for multiple procedures apply, 150% payment adjustment for bilateral procedures applies, assistant surgeon may be paid

35302   **Rechannel artery**   ~ follow-up period is 90 days, standard payment adjustment rules for multiple procedures apply, 150% payment adjustment for bilateral procedures applies, assistant surgeon may be paid

35303   **Rechannel artery**   ~ follow-up period is 90 days, standard payment adjustment rules for multiple procedures apply, 150% payment adjustment for bilateral procedures applies, assistant surgeon may be paid

35304   **Rechannel artery**   ~ follow-up period is 90 days, standard payment adjustment rules for multiple procedures apply, 150% payment adjustment for bilateral procedures applies, assistant surgeon may be paid

35305   **Rechannel artery**   ~ follow-up period is 90 days, standard payment adjustment rules for multiple procedures apply, 150% payment adjustment for bilateral procedures applies, assistant surgeon may be paid

35306   **Rechannel artery**   ~ follow-up period included in another service, no payment adjustment rules for multiple procedures apply, 150% payment adjustment for bilateral procedures does not apply, assistant surgeon may be paid

35311   **Rechannel artery**   ~ follow-up period is 90 days, standard payment adjustment rules for multiple procedures apply, 150% payment adjustment for bilateral procedures applies, assistant surgeon may be paid

35321   **Rechannel artery**   ~ follow-up period is 90 days, standard payment adjustment rules for multiple procedures apply, 150% payment adjustment for bilateral procedures applies, assistant surgeon may be paid

35331   **Rechannel artery**   ~ follow-up period is 90 days, standard payment adjustment rules for multiple procedures apply, 150% payment adjustment for bilateral procedures applies, assistant surgeon may be paid

35341   **Rechannel artery**   ~ follow-up period is 90 days, standard payment adjustment rules for multiple procedures apply, 150% payment adjustment for bilateral procedures applies, assistant surgeon may be paid

35351   **Rechannel artery**   ~ follow-up period is 90 days, standard payment adjustment rules for multiple procedures apply, 150% payment adjustment for bilateral procedures applies, assistant surgeon may be paid

35355   **Rechannel artery**   ~ follow-up period is 90 days, standard payment adjustment rules for multiple procedures apply, 150% payment adjustment for bilateral procedures applies, assistant surgeon may be paid

35361   **Rechannel artery**   ~ follow-up period is 90 days, standard payment adjustment rules for multiple procedures apply, 150% payment adjustment for bilateral procedures applies, assistant surgeon may be paid

35363   **Rechannel artery**   ~ follow-up period is 90 days, standard payment adjustment rules for multiple procedures apply, 150% payment adjustment for bilateral procedures applies, assistant surgeon may be paid

35371   **Rechannel artery**   ~ follow-up period is 90 days, standard payment adjustment rules for multiple procedures apply, 150% payment adjustment for bilateral procedures applies, assistant surgeon may be paid

35372   **Rechannel artery**   ~ follow-up period is 90 days, standard payment adjustment rules for multiple procedures apply, 150% payment adjustment for bilateral procedures applies, assistant surgeon may be paid

35390   **Reoperation, carotid, add-on**   ~ follow-up period included in another service, no payment adjustment rules for multiple procedures apply, 150% payment adjustment for

---

bilateral procedures does not apply, assistant surgeon may be paid, +add-on code (list separately in addition to primary procedure)

35400   **Angioscopy**   ~ follow-up period included in another service, no payment adjustment rules for multiple procedures apply, 150% payment adjustment for bilateral procedures does not apply, payment for assistant surgeon subject to documentation of medical necessity

35450   **Repair arterial blockage**   ~ endoscopies or minor procedure - E/M services on the same day generally not paid, standard payment adjustment rules for multiple procedures apply, 150% payment adjustment for bilateral procedures applies, assistant surgeon may be paid

35452   **Repair arterial blockage**   ~ endoscopies or minor procedure - E/M services on the same day generally not paid, standard payment adjustment rules for multiple procedures apply, 150% payment adjustment for bilateral procedures applies, assistant surgeon may be paid

35454   **Repair arterial blockage**   ~ endoscopies or minor procedure - E/M services on the same day generally not paid, standard payment adjustment rules for multiple procedures apply, 150% payment adjustment for bilateral procedures applies, assistant surgeon may be paid

35456   **Repair arterial blockage**   ~ endoscopies or minor procedure - E/M services on the same day generally not paid, standard payment adjustment rules for multiple procedures apply, 150% payment adjustment for bilateral procedures applies, assistant surgeon may be paid

35458   **Repair arterial blockage**   ~ endoscopies or minor procedure - E/M services on the same day generally not paid, standard payment adjustment rules for multiple procedures apply, 150% payment adjustment for bilateral procedures applies, assistant surgeon may be paid

35459   **Repair arterial blockage**   ~ endoscopies or minor procedure - E/M services on the same day generally not paid, standard payment adjustment rules for multiple procedures apply, 150% payment adjustment for bilateral procedures applies, assistant surgeon may be paid

35460   **Repair venous blockage**   ~ endoscopies or minor procedure - E/M services on the same day generally not paid, standard payment adjustment rules for multiple procedures apply, 150% payment adjustment for bilateral procedures applies, assistant surgeon may not be paid

35470   **Repair arterial blockage**   ~ endoscopies or minor procedure - E/M services on the same day generally not paid, standard payment adjustment rules for multiple procedures apply, 150% payment adjustment for bilateral procedures applies, assistant surgeon may not be paid

35471 **Repair arterial blockage** ~ endoscopies or minor procedure - E/M services on the same day generally not paid, standard payment adjustment rules for multiple procedures apply, 150% payment adjustment for bilateral procedures applies, assistant surgeon may not be paid

35472 **Repair arterial blockage** ~ endoscopies or minor procedure - E/M services on the same day generally not paid, standard payment adjustment rules for multiple procedures apply, 150% payment adjustment for bilateral procedures applies, payment for assistant surgeon subject to documentation of medical necessity

35473 **Repair arterial blockage** ~ endoscopies or minor procedure - E/M services on the same day generally not paid, standard payment adjustment rules for multiple procedures apply, 150% payment adjustment for bilateral procedures applies, assistant surgeon may not be paid

35474 **Repair arterial blockage** ~ endoscopies or minor procedure - E/M services on the same day generally not paid, standard payment adjustment rules for multiple procedures apply, 150% payment adjustment for bilateral procedures applies, assistant surgeon may not be paid

35475 **Repair arterial blockage** ~ restricted coverage - special coverage rules apply, endoscopies or minor procedure - E/M services on the same day generally not paid, standard payment adjustment rules for multiple procedures apply, 150% payment adjustment for bilateral procedures applies, assistant surgeon may not be paid

35476 **Repair venous blockage** ~ endoscopies or minor procedure - E/M services on the same day generally not paid, standard payment adjustment rules for multiple procedures apply, 150% payment adjustment for bilateral procedures applies, assistant surgeon may not be paid

35480 **Atherectomy, open** ~ endoscopies or minor procedure - E/M services on the same day generally not paid, standard payment adjustment rules for multiple procedures apply, 150% payment adjustment for bilateral procedures does not apply, assistant surgeon may be paid

35481 **Atherectomy, open** ~ endoscopies or minor procedure - E/M services on the same day generally not paid, standard payment adjustment rules for multiple procedures apply, 150% payment adjustment for bilateral procedures does not apply, assistant surgeon may be paid

35482 **Atherectomy, open** ~ endoscopies or minor procedure - E/M services on the same day generally not paid, standard payment adjustment rules for multiple procedures apply, 150% payment adjustment for bilateral procedures does not apply, assistant surgeon may be paid

35483 **Atherectomy, open** ~ endoscopies or minor procedure - E/M services on the same day generally not paid, standard payment adjustment rules for multiple

procedures apply, 150% payment adjustment for bilateral procedures does not apply, assistant surgeon may be paid

35484   **Atherectomy, open**   ~ endoscopies or minor procedure - E/M services on the same day generally not paid, standard payment adjustment rules for multiple procedures apply, 150% payment adjustment for bilateral procedures does not apply, assistant surgeon may be paid

35485   **Atherectomy, open**   ~ endoscopies or minor procedure - E/M services on the same day generally not paid, standard payment adjustment rules for multiple procedures apply, 150% payment adjustment for bilateral procedures does not apply, assistant surgeon may be paid

35490   **Atherectomy, percutaneous**   ~ endoscopies or minor procedure - E/M services on the same day generally not paid, standard payment adjustment rules for multiple procedures apply, 150% payment adjustment for bilateral procedures does not apply, assistant surgeon may be paid

35491   **Atherectomy, percutaneous**   ~ endoscopies or minor procedure - E/M services on the same day generally not paid, standard payment adjustment rules for multiple procedures apply, 150% payment adjustment for bilateral procedures does not apply, assistant surgeon may be paid

35492   **Atherectomy, percutaneous**   ~ endoscopies or minor procedure - E/M services on the same day generally not paid, standard payment adjustment rules for multiple procedures apply, 150% payment adjustment for bilateral procedures does not apply, assistant surgeon may be paid

35493   **Atherectomy, percutaneous**   ~ endoscopies or minor procedure - E/M services on the same day generally not paid, standard payment adjustment rules for multiple procedures apply, 150% payment adjustment for bilateral procedures does not apply, assistant surgeon may not be paid

35494   **Atherectomy, percutaneous**   ~ endoscopies or minor procedure - E/M services on the same day generally not paid, standard payment adjustment rules for multiple procedures apply, 150% payment adjustment for bilateral procedures does not apply, assistant surgeon may not be paid

35495   **Atherectomy, percutaneous**   ~ endoscopies or minor procedure - E/M services on the same day generally not paid, standard payment adjustment rules for multiple procedures apply, 150% payment adjustment for bilateral procedures does not apply, payment for assistant surgeon subject to documentation of medical necessity

35500   **Harvest vein for bypass**   ~ follow-up period included in another service, no payment adjustment rules for multiple procedures apply, 150% payment adjustment for bilateral procedures does not apply, assistant surgeon may be paid

35501 **Artery bypass graft** ~ follow-up period is 90 days, standard payment adjustment rules for multiple procedures apply, 150% payment adjustment for bilateral procedures applies, assistant surgeon may be paid

35506 **Artery bypass graft** ~ follow-up period is 90 days, standard payment adjustment rules for multiple procedures apply, 150% payment adjustment for bilateral procedures applies, assistant surgeon may be paid

35508 **Artery bypass graft** ~ follow-up period is 90 days, standard payment adjustment rules for multiple procedures apply, 150% payment adjustment for bilateral procedures applies, assistant surgeon may be paid

35509 **Artery bypass graft** ~ follow-up period is 90 days, standard payment adjustment rules for multiple procedures apply, 150% payment adjustment for bilateral procedures applies, assistant surgeon may be paid

35510 **Artery bypass graft** ~ follow-up period is 90 days, standard payment adjustment rules for multiple procedures apply, 150% payment adjustment for bilateral procedures applies, assistant surgeon may be paid

35511 **Artery bypass graft** ~ follow-up period is 90 days, standard payment adjustment rules for multiple procedures apply, 150% payment adjustment for bilateral procedures applies, assistant surgeon may be paid

35512 **Artery bypass graft** ~ follow-up period is 90 days, standard payment adjustment rules for multiple procedures apply, 150% payment adjustment for bilateral procedures applies, assistant surgeon may be paid

35515 **Artery bypass graft** ~ follow-up period is 90 days, standard payment adjustment rules for multiple procedures apply, 150% payment adjustment for bilateral procedures applies, assistant surgeon may be paid

35516 **Artery bypass graft** ~ follow-up period is 90 days, standard payment adjustment rules for multiple procedures apply, 150% payment adjustment for bilateral procedures applies, assistant surgeon may be paid

35518 **Artery bypass graft** ~ follow-up period is 90 days, standard payment adjustment rules for multiple procedures apply, 150% payment adjustment for bilateral procedures applies, assistant surgeon may be paid

35521 **Artery bypass graft** ~ follow-up period is 90 days, standard payment adjustment rules for multiple procedures apply, 150% payment adjustment for bilateral procedures applies, assistant surgeon may be paid

35522 **Artery bypass graft** ~ follow-up period is 90 days, standard payment adjustment rules for multiple procedures apply, 150% payment adjustment for bilateral procedures applies, assistant surgeon may be paid

35525   **Artery bypass graft**   ~ follow-up period is 90 days, standard payment adjustment rules for multiple procedures apply, 150% payment adjustment for bilateral procedures applies, assistant surgeon may be paid

35526   **Artery bypass graft**   ~ follow-up period is 90 days, standard payment adjustment rules for multiple procedures apply, 150% payment adjustment for bilateral procedures applies, assistant surgeon may be paid

35531   **Artery bypass graft**   ~ follow-up period is 90 days, standard payment adjustment rules for multiple procedures apply, 150% payment adjustment for bilateral procedures applies, assistant surgeon may be paid

35533   **Artery bypass graft**   ~ follow-up period is 90 days, standard payment adjustment rules for multiple procedures apply, 150% payment adjustment for bilateral procedures applies, assistant surgeon may be paid

35536   **Artery bypass graft**   ~ follow-up period is 90 days, standard payment adjustment rules for multiple procedures apply, 150% payment adjustment for bilateral procedures applies, assistant surgeon may be paid

35537   **Artery bypass graft**   ~ follow-up period is 90 days, standard payment adjustment rules for multiple procedures apply, 150% payment adjustment for bilateral procedures does not apply, assistant surgeon may be paid

35538   **Artery bypass graft**   ~ follow-up period is 90 days, standard payment adjustment rules for multiple procedures apply, 150% payment adjustment for bilateral procedures does not apply, assistant surgeon may be paid

35539   **Artery bypass graft**   ~ follow-up period is 90 days, standard payment adjustment rules for multiple procedures apply, 150% payment adjustment for bilateral procedures applies, assistant surgeon may be paid

35540   **Artery bypass graft**   ~ follow-up period is 90 days, standard payment adjustment rules for multiple procedures apply, 150% payment adjustment for bilateral procedures applies, assistant surgeon may not be paid

35548   **Artery bypass graft**   ~ follow-up period is 90 days, standard payment adjustment rules for multiple procedures apply, 150% payment adjustment for bilateral procedures does not apply, assistant surgeon may be paid

35549   **Artery bypass graft**   ~ follow-up period is 90 days, standard payment adjustment rules for multiple procedures apply, 150% payment adjustment does not apply - RVUs based on bilateral procedure, assistant surgeon may be paid

35551   **Artery bypass graft**   ~ follow-up period is 90 days, standard payment adjustment rules for multiple procedures apply, 150% payment adjustment for bilateral procedures applies, assistant surgeon may be paid

35556   **Artery bypass graft**   ~ follow-up period is 90 days, standard payment adjustment rules for multiple procedures apply, 150% payment adjustment for bilateral procedures applies, assistant surgeon may be paid

35558   **Artery bypass graft**   ~ follow-up period is 90 days, standard payment adjustment rules for multiple procedures apply, 150% payment adjustment for bilateral procedures applies, assistant surgeon may be paid

35560   **Artery bypass graft**   ~ follow-up period is 90 days, standard payment adjustment rules for multiple procedures apply, 150% payment adjustment for bilateral procedures applies, assistant surgeon may be paid

35563   **Artery bypass graft**   ~ follow-up period is 90 days, standard payment adjustment rules for multiple procedures apply, 150% payment adjustment for bilateral procedures applies, assistant surgeon may be paid

35565   **Artery bypass graft**   ~ follow-up period is 90 days, standard payment adjustment rules for multiple procedures apply, 150% payment adjustment for bilateral procedures applies, assistant surgeon may be paid

35566   **Artery bypass graft**   ~ follow-up period is 90 days, standard payment adjustment rules for multiple procedures apply, 150% payment adjustment for bilateral procedures applies, assistant surgeon may be paid

35571   **Artery bypass graft**   ~ follow-up period is 90 days, standard payment adjustment rules for multiple procedures apply, 150% payment adjustment for bilateral procedures applies, assistant surgeon may be paid

35572   **Harvest femoropopliteal vein**   ~ follow-up period included in another service, no payment adjustment rules for multiple procedures apply, 150% payment adjustment for bilateral procedures does not apply, assistant surgeon may be paid

35583   **Vein bypass graft**   ~ follow-up period is 90 days, standard payment adjustment rules for multiple procedures apply, 150% payment adjustment for bilateral procedures applies, assistant surgeon may be paid

35585   **Vein bypass graft**   ~ follow-up period is 90 days, standard payment adjustment rules for multiple procedures apply, 150% payment adjustment for bilateral procedures applies, assistant surgeon may be paid

35587   **Vein bypass graft**   ~ follow-up period is 90 days, standard payment adjustment rules for multiple procedures apply, 150% payment adjustment for bilateral procedures applies, assistant surgeon may be paid

35600   **Harvest artery for CABG**   ~ follow-up period included in another service, no payment adjustment rules for multiple procedures apply, 150% payment adjustment for bilateral procedures does not apply, assistant surgeon may be paid

35601   **Artery bypass graft**   ~ follow-up period is 90 days, standard payment adjustment rules for multiple procedures apply, 150% payment adjustment for bilateral procedures applies, assistant surgeon may be paid

35606   **Artery bypass graft**   ~ follow-up period is 90 days, standard payment adjustment rules for multiple procedures apply, 150% payment adjustment for bilateral procedures applies, assistant surgeon may be paid

35612   **Artery bypass graft**   ~ follow-up period is 90 days, standard payment adjustment rules for multiple procedures apply, 150% payment adjustment for bilateral procedures applies, assistant surgeon may be paid

35616   **Artery bypass graft**   ~ follow-up period is 90 days, standard payment adjustment rules for multiple procedures apply, 150% payment adjustment for bilateral procedures applies, assistant surgeon may be paid

35621   **Artery bypass graft**   ~ follow-up period is 90 days, standard payment adjustment rules for multiple procedures apply, 150% payment adjustment for bilateral procedures applies, assistant surgeon may be paid

35623   **Bypass graft, not vein**   ~ follow-up period is 90 days, standard payment adjustment rules for multiple procedures apply, 150% payment adjustment for bilateral procedures applies, assistant surgeon may be paid

35626   **Artery bypass graft**   ~ follow-up period is 90 days, standard payment adjustment rules for multiple procedures apply, 150% payment adjustment for bilateral procedures applies, assistant surgeon may be paid

35631   **Artery bypass graft**   ~ follow-up period is 90 days, standard payment adjustment rules for multiple procedures apply, 150% payment adjustment for bilateral procedures applies, assistant surgeon may be paid

35636   **Artery bypass graft**   ~ follow-up period is 90 days, standard payment adjustment rules for multiple procedures apply, 150% payment adjustment for bilateral procedures applies, assistant surgeon may be paid

35637   **Artery bypass graft**   ~ follow-up period is 90 days, standard payment adjustment rules for multiple procedures apply, 150% payment adjustment for bilateral procedures does not apply, assistant surgeon may be paid

35638   **Artery bypass graft**   ~ follow-up period is 90 days, standard payment adjustment rules for multiple procedures apply, 150% payment adjustment for bilateral procedures does not apply, assistant surgeon may be paid

35642   **Artery bypass graft**   ~ follow-up period is 90 days, standard payment adjustment rules for multiple procedures apply, 150% payment adjustment for bilateral procedures applies, assistant surgeon may be paid

35645 **Artery bypass graft** ~ follow-up period is 90 days, standard payment adjustment rules for multiple procedures apply, 150% payment adjustment for bilateral procedures applies, assistant surgeon may be paid

35646 **Artery bypass graft** ~ follow-up period is 90 days, standard payment adjustment rules for multiple procedures apply, 150% payment adjustment for bilateral procedures does not apply, assistant surgeon may be paid

35647 **Artery bypass graft** ~ follow-up period is 90 days, standard payment adjustment rules for multiple procedures apply, 150% payment adjustment for bilateral procedures applies, assistant surgeon may be paid

35650 **Artery bypass graft** ~ follow-up period is 90 days, standard payment adjustment rules for multiple procedures apply, 150% payment adjustment for bilateral procedures applies, assistant surgeon may be paid

35651 **Artery bypass graft** ~ follow-up period is 90 days, standard payment adjustment rules for multiple procedures apply, 150% payment adjustment for bilateral procedures applies, assistant surgeon may be paid

35654 **Artery bypass graft** ~ follow-up period is 90 days, standard payment adjustment rules for multiple procedures apply, 150% payment adjustment for bilateral procedures does not apply, assistant surgeon may be paid

35656 **Artery bypass graft** ~ follow-up period is 90 days, standard payment adjustment rules for multiple procedures apply, 150% payment adjustment for bilateral procedures applies, assistant surgeon may be paid

35661 **Artery bypass graft** ~ follow-up period is 90 days, standard payment adjustment rules for multiple procedures apply, 150% payment adjustment for bilateral procedures applies, assistant surgeon may be paid

35663 **Artery bypass graft** ~ follow-up period is 90 days, standard payment adjustment rules for multiple procedures apply, 150% payment adjustment for bilateral procedures applies, assistant surgeon may be paid

35665 **Artery bypass graft** ~ follow-up period is 90 days, standard payment adjustment rules for multiple procedures apply, 150% payment adjustment for bilateral procedures applies, assistant surgeon may be paid

35666 **Artery bypass graft** ~ follow-up period is 90 days, standard payment adjustment rules for multiple procedures apply, 150% payment adjustment for bilateral procedures applies, assistant surgeon may be paid

35671 **Artery bypass graft** ~ follow-up period is 90 days, standard payment adjustment rules for multiple procedures apply, 150% payment adjustment for bilateral procedures applies, assistant surgeon may be paid

35681   **Composite bypass graft**   ~ follow-up period included in another service, no payment adjustment rules for multiple procedures apply, 150% payment adjustment for bilateral procedures does not apply, assistant surgeon may be paid

35682   **Composite bypass graft**   ~ follow-up period included in another service, no payment adjustment rules for multiple procedures apply, 150% payment adjustment for bilateral procedures does not apply, payment for assistant surgeon subject to documentation of medical necessity

35683   **Composite bypass graft**   ~ follow-up period included in another service, no payment adjustment rules for multiple procedures apply, 150% payment adjustment for bilateral procedures does not apply, payment for assistant surgeon subject to documentation of medical necessity

35685   **Bypass graft patency/patch**   ~ follow-up period included in another service, no payment adjustment rules for multiple procedures apply, 150% payment adjustment for bilateral procedures does not apply, assistant surgeon may be paid

35686   **Bypass graft/av fist patency**   ~ follow-up period included in another service, no payment adjustment rules for multiple procedures apply, 150% payment adjustment for bilateral procedures does not apply, assistant surgeon may be paid

35691   **Arterial transposition**   ~ follow-up period is 90 days, standard payment adjustment rules for multiple procedures apply, 150% payment adjustment for bilateral procedures applies, assistant surgeon may be paid

35693   **Arterial transposition**   ~ follow-up period is 90 days, standard payment adjustment rules for multiple procedures apply, 150% payment adjustment for bilateral procedures applies, assistant surgeon may be paid

35694   **Arterial transposition**   ~ follow-up period is 90 days, standard payment adjustment rules for multiple procedures apply, 150% payment adjustment for bilateral procedures applies, assistant surgeon may be paid

35695   **Arterial transposition**   ~ follow-up period is 90 days, standard payment adjustment rules for multiple procedures apply, 150% payment adjustment for bilateral procedures applies, assistant surgeon may be paid

35697   **Reimplant artery each**   ~ follow-up period included in another service, no payment adjustment rules for multiple procedures apply, 150% payment adjustment for bilateral procedures does not apply, assistant surgeon may be paid

35700   **Reoperation, bypass graft**   ~ follow-up period included in another service, no payment adjustment rules for multiple procedures apply, 150% payment adjustment for bilateral procedures does not apply, assistant surgeon may be paid

35701   **Explore carotid artery**   ~ follow-up period is 90 days, standard payment adjustment rules for multiple procedures apply, 150% payment adjustment for bilateral procedures applies, assistant surgeon may be paid

35721   **Explore femoral artery**   ~ follow-up period is 90 days, standard payment adjustment rules for multiple procedures apply, 150% payment adjustment for bilateral procedures applies, assistant surgeon may be paid

35741   **Explore popliteal artery**   ~ follow-up period is 90 days, standard payment adjustment rules for multiple procedures apply, 150% payment adjustment for bilateral procedures applies, assistant surgeon may be paid

35761   **Explore artery/vein**   ~ follow-up period is 90 days, standard payment adjustment rules for multiple procedures apply, 150% payment adjustment for bilateral procedures applies, assistant surgeon may be paid

35800   **Explore neck vessels**   ~ follow-up period is 90 days, standard payment adjustment rules for multiple procedures apply, 150% payment adjustment for bilateral procedures does not apply, assistant surgeon may be paid

35820   **Explore chest vessels**   ~ follow-up period is 90 days, standard payment adjustment rules for multiple procedures apply, 150% payment adjustment for bilateral procedures does not apply, assistant surgeon may be paid

35840   **Explore abdominal vessels**   ~ follow-up period is 90 days, standard payment adjustment rules for multiple procedures apply, 150% payment adjustment for bilateral procedures does not apply, assistant surgeon may be paid

35860   **Explore limb vessels**   ~ follow-up period is 90 days, standard payment adjustment rules for multiple procedures apply, 150% payment adjustment for bilateral procedures does not apply, assistant surgeon may be paid

35870   **Repair vessel graft defect**   ~ follow-up period is 90 days, standard payment adjustment rules for multiple procedures apply, 150% payment adjustment for bilateral procedures does not apply, assistant surgeon may be paid

35875   **Remove clot in graft**   ~ follow-up period is 90 days, standard payment adjustment rules for multiple procedures apply, 150% payment adjustment for bilateral procedures does not apply, assistant surgeon may not be paid

35876   **Remove clot in graft**   ~ follow-up period is 90 days, standard payment adjustment rules for multiple procedures apply, 150% payment adjustment for bilateral procedures does not apply, assistant surgeon may be paid

35879   **Revise graft w/vein**   ~ follow-up period is 90 days, standard payment adjustment rules for multiple procedures apply, 150% payment adjustment for bilateral procedures applies, assistant surgeon may be paid

---

35881   **Revise graft w/vein**   ~ follow-up period is 90 days, standard payment adjustment rules for multiple procedures apply, 150% payment adjustment for bilateral procedures applies, assistant surgeon may be paid

35883   **Revise graft w/nonautograft**   ~ follow-up period is 90 days, standard payment adjustment rules for multiple procedures apply, 150% payment adjustment for bilateral procedures applies, assistant surgeon may be paid

35884   **Revise graft w/vein**   ~ follow-up period is 90 days, standard payment adjustment rules for multiple procedures apply, 150% payment adjustment for bilateral procedures applies, assistant surgeon may be paid

35901   **Excise graft, neck**   ~ follow-up period is 90 days, standard payment adjustment rules for multiple procedures apply, 150% payment adjustment for bilateral procedures does not apply, assistant surgeon may be paid

35903   **Excise graft, extremity**   ~ follow-up period is 90 days, standard payment adjustment rules for multiple procedures apply, 150% payment adjustment for bilateral procedures does not apply, assistant surgeon may be paid

35905   **Excise graft, thorax**   ~ follow-up period is 90 days, standard payment adjustment rules for multiple procedures apply, 150% payment adjustment for bilateral procedures does not apply, assistant surgeon may be paid

35907   **Excise graft, abdomen**   ~ follow-up period is 90 days, standard payment adjustment rules for multiple procedures apply, 150% payment adjustment for bilateral procedures does not apply, assistant surgeon may be paid

36000   **Place needle in vein**   ~ standard payment adjustment rules for multiple procedures apply, 150% payment adjustment for bilateral procedures applies, assistant surgeon may not be paid

36002   **Pseudoaneurysm injection treatment**   ~ endoscopies or minor procedure - E/M services on the same day generally not paid, standard payment adjustment rules for multiple procedures apply, 150% payment adjustment for bilateral procedures applies, assistant surgeon may not be paid

36005   **Injection ext venography**   ~ endoscopies or minor procedure - E/M services on the same day generally not paid, standard payment adjustment rules for multiple procedures apply, 150% payment adjustment for bilateral procedures applies, payment for assistant surgeon subject to documentation of medical necessity

36010   **Place catheter in vein**   ~ standard payment adjustment rules for multiple procedures apply, 150% payment adjustment for bilateral procedures applies, assistant surgeon may not be paid

36011 **Place catheter in vein** ~ standard payment adjustment rules for multiple procedures apply, 150% payment adjustment for bilateral procedures applies, assistant surgeon may not be paid

36012 **Place catheter in vein** ~ standard payment adjustment rules for multiple procedures apply, 150% payment adjustment for bilateral procedures applies, assistant surgeon may not be paid

36013 **Place catheter in artery** ~ standard payment adjustment rules for multiple procedures apply, 150% payment adjustment for bilateral procedures does not apply, assistant surgeon may not be paid

36014 **Place catheter in artery** ~ standard payment adjustment rules for multiple procedures apply, 150% payment adjustment for bilateral procedures applies, assistant surgeon may not be paid

36015 **Place catheter in artery** ~ standard payment adjustment rules for multiple procedures apply, 150% payment adjustment for bilateral procedures applies, assistant surgeon may not be paid

36100 **Establish access to artery** ~ standard payment adjustment rules for multiple procedures apply, 150% payment adjustment for bilateral procedures applies, assistant surgeon may not be paid

36120 **Establish access to artery** ~ standard payment adjustment rules for multiple procedures apply, 150% payment adjustment for bilateral procedures does not apply, assistant surgeon may not be paid

36140 **Establish access to artery** ~ standard payment adjustment rules for multiple procedures apply, 150% payment adjustment for bilateral procedures does not apply, assistant surgeon may not be paid

36145 **Artery to vein shunt** ~ standard payment adjustment rules for multiple procedures apply, 150% payment adjustment for bilateral procedures does not apply, assistant surgeon may not be paid

36160 **Establish access to aorta** ~ standard payment adjustment rules for multiple procedures apply, 150% payment adjustment for bilateral procedures does not apply, assistant surgeon may not be paid

36200 **Place catheter in aorta** ~ standard payment adjustment rules for multiple procedures apply, 150% payment adjustment for bilateral procedures applies, assistant surgeon may not be paid

36215 **Place catheter in artery** ~ standard payment adjustment rules for multiple procedures apply, 150% payment adjustment for bilateral procedures does not apply, assistant surgeon may not be paid

36216	**Place catheter in artery**	~ standard payment adjustment rules for multiple procedures apply, 150% payment adjustment for bilateral procedures does not apply, assistant surgeon may not be paid

36217	**Place catheter in artery**	~ standard payment adjustment rules for multiple procedures apply, 150% payment adjustment for bilateral procedures does not apply, assistant surgeon may not be paid

36218	**Place catheter in artery**	~ follow-up period included in another service, no payment adjustment rules for multiple procedures apply, 150% payment adjustment for bilateral procedures does not apply, assistant surgeon may not be paid

36245	**Place catheter in artery**	~ standard payment adjustment rules for multiple procedures apply, 150% payment adjustment for bilateral procedures applies, assistant surgeon may not be paid

36246	**Place catheter in artery**	~ standard payment adjustment rules for multiple procedures apply, 150% payment adjustment for bilateral procedures applies, assistant surgeon may not be paid

36247	**Place catheter in artery**	~ standard payment adjustment rules for multiple procedures apply, 150% payment adjustment for bilateral procedures applies, assistant surgeon may not be paid

36248	**Place catheter in artery**	~ follow-up period included in another service, no payment adjustment rules for multiple procedures apply, 150% payment adjustment for bilateral procedures does not apply, assistant surgeon may not be paid

36260	**Insert infuse pump**	~ follow-up period is 90 days, standard payment adjustment rules for multiple procedures apply, 150% payment adjustment for bilateral procedures does not apply, assistant surgeon may not be paid

36261	**Revise infuse pump**	~ follow-up period is 90 days, standard payment adjustment rules for multiple procedures apply, 150% payment adjustment for bilateral procedures does not apply, assistant surgeon may be paid

36262	**Remove infuse pump**	~ follow-up period is 90 days, standard payment adjustment rules for multiple procedures apply, 150% payment adjustment for bilateral procedures does not apply, assistant surgeon may not be paid

36299	**Vessel injection procedure**	~ medicare carrier determines global period, standard payment adjustment rules for multiple procedures apply, 150% payment adjustment for bilateral procedures does not apply, payment for assistant surgeon subject to documentation of medical necessity

36400   **Blood draw < 3 yrs fem/jugular**   ~ standard payment adjustment rules for multiple procedures apply, 150% payment adjustment for bilateral procedures does not apply, assistant surgeon may not be paid

36405   **Blood draw < 3 yrs scalp vein**   ~ standard payment adjustment rules for multiple procedures apply, 150% payment adjustment for bilateral procedures does not apply, assistant surgeon may not be paid

36406   **Blood draw < 3 yrs other vein**   ~ standard payment adjustment rules for multiple procedures apply, 150% payment adjustment for bilateral procedures does not apply, assistant surgeon may not be paid

36410   **Non-routine blood draw > 3 yrs**   ~ standard payment adjustment rules for multiple procedures apply, 150% payment adjustment for bilateral procedures does not apply, assistant surgeon may not be paid

36415   **Routine venipuncture**   ~ multiple procedure concept does not apply, bilateral surgery concept does not apply, assistant surgery concept does not apply

36416   **Capillary blood draw**   ~ bundled code - no separate payment made, multiple procedure concept does not apply, bilateral surgery concept does not apply, assistant surgery concept does not apply

36420   **Vein access cutdown < 1 yr**   ~ standard payment adjustment rules for multiple procedures apply, 150% payment adjustment for bilateral procedures does not apply, payment for assistant surgeon subject to documentation of medical necessity

36425   **Vein access cutdown > 1 yr**   ~ standard payment adjustment rules for multiple procedures apply, 150% payment adjustment for bilateral procedures does not apply, assistant surgeon may not be paid

36430   **Blood transfuse service**   ~ no payment adjustment rules for multiple procedures apply, 150% payment adjustment for bilateral procedures does not apply, assistant surgeon may not be paid

36440   **Blood push transfuse, 2 yr or <**   ~ standard payment adjustment rules for multiple procedures apply, 150% payment adjustment for bilateral procedures does not apply, payment for assistant surgeon subject to documentation of medical necessity

36450   **Blood exchange/transfuse, nb**   ~ standard payment adjustment rules for multiple procedures apply, 150% payment adjustment for bilateral procedures does not apply, payment for assistant surgeon subject to documentation of medical necessity

36455   **Blood exchange/transfuse non-nb**   ~ standard payment adjustment rules for multiple procedures apply, 150% payment adjustment for bilateral procedures does not apply, assistant surgeon may not be paid

36460   **Transfuse service, fetal**   ~ standard payment adjustment rules for multiple procedures apply, 150% payment adjustment for bilateral procedures does not apply, assistant surgeon may be paid

36468   **Injection(s), spider veins**   ~ restricted coverage - special coverage rules apply, endoscopies or minor procedure - E/M services on the same day generally not paid, standard payment adjustment rules for multiple procedures apply, 150% payment adjustment for bilateral procedures does not apply, payment for assistant surgeon subject to documentation of medical necessity

36469   **Injection(s), spider veins**   ~ restricted coverage - special coverage rules apply, endoscopies or minor procedure - E/M services on the same day generally not paid, standard payment adjustment rules for multiple procedures apply, 150% payment adjustment for bilateral procedures does not apply, payment for assistant surgeon subject to documentation of medical necessity

36470   **Injection therapy of vein**   ~ follow-up period is 10 days, standard payment adjustment rules for multiple procedures apply, 150% payment adjustment for bilateral procedures applies, assistant surgeon may not be paid

36471   **Injection therapy of veins**   ~ follow-up period is 10 days, standard payment adjustment rules for multiple procedures apply, 150% payment adjustment for bilateral procedures applies, assistant surgeon may not be paid

36475   **Endovenous rf, 1st vein**   ~ endoscopies or minor procedure - E/M services on the same day generally not paid, standard payment adjustment rules for multiple procedures apply, 150% payment adjustment for bilateral procedures applies, assistant surgeon may not be paid

36476   **Endovenous rf, vein, add-on**   ~ follow-up period included in another service, no payment adjustment rules for multiple procedures apply, 150% payment adjustment for bilateral procedures applies, assistant surgeon may not be paid, +add-on code (list separately in addition to primary procedure)

36478   **Endovenous laser, 1st vein**   ~ endoscopies or minor procedure - E/M services on the same day generally not paid, standard payment adjustment rules for multiple procedures apply, 150% payment adjustment for bilateral procedures applies, assistant surgeon may not be paid

36479   **Endovenous laser vein add on**   ~ follow-up period included in another service, no payment adjustment rules for multiple procedures apply, 150% payment adjustment for bilateral procedures applies, assistant surgeon may not be paid, +add-on code (list separately in addition to primary procedure)

36481   **Insert catheter, vein**   ~ endoscopies or minor procedure - E/M services on the same day generally not paid, standard payment adjustment rules for multiple

procedures apply, 150% payment adjustment for bilateral procedures does not apply, assistant surgeon may not be paid

36500 **Insert catheter, vein** ~ endoscopies or minor procedure - E/M services on the same day generally not paid, standard payment adjustment rules for multiple procedures apply, 150% payment adjustment for bilateral procedures does not apply, assistant surgeon may not be paid

36510 **Insert catheter, vein** ~ endoscopies or minor procedure - E/M services on the same day generally not paid, standard payment adjustment rules for multiple procedures apply, 150% payment adjustment for bilateral procedures does not apply, payment for assistant surgeon subject to documentation of medical necessity

36511 **Apheresis wbc** ~ endoscopies or minor procedure - E/M services on the same day generally not paid, standard payment adjustment rules for multiple procedures apply, 150% payment adjustment for bilateral procedures does not apply, assistant surgeon may not be paid

36512 **Apheresis rbc** ~ endoscopies or minor procedure - E/M services on the same day generally not paid, standard payment adjustment rules for multiple procedures apply, 150% payment adjustment for bilateral procedures does not apply, assistant surgeon may not be paid

36513 **Apheresis platelets** ~ endoscopies or minor procedure - E/M services on the same day generally not paid, standard payment adjustment rules for multiple procedures apply, 150% payment adjustment for bilateral procedures does not apply, assistant surgeon may not be paid

36514 **Apheresis plasma** ~ endoscopies or minor procedure - E/M services on the same day generally not paid, standard payment adjustment rules for multiple procedures apply, 150% payment adjustment for bilateral procedures does not apply, assistant surgeon may not be paid

36515 **Apheresis, adsorp/reinfuse** ~ endoscopies or minor procedure - E/M services on the same day generally not paid, standard payment adjustment rules for multiple procedures apply, 150% payment adjustment for bilateral procedures does not apply, assistant surgeon may not be paid

36516 **Apheresis, selective** ~ endoscopies or minor procedure - E/M services on the same day generally not paid, standard payment adjustment rules for multiple procedures apply, 150% payment adjustment for bilateral procedures does not apply, assistant surgeon may not be paid

36522 **Photopheresis** ~ endoscopies or minor procedure - E/M services on the same day generally not paid, standard payment adjustment rules for multiple procedures apply, 150% payment adjustment for bilateral procedures does not apply, assistant surgeon may not be paid

36540   **Collect blood venous device**   ~ bundled code - no separate payment made, multiple procedure concept does not apply, bilateral surgery concept does not apply, assistant surgery concept does not apply

36550   **Declot vascular device**   ~ no payment adjustment rules for multiple procedures apply, 150% payment adjustment for bilateral procedures does not apply, payment for assistant surgeon subject to documentation of medical necessity

36555   **Insert non-tunnel cv cath**   ~ endoscopies or minor procedure - E/M services on the same day generally not paid, no payment adjustment rules for multiple procedures apply, 150% payment adjustment for bilateral procedures does not apply, assistant surgeon may not be paid

36556   **Insert non-tunnel cv cath**   ~ endoscopies or minor procedure - E/M services on the same day generally not paid, no payment adjustment rules for multiple procedures apply, 150% payment adjustment for bilateral procedures does not apply, assistant surgeon may not be paid

36557   **Insert tunneled cv cath**   ~ follow-up period is 10 days, standard payment adjustment rules for multiple procedures apply, 150% payment adjustment for bilateral procedures applies, payment for assistant surgeon subject to documentation of medical necessity

36558   **Insert tunneled cv cath**   ~ follow-up period is 10 days, standard payment adjustment rules for multiple procedures apply, 150% payment adjustment for bilateral procedures applies, payment for assistant surgeon subject to documentation of medical necessity

36560   **Insert tunneled cv cath**   ~ follow-up period is 10 days, standard payment adjustment rules for multiple procedures apply, 150% payment adjustment for bilateral procedures applies, payment for assistant surgeon subject to documentation of medical necessity

36561   **Insert tunneled cv cath**   ~ follow-up period is 10 days, standard payment adjustment rules for multiple procedures apply, 150% payment adjustment for bilateral procedures applies, payment for assistant surgeon subject to documentation of medical necessity

36563   **Insert tunneled cv cath**   ~ follow-up period is 10 days, standard payment adjustment rules for multiple procedures apply, 150% payment adjustment for bilateral procedures does not apply, payment for assistant surgeon subject to documentation of medical necessity

36565   **Insert tunneled cv cath**   ~ follow-up period is 10 days, standard payment adjustment rules for multiple procedures apply, 150% payment adjustment for bilateral procedures applies, payment for assistant surgeon subject to documentation of medical necessity

36566 **Insert tunneled cv cath** ~ follow-up period is 10 days, standard payment adjustment rules for multiple procedures apply, 150% payment adjustment for bilateral procedures applies, payment for assistant surgeon subject to documentation of medical necessity

36568 **Insert picc cath** ~ endoscopies or minor procedure - E/M services on the same day generally not paid, no payment adjustment rules for multiple procedures apply, 150% payment adjustment for bilateral procedures does not apply, assistant surgeon may not be paid

36569 **Insert picc cath** ~ endoscopies or minor procedure - E/M services on the same day generally not paid, no payment adjustment rules for multiple procedures apply, 150% payment adjustment for bilateral procedures does not apply, assistant surgeon may not be paid

36570 **Insert picvad cath** ~ follow-up period is 10 days, standard payment adjustment rules for multiple procedures apply, 150% payment adjustment for bilateral procedures applies, payment for assistant surgeon subject to documentation of medical necessity

36571 **Insert picvad cath** ~ follow-up period is 10 days, standard payment adjustment rules for multiple procedures apply, 150% payment adjustment for bilateral procedures applies, payment for assistant surgeon subject to documentation of medical necessity

36575 **Repair tunneled cv cath** ~ endoscopies or minor procedure - E/M services on the same day generally not paid, standard payment adjustment rules for multiple procedures apply, 150% payment adjustment for bilateral procedures does not apply, payment for assistant surgeon subject to documentation of medical necessity

36576 **Repair tunneled cv cath** ~ follow-up period is 10 days, standard payment adjustment rules for multiple procedures apply, 150% payment adjustment for bilateral procedures does not apply, payment for assistant surgeon subject to documentation of medical necessity

36578 **Replace tunneled cv cath** ~ follow-up period is 10 days, standard payment adjustment rules for multiple procedures apply, 150% payment adjustment for bilateral procedures does not apply, payment for assistant surgeon subject to documentation of medical necessity

36580 **Replace cvad cath** ~ endoscopies or minor procedure - E/M services on the same day generally not paid, no payment adjustment rules for multiple procedures apply, 150% payment adjustment for bilateral procedures does not apply, assistant surgeon may not be paid

36581 **Replace tunneled cv cath** ~ follow-up period is 10 days, standard payment adjustment rules for multiple procedures apply, 150% payment adjustment for

bilateral procedures does not apply, payment for assistant surgeon subject to documentation of medical necessity

36582   **Replace tunneled cv cath**   ~ follow-up period is 10 days, standard payment adjustment rules for multiple procedures apply, 150% payment adjustment for bilateral procedures does not apply, payment for assistant surgeon subject to documentation of medical necessity

36583   **Replace tunneled cv cath**   ~ follow-up period is 10 days, standard payment adjustment rules for multiple procedures apply, 150% payment adjustment for bilateral procedures does not apply, payment for assistant surgeon subject to documentation of medical necessity

36584   **Replace picc cath**   ~ endoscopies or minor procedure - E/M services on the same day generally not paid, no payment adjustment rules for multiple procedures apply, 150% payment adjustment for bilateral procedures does not apply, assistant surgeon may not be paid

36585   **Replace picvad cath**   ~ follow-up period is 10 days, standard payment adjustment rules for multiple procedures apply, 150% payment adjustment for bilateral procedures does not apply, payment for assistant surgeon subject to documentation of medical necessity

36589   **Remove tunneled cv cath**   ~ follow-up period is 10 days, standard payment adjustment rules for multiple procedures apply, 150% payment adjustment for bilateral procedures applies, payment for assistant surgeon subject to documentation of medical necessity

36590   **Remove tunneled cv cath**   ~ follow-up period is 10 days, standard payment adjustment rules for multiple procedures apply, 150% payment adjustment for bilateral procedures does not apply, payment for assistant surgeon subject to documentation of medical necessity

36595   **Mechanical remove tunneled cv cath**   ~ endoscopies or minor procedure - E/M services on the same day generally not paid, standard payment adjustment rules for multiple procedures apply, 150% payment adjustment for bilateral procedures does not apply, assistant surgeon may not be paid

36596   **Mechanical remove tunneled cv cath**   ~ endoscopies or minor procedure - E/M services on the same day generally not paid, standard payment adjustment rules for multiple procedures apply, 150% payment adjustment for bilateral procedures does not apply, assistant surgeon may not be paid

36597   **Reposition venous catheter**   ~ endoscopies or minor procedure - E/M services on the same day generally not paid, standard payment adjustment rules for multiple procedures apply, 150% payment adjustment for bilateral procedures does not apply, assistant surgeon may not be paid

36598 **Inject w/fluor, evaluate cv device** ~ endoscopies or minor procedure - E/M services on the same day generally not paid, standard payment adjustment rules for multiple procedures apply, 150% payment adjustment for bilateral procedures applies, payment for assistant surgeon subject to documentation of medical necessity

36600 **Withdrawal of arterial blood** ~ standard payment adjustment rules for multiple procedures apply, 150% payment adjustment for bilateral procedures does not apply, assistant surgeon may not be paid

36620 **Insert catheter, artery** ~ endoscopies or minor procedure - E/M services on the same day generally not paid, no payment adjustment rules for multiple procedures apply, 150% payment adjustment for bilateral procedures does not apply, assistant surgeon may not be paid

36625 **Insert catheter, artery** ~ endoscopies or minor procedure - E/M services on the same day generally not paid, no payment adjustment rules for multiple procedures apply, 150% payment adjustment for bilateral procedures does not apply, assistant surgeon may not be paid

36640 **Insert catheter, artery** ~ endoscopies or minor procedure - E/M services on the same day generally not paid, standard payment adjustment rules for multiple procedures apply, 150% payment adjustment for bilateral procedures does not apply, assistant surgeon may not be paid

36660 **Insert catheter, artery** ~ endoscopies or minor procedure - E/M services on the same day generally not paid, no payment adjustment rules for multiple procedures apply, 150% payment adjustment for bilateral procedures does not apply, payment for assistant surgeon subject to documentation of medical necessity

36680 **Insert needle, bone cavity** ~ endoscopies or minor procedure - E/M services on the same day generally not paid, standard payment adjustment rules for multiple procedures apply, 150% payment adjustment for bilateral procedures does not apply, payment for assistant surgeon subject to documentation of medical necessity

36800 **Insert cannula** ~ endoscopies or minor procedure - E/M services on the same day generally not paid, standard payment adjustment rules for multiple procedures apply, 150% payment adjustment for bilateral procedures does not apply, assistant surgeon may not be paid

36810 **Insert cannula** ~ endoscopies or minor procedure - E/M services on the same day generally not paid, standard payment adjustment rules for multiple procedures apply, 150% payment adjustment for bilateral procedures does not apply, assistant surgeon may not be paid

36815 **Insert cannula** ~ endoscopies or minor procedure - E/M services on the same day generally not paid, standard payment adjustment rules for multiple

procedures apply, 150% payment adjustment for bilateral procedures does not apply, assistant surgeon may not be paid

36818 **Av fuse, upper arm, cephalic** ~ follow-up period is 90 days, standard payment adjustment rules for multiple procedures apply, 150% payment adjustment for bilateral procedures does not apply, assistant surgeon may be paid

36819 **Av fuse, upper arm, basilic** ~ follow-up period is 90 days, standard payment adjustment rules for multiple procedures apply, 150% payment adjustment for bilateral procedures does not apply, assistant surgeon may be paid

36820 **Av fuse/forearm vein** ~ follow-up period is 90 days, standard payment adjustment rules for multiple procedures apply, 150% payment adjustment for bilateral procedures applies, assistant surgeon may be paid

36821 **Av fuse direct any site** ~ follow-up period is 90 days, standard payment adjustment rules for multiple procedures apply, 150% payment adjustment for bilateral procedures does not apply, assistant surgeon may be paid

36822 **Insert cannula(s)** ~ follow-up period is 90 days, standard payment adjustment rules for multiple procedures apply, 150% payment adjustment for bilateral procedures does not apply, assistant surgeon may not be paid

36823 **Insert cannula(s)** ~ follow-up period is 90 days, standard payment adjustment rules for multiple procedures apply, 150% payment adjustment for bilateral procedures does not apply, assistant surgeon may not be paid

36825 **Artery-vein autograft** ~ follow-up period is 90 days, standard payment adjustment rules for multiple procedures apply, 150% payment adjustment for bilateral procedures does not apply, assistant surgeon may be paid

36830 **Artery-vein nonautograft** ~ follow-up period is 90 days, standard payment adjustment rules for multiple procedures apply, 150% payment adjustment for bilateral procedures does not apply, assistant surgeon may be paid

36831 **Open thrombectomy av fistula** ~ follow-up period is 90 days, standard payment adjustment rules for multiple procedures apply, 150% payment adjustment for bilateral procedures does not apply, assistant surgeon may be paid

36832 **Av fistula revise open** ~ follow-up period is 90 days, standard payment adjustment rules for multiple procedures apply, 150% payment adjustment for bilateral procedures does not apply, assistant surgeon may be paid

36833 **Av fistula revision** ~ follow-up period is 90 days, standard payment adjustment rules for multiple procedures apply, 150% payment adjustment for bilateral procedures does not apply, assistant surgeon may be paid

36834   **Repair a-v aneurysm**   ~ follow-up period is 90 days, standard payment adjustment rules for multiple procedures apply, 150% payment adjustment for bilateral procedures does not apply, assistant surgeon may be paid

36835   **Artery to vein shunt**   ~ follow-up period is 90 days, standard payment adjustment rules for multiple procedures apply, 150% payment adjustment for bilateral procedures does not apply, assistant surgeon may not be paid

36838   **Dist revasc ligate hemo**   ~ follow-up period is 90 days, standard payment adjustment rules for multiple procedures apply, 150% payment adjustment for bilateral procedures applies, assistant surgeon may be paid

36860   **External cannula declotting**   ~ endoscopies or minor procedure - E/M services on the same day generally not paid, standard payment adjustment rules for multiple procedures apply, 150% payment adjustment for bilateral procedures does not apply, assistant surgeon may not be paid

36861   **Cannula declotting**   ~ endoscopies or minor procedure - E/M services on the same day generally not paid, standard payment adjustment rules for multiple procedures apply, 150% payment adjustment for bilateral procedures does not apply, assistant surgeon may not be paid

36870   **Percutaneous thrombectomy av fistula**   ~ follow-up period is 90 days, standard payment adjustment rules for multiple procedures apply, 150% payment adjustment for bilateral procedures applies, assistant surgeon may not be paid

37140   **Revise circulation**   ~ follow-up period is 90 days, standard payment adjustment rules for multiple procedures apply, 150% payment adjustment for bilateral procedures does not apply, assistant surgeon may not be paid

37145   **Revise circulation**   ~ follow-up period is 90 days, standard payment adjustment rules for multiple procedures apply, 150% payment adjustment for bilateral procedures does not apply, assistant surgeon may be paid

37160   **Revise circulation**   ~ follow-up period is 90 days, standard payment adjustment rules for multiple procedures apply, 150% payment adjustment for bilateral procedures does not apply, assistant surgeon may be paid

37180   **Revise circulation**   ~ follow-up period is 90 days, standard payment adjustment rules for multiple procedures apply, 150% payment adjustment for bilateral procedures does not apply, assistant surgeon may be paid

37181   **Splice spleen/kidney veins**   ~ follow-up period is 90 days, standard payment adjustment rules for multiple procedures apply, 150% payment adjustment for bilateral procedures does not apply, assistant surgeon may be paid

37182   **Insert hepatic shunt (tips)**   ~ endoscopies or minor procedure - E/M services on the same day generally not paid, standard payment adjustment rules for multiple procedures apply, 150% payment adjustment for bilateral procedures does not apply, payment for assistant surgeon subject to documentation of medical necessity

37183   **Remove hepatic shunt (tips)**   ~ endoscopies or minor procedure - E/M services on the same day generally not paid, standard payment adjustment rules for multiple procedures apply, 150% payment adjustment for bilateral procedures does not apply, payment for assistant surgeon subject to documentation of medical necessity

37184   **Prim art mechanical thrombectomy**   ~ endoscopies or minor procedure - E/M services on the same day generally not paid, standard payment adjustment rules for multiple procedures apply, 150% payment adjustment for bilateral procedures applies, assistant surgeon may not be paid

37185   **Prim art m-thrombectomy, add-on**   ~ follow-up period included in another service, no payment adjustment rules for multiple procedures apply, 150% payment adjustment does not apply - RVUs based on bilateral procedure, assistant surgeon may not be paid, +add-on code (list separately in addition to primary procedure)

37186   **Sec art m-thrombectomy, add-on**   ~ follow-up period included in another service, no payment adjustment rules for multiple procedures apply, 150% payment adjustment does not apply - RVUs based on bilateral procedure, assistant surgeon may not be paid, +add-on code (list separately in addition to primary procedure)

37187   **Venous mechanical thrombectomy**   ~ endoscopies or minor procedure - E/M services on the same day generally not paid, standard payment adjustment rules for multiple procedures apply, 150% payment adjustment for bilateral procedures applies, assistant surgeon may not be paid

37188   **Venous m-thrombectomy, add-on**   ~ endoscopies or minor procedure - E/M services on the same day generally not paid, standard payment adjustment rules for multiple procedures apply, 150% payment adjustment for bilateral procedures applies, assistant surgeon may not be paid, +add-on code (list separately in addition to primary procedure)

37195   **Thrombolytic therapy, stroke**   ~ no payment adjustment rules for multiple procedures apply, 150% payment adjustment for bilateral procedures does not apply, payment for assistant surgeon subject to documentation of medical necessity

37200   **Transcatheter biopsy**   ~ endoscopies or minor procedure - E/M services on the same day generally not paid, standard payment adjustment rules for multiple procedures apply, 150% payment adjustment for bilateral procedures does not apply, assistant surgeon may not be paid

37201   **Transcatheter therapy infuse**   ~ endoscopies or minor procedure - E/M services on the same day generally not paid, standard payment adjustment rules for multiple

procedures apply, 150% payment adjustment for bilateral procedures does not apply, assistant surgeon may not be paid

37202 Transcatheter therapy infuse ~ endoscopies or minor procedure - E/M services on the same day generally not paid, standard payment adjustment rules for multiple procedures apply, 150% payment adjustment for bilateral procedures does not apply, assistant surgeon may not be paid

37203 Transcatheter retrieval ~ endoscopies or minor procedure - E/M services on the same day generally not paid, standard payment adjustment rules for multiple procedures apply, 150% payment adjustment for bilateral procedures does not apply, assistant surgeon may not be paid

37204 Transcatheter occlusion ~ endoscopies or minor procedure - E/M services on the same day generally not paid, standard payment adjustment rules for multiple procedures apply, 150% payment adjustment for bilateral procedures does not apply, assistant surgeon may not be paid

37205 Transcatheter iv stent, percutaneous ~ endoscopies or minor procedure - E/M services on the same day generally not paid, standard payment adjustment rules for multiple procedures apply, 150% payment adjustment for bilateral procedures does not apply, payment for assistant surgeon subject to documentation of medical necessity

37206 Transcatheter iv stent/perc added ~ follow-up period included in another service, no payment adjustment rules for multiple procedures apply, 150% payment adjustment for bilateral procedures does not apply, payment for assistant surgeon subject to documentation of medical necessity, +add-on code (list separately in addition to primary procedure)

37207 Transcatheter iv stent, open ~ endoscopies or minor procedure - E/M services on the same day generally not paid, standard payment adjustment rules for multiple procedures apply, 150% payment adjustment for bilateral procedures applies, assistant surgeon may be paid

37208 Transcatheter iv stent/open added ~ follow-up period included in another service, no payment adjustment rules for multiple procedures apply, 150% payment adjustment for bilateral procedures does not apply, assistant surgeon may be paid, +add-on code (list separately in addition to primary procedure)

37209 Change iv cath at thrombectomy tx ~ endoscopies or minor procedure - E/M services on the same day generally not paid, standard payment adjustment rules for multiple procedures apply, 150% payment adjustment for bilateral procedures does not apply, assistant surgeon may not be paid

37210 Embolization uterine fibroid ~ endoscopies or minor procedure - E/M services on the same day generally not paid, standard payment adjustment rules for multiple

procedures apply, 150% payment adjustment for bilateral procedures does not apply, assistant surgeon may not be paid

37215   **Transcatheter stent, cca w/eps**   ~ restricted coverage - special coverage rules apply, follow-up period is 90 days, standard payment adjustment rules for multiple procedures apply, 150% payment adjustment for bilateral procedures does not apply, payment for assistant surgeon subject to documentation of medical necessity

37216   **Transcatheter stent, cca w/o eps**   non-covered service, follow-up period is 90 days, multiple procedure concept does not apply, bilateral surgery concept does not apply, assistant surgery concept does not apply

37250   **Iv us first vessel, add-on**   ~ follow-up period included in another service, no payment adjustment rules for multiple procedures apply, 150% payment adjustment for bilateral procedures does not apply, payment for assistant surgeon subject to documentation of medical necessity, +add-on code (list separately in addition to primary procedure)

37251   **Iv us each add vessel, add-on**   ~ follow-up period included in another service, no payment adjustment rules for multiple procedures apply, 150% payment adjustment for bilateral procedures does not apply, payment for assistant surgeon subject to documentation of medical necessity, +add-on code (list separately in addition to primary procedure)

37500   **Endoscopy ligate perforate veins**   ~ follow-up period is 90 days, standard payment adjustment rules for multiple procedures apply, 150% payment adjustment for bilateral procedures applies, assistant surgeon may not be paid

37501   **Vascular endoscopy procedure**   ~ medicare carrier determines global period, standard payment adjustment rules for multiple procedures apply, 150% payment adjustment for bilateral procedures applies, assistant surgeon may not be paid

37565   **Ligate neck vein**   ~ follow-up period is 90 days, standard payment adjustment rules for multiple procedures apply, 150% payment adjustment for bilateral procedures does not apply, payment for assistant surgeon subject to documentation of medical necessity

37600   **Ligate neck artery**   ~ follow-up period is 90 days, standard payment adjustment rules for multiple procedures apply, 150% payment adjustment for bilateral procedures does not apply, assistant surgeon may be paid

37605   **Ligate neck artery**   ~ follow-up period is 90 days, standard payment adjustment rules for multiple procedures apply, 150% payment adjustment for bilateral procedures does not apply, assistant surgeon may be paid

37606   **Ligate neck artery**   ~ follow-up period is 90 days, standard payment adjustment rules for multiple procedures apply, 150% payment adjustment for bilateral procedures does not apply, assistant surgeon may be paid

37607   **Ligate a-v fistula**   ~ follow-up period is 90 days, standard payment adjustment rules for multiple procedures apply, 150% payment adjustment for bilateral procedures does not apply, assistant surgeon may not be paid

37609   **Temporal artery procedure**   ~ follow-up period is 10 days, standard payment adjustment rules for multiple procedures apply, 150% payment adjustment for bilateral procedures applies, assistant surgeon may not be paid

37615   **Ligate neck artery**   ~ follow-up period is 90 days, standard payment adjustment rules for multiple procedures apply, 150% payment adjustment for bilateral procedures does not apply, assistant surgeon may be paid

37616   **Ligate chest artery**   ~ follow-up period is 90 days, standard payment adjustment rules for multiple procedures apply, 150% payment adjustment for bilateral procedures does not apply, assistant surgeon may be paid

37617   **Ligate abdomen artery**   ~ follow-up period is 90 days, standard payment adjustment rules for multiple procedures apply, 150% payment adjustment for bilateral procedures does not apply, assistant surgeon may be paid

37618   **Ligate extremity artery**   ~ follow-up period is 90 days, standard payment adjustment rules for multiple procedures apply, 150% payment adjustment for bilateral procedures does not apply, assistant surgeon may be paid

37620   **Revise major vein**   ~ follow-up period is 90 days, standard payment adjustment rules for multiple procedures apply, 150% payment adjustment for bilateral procedures does not apply, assistant surgeon may not be paid

37650   **Revise major vein**   ~ follow-up period is 90 days, standard payment adjustment rules for multiple procedures apply, 150% payment adjustment for bilateral procedures applies, assistant surgeon may not be paid

37660   **Revise major vein**   ~ follow-up period is 90 days, standard payment adjustment rules for multiple procedures apply, 150% payment adjustment for bilateral procedures does not apply, assistant surgeon may be paid

37700   **Revise leg vein**   ~ follow-up period is 90 days, standard payment adjustment rules for multiple procedures apply, 150% payment adjustment for bilateral procedures applies, assistant surgeon may not be paid

37718   **Ligate/strip short leg vein**   ~ follow-up period is 90 days, standard payment adjustment rules for multiple procedures apply, 150% payment adjustment for bilateral procedures applies, assistant surgeon may not be paid

37722   **Ligate/strip long leg vein**   ~ follow-up period is 90 days, standard payment adjustment rules for multiple procedures apply, 150% payment adjustment for bilateral procedures applies, assistant surgeon may not be paid

37735   **Remove leg veins/lesion**   ~ follow-up period is 90 days, standard payment adjustment rules for multiple procedures apply, 150% payment adjustment for bilateral procedures applies, assistant surgeon may be paid

37760   **Ligate leg veins, open**   ~ follow-up period is 90 days, standard payment adjustment rules for multiple procedures apply, 150% payment adjustment for bilateral procedures does not apply, assistant surgeon may be paid

37765   **Phlebectomy veins - extremity - to 20**   ~ follow-up period is 90 days, standard payment adjustment rules for multiple procedures apply, 150% payment adjustment for bilateral procedures applies, assistant surgeon may not be paid

37766   **Phlebectomy veins - extremity 20+**   ~ follow-up period is 90 days, standard payment adjustment rules for multiple procedures apply, 150% payment adjustment for bilateral procedures applies, assistant surgeon may not be paid

37780   **Revise leg vein**   ~ follow-up period is 90 days, standard payment adjustment rules for multiple procedures apply, 150% payment adjustment for bilateral procedures applies, assistant surgeon may not be paid

37785   **Ligate/divide/excise vein**   ~ follow-up period is 90 days, standard payment adjustment rules for multiple procedures apply, 150% payment adjustment for bilateral procedures applies, assistant surgeon may not be paid

37788   **Revascularization, penis**   ~ follow-up period is 90 days, standard payment adjustment rules for multiple procedures apply, 150% payment adjustment for bilateral procedures does not apply, assistant surgeon may be paid

37790   **Penile venous occlusion**   ~ follow-up period is 90 days, standard payment adjustment rules for multiple procedures apply, 150% payment adjustment for bilateral procedures does not apply, payment for assistant surgeon subject to documentation of medical necessity

37799   **Vascular surgery procedure**   ~ medicare carrier determines global period, standard payment adjustment rules for multiple procedures apply, 150% payment adjustment for bilateral procedures does not apply, payment for assistant surgeon subject to documentation of medical necessity

HEMIC AND LYMPHATIC SYSTEMS

Spleen

38100   **Remove spleen, total**   ~ follow-up period is 90 days, standard payment adjustment rules for multiple procedures apply, 150% payment adjustment for bilateral procedures does not apply, assistant surgeon may be paid

38101   **Remove spleen, partial**   ~ follow-up period is 90 days, standard payment adjustment rules for multiple procedures apply, 150% payment adjustment for bilateral procedures does not apply, assistant surgeon may be paid

38102   **Remove spleen, total**   ~ follow-up period included in another service, no payment adjustment rules for multiple procedures apply, 150% payment adjustment for bilateral procedures does not apply, assistant surgeon may be paid

38115   **Repair ruptured spleen**   ~ follow-up period is 90 days, standard payment adjustment rules for multiple procedures apply, 150% payment adjustment for bilateral procedures does not apply, assistant surgeon may be paid

38120   **Laparoscopy, splenectomy**   ~ follow-up period is 90 days, standard payment adjustment rules for multiple procedures apply, 150% payment adjustment for bilateral procedures does not apply, assistant surgeon may be paid

38129   **Laparoscope proc, spleen**   ~ medicare carrier determines global period, standard payment adjustment rules for multiple procedures apply, 150% payment adjustment for bilateral procedures does not apply, assistant surgeon may be paid

General

38200   **Inject for spleen x-ray**   ~ endoscopies or minor procedure - E/M services on the same day generally not paid, standard payment adjustment rules for multiple procedures apply, 150% payment adjustment for bilateral procedures does not apply, payment for assistant surgeon subject to documentation of medical necessity

38204   **Blood donor search management**   ~ bundled code - no separate payment made, multiple procedure concept does not apply, bilateral surgery concept does not apply, assistant surgery concept does not apply

38205   **Harvest allogenic stem cells**   ~ restricted coverage - special coverage rules apply, endoscopies or minor procedure - E/M services on the same day generally not paid, standard payment adjustment rules for multiple procedures apply, 150% payment adjustment for bilateral procedures does not apply, payment for assistant surgeon subject to documentation of medical necessity

38206   **Harvest auto stem cells**   ~ restricted coverage - special coverage rules apply, endoscopies or minor procedure - E/M services on the same day generally not paid, standard payment adjustment rules for multiple procedures apply, 150% payment adjustment for bilateral procedures does not apply, payment for assistant surgeon subject to documentation of medical necessity

38207   **Cryopreserve stem cells**   ~ not valid for Medicare, multiple procedure concept does not apply, bilateral surgery concept does not apply, assistant surgery concept does not apply

38208   **Thaw preserved stem cells**   ~ not valid for Medicare, multiple procedure concept does not apply, bilateral surgery concept does not apply, assistant surgery concept does not apply

38209   **Wash harvest stem cells**   ~ not valid for Medicare, multiple procedure concept does not apply, bilateral surgery concept does not apply, assistant surgery concept does not apply

38210   **T-cell depletion of harvest**   ~ not valid for Medicare, multiple procedure concept does not apply, bilateral surgery concept does not apply, assistant surgery concept does not apply

38211   **Tumor cell deplete of harvest**   ~ not valid for Medicare, multiple procedure concept does not apply, bilateral surgery concept does not apply, assistant surgery concept does not apply

38212   **Rbc depletion of harvest**   ~ not valid for Medicare, multiple procedure concept does not apply, bilateral surgery concept does not apply, assistant surgery concept does not apply

38213   **Platelet deplete of harvest**   ~ not valid for Medicare, multiple procedure concept does not apply, bilateral surgery concept does not apply, assistant surgery concept does not apply

38214   **Volume deplete of harvest**   ~ not valid for Medicare, multiple procedure concept does not apply, bilateral surgery concept does not apply, assistant surgery concept does not apply

38215   **Harvest stem cell concentrate**   ~ not valid for Medicare, multiple procedure concept does not apply, bilateral surgery concept does not apply, assistant surgery concept does not apply

38220   **Bone marrow aspiration**   ~ standard payment adjustment rules for multiple procedures apply, 150% payment adjustment for bilateral procedures applies, payment for assistant surgeon subject to documentation of medical necessity

38221 **Bone marrow biopsy** ~ standard payment adjustment rules for multiple procedures apply, 150% payment adjustment for bilateral procedures applies, payment for assistant surgeon subject to documentation of medical necessity

38230 **Bone marrow collection** ~ restricted coverage - special coverage rules apply, follow-up period is 10 days, standard payment adjustment rules for multiple procedures apply, 150% payment adjustment for bilateral procedures does not apply, payment for assistant surgeon subject to documentation of medical necessity

38240 **Bone marrow/stem transplant** ~ restricted coverage - special coverage rules apply, standard payment adjustment rules for multiple procedures apply, 150% payment adjustment for bilateral procedures does not apply, payment for assistant surgeon subject to documentation of medical necessity

38241 **Bone marrow/stem transplant** ~ restricted coverage - special coverage rules apply, standard payment adjustment rules for multiple procedures apply, 150% payment adjustment for bilateral procedures does not apply, payment for assistant surgeon subject to documentation of medical necessity

38242 **Lymphocyte infuse transplant** ~ endoscopies or minor procedure - E/M services on the same day generally not paid, standard payment adjustment rules for multiple procedures apply, 150% payment adjustment for bilateral procedures does not apply, payment for assistant surgeon subject to documentation of medical necessity

Lymph Nodes and Lymphatic Channels

38300 **Drain lymph node lesion** ~ follow-up period is 10 days, standard payment adjustment rules for multiple procedures apply, 150% payment adjustment for bilateral procedures does not apply, assistant surgeon may not be paid

38305 **Drain lymph node lesion** ~ follow-up period is 90 days, standard payment adjustment rules for multiple procedures apply, 150% payment adjustment for bilateral procedures does not apply, assistant surgeon may not be paid

38308 **Incise lymph channels** ~ follow-up period is 90 days, standard payment adjustment rules for multiple procedures apply, 150% payment adjustment for bilateral procedures does not apply, assistant surgeon may be paid

38380 **Thoracic duct procedure** ~ follow-up period is 90 days, standard payment adjustment rules for multiple procedures apply, 150% payment adjustment for bilateral procedures does not apply, assistant surgeon may be paid

38381 **Thoracic duct procedure** ~ follow-up period is 90 days, standard payment adjustment rules for multiple procedures apply, 150% payment adjustment for bilateral procedures does not apply, assistant surgeon may be paid

---

38382 **Thoracic duct procedure** ~ follow-up period is 90 days, standard payment adjustment rules for multiple procedures apply, 150% payment adjustment for bilateral procedures does not apply, assistant surgeon may be paid

38500 **Biopsy/remove lymph nodes** ~ follow-up period is 10 days, standard payment adjustment rules for multiple procedures apply, 150% payment adjustment for bilateral procedures applies, assistant surgeon may not be paid

38505 **Needle biopsy lymph nodes** ~ endoscopies or minor procedure - E/M services on the same day generally not paid, standard payment adjustment rules for multiple procedures apply, 150% payment adjustment for bilateral procedures applies, assistant surgeon may not be paid

38510 **Biopsy/remove lymph nodes** ~ follow-up period is 10 days, standard payment adjustment rules for multiple procedures apply, 150% payment adjustment for bilateral procedures applies, assistant surgeon may not be paid

38520 **Biopsy/remove lymph nodes** ~ follow-up period is 90 days, standard payment adjustment rules for multiple procedures apply, 150% payment adjustment for bilateral procedures applies, assistant surgeon may not be paid

38525 **Biopsy/remove lymph nodes** ~ follow-up period is 90 days, standard payment adjustment rules for multiple procedures apply, 150% payment adjustment for bilateral procedures applies, assistant surgeon may not be paid

38530 **Biopsy/remove lymph nodes** ~ follow-up period is 90 days, standard payment adjustment rules for multiple procedures apply, 150% payment adjustment for bilateral procedures applies, assistant surgeon may be paid

38542 **Explore deep node(s), neck** ~ follow-up period is 90 days, standard payment adjustment rules for multiple procedures apply, 150% payment adjustment for bilateral procedures applies, assistant surgeon may be paid

38550 **Remove neck/armpit lesion** ~ follow-up period is 90 days, standard payment adjustment rules for multiple procedures apply, 150% payment adjustment for bilateral procedures does not apply, payment for assistant surgeon subject to documentation of medical necessity

38555 **Remove neck/armpit lesion** ~ follow-up period is 90 days, standard payment adjustment rules for multiple procedures apply, 150% payment adjustment for bilateral procedures does not apply, assistant surgeon may be paid

38562 **Remove pelvic lymph nodes** ~ follow-up period is 90 days, standard payment adjustment rules for multiple procedures apply, 150% payment adjustment does not apply - RVUs based on bilateral procedure, assistant surgeon may be paid

38564   **Remove abdomen lymph nodes**   ~ follow-up period is 90 days, standard payment adjustment rules for multiple procedures apply, 150% payment adjustment for bilateral procedures does not apply, assistant surgeon may be paid

38570   **Laparoscopy, lymph node biopsy**   ~ follow-up period is 10 days, special rules for multiple endoscopic procedures apply if billed with another endoscopy in the same family, 150% payment adjustment for bilateral procedures does not apply, assistant surgeon may be paid

38571   **Laparoscopy, lymphadenectomy**   ~ follow-up period is 10 days, standard payment adjustment rules for multiple procedures apply, 150% payment adjustment does not apply - RVUs based on bilateral procedure, assistant surgeon may be paid

38572   **Laparoscopy, lymphadenectomy**   ~ follow-up period is 10 days, standard payment adjustment rules for multiple procedures apply, 150% payment adjustment does not apply - RVUs based on bilateral procedure, assistant surgeon may be paid

38589   **Laparoscope proc, lymphatic**   ~ medicare carrier determines global period, standard payment adjustment rules for multiple procedures apply, 150% payment adjustment for bilateral procedures applies, assistant surgeon may be paid

38700   **Remove lymph nodes, neck**   ~ follow-up period is 90 days, standard payment adjustment rules for multiple procedures apply, 150% payment adjustment for bilateral procedures applies, assistant surgeon may be paid

38720   **Remove lymph nodes, neck**   ~ follow-up period is 90 days, standard payment adjustment rules for multiple procedures apply, 150% payment adjustment for bilateral procedures applies, assistant surgeon may be paid

38724   **Remove lymph nodes, neck**   ~ follow-up period is 90 days, standard payment adjustment rules for multiple procedures apply, 150% payment adjustment for bilateral procedures applies, assistant surgeon may be paid

38740   **Remove armpit lymph nodes**   ~ follow-up period is 90 days, standard payment adjustment rules for multiple procedures apply, 150% payment adjustment for bilateral procedures does not apply, assistant surgeon may be paid

38745   **Remove armpit lymph nodes**   ~ follow-up period is 90 days, standard payment adjustment rules for multiple procedures apply, 150% payment adjustment for bilateral procedures does not apply, assistant surgeon may be paid

38746   **Remove thoracic lymph nodes**   ~ follow-up period included in another service, no payment adjustment rules for multiple procedures apply, 150% payment adjustment for bilateral procedures does not apply, assistant surgeon may be paid

38747   **Remove abdominal lymph nodes**   ~ follow-up period included in another service, no payment adjustment rules for multiple procedures apply, 150% payment adjustment for bilateral procedures does not apply, assistant surgeon may be paid

38760   **Remove groin lymph nodes**   ~ follow-up period is 90 days, standard payment adjustment rules for multiple procedures apply, 150% payment adjustment for bilateral procedures applies, assistant surgeon may be paid

38765   **Remove groin lymph nodes**   ~ follow-up period is 90 days, standard payment adjustment rules for multiple procedures apply, 150% payment adjustment for bilateral procedures applies, assistant surgeon may be paid

38770   **Remove pelvis lymph nodes**   ~ follow-up period is 90 days, standard payment adjustment rules for multiple procedures apply, 150% payment adjustment for bilateral procedures applies, assistant surgeon may be paid

38780   **Remove abdomen lymph nodes**   ~ follow-up period is 90 days, standard payment adjustment rules for multiple procedures apply, 150% payment adjustment for bilateral procedures does not apply, assistant surgeon may be paid

38790   **Inject for lymphatic x-ray**   ~ endoscopies or minor procedure - E/M services on the same day generally not paid, standard payment adjustment rules for multiple procedures apply, 150% payment adjustment for bilateral procedures applies, assistant surgeon may not be paid

38792   **Identify sentinel node**   ~ endoscopies or minor procedure - E/M services on the same day generally not paid, standard payment adjustment rules for multiple procedures apply, 150% payment adjustment for bilateral procedures applies, assistant surgeon may not be paid

38794   **Access thoracic lymph duct**   ~ follow-up period is 90 days, standard payment adjustment rules for multiple procedures apply, 150% payment adjustment for bilateral procedures does not apply, payment for assistant surgeon subject to documentation of medical necessity

38999   **Blood/lymph system procedure**   ~ medicare carrier determines global period, standard payment adjustment rules for multiple procedures apply, 150% payment adjustment for bilateral procedures does not apply, assistant surgeon may be paid

MEDIASTINUM AND DIAPHRAGM

Mediastinum

39000   **Explore chest**   ~ follow-up period is 90 days, standard payment adjustment rules for multiple procedures apply, 150% payment adjustment for bilateral procedures does not apply, assistant surgeon may be paid

39010   **Explore chest**   ~ follow-up period is 90 days, standard payment adjustment rules for multiple procedures apply, 150% payment adjustment for bilateral procedures does not apply, assistant surgeon may be paid

39200   **Remove chest lesion**   ~ follow-up period is 90 days, standard payment adjustment rules for multiple procedures apply, 150% payment adjustment for bilateral procedures does not apply, assistant surgeon may be paid

39220   **Remove chest lesion**   ~ follow-up period is 90 days, standard payment adjustment rules for multiple procedures apply, 150% payment adjustment for bilateral procedures does not apply, assistant surgeon may be paid

39400   **Visualization of chest**   ~ follow-up period is 10 days, standard payment adjustment rules for multiple procedures apply, 150% payment adjustment for bilateral procedures does not apply, assistant surgeon may not be paid

39499   **Chest procedure**   ~ medicare carrier determines global period, standard payment adjustment rules for multiple procedures apply, 150% payment adjustment for bilateral procedures does not apply, assistant surgeon may be paid

Diaphragm

39501   **Repair diaphragm laceration**   ~ follow-up period is 90 days, standard payment adjustment rules for multiple procedures apply, 150% payment adjustment for bilateral procedures does not apply, assistant surgeon may be paid

39502   **Repair paraesophageal hernia**   ~ follow-up period is 90 days, standard payment adjustment rules for multiple procedures apply, 150% payment adjustment for bilateral procedures does not apply, assistant surgeon may be paid

39503   **Repair diaphragm hernia**   ~ follow-up period is 90 days, standard payment adjustment rules for multiple procedures apply, 150% payment adjustment for bilateral procedures does not apply, assistant surgeon may be paid

39520   **Repair diaphragm hernia**   ~ follow-up period is 90 days, standard payment adjustment rules for multiple procedures apply, 150% payment adjustment for bilateral procedures does not apply, assistant surgeon may be paid

39530   **Repair diaphragm hernia**   ~ follow-up period is 90 days, standard payment adjustment rules for multiple procedures apply, 150% payment adjustment for bilateral procedures does not apply, assistant surgeon may be paid

39531   **Repair diaphragm hernia**   ~ follow-up period is 90 days, standard payment adjustment rules for multiple procedures apply, 150% payment adjustment for bilateral procedures does not apply, assistant surgeon may be paid

39540   **Repair diaphragm hernia**   ~ follow-up period is 90 days, standard payment adjustment rules for multiple procedures apply, 150% payment adjustment for bilateral procedures does not apply, assistant surgeon may be paid

39541   **Repair diaphragm hernia**   ~ follow-up period is 90 days, standard payment adjustment rules for multiple procedures apply, 150% payment adjustment for bilateral procedures does not apply, assistant surgeon may be paid

39545   **Revise diaphragm**   ~ follow-up period is 90 days, standard payment adjustment rules for multiple procedures apply, 150% payment adjustment for bilateral procedures does not apply, assistant surgeon may be paid

39560   **Resect diaphragm, simple**   ~ follow-up period is 90 days, standard payment adjustment rules for multiple procedures apply, 150% payment adjustment for bilateral procedures does not apply, assistant surgeon may be paid

39561   **Resect diaphragm, complex**   ~ follow-up period is 90 days, standard payment adjustment rules for multiple procedures apply, 150% payment adjustment for bilateral procedures does not apply, assistant surgeon may be paid

39599   **Diaphragm surgery procedure**   ~ medicare carrier determines global period, standard payment adjustment rules for multiple procedures apply, 150% payment adjustment for bilateral procedures does not apply, assistant surgeon may be paid

DIGESTIVE SYSTEM

Lips

40490   **Biopsy lip**   ~ endoscopies or minor procedure - E/M services on the same day generally not paid, standard payment adjustment rules for multiple procedures apply, 150% payment adjustment for bilateral procedures does not apply, assistant surgeon may not be paid

40500   **Partial excise lip**   ~ follow-up period is 90 days, standard payment adjustment rules for multiple procedures apply, 150% payment adjustment for bilateral procedures does not apply, assistant surgeon may not be paid

40510   **Partial excise lip**   ~ follow-up period is 90 days, standard payment adjustment rules for multiple procedures apply, 150% payment adjustment for bilateral procedures does not apply, assistant surgeon may not be paid

40520   **Partial excise lip**   ~ follow-up period is 90 days, standard payment adjustment rules for multiple procedures apply, 150% payment adjustment for bilateral procedures does not apply, assistant surgeon may not be paid

40525   **Reconstruct lip with flap**   ~ follow-up period is 90 days, standard payment adjustment rules for multiple procedures apply, 150% payment adjustment for bilateral procedures does not apply, assistant surgeon may not be paid

40527   **Reconstruct lip with flap**   ~ follow-up period is 90 days, standard payment adjustment rules for multiple procedures apply, 150% payment adjustment for bilateral procedures does not apply, payment for assistant surgeon subject to documentation of medical necessity

40530   **Partial remove lip**   ~ follow-up period is 90 days, standard payment adjustment rules for multiple procedures apply, 150% payment adjustment for bilateral procedures does not apply, assistant surgeon may not be paid

40650   **Repair lip**   ~ follow-up period is 90 days, standard payment adjustment rules for multiple procedures apply, 150% payment adjustment for bilateral procedures does not apply, payment for assistant surgeon subject to documentation of medical necessity

40652   **Repair lip**   ~ follow-up period is 90 days, standard payment adjustment rules for multiple procedures apply, 150% payment adjustment for bilateral procedures does not apply, payment for assistant surgeon subject to documentation of medical necessity

40654   **Repair lip**   ~ follow-up period is 90 days, standard payment adjustment rules for multiple procedures apply, 150% payment adjustment for bilateral procedures does not apply, assistant surgeon may not be paid

40700   **Repair cleft lip/nasal**   ~ follow-up period is 90 days, standard payment adjustment rules for multiple procedures apply, 150% payment adjustment for bilateral procedures does not apply, payment for assistant surgeon subject to documentation of medical necessity

40701   **Repair cleft lip/nasal**   ~ follow-up period is 90 days, standard payment adjustment rules for multiple procedures apply, 150% payment adjustment does not apply - RVUs based on bilateral procedure, assistant surgeon may be paid

40702   **Repair cleft lip/nasal**   ~ follow-up period is 90 days, standard payment adjustment rules for multiple procedures apply, 150% payment adjustment does not apply - RVUs based on bilateral procedure, assistant surgeon may be paid

40720   **Repair cleft lip/nasal**   ~ follow-up period is 90 days, standard payment adjustment rules for multiple procedures apply, 150% payment adjustment for bilateral procedures applies, payment for assistant surgeon subject to documentation of medical necessity

40761   **Repair cleft lip/nasal**   ~ follow-up period is 90 days, standard payment adjustment rules for multiple procedures apply, 150% payment adjustment for bilateral procedures does not apply, assistant surgeon may not be paid

40799   **Lip surgery procedure**   ~ medicare carrier determines global period, standard payment adjustment rules for multiple procedures apply, 150% payment adjustment for bilateral procedures does not apply, assistant surgeon may be paid

Vestibule of Mouth

40800   **Drain mouth lesion**   ~ follow-up period is 10 days, standard payment adjustment rules for multiple procedures apply, 150% payment adjustment for bilateral procedures does not apply, assistant surgeon may not be paid

40801   **Drain mouth lesion**   ~ follow-up period is 10 days, standard payment adjustment rules for multiple procedures apply, 150% payment adjustment for bilateral procedures does not apply, assistant surgeon may not be paid

40804   **Remove foreign body mouth**   ~ follow-up period is 10 days, standard payment adjustment rules for multiple procedures apply, 150% payment adjustment for bilateral procedures does not apply, payment for assistant surgeon subject to documentation of medical necessity

40805   **Remove foreign body mouth**   ~ follow-up period is 10 days, standard payment adjustment rules for multiple procedures apply, 150% payment adjustment for bilateral procedures does not apply, payment for assistant surgeon subject to documentation of medical necessity

40806   **Incise lip fold**   ~ endoscopies or minor procedure - E/M services on the same day generally not paid, standard payment adjustment rules for multiple procedures apply, 150% payment adjustment for bilateral procedures does not apply, payment for assistant surgeon subject to documentation of medical necessity

40808   **Biopsy mouth lesion**   ~ follow-up period is 10 days, standard payment adjustment rules for multiple procedures apply, 150% payment adjustment for bilateral procedures does not apply, assistant surgeon may not be paid

40810   **Excise mouth lesion**   ~ follow-up period is 10 days, standard payment adjustment rules for multiple procedures apply, 150% payment adjustment for bilateral procedures does not apply, assistant surgeon may not be paid

40812   **Excise/repair mouth lesion**   ~ follow-up period is 10 days, standard payment adjustment rules for multiple procedures apply, 150% payment adjustment for bilateral procedures does not apply, assistant surgeon may not be paid

40814   **Excise/repair mouth lesion**   ~ follow-up period is 90 days, standard payment adjustment rules for multiple procedures apply, 150% payment adjustment for bilateral procedures does not apply, assistant surgeon may not be paid

40816   **Excise mouth lesion**   ~ follow-up period is 90 days, standard payment adjustment rules for multiple procedures apply, 150% payment adjustment for bilateral procedures does not apply, assistant surgeon may not be paid

40818   **Excise oral mucosa for graft**   ~ follow-up period is 90 days, standard payment adjustment rules for multiple procedures apply, 150% payment adjustment for bilateral procedures does not apply, payment for assistant surgeon subject to documentation of medical necessity

40819   **Excise lip or cheek fold**   ~ follow-up period is 90 days, standard payment adjustment rules for multiple procedures apply, 150% payment adjustment for bilateral procedures does not apply, payment for assistant surgeon subject to documentation of medical necessity

40820   **Treat mouth lesion**   ~ follow-up period is 10 days, standard payment adjustment rules for multiple procedures apply, 150% payment adjustment for bilateral procedures does not apply, assistant surgeon may not be paid

40830   **Repair mouth laceration**   ~ follow-up period is 10 days, standard payment adjustment rules for multiple procedures apply, 150% payment adjustment for bilateral procedures does not apply, payment for assistant surgeon subject to documentation of medical necessity

40831   **Repair mouth laceration**   ~ follow-up period is 10 days, standard payment adjustment rules for multiple procedures apply, 150% payment adjustment for bilateral procedures does not apply, payment for assistant surgeon subject to documentation of medical necessity

40840   **Reconstruct mouth**   ~ restricted coverage - special coverage rules apply, follow-up period is 90 days, standard payment adjustment rules for multiple procedures apply, 150% payment adjustment for bilateral procedures does not apply, assistant surgeon may be paid

40842   **Reconstruct mouth**   ~ restricted coverage - special coverage rules apply, follow-up period is 90 days, standard payment adjustment rules for multiple procedures apply, 150% payment adjustment for bilateral procedures does not apply, payment for assistant surgeon subject to documentation of medical necessity

40843   **Reconstruct mouth**   ~ restricted coverage - special coverage rules apply, follow-up period is 90 days, standard payment adjustment rules for multiple procedures apply, 150% payment adjustment does not apply - RVUs based on bilateral procedure, assistant surgeon may be paid

40844   **Reconstruct mouth**   ~ restricted coverage - special coverage rules apply, follow-up period is 90 days, standard payment adjustment rules for multiple procedures apply, 150% payment adjustment for bilateral procedures does not apply, assistant surgeon may be paid

40845   **Reconstruct mouth**   ~ restricted coverage - special coverage rules apply, follow-up period is 90 days, standard payment adjustment rules for multiple procedures apply, 150% payment adjustment for bilateral procedures does not apply, payment for assistant surgeon subject to documentation of medical necessity

40899   **Mouth surgery procedure**   ~ medicare carrier determines global period, standard payment adjustment rules for multiple procedures apply, 150% payment adjustment for bilateral procedures does not apply, payment for assistant surgeon subject to documentation of medical necessity

Tongue and Floor Of Mouth

41000   **Drain mouth lesion**   ~ follow-up period is 10 days, standard payment adjustment rules for multiple procedures apply, 150% payment adjustment for bilateral procedures does not apply, assistant surgeon may not be paid

41005   **Drain mouth lesion**   ~ follow-up period is 10 days, standard payment adjustment rules for multiple procedures apply, 150% payment adjustment for bilateral procedures does not apply, payment for assistant surgeon subject to documentation of medical necessity

41006   **Drain mouth lesion**   ~ follow-up period is 90 days, standard payment adjustment rules for multiple procedures apply, 150% payment adjustment for bilateral procedures does not apply, payment for assistant surgeon subject to documentation of medical necessity

41007   **Drain mouth lesion**   ~ follow-up period is 90 days, standard payment adjustment rules for multiple procedures apply, 150% payment adjustment for bilateral procedures does not apply, payment for assistant surgeon subject to documentation of medical necessity

41008   **Drain mouth lesion**   ~ follow-up period is 90 days, standard payment adjustment rules for multiple procedures apply, 150% payment adjustment for bilateral procedures does not apply, payment for assistant surgeon subject to documentation of medical necessity

41009   **Drain mouth lesion**   ~ follow-up period is 90 days, standard payment adjustment rules for multiple procedures apply, 150% payment adjustment for bilateral procedures does not apply, payment for assistant surgeon subject to documentation of medical necessity

41010   **Incise tongue fold**   ~ follow-up period is 10 days, standard payment adjustment rules for multiple procedures apply, 150% payment adjustment for bilateral procedures does not apply, payment for assistant surgeon subject to documentation of medical necessity

41015   **Drain mouth lesion**   ~ follow-up period is 90 days, standard payment adjustment rules for multiple procedures apply, 150% payment adjustment for bilateral procedures does not apply, payment for assistant surgeon subject to documentation of medical necessity

41016   **Drain mouth lesion**   ~ follow-up period is 90 days, standard payment adjustment rules for multiple procedures apply, 150% payment adjustment for bilateral procedures does not apply, payment for assistant surgeon subject to documentation of medical necessity

41017   **Drain mouth lesion**   ~ follow-up period is 90 days, standard payment adjustment rules for multiple procedures apply, 150% payment adjustment for bilateral procedures does not apply, payment for assistant surgeon subject to documentation of medical necessity

41018   **Drain mouth lesion**   ~ follow-up period is 90 days, standard payment adjustment rules for multiple procedures apply, 150% payment adjustment for bilateral procedures does not apply, payment for assistant surgeon subject to documentation of medical necessity

41100   **Biopsy tongue**   ~ follow-up period is 10 days, standard payment adjustment rules for multiple procedures apply, 150% payment adjustment for bilateral procedures does not apply, assistant surgeon may not be paid

41105   **Biopsy tongue**   ~ follow-up period is 10 days, standard payment adjustment rules for multiple procedures apply, 150% payment adjustment for bilateral procedures does not apply, assistant surgeon may not be paid

41108   **Biopsy floor of mouth**   ~ follow-up period is 10 days, standard payment adjustment rules for multiple procedures apply, 150% payment adjustment for bilateral procedures does not apply, assistant surgeon may not be paid

41110   **Excise tongue lesion**   ~ follow-up period is 10 days, standard payment adjustment rules for multiple procedures apply, 150% payment adjustment for bilateral procedures does not apply, assistant surgeon may not be paid

41112   **Excise tongue lesion**   ~ follow-up period is 90 days, standard payment adjustment rules for multiple procedures apply, 150% payment adjustment for bilateral procedures does not apply, assistant surgeon may not be paid

41113   **Excise tongue lesion**   ~ follow-up period is 90 days, standard payment adjustment rules for multiple procedures apply, 150% payment adjustment for bilateral procedures does not apply, assistant surgeon may not be paid

41114   **Excise tongue lesion**   ~ follow-up period is 90 days, standard payment adjustment rules for multiple procedures apply, 150% payment adjustment for

bilateral procedures does not apply, payment for assistant surgeon subject to documentation of medical necessity

41115 **Excise tongue fold** ~ follow-up period is 10 days, standard payment adjustment rules for multiple procedures apply, 150% payment adjustment for bilateral procedures does not apply, payment for assistant surgeon subject to documentation of medical necessity

41116 **Excise mouth lesion** ~ follow-up period is 90 days, standard payment adjustment rules for multiple procedures apply, 150% payment adjustment for bilateral procedures does not apply, assistant surgeon may not be paid

41120 **Partial remove tongue** ~ follow-up period is 90 days, standard payment adjustment rules for multiple procedures apply, 150% payment adjustment for bilateral procedures does not apply, assistant surgeon may be paid

41130 **Partial remove tongue** ~ follow-up period is 90 days, standard payment adjustment rules for multiple procedures apply, 150% payment adjustment for bilateral procedures does not apply, assistant surgeon may be paid

41135 **Tongue and neck surgery** ~ follow-up period is 90 days, standard payment adjustment rules for multiple procedures apply, 150% payment adjustment for bilateral procedures does not apply, assistant surgeon may be paid

41140 **Remove tongue** ~ follow-up period is 90 days, standard payment adjustment rules for multiple procedures apply, 150% payment adjustment for bilateral procedures does not apply, assistant surgeon may be paid

41145 **Tongue remove neck surgery** ~ follow-up period is 90 days, standard payment adjustment rules for multiple procedures apply, 150% payment adjustment for bilateral procedures does not apply, assistant surgeon may be paid

41150 **Tongue, mouth, jaw surgery** ~ follow-up period is 90 days, standard payment adjustment rules for multiple procedures apply, 150% payment adjustment for bilateral procedures does not apply, assistant surgeon may be paid

41153 **Tongue, mouth, neck surgery** ~ follow-up period is 90 days, standard payment adjustment rules for multiple procedures apply, 150% payment adjustment for bilateral procedures does not apply, assistant surgeon may be paid

41155 **Tongue, jaw, & neck surgery** ~ follow-up period is 90 days, standard payment adjustment rules for multiple procedures apply, 150% payment adjustment for bilateral procedures does not apply, assistant surgeon may be paid

41250 **Repair tongue laceration** ~ follow-up period is 10 days, standard payment adjustment rules for multiple procedures apply, 150% payment adjustment for

bilateral procedures does not apply, payment for assistant surgeon subject to documentation of medical necessity

41251   **Repair tongue laceration**   ~ follow-up period is 10 days, standard payment adjustment rules for multiple procedures apply, 150% payment adjustment for bilateral procedures does not apply, payment for assistant surgeon subject to documentation of medical necessity

41252   **Repair tongue laceration**   ~ follow-up period is 10 days, standard payment adjustment rules for multiple procedures apply, 150% payment adjustment for bilateral procedures does not apply, payment for assistant surgeon subject to documentation of medical necessity

41500   **Fixate tongue**   ~ follow-up period is 90 days, standard payment adjustment rules for multiple procedures apply, 150% payment adjustment for bilateral procedures does not apply, payment for assistant surgeon subject to documentation of medical necessity

41510   **Tongue to lip surgery**   ~ follow-up period is 90 days, standard payment adjustment rules for multiple procedures apply, 150% payment adjustment for bilateral procedures does not apply, payment for assistant surgeon subject to documentation of medical necessity

41520   **Reconstruct tongue fold**   ~ follow-up period is 90 days, standard payment adjustment rules for multiple procedures apply, 150% payment adjustment for bilateral procedures does not apply, payment for assistant surgeon subject to documentation of medical necessity

41599   **Tongue and mouth surgery**   ~ medicare carrier determines global period, standard payment adjustment rules for multiple procedures apply, 150% payment adjustment for bilateral procedures does not apply, payment for assistant surgeon subject to documentation of medical necessity

Dentoalveolar Structures

41800   **Drain gum lesion**   ~ follow-up period is 10 days, standard payment adjustment rules for multiple procedures apply, 150% payment adjustment for bilateral procedures does not apply, assistant surgeon may not be paid

41805   **Remove foreign body gum**   ~ follow-up period is 10 days, standard payment adjustment rules for multiple procedures apply, 150% payment adjustment for bilateral procedures does not apply, payment for assistant surgeon subject to documentation of medical necessity

41806   **Remove foreign body jawbone**   ~ follow-up period is 10 days, standard payment adjustment rules for multiple procedures apply, 150% payment adjustment for

bilateral procedures does not apply, payment for assistant surgeon subject to documentation of medical necessity

41820   **Excise gum, each quadrant**   ~ restricted coverage - special coverage rules apply, endoscopies or minor procedure - E/M services on the same day generally not paid, standard payment adjustment rules for multiple procedures apply, 150% payment adjustment for bilateral procedures does not apply, payment for assistant surgeon subject to documentation of medical necessity

41821   **Excise gum flap**   ~ restricted coverage - special coverage rules apply, endoscopies or minor procedure - E/M services on the same day generally not paid, standard payment adjustment rules for multiple procedures apply, 150% payment adjustment for bilateral procedures does not apply, payment for assistant surgeon subject to documentation of medical necessity

41822   **Excise gum lesion**   ~ restricted coverage - special coverage rules apply, follow-up period is 10 days, standard payment adjustment rules for multiple procedures apply, 150% payment adjustment for bilateral procedures does not apply, payment for assistant surgeon subject to documentation of medical necessity

41823   **Excise gum lesion**   ~ restricted coverage - special coverage rules apply, follow-up period is 90 days, standard payment adjustment rules for multiple procedures apply, 150% payment adjustment for bilateral procedures does not apply, payment for assistant surgeon subject to documentation of medical necessity

41825   **Excise gum lesion**   ~ follow-up period is 10 days, standard payment adjustment rules for multiple procedures apply, 150% payment adjustment for bilateral procedures does not apply, assistant surgeon may not be paid

41826   **Excise gum lesion**   ~ follow-up period is 10 days, standard payment adjustment rules for multiple procedures apply, 150% payment adjustment for bilateral procedures does not apply, assistant surgeon may not be paid

41827   **Excise gum lesion**   ~ follow-up period is 90 days, standard payment adjustment rules for multiple procedures apply, 150% payment adjustment for bilateral procedures does not apply, assistant surgeon may not be paid

41828   **Excise gum lesion**   ~ restricted coverage - special coverage rules apply, follow-up period is 10 days, standard payment adjustment rules for multiple procedures apply, 150% payment adjustment for bilateral procedures does not apply, payment for assistant surgeon subject to documentation of medical necessity

41830   **Remove gum tissue**   ~ restricted coverage - special coverage rules apply, follow-up period is 10 days, standard payment adjustment rules for multiple procedures apply, 150% payment adjustment for bilateral procedures does not apply, payment for assistant surgeon subject to documentation of medical necessity

41850   **Treat gum lesion**   ~ restricted coverage - special coverage rules apply, endoscopies or minor procedure - E/M services on the same day generally not paid, standard payment adjustment rules for multiple procedures apply, 150% payment adjustment for bilateral procedures does not apply, payment for assistant surgeon subject to documentation of medical necessity

41870   **Gum graft**   ~ restricted coverage - special coverage rules apply, endoscopies or minor procedure - E/M services on the same day generally not paid, standard payment adjustment rules for multiple procedures apply, 150% payment adjustment for bilateral procedures does not apply, payment for assistant surgeon subject to documentation of medical necessity

41872   **Repair gum**   ~ restricted coverage - special coverage rules apply, follow-up period is 90 days, standard payment adjustment rules for multiple procedures apply, 150% payment adjustment for bilateral procedures does not apply, payment for assistant surgeon subject to documentation of medical necessity

41874   **Repair tooth socket**   ~ restricted coverage - special coverage rules apply, follow-up period is 90 days, standard payment adjustment rules for multiple procedures apply, 150% payment adjustment for bilateral procedures does not apply, payment for assistant surgeon subject to documentation of medical necessity

41899   **Dental surgery procedure**   ~ medicare carrier determines global period, standard payment adjustment rules for multiple procedures apply, 150% payment adjustment for bilateral procedures does not apply, payment for assistant surgeon subject to documentation of medical necessity

Palate and Uvula

42000   **Drain mouth roof lesion**   ~ follow-up period is 10 days, standard payment adjustment rules for multiple procedures apply, 150% payment adjustment for bilateral procedures does not apply, payment for assistant surgeon subject to documentation of medical necessity

42100   **Biopsy roof of mouth**   ~ follow-up period is 10 days, standard payment adjustment rules for multiple procedures apply, 150% payment adjustment for bilateral procedures does not apply, assistant surgeon may not be paid

42104   **Excise lesion, mouth roof**   ~ follow-up period is 10 days, standard payment adjustment rules for multiple procedures apply, 150% payment adjustment for bilateral procedures does not apply, assistant surgeon may not be paid

42106   **Excise lesion, mouth roof**   ~ follow-up period is 10 days, standard payment adjustment rules for multiple procedures apply, 150% payment adjustment for bilateral procedures does not apply, assistant surgeon may not be paid

42107   **Excise lesion, mouth roof**   ~ follow-up period is 90 days, standard payment adjustment rules for multiple procedures apply, 150% payment adjustment for bilateral procedures does not apply, assistant surgeon may not be paid

42120   **Remove palate/lesion**   ~ follow-up period is 90 days, standard payment adjustment rules for multiple procedures apply, 150% payment adjustment for bilateral procedures does not apply, assistant surgeon may be paid

42140   **Excise uvula**   ~ follow-up period is 90 days, standard payment adjustment rules for multiple procedures apply, 150% payment adjustment for bilateral procedures does not apply, assistant surgeon may not be paid

42145   **Repair palate, pharynx/uvula**   ~ follow-up period is 90 days, standard payment adjustment rules for multiple procedures apply, 150% payment adjustment for bilateral procedures does not apply, assistant surgeon may not be paid

42160   **Treatment mouth roof lesion**   ~ follow-up period is 10 days, standard payment adjustment rules for multiple procedures apply, 150% payment adjustment for bilateral procedures does not apply, payment for assistant surgeon subject to documentation of medical necessity

42180   **Repair palate**   ~ follow-up period is 10 days, standard payment adjustment rules for multiple procedures apply, 150% payment adjustment for bilateral procedures does not apply, payment for assistant surgeon subject to documentation of medical necessity

42182   **Repair palate**   ~ follow-up period is 10 days, standard payment adjustment rules for multiple procedures apply, 150% payment adjustment for bilateral procedures does not apply, payment for assistant surgeon subject to documentation of medical necessity

42200   **Reconstruct cleft palate**   ~ follow-up period is 90 days, standard payment adjustment rules for multiple procedures apply, 150% payment adjustment for bilateral procedures does not apply, assistant surgeon may be paid

42205   **Reconstruct cleft palate**   ~ follow-up period is 90 days, standard payment adjustment rules for multiple procedures apply, 150% payment adjustment for bilateral procedures does not apply, assistant surgeon may be paid

42210   **Reconstruct cleft palate**   ~ follow-up period is 90 days, standard payment adjustment rules for multiple procedures apply, 150% payment adjustment for bilateral procedures does not apply, assistant surgeon may be paid

42215   **Reconstruct cleft palate**   ~ follow-up period is 90 days, standard payment adjustment rules for multiple procedures apply, 150% payment adjustment for bilateral procedures does not apply, assistant surgeon may be paid

42220   **Reconstruct cleft palate**   ~ follow-up period is 90 days, standard payment adjustment rules for multiple procedures apply, 150% payment adjustment for bilateral procedures does not apply, assistant surgeon may be paid

42225   **Reconstruct cleft palate**   ~ follow-up period is 90 days, standard payment adjustment rules for multiple procedures apply, 150% payment adjustment for bilateral procedures does not apply, assistant surgeon may be paid

42226   **Lengthening of palate**   ~ follow-up period is 90 days, standard payment adjustment rules for multiple procedures apply, 150% payment adjustment for bilateral procedures does not apply, assistant surgeon may be paid

42227   **Lengthening of palate**   ~ follow-up period is 90 days, standard payment adjustment rules for multiple procedures apply, 150% payment adjustment for bilateral procedures does not apply, assistant surgeon may be paid

42235   **Repair palate**   ~ follow-up period is 90 days, standard payment adjustment rules for multiple procedures apply, 150% payment adjustment for bilateral procedures does not apply, assistant surgeon may be paid

42260   **Repair nose to lip fistula**   ~ follow-up period is 90 days, standard payment adjustment rules for multiple procedures apply, 150% payment adjustment for bilateral procedures does not apply, assistant surgeon may be paid

42280   **Prepare palate mold**   ~ follow-up period is 10 days, standard payment adjustment rules for multiple procedures apply, 150% payment adjustment for bilateral procedures does not apply, payment for assistant surgeon subject to documentation of medical necessity

42281   **Insert palate prosthesis**   ~ follow-up period is 10 days, standard payment adjustment rules for multiple procedures apply, 150% payment adjustment for bilateral procedures does not apply, payment for assistant surgeon subject to documentation of medical necessity

42299   **Palate/uvula surgery**   ~ medicare carrier determines global period, standard payment adjustment rules for multiple procedures apply, 150% payment adjustment for bilateral procedures does not apply, assistant surgeon may be paid

Salivary Gland and Ducts

42300   **Drain salivary gland**   ~ follow-up period is 10 days, standard payment adjustment rules for multiple procedures apply, 150% payment adjustment for bilateral procedures does not apply, assistant surgeon may not be paid

42305   **Drain salivary gland**   ~ follow-up period is 90 days, standard payment adjustment rules for multiple procedures apply, 150% payment adjustment for

bilateral procedures does not apply, payment for assistant surgeon subject to documentation of medical necessity

42310 **Drain salivary gland** ~ follow-up period is 10 days, standard payment adjustment rules for multiple procedures apply, 150% payment adjustment for bilateral procedures does not apply, payment for assistant surgeon subject to documentation of medical necessity

42320 **Drain salivary gland** ~ follow-up period is 10 days, standard payment adjustment rules for multiple procedures apply, 150% payment adjustment for bilateral procedures does not apply, payment for assistant surgeon subject to documentation of medical necessity

42330 **Remove salivary stone** ~ follow-up period is 10 days, standard payment adjustment rules for multiple procedures apply, 150% payment adjustment for bilateral procedures does not apply, assistant surgeon may not be paid

42335 **Remove salivary stone** ~ follow-up period is 90 days, standard payment adjustment rules for multiple procedures apply, 150% payment adjustment for bilateral procedures does not apply, assistant surgeon may not be paid

42340 **Remove salivary stone** ~ follow-up period is 90 days, standard payment adjustment rules for multiple procedures apply, 150% payment adjustment for bilateral procedures does not apply, payment for assistant surgeon subject to documentation of medical necessity

42400 **Biopsy salivary gland** ~ endoscopies or minor procedure - E/M services on the same day generally not paid, standard payment adjustment rules for multiple procedures apply, 150% payment adjustment for bilateral procedures does not apply, assistant surgeon may not be paid

42405 **Biopsy salivary gland** ~ follow-up period is 10 days, standard payment adjustment rules for multiple procedures apply, 150% payment adjustment for bilateral procedures does not apply, assistant surgeon may not be paid

42408 **Excise salivary cyst** ~ follow-up period is 90 days, standard payment adjustment rules for multiple procedures apply, 150% payment adjustment for bilateral procedures does not apply, payment for assistant surgeon subject to documentation of medical necessity

42409 **Drain salivary cyst** ~ follow-up period is 90 days, standard payment adjustment rules for multiple procedures apply, 150% payment adjustment for bilateral procedures does not apply, assistant surgeon may be paid

42410 **Excise parotid gland/lesion** ~ follow-up period is 90 days, standard payment adjustment rules for multiple procedures apply, 150% payment adjustment for bilateral procedures does not apply, assistant surgeon may be paid

42415 **Excise parotid gland/lesion** ~ follow-up period is 90 days, standard payment adjustment rules for multiple procedures apply, 150% payment adjustment for bilateral procedures does not apply, assistant surgeon may be paid

42420 **Excise parotid gland/lesion** ~ follow-up period is 90 days, standard payment adjustment rules for multiple procedures apply, 150% payment adjustment for bilateral procedures does not apply, assistant surgeon may be paid

42425 **Excise parotid gland/lesion** ~ follow-up period is 90 days, standard payment adjustment rules for multiple procedures apply, 150% payment adjustment for bilateral procedures does not apply, assistant surgeon may be paid

42426 **Excise parotid gland/lesion** ~ follow-up period is 90 days, standard payment adjustment rules for multiple procedures apply, 150% payment adjustment for bilateral procedures does not apply, assistant surgeon may be paid

42440 **Excise submaxillary gland** ~ follow-up period is 90 days, standard payment adjustment rules for multiple procedures apply, 150% payment adjustment for bilateral procedures does not apply, assistant surgeon may be paid

42450 **Excise sublingual gland** ~ follow-up period is 90 days, standard payment adjustment rules for multiple procedures apply, 150% payment adjustment for bilateral procedures does not apply, payment for assistant surgeon subject to documentation of medical necessity

42500 **Repair salivary duct** ~ follow-up period is 90 days, standard payment adjustment rules for multiple procedures apply, 150% payment adjustment for bilateral procedures does not apply, payment for assistant surgeon subject to documentation of medical necessity

42505 **Repair salivary duct** ~ follow-up period is 90 days, standard payment adjustment rules for multiple procedures apply, 150% payment adjustment for bilateral procedures does not apply, assistant surgeon may not be paid

42507 **Parotid duct diversion** ~ follow-up period is 90 days, standard payment adjustment rules for multiple procedures apply, 150% payment adjustment does not apply - RVUs based on bilateral procedure, assistant surgeon may be paid

42508 **Parotid duct diversion** ~ follow-up period is 90 days, standard payment adjustment rules for multiple procedures apply, 150% payment adjustment does not apply - RVUs based on bilateral procedure, assistant surgeon may be paid

42509 **Parotid duct diversion** ~ follow-up period is 90 days, standard payment adjustment rules for multiple procedures apply, 150% payment adjustment does not apply - RVUs based on bilateral procedure, payment for assistant surgeon subject to documentation of medical necessity

42510 **Parotid duct diversion** ~ follow-up period is 90 days, standard payment adjustment rules for multiple procedures apply, 150% payment adjustment does not apply - RVUs based on bilateral procedure, assistant surgeon may be paid

42550 **Inject for salivary x-ray** ~ endoscopies or minor procedure - E/M services on the same day generally not paid, standard payment adjustment rules for multiple procedures apply, 150% payment adjustment for bilateral procedures does not apply, assistant surgeon may not be paid

42600 **Closure salivary fistula** ~ follow-up period is 90 days, standard payment adjustment rules for multiple procedures apply, 150% payment adjustment for bilateral procedures does not apply, payment for assistant surgeon subject to documentation of medical necessity

42650 **Dilate salivary duct** ~ endoscopies or minor procedure - E/M services on the same day generally not paid, standard payment adjustment rules for multiple procedures apply, 150% payment adjustment for bilateral procedures does not apply, assistant surgeon may not be paid

42660 **Dilate salivary duct** ~ endoscopies or minor procedure - E/M services on the same day generally not paid, standard payment adjustment rules for multiple procedures apply, 150% payment adjustment for bilateral procedures does not apply, payment for assistant surgeon subject to documentation of medical necessity

42665 **Ligate salivary duct** ~ follow-up period is 90 days, standard payment adjustment rules for multiple procedures apply, 150% payment adjustment for bilateral procedures does not apply, payment for assistant surgeon subject to documentation of medical necessity

42699 **Salivary surgery procedure** ~ medicare carrier determines global period, standard payment adjustment rules for multiple procedures apply, 150% payment adjustment for bilateral procedures does not apply, assistant surgeon may be paid

Pharynx, Adenoids and Tonsils

42700 **Drain tonsil abscess** ~ follow-up period is 10 days, standard payment adjustment rules for multiple procedures apply, 150% payment adjustment for bilateral procedures does not apply, assistant surgeon may not be paid

42720 **Drain throat abscess** ~ follow-up period is 10 days, standard payment adjustment rules for multiple procedures apply, 150% payment adjustment for bilateral procedures does not apply, payment for assistant surgeon subject to documentation of medical necessity

42725 **Drain throat abscess** ~ follow-up period is 90 days, standard payment adjustment rules for multiple procedures apply, 150% payment adjustment for bilateral procedures does not apply, assistant surgeon may be paid

42800   **Biopsy throat** ~ follow-up period is 10 days, standard payment adjustment rules for multiple procedures apply, 150% payment adjustment for bilateral procedures does not apply, assistant surgeon may not be paid

42802   **Biopsy throat** ~ follow-up period is 10 days, standard payment adjustment rules for multiple procedures apply, 150% payment adjustment for bilateral procedures does not apply, assistant surgeon may not be paid

42804   **Biopsy upper nose/throat** ~ follow-up period is 10 days, standard payment adjustment rules for multiple procedures apply, 150% payment adjustment for bilateral procedures does not apply, assistant surgeon may not be paid

42806   **Biopsy upper nose/throat** ~ follow-up period is 10 days, standard payment adjustment rules for multiple procedures apply, 150% payment adjustment for bilateral procedures does not apply, assistant surgeon may not be paid

42808   **Excise pharynx lesion** ~ follow-up period is 10 days, standard payment adjustment rules for multiple procedures apply, 150% payment adjustment for bilateral procedures does not apply, assistant surgeon may not be paid

42809   **Remove pharynx foreign body** ~ follow-up period is 10 days, standard payment adjustment rules for multiple procedures apply, 150% payment adjustment for bilateral procedures does not apply, assistant surgeon may not be paid

42810   **Excise neck cyst** ~ follow-up period is 90 days, standard payment adjustment rules for multiple procedures apply, 150% payment adjustment for bilateral procedures does not apply, assistant surgeon may be paid

42815   **Excise neck cyst** ~ follow-up period is 90 days, standard payment adjustment rules for multiple procedures apply, 150% payment adjustment for bilateral procedures does not apply, assistant surgeon may be paid

42820   **Remove tonsils and adenoids** ~ follow-up period is 90 days, standard payment adjustment rules for multiple procedures apply, 150% payment adjustment for bilateral procedures does not apply, payment for assistant surgeon subject to documentation of medical necessity

42821   **Remove tonsils and adenoids** ~ follow-up period is 90 days, standard payment adjustment rules for multiple procedures apply, 150% payment adjustment for bilateral procedures does not apply, payment for assistant surgeon subject to documentation of medical necessity

42825   **Remove tonsils** ~ follow-up period is 90 days, standard payment adjustment rules for multiple procedures apply, 150% payment adjustment for bilateral procedures does not apply, payment for assistant surgeon subject to documentation of medical necessity

42826 **Remove tonsils** ~ follow-up period is 90 days, standard payment adjustment rules for multiple procedures apply, 150% payment adjustment for bilateral procedures does not apply, assistant surgeon may not be paid

42830 **Remove adenoids** ~ follow-up period is 90 days, standard payment adjustment rules for multiple procedures apply, 150% payment adjustment for bilateral procedures does not apply, payment for assistant surgeon subject to documentation of medical necessity

42831 **Remove adenoids** ~ follow-up period is 90 days, standard payment adjustment rules for multiple procedures apply, 150% payment adjustment for bilateral procedures does not apply, payment for assistant surgeon subject to documentation of medical necessity

42835 **Remove adenoids** ~ follow-up period is 90 days, standard payment adjustment rules for multiple procedures apply, 150% payment adjustment for bilateral procedures does not apply, payment for assistant surgeon subject to documentation of medical necessity

42836 **Remove adenoids** ~ follow-up period is 90 days, standard payment adjustment rules for multiple procedures apply, 150% payment adjustment for bilateral procedures does not apply, payment for assistant surgeon subject to documentation of medical necessity

42842 **Extensive surgery throat** ~ follow-up period is 90 days, standard payment adjustment rules for multiple procedures apply, 150% payment adjustment for bilateral procedures does not apply, payment for assistant surgeon subject to documentation of medical necessity

42844 **Extensive surgery throat** ~ follow-up period is 90 days, standard payment adjustment rules for multiple procedures apply, 150% payment adjustment for bilateral procedures does not apply, assistant surgeon may be paid

42845 **Extensive surgery throat** ~ follow-up period is 90 days, standard payment adjustment rules for multiple procedures apply, 150% payment adjustment for bilateral procedures does not apply, assistant surgeon may be paid

42860 **Excise tonsil tags** ~ follow-up period is 90 days, standard payment adjustment rules for multiple procedures apply, 150% payment adjustment for bilateral procedures does not apply, payment for assistant surgeon subject to documentation of medical necessity

42870 **Excise lingual tonsil** ~ follow-up period is 90 days, standard payment adjustment rules for multiple procedures apply, 150% payment adjustment for bilateral procedures does not apply, payment for assistant surgeon subject to documentation of medical necessity

| 42890 | **Partial remove pharynx** | ~ follow-up period is 90 days, standard payment adjustment rules for multiple procedures apply, 150% payment adjustment for bilateral procedures does not apply, assistant surgeon may be paid |

| 42892 | **Revise pharyngeal walls** | ~ follow-up period is 90 days, standard payment adjustment rules for multiple procedures apply, 150% payment adjustment for bilateral procedures does not apply, assistant surgeon may be paid |

| 42894 | **Revise pharyngeal walls** | ~ follow-up period is 90 days, standard payment adjustment rules for multiple procedures apply, 150% payment adjustment for bilateral procedures does not apply, assistant surgeon may be paid |

| 42900 | **Repair throat wound** | ~ follow-up period is 10 days, standard payment adjustment rules for multiple procedures apply, 150% payment adjustment for bilateral procedures does not apply, payment for assistant surgeon subject to documentation of medical necessity |

| 42950 | **Reconstruct throat** | ~ follow-up period is 90 days, standard payment adjustment rules for multiple procedures apply, 150% payment adjustment for bilateral procedures does not apply, assistant surgeon may be paid |

| 42953 | **Repair throat, esophagus** | ~ follow-up period is 90 days, standard payment adjustment rules for multiple procedures apply, 150% payment adjustment for bilateral procedures does not apply, assistant surgeon may be paid |

| 42955 | **Surgical opening of throat** | ~ follow-up period is 90 days, standard payment adjustment rules for multiple procedures apply, 150% payment adjustment for bilateral procedures does not apply, assistant surgeon may be paid |

| 42960 | **Control throat bleeding** | ~ follow-up period is 10 days, standard payment adjustment rules for multiple procedures apply, 150% payment adjustment for bilateral procedures does not apply, payment for assistant surgeon subject to documentation of medical necessity |

| 42961 | **Control throat bleeding** | ~ follow-up period is 90 days, standard payment adjustment rules for multiple procedures apply, 150% payment adjustment for bilateral procedures does not apply, assistant surgeon may be paid |

| 42962 | **Control throat bleeding** | ~ follow-up period is 90 days, standard payment adjustment rules for multiple procedures apply, 150% payment adjustment for bilateral procedures does not apply, assistant surgeon may be paid |

| 42970 | **Control nose/throat bleeding** | ~ follow-up period is 90 days, standard payment adjustment rules for multiple procedures apply, 150% payment adjustment for bilateral procedures does not apply, assistant surgeon may not be paid |

42971   **Control nose/throat bleeding**   ~ follow-up period is 90 days, standard payment adjustment rules for multiple procedures apply, 150% payment adjustment for bilateral procedures does not apply, assistant surgeon may be paid

42972   **Control nose/throat bleeding**   ~ follow-up period is 90 days, standard payment adjustment rules for multiple procedures apply, 150% payment adjustment for bilateral procedures does not apply, assistant surgeon may be paid

42999   **Throat surgery procedure**   ~ medicare carrier determines global period, standard payment adjustment rules for multiple procedures apply, 150% payment adjustment for bilateral procedures does not apply, payment for assistant surgeon subject to documentation of medical necessity

Esophagus

43020   **Incise esophagus**   ~ follow-up period is 90 days, standard payment adjustment rules for multiple procedures apply, 150% payment adjustment for bilateral procedures does not apply, assistant surgeon may be paid

43030   **Throat muscle surgery**   ~ follow-up period is 90 days, standard payment adjustment rules for multiple procedures apply, 150% payment adjustment for bilateral procedures does not apply, assistant surgeon may be paid

43045   **Incise esophagus**   ~ follow-up period is 90 days, standard payment adjustment rules for multiple procedures apply, 150% payment adjustment for bilateral procedures does not apply, assistant surgeon may be paid

43100   **Excise esophagus lesion**   ~ follow-up period is 90 days, standard payment adjustment rules for multiple procedures apply, 150% payment adjustment for bilateral procedures does not apply, assistant surgeon may be paid

43101   **Excise esophagus lesion**   ~ follow-up period is 90 days, standard payment adjustment rules for multiple procedures apply, 150% payment adjustment for bilateral procedures does not apply, assistant surgeon may be paid

43107   **Remove esophagus**   ~ follow-up period is 90 days, standard payment adjustment rules for multiple procedures apply, 150% payment adjustment for bilateral procedures does not apply, assistant surgeon may be paid

43108   **Remove esophagus**   ~ follow-up period is 90 days, standard payment adjustment rules for multiple procedures apply, 150% payment adjustment for bilateral procedures does not apply, assistant surgeon may be paid

43112   **Remove esophagus**   ~ follow-up period is 90 days, standard payment adjustment rules for multiple procedures apply, 150% payment adjustment for bilateral procedures does not apply, assistant surgeon may be paid

43113   **Remove esophagus**   ~ follow-up period is 90 days, standard payment adjustment rules for multiple procedures apply, 150% payment adjustment for bilateral procedures does not apply, assistant surgeon may be paid

43116   **Partial remove esophagus**   ~ follow-up period is 90 days, standard payment adjustment rules for multiple procedures apply, 150% payment adjustment for bilateral procedures does not apply, assistant surgeon may be paid

43117   **Partial remove esophagus**   ~ follow-up period is 90 days, standard payment adjustment rules for multiple procedures apply, 150% payment adjustment for bilateral procedures does not apply, assistant surgeon may be paid

43118   **Partial remove esophagus**   ~ follow-up period is 90 days, standard payment adjustment rules for multiple procedures apply, 150% payment adjustment for bilateral procedures does not apply, assistant surgeon may be paid

43121   **Partial remove esophagus**   ~ follow-up period is 90 days, standard payment adjustment rules for multiple procedures apply, 150% payment adjustment for bilateral procedures does not apply, assistant surgeon may be paid

43122   **Partial remove esophagus**   ~ follow-up period is 90 days, standard payment adjustment rules for multiple procedures apply, 150% payment adjustment for bilateral procedures does not apply, assistant surgeon may be paid

43123   **Partial remove esophagus**   ~ follow-up period is 90 days, standard payment adjustment rules for multiple procedures apply, 150% payment adjustment for bilateral procedures does not apply, assistant surgeon may be paid

43124   **Remove esophagus**   ~ follow-up period is 90 days, standard payment adjustment rules for multiple procedures apply, 150% payment adjustment for bilateral procedures does not apply, assistant surgeon may be paid

43130   **Remove esophagus pouch**   ~ follow-up period is 90 days, standard payment adjustment rules for multiple procedures apply, 150% payment adjustment for bilateral procedures does not apply, assistant surgeon may be paid

43135   **Remove esophagus pouch**   ~ follow-up period is 90 days, standard payment adjustment rules for multiple procedures apply, 150% payment adjustment for bilateral procedures does not apply, assistant surgeon may be paid

43200   **Esophagus endoscopy**   ~ endoscopies or minor procedure - E/M services on the same day generally not paid, standard payment adjustment rules for multiple procedures apply, 150% payment adjustment for bilateral procedures does not apply, assistant surgeon may not be paid

43201   **Esophagus scope w/submucous inject**   ~ endoscopies or minor procedure - E/M services on the same day generally not paid, special rules for multiple endoscopic

---

procedures apply if billed with another endoscopy in the same family, 150% payment adjustment for bilateral procedures does not apply, assistant surgeon may not be paid

43202   **Esophagus endoscopy, biopsy**   ~ endoscopies or minor procedure - E/M services on the same day generally not paid, special rules for multiple endoscopic procedures apply if billed with another endoscopy in the same family, 150% payment adjustment for bilateral procedures does not apply, assistant surgeon may not be paid

43204   **Esophagus scope w/sclerosis inject**   ~ endoscopies or minor procedure - E/M services on the same day generally not paid, special rules for multiple endoscopic procedures apply if billed with another endoscopy in the same family, 150% payment adjustment for bilateral procedures does not apply, assistant surgeon may not be paid

43205   **Esophagus endoscopy/ligation**   ~ endoscopies or minor procedure - E/M services on the same day generally not paid, special rules for multiple endoscopic procedures apply if billed with another endoscopy in the same family, 150% payment adjustment for bilateral procedures does not apply, payment for assistant surgeon subject to documentation of medical necessity

43215   **Esophagus endoscopy**   ~ endoscopies or minor procedure - E/M services on the same day generally not paid, special rules for multiple endoscopic procedures apply if billed with another endoscopy in the same family, 150% payment adjustment for bilateral procedures does not apply, assistant surgeon may not be paid

43216   **Esophagus endoscopy/lesion**   ~ endoscopies or minor procedure - E/M services on the same day generally not paid, special rules for multiple endoscopic procedures apply if billed with another endoscopy in the same family, 150% payment adjustment for bilateral procedures does not apply, payment for assistant surgeon subject to documentation of medical necessity

43217   **Esophagus endoscopy**   ~ endoscopies or minor procedure - E/M services on the same day generally not paid, special rules for multiple endoscopic procedures apply if billed with another endoscopy in the same family, 150% payment adjustment for bilateral procedures does not apply, assistant surgeon may not be paid

43219   **Esophagus endoscopy**   ~ endoscopies or minor procedure - E/M services on the same day generally not paid, special rules for multiple endoscopic procedures apply if billed with another endoscopy in the same family, 150% payment adjustment for bilateral procedures does not apply, assistant surgeon may not be paid

43220   **Esophagus endoscopy, dilate**   ~ endoscopies or minor procedure - E/M services on the same day generally not paid, special rules for multiple endoscopic procedures apply if billed with another endoscopy in the same family, 150% payment adjustment for bilateral procedures does not apply, assistant surgeon may not be paid

43226   **Esophagus endoscopy, dilate**   ~ endoscopies or minor procedure - E/M services on the same day generally not paid, special rules for multiple endoscopic

procedures apply if billed with another endoscopy in the same family, 150% payment adjustment for bilateral procedures does not apply, assistant surgeon may not be paid

43227 **Esophagus endoscopy, repair** ~ endoscopies or minor procedure - E/M services on the same day generally not paid, special rules for multiple endoscopic procedures apply if billed with another endoscopy in the same family, 150% payment adjustment for bilateral procedures does not apply, assistant surgeon may not be paid

43228 **Esophagus endoscopy, ablation** ~ endoscopies or minor procedure - E/M services on the same day generally not paid, special rules for multiple endoscopic procedures apply if billed with another endoscopy in the same family, 150% payment adjustment for bilateral procedures does not apply, assistant surgeon may not be paid

43231 **Esophagus endoscopy w/us exam** ~ endoscopies or minor procedure - E/M services on the same day generally not paid, special rules for multiple endoscopic procedures apply if billed with another endoscopy in the same family, 150% payment adjustment for bilateral procedures does not apply, payment for assistant surgeon subject to documentation of medical necessity

43232 **Esophagus endoscopy w/us fn biopsy** ~ endoscopies or minor procedure - E/M services on the same day generally not paid, special rules for multiple endoscopic procedures apply if billed with another endoscopy in the same family, 150% payment adjustment for bilateral procedures does not apply, payment for assistant surgeon subject to documentation of medical necessity

43234 **Upper gi endoscopy, exam** ~ endoscopies or minor procedure - E/M services on the same day generally not paid, standard payment adjustment rules for multiple procedures apply, 150% payment adjustment for bilateral procedures does not apply, assistant surgeon may not be paid

43235 **Upper gi endoscopy, diagnosis** ~ endoscopies or minor procedure - E/M services on the same day generally not paid, standard payment adjustment rules for multiple procedures apply, 150% payment adjustment for bilateral procedures does not apply, assistant surgeon may not be paid

43236 **Upper gi scope w/submucosa inject** ~ endoscopies or minor procedure - E/M services on the same day generally not paid, special rules for multiple endoscopic procedures apply if billed with another endoscopy in the same family, 150% payment adjustment for bilateral procedures does not apply, assistant surgeon may not be paid

43237 **Endoscopic us exam esophagus** ~ endoscopies or minor procedure - E/M services on the same day generally not paid, special rules for multiple endoscopic procedures apply if billed with another endoscopy in the same family, 150% payment adjustment for bilateral procedures does not apply, payment for assistant surgeon subject to documentation of medical necessity

43238 **Upper gi endoscopy w/us fn biopsy** ~ endoscopies or minor procedure - E/M services on the same day generally not paid, special rules for multiple endoscopic procedures apply if billed with another endoscopy in the same family, 150% payment adjustment for bilateral procedures does not apply, payment for assistant surgeon subject to documentation of medical necessity

43239 **Upper gi endoscopy, biopsy** ~ endoscopies or minor procedure - E/M services on the same day generally not paid, special rules for multiple endoscopic procedures apply if billed with another endoscopy in the same family, 150% payment adjustment for bilateral procedures does not apply, assistant surgeon may not be paid

43240 **Esophagus endoscope w/drain cyst** ~ endoscopies or minor procedure - E/M services on the same day generally not paid, special rules for multiple endoscopic procedures apply if billed with another endoscopy in the same family, 150% payment adjustment for bilateral procedures does not apply, assistant surgeon may not be paid

43241 **Upper gi endoscopy with tube** ~ endoscopies or minor procedure - E/M services on the same day generally not paid, special rules for multiple endoscopic procedures apply if billed with another endoscopy in the same family, 150% payment adjustment for bilateral procedures does not apply, assistant surgeon may not be paid

43242 **Upper gi endoscopy w/us fn biopsy** ~ endoscopies or minor procedure - E/M services on the same day generally not paid, special rules for multiple endoscopic procedures apply if billed with another endoscopy in the same family, 150% payment adjustment for bilateral procedures does not apply, payment for assistant surgeon subject to documentation of medical necessity

43243 **Upper gi endoscopy & inject** ~ endoscopies or minor procedure - E/M services on the same day generally not paid, special rules for multiple endoscopic procedures apply if billed with another endoscopy in the same family, 150% payment adjustment for bilateral procedures does not apply, assistant surgeon may not be paid

43244 **Upper gi endoscopy/ligation** ~ endoscopies or minor procedure - E/M services on the same day generally not paid, special rules for multiple endoscopic procedures apply if billed with another endoscopy in the same family, 150% payment adjustment for bilateral procedures does not apply, payment for assistant surgeon subject to documentation of medical necessity

43245 **Upper gi scope dilate stricture** ~ endoscopies or minor procedure - E/M services on the same day generally not paid, special rules for multiple endoscopic procedures apply if billed with another endoscopy in the same family, 150% payment adjustment for bilateral procedures does not apply, assistant surgeon may not be paid

43246 **Place gastrostomy tube** ~ endoscopies or minor procedure - E/M services on the same day generally not paid, special rules for multiple endoscopic procedures apply if billed with another endoscopy in the same family, 150% payment

adjustment for bilateral procedures does not apply, payment for assistant surgeon subject to documentation of medical necessity

43247   **Operative upper gi endoscopy**   ~ endoscopies or minor procedure - E/M services on the same day generally not paid, special rules for multiple endoscopic procedures apply if billed with another endoscopy in the same family, 150% payment adjustment for bilateral procedures does not apply, assistant surgeon may not be paid

43248   **Upper gi endoscopy/guide wire**   ~ endoscopies or minor procedure - E/M services on the same day generally not paid, special rules for multiple endoscopic procedures apply if billed with another endoscopy in the same family, 150% payment adjustment for bilateral procedures does not apply, assistant surgeon may not be paid

43249   **Esophagus endoscopy, dilate**   ~ endoscopies or minor procedure - E/M services on the same day generally not paid, special rules for multiple endoscopic procedures apply if billed with another endoscopy in the same family, 150% payment adjustment for bilateral procedures does not apply, assistant surgeon may not be paid

43250   **Upper gi endoscopy/tumor**   ~ endoscopies or minor procedure - E/M services on the same day generally not paid, special rules for multiple endoscopic procedures apply if billed with another endoscopy in the same family, 150% payment adjustment for bilateral procedures does not apply, assistant surgeon may not be paid

43251   **Operative upper gi endoscopy**   ~ endoscopies or minor procedure - E/M services on the same day generally not paid, special rules for multiple endoscopic procedures apply if billed with another endoscopy in the same family, 150% payment adjustment for bilateral procedures does not apply, assistant surgeon may not be paid

43255   **Operative upper gi endoscopy**   ~ endoscopies or minor procedure - E/M services on the same day generally not paid, special rules for multiple endoscopic procedures apply if billed with another endoscopy in the same family, 150% payment adjustment for bilateral procedures does not apply, assistant surgeon may not be paid

43256   **Upper gi endoscopy w/stent**   ~ endoscopies or minor procedure - E/M services on the same day generally not paid, special rules for multiple endoscopic procedures apply if billed with another endoscopy in the same family, 150% payment adjustment for bilateral procedures does not apply, assistant surgeon may not be paid

43257   **Upper gi scope w/thermal treat**   ~ endoscopies or minor procedure - E/M services on the same day generally not paid, special rules for multiple endoscopic procedures apply if billed with another endoscopy in the same family, 150% payment adjustment for bilateral procedures does not apply, assistant surgeon may not be paid

43258   **Operative upper gi endoscopy**   ~ endoscopies or minor procedure - E/M services on the same day generally not paid, special rules for multiple endoscopic procedures apply if billed with another endoscopy in the same family, 150% payment adjustment for bilateral procedures does not apply, assistant surgeon may not be paid

43259   **Endoscopic ultrasound exam**   ~ endoscopies or minor procedure - E/M services on the same day generally not paid, special rules for multiple endoscopic procedures apply if billed with another endoscopy in the same family, 150% payment adjustment for bilateral procedures does not apply, payment for assistant surgeon subject to documentation of medical necessity

43260   **Endo cholangiopancreatography**   ~ endoscopies or minor procedure - E/M services on the same day generally not paid, standard payment adjustment rules for multiple procedures apply, 150% payment adjustment for bilateral procedures does not apply, assistant surgeon may not be paid

43261   **Endo cholangiopancreatography**   ~ endoscopies or minor procedure - E/M services on the same day generally not paid, special rules for multiple endoscopic procedures apply if billed with another endoscopy in the same family, 150% payment adjustment for bilateral procedures does not apply, assistant surgeon may not be paid

43262   **Endo cholangiopancreatography**   ~ endoscopies or minor procedure - E/M services on the same day generally not paid, special rules for multiple endoscopic procedures apply if billed with another endoscopy in the same family, 150% payment adjustment for bilateral procedures does not apply, assistant surgeon may not be paid

43263   **Endo cholangiopancreatography**   ~ endoscopies or minor procedure - E/M services on the same day generally not paid, special rules for multiple endoscopic procedures apply if billed with another endoscopy in the same family, 150% payment adjustment for bilateral procedures does not apply, assistant surgeon may not be paid

43264   **Endo cholangiopancreatography**   ~ endoscopies or minor procedure - E/M services on the same day generally not paid, special rules for multiple endoscopic procedures apply if billed with another endoscopy in the same family, 150% payment adjustment for bilateral procedures does not apply, assistant surgeon may not be paid

43265   **Endo cholangiopancreatography**   ~ endoscopies or minor procedure - E/M services on the same day generally not paid, special rules for multiple endoscopic procedures apply if billed with another endoscopy in the same family, 150% payment adjustment for bilateral procedures does not apply, assistant surgeon may not be paid

43267   **Endo cholangiopancreatography**   ~ endoscopies or minor procedure - E/M services on the same day generally not paid, special rules for multiple endoscopic procedures apply if billed with another endoscopy in the same family, 150% payment adjustment for bilateral procedures does not apply, assistant surgeon may not be paid

43268   **Endo cholangiopancreatography**   ~ endoscopies or minor procedure - E/M services on the same day generally not paid, special rules for multiple endoscopic procedures apply if billed with another endoscopy in the same family, 150% payment adjustment for bilateral procedures does not apply, assistant surgeon may not be paid

43269   **Endo cholangiopancreatography**   ~ endoscopies or minor procedure - E/M services on the same day generally not paid, special rules for multiple endoscopic procedures apply if billed with another endoscopy in the same family, 150% payment adjustment for bilateral procedures does not apply, assistant surgeon may not be paid

43271   **Endo cholangiopancreatography**   ~ endoscopies or minor procedure - E/M services on the same day generally not paid, special rules for multiple endoscopic procedures apply if billed with another endoscopy in the same family, 150% payment adjustment for bilateral procedures does not apply, assistant surgeon may not be paid

43272   **Endo cholangiopancreatography**   ~ endoscopies or minor procedure - E/M services on the same day generally not paid, special rules for multiple endoscopic procedures apply if billed with another endoscopy in the same family, 150% payment adjustment for bilateral procedures does not apply, payment for assistant surgeon subject to documentation of medical necessity

43280   **Laparoscopy, fundoplasty**   ~ follow-up period is 90 days, standard payment adjustment rules for multiple procedures apply, 150% payment adjustment for bilateral procedures does not apply, assistant surgeon may be paid

43289   **Laparoscope proc, esophagus**   ~ medicare carrier determines global period, standard payment adjustment rules for multiple procedures apply, 150% payment adjustment for bilateral procedures applies, assistant surgeon may be paid

43300   **Repair esophagus**   ~ follow-up period is 90 days, standard payment adjustment rules for multiple procedures apply, 150% payment adjustment for bilateral procedures does not apply, assistant surgeon may be paid

43305   **Repair esophagus and fistula**   ~ follow-up period is 90 days, standard payment adjustment rules for multiple procedures apply, 150% payment adjustment for bilateral procedures does not apply, assistant surgeon may be paid

43310   **Repair esophagus**   ~ follow-up period is 90 days, standard payment adjustment rules for multiple procedures apply, 150% payment adjustment for bilateral procedures does not apply, assistant surgeon may be paid

43312   **Repair esophagus and fistula**   ~ follow-up period is 90 days, standard payment adjustment rules for multiple procedures apply, 150% payment adjustment for bilateral procedures does not apply, assistant surgeon may be paid

43313   **Esophagoplasty congenital**   ~ follow-up period is 90 days, standard payment adjustment rules for multiple procedures apply, 150% payment adjustment for bilateral procedures does not apply, assistant surgeon may be paid

43314   **Tracheo-esophagoplasty cong**   ~ follow-up period is 90 days, standard payment adjustment rules for multiple procedures apply, 150% payment adjustment for bilateral procedures does not apply, assistant surgeon may be paid

43320   **Fuse esophagus & stomach**   ~ follow-up period is 90 days, standard payment adjustment rules for multiple procedures apply, 150% payment adjustment for bilateral procedures does not apply, assistant surgeon may be paid

43324   **Revise esophagus & stomach**   ~ follow-up period is 90 days, standard payment adjustment rules for multiple procedures apply, 150% payment adjustment for bilateral procedures does not apply, assistant surgeon may be paid

43325   **Revise esophagus & stomach**   ~ follow-up period is 90 days, standard payment adjustment rules for multiple procedures apply, 150% payment adjustment for bilateral procedures does not apply, assistant surgeon may be paid

43326   **Revise esophagus & stomach**   ~ follow-up period is 90 days, standard payment adjustment rules for multiple procedures apply, 150% payment adjustment for bilateral procedures does not apply, assistant surgeon may be paid

43330   **Repair esophagus**   ~ follow-up period is 90 days, standard payment adjustment rules for multiple procedures apply, 150% payment adjustment for bilateral procedures does not apply, assistant surgeon may be paid

43331   **Repair esophagus**   ~ follow-up period is 90 days, standard payment adjustment rules for multiple procedures apply, 150% payment adjustment for bilateral procedures does not apply, assistant surgeon may be paid

43340   **Fuse esophagus & intestine**   ~ follow-up period is 90 days, standard payment adjustment rules for multiple procedures apply, 150% payment adjustment for bilateral procedures does not apply, assistant surgeon may be paid

43341   **Fuse esophagus & intestine**   ~ follow-up period is 90 days, standard payment adjustment rules for multiple procedures apply, 150% payment adjustment for bilateral procedures does not apply, assistant surgeon may be paid

43350   **Surgical opening, esophagus**   ~ follow-up period is 90 days, standard payment adjustment rules for multiple procedures apply, 150% payment adjustment for bilateral procedures does not apply, assistant surgeon may be paid

43351   **Surgical opening, esophagus**   ~ follow-up period is 90 days, standard payment adjustment rules for multiple procedures apply, 150% payment adjustment for bilateral procedures does not apply, assistant surgeon may be paid

43352   **Surgical opening, esophagus**   ~ follow-up period is 90 days, standard payment adjustment rules for multiple procedures apply, 150% payment adjustment for bilateral procedures does not apply, assistant surgeon may be paid

43360   **Gastrointestinal repair**   ~ follow-up period is 90 days, standard payment adjustment rules for multiple procedures apply, 150% payment adjustment for bilateral procedures does not apply, assistant surgeon may be paid

43361   **Gastrointestinal repair**   ~ follow-up period is 90 days, standard payment adjustment rules for multiple procedures apply, 150% payment adjustment for bilateral procedures does not apply, assistant surgeon may be paid

43400   **Ligate esophagus veins**   ~ follow-up period is 90 days, standard payment adjustment rules for multiple procedures apply, 150% payment adjustment for bilateral procedures does not apply, assistant surgeon may be paid

43401   **Esophagus surgery for veins**   ~ follow-up period is 90 days, standard payment adjustment rules for multiple procedures apply, 150% payment adjustment for bilateral procedures does not apply, assistant surgeon may be paid

43405   **Ligate/staple esophagus**   ~ follow-up period is 90 days, standard payment adjustment rules for multiple procedures apply, 150% payment adjustment for bilateral procedures does not apply, assistant surgeon may be paid

43410   **Repair esophagus wound**   ~ follow-up period is 90 days, standard payment adjustment rules for multiple procedures apply, 150% payment adjustment for bilateral procedures does not apply, assistant surgeon may be paid

43415   **Repair esophagus wound**   ~ follow-up period is 90 days, standard payment adjustment rules for multiple procedures apply, 150% payment adjustment for bilateral procedures does not apply, assistant surgeon may be paid

43420   **Repair esophagus opening**   ~ follow-up period is 90 days, standard payment adjustment rules for multiple procedures apply, 150% payment adjustment for bilateral procedures does not apply, payment for assistant surgeon subject to documentation of medical necessity

43425   **Repair esophagus opening**   ~ follow-up period is 90 days, standard payment adjustment rules for multiple procedures apply, 150% payment adjustment for bilateral procedures does not apply, assistant surgeon may be paid

43450   **Dilate esophagus**   ~ endoscopies or minor procedure - E/M services on the same day generally not paid, standard payment adjustment rules for multiple procedures apply, 150% payment adjustment for bilateral procedures does not apply, assistant surgeon may not be paid

43453   **Dilate esophagus**   ~ endoscopies or minor procedure - E/M services on the same day generally not paid, standard payment adjustment rules for multiple procedures apply, 150% payment adjustment for bilateral procedures does not apply, assistant surgeon may not be paid

43456   **Dilate esophagus**   ~ endoscopies or minor procedure - E/M services on the same day generally not paid, standard payment adjustment rules for multiple procedures apply, 150% payment adjustment for bilateral procedures does not apply, assistant surgeon may not be paid

43458   **Dilate esophagus**   ~ endoscopies or minor procedure - E/M services on the same day generally not paid, standard payment adjustment rules for multiple procedures apply, 150% payment adjustment for bilateral procedures does not apply, assistant surgeon may not be paid

43460   **Pressure treatment esophagus**   ~ endoscopies or minor procedure - E/M services on the same day generally not paid, standard payment adjustment rules for multiple procedures apply, 150% payment adjustment for bilateral procedures does not apply, assistant surgeon may not be paid

43496   **Free jejunum flap, microvasc**   ~ follow-up period is 90 days, standard payment adjustment rules for multiple procedures apply, 150% payment adjustment for bilateral procedures does not apply, assistant surgeon may be paid

43499   **Esophagus surgery procedure**   ~ medicare carrier determines global period, standard payment adjustment rules for multiple procedures apply, 150% payment adjustment for bilateral procedures does not apply, assistant surgeon may be paid

Stomach

43500   **Surgical opening of stomach**   ~ follow-up period is 90 days, standard payment adjustment rules for multiple procedures apply, 150% payment adjustment for bilateral procedures does not apply, assistant surgeon may be paid

43501   **Surgical repair stomach**   ~ follow-up period is 90 days, standard payment adjustment rules for multiple procedures apply, 150% payment adjustment for bilateral procedures does not apply, assistant surgeon may be paid

43502   **Surgical repair stomach**   ~ follow-up period is 90 days, standard payment adjustment rules for multiple procedures apply, 150% payment adjustment for bilateral procedures does not apply, assistant surgeon may be paid

43510   **Surgical opening of stomach**   ~ follow-up period is 90 days, standard payment adjustment rules for multiple procedures apply, 150% payment adjustment for bilateral procedures does not apply, assistant surgeon may be paid

43520   **Incise pyloric muscle**   ~ follow-up period is 90 days, standard payment adjustment rules for multiple procedures apply, 150% payment adjustment for bilateral procedures does not apply, assistant surgeon may be paid

43600   **Biopsy stomach**   ~ endoscopies or minor procedure - E/M services on the same day generally not paid, standard payment adjustment rules for multiple procedures apply, 150% payment adjustment for bilateral procedures does not apply, assistant surgeon may not be paid

43605 **Biopsy stomach** ~ follow-up period is 90 days, standard payment adjustment rules for multiple procedures apply, 150% payment adjustment for bilateral procedures does not apply, assistant surgeon may be paid

43610 **Excise stomach lesion** ~ follow-up period is 90 days, standard payment adjustment rules for multiple procedures apply, 150% payment adjustment for bilateral procedures does not apply, assistant surgeon may be paid

43611 **Excise stomach lesion** ~ follow-up period is 90 days, standard payment adjustment rules for multiple procedures apply, 150% payment adjustment for bilateral procedures does not apply, assistant surgeon may be paid

43620 **Remove stomach** ~ follow-up period is 90 days, standard payment adjustment rules for multiple procedures apply, 150% payment adjustment for bilateral procedures does not apply, assistant surgeon may be paid

43621 **Remove stomach** ~ follow-up period is 90 days, standard payment adjustment rules for multiple procedures apply, 150% payment adjustment for bilateral procedures does not apply, assistant surgeon may be paid

43622 **Remove stomach** ~ follow-up period is 90 days, standard payment adjustment rules for multiple procedures apply, 150% payment adjustment for bilateral procedures does not apply, assistant surgeon may be paid

43631 **Remove stomach, partial** ~ follow-up period is 90 days, standard payment adjustment rules for multiple procedures apply, 150% payment adjustment for bilateral procedures does not apply, assistant surgeon may be paid

43632 **Remove stomach, partial** ~ follow-up period is 90 days, standard payment adjustment rules for multiple procedures apply, 150% payment adjustment for bilateral procedures does not apply, assistant surgeon may be paid

43633 **Remove stomach, partial** ~ follow-up period is 90 days, standard payment adjustment rules for multiple procedures apply, 150% payment adjustment for bilateral procedures does not apply, assistant surgeon may be paid

43634 **Remove stomach, partial** ~ follow-up period is 90 days, standard payment adjustment rules for multiple procedures apply, 150% payment adjustment for bilateral procedures does not apply, assistant surgeon may be paid

43635 **Remove stomach, partial** ~ follow-up period included in another service, no payment adjustment rules for multiple procedures apply, 150% payment adjustment for bilateral procedures does not apply, assistant surgeon may be paid

43640 **Vagotomy & pylorus repair** ~ follow-up period is 90 days, standard payment adjustment rules for multiple procedures apply, 150% payment adjustment for bilateral procedures does not apply, assistant surgeon may be paid

43641 **Vagotomy & pylorus repair** ~ follow-up period is 90 days, standard payment adjustment rules for multiple procedures apply, 150% payment adjustment for bilateral procedures does not apply, assistant surgeon may be paid

43644 **Laparoscopy gastric bypass/roux-en-y** ~ follow-up period is 90 days, standard payment adjustment rules for multiple procedures apply, 150% payment adjustment for bilateral procedures does not apply, assistant surgeon may be paid

43645 **Laparoscopy gastric bypass including small i** ~ follow-up period is 90 days, standard payment adjustment rules for multiple procedures apply, 150% payment adjustment for bilateral procedures does not apply, assistant surgeon may be paid

43647 **Laparoscopy implant electrode, antrum** ~ medicare carrier determines global period, standard payment adjustment rules for multiple procedures apply, 150% payment adjustment for bilateral procedures does not apply, assistant surgeon may be paid

43648 **Laparoscopy revise/remove electrode antrum** ~ medicare carrier determines global period, standard payment adjustment rules for multiple procedures apply, 150% payment adjustment for bilateral procedures does not apply, assistant surgeon may be paid

43651 **Laparoscopy, vagus nerve** ~ follow-up period is 90 days, standard payment adjustment rules for multiple procedures apply, 150% payment adjustment for bilateral procedures does not apply, assistant surgeon may be paid

43652 **Laparoscopy, vagus nerve** ~ follow-up period is 90 days, standard payment adjustment rules for multiple procedures apply, 150% payment adjustment for bilateral procedures does not apply, assistant surgeon may be paid

43653 **Laparoscopy, gastrostomy** ~ follow-up period is 90 days, standard payment adjustment rules for multiple procedures apply, 150% payment adjustment for bilateral procedures does not apply, assistant surgeon may be paid

43659 **Laparoscope proc, stomach** ~ medicare carrier determines global period, standard payment adjustment rules for multiple procedures apply, 150% payment adjustment for bilateral procedures applies, assistant surgeon may be paid

43750 **Place gastrostomy tube** ~ follow-up period is 10 days, standard payment adjustment rules for multiple procedures apply, 150% payment adjustment for bilateral procedures does not apply, assistant surgeon may not be paid

43752 **Nasal/orogastric w/stent** ~ endoscopies or minor procedure - E/M services on the same day generally not paid, no payment adjustment rules for multiple procedures apply, 150% payment adjustment for bilateral procedures does not apply, assistant surgeon may not be paid

43760 **Change gastrostomy tube** ~ endoscopies or minor procedure - E/M services on the same day generally not paid, standard payment adjustment rules for multiple

procedures apply, 150% payment adjustment for bilateral procedures does not apply, assistant surgeon may not be paid

43761 **Reposition gastrostomy tube** ~ endoscopies or minor procedure - E/M services on the same day generally not paid, standard payment adjustment rules for multiple procedures apply, 150% payment adjustment for bilateral procedures does not apply, assistant surgeon may not be paid

43770 **Laparoscopy, place gastric adjust band** ~ follow-up period is 90 days, standard payment adjustment rules for multiple procedures apply, 150% payment adjustment for bilateral procedures does not apply, assistant surgeon may be paid

43771 **Laparoscopy, revise adjust gastric band** ~ follow-up period is 90 days, standard payment adjustment rules for multiple procedures apply, 150% payment adjustment for bilateral procedures does not apply, assistant surgeon may be paid

43772 **Laparoscopy, remove adjust gastric band** ~ follow-up period is 90 days, standard payment adjustment rules for multiple procedures apply, 150% payment adjustment for bilateral procedures does not apply, assistant surgeon may be paid

43773 **Laparoscopy, change adjust gastric band** ~ follow-up period is 90 days, standard payment adjustment rules for multiple procedures apply, 150% payment adjustment for bilateral procedures does not apply, assistant surgeon may be paid

43774 **Laparoscopy remove adjust gastric band/port** ~ follow-up period is 90 days, standard payment adjustment rules for multiple procedures apply, 150% payment adjustment for bilateral procedures does not apply, assistant surgeon may be paid

43800 **Reconstruct pylorus** ~ follow-up period is 90 days, standard payment adjustment rules for multiple procedures apply, 150% payment adjustment for bilateral procedures does not apply, assistant surgeon may be paid

43810 **Fuse stomach and bowel** ~ follow-up period is 90 days, standard payment adjustment rules for multiple procedures apply, 150% payment adjustment for bilateral procedures does not apply, assistant surgeon may be paid

43820 **Fuse stomach and bowel** ~ follow-up period is 90 days, standard payment adjustment rules for multiple procedures apply, 150% payment adjustment for bilateral procedures does not apply, assistant surgeon may be paid

43825 **Fuse stomach and bowel** ~ follow-up period is 90 days, standard payment adjustment rules for multiple procedures apply, 150% payment adjustment for bilateral procedures does not apply, assistant surgeon may be paid

43830 **Place gastrostomy tube** ~ follow-up period is 90 days, standard payment adjustment rules for multiple procedures apply, 150% payment adjustment for bilateral procedures does not apply, assistant surgeon may be paid

43831 **Place gastrostomy tube**   ~ follow-up period is 90 days, standard payment adjustment rules for multiple procedures apply, 150% payment adjustment for bilateral procedures does not apply, assistant surgeon may be paid

43832 **Place gastrostomy tube**   ~ follow-up period is 90 days, standard payment adjustment rules for multiple procedures apply, 150% payment adjustment for bilateral procedures does not apply, assistant surgeon may be paid

43840 **Repair stomach lesion**   ~ follow-up period is 90 days, standard payment adjustment rules for multiple procedures apply, 150% payment adjustment for bilateral procedures does not apply, assistant surgeon may be paid

43842 **V-band gastroplasty**   non-covered service, follow-up period is 90 days, multiple procedure concept does not apply, bilateral surgery concept does not apply, assistant surgery concept does not apply

43843 **Gastroplasty w/o v-band**   ~ follow-up period is 90 days, standard payment adjustment rules for multiple procedures apply, 150% payment adjustment for bilateral procedures does not apply, assistant surgeon may be paid

43845 **Gastroplasty duodenal switch**   ~ follow-up period is 90 days, standard payment adjustment rules for multiple procedures apply, 150% payment adjustment for bilateral procedures does not apply, assistant surgeon may be paid

43846 **Gastric bypass for obesity**   ~ follow-up period is 90 days, standard payment adjustment rules for multiple procedures apply, 150% payment adjustment for bilateral procedures does not apply, assistant surgeon may be paid

43847 **Gastric bypass including small i**   ~ follow-up period is 90 days, standard payment adjustment rules for multiple procedures apply, 150% payment adjustment for bilateral procedures does not apply, assistant surgeon may be paid

43848 **Revision gastroplasty**   ~ follow-up period is 90 days, standard payment adjustment rules for multiple procedures apply, 150% payment adjustment for bilateral procedures does not apply, assistant surgeon may be paid

43850 **Revise stomach-bowel fusion**   ~ follow-up period is 90 days, standard payment adjustment rules for multiple procedures apply, 150% payment adjustment for bilateral procedures does not apply, assistant surgeon may be paid

43855 **Revise stomach-bowel fusion**   ~ follow-up period is 90 days, standard payment adjustment rules for multiple procedures apply, 150% payment adjustment for bilateral procedures does not apply, assistant surgeon may be paid

43860 **Revise stomach-bowel fusion**   ~ follow-up period is 90 days, standard payment adjustment rules for multiple procedures apply, 150% payment adjustment for bilateral procedures does not apply, assistant surgeon may be paid

43865 **Revise stomach-bowel fusion** ~ follow-up period is 90 days, standard payment adjustment rules for multiple procedures apply, 150% payment adjustment for bilateral procedures does not apply, assistant surgeon may be paid

43870 **Repair stomach opening** ~ follow-up period is 90 days, standard payment adjustment rules for multiple procedures apply, 150% payment adjustment for bilateral procedures does not apply, assistant surgeon may be paid

43880 **Repair stomach-bowel fistula** ~ follow-up period is 90 days, standard payment adjustment rules for multiple procedures apply, 150% payment adjustment for bilateral procedures does not apply, assistant surgeon may be paid

43881 **Implant/redo electrode, antrum** ~ medicare carrier determines global period, standard payment adjustment rules for multiple procedures apply, 150% payment adjustment for bilateral procedures does not apply, assistant surgeon may be paid

43882 **Revise/remove electrode antrum** ~ medicare carrier determines global period, standard payment adjustment rules for multiple procedures apply, 150% payment adjustment for bilateral procedures does not apply, assistant surgeon may be paid

43886 **Revise gastric port, open** ~ follow-up period is 90 days, standard payment adjustment rules for multiple procedures apply, 150% payment adjustment for bilateral procedures does not apply, assistant surgeon may be paid

43887 **Remove gastric port, open** ~ follow-up period is 90 days, standard payment adjustment rules for multiple procedures apply, 150% payment adjustment for bilateral procedures does not apply, assistant surgeon may be paid

43888 **Change gastric port, open** ~ follow-up period is 90 days, standard payment adjustment rules for multiple procedures apply, 150% payment adjustment for bilateral procedures does not apply, assistant surgeon may be paid

43999 **Stomach surgery procedure** ~ medicare carrier determines global period, standard payment adjustment rules for multiple procedures apply, 150% payment adjustment for bilateral procedures does not apply, payment for assistant surgeon subject to documentation of medical necessity

Intestines (Except Rectum)

44005 **Freeing of bowel adhesion** ~ follow-up period is 90 days, standard payment adjustment rules for multiple procedures apply, 150% payment adjustment for bilateral procedures does not apply, assistant surgeon may be paid

44010 **Incise small bowel** ~ follow-up period is 90 days, standard payment adjustment rules for multiple procedures apply, 150% payment adjustment for bilateral procedures does not apply, assistant surgeon may be paid

44015   **Insert needle cath bowel**   ~ follow-up period included in another service, no payment adjustment rules for multiple procedures apply, 150% payment adjustment for bilateral procedures does not apply, assistant surgeon may be paid

44020   **Explore small intestine**   ~ follow-up period is 90 days, standard payment adjustment rules for multiple procedures apply, 150% payment adjustment for bilateral procedures does not apply, assistant surgeon may be paid

44021   **Decompress small bowel**   ~ follow-up period is 90 days, standard payment adjustment rules for multiple procedures apply, 150% payment adjustment for bilateral procedures does not apply, assistant surgeon may be paid

44025   **Incise large bowel**   ~ follow-up period is 90 days, standard payment adjustment rules for multiple procedures apply, 150% payment adjustment for bilateral procedures does not apply, assistant surgeon may be paid

44050   **Reduce bowel obstruction**   ~ follow-up period is 90 days, standard payment adjustment rules for multiple procedures apply, 150% payment adjustment for bilateral procedures does not apply, assistant surgeon may be paid

44055   **Correct malrotation of bowel**   ~ follow-up period is 90 days, standard payment adjustment rules for multiple procedures apply, 150% payment adjustment for bilateral procedures does not apply, assistant surgeon may be paid

44100   **Biopsy bowel**   ~ endoscopies or minor procedure - E/M services on the same day generally not paid, standard payment adjustment rules for multiple procedures apply, 150% payment adjustment for bilateral procedures does not apply, assistant surgeon may not be paid

44110   **Excise intestine lesion(s)**   ~ follow-up period is 90 days, standard payment adjustment rules for multiple procedures apply, 150% payment adjustment for bilateral procedures does not apply, assistant surgeon may be paid

44111   **Excise bowel lesion(s)**   ~ follow-up period is 90 days, standard payment adjustment rules for multiple procedures apply, 150% payment adjustment for bilateral procedures does not apply, assistant surgeon may be paid

44120   **Remove small intestine**   ~ follow-up period is 90 days, standard payment adjustment rules for multiple procedures apply, 150% payment adjustment for bilateral procedures does not apply, assistant surgeon may be paid

44121   **Remove small intestine**   ~ follow-up period included in another service, no payment adjustment rules for multiple procedures apply, 150% payment adjustment for bilateral procedures does not apply, assistant surgeon may be paid

44125   **Remove small intestine** ~ follow-up period is 90 days, standard payment adjustment rules for multiple procedures apply, 150% payment adjustment for bilateral procedures does not apply, assistant surgeon may be paid

44126   **Enterectomy w/o taper, cong** ~ follow-up period is 90 days, standard payment adjustment rules for multiple procedures apply, 150% payment adjustment for bilateral procedures does not apply, assistant surgeon may be paid

44127   **Enterectomy w/taper, cong** ~ follow-up period is 90 days, standard payment adjustment rules for multiple procedures apply, 150% payment adjustment for bilateral procedures does not apply, assistant surgeon may be paid

44128   **Enterectomy cong, add-on** ~ follow-up period included in another service, no payment adjustment rules for multiple procedures apply, 150% payment adjustment for bilateral procedures does not apply, assistant surgeon may be paid, +add-on code (list separately in addition to primary procedure)

44130   **Bowel to bowel fusion** ~ follow-up period is 90 days, standard payment adjustment rules for multiple procedures apply, 150% payment adjustment for bilateral procedures does not apply, assistant surgeon may be paid

44132   **Enterectomy, cadaver donor** ~ restricted coverage - special coverage rules apply, no payment adjustment rules for multiple procedures apply, 150% payment adjustment for bilateral procedures does not apply, payment for assistant surgeon subject to documentation of medical necessity

44133   **Enterectomy, live donor** ~ restricted coverage - special coverage rules apply, no payment adjustment rules for multiple procedures apply, 150% payment adjustment for bilateral procedures does not apply, payment for assistant surgeon subject to documentation of medical necessity

44135   **Intestine transplant, cadaver** ~ restricted coverage - special coverage rules apply, no payment adjustment rules for multiple procedures apply, 150% payment adjustment for bilateral procedures does not apply, payment for assistant surgeon subject to documentation of medical necessity

44136   **Intestine transplant, live** ~ restricted coverage - special coverage rules apply, no payment adjustment rules for multiple procedures apply, 150% payment adjustment for bilateral procedures does not apply, payment for assistant surgeon subject to documentation of medical necessity

44137   **Remove intestinal allograft** ~ standard payment adjustment rules for multiple procedures apply, 150% payment adjustment for bilateral procedures does not apply, assistant surgeon may be paid

44139   **Mobilization of colon**   ~ follow-up period included in another service, no payment adjustment rules for multiple procedures apply, 150% payment adjustment for bilateral procedures does not apply, assistant surgeon may be paid

44140   **Partial remove colon**   ~ follow-up period is 90 days, standard payment adjustment rules for multiple procedures apply, 150% payment adjustment for bilateral procedures does not apply, assistant surgeon may be paid

44141   **Partial remove colon**   ~ follow-up period is 90 days, standard payment adjustment rules for multiple procedures apply, 150% payment adjustment for bilateral procedures does not apply, assistant surgeon may be paid

44143   **Partial remove colon**   ~ follow-up period is 90 days, standard payment adjustment rules for multiple procedures apply, 150% payment adjustment for bilateral procedures does not apply, assistant surgeon may be paid

44144   **Partial remove colon**   ~ follow-up period is 90 days, standard payment adjustment rules for multiple procedures apply, 150% payment adjustment for bilateral procedures does not apply, assistant surgeon may be paid

44145   **Partial remove colon**   ~ follow-up period is 90 days, standard payment adjustment rules for multiple procedures apply, 150% payment adjustment for bilateral procedures does not apply, assistant surgeon may be paid

44146   **Partial remove colon**   ~ follow-up period is 90 days, standard payment adjustment rules for multiple procedures apply, 150% payment adjustment for bilateral procedures does not apply, assistant surgeon may be paid

44147   **Partial remove colon**   ~ follow-up period is 90 days, standard payment adjustment rules for multiple procedures apply, 150% payment adjustment for bilateral procedures does not apply, assistant surgeon may be paid

44150   **Remove colon**   ~ follow-up period is 90 days, standard payment adjustment rules for multiple procedures apply, 150% payment adjustment for bilateral procedures does not apply, assistant surgeon may be paid

44151   **Remove colon/ileostomy**   ~ follow-up period is 90 days, standard payment adjustment rules for multiple procedures apply, 150% payment adjustment for bilateral procedures does not apply, assistant surgeon may be paid

44155   **Remove colon/ileostomy**   ~ follow-up period is 90 days, standard payment adjustment rules for multiple procedures apply, 150% payment adjustment for bilateral procedures does not apply, assistant surgeon may be paid

44156   **Remove colon/ileostomy**   ~ follow-up period is 90 days, standard payment adjustment rules for multiple procedures apply, 150% payment adjustment for bilateral procedures does not apply, assistant surgeon may be paid

44157   **Colectomy w/ileoanal anastomosis**   ~ follow-up period is 90 days, standard payment adjustment rules for multiple procedures apply, 150% payment adjustment for bilateral procedures does not apply, assistant surgeon may be paid

44158   **Colectomy w/neo-rectum pouch**   ~ follow-up period is 90 days, standard payment adjustment rules for multiple procedures apply, 150% payment adjustment for bilateral procedures does not apply, assistant surgeon may be paid

44160   **Remove colon**   ~ follow-up period is 90 days, standard payment adjustment rules for multiple procedures apply, 150% payment adjustment for bilateral procedures does not apply, assistant surgeon may be paid

44180   **Laparoscopy, enterolysis**   ~ follow-up period is 90 days, standard payment adjustment rules for multiple procedures apply, 150% payment adjustment for bilateral procedures does not apply, assistant surgeon may be paid

44186   **Laparoscopy, jejunostomy**   ~ follow-up period is 90 days, standard payment adjustment rules for multiple procedures apply, 150% payment adjustment for bilateral procedures does not apply, assistant surgeon may be paid

44187   **Laparoscopy, ileo/jejunostomy**   ~ follow-up period is 90 days, standard payment adjustment rules for multiple procedures apply, 150% payment adjustment for bilateral procedures does not apply, assistant surgeon may be paid

44188   **Laparoscopy, colostomy**   ~ follow-up period is 90 days, standard payment adjustment rules for multiple procedures apply, 150% payment adjustment for bilateral procedures does not apply, assistant surgeon may be paid

44202   **Laparoscopy, enterectomy**   ~ follow-up period is 90 days, standard payment adjustment rules for multiple procedures apply, 150% payment adjustment for bilateral procedures does not apply, assistant surgeon may be paid

44203   **Laparoscopy resect s/intestine, added**   ~ follow-up period included in another service, no payment adjustment rules for multiple procedures apply, 150% payment adjustment for bilateral procedures does not apply, assistant surgeon may be paid, +add-on code (list separately in addition to primary procedure)

44204   **Laparo partial colectomy**   ~ follow-up period is 90 days, standard payment adjustment rules for multiple procedures apply, 150% payment adjustment for bilateral procedures does not apply, assistant surgeon may be paid

44205   **Laparoscopy colectomy part w/ileum**   ~ follow-up period is 90 days, standard payment adjustment rules for multiple procedures apply, 150% payment adjustment for bilateral procedures does not apply, assistant surgeon may be paid

44206 **Laparoscopy part colectomy w/stoma** ~ follow-up period is 90 days, standard payment adjustment rules for multiple procedures apply, 150% payment adjustment for bilateral procedures does not apply, assistant surgeon may be paid

44207 **L colectomy/coloproctostomy** ~ follow-up period is 90 days, standard payment adjustment rules for multiple procedures apply, 150% payment adjustment for bilateral procedures does not apply, assistant surgeon may be paid

44208 **L colectomy/coloproctostomy** ~ follow-up period is 90 days, standard payment adjustment rules for multiple procedures apply, 150% payment adjustment for bilateral procedures does not apply, assistant surgeon may be paid

44210 **Laparo total proctocolectomy** ~ follow-up period is 90 days, standard payment adjustment rules for multiple procedures apply, 150% payment adjustment for bilateral procedures does not apply, assistant surgeon may be paid

44211 **Laparoscopy colectomy w/proctectomy** ~ follow-up period is 90 days, standard payment adjustment rules for multiple procedures apply, 150% payment adjustment for bilateral procedures does not apply, assistant surgeon may be paid

44212 **Laparo total proctocolectomy** ~ follow-up period is 90 days, standard payment adjustment rules for multiple procedures apply, 150% payment adjustment for bilateral procedures does not apply, assistant surgeon may be paid

44213 **Laparoscopy, mobile splenic fl, add-on** ~ follow-up period included in another service, no payment adjustment rules for multiple procedures apply, 150% payment adjustment for bilateral procedures does not apply, assistant surgeon may be paid, +add-on code (list separately in addition to primary procedure)

44227 **Laparoscopy, close enterostomy** ~ follow-up period is 90 days, standard payment adjustment rules for multiple procedures apply, 150% payment adjustment for bilateral procedures does not apply, assistant surgeon may be paid

44238 **Laparoscope proc, intestine** ~ medicare carrier determines global period, standard payment adjustment rules for multiple procedures apply, 150% payment adjustment for bilateral procedures applies, assistant surgeon may be paid

44300 **Open bowel to skin** ~ follow-up period is 90 days, standard payment adjustment rules for multiple procedures apply, 150% payment adjustment for bilateral procedures does not apply, assistant surgeon may be paid

44310 **Ileostomy/jejunostomy** ~ follow-up period is 90 days, standard payment adjustment rules for multiple procedures apply, 150% payment adjustment for bilateral procedures does not apply, assistant surgeon may be paid

44312 **Revise ileostomy** ~ follow-up period is 90 days, standard payment adjustment rules for multiple procedures apply, 150% payment adjustment for

bilateral procedures does not apply, payment for assistant surgeon subject to documentation of medical necessity

44314   **Revise ileostomy**   ~ follow-up period is 90 days, standard payment adjustment rules for multiple procedures apply, 150% payment adjustment for bilateral procedures does not apply, assistant surgeon may be paid

44316   **Devise bowel pouch**   ~ follow-up period is 90 days, standard payment adjustment rules for multiple procedures apply, 150% payment adjustment for bilateral procedures does not apply, assistant surgeon may be paid

44320   **Colostomy**   ~ follow-up period is 90 days, standard payment adjustment rules for multiple procedures apply, 150% payment adjustment for bilateral procedures does not apply, assistant surgeon may be paid

44322   **Colostomy with biopsies**   ~ follow-up period is 90 days, standard payment adjustment rules for multiple procedures apply, 150% payment adjustment for bilateral procedures does not apply, assistant surgeon may be paid

44340   **Revise colostomy**   ~ follow-up period is 90 days, standard payment adjustment rules for multiple procedures apply, 150% payment adjustment for bilateral procedures does not apply, assistant surgeon may not be paid

44345   **Revise colostomy**   ~ follow-up period is 90 days, standard payment adjustment rules for multiple procedures apply, 150% payment adjustment for bilateral procedures does not apply, assistant surgeon may be paid

44346   **Revise colostomy**   ~ follow-up period is 90 days, standard payment adjustment rules for multiple procedures apply, 150% payment adjustment for bilateral procedures does not apply, assistant surgeon may be paid

44360   **Small bowel endoscopy**   ~ endoscopies or minor procedure - E/M services on the same day generally not paid, standard payment adjustment rules for multiple procedures apply, 150% payment adjustment for bilateral procedures does not apply, assistant surgeon may not be paid

44361   **Small bowel endoscopy/biopsy**   ~ endoscopies or minor procedure - E/M services on the same day generally not paid, special rules for multiple endoscopic procedures apply if billed with another endoscopy in the same family, 150% payment adjustment for bilateral procedures does not apply, assistant surgeon may not be paid

44363   **Small bowel endoscopy**   ~ endoscopies or minor procedure - E/M services on the same day generally not paid, special rules for multiple endoscopic procedures apply if billed with another endoscopy in the same family, 150% payment adjustment for bilateral procedures does not apply, payment for assistant surgeon subject to documentation of medical necessity

44364   **Small bowel endoscopy**   ~ endoscopies or minor procedure - E/M services on the same day generally not paid, special rules for multiple endoscopic procedures apply if billed with another endoscopy in the same family, 150% payment adjustment for bilateral procedures does not apply, payment for assistant surgeon subject to documentation of medical necessity

44365   **Small bowel endoscopy**   ~ endoscopies or minor procedure - E/M services on the same day generally not paid, special rules for multiple endoscopic procedures apply if billed with another endoscopy in the same family, 150% payment adjustment for bilateral procedures does not apply, payment for assistant surgeon subject to documentation of medical necessity

44366   **Small bowel endoscopy**   ~ endoscopies or minor procedure - E/M services on the same day generally not paid, special rules for multiple endoscopic procedures apply if billed with another endoscopy in the same family, 150% payment adjustment for bilateral procedures does not apply, assistant surgeon may not be paid

44369   **Small bowel endoscopy**   ~ endoscopies or minor procedure - E/M services on the same day generally not paid, special rules for multiple endoscopic procedures apply if billed with another endoscopy in the same family, 150% payment adjustment for bilateral procedures does not apply, payment for assistant surgeon subject to documentation of medical necessity

44370   **Small bowel endoscopy/stent**   ~ endoscopies or minor procedure - E/M services on the same day generally not paid, special rules for multiple endoscopic procedures apply if billed with another endoscopy in the same family, 150% payment adjustment for bilateral procedures does not apply, payment for assistant surgeon subject to documentation of medical necessity

44372   **Small bowel endoscopy**   ~ endoscopies or minor procedure - E/M services on the same day generally not paid, special rules for multiple endoscopic procedures apply if billed with another endoscopy in the same family, 150% payment adjustment for bilateral procedures does not apply, assistant surgeon may not be paid

44373   **Small bowel endoscopy**   ~ endoscopies or minor procedure - E/M services on the same day generally not paid, special rules for multiple endoscopic procedures apply if billed with another endoscopy in the same family, 150% payment adjustment for bilateral procedures does not apply, assistant surgeon may not be paid

44376   **Small bowel endoscopy**   ~ endoscopies or minor procedure - E/M services on the same day generally not paid, standard payment adjustment rules for multiple procedures apply, 150% payment adjustment for bilateral procedures does not apply, payment for assistant surgeon subject to documentation of medical necessity

44377   **Small bowel endoscopy/biopsy**   ~ endoscopies or minor procedure - E/M services on the same day generally not paid, special rules for multiple endoscopic procedures apply if billed with another endoscopy in the same family, 150% payment

      CPT codes and descriptions only copyright American Medical Association

adjustment for bilateral procedures does not apply, payment for assistant surgeon subject to documentation of medical necessity

44378   **Small bowel endoscopy**   ~ endoscopies or minor procedure - E/M services on the same day generally not paid, special rules for multiple endoscopic procedures apply if billed with another endoscopy in the same family, 150% payment adjustment for bilateral procedures does not apply, payment for assistant surgeon subject to documentation of medical necessity

44379   **S bowel endoscope w/stent**   ~ endoscopies or minor procedure - E/M services on the same day generally not paid, special rules for multiple endoscopic procedures apply if billed with another endoscopy in the same family, 150% payment adjustment for bilateral procedures does not apply, payment for assistant surgeon subject to documentation of medical necessity

44380   **Small bowel endoscopy**   ~ endoscopies or minor procedure - E/M services on the same day generally not paid, standard payment adjustment rules for multiple procedures apply, 150% payment adjustment for bilateral procedures does not apply, assistant surgeon may not be paid

44382   **Small bowel endoscopy**   ~ endoscopies or minor procedure - E/M services on the same day generally not paid, standard payment adjustment rules for multiple procedures apply, 150% payment adjustment for bilateral procedures does not apply, assistant surgeon may not be paid

44383   **Ileoscopy w/stent**   ~ endoscopies or minor procedure - E/M services on the same day generally not paid, standard payment adjustment rules for multiple procedures apply, 150% payment adjustment for bilateral procedures does not apply, assistant surgeon may not be paid

44385   **Endoscopy of bowel pouch**   ~ endoscopies or minor procedure - E/M services on the same day generally not paid, standard payment adjustment rules for multiple procedures apply, 150% payment adjustment for bilateral procedures does not apply, assistant surgeon may not be paid

44386   **Endoscopy, bowel pouch/biopsy**   ~ endoscopies or minor procedure - E/M services on the same day generally not paid, standard payment adjustment rules for multiple procedures apply, 150% payment adjustment for bilateral procedures does not apply, payment for assistant surgeon subject to documentation of medical necessity

44388   **Colonoscopy**   ~ endoscopies or minor procedure - E/M services on the same day generally not paid, standard payment adjustment rules for multiple procedures apply, 150% payment adjustment for bilateral procedures does not apply, assistant surgeon may not be paid

44389   **Colonoscopy with biopsy**   ~ endoscopies or minor procedure - E/M services on the same day generally not paid, special rules for multiple endoscopic

procedures apply if billed with another endoscopy in the same family, 150% payment adjustment for bilateral procedures does not apply, assistant surgeon may not be paid

44390   **Colonoscopy for foreign body**   ~ endoscopies or minor procedure - E/M services on the same day generally not paid, special rules for multiple endoscopic procedures apply if billed with another endoscopy in the same family, 150% payment adjustment for bilateral procedures does not apply, payment for assistant surgeon subject to documentation of medical necessity

44391   **Colonoscopy for bleeding**   ~ endoscopies or minor procedure - E/M services on the same day generally not paid, special rules for multiple endoscopic procedures apply if billed with another endoscopy in the same family, 150% payment adjustment for bilateral procedures does not apply, payment for assistant surgeon subject to documentation of medical necessity

44392   **Colonoscopy & polypectomy**   ~ endoscopies or minor procedure - E/M services on the same day generally not paid, special rules for multiple endoscopic procedures apply if billed with another endoscopy in the same family, 150% payment adjustment for bilateral procedures does not apply, assistant surgeon may not be paid

44393   **Colonoscopy, lesion remove**   ~ endoscopies or minor procedure - E/M services on the same day generally not paid, special rules for multiple endoscopic procedures apply if billed with another endoscopy in the same family, 150% payment adjustment for bilateral procedures does not apply, assistant surgeon may not be paid

44394   **Colonoscopy w/snare**   ~ endoscopies or minor procedure - E/M services on the same day generally not paid, special rules for multiple endoscopic procedures apply if billed with another endoscopy in the same family, 150% payment adjustment for bilateral procedures does not apply, assistant surgeon may not be paid

44397   **Colonoscopy w/stent**   ~ endoscopies or minor procedure - E/M services on the same day generally not paid, special rules for multiple endoscopic procedures apply if billed with another endoscopy in the same family, 150% payment adjustment for bilateral procedures does not apply, assistant surgeon may not be paid

44500   **Intro, gastrointestinal tube**   ~ endoscopies or minor procedure - E/M services on the same day generally not paid, no payment adjustment rules for multiple procedures apply, 150% payment adjustment for bilateral procedures does not apply, payment for assistant surgeon subject to documentation of medical necessity

44602   **Suture small intestine**   ~ follow-up period is 90 days, standard payment adjustment rules for multiple procedures apply, 150% payment adjustment for bilateral procedures does not apply, assistant surgeon may be paid

44603   **Suture small intestine**   ~ follow-up period is 90 days, standard payment adjustment rules for multiple procedures apply, 150% payment adjustment for bilateral procedures does not apply, assistant surgeon may be paid

44604   **Suture large intestine**   ~ follow-up period is 90 days, standard payment adjustment rules for multiple procedures apply, 150% payment adjustment for bilateral procedures does not apply, assistant surgeon may be paid

44605   **Repair bowel lesion**   ~ follow-up period is 90 days, standard payment adjustment rules for multiple procedures apply, 150% payment adjustment for bilateral procedures does not apply, assistant surgeon may be paid

44615   **Intestinal stricturoplasty**   ~ follow-up period is 90 days, standard payment adjustment rules for multiple procedures apply, 150% payment adjustment for bilateral procedures does not apply, assistant surgeon may be paid

44620   **Repair bowel opening**   ~ follow-up period is 90 days, standard payment adjustment rules for multiple procedures apply, 150% payment adjustment for bilateral procedures does not apply, assistant surgeon may be paid

44625   **Repair bowel opening**   ~ follow-up period is 90 days, standard payment adjustment rules for multiple procedures apply, 150% payment adjustment for bilateral procedures does not apply, assistant surgeon may be paid

44626   **Repair bowel opening**   ~ follow-up period is 90 days, standard payment adjustment rules for multiple procedures apply, 150% payment adjustment for bilateral procedures does not apply, assistant surgeon may be paid

44640   **Repair bowel-skin fistula**   ~ follow-up period is 90 days, standard payment adjustment rules for multiple procedures apply, 150% payment adjustment for bilateral procedures does not apply, assistant surgeon may be paid

44650   **Repair bowel fistula**   ~ follow-up period is 90 days, standard payment adjustment rules for multiple procedures apply, 150% payment adjustment for bilateral procedures does not apply, assistant surgeon may be paid

44660   **Repair bowel-bladder fistula**   ~ follow-up period is 90 days, standard payment adjustment rules for multiple procedures apply, 150% payment adjustment for bilateral procedures does not apply, assistant surgeon may be paid

44661   **Repair bowel-bladder fistula**   ~ follow-up period is 90 days, standard payment adjustment rules for multiple procedures apply, 150% payment adjustment for bilateral procedures does not apply, assistant surgeon may be paid

44680   **Surgical revise intestine**   ~ follow-up period is 90 days, standard payment adjustment rules for multiple procedures apply, 150% payment adjustment for bilateral procedures does not apply, assistant surgeon may be paid

44700   **Suspend bowel w/prosthesis**   ~ follow-up period is 90 days, standard payment adjustment rules for multiple procedures apply, 150% payment adjustment for bilateral procedures does not apply, assistant surgeon may be paid

44701   **Intraop colon lavage, add-on**   ~ follow-up period included in another service, no payment adjustment rules for multiple procedures apply, 150% payment adjustment for bilateral procedures does not apply, assistant surgeon may be paid, +add-on code (list separately in addition to primary procedure)

44715   **Prepare donor intestine**   ~ standard payment adjustment rules for multiple procedures apply, 150% payment adjustment for bilateral procedures does not apply, assistant surgeon may be paid

44720   **Prepare donor intestine/venous**   ~ standard payment adjustment rules for multiple procedures apply, 150% payment adjustment for bilateral procedures does not apply, assistant surgeon may be paid

44721   **Prepare donor intestine/artery**   ~ standard payment adjustment rules for multiple procedures apply, 150% payment adjustment for bilateral procedures does not apply, assistant surgeon may be paid

44799   **Unlisted procedure intestine**   ~ medicare carrier determines global period, standard payment adjustment rules for multiple procedures apply, 150% payment adjustment for bilateral procedures does not apply, assistant surgeon may be paid

Meckel's Diverticulum and The Mesentery

44800   **Excise bowel pouch**   ~ follow-up period is 90 days, standard payment adjustment rules for multiple procedures apply, 150% payment adjustment for bilateral procedures does not apply, assistant surgeon may be paid

44820   **Excise mesentery lesion**   ~ follow-up period is 90 days, standard payment adjustment rules for multiple procedures apply, 150% payment adjustment for bilateral procedures does not apply, assistant surgeon may be paid

44850   **Repair mesentery**   ~ follow-up period is 90 days, standard payment adjustment rules for multiple procedures apply, 150% payment adjustment for bilateral procedures does not apply, assistant surgeon may be paid

44899   **Bowel surgery procedure**   ~ medicare carrier determines global period, standard payment adjustment rules for multiple procedures apply, 150% payment adjustment for bilateral procedures does not apply, assistant surgeon may be paid

Appendix

44900   **Drain app abscess, open**   ~ follow-up period is 90 days, standard payment adjustment rules for multiple procedures apply, 150% payment adjustment for bilateral procedures does not apply, assistant surgeon may be paid

44901   **Drain app abscess, percutaneous**   ~ endoscopies or minor procedure - E/M services on the same day generally not paid, standard payment adjustment rules for multiple

procedures apply, 150% payment adjustment for bilateral procedures does not apply, assistant surgeon may be paid

44950   **Appendectomy**   ~ follow-up period is 90 days, standard payment adjustment rules for multiple procedures apply, 150% payment adjustment for bilateral procedures does not apply, assistant surgeon may be paid

44955   **Appendectomy, add-on**   ~ follow-up period included in another service, no payment adjustment rules for multiple procedures apply, 150% payment adjustment for bilateral procedures does not apply, assistant surgeon may be paid, +add-on code (list separately in addition to primary procedure)

44960   **Appendectomy**   ~ follow-up period is 90 days, standard payment adjustment rules for multiple procedures apply, 150% payment adjustment for bilateral procedures does not apply, assistant surgeon may be paid

44970   **Laparoscopy, appendectomy**   ~ follow-up period is 90 days, standard payment adjustment rules for multiple procedures apply, 150% payment adjustment for bilateral procedures does not apply, assistant surgeon may be paid

44979   **Laparoscope proc, app**   ~ medicare carrier determines global period, standard payment adjustment rules for multiple procedures apply, 150% payment adjustment for bilateral procedures applies, assistant surgeon may be paid

Rectum

45000   **Drain pelvic abscess**   ~ follow-up period is 90 days, standard payment adjustment rules for multiple procedures apply, 150% payment adjustment for bilateral procedures does not apply, assistant surgeon may not be paid

45005   **Drain rectal abscess**   ~ follow-up period is 10 days, standard payment adjustment rules for multiple procedures apply, 150% payment adjustment for bilateral procedures does not apply, assistant surgeon may not be paid

45020   **Drain rectal abscess**   ~ follow-up period is 90 days, standard payment adjustment rules for multiple procedures apply, 150% payment adjustment for bilateral procedures does not apply, assistant surgeon may not be paid

45100   **Biopsy rectum**   ~ follow-up period is 90 days, standard payment adjustment rules for multiple procedures apply, 150% payment adjustment for bilateral procedures does not apply, assistant surgeon may not be paid

45108   **Remove anorectal lesion**   ~ follow-up period is 90 days, standard payment adjustment rules for multiple procedures apply, 150% payment adjustment for bilateral procedures does not apply, assistant surgeon may not be paid

45110 **Remove rectum** ~ follow-up period is 90 days, standard payment adjustment rules for multiple procedures apply, 150% payment adjustment for bilateral procedures does not apply, assistant surgeon may be paid

45111 **Partial remove rectum** ~ follow-up period is 90 days, standard payment adjustment rules for multiple procedures apply, 150% payment adjustment for bilateral procedures does not apply, assistant surgeon may be paid

45112 **Remove rectum** ~ follow-up period is 90 days, standard payment adjustment rules for multiple procedures apply, 150% payment adjustment for bilateral procedures does not apply, assistant surgeon may be paid

45113 **Partial proctectomy** ~ follow-up period is 90 days, standard payment adjustment rules for multiple procedures apply, 150% payment adjustment for bilateral procedures does not apply, assistant surgeon may be paid

45114 **Partial remove rectum** ~ follow-up period is 90 days, standard payment adjustment rules for multiple procedures apply, 150% payment adjustment for bilateral procedures does not apply, assistant surgeon may be paid

45116 **Partial remove rectum** ~ follow-up period is 90 days, standard payment adjustment rules for multiple procedures apply, 150% payment adjustment for bilateral procedures does not apply, assistant surgeon may be paid

45119 **Remove rectum w/reservoir** ~ follow-up period is 90 days, standard payment adjustment rules for multiple procedures apply, 150% payment adjustment for bilateral procedures does not apply, assistant surgeon may be paid

45120 **Remove rectum** ~ follow-up period is 90 days, standard payment adjustment rules for multiple procedures apply, 150% payment adjustment for bilateral procedures does not apply, assistant surgeon may be paid

45121 **Remove rectum and colon** ~ follow-up period is 90 days, standard payment adjustment rules for multiple procedures apply, 150% payment adjustment for bilateral procedures does not apply, assistant surgeon may be paid

45123 **Partial proctectomy** ~ follow-up period is 90 days, standard payment adjustment rules for multiple procedures apply, 150% payment adjustment for bilateral procedures does not apply, assistant surgeon may be paid

45126 **Pelvic exenteration** ~ follow-up period is 90 days, standard payment adjustment rules for multiple procedures apply, 150% payment adjustment for bilateral procedures does not apply, assistant surgeon may be paid

45130 **Excise rectal prolapse** ~ follow-up period is 90 days, standard payment adjustment rules for multiple procedures apply, 150% payment adjustment for bilateral procedures does not apply, assistant surgeon may be paid

45135   **Excise rectal prolapse**   ~ follow-up period is 90 days, standard payment adjustment rules for multiple procedures apply, 150% payment adjustment for bilateral procedures does not apply, assistant surgeon may be paid

45136   **Excise ileoanal reservoir**   ~ follow-up period is 90 days, standard payment adjustment rules for multiple procedures apply, 150% payment adjustment for bilateral procedures does not apply, assistant surgeon may be paid

45150   **Excise rectal stricture**   ~ follow-up period is 90 days, standard payment adjustment rules for multiple procedures apply, 150% payment adjustment for bilateral procedures does not apply, payment for assistant surgeon subject to documentation of medical necessity

45160   **Excise rectal lesion**   ~ follow-up period is 90 days, standard payment adjustment rules for multiple procedures apply, 150% payment adjustment for bilateral procedures does not apply, assistant surgeon may be paid

45170   **Excise rectal lesion**   ~ follow-up period is 90 days, standard payment adjustment rules for multiple procedures apply, 150% payment adjustment for bilateral procedures does not apply, assistant surgeon may be paid

45190   **Destroy rectal tumor**   ~ follow-up period is 90 days, standard payment adjustment rules for multiple procedures apply, 150% payment adjustment for bilateral procedures does not apply, assistant surgeon may be paid

45300   **Proctosigmoidoscopy dx**   ~ endoscopies or minor procedure - E/M services on the same day generally not paid, standard payment adjustment rules for multiple procedures apply, 150% payment adjustment for bilateral procedures does not apply, assistant surgeon may not be paid

45303   **Proctosigmoidoscopy dilate**   ~ endoscopies or minor procedure - E/M services on the same day generally not paid, special rules for multiple endoscopic procedures apply if billed with another endoscopy in the same family, 150% payment adjustment for bilateral procedures does not apply, assistant surgeon may not be paid

45305   **Proctosigmoidoscopy w/biopsy**   ~ endoscopies or minor procedure - E/M services on the same day generally not paid, special rules for multiple endoscopic procedures apply if billed with another endoscopy in the same family, 150% payment adjustment for bilateral procedures does not apply, assistant surgeon may not be paid

45307   **Proctosigmoidoscopy foreign body**   ~ endoscopies or minor procedure - E/M services on the same day generally not paid, special rules for multiple endoscopic procedures apply if billed with another endoscopy in the same family, 150% payment adjustment for bilateral procedures does not apply, payment for assistant surgeon subject to documentation of medical necessity

45308   **Proctosigmoidoscopy remove**   ~ endoscopies or minor procedure - E/M services on the same day generally not paid, special rules for multiple endoscopic procedures apply if billed with another endoscopy in the same family, 150% payment adjustment for bilateral procedures does not apply, assistant surgeon may not be paid

45309   **Proctosigmoidoscopy remove**   ~ endoscopies or minor procedure - E/M services on the same day generally not paid, special rules for multiple endoscopic procedures apply if billed with another endoscopy in the same family, 150% payment adjustment for bilateral procedures does not apply, assistant surgeon may not be paid

45315   **Proctosigmoidoscopy remove**   ~ endoscopies or minor procedure - E/M services on the same day generally not paid, special rules for multiple endoscopic procedures apply if billed with another endoscopy in the same family, 150% payment adjustment for bilateral procedures does not apply, assistant surgeon may not be paid

45317   **Proctosigmoidoscopy bleed**   ~ endoscopies or minor procedure - E/M services on the same day generally not paid, special rules for multiple endoscopic procedures apply if billed with another endoscopy in the same family, 150% payment adjustment for bilateral procedures does not apply, assistant surgeon may not be paid

45320   **Proctosigmoidoscopy ablate**   ~ endoscopies or minor procedure - E/M services on the same day generally not paid, special rules for multiple endoscopic procedures apply if billed with another endoscopy in the same family, 150% payment adjustment for bilateral procedures does not apply, assistant surgeon may not be paid

45321   **Proctosigmoidoscopy volvulus**   ~ endoscopies or minor procedure - E/M services on the same day generally not paid, special rules for multiple endoscopic procedures apply if billed with another endoscopy in the same family, 150% payment adjustment for bilateral procedures does not apply, assistant surgeon may not be paid

45327   **Proctosigmoidoscopy w/stent**   ~ endoscopies or minor procedure - E/M services on the same day generally not paid, special rules for multiple endoscopic procedures apply if billed with another endoscopy in the same family, 150% payment adjustment for bilateral procedures does not apply, assistant surgeon may not be paid

45330   **Diagnostic sigmoidoscopy**   ~ endoscopies or minor procedure - E/M services on the same day generally not paid, standard payment adjustment rules for multiple procedures apply, 150% payment adjustment for bilateral procedures does not apply, assistant surgeon may not be paid

45331   **Sigmoidoscopy and biopsy**   ~ endoscopies or minor procedure - E/M services on the same day generally not paid, special rules for multiple endoscopic procedures apply if billed with another endoscopy in the same family, 150% payment adjustment for bilateral procedures does not apply, assistant surgeon may not be paid

45332   **Sigmoidoscopy w/foreign body remove**   ~ endoscopies or minor procedure - E/M services on the same day generally not paid, special rules for multiple endoscopic

procedures apply if billed with another endoscopy in the same family, 150% payment adjustment for bilateral procedures does not apply, assistant surgeon may not be paid

45333   **Sigmoidoscopy & polypectomy**   ~ endoscopies or minor procedure - E/M services on the same day generally not paid, special rules for multiple endoscopic procedures apply if billed with another endoscopy in the same family, 150% payment adjustment for bilateral procedures does not apply, assistant surgeon may not be paid

45334   **Sigmoidoscopy for bleeding**   ~ endoscopies or minor procedure - E/M services on the same day generally not paid, special rules for multiple endoscopic procedures apply if billed with another endoscopy in the same family, 150% payment adjustment for bilateral procedures does not apply, assistant surgeon may not be paid

45335   **Sigmoidoscopy w/submucosa inject**   ~ endoscopies or minor procedure - E/M services on the same day generally not paid, special rules for multiple endoscopic procedures apply if billed with another endoscopy in the same family, 150% payment adjustment for bilateral procedures does not apply, assistant surgeon may not be paid

45337   **Sigmoidoscopy & decompress**   ~ endoscopies or minor procedure - E/M services on the same day generally not paid, special rules for multiple endoscopic procedures apply if billed with another endoscopy in the same family, 150% payment adjustment for bilateral procedures does not apply, assistant surgeon may not be paid

45338   **Sigmoidoscopy w/tumor remove**   ~ endoscopies or minor procedure - E/M services on the same day generally not paid, special rules for multiple endoscopic procedures apply if billed with another endoscopy in the same family, 150% payment adjustment for bilateral procedures does not apply, assistant surgeon may not be paid

45339   **Sigmoidoscopy w/ablate tumor**   ~ endoscopies or minor procedure - E/M services on the same day generally not paid, special rules for multiple endoscopic procedures apply if billed with another endoscopy in the same family, 150% payment adjustment for bilateral procedures does not apply, assistant surgeon may not be paid

45340   **Sig w/balloon dilate**   ~ endoscopies or minor procedure - E/M services on the same day generally not paid, special rules for multiple endoscopic procedures apply if billed with another endoscopy in the same family, 150% payment adjustment for bilateral procedures does not apply, assistant surgeon may not be paid

45341   **Sigmoidoscopy w/ultrasound**   ~ endoscopies or minor procedure - E/M services on the same day generally not paid, standard payment adjustment rules for multiple procedures apply, 150% payment adjustment for bilateral procedures does not apply, assistant surgeon may not be paid

45342   **Sigmoidoscopy w/us guide biopsy**   ~ endoscopies or minor procedure - E/M services on the same day generally not paid, standard payment adjustment rules for multiple procedures apply, 150% payment adjustment for bilateral procedures does not apply, assistant surgeon may not be paid

---

45345   **Sigmoidoscopy w/stent**   ~ endoscopies or minor procedure - E/M services on the same day generally not paid, special rules for multiple endoscopic procedures apply if billed with another endoscopy in the same family, 150% payment adjustment for bilateral procedures does not apply, assistant surgeon may not be paid

45355   **Surgical colonoscopy**   ~ endoscopies or minor procedure - E/M services on the same day generally not paid, standard payment adjustment rules for multiple procedures apply, 150% payment adjustment for bilateral procedures does not apply, assistant surgeon may not be paid

45378   **Diagnostic colonoscopy**   ~ endoscopies or minor procedure - E/M services on the same day generally not paid, standard payment adjustment rules for multiple procedures apply, 150% payment adjustment for bilateral procedures does not apply, assistant surgeon may not be paid

45379   **Colonoscopy w/foreign body remove**   ~ endoscopies or minor procedure - E/M services on the same day generally not paid, special rules for multiple endoscopic procedures apply if billed with another endoscopy in the same family, 150% payment adjustment for bilateral procedures does not apply, assistant surgeon may not be paid

45380   **Colonoscopy and biopsy**   ~ endoscopies or minor procedure - E/M services on the same day generally not paid, special rules for multiple endoscopic procedures apply if billed with another endoscopy in the same family, 150% payment adjustment for bilateral procedures does not apply, assistant surgeon may not be paid

45381   **Colonoscopy, submucous inject**   ~ endoscopies or minor procedure - E/M services on the same day generally not paid, special rules for multiple endoscopic procedures apply if billed with another endoscopy in the same family, 150% payment adjustment for bilateral procedures does not apply, assistant surgeon may not be paid

45382   **Colonoscopy/control bleeding**   ~ endoscopies or minor procedure - E/M services on the same day generally not paid, special rules for multiple endoscopic procedures apply if billed with another endoscopy in the same family, 150% payment adjustment for bilateral procedures does not apply, assistant surgeon may not be paid

45383   **Lesion remove colonoscopy**   ~ endoscopies or minor procedure - E/M services on the same day generally not paid, special rules for multiple endoscopic procedures apply if billed with another endoscopy in the same family, 150% payment adjustment for bilateral procedures does not apply, assistant surgeon may not be paid

45384   **Lesion remove colonoscopy**   ~ endoscopies or minor procedure - E/M services on the same day generally not paid, special rules for multiple endoscopic procedures apply if billed with another endoscopy in the same family, 150% payment adjustment for bilateral procedures does not apply, assistant surgeon may not be paid

45385   **Lesion remove colonoscopy**   ~ endoscopies or minor procedure - E/M services on the same day generally not paid, special rules for multiple endoscopic

      CPT codes and descriptions only copyright American Medical Association

procedures apply if billed with another endoscopy in the same family, 150% payment adjustment for bilateral procedures does not apply, assistant surgeon may not be paid

45386 **Colonoscopy dilate stricture** ~ endoscopies or minor procedure - E/M services on the same day generally not paid, special rules for multiple endoscopic procedures apply if billed with another endoscopy in the same family, 150% payment adjustment for bilateral procedures does not apply, assistant surgeon may not be paid

45387 **Colonoscopy w/stent** ~ endoscopies or minor procedure - E/M services on the same day generally not paid, special rules for multiple endoscopic procedures apply if billed with another endoscopy in the same family, 150% payment adjustment for bilateral procedures does not apply, assistant surgeon may not be paid

45391 **Colonoscopy w/endoscope us** ~ endoscopies or minor procedure - E/M services on the same day generally not paid, special rules for multiple endoscopic procedures apply if billed with another endoscopy in the same family, 150% payment adjustment for bilateral procedures does not apply, assistant surgeon may not be paid

45392 **Colonoscopy w/endoscopic fnb** ~ endoscopies or minor procedure - E/M services on the same day generally not paid, special rules for multiple endoscopic procedures apply if billed with another endoscopy in the same family, 150% payment adjustment for bilateral procedures does not apply, assistant surgeon may not be paid

45395 **Laparoscopy, remove rectum** ~ follow-up period is 90 days, standard payment adjustment rules for multiple procedures apply, 150% payment adjustment for bilateral procedures does not apply, assistant surgeon may be paid

45397 **Laparoscopy, remove rectum w/pouch** ~ follow-up period is 90 days, standard payment adjustment rules for multiple procedures apply, 150% payment adjustment for bilateral procedures does not apply, assistant surgeon may be paid

45400 **Laparoscopic proc** ~ follow-up period is 90 days, standard payment adjustment rules for multiple procedures apply, 150% payment adjustment for bilateral procedures does not apply, assistant surgeon may be paid

45402 **Laparoscopy proctopexy w/sig resect** ~ follow-up period is 90 days, standard payment adjustment rules for multiple procedures apply, 150% payment adjustment for bilateral procedures does not apply, assistant surgeon may be paid

45499 **Laparoscope proc, rectum** ~ medicare carrier determines global period, standard payment adjustment rules for multiple procedures apply, 150% payment adjustment for bilateral procedures does not apply, assistant surgeon may be paid

45500 **Repair rectum** ~ follow-up period is 90 days, standard payment adjustment rules for multiple procedures apply, 150% payment adjustment for bilateral procedures does not apply, payment for assistant surgeon subject to documentation of medical necessity

45505 **Repair rectum** ~ follow-up period is 90 days, standard payment adjustment rules for multiple procedures apply, 150% payment adjustment for bilateral procedures does not apply, assistant surgeon may not be paid

45520 **Treat rectal prolapse** ~ endoscopies or minor procedure - E/M services on the same day generally not paid, standard payment adjustment rules for multiple procedures apply, 150% payment adjustment for bilateral procedures does not apply, assistant surgeon may not be paid

45540 **Correct rectal prolapse** ~ follow-up period is 90 days, standard payment adjustment rules for multiple procedures apply, 150% payment adjustment for bilateral procedures does not apply, assistant surgeon may be paid

45541 **Correct rectal prolapse** ~ follow-up period is 90 days, standard payment adjustment rules for multiple procedures apply, 150% payment adjustment for bilateral procedures does not apply, assistant surgeon may be paid

45550 **Repair rectum/remove sigmoid** ~ follow-up period is 90 days, standard payment adjustment rules for multiple procedures apply, 150% payment adjustment for bilateral procedures does not apply, assistant surgeon may be paid

45560 **Repair rectocele** ~ follow-up period is 90 days, standard payment adjustment rules for multiple procedures apply, 150% payment adjustment for bilateral procedures does not apply, assistant surgeon may be paid

45562 **Explore/repair rectum** ~ follow-up period is 90 days, standard payment adjustment rules for multiple procedures apply, 150% payment adjustment for bilateral procedures does not apply, assistant surgeon may be paid

45563 **Explore/repair rectum** ~ follow-up period is 90 days, standard payment adjustment rules for multiple procedures apply, 150% payment adjustment for bilateral procedures does not apply, assistant surgeon may be paid

45800 **Repair rectal/bladder fistula** ~ follow-up period is 90 days, standard payment adjustment rules for multiple procedures apply, 150% payment adjustment for bilateral procedures does not apply, assistant surgeon may be paid

45805 **Repair fistula w/colostomy** ~ follow-up period is 90 days, standard payment adjustment rules for multiple procedures apply, 150% payment adjustment for bilateral procedures does not apply, assistant surgeon may be paid

45820 **Repair rectourethral fistula** ~ follow-up period is 90 days, standard payment adjustment rules for multiple procedures apply, 150% payment adjustment for bilateral procedures does not apply, assistant surgeon may be paid

45825   **Repair fistula w/colostomy**   ~ follow-up period is 90 days, standard payment adjustment rules for multiple procedures apply, 150% payment adjustment for bilateral procedures does not apply, assistant surgeon may be paid

45900   **Reduce rectal prolapse**   ~ follow-up period is 10 days, standard payment adjustment rules for multiple procedures apply, 150% payment adjustment for bilateral procedures does not apply, payment for assistant surgeon subject to documentation of medical necessity

45905   **Dilate anal sphincter**   ~ follow-up period is 10 days, standard payment adjustment rules for multiple procedures apply, 150% payment adjustment for bilateral procedures does not apply, assistant surgeon may not be paid

45910   **Dilate rectal narrowing**   ~ follow-up period is 10 days, standard payment adjustment rules for multiple procedures apply, 150% payment adjustment for bilateral procedures does not apply, assistant surgeon may not be paid

45915   **Remove rectal obstruction**   ~ follow-up period is 10 days, standard payment adjustment rules for multiple procedures apply, 150% payment adjustment for bilateral procedures does not apply, assistant surgeon may not be paid

45990   **Surg dx exam anorectal**   ~ endoscopies or minor procedure - E/M services on the same day generally not paid, standard payment adjustment rules for multiple procedures apply, 150% payment adjustment for bilateral procedures does not apply, payment for assistant surgeon subject to documentation of medical necessity

45999   **Rectum surgery procedure**   ~ medicare carrier determines global period, standard payment adjustment rules for multiple procedures apply, 150% payment adjustment for bilateral procedures does not apply, payment for assistant surgeon subject to documentation of medical necessity

Anus

46020   **Placement of seton**   ~ follow-up period is 10 days, standard payment adjustment rules for multiple procedures apply, 150% payment adjustment for bilateral procedures does not apply, assistant surgeon may not be paid

46030   **Remove rectal marker**   ~ follow-up period is 10 days, standard payment adjustment rules for multiple procedures apply, 150% payment adjustment for bilateral procedures does not apply, payment for assistant surgeon subject to documentation of medical necessity

46040   **Incise rectal abscess**   ~ follow-up period is 90 days, standard payment adjustment rules for multiple procedures apply, 150% payment adjustment for bilateral procedures does not apply, assistant surgeon may not be paid

46045   **Incise rectal abscess**   ~ follow-up period is 90 days, standard payment adjustment rules for multiple procedures apply, 150% payment adjustment for bilateral procedures does not apply, assistant surgeon may not be paid

46050   **Incise anal abscess**   ~ follow-up period is 10 days, standard payment adjustment rules for multiple procedures apply, 150% payment adjustment for bilateral procedures does not apply, assistant surgeon may not be paid

46060   **Incise rectal abscess**   ~ follow-up period is 90 days, standard payment adjustment rules for multiple procedures apply, 150% payment adjustment for bilateral procedures does not apply, assistant surgeon may not be paid

46070   **Incise anal septum**   ~ follow-up period is 90 days, standard payment adjustment rules for multiple procedures apply, 150% payment adjustment for bilateral procedures does not apply, payment for assistant surgeon subject to documentation of medical necessity

46080   **Incise anal sphincter**   ~ follow-up period is 10 days, standard payment adjustment rules for multiple procedures apply, 150% payment adjustment for bilateral procedures does not apply, assistant surgeon may not be paid

;083   **Incise external hemorrhoid**   ~ follow-up period is 10 days, standard payment adjustment rules for multiple procedures apply, 150% payment adjustment for bilateral procedures does not apply, assistant surgeon may not be paid

:00   **Remove anal fissure**   ~ follow-up period is 90 days, standard payment adjustment rules for multiple procedures apply, 150% payment adjustment for bilateral procedures does not apply, assistant surgeon may not be paid

210   **Remove anal crypt**   ~ follow-up period is 90 days, standard payment adjustment rules for multiple procedures apply, 150% payment adjustment for bilateral procedures does not apply, payment for assistant surgeon subject to documentation of medical necessity

;211   **Remove anal crypts**   ~ follow-up period is 90 days, standard payment adjustment rules for multiple procedures apply, 150% payment adjustment for bilateral procedures does not apply, payment for assistant surgeon subject to documentation of medical necessity

46220   **Remove anal tag**   ~ follow-up period is 10 days, standard payment adjustment rules for multiple procedures apply, 150% payment adjustment for bilateral procedures does not apply, assistant surgeon may not be paid

46221   **Ligate hemorrhoid(s)**   ~ follow-up period is 10 days, standard payment adjustment rules for multiple procedures apply, 150% payment adjustment for bilateral procedures does not apply, assistant surgeon may not be paid

46230   **Remove anal tags**   ~ follow-up period is 10 days, standard payment adjustment rules for multiple procedures apply, 150% payment adjustment for bilateral procedures does not apply, assistant surgeon may not be paid

46250   **Hemorrhoidectomy**   ~ follow-up period is 90 days, standard payment adjustment rules for multiple procedures apply, 150% payment adjustment for bilateral procedures does not apply, assistant surgeon may not be paid

46255   **Hemorrhoidectomy**   ~ follow-up period is 90 days, standard payment adjustment rules for multiple procedures apply, 150% payment adjustment for bilateral procedures does not apply, assistant surgeon may not be paid

46257   **Remove hemorrhoids & fissure**   ~ follow-up period is 90 days, standard payment adjustment rules for multiple procedures apply, 150% payment adjustment for bilateral procedures does not apply, assistant surgeon may not be paid

46258   **Remove hemorrhoids & fistula**   ~ follow-up period is 90 days, standard payment adjustment rules for multiple procedures apply, 150% payment adjustment for bilateral procedures does not apply, payment for assistant surgeon subject to documentation of medical necessity

46260   **Hemorrhoidectomy**   ~ follow-up period is 90 days, standard payment adjustment rules for multiple procedures apply, 150% payment adjustment for bilateral procedures does not apply, assistant surgeon may not be paid

46261   **Remove hemorrhoids & fissure**   ~ follow-up period is 90 days, standard payment adjustment rules for multiple procedures apply, 150% payment adjustment for bilateral procedures does not apply, assistant surgeon may not be paid

46262   **Remove hemorrhoids & fistula**   ~ follow-up period is 90 days, standard payment adjustment rules for multiple procedures apply, 150% payment adjustment for bilateral procedures does not apply, assistant surgeon may not be paid

46270   **Remove anal fistula**   ~ follow-up period is 90 days, standard payment adjustment rules for multiple procedures apply, 150% payment adjustment for bilateral procedures does not apply, assistant surgeon may not be paid

46275   **Remove anal fistula**   ~ follow-up period is 90 days, standard payment adjustment rules for multiple procedures apply, 150% payment adjustment for bilateral procedures does not apply, assistant surgeon may not be paid

46280   **Remove anal fistula**   ~ follow-up period is 90 days, standard payment adjustment rules for multiple procedures apply, 150% payment adjustment for bilateral procedures does not apply, assistant surgeon may not be paid

| 46285 | **Remove anal fistula** | ~ follow-up period is 90 days, standard payment adjustment rules for multiple procedures apply, 150% payment adjustment for bilateral procedures does not apply, assistant surgeon may not be paid |

46285   **Remove anal fistula**   ~ follow-up period is 90 days, standard payment adjustment rules for multiple procedures apply, 150% payment adjustment for bilateral procedures does not apply, assistant surgeon may not be paid

46288   **Repair anal fistula**   ~ follow-up period is 90 days, standard payment adjustment rules for multiple procedures apply, 150% payment adjustment for bilateral procedures does not apply, assistant surgeon may not be paid

46320   **Remove hemorrhoid clot**   ~ follow-up period is 10 days, standard payment adjustment rules for multiple procedures apply, 150% payment adjustment for bilateral procedures does not apply, assistant surgeon may not be paid

46500   **Inject into hemorrhoid(s)**   ~ follow-up period is 10 days, standard payment adjustment rules for multiple procedures apply, 150% payment adjustment for bilateral procedures does not apply, assistant surgeon may not be paid

46505   **Chemodenervation anal muscle**   ~ follow-up period is 10 days, standard payment adjustment rules for multiple procedures apply, 150% payment adjustment for bilateral procedures applies, assistant surgeon may not be paid

46600   **Diagnostic anoscopy**   ~ endoscopies or minor procedure - E/M services on the same day generally not paid, standard payment adjustment rules for multiple procedures apply, 150% payment adjustment for bilateral procedures does not apply, assistant surgeon may not be paid

46604   **Anoscopy and dilate**   ~ endoscopies or minor procedure - E/M services on the same day generally not paid, special rules for multiple endoscopic procedures apply if billed with another endoscopy in the same family, 150% payment adjustment for bilateral procedures does not apply, assistant surgeon may not be paid

46606   **Anoscopy and biopsy**   ~ endoscopies or minor procedure - E/M services on the same day generally not paid, special rules for multiple endoscopic procedures apply if billed with another endoscopy in the same family, 150% payment adjustment for bilateral procedures does not apply, assistant surgeon may not be paid

46608   **Anoscopy, remove for body**   ~ endoscopies or minor procedure - E/M services on the same day generally not paid, special rules for multiple endoscopic procedures apply if billed with another endoscopy in the same family, 150% payment adjustment for bilateral procedures does not apply, payment for assistant surgeon subject to documentation of medical necessity

46610   **Anoscopy, remove lesion**   ~ endoscopies or minor procedure - E/M services on the same day generally not paid, special rules for multiple endoscopic procedures apply if billed with another endoscopy in the same family, 150% payment adjustment for bilateral procedures does not apply, assistant surgeon may not be paid

46611   **Anoscopy**   ~ endoscopies or minor procedure - E/M services on the same day generally not paid, special rules for multiple endoscopic procedures apply if billed with another endoscopy in the same family, 150% payment adjustment for bilateral procedures does not apply, payment for assistant surgeon subject to documentation of medical necessity

46612   **Anoscopy, remove lesions**   ~ endoscopies or minor procedure - E/M services on the same day generally not paid, special rules for multiple endoscopic procedures apply if billed with another endoscopy in the same family, 150% payment adjustment for bilateral procedures does not apply, payment for assistant surgeon subject to documentation of medical necessity

46614   **Anoscopy, control bleeding**   ~ endoscopies or minor procedure - E/M services on the same day generally not paid, special rules for multiple endoscopic procedures apply if billed with another endoscopy in the same family, 150% payment adjustment for bilateral procedures does not apply, assistant surgeon may not be paid

46615   **Anoscopy**   ~ endoscopies or minor procedure - E/M services on the same day generally not paid, special rules for multiple endoscopic procedures apply if billed with another endoscopy in the same family, 150% payment adjustment for bilateral procedures does not apply, payment for assistant surgeon subject to documentation of medical necessity

46700   **Repair anal stricture**   ~ follow-up period is 90 days, standard payment adjustment rules for multiple procedures apply, 150% payment adjustment for bilateral procedures does not apply, assistant surgeon may not be paid

46705   **Repair anal stricture**   ~ follow-up period is 90 days, standard payment adjustment rules for multiple procedures apply, 150% payment adjustment for bilateral procedures does not apply, assistant surgeon may be paid

46706   **Repair of anal fistula w/glue**   ~ follow-up period is 10 days, standard payment adjustment rules for multiple procedures apply, 150% payment adjustment for bilateral procedures does not apply, assistant surgeon may not be paid

46710   **Repair per/vaginal pouch single proc**   ~ follow-up period is 90 days, standard payment adjustment rules for multiple procedures apply, 150% payment adjustment for bilateral procedures does not apply, assistant surgeon may be paid

46712   **Repair per/vaginal pouch dbl proc**   ~ follow-up period is 90 days, standard payment adjustment rules for multiple procedures apply, 150% payment adjustment for bilateral procedures does not apply, assistant surgeon may be paid

46715   **Rep perforate anoperineal fistula**   ~ follow-up period is 90 days, standard payment adjustment rules for multiple procedures apply, 150% payment adjustment for bilateral procedures does not apply, assistant surgeon may be paid

---

THE CODER'S HANDBOOK 2007

46716 **Rep perforate anoperineal/vestibular fistula** ~ follow-up period is 90 days, standard payment adjustment rules for multiple procedures apply, 150% payment adjustment for bilateral procedures does not apply, assistant surgeon may be paid

46730 **Construct absent anus** ~ follow-up period is 90 days, standard payment adjustment rules for multiple procedures apply, 150% payment adjustment for bilateral procedures does not apply, assistant surgeon may be paid

46735 **Construct absent anus** ~ follow-up period is 90 days, standard payment adjustment rules for multiple procedures apply, 150% payment adjustment for bilateral procedures does not apply, assistant surgeon may be paid

46740 **Construct absent anus** ~ follow-up period is 90 days, standard payment adjustment rules for multiple procedures apply, 150% payment adjustment for bilateral procedures does not apply, assistant surgeon may be paid

46742 **Repair imperforated anus** ~ follow-up period is 90 days, standard payment adjustment rules for multiple procedures apply, 150% payment adjustment for bilateral procedures does not apply, assistant surgeon may be paid

46744 **Repair cloacal anomaly** ~ follow-up period is 90 days, standard payment adjustment rules for multiple procedures apply, 150% payment adjustment for bilateral procedures does not apply, assistant surgeon may be paid

46746 **Repair cloacal anomaly** ~ follow-up period is 90 days, standard payment adjustment rules for multiple procedures apply, 150% payment adjustment for bilateral procedures does not apply, assistant surgeon may be paid

46748 **Repair cloacal anomaly** ~ follow-up period is 90 days, standard payment adjustment rules for multiple procedures apply, 150% payment adjustment for bilateral procedures does not apply, assistant surgeon may be paid

46750 **Repair anal sphincter** ~ follow-up period is 90 days, standard payment adjustment rules for multiple procedures apply, 150% payment adjustment for bilateral procedures does not apply, assistant surgeon may be paid

46751 **Repair anal sphincter** ~ follow-up period is 90 days, standard payment adjustment rules for multiple procedures apply, 150% payment adjustment for bilateral procedures does not apply, assistant surgeon may be paid

46753 **Reconstruct anus** ~ follow-up period is 90 days, standard payment adjustment rules for multiple procedures apply, 150% payment adjustment for bilateral procedures does not apply, assistant surgeon may not be paid

46754 **Remove suture from anus** ~ follow-up period is 10 days, standard payment adjustment rules for multiple procedures apply, 150% payment adjustment for

bilateral procedures does not apply, payment for assistant surgeon subject to documentation of medical necessity

46760   **Repair anal sphincter**   ~ follow-up period is 90 days, standard payment adjustment rules for multiple procedures apply, 150% payment adjustment for bilateral procedures does not apply, assistant surgeon may be paid

46761   **Repair anal sphincter**   ~ follow-up period is 90 days, standard payment adjustment rules for multiple procedures apply, 150% payment adjustment for bilateral procedures does not apply, assistant surgeon may be paid

46762   **Implant artificial sphincter**   ~ follow-up period is 90 days, standard payment adjustment rules for multiple procedures apply, 150% payment adjustment for bilateral procedures does not apply, assistant surgeon may be paid

46900   **Destroy anal lesion(s)**   ~ follow-up period is 10 days, standard payment adjustment rules for multiple procedures apply, 150% payment adjustment for bilateral procedures does not apply, assistant surgeon may not be paid

46910   **Destroy anal lesion(s)**   ~ follow-up period is 10 days, standard payment adjustment rules for multiple procedures apply, 150% payment adjustment for bilateral procedures does not apply, assistant surgeon may not be paid

46916   **Cryosurgery, anal lesion(s)**   ~ follow-up period is 10 days, standard payment adjustment rules for multiple procedures apply, 150% payment adjustment for bilateral procedures does not apply, assistant surgeon may not be paid

46917   **Laser surgery, anal lesions**   ~ follow-up period is 10 days, standard payment adjustment rules for multiple procedures apply, 150% payment adjustment for bilateral procedures does not apply, assistant surgeon may not be paid

46922   **Excise anal lesion(s)**   ~ follow-up period is 10 days, standard payment adjustment rules for multiple procedures apply, 150% payment adjustment for bilateral procedures does not apply, assistant surgeon may not be paid

46924   **Destroy anal lesion(s)**   ~ follow-up period is 10 days, standard payment adjustment rules for multiple procedures apply, 150% payment adjustment for bilateral procedures does not apply, assistant surgeon may not be paid

46934   **Destroy hemorrhoids**   ~ follow-up period is 90 days, standard payment adjustment rules for multiple procedures apply, 150% payment adjustment for bilateral procedures does not apply, assistant surgeon may not be paid

46935   **Destroy hemorrhoids**   ~ follow-up period is 10 days, standard payment adjustment rules for multiple procedures apply, 150% payment adjustment for bilateral procedures does not apply, assistant surgeon may not be paid

46936   **Destroy hemorrhoids** ~ follow-up period is 90 days, standard payment adjustment rules for multiple procedures apply, 150% payment adjustment for bilateral procedures does not apply, assistant surgeon may not be paid

46937   **Cryotherapy of rectal lesion** ~ follow-up period is 10 days, standard payment adjustment rules for multiple procedures apply, 150% payment adjustment for bilateral procedures does not apply, payment for assistant surgeon subject to documentation of medical necessity

46938   **Cryotherapy of rectal lesion** ~ follow-up period is 90 days, standard payment adjustment rules for multiple procedures apply, 150% payment adjustment for bilateral procedures does not apply, payment for assistant surgeon subject to documentation of medical necessity

46940   **Treat anal fissure** ~ follow-up period is 10 days, standard payment adjustment rules for multiple procedures apply, 150% payment adjustment for bilateral procedures does not apply, assistant surgeon may not be paid

46942   **Treat anal fissure** ~ follow-up period is 10 days, standard payment adjustment rules for multiple procedures apply, 150% payment adjustment for bilateral procedures does not apply, payment for assistant surgeon subject to documentation of medical necessity

46945   **Ligate hemorrhoids** ~ follow-up period is 90 days, standard payment adjustment rules for multiple procedures apply, 150% payment adjustment for bilateral procedures does not apply, assistant surgeon may not be paid

46946   **Ligate hemorrhoids** ~ follow-up period is 90 days, standard payment adjustment rules for multiple procedures apply, 150% payment adjustment for bilateral procedures does not apply, assistant surgeon may not be paid

46947   **Hemorrhoidopexy by stapling** ~ follow-up period is 90 days, standard payment adjustment rules for multiple procedures apply, 150% payment adjustment for bilateral procedures does not apply, assistant surgeon may not be paid

46999   **Anus surgery procedure** ~ medicare carrier determines global period, standard payment adjustment rules for multiple procedures apply, 150% payment adjustment for bilateral procedures does not apply, payment for assistant surgeon subject to documentation of medical necessity

Liver

47000   **Needle biopsy liver** ~ endoscopies or minor procedure - E/M services on the same day generally not paid, standard payment adjustment rules for multiple procedures apply, 150% payment adjustment for bilateral procedures does not apply, assistant surgeon may not be paid

47001 **Needle biopsy liver, add-on** ~ follow-up period included in another service, no payment adjustment rules for multiple procedures apply, 150% payment adjustment for bilateral procedures does not apply, assistant surgeon may not be paid, +add-on code (list separately in addition to primary procedure)

47010 **Open drain liver lesion** ~ follow-up period is 90 days, standard payment adjustment rules for multiple procedures apply, 150% payment adjustment for bilateral procedures does not apply, assistant surgeon may be paid

47011 **Percutaneous drain, liver lesion** ~ endoscopies or minor procedure - E/M services on the same day generally not paid, standard payment adjustment rules for multiple procedures apply, 150% payment adjustment for bilateral procedures does not apply, assistant surgeon may be paid

47015 **Inject/aspirate liver cyst** ~ follow-up period is 90 days, standard payment adjustment rules for multiple procedures apply, 150% payment adjustment for bilateral procedures does not apply, assistant surgeon may be paid

47100 **Wedge biopsy liver** ~ follow-up period is 90 days, standard payment adjustment rules for multiple procedures apply, 150% payment adjustment for bilateral procedures does not apply, assistant surgeon may be paid

47120 **Partial remove liver** ~ follow-up period is 90 days, standard payment adjustment rules for multiple procedures apply, 150% payment adjustment for bilateral procedures does not apply, assistant surgeon may be paid

47122 **Extensive remove liver** ~ follow-up period is 90 days, standard payment adjustment rules for multiple procedures apply, 150% payment adjustment for bilateral procedures does not apply, assistant surgeon may be paid

47125 **Partial remove liver** ~ follow-up period is 90 days, standard payment adjustment rules for multiple procedures apply, 150% payment adjustment for bilateral procedures does not apply, assistant surgeon may be paid

47130 **Partial remove liver** ~ follow-up period is 90 days, standard payment adjustment rules for multiple procedures apply, 150% payment adjustment for bilateral procedures does not apply, assistant surgeon may be paid

47133 **Remove donor liver** ~ multiple procedure concept does not apply, bilateral surgery concept does not apply, assistant surgery concept does not apply

47135 **Transplant liver** ~ restricted coverage - special coverage rules apply, follow-up period is 90 days, standard payment adjustment rules for multiple procedures apply, 150% payment adjustment for bilateral procedures does not apply, assistant surgeon may be paid

47136   **Transplant liver**   ~ restricted coverage - special coverage rules apply, follow-up period is 90 days, standard payment adjustment rules for multiple procedures apply, 150% payment adjustment for bilateral procedures does not apply, assistant surgeon may be paid

47140   **Partial remove donor liver**   ~ follow-up period is 90 days, standard payment adjustment rules for multiple procedures apply, 150% payment adjustment for bilateral procedures does not apply, assistant surgeon may be paid

47141   **Partial remove donor liver**   ~ follow-up period is 90 days, standard payment adjustment rules for multiple procedures apply, 150% payment adjustment for bilateral procedures does not apply, assistant surgeon may be paid

47142   **Partial remove donor liver**   ~ follow-up period is 90 days, standard payment adjustment rules for multiple procedures apply, 150% payment adjustment for bilateral procedures does not apply, assistant surgeon may be paid

47143   **Prepare donor liver, whole**   ~ standard payment adjustment rules for multiple procedures apply, 150% payment adjustment for bilateral procedures does not apply, assistant surgeon may be paid

47144   **Prepare donor liver, 3-segment**   ~ follow-up period is 90 days, standard payment adjustment rules for multiple procedures apply, 150% payment adjustment for bilateral procedures does not apply, assistant surgeon may be paid

47145   **Prepare donor liver, lobe split**   ~ standard payment adjustment rules for multiple procedures apply, 150% payment adjustment for bilateral procedures does not apply, assistant surgeon may be paid

47146   **Prepare donor liver/venous**   ~ standard payment adjustment rules for multiple procedures apply, 150% payment adjustment for bilateral procedures does not apply, assistant surgeon may be paid

47147   **Prepare donor liver/arterial**   ~ standard payment adjustment rules for multiple procedures apply, 150% payment adjustment for bilateral procedures does not apply, assistant surgeon may be paid

47300   **Surgery for liver lesion**   ~ follow-up period is 90 days, standard payment adjustment rules for multiple procedures apply, 150% payment adjustment for bilateral procedures does not apply, assistant surgeon may be paid

47350   **Repair liver wound**   ~ follow-up period is 90 days, standard payment adjustment rules for multiple procedures apply, 150% payment adjustment for bilateral procedures does not apply, assistant surgeon may be paid

47360   **Repair liver wound**   ~ follow-up period is 90 days, standard payment adjustment rules for multiple procedures apply, 150% payment adjustment for bilateral procedures does not apply, assistant surgeon may be paid

47361   **Repair liver wound**   ~ follow-up period is 90 days, standard payment adjustment rules for multiple procedures apply, 150% payment adjustment for bilateral procedures does not apply, assistant surgeon may be paid

47362   **Repair liver wound**   ~ follow-up period is 90 days, standard payment adjustment rules for multiple procedures apply, 150% payment adjustment for bilateral procedures does not apply, assistant surgeon may be paid

47370   **Laparo ablate liver tumor rf**   ~ follow-up period is 90 days, standard payment adjustment rules for multiple procedures apply, 150% payment adjustment for bilateral procedures does not apply, assistant surgeon may be paid

47371   **Laparo ablate liver cryosurgery**   ~ follow-up period is 90 days, standard payment adjustment rules for multiple procedures apply, 150% payment adjustment for bilateral procedures does not apply, assistant surgeon may be paid

47379   **Laparoscope procedure, liver**   ~ medicare carrier determines global period, standard payment adjustment rules for multiple procedures apply, 150% payment adjustment for bilateral procedures does not apply, assistant surgeon may be paid

47380   **Open ablate liver tumor rf**   ~ follow-up period is 90 days, standard payment adjustment rules for multiple procedures apply, 150% payment adjustment for bilateral procedures does not apply, assistant surgeon may be paid

47381   **Open ablate liver tumor cryo**   ~ follow-up period is 90 days, standard payment adjustment rules for multiple procedures apply, 150% payment adjustment for bilateral procedures does not apply, assistant surgeon may be paid

47382   **Percutaneous ablate liver rf**   ~ follow-up period is 10 days, standard payment adjustment rules for multiple procedures apply, 150% payment adjustment for bilateral procedures does not apply, assistant surgeon may be paid

47399   **Liver surgery procedure**   ~ medicare carrier determines global period, standard payment adjustment rules for multiple procedures apply, 150% payment adjustment for bilateral procedures does not apply, assistant surgeon may be paid

Biliary Tract

47400   **Incise liver duct**   ~ follow-up period is 90 days, standard payment adjustment rules for multiple procedures apply, 150% payment adjustment for bilateral procedures does not apply, assistant surgeon may be paid

---

47420   **Incise bile duct**   ~ follow-up period is 90 days, standard payment adjustment rules for multiple procedures apply, 150% payment adjustment for bilateral procedures does not apply, assistant surgeon may be paid

47425   **Incise bile duct**   ~ follow-up period is 90 days, standard payment adjustment rules for multiple procedures apply, 150% payment adjustment for bilateral procedures does not apply, assistant surgeon may be paid

47460   **Incise bile duct sphincter**   ~ follow-up period is 90 days, standard payment adjustment rules for multiple procedures apply, 150% payment adjustment for bilateral procedures does not apply, assistant surgeon may be paid

47480   **Incise gallbladder**   ~ follow-up period is 90 days, standard payment adjustment rules for multiple procedures apply, 150% payment adjustment for bilateral procedures does not apply, assistant surgeon may be paid

47490   **Incise gallbladder**   ~ follow-up period is 90 days, standard payment adjustment rules for multiple procedures apply, 150% payment adjustment for bilateral procedures does not apply, assistant surgeon may not be paid

47500   **Inject for liver x-rays**   ~ endoscopies or minor procedure - E/M services on the same day generally not paid, standard payment adjustment rules for multiple procedures apply, 150% payment adjustment for bilateral procedures does not apply, assistant surgeon may not be paid

47505   **Inject for liver x-rays**   ~ endoscopies or minor procedure - E/M services on the same day generally not paid, standard payment adjustment rules for multiple procedures apply, 150% payment adjustment for bilateral procedures does not apply, payment for assistant surgeon subject to documentation of medical necessity

47510   **Insert catheter, bile duct**   ~ follow-up period is 90 days, standard payment adjustment rules for multiple procedures apply, 150% payment adjustment for bilateral procedures does not apply, assistant surgeon may not be paid

47511   **Insert bile duct drain**   ~ follow-up period is 90 days, standard payment adjustment rules for multiple procedures apply, 150% payment adjustment for bilateral procedures applies, assistant surgeon may not be paid

47525   **Change bile duct catheter**   ~ follow-up period is 10 days, standard payment adjustment rules for multiple procedures apply, 150% payment adjustment for bilateral procedures applies, assistant surgeon may not be paid

47530   **Revise/reinsert bile tube**   ~ follow-up period is 90 days, standard payment adjustment rules for multiple procedures apply, 150% payment adjustment for bilateral procedures does not apply, assistant surgeon may not be paid

47550 **Bile duct endoscopy, add-on** ~ follow-up period included in another service, no payment adjustment rules for multiple procedures apply, 150% payment adjustment for bilateral procedures does not apply, assistant surgeon may be paid, +add-on code (list separately in addition to primary procedure)

47552 **Biliary endoscopy thru skin** ~ endoscopies or minor procedure - E/M services on the same day generally not paid, standard payment adjustment rules for multiple procedures apply, 150% payment adjustment for bilateral procedures does not apply, assistant surgeon may not be paid

47553 **Biliary endoscopy thru skin** ~ endoscopies or minor procedure - E/M services on the same day generally not paid, special rules for multiple endoscopic procedures apply if billed with another endoscopy in the same family, 150% payment adjustment for bilateral procedures does not apply, assistant surgeon may not be paid

47554 **Biliary endoscopy thru skin** ~ endoscopies or minor procedure - E/M services on the same day generally not paid, special rules for multiple endoscopic procedures apply if billed with another endoscopy in the same family, 150% payment adjustment for bilateral procedures does not apply, assistant surgeon may not be paid

47555 **Biliary endoscopy thru skin** ~ endoscopies or minor procedure - E/M services on the same day generally not paid, special rules for multiple endoscopic procedures apply if billed with another endoscopy in the same family, 150% payment adjustment for bilateral procedures does not apply, assistant surgeon may not be paid

47556 **Biliary endoscopy thru skin** ~ endoscopies or minor procedure - E/M services on the same day generally not paid, special rules for multiple endoscopic procedures apply if billed with another endoscopy in the same family, 150% payment adjustment for bilateral procedures does not apply, assistant surgeon may not be paid

47560 **Laparoscopy w/cholangiogram** ~ endoscopies or minor procedure - E/M services on the same day generally not paid, standard payment adjustment rules for multiple procedures apply, 150% payment adjustment for bilateral procedures does not apply, payment for assistant surgeon subject to documentation of medical necessity

47561 **Laparo w/cholangiogram/biopsy** ~ endoscopies or minor procedure - E/M services on the same day generally not paid, standard payment adjustment rules for multiple procedures apply, 150% payment adjustment for bilateral procedures does not apply, payment for assistant surgeon subject to documentation of medical necessity

47562 **Laparoscopic cholecystectomy** ~ follow-up period is 90 days, standard payment adjustment rules for multiple procedures apply, 150% payment adjustment for bilateral procedures does not apply, assistant surgeon may be paid

47563 **Laparo cholecystectomy/graph** ~ follow-up period is 90 days, standard payment adjustment rules for multiple procedures apply, 150% payment adjustment for bilateral procedures does not apply, assistant surgeon may be paid

---

47564   **Laparo cholecystectomy/explore**   ~ follow-up period is 90 days, standard payment adjustment rules for multiple procedures apply, 150% payment adjustment for bilateral procedures does not apply, assistant surgeon may be paid

47570   **Laparo cholecystoenterostomy**   ~ follow-up period is 90 days, standard payment adjustment rules for multiple procedures apply, 150% payment adjustment for bilateral procedures does not apply, assistant surgeon may be paid

47579   **Laparoscope proc, biliary**   ~ medicare carrier determines global period, standard payment adjustment rules for multiple procedures apply, 150% payment adjustment for bilateral procedures applies, assistant surgeon may be paid

47600   **Remove gallbladder**   ~ follow-up period is 90 days, standard payment adjustment rules for multiple procedures apply, 150% payment adjustment for bilateral procedures does not apply, assistant surgeon may be paid

47605   **Remove gallbladder**   ~ follow-up period is 90 days, standard payment adjustment rules for multiple procedures apply, 150% payment adjustment for bilateral procedures does not apply, assistant surgeon may be paid

47610   **Remove gallbladder**   ~ follow-up period is 90 days, standard payment adjustment rules for multiple procedures apply, 150% payment adjustment for bilateral procedures does not apply, assistant surgeon may be paid

47612   **Remove gallbladder**   ~ follow-up period is 90 days, standard payment adjustment rules for multiple procedures apply, 150% payment adjustment for bilateral procedures does not apply, assistant surgeon may be paid

47620   **Remove gallbladder**   ~ follow-up period is 90 days, standard payment adjustment rules for multiple procedures apply, 150% payment adjustment for bilateral procedures does not apply, assistant surgeon may be paid

47630   **Remove bile duct stone**   ~ follow-up period is 90 days, standard payment adjustment rules for multiple procedures apply, 150% payment adjustment for bilateral procedures does not apply, assistant surgeon may not be paid

47700   **Explore bile ducts**   ~ follow-up period is 90 days, standard payment adjustment rules for multiple procedures apply, 150% payment adjustment for bilateral procedures does not apply, assistant surgeon may be paid

47701   **Bile duct revision**   ~ follow-up period is 90 days, standard payment adjustment rules for multiple procedures apply, 150% payment adjustment for bilateral procedures does not apply, payment for assistant surgeon subject to documentation of medical necessity

47711   **Excise bile duct tumor**   ~ follow-up period is 90 days, standard payment adjustment rules for multiple procedures apply, 150% payment adjustment for bilateral procedures does not apply, assistant surgeon may be paid

47712   **Excise bile duct tumor**   ~ follow-up period is 90 days, standard payment adjustment rules for multiple procedures apply, 150% payment adjustment for bilateral procedures does not apply, assistant surgeon may be paid

47715   **Excise bile duct cyst**   ~ follow-up period is 90 days, standard payment adjustment rules for multiple procedures apply, 150% payment adjustment for bilateral procedures does not apply, assistant surgeon may be paid

47719   **Fuse bile duct cyst**   ~ follow-up period is 90 days, standard payment adjustment rules for multiple procedures apply, 150% payment adjustment for bilateral procedures does not apply, assistant surgeon may be paid

47720   **Fuse gallbladder & bowel**   ~ follow-up period is 90 days, standard payment adjustment rules for multiple procedures apply, 150% payment adjustment for bilateral procedures does not apply, assistant surgeon may be paid

47721   **Fuse upper gi structures**   ~ follow-up period is 90 days, standard payment adjustment rules for multiple procedures apply, 150% payment adjustment for bilateral procedures does not apply, assistant surgeon may be paid

47740   **Fuse gallbladder & bowel**   ~ follow-up period is 90 days, standard payment adjustment rules for multiple procedures apply, 150% payment adjustment for bilateral procedures does not apply, assistant surgeon may be paid

47741   **Fuse gallbladder & bowel**   ~ follow-up period is 90 days, standard payment adjustment rules for multiple procedures apply, 150% payment adjustment for bilateral procedures does not apply, assistant surgeon may be paid

47760   **Fuse bile ducts and bowel**   ~ follow-up period is 90 days, standard payment adjustment rules for multiple procedures apply, 150% payment adjustment for bilateral procedures does not apply, assistant surgeon may be paid

47765   **Fuse liver ducts & bowel**   ~ follow-up period is 90 days, standard payment adjustment rules for multiple procedures apply, 150% payment adjustment for bilateral procedures does not apply, assistant surgeon may be paid

47780   **Fuse bile ducts and bowel**   ~ follow-up period is 90 days, standard payment adjustment rules for multiple procedures apply, 150% payment adjustment for bilateral procedures does not apply, assistant surgeon may be paid

47785   **Fuse bile ducts and bowel**   ~ follow-up period is 90 days, standard payment adjustment rules for multiple procedures apply, 150% payment adjustment for bilateral procedures does not apply, assistant surgeon may be paid

47800   **Reconstruct bile ducts**   ~ follow-up period is 90 days, standard payment adjustment rules for multiple procedures apply, 150% payment adjustment for bilateral procedures does not apply, assistant surgeon may be paid

47801   **Placement, bile duct support**   ~ follow-up period is 90 days, standard payment adjustment rules for multiple procedures apply, 150% payment adjustment for bilateral procedures does not apply, assistant surgeon may be paid

47802   **Fuse liver duct & intestine**   ~ follow-up period is 90 days, standard payment adjustment rules for multiple procedures apply, 150% payment adjustment for bilateral procedures does not apply, assistant surgeon may be paid

47900   **Suture bile duct injury**   ~ follow-up period is 90 days, standard payment adjustment rules for multiple procedures apply, 150% payment adjustment for bilateral procedures does not apply, assistant surgeon may be paid

47999   **Bile tract surgery procedure**   ~ medicare carrier determines global period, standard payment adjustment rules for multiple procedures apply, 150% payment adjustment for bilateral procedures does not apply, assistant surgeon may be paid

Pancreas

48000   **Drain abdomen**   ~ follow-up period is 90 days, standard payment adjustment rules for multiple procedures apply, 150% payment adjustment for bilateral procedures does not apply, assistant surgeon may be paid

48001   **Placement of drain, pancreas**   ~ follow-up period is 90 days, standard payment adjustment rules for multiple procedures apply, 150% payment adjustment for bilateral procedures does not apply, assistant surgeon may be paid

48020   **Remove pancreatic stone**   ~ follow-up period is 90 days, standard payment adjustment rules for multiple procedures apply, 150% payment adjustment for bilateral procedures does not apply, assistant surgeon may be paid

48100   **Biopsy pancreas, open**   ~ follow-up period is 90 days, standard payment adjustment rules for multiple procedures apply, 150% payment adjustment for bilateral procedures does not apply, assistant surgeon may be paid

48102   **Needle biopsy pancreas**   ~ follow-up period is 10 days, standard payment adjustment rules for multiple procedures apply, 150% payment adjustment for bilateral procedures does not apply, assistant surgeon may not be paid

48105   **Resect/debride pancreas**   ~ follow-up period is 90 days, standard payment adjustment rules for multiple procedures apply, 150% payment adjustment for bilateral procedures does not apply, assistant surgeon may be paid

48120   **Remove pancreas lesion**   ~ follow-up period is 90 days, standard payment adjustment rules for multiple procedures apply, 150% payment adjustment for bilateral procedures does not apply, assistant surgeon may be paid

48140   **Partial remove pancreas**   ~ follow-up period is 90 days, standard payment adjustment rules for multiple procedures apply, 150% payment adjustment for bilateral procedures does not apply, assistant surgeon may be paid

48145   **Partial remove pancreas**   ~ follow-up period is 90 days, standard payment adjustment rules for multiple procedures apply, 150% payment adjustment for bilateral procedures does not apply, assistant surgeon may be paid

48146   **Pancreatectomy**   ~ follow-up period is 90 days, standard payment adjustment rules for multiple procedures apply, 150% payment adjustment for bilateral procedures does not apply, assistant surgeon may be paid

48148   **Remove pancreatic duct**   ~ follow-up period is 90 days, standard payment adjustment rules for multiple procedures apply, 150% payment adjustment for bilateral procedures does not apply, assistant surgeon may be paid

48150   **Partial remove pancreas**   ~ follow-up period is 90 days, standard payment adjustment rules for multiple procedures apply, 150% payment adjustment for bilateral procedures does not apply, assistant surgeon may be paid

48152   **Pancreatectomy**   ~ follow-up period is 90 days, standard payment adjustment rules for multiple procedures apply, 150% payment adjustment for bilateral procedures does not apply, assistant surgeon may be paid

48153   **Pancreatectomy**   ~ follow-up period is 90 days, standard payment adjustment rules for multiple procedures apply, 150% payment adjustment for bilateral procedures does not apply, assistant surgeon may be paid

48154   **Pancreatectomy**   ~ follow-up period is 90 days, standard payment adjustment rules for multiple procedures apply, 150% payment adjustment for bilateral procedures does not apply, assistant surgeon may be paid

48155   **Remove pancreas**   ~ follow-up period is 90 days, standard payment adjustment rules for multiple procedures apply, 150% payment adjustment for bilateral procedures does not apply, assistant surgeon may be paid

48160   **Pancreas remove/transplant**   non-covered service, multiple procedure concept does not apply, bilateral surgery concept does not apply, assistant surgery concept does not apply, +add-on code (list separately in addition to primary procedure)

48400   **Injection, intraop, add-on**   ~ follow-up period included in another service, no payment adjustment rules for multiple procedures apply, 150% payment adjustment for bilateral procedures does not apply, payment for assistant surgeon subject to

---

documentation of medical necessity, +add-on code (list separately in addition to primary procedure)

48500   **Surgery pancreatic cyst**   ~ follow-up period is 90 days, standard payment adjustment rules for multiple procedures apply, 150% payment adjustment for bilateral procedures does not apply, assistant surgeon may be paid

48510   **Drain pancreatic pseudocyst**   ~ follow-up period is 90 days, standard payment adjustment rules for multiple procedures apply, 150% payment adjustment for bilateral procedures does not apply, assistant surgeon may be paid

48511   **Drain pancreatic pseudocyst**   ~ endoscopies or minor procedure - E/M services on the same day generally not paid, standard payment adjustment rules for multiple procedures apply, 150% payment adjustment for bilateral procedures does not apply, assistant surgeon may be paid

48520   **Fuse pancreas cyst and bowel**   ~ follow-up period is 90 days, standard payment adjustment rules for multiple procedures apply, 150% payment adjustment for bilateral procedures does not apply, assistant surgeon may be paid

48540   **Fuse pancreas cyst and bowel**   ~ follow-up period is 90 days, standard payment adjustment rules for multiple procedures apply, 150% payment adjustment for bilateral procedures does not apply, assistant surgeon may be paid

48545   **Pancreatorrhaphy**   ~ follow-up period is 90 days, standard payment adjustment rules for multiple procedures apply, 150% payment adjustment for bilateral procedures does not apply, assistant surgeon may be paid

48547   **Duodenal exclusion**   ~ follow-up period is 90 days, standard payment adjustment rules for multiple procedures apply, 150% payment adjustment for bilateral procedures does not apply, assistant surgeon may be paid

48548   **Fuse pancreas and bowel**   ~ follow-up period is 90 days, standard payment adjustment rules for multiple procedures apply, 150% payment adjustment for bilateral procedures does not apply, assistant surgeon may be paid

48550   **Donor pancreatectomy**   ~ multiple procedure concept does not apply, bilateral surgery concept does not apply, assistant surgery concept does not apply

48551   **Prepare donor pancreas**   ~ standard payment adjustment rules for multiple procedures apply, 150% payment adjustment for bilateral procedures does not apply, assistant surgeon may be paid

48552   **Prepare donor pancreas/venous**   ~ standard payment adjustment rules for multiple procedures apply, 150% payment adjustment for bilateral procedures does not apply, assistant surgeon may be paid

48554   **Transplant allograft pancreas**   ~ restricted coverage - special coverage rules apply, follow-up period is 90 days, standard payment adjustment rules for multiple procedures apply, 150% payment adjustment for bilateral procedures does not apply, assistant surgeon may be paid

48556   **Remove allograft pancreas**   ~ follow-up period is 90 days, standard payment adjustment rules for multiple procedures apply, 150% payment adjustment for bilateral procedures does not apply, assistant surgeon may be paid

48999   **Pancreas surgery procedure**   ~ medicare carrier determines global period, standard payment adjustment rules for multiple procedures apply, 150% payment adjustment for bilateral procedures does not apply, assistant surgeon may be paid

Abdomen, Peritoneum, and Omentum

49000   **Explore abdomen**   ~ follow-up period is 90 days, standard payment adjustment rules for multiple procedures apply, 150% payment adjustment for bilateral procedures does not apply, assistant surgeon may be paid

49002   **Reopening of abdomen**   ~ follow-up period is 90 days, standard payment adjustment rules for multiple procedures apply, 150% payment adjustment for bilateral procedures does not apply, assistant surgeon may be paid

49010   **Explore behind abdomen**   ~ follow-up period is 90 days, standard payment adjustment rules for multiple procedures apply, 150% payment adjustment for bilateral procedures does not apply, assistant surgeon may be paid

49020   **Drain abdominal abscess**   ~ follow-up period is 90 days, standard payment adjustment rules for multiple procedures apply, 150% payment adjustment for bilateral procedures does not apply, assistant surgeon may be paid

49021   **Drain abdominal abscess**   ~ endoscopies or minor procedure - E/M services on the same day generally not paid, standard payment adjustment rules for multiple procedures apply, 150% payment adjustment for bilateral procedures does not apply, assistant surgeon may not be paid

49040   **Drain, open, abdom abscess**   ~ follow-up period is 90 days, standard payment adjustment rules for multiple procedures apply, 150% payment adjustment for bilateral procedures does not apply, assistant surgeon may be paid

49041   **Drain, percutaneous, abdom abscess**   ~ endoscopies or minor procedure - E/M services on the same day generally not paid, standard payment adjustment rules for multiple procedures apply, 150% payment adjustment for bilateral procedures does not apply, assistant surgeon may be paid

49060   **Drain, open, retroperitoneal abscess**   ~ follow-up period is 90 days, standard payment adjustment rules for multiple procedures apply, 150% payment adjustment for bilateral procedures does not apply, assistant surgeon may not be paid

49061   **Drain, percutaneous, retroperitoneal abscess** ~ endoscopies or minor procedure - E/M services on the same day generally not paid, standard payment adjustment rules for multiple procedures apply, 150% payment adjustment for bilateral procedures does not apply, assistant surgeon may be paid

49062   **Drain to peritoneal cavity**   ~ follow-up period is 90 days, standard payment adjustment rules for multiple procedures apply, 150% payment adjustment for bilateral procedures does not apply, assistant surgeon may be paid

49080   **Puncture, peritoneal cavity**   ~ endoscopies or minor procedure - E/M services on the same day generally not paid, standard payment adjustment rules for multiple procedures apply, 150% payment adjustment for bilateral procedures does not apply, assistant surgeon may not be paid

49081   **Remove abdominal fluid**   ~ endoscopies or minor procedure - E/M services on the same day generally not paid, standard payment adjustment rules for multiple procedures apply, 150% payment adjustment for bilateral procedures does not apply, assistant surgeon may not be paid

49180   **Biopsy abdominal mass**   ~ endoscopies or minor procedure - E/M services on the same day generally not paid, standard payment adjustment rules for multiple procedures apply, 150% payment adjustment for bilateral procedures does not apply, assistant surgeon may not be paid

49200   **Remove abdominal lesion**   ~ follow-up period is 90 days, standard payment adjustment rules for multiple procedures apply, 150% payment adjustment for bilateral procedures does not apply, assistant surgeon may be paid

49201   **Remove abdom lesion, complex**   ~ follow-up period is 90 days, standard payment adjustment rules for multiple procedures apply, 150% payment adjustment for bilateral procedures does not apply, assistant surgeon may be paid

49215   **Excise sacral spine tumor**   ~ follow-up period is 90 days, standard payment adjustment rules for multiple procedures apply, 150% payment adjustment for bilateral procedures does not apply, assistant surgeon may be paid

49220   **Multiple surgery, abdomen**   ~ follow-up period is 90 days, standard payment adjustment rules for multiple procedures apply, 150% payment adjustment for bilateral procedures does not apply, assistant surgeon may be paid

49250   **Excise umbilicus**   ~ follow-up period is 90 days, standard payment adjustment rules for multiple procedures apply, 150% payment adjustment for bilateral procedures does not apply, assistant surgeon may not be paid

49255   **Remove omentum**   ~ follow-up period is 90 days, standard payment adjustment rules for multiple procedures apply, 150% payment adjustment for bilateral procedures does not apply, assistant surgeon may be paid

49320   **Diag laparo separate proc**   ~ follow-up period is 10 days, standard payment adjustment rules for multiple procedures apply, 150% payment adjustment for bilateral procedures does not apply, assistant surgeon may be paid

49321   **Laparoscopy, biopsy**   ~ follow-up period is 10 days, special rules for multiple endoscopic procedures apply if billed with another endoscopy in the same family, 150% payment adjustment for bilateral procedures does not apply, assistant surgeon may be paid

49322   **Laparoscopy, aspiration**   ~ follow-up period is 10 days, special rules for multiple endoscopic procedures apply if billed with another endoscopy in the same family, 150% payment adjustment for bilateral procedures does not apply, assistant surgeon may be paid

49323   **Laparo drain lymphocele**   ~ follow-up period is 90 days, special rules for multiple endoscopic procedures apply if billed with another endoscopy in the same family, 150% payment adjustment for bilateral procedures does not apply, assistant surgeon may be paid

49324   **Laparoscopy insert perm ip cath**   ~ follow-up period is 10 days, special rules for multiple endoscopic procedures apply if billed with another endoscopy in the same family, 150% payment adjustment for bilateral procedures does not apply, assistant surgeon may be paid

49325   **Laparoscopy revision perm ip cath**   ~ follow-up period is 10 days, special rules for multiple endoscopic procedures apply if billed with another endoscopy in the same family, 150% payment adjustment for bilateral procedures does not apply, assistant surgeon may be paid

49326   **Laparoscopy w/omentopexy, add-on**   ~ follow-up period included in another service, no payment adjustment rules for multiple procedures apply, 150% payment adjustment for bilateral procedures does not apply, assistant surgeon may be paid, +add-on code (list separately in addition to primary procedure)

49329   **Laparo proc, abdomen/peritoneum/omentum** ~ medicare carrier determines global period, standard payment adjustment rules for multiple procedures apply, 150% payment adjustment for bilateral procedures applies, assistant surgeon may be paid

49400   **Air inject into abdomen**   ~ endoscopies or minor procedure - E/M services on the same day generally not paid, standard payment adjustment rules for multiple procedures apply, 150% payment adjustment for bilateral procedures does not apply, assistant surgeon may not be paid

49402 **Remove foreign body abdomen** ~ follow-up period is 90 days, standard payment adjustment rules for multiple procedures apply, 150% payment adjustment for bilateral procedures does not apply, assistant surgeon may not be paid

49419 **Insert abdom cath for chemotherapy** ~ follow-up period is 90 days, standard payment adjustment rules for multiple procedures apply, 150% payment adjustment for bilateral procedures does not apply, assistant surgeon may not be paid

49420 **Insert abdom drain, temp** ~ endoscopies or minor procedure - E/M services on the same day generally not paid, standard payment adjustment rules for multiple procedures apply, 150% payment adjustment for bilateral procedures does not apply, assistant surgeon may not be paid

49421 **Insert abdom drain, perm** ~ follow-up period is 90 days, standard payment adjustment rules for multiple procedures apply, 150% payment adjustment for bilateral procedures does not apply, assistant surgeon may not be paid

49422 **Remove perm cannula/catheter** ~ follow-up period is 10 days, standard payment adjustment rules for multiple procedures apply, 150% payment adjustment for bilateral procedures does not apply, assistant surgeon may not be paid

49423 **Exchange drain catheter** ~ endoscopies or minor procedure - E/M services on the same day generally not paid, standard payment adjustment rules for multiple procedures apply, 150% payment adjustment for bilateral procedures does not apply, payment for assistant surgeon subject to documentation of medical necessity

49424 **Assess cyst, contrast inject** ~ endoscopies or minor procedure - E/M services on the same day generally not paid, standard payment adjustment rules for multiple procedures apply, 150% payment adjustment for bilateral procedures does not apply, payment for assistant surgeon subject to documentation of medical necessity

49425 **Insert abdomen-venous drain** ~ follow-up period is 90 days, standard payment adjustment rules for multiple procedures apply, 150% payment adjustment for bilateral procedures does not apply, assistant surgeon may be paid

49426 **Revise abdomen-venous shunt** ~ follow-up period is 90 days, standard payment adjustment rules for multiple procedures apply, 150% payment adjustment for bilateral procedures does not apply, assistant surgeon may not be paid

49427 **Injection, abdominal shunt** ~ endoscopies or minor procedure - E/M services on the same day generally not paid, standard payment adjustment rules for multiple procedures apply, 150% payment adjustment for bilateral procedures does not apply, payment for assistant surgeon subject to documentation of medical necessity

49428 **Ligate shunt** ~ follow-up period is 10 days, standard payment adjustment rules for multiple procedures apply, 150% payment adjustment for bilateral procedures does not apply, assistant surgeon may not be paid

49429   **Remove shunt**   ~ follow-up period is 10 days, standard payment adjustment rules for multiple procedures apply, 150% payment adjustment for bilateral procedures does not apply, assistant surgeon may not be paid

49435   **Insert subcutaneous extensive to ip cath**   ~ follow-up period included in another service, no payment adjustment rules for multiple procedures apply, 150% payment adjustment for bilateral procedures does not apply, assistant surgeon may be paid

49436   **Embedded ip cath exit-site**   ~ follow-up period is 10 days, standard payment adjustment rules for multiple procedures apply, 150% payment adjustment for bilateral procedures does not apply, assistant surgeon may be paid

49491   **Repair hernia preemie reduce**   ~ follow-up period is 90 days, standard payment adjustment rules for multiple procedures apply, 150% payment adjustment for bilateral procedures applies, assistant surgeon may be paid

49492   **Repair inguinal hernia preemie, blocked**   ~ follow-up period is 90 days, standard payment adjustment rules for multiple procedures apply, 150% payment adjustment for bilateral procedures applies, assistant surgeon may be paid

49495   **Repair inguinal hernia baby, reduce**   ~ follow-up period is 90 days, standard payment adjustment rules for multiple procedures apply, 150% payment adjustment for bilateral procedures applies, assistant surgeon may be paid

49496   **Repair inguinal hernia baby, blocked**   ~ follow-up period is 90 days, standard payment adjustment rules for multiple procedures apply, 150% payment adjustment for bilateral procedures applies, assistant surgeon may be paid

49500   **Repair inguinal hernia, init, reduce**   ~ follow-up period is 90 days, standard payment adjustment rules for multiple procedures apply, 150% payment adjustment for bilateral procedures applies, assistant surgeon may be paid

49501   **Repair inguinal hernia, initial blocked**   ~ follow-up period is 90 days, standard payment adjustment rules for multiple procedures apply, 150% payment adjustment for bilateral procedures applies, assistant surgeon may be paid

49505   **Repair i/hernia initial reduce >5 yr**   ~ follow-up period is 90 days, standard payment adjustment rules for multiple procedures apply, 150% payment adjustment for bilateral procedures applies, assistant surgeon may be paid

49507   **Repair i/hernia initial block >5 yr**   ~ follow-up period is 90 days, standard payment adjustment rules for multiple procedures apply, 150% payment adjustment for bilateral procedures applies, assistant surgeon may be paid

49520   **Rerepair inguinal hernia, reduce**   ~ follow-up period is 90 days, standard payment adjustment rules for multiple procedures apply, 150% payment adjustment for bilateral procedures applies, assistant surgeon may be paid

49521   **Rerepair inguinal hernia, blocked**   ~ follow-up period is 90 days, standard payment adjustment rules for multiple procedures apply, 150% payment adjustment for bilateral procedures applies, assistant surgeon may be paid

49525   **Repair inguinal hernia, sliding**   ~ follow-up period is 90 days, standard payment adjustment rules for multiple procedures apply, 150% payment adjustment for bilateral procedures applies, assistant surgeon may be paid

49540   **Repair lumbar hernia**   ~ follow-up period is 90 days, standard payment adjustment rules for multiple procedures apply, 150% payment adjustment for bilateral procedures applies, assistant surgeon may be paid

49550   **Repair rem hernia, init, reduce**   ~ follow-up period is 90 days, standard payment adjustment rules for multiple procedures apply, 150% payment adjustment for bilateral procedures applies, assistant surgeon may be paid

49553   **Repair fem hernia, initial blocked**   ~ follow-up period is 90 days, standard payment adjustment rules for multiple procedures apply, 150% payment adjustment for bilateral procedures applies, assistant surgeon may be paid

49555   **Rerepair fem hernia, reduce**   ~ follow-up period is 90 days, standard payment adjustment rules for multiple procedures apply, 150% payment adjustment for bilateral procedures applies, assistant surgeon may be paid

49557   **Rerepair fem hernia, blocked**   ~ follow-up period is 90 days, standard payment adjustment rules for multiple procedures apply, 150% payment adjustment for bilateral procedures applies, assistant surgeon may be paid

49560   **Repair ventral hernia init, reduce**   ~ follow-up period is 90 days, standard payment adjustment rules for multiple procedures apply, 150% payment adjustment for bilateral procedures applies, assistant surgeon may be paid

49561   **Repair ventral hernia init, block**   ~ follow-up period is 90 days, standard payment adjustment rules for multiple procedures apply, 150% payment adjustment for bilateral procedures applies, assistant surgeon may be paid

49565   **Rerepair ventral hernia, reduce**   ~ follow-up period is 90 days, standard payment adjustment rules for multiple procedures apply, 150% payment adjustment for bilateral procedures applies, assistant surgeon may be paid

49566   **Rerepair ventral hernia, block**   ~ follow-up period is 90 days, standard payment adjustment rules for multiple procedures apply, 150% payment adjustment for bilateral procedures applies, assistant surgeon may be paid

49568   **Hernia repair w/mesh**   ~ follow-up period included in another service, no payment adjustment rules for multiple procedures apply, 150% payment adjustment for bilateral procedures does not apply, assistant surgeon may be paid

49570   **Repair epigastric hernia, reduce**   ~ follow-up period is 90 days, standard payment adjustment rules for multiple procedures apply, 150% payment adjustment for bilateral procedures applies, assistant surgeon may be paid

49572   **Repair epigastric hernia, blocked**   ~ follow-up period is 90 days, standard payment adjustment rules for multiple procedures apply, 150% payment adjustment for bilateral procedures applies, assistant surgeon may be paid

49580   **Repair umbilical hernia, reduce < 5 yr**   ~ follow-up period is 90 days, standard payment adjustment rules for multiple procedures apply, 150% payment adjustment for bilateral procedures does not apply, assistant surgeon may be paid

49582   **Repair umbilical hernia, block < 5 yr**   ~ follow-up period is 90 days, standard payment adjustment rules for multiple procedures apply, 150% payment adjustment for bilateral procedures does not apply, assistant surgeon may be paid

49585   **Repair umbilical hernia, reduce > 5 yr**   ~ follow-up period is 90 days, standard payment adjustment rules for multiple procedures apply, 150% payment adjustment for bilateral procedures does not apply, assistant surgeon may be paid

49587   **Repair umbilical hernia, block > 5 yr**   ~ follow-up period is 90 days, standard payment adjustment rules for multiple procedures apply, 150% payment adjustment for bilateral procedures does not apply, assistant surgeon may be paid

49590   **Repair spigelian hernia**   ~ follow-up period is 90 days, standard payment adjustment rules for multiple procedures apply, 150% payment adjustment for bilateral procedures applies, assistant surgeon may be paid

49600   **Repair umbilical lesion**   ~ follow-up period is 90 days, standard payment adjustment rules for multiple procedures apply, 150% payment adjustment for bilateral procedures does not apply, assistant surgeon may be paid

49605   **Repair umbilical lesion**   ~ follow-up period is 90 days, standard payment adjustment rules for multiple procedures apply, 150% payment adjustment for bilateral procedures does not apply, assistant surgeon may be paid

49606   **Repair umbilical lesion**   ~ follow-up period is 90 days, standard payment adjustment rules for multiple procedures apply, 150% payment adjustment for bilateral procedures does not apply, assistant surgeon may be paid

49610   **Repair umbilical lesion**   ~ follow-up period is 90 days, standard payment adjustment rules for multiple procedures apply, 150% payment adjustment for bilateral procedures does not apply, assistant surgeon may be paid

49611   **Repair umbilical lesion**   ~ follow-up period is 90 days, standard payment adjustment rules for multiple procedures apply, 150% payment adjustment for bilateral procedures does not apply, assistant surgeon may be paid

49650   **Laparo hernia repair initial**   ~ follow-up period is 90 days, standard payment adjustment rules for multiple procedures apply, 150% payment adjustment for bilateral procedures applies, assistant surgeon may be paid

49651   **Laparo hernia repair recur**   ~ follow-up period is 90 days, standard payment adjustment rules for multiple procedures apply, 150% payment adjustment for bilateral procedures applies, assistant surgeon may be paid

49659   **Laparo proc, hernia repair**   ~ medicare carrier determines global period, standard payment adjustment rules for multiple procedures apply, 150% payment adjustment for bilateral procedures applies, assistant surgeon may be paid

49900   **Repair abdominal wall**   ~ follow-up period is 90 days, standard payment adjustment rules for multiple procedures apply, 150% payment adjustment for bilateral procedures does not apply, assistant surgeon may be paid

49904   **Omental flap, extra-abdom**   ~ follow-up period is 90 days, standard payment adjustment rules for multiple procedures apply, 150% payment adjustment for bilateral procedures does not apply, assistant surgeon may not be paid

49905   **Omental flap, intra-abdom**   ~ follow-up period included in another service, no payment adjustment rules for multiple procedures apply, 150% payment adjustment for bilateral procedures does not apply, assistant surgeon may be paid

49906   **Free omental flap, microvasc**   ~ follow-up period is 90 days, standard payment adjustment rules for multiple procedures apply, 150% payment adjustment for bilateral procedures does not apply, assistant surgeon may not be paid

49999   **Abdomen surgery procedure**   ~ medicare carrier determines global period, standard payment adjustment rules for multiple procedures apply, 150% payment adjustment for bilateral procedures does not apply, assistant surgeon may be paid

URINARY SYSTEM

Kidney

50010   **Explore kidney**   ~ follow-up period is 90 days, standard payment adjustment rules for multiple procedures apply, 150% payment adjustment for bilateral procedures does not apply, assistant surgeon may be paid

50020   **Renal abscess, open drain**   ~ follow-up period is 90 days, standard payment adjustment rules for multiple procedures apply, 150% payment adjustment for bilateral procedures does not apply, assistant surgeon may not be paid

50021   **Renal abscess, percutaneous drain**   ~ endoscopies or minor procedure - E/M services on the same day generally not paid, standard payment adjustment rules for multiple

procedures apply, 150% payment adjustment for bilateral procedures does not apply, assistant surgeon may be paid

50040 **Drain kidney** ~ follow-up period is 90 days, standard payment adjustment rules for multiple procedures apply, 150% payment adjustment for bilateral procedures does not apply, assistant surgeon may not be paid

50045 **Explore kidney** ~ follow-up period is 90 days, standard payment adjustment rules for multiple procedures apply, 150% payment adjustment for bilateral procedures does not apply, assistant surgeon may be paid

50060 **Remove kidney stone** ~ follow-up period is 90 days, standard payment adjustment rules for multiple procedures apply, 150% payment adjustment for bilateral procedures does not apply, assistant surgeon may be paid

50065 **Incise kidney** ~ follow-up period is 90 days, standard payment adjustment rules for multiple procedures apply, 150% payment adjustment for bilateral procedures does not apply, assistant surgeon may be paid

50070 **Incise kidney** ~ follow-up period is 90 days, standard payment adjustment rules for multiple procedures apply, 150% payment adjustment for bilateral procedures does not apply, assistant surgeon may be paid

50075 **Remove kidney stone** ~ follow-up period is 90 days, standard payment adjustment rules for multiple procedures apply, 150% payment adjustment for bilateral procedures does not apply, assistant surgeon may be paid

50080 **Remove kidney stone** ~ follow-up period is 90 days, standard payment adjustment rules for multiple procedures apply, 150% payment adjustment for bilateral procedures applies, assistant surgeon may not be paid

50081 **Remove kidney stone** ~ follow-up period is 90 days, standard payment adjustment rules for multiple procedures apply, 150% payment adjustment for bilateral procedures applies, assistant surgeon may be paid

50100 **Revise kidney blood vessels** ~ follow-up period is 90 days, standard payment adjustment rules for multiple procedures apply, 150% payment adjustment for bilateral procedures does not apply, assistant surgeon may be paid

50120 **Explore kidney** ~ follow-up period is 90 days, standard payment adjustment rules for multiple procedures apply, 150% payment adjustment for bilateral procedures applies, assistant surgeon may be paid

50125 **Explore and drain kidney** ~ follow-up period is 90 days, standard payment adjustment rules for multiple procedures apply, 150% payment adjustment for bilateral procedures applies, assistant surgeon may be paid

50130 **Remove kidney stone** ~ follow-up period is 90 days, standard payment adjustment rules for multiple procedures apply, 150% payment adjustment for bilateral procedures applies, assistant surgeon may be paid

50135 **Explore kidney** ~ follow-up period is 90 days, standard payment adjustment rules for multiple procedures apply, 150% payment adjustment for bilateral procedures applies, assistant surgeon may be paid

50200 **Biopsy kidney** ~ endoscopies or minor procedure - E/M services on the same day generally not paid, standard payment adjustment rules for multiple procedures apply, 150% payment adjustment for bilateral procedures applies, assistant surgeon may not be paid

50205 **Biopsy kidney** ~ follow-up period is 90 days, standard payment adjustment rules for multiple procedures apply, 150% payment adjustment for bilateral procedures applies, assistant surgeon may be paid

50220 **Remove kidney, open** ~ follow-up period is 90 days, standard payment adjustment rules for multiple procedures apply, 150% payment adjustment for bilateral procedures applies, assistant surgeon may be paid

50225 **Remove kidney open, complex** ~ follow-up period is 90 days, standard payment adjustment rules for multiple procedures apply, 150% payment adjustment for bilateral procedures applies, assistant surgeon may be paid

50230 **Remove kidney open, radical** ~ follow-up period is 90 days, standard payment adjustment rules for multiple procedures apply, 150% payment adjustment for bilateral procedures applies, assistant surgeon may be paid

50234 **Remove kidney & ureter** ~ follow-up period is 90 days, standard payment adjustment rules for multiple procedures apply, 150% payment adjustment for bilateral procedures does not apply, assistant surgeon may be paid

50236 **Remove kidney & ureter** ~ follow-up period is 90 days, standard payment adjustment rules for multiple procedures apply, 150% payment adjustment for bilateral procedures does not apply, assistant surgeon may be paid

50240 **Partial remove kidney** ~ follow-up period is 90 days, standard payment adjustment rules for multiple procedures apply, 150% payment adjustment for bilateral procedures does not apply, assistant surgeon may be paid

50250 **Cryoablate renal mass open** ~ follow-up period is 90 days, standard payment adjustment rules for multiple procedures apply, 150% payment adjustment for bilateral procedures does not apply, assistant surgeon may be paid

50280 **Remove kidney lesion** ~ follow-up period is 90 days, standard payment adjustment rules for multiple procedures apply, 150% payment adjustment for bilateral procedures does not apply, assistant surgeon may be paid

50290 **Remove kidney lesion** ~ follow-up period is 90 days, standard payment adjustment rules for multiple procedures apply, 150% payment adjustment for bilateral procedures does not apply, assistant surgeon may be paid

50300 **Remove cadaver donor kidney** ~ multiple procedure concept does not apply, bilateral surgery concept does not apply, assistant surgery concept does not apply

50320 **Remove kidney, living donor** ~ follow-up period is 90 days, standard payment adjustment rules for multiple procedures apply, 150% payment adjustment for bilateral procedures applies, assistant surgeon may be paid

50323 **Prepare cadaver renal allograft** ~ standard payment adjustment rules for multiple procedures apply, 150% payment adjustment for bilateral procedures does not apply, assistant surgeon may be paid

50325 **Prepare donor renal graft** ~ standard payment adjustment rules for multiple procedures apply, 150% payment adjustment for bilateral procedures does not apply, assistant surgeon may be paid

50327 **Prepare renal graft/venous** ~ standard payment adjustment rules for multiple procedures apply, 150% payment adjustment for bilateral procedures does not apply, assistant surgeon may be paid

50328 **Prepare renal graft/arterial** ~ standard payment adjustment rules for multiple procedures apply, 150% payment adjustment for bilateral procedures does not apply, assistant surgeon may be paid

50329 **Prepare renal graft/ureteral** ~ standard payment adjustment rules for multiple procedures apply, 150% payment adjustment for bilateral procedures does not apply, assistant surgeon may be paid

50340 **Remove kidney** ~ follow-up period is 90 days, standard payment adjustment rules for multiple procedures apply, 150% payment adjustment for bilateral procedures applies, assistant surgeon may be paid

50360 **Transplant kidney** ~ follow-up period is 90 days, standard payment adjustment rules for multiple procedures apply, 150% payment adjustment for bilateral procedures does not apply, assistant surgeon may be paid

50365 **Transplant kidney** ~ follow-up period is 90 days, standard payment adjustment rules for multiple procedures apply, 150% payment adjustment for bilateral procedures applies, assistant surgeon may be paid

---

50370   **Remove transplanted kidney**   ~ follow-up period is 90 days, standard payment adjustment rules for multiple procedures apply, 150% payment adjustment for bilateral procedures does not apply, assistant surgeon may be paid

50380   **Reimplantation of kidney**   ~ follow-up period is 90 days, standard payment adjustment rules for multiple procedures apply, 150% payment adjustment for bilateral procedures does not apply, assistant surgeon may be paid

50382   **Change ureter stent, percutaneous**   ~ endoscopies or minor procedure - E/M services on the same day generally not paid, standard payment adjustment rules for multiple procedures apply, 150% payment adjustment for bilateral procedures applies, assistant surgeon may not be paid

50384   **Remove ureter stent, percutaneous**   ~ endoscopies or minor procedure - E/M services on the same day generally not paid, standard payment adjustment rules for multiple procedures apply, 150% payment adjustment for bilateral procedures applies, assistant surgeon may not be paid

50387   **Change ext/internal ureter stent**   ~ endoscopies or minor procedure - E/M services on the same day generally not paid, standard payment adjustment rules for multiple procedures apply, 150% payment adjustment for bilateral procedures applies, payment for assistant surgeon subject to documentation of medical necessity

50389   **Remove renal tube w/fluoroscope**   ~ endoscopies or minor procedure - E/M services on the same day generally not paid, standard payment adjustment rules for multiple procedures apply, 150% payment adjustment for bilateral procedures applies, assistant surgeon may not be paid

50390   **Drain kidney lesion**   ~ endoscopies or minor procedure - E/M services on the same day generally not paid, standard payment adjustment rules for multiple procedures apply, 150% payment adjustment for bilateral procedures applies, assistant surgeon may not be paid

50391   **Instill rx agent into renal tub**   ~ endoscopies or minor procedure - E/M services on the same day generally not paid, standard payment adjustment rules for multiple procedures apply, 150% payment adjustment for bilateral procedures does not apply, assistant surgeon may not be paid

50392   **Insert kidney drain**   ~ endoscopies or minor procedure - E/M services on the same day generally not paid, standard payment adjustment rules for multiple procedures apply, 150% payment adjustment for bilateral procedures applies, assistant surgeon may not be paid

50393   **Insert ureteral tube**   ~ endoscopies or minor procedure - E/M services on the same day generally not paid, standard payment adjustment rules for multiple procedures apply, 150% payment adjustment for bilateral procedures applies, assistant surgeon may not be paid

50394   **Inject for kidney x-ray**   ~ endoscopies or minor procedure - E/M services on the same day generally not paid, standard payment adjustment rules for multiple procedures apply, 150% payment adjustment for bilateral procedures applies, assistant surgeon may not be paid

50395   **Create passage to kidney**   ~ endoscopies or minor procedure - E/M services on the same day generally not paid, standard payment adjustment rules for multiple procedures apply, 150% payment adjustment for bilateral procedures applies, assistant surgeon may not be paid

50396   **Measure kidney pressure**   ~ endoscopies or minor procedure - E/M services on the same day generally not paid, standard payment adjustment rules for multiple procedures apply, 150% payment adjustment for bilateral procedures applies, payment for assistant surgeon subject to documentation of medical necessity

50398   **Change kidney tube**   ~ endoscopies or minor procedure - E/M services on the same day generally not paid, standard payment adjustment rules for multiple procedures apply, 150% payment adjustment for bilateral procedures applies, assistant surgeon may not be paid

50400   **Revise kidney/ureter**   ~ follow-up period is 90 days, standard payment adjustment rules for multiple procedures apply, 150% payment adjustment for bilateral procedures does not apply, assistant surgeon may be paid

50405   **Revise kidney/ureter**   ~ follow-up period is 90 days, standard payment adjustment rules for multiple procedures apply, 150% payment adjustment for bilateral procedures does not apply, assistant surgeon may be paid

50500   **Repair kidney wound**   ~ follow-up period is 90 days, standard payment adjustment rules for multiple procedures apply, 150% payment adjustment for bilateral procedures does not apply, assistant surgeon may be paid

50520   **Close kidney-skin fistula**   ~ follow-up period is 90 days, standard payment adjustment rules for multiple procedures apply, 150% payment adjustment for bilateral procedures does not apply, assistant surgeon may be paid

50525   **Repair renal-abdomen fistula**   ~ follow-up period is 90 days, standard payment adjustment rules for multiple procedures apply, 150% payment adjustment for bilateral procedures does not apply, assistant surgeon may be paid

50526   **Repair renal-abdomen fistula**   ~ follow-up period is 90 days, standard payment adjustment rules for multiple procedures apply, 150% payment adjustment for bilateral procedures does not apply, assistant surgeon may be paid

50540   **Revise horseshoe kidney**   ~ follow-up period is 90 days, standard payment adjustment rules for multiple procedures apply, 150% payment adjustment does not apply - RVUs based on bilateral procedure, assistant surgeon may be paid

50541   **Laparo ablate renal cyst**   ~ follow-up period is 90 days, standard payment adjustment rules for multiple procedures apply, 150% payment adjustment for bilateral procedures does not apply, assistant surgeon may be paid

50542   **Laparo ablate renal mass**   ~ follow-up period is 90 days, standard payment adjustment rules for multiple procedures apply, 150% payment adjustment for bilateral procedures does not apply, assistant surgeon may be paid

50543   **Laparo partial nephrectomy**   ~ follow-up period is 90 days, standard payment adjustment rules for multiple procedures apply, 150% payment adjustment for bilateral procedures does not apply, assistant surgeon may be paid

50544   **Laparoscopy, pyeloplasty**   ~ follow-up period is 90 days, standard payment adjustment rules for multiple procedures apply, 150% payment adjustment for bilateral procedures does not apply, assistant surgeon may be paid

50545   **Laparo radical nephrectomy**   ~ follow-up period is 90 days, standard payment adjustment rules for multiple procedures apply, 150% payment adjustment for bilateral procedures applies, assistant surgeon may be paid

50546   **Laparoscopic nephrectomy**   ~ follow-up period is 90 days, standard payment adjustment rules for multiple procedures apply, 150% payment adjustment for bilateral procedures does not apply, assistant surgeon may be paid

50547   **Laparo remove donor kidney**   ~ follow-up period is 90 days, standard payment adjustment rules for multiple procedures apply, 150% payment adjustment for bilateral procedures applies, assistant surgeon may be paid

50548   **Laparo remove w/ureter**   ~ follow-up period is 90 days, standard payment adjustment rules for multiple procedures apply, 150% payment adjustment for bilateral procedures does not apply, assistant surgeon may be paid

50549   **Laparoscope proc, renal**   ~ medicare carrier determines global period, standard payment adjustment rules for multiple procedures apply, 150% payment adjustment for bilateral procedures applies, assistant surgeon may be paid

50551   **Kidney endoscopy**   ~ endoscopies or minor procedure - E/M services on the same day generally not paid, standard payment adjustment rules for multiple procedures apply, 150% payment adjustment for bilateral procedures applies, payment for assistant surgeon subject to documentation of medical necessity

50553   **Kidney endoscopy**   ~ endoscopies or minor procedure - E/M services on the same day generally not paid, standard payment adjustment rules for multiple procedures apply, 150% payment adjustment for bilateral procedures applies, assistant surgeon may not be paid

50555   **Kidney endoscopy & biopsy**   ~ endoscopies or minor procedure - E/M services on the same day generally not paid, special rules for multiple endoscopic procedures apply if billed with another endoscopy in the same family, 150% payment adjustment for bilateral procedures applies, payment for assistant surgeon subject to documentation of medical necessity

50557   **Kidney endoscopy & treatment**   ~ endoscopies or minor procedure - E/M services on the same day generally not paid, special rules for multiple endoscopic procedures apply if billed with another endoscopy in the same family, 150% payment adjustment for bilateral procedures applies, payment for assistant surgeon subject to documentation of medical necessity

50561   **Kidney endoscopy & treatment**   ~ endoscopies or minor procedure - E/M services on the same day generally not paid, special rules for multiple endoscopic procedures apply if billed with another endoscopy in the same family, 150% payment adjustment for bilateral procedures applies, payment for assistant surgeon subject to documentation of medical necessity

50562   **Renal scope w/tumor resect**   ~ follow-up period is 90 days, standard payment adjustment rules for multiple procedures apply, 150% payment adjustment for bilateral procedures does not apply, assistant surgeon may be paid

50570   **Kidney endoscopy**   ~ endoscopies or minor procedure - E/M services on the same day generally not paid, standard payment adjustment rules for multiple procedures apply, 150% payment adjustment for bilateral procedures applies, payment for assistant surgeon subject to documentation of medical necessity

50572   **Kidney endoscopy**   ~ endoscopies or minor procedure - E/M services on the same day generally not paid, special rules for multiple endoscopic procedures apply if billed with another endoscopy in the same family, 150% payment adjustment for bilateral procedures applies, payment for assistant surgeon subject to documentation of medical necessity

50574   **Kidney endoscopy & biopsy**   ~ endoscopies or minor procedure - E/M services on the same day generally not paid, special rules for multiple endoscopic procedures apply if billed with another endoscopy in the same family, 150% payment adjustment for bilateral procedures applies, payment for assistant surgeon subject to documentation of medical necessity

50575   **Kidney endoscopy**   ~ endoscopies or minor procedure - E/M services on the same day generally not paid, special rules for multiple endoscopic procedures apply if billed with another endoscopy in the same family, 150% payment adjustment for bilateral procedures applies, assistant surgeon may not be paid

50576   **Kidney endoscopy & treatment**   ~ endoscopies or minor procedure - E/M services on the same day generally not paid, special rules for multiple endoscopic procedures apply if billed with another endoscopy in the same family, 150% payment adjustment for bilateral procedures applies, payment for assistant surgeon subject to documentation of medical necessity

50580   **Kidney endoscopy & treatment**   ~ endoscopies or minor procedure - E/M services on the same day generally not paid, special rules for multiple endoscopic procedures apply if billed with another endoscopy in the same family, 150% payment adjustment for bilateral procedures applies, payment for assistant surgeon subject to documentation of medical necessity

50590   **Fragmenting of kidney stone**   ~ follow-up period is 90 days, standard payment adjustment rules for multiple procedures apply, 150% payment adjustment for bilateral procedures applies, assistant surgeon may not be paid

50592   **Perc rf ablate renal tumor**   ~ follow-up period is 10 days, standard payment adjustment rules for multiple procedures apply, 150% payment adjustment for bilateral procedures applies, assistant surgeon may be paid

Ureter

50600   **Explore ureter**   ~ follow-up period is 90 days, standard payment adjustment rules for multiple procedures apply, 150% payment adjustment for bilateral procedures applies, assistant surgeon may be paid

50605   **Insert ureteral support**   ~ follow-up period is 90 days, standard payment adjustment rules for multiple procedures apply, 150% payment adjustment for bilateral procedures applies, assistant surgeon may be paid

50610   **Remove ureter stone**   ~ follow-up period is 90 days, standard payment adjustment rules for multiple procedures apply, 150% payment adjustment for bilateral procedures applies, assistant surgeon may be paid

50620   **Remove ureter stone**   ~ follow-up period is 90 days, standard payment adjustment rules for multiple procedures apply, 150% payment adjustment for bilateral procedures applies, assistant surgeon may be paid

50630   **Remove ureter stone**   ~ follow-up period is 90 days, standard payment adjustment rules for multiple procedures apply, 150% payment adjustment for bilateral procedures applies, assistant surgeon may be paid

50650   **Remove ureter**   ~ follow-up period is 90 days, standard payment adjustment rules for multiple procedures apply, 150% payment adjustment for bilateral procedures does not apply, assistant surgeon may be paid

50660   **Remove ureter**   ~ follow-up period is 90 days, standard payment adjustment rules for multiple procedures apply, 150% payment adjustment for bilateral procedures does not apply, assistant surgeon may be paid

50684 **Inject for ureter x-ray** ~ endoscopies or minor procedure - E/M services on the same day generally not paid, standard payment adjustment rules for multiple procedures apply, 150% payment adjustment for bilateral procedures applies, assistant surgeon may not be paid

50686 **Measure ureter pressure** ~ endoscopies or minor procedure - E/M services on the same day generally not paid, standard payment adjustment rules for multiple procedures apply, 150% payment adjustment for bilateral procedures does not apply, payment for assistant surgeon subject to documentation of medical necessity

50688 **Change of ureter tube/stent** ~ follow-up period is 10 days, standard payment adjustment rules for multiple procedures apply, 150% payment adjustment for bilateral procedures does not apply, assistant surgeon may not be paid

50690 **Inject for ureter x-ray** ~ endoscopies or minor procedure - E/M services on the same day generally not paid, standard payment adjustment rules for multiple procedures apply, 150% payment adjustment for bilateral procedures does not apply, assistant surgeon may not be paid

50700 **Revise ureter** ~ follow-up period is 90 days, standard payment adjustment rules for multiple procedures apply, 150% payment adjustment for bilateral procedures does not apply, assistant surgeon may be paid

50715 **Release ureter** ~ follow-up period is 90 days, standard payment adjustment rules for multiple procedures apply, 150% payment adjustment for bilateral procedures applies, assistant surgeon may be paid

50722 **Release ureter** ~ follow-up period is 90 days, standard payment adjustment rules for multiple procedures apply, 150% payment adjustment for bilateral procedures does not apply, assistant surgeon may be paid

50725 **Release/revise ureter** ~ follow-up period is 90 days, standard payment adjustment rules for multiple procedures apply, 150% payment adjustment for bilateral procedures does not apply, assistant surgeon may be paid

50727 **Revise ureter** ~ follow-up period is 90 days, standard payment adjustment rules for multiple procedures apply, 150% payment adjustment for bilateral procedures does not apply, assistant surgeon may be paid

50728 **Revise ureter** ~ follow-up period is 90 days, standard payment adjustment rules for multiple procedures apply, 150% payment adjustment for bilateral procedures does not apply, assistant surgeon may be paid

50740 **Fuse ureter & kidney** ~ follow-up period is 90 days, standard payment adjustment rules for multiple procedures apply, 150% payment adjustment for bilateral procedures does not apply, assistant surgeon may be paid

---

50750   **Fuse ureter & kidney**   ~ follow-up period is 90 days, standard payment adjustment rules for multiple procedures apply, 150% payment adjustment for bilateral procedures does not apply, assistant surgeon may be paid

50760   **Fuse ureters**   ~ follow-up period is 90 days, standard payment adjustment rules for multiple procedures apply, 150% payment adjustment for bilateral procedures does not apply, assistant surgeon may be paid

50770   **Splicing of ureters**   ~ follow-up period is 90 days, standard payment adjustment rules for multiple procedures apply, 150% payment adjustment for bilateral procedures does not apply, assistant surgeon may be paid

50780   **Reimplant ureter in bladder**   ~ follow-up period is 90 days, standard payment adjustment rules for multiple procedures apply, 150% payment adjustment for bilateral procedures applies, assistant surgeon may be paid

50782   **Reimplant ureter in bladder**   ~ follow-up period is 90 days, standard payment adjustment rules for multiple procedures apply, 150% payment adjustment for bilateral procedures applies, assistant surgeon may be paid

50783   **Reimplant ureter in bladder**   ~ follow-up period is 90 days, standard payment adjustment rules for multiple procedures apply, 150% payment adjustment for bilateral procedures applies, assistant surgeon may be paid

50785   **Reimplant ureter in bladder**   ~ follow-up period is 90 days, standard payment adjustment rules for multiple procedures apply, 150% payment adjustment for bilateral procedures applies, assistant surgeon may be paid

50800   **Implant ureter in bowel**   ~ follow-up period is 90 days, standard payment adjustment rules for multiple procedures apply, 150% payment adjustment for bilateral procedures applies, assistant surgeon may be paid

50810   **Fuse ureter & bowel**   ~ follow-up period is 90 days, standard payment adjustment rules for multiple procedures apply, 150% payment adjustment for bilateral procedures does not apply, assistant surgeon may be paid

50815   **Urine shunt to intestine**   ~ follow-up period is 90 days, standard payment adjustment rules for multiple procedures apply, 150% payment adjustment for bilateral procedures applies, assistant surgeon may be paid

50820   **Construct bowel bladder**   ~ follow-up period is 90 days, standard payment adjustment rules for multiple procedures apply, 150% payment adjustment for bilateral procedures applies, assistant surgeon may be paid

50825   **Construct bowel bladder**   ~ follow-up period is 90 days, standard payment adjustment rules for multiple procedures apply, 150% payment adjustment for bilateral procedures does not apply, assistant surgeon may be paid

50830 **Revise urine flow** ~ follow-up period is 90 days, standard payment adjustment rules for multiple procedures apply, 150% payment adjustment for bilateral procedures does not apply, assistant surgeon may be paid

50840 **Replace ureter by bowel** ~ follow-up period is 90 days, standard payment adjustment rules for multiple procedures apply, 150% payment adjustment for bilateral procedures applies, assistant surgeon may be paid

50845 **Appendico-vesicostomy** ~ follow-up period is 90 days, standard payment adjustment rules for multiple procedures apply, 150% payment adjustment for bilateral procedures does not apply, assistant surgeon may be paid

50860 **Transplant ureter to skin** ~ follow-up period is 90 days, standard payment adjustment rules for multiple procedures apply, 150% payment adjustment for bilateral procedures applies, assistant surgeon may be paid

50900 **Repair ureter** ~ follow-up period is 90 days, standard payment adjustment rules for multiple procedures apply, 150% payment adjustment for bilateral procedures does not apply, assistant surgeon may be paid

50920 **Closure ureter/skin fistula** ~ follow-up period is 90 days, standard payment adjustment rules for multiple procedures apply, 150% payment adjustment for bilateral procedures does not apply, assistant surgeon may be paid

50930 **Closure ureter/bowel fistula** ~ follow-up period is 90 days, standard payment adjustment rules for multiple procedures apply, 150% payment adjustment for bilateral procedures does not apply, assistant surgeon may be paid

50940 **Release ureter** ~ follow-up period is 90 days, standard payment adjustment rules for multiple procedures apply, 150% payment adjustment for bilateral procedures applies, assistant surgeon may be paid

50945 **Laparoscopy ureterolithotomy** ~ follow-up period is 90 days, standard payment adjustment rules for multiple procedures apply, 150% payment adjustment for bilateral procedures applies, assistant surgeon may be paid

50947 **Laparo new ureter/bladder** ~ follow-up period is 90 days, standard payment adjustment rules for multiple procedures apply, 150% payment adjustment for bilateral procedures applies, assistant surgeon may be paid

50948 **Laparo new ureter/bladder** ~ follow-up period is 90 days, standard payment adjustment rules for multiple procedures apply, 150% payment adjustment for bilateral procedures applies, assistant surgeon may be paid

50949 **Laparoscope proc, ureter** ~ medicare carrier determines global period, standard payment adjustment rules for multiple procedures apply, 150% payment adjustment for bilateral procedures applies, assistant surgeon may be paid

50951   **Endoscopy of ureter**   ~ endoscopies or minor procedure - E/M services on the same day generally not paid, standard payment adjustment rules for multiple procedures apply, 150% payment adjustment for bilateral procedures applies, payment for assistant surgeon subject to documentation of medical necessity

50953   **Endoscopy of ureter**   ~ endoscopies or minor procedure - E/M services on the same day generally not paid, special rules for multiple endoscopic procedures apply if billed with another endoscopy in the same family, 150% payment adjustment for bilateral procedures applies, payment for assistant surgeon subject to documentation of medical necessity

50955   **Ureter endoscopy & biopsy**   ~ endoscopies or minor procedure - E/M services on the same day generally not paid, special rules for multiple endoscopic procedures apply if billed with another endoscopy in the same family, 150% payment adjustment for bilateral procedures applies, payment for assistant surgeon subject to documentation of medical necessity

50957   **Ureter endoscopy & treatment**   ~ endoscopies or minor procedure - E/M services on the same day generally not paid, special rules for multiple endoscopic procedures apply if billed with another endoscopy in the same family, 150% payment adjustment for bilateral procedures applies, payment for assistant surgeon subject to documentation of medical necessity

50961   **Ureter endoscopy & treatment**   ~ endoscopies or minor procedure - E/M services on the same day generally not paid, special rules for multiple endoscopic procedures apply if billed with another endoscopy in the same family, 150% payment adjustment for bilateral procedures applies, payment for assistant surgeon subject to documentation of medical necessity

50970   **Ureter endoscopy**   ~ endoscopies or minor procedure - E/M services on the same day generally not paid, standard payment adjustment rules for multiple procedures apply, 150% payment adjustment for bilateral procedures applies, payment for assistant surgeon subject to documentation of medical necessity

50972   **Ureter endoscopy & catheter**   ~ endoscopies or minor procedure - E/M services on the same day generally not paid, standard payment adjustment rules for multiple procedures apply, 150% payment adjustment for bilateral procedures applies, payment for assistant surgeon subject to documentation of medical necessity

50974   **Ureter endoscopy & biopsy**   ~ endoscopies or minor procedure - E/M services on the same day generally not paid, special rules for multiple endoscopic procedures apply if billed with another endoscopy in the same family, 150% payment adjustment for bilateral procedures applies, payment for assistant surgeon subject to documentation of medical necessity

50976   **Ureter endoscopy & treatment**   ~ endoscopies or minor procedure - E/M services on the same day generally not paid, special rules for multiple endoscopic procedures apply if billed with another endoscopy in the same family, 150% payment adjustment for bilateral procedures applies, payment for assistant surgeon subject to documentation of medical necessity

50980   **Ureter endoscopy & treatment**   ~ endoscopies or minor procedure - E/M services on the same day generally not paid, standard payment adjustment rules for multiple procedures apply, 150% payment adjustment for bilateral procedures applies, payment for assistant surgeon subject to documentation of medical necessity

Bladder

51000   **Drain bladder**   ~ endoscopies or minor procedure - E/M services on the same day generally not paid, standard payment adjustment rules for multiple procedures apply, 150% payment adjustment for bilateral procedures does not apply, assistant surgeon may not be paid

51005   **Drain bladder**   ~ endoscopies or minor procedure - E/M services on the same day generally not paid, standard payment adjustment rules for multiple procedures apply, 150% payment adjustment for bilateral procedures does not apply, assistant surgeon may not be paid

51010   **Drain bladder**   ~ follow-up period is 10 days, standard payment adjustment rules for multiple procedures apply, 150% payment adjustment for bilateral procedures does not apply, assistant surgeon may not be paid

51020   **Incise & treat bladder**   ~ follow-up period is 90 days, standard payment adjustment rules for multiple procedures apply, 150% payment adjustment for bilateral procedures does not apply, assistant surgeon may be paid

51030   **Incise & treat bladder**   ~ follow-up period is 90 days, standard payment adjustment rules for multiple procedures apply, 150% payment adjustment for bilateral procedures does not apply, payment for assistant surgeon subject to documentation of medical necessity

51040   **Incise & drain bladder**   ~ follow-up period is 90 days, standard payment adjustment rules for multiple procedures apply, 150% payment adjustment for bilateral procedures does not apply, assistant surgeon may be paid

51045   **Incise bladder/drain ureter**   ~ follow-up period is 90 days, standard payment adjustment rules for multiple procedures apply, 150% payment adjustment for bilateral procedures does not apply, assistant surgeon may be paid

51050   **Remove bladder stone**   ~ follow-up period is 90 days, standard payment adjustment rules for multiple procedures apply, 150% payment adjustment for bilateral procedures does not apply, assistant surgeon may be paid

51060 **Remove ureter stone** ~ follow-up period is 90 days, standard payment adjustment rules for multiple procedures apply, 150% payment adjustment for bilateral procedures does not apply, assistant surgeon may be paid

51065 **Remove ureter calculus** ~ follow-up period is 90 days, standard payment adjustment rules for multiple procedures apply, 150% payment adjustment for bilateral procedures does not apply, payment for assistant surgeon subject to documentation of medical necessity

51080 **Drain bladder abscess** ~ follow-up period is 90 days, standard payment adjustment rules for multiple procedures apply, 150% payment adjustment for bilateral procedures does not apply, assistant surgeon may be paid

51500 **Remove bladder cyst** ~ follow-up period is 90 days, standard payment adjustment rules for multiple procedures apply, 150% payment adjustment for bilateral procedures does not apply, assistant surgeon may be paid

51520 **Remove bladder lesion** ~ follow-up period is 90 days, standard payment adjustment rules for multiple procedures apply, 150% payment adjustment for bilateral procedures does not apply, assistant surgeon may be paid

51525 **Remove bladder lesion** ~ follow-up period is 90 days, standard payment adjustment rules for multiple procedures apply, 150% payment adjustment for bilateral procedures does not apply, assistant surgeon may be paid

51530 **Remove bladder lesion** ~ follow-up period is 90 days, standard payment adjustment rules for multiple procedures apply, 150% payment adjustment for bilateral procedures does not apply, assistant surgeon may be paid

51535 **Repair ureter lesion** ~ follow-up period is 90 days, standard payment adjustment rules for multiple procedures apply, 150% payment adjustment for bilateral procedures applies, assistant surgeon may be paid

51550 **Partial remove bladder** ~ follow-up period is 90 days, standard payment adjustment rules for multiple procedures apply, 150% payment adjustment for bilateral procedures does not apply, assistant surgeon may be paid

51555 **Partial remove bladder** ~ follow-up period is 90 days, standard payment adjustment rules for multiple procedures apply, 150% payment adjustment for bilateral procedures does not apply, assistant surgeon may be paid

51565 **Revise bladder & ureter(s)** ~ follow-up period is 90 days, standard payment adjustment rules for multiple procedures apply, 150% payment adjustment for bilateral procedures does not apply, assistant surgeon may be paid

51570   **Remove bladder**   ~ follow-up period is 90 days, standard payment adjustment rules for multiple procedures apply, 150% payment adjustment for bilateral procedures does not apply, assistant surgeon may be paid

51575   **Remove bladder & nodes**   ~ follow-up period is 90 days, standard payment adjustment rules for multiple procedures apply, 150% payment adjustment does not apply - RVUs based on bilateral procedure, assistant surgeon may be paid

51580   **Remove bladder/revise tract**   ~ follow-up period is 90 days, standard payment adjustment rules for multiple procedures apply, 150% payment adjustment for bilateral procedures does not apply, assistant surgeon may be paid

51585   **Remove bladder & nodes**   ~ follow-up period is 90 days, standard payment adjustment rules for multiple procedures apply, 150% payment adjustment does not apply - RVUs based on bilateral procedure, assistant surgeon may be paid

51590   **Remove bladder/revise tract**   ~ follow-up period is 90 days, standard payment adjustment rules for multiple procedures apply, 150% payment adjustment for bilateral procedures does not apply, assistant surgeon may be paid

51595   **Remove bladder/revise tract**   ~ follow-up period is 90 days, standard payment adjustment rules for multiple procedures apply, 150% payment adjustment does not apply - RVUs based on bilateral procedure, assistant surgeon may be paid

51596   **Remove bladder/create pouch**   ~ follow-up period is 90 days, standard payment adjustment rules for multiple procedures apply, 150% payment adjustment for bilateral procedures does not apply, assistant surgeon may be paid

51597   **Remove pelvic structures**   ~ follow-up period is 90 days, standard payment adjustment rules for multiple procedures apply, 150% payment adjustment for bilateral procedures does not apply, assistant surgeon may be paid

51600   **Inject for bladder x-ray**   ~ endoscopies or minor procedure - E/M services on the same day generally not paid, standard payment adjustment rules for multiple procedures apply, 150% payment adjustment for bilateral procedures does not apply, assistant surgeon may not be paid

51605   **Prepare for bladder x-ray**   ~ endoscopies or minor procedure - E/M services on the same day generally not paid, standard payment adjustment rules for multiple procedures apply, 150% payment adjustment for bilateral procedures does not apply, assistant surgeon may not be paid

51610   **Inject for bladder x-ray**   ~ endoscopies or minor procedure - E/M services on the same day generally not paid, standard payment adjustment rules for multiple procedures apply, 150% payment adjustment for bilateral procedures does not apply, assistant surgeon may not be paid

51700   **Irrigation of bladder**   ~ endoscopies or minor procedure - E/M services on the same day generally not paid, standard payment adjustment rules for multiple procedures apply, 150% payment adjustment for bilateral procedures does not apply, assistant surgeon may not be paid

51701   **Insert bladder catheter**   ~ endoscopies or minor procedure - E/M services on the same day generally not paid, standard payment adjustment rules for multiple procedures apply, 150% payment adjustment for bilateral procedures does not apply, assistant surgeon may not be paid

51702   **Insert temp bladder cath**   ~ endoscopies or minor procedure - E/M services on the same day generally not paid, standard payment adjustment rules for multiple procedures apply, 150% payment adjustment for bilateral procedures does not apply, assistant surgeon may not be paid

51703   **Insert bladder cath, complex**   ~ endoscopies or minor procedure - E/M services on the same day generally not paid, standard payment adjustment rules for multiple procedures apply, 150% payment adjustment for bilateral procedures does not apply, assistant surgeon may not be paid

51705   **Change of bladder tube**   ~ follow-up period is 10 days, standard payment adjustment rules for multiple procedures apply, 150% payment adjustment for bilateral procedures does not apply, assistant surgeon may not be paid

51710   **Change of bladder tube**   ~ follow-up period is 10 days, standard payment adjustment rules for multiple procedures apply, 150% payment adjustment for bilateral procedures does not apply, assistant surgeon may not be paid

51715   **Endoscopic injection/implant**   ~ endoscopies or minor procedure - E/M services on the same day generally not paid, standard payment adjustment rules for multiple procedures apply, 150% payment adjustment for bilateral procedures does not apply, payment for assistant surgeon subject to documentation of medical necessity

51720   **Treat bladder lesion**   ~ endoscopies or minor procedure - E/M services on the same day generally not paid, standard payment adjustment rules for multiple procedures apply, 150% payment adjustment for bilateral procedures does not apply, assistant surgeon may not be paid

51725   **Simple cystometrogram**   ~ endoscopies or minor procedure - E/M services on the same day generally not paid, standard payment adjustment rules for multiple procedures apply, 150% payment adjustment for bilateral procedures does not apply, payment for assistant surgeon subject to documentation of medical necessity

51726   **Complex cystometrogram**   ~ endoscopies or minor procedure - E/M services on the same day generally not paid, standard payment adjustment rules for multiple procedures apply, 150% payment adjustment for bilateral procedures does not apply, assistant surgeon may not be paid

51736 **Urine flow measurement** ~ endoscopies or minor procedure - E/M services on the same day generally not paid, standard payment adjustment rules for multiple procedures apply, 150% payment adjustment for bilateral procedures does not apply, payment for assistant surgeon subject to documentation of medical necessity

51741 **Electro-uroflowmetry, first** ~ endoscopies or minor procedure - E/M services on the same day generally not paid, standard payment adjustment rules for multiple procedures apply, 150% payment adjustment for bilateral procedures does not apply, assistant surgeon may not be paid

51772 **Urethra pressure profile** ~ endoscopies or minor procedure - E/M services on the same day generally not paid, standard payment adjustment rules for multiple procedures apply, 150% payment adjustment for bilateral procedures does not apply, payment for assistant surgeon subject to documentation of medical necessity

51784 **Anal/urinary muscle study** ~ endoscopies or minor procedure - E/M services on the same day generally not paid, standard payment adjustment rules for multiple procedures apply, 150% payment adjustment for bilateral procedures does not apply, assistant surgeon may not be paid

51785 **Anal/urinary muscle study** ~ endoscopies or minor procedure - E/M services on the same day generally not paid, standard payment adjustment rules for multiple procedures apply, 150% payment adjustment for bilateral procedures does not apply, payment for assistant surgeon subject to documentation of medical necessity

51792 **Urinary reflex study** ~ endoscopies or minor procedure - E/M services on the same day generally not paid, standard payment adjustment rules for multiple procedures apply, 150% payment adjustment for bilateral procedures does not apply, payment for assistant surgeon subject to documentation of medical necessity

51795 **Urine voiding pressure study** ~ endoscopies or minor procedure - E/M services on the same day generally not paid, standard payment adjustment rules for multiple procedures apply, 150% payment adjustment for bilateral procedures does not apply, payment for assistant surgeon subject to documentation of medical necessity

51797 **Intraabdominal pressure test** ~ endoscopies or minor procedure - E/M services on the same day generally not paid, standard payment adjustment rules for multiple procedures apply, 150% payment adjustment for bilateral procedures does not apply, payment for assistant surgeon subject to documentation of medical necessity

51798 **Us urine capacity measure** ~ no payment adjustment rules for multiple procedures apply, 150% payment adjustment for bilateral procedures does not apply, payment for assistant surgeon subject to documentation of medical necessity

51800 **Revise bladder/urethra** ~ follow-up period is 90 days, standard payment adjustment rules for multiple procedures apply, 150% payment adjustment for bilateral procedures does not apply, assistant surgeon may be paid

---

51820   **Revise urinary tract**   ~ follow-up period is 90 days, standard payment adjustment rules for multiple procedures apply, 150% payment adjustment does not apply - RVUs based on bilateral procedure, assistant surgeon may be paid

51840   **Attach bladder/urethra**   ~ follow-up period is 90 days, standard payment adjustment rules for multiple procedures apply, 150% payment adjustment for bilateral procedures does not apply, assistant surgeon may be paid

51841   **Attach bladder/urethra**   ~ follow-up period is 90 days, standard payment adjustment rules for multiple procedures apply, 150% payment adjustment for bilateral procedures does not apply, assistant surgeon may be paid

51845   **Repair bladder neck**   ~ follow-up period is 90 days, standard payment adjustment rules for multiple procedures apply, 150% payment adjustment for bilateral procedures does not apply, assistant surgeon may be paid

51860   **Repair bladder wound**   ~ follow-up period is 90 days, standard payment adjustment rules for multiple procedures apply, 150% payment adjustment for bilateral procedures does not apply, assistant surgeon may be paid

51865   **Repair bladder wound**   ~ follow-up period is 90 days, standard payment adjustment rules for multiple procedures apply, 150% payment adjustment for bilateral procedures does not apply, assistant surgeon may be paid

51880   **Repair bladder opening**   ~ follow-up period is 90 days, standard payment adjustment rules for multiple procedures apply, 150% payment adjustment for bilateral procedures does not apply, assistant surgeon may be paid

51900   **Repair bladder/vagina lesion**   ~ follow-up period is 90 days, standard payment adjustment rules for multiple procedures apply, 150% payment adjustment for bilateral procedures does not apply, assistant surgeon may be paid

51920   **Close bladder-uterus fistula**   ~ follow-up period is 90 days, standard payment adjustment rules for multiple procedures apply, 150% payment adjustment for bilateral procedures does not apply, assistant surgeon may be paid

51925   **Hysterectomy/bladder repair**   ~ follow-up period is 90 days, standard payment adjustment rules for multiple procedures apply, 150% payment adjustment for bilateral procedures does not apply, assistant surgeon may be paid

51940   **Correct bladder defect**   ~ follow-up period is 90 days, standard payment adjustment rules for multiple procedures apply, 150% payment adjustment for bilateral procedures does not apply, assistant surgeon may be paid

51960   **Revise bladder & bowel**   ~ follow-up period is 90 days, standard payment adjustment rules for multiple procedures apply, 150% payment adjustment for bilateral procedures does not apply, assistant surgeon may be paid

51980 **Construct bladder opening** ~ follow-up period is 90 days, standard payment adjustment rules for multiple procedures apply, 150% payment adjustment for bilateral procedures does not apply, assistant surgeon may be paid

51990 **Laparo urethral suspension** ~ follow-up period is 90 days, standard payment adjustment rules for multiple procedures apply, 150% payment adjustment for bilateral procedures does not apply, assistant surgeon may be paid

51992 **Laparo sling operation** ~ follow-up period is 90 days, standard payment adjustment rules for multiple procedures apply, 150% payment adjustment for bilateral procedures does not apply, assistant surgeon may be paid

51999 **Laparoscope proc, bla** ~ medicare carrier determines global period, no payment adjustment rules for multiple procedures apply, 150% payment adjustment for bilateral procedures does not apply, payment for assistant surgeon subject to documentation of medical necessity

52000 **Cystoscopy** ~ endoscopies or minor procedure - E/M services on the same day generally not paid, standard payment adjustment rules for multiple procedures apply, 150% payment adjustment for bilateral procedures does not apply, assistant surgeon may not be paid

52001 **Cystoscopy, remove clots** ~ endoscopies or minor procedure - E/M services on the same day generally not paid, special rules for multiple endoscopic procedures apply if billed with another endoscopy in the same family, 150% payment adjustment for bilateral procedures does not apply, assistant surgeon may not be paid

52005 **Cystoscopy & ureter catheter** ~ endoscopies or minor procedure - E/M services on the same day generally not paid, special rules for multiple endoscopic procedures apply if billed with another endoscopy in the same family, 150% payment adjustment for bilateral procedures does not apply, assistant surgeon may not be paid

52007 **Cystoscopy and biopsy** ~ endoscopies or minor procedure - E/M services on the same day generally not paid, special rules for multiple endoscopic procedures apply if billed with another endoscopy in the same family, 150% payment adjustment for bilateral procedures applies, assistant surgeon may not be paid

52010 **Cystoscopy & duct catheter** ~ endoscopies or minor procedure - E/M services on the same day generally not paid, special rules for multiple endoscopic procedures apply if billed with another endoscopy in the same family, 150% payment adjustment for bilateral procedures does not apply, assistant surgeon may not be paid

52204 **Cystoscopy w/biopsy(s)** ~ endoscopies or minor procedure - E/M services on the same day generally not paid, special rules for multiple endoscopic procedures apply if billed with another endoscopy in the same family, 150% payment adjustment for bilateral procedures does not apply, assistant surgeon may not be paid

52214   **Cystoscopy and treatment**   ~ endoscopies or minor procedure - E/M services on the same day generally not paid, special rules for multiple endoscopic procedures apply if billed with another endoscopy in the same family, 150% payment adjustment for bilateral procedures does not apply, assistant surgeon may not be paid

52224   **Cystoscopy and treatment**   ~ endoscopies or minor procedure - E/M services on the same day generally not paid, special rules for multiple endoscopic procedures apply if billed with another endoscopy in the same family, 150% payment adjustment for bilateral procedures does not apply, assistant surgeon may not be paid

52234   **Cystoscopy and treatment**   ~ endoscopies or minor procedure - E/M services on the same day generally not paid, special rules for multiple endoscopic procedures apply if billed with another endoscopy in the same family, 150% payment adjustment for bilateral procedures does not apply, assistant surgeon may not be paid

52235   **Cystoscopy and treatment**   ~ endoscopies or minor procedure - E/M services on the same day generally not paid, special rules for multiple endoscopic procedures apply if billed with another endoscopy in the same family, 150% payment adjustment for bilateral procedures does not apply, assistant surgeon may not be paid

52240   **Cystoscopy and treatment**   ~ endoscopies or minor procedure - E/M services on the same day generally not paid, special rules for multiple endoscopic procedures apply if billed with another endoscopy in the same family, 150% payment adjustment for bilateral procedures does not apply, assistant surgeon may not be paid

52250   **Cystoscopy and radiotracer**   ~ endoscopies or minor procedure - E/M services on the same day generally not paid, special rules for multiple endoscopic procedures apply if billed with another endoscopy in the same family, 150% payment adjustment for bilateral procedures does not apply, assistant surgeon may not be paid

52260   **Cystoscopy and treatment**   ~ endoscopies or minor procedure - E/M services on the same day generally not paid, special rules for multiple endoscopic procedures apply if billed with another endoscopy in the same family, 150% payment adjustment for bilateral procedures does not apply, assistant surgeon may not be paid

52265   **Cystoscopy and treatment**   ~ endoscopies or minor procedure - E/M services on the same day generally not paid, special rules for multiple endoscopic procedures apply if billed with another endoscopy in the same family, 150% payment adjustment for bilateral procedures does not apply, assistant surgeon may not be paid

52270   **Cystoscopy & revise urethra**   ~ endoscopies or minor procedure - E/M services on the same day generally not paid, special rules for multiple endoscopic procedures apply if billed with another endoscopy in the same family, 150% payment adjustment for bilateral procedures does not apply, assistant surgeon may not be paid

52275   **Cystoscopy & revise urethra**   ~ endoscopies or minor procedure - E/M services on the same day generally not paid, special rules for multiple endoscopic

procedures apply if billed with another endoscopy in the same family, 150% payment adjustment for bilateral procedures does not apply, assistant surgeon may not be paid

52276 **Cystoscopy and treatment** ~ endoscopies or minor procedure - E/M services on the same day generally not paid, special rules for multiple endoscopic procedures apply if billed with another endoscopy in the same family, 150% payment adjustment for bilateral procedures does not apply, assistant surgeon may not be paid

52277 **Cystoscopy and treatment** ~ endoscopies or minor procedure - E/M services on the same day generally not paid, special rules for multiple endoscopic procedures apply if billed with another endoscopy in the same family, 150% payment adjustment for bilateral procedures does not apply, payment for assistant surgeon subject to documentation of medical necessity

52281 **Cystoscopy and treatment** ~ endoscopies or minor procedure - E/M services on the same day generally not paid, special rules for multiple endoscopic procedures apply if billed with another endoscopy in the same family, 150% payment adjustment for bilateral procedures does not apply, assistant surgeon may not be paid

52282 **Cystoscopy, implant stent** ~ endoscopies or minor procedure - E/M services on the same day generally not paid, special rules for multiple endoscopic procedures apply if billed with another endoscopy in the same family, 150% payment adjustment for bilateral procedures does not apply, assistant surgeon may not be paid

52283 **Cystoscopy and treatment** ~ endoscopies or minor procedure - E/M services on the same day generally not paid, special rules for multiple endoscopic procedures apply if billed with another endoscopy in the same family, 150% payment adjustment for bilateral procedures does not apply, assistant surgeon may not be paid

52285 **Cystoscopy and treatment** ~ endoscopies or minor procedure - E/M services on the same day generally not paid, special rules for multiple endoscopic procedures apply if billed with another endoscopy in the same family, 150% payment adjustment for bilateral procedures does not apply, assistant surgeon may not be paid

52290 **Cystoscopy and treatment** ~ endoscopies or minor procedure - E/M services on the same day generally not paid, special rules for multiple endoscopic procedures apply if billed with another endoscopy in the same family, 150% payment adjustment does not apply - RVUs based on bilateral procedure, assistant surgeon may not be paid

52300 **Cystoscopy and treatment** ~ endoscopies or minor procedure - E/M services on the same day generally not paid, special rules for multiple endoscopic procedures apply if billed with another endoscopy in the same family, 150% payment adjustment does not apply - RVUs based on bilateral procedure, payment for assistant surgeon subject to documentation of medical necessity

52301   **Cystoscopy and treatment**   ~ endoscopies or minor procedure - E/M services on the same day generally not paid, special rules for multiple endoscopic procedures apply if billed with another endoscopy in the same family, 150% payment adjustment does not apply - RVUs based on bilateral procedure, payment for assistant surgeon subject to documentation of medical necessity

52305   **Cystoscopy and treatment**   ~ endoscopies or minor procedure - E/M services on the same day generally not paid, special rules for multiple endoscopic procedures apply if billed with another endoscopy in the same family, 150% payment adjustment for bilateral procedures does not apply, assistant surgeon may not be paid

52310   **Cystoscopy and treatment**   ~ endoscopies or minor procedure - E/M services on the same day generally not paid, special rules for multiple endoscopic procedures apply if billed with another endoscopy in the same family, 150% payment adjustment for bilateral procedures does not apply, assistant surgeon may not be paid

52315   **Cystoscopy and treatment**   ~ endoscopies or minor procedure - E/M services on the same day generally not paid, special rules for multiple endoscopic procedures apply if billed with another endoscopy in the same family, 150% payment adjustment for bilateral procedures does not apply, assistant surgeon may not be paid

52317   **Remove bladder stone**   ~ endoscopies or minor procedure - E/M services on the same day generally not paid, special rules for multiple endoscopic procedures apply if billed with another endoscopy in the same family, 150% payment adjustment for bilateral procedures does not apply, assistant surgeon may not be paid

52318   **Remove bladder stone**   ~ endoscopies or minor procedure - E/M services on the same day generally not paid, special rules for multiple endoscopic procedures apply if billed with another endoscopy in the same family, 150% payment adjustment for bilateral procedures does not apply, assistant surgeon may not be paid

52320   **Cystoscopy and treatment**   ~ endoscopies or minor procedure - E/M services on the same day generally not paid, special rules for multiple endoscopic procedures apply if billed with another endoscopy in the same family, 150% payment adjustment for bilateral procedures applies, assistant surgeon may not be paid

52325   **Cystoscopy, stone remove**   ~ endoscopies or minor procedure - E/M services on the same day generally not paid, special rules for multiple endoscopic procedures apply if billed with another endoscopy in the same family, 150% payment adjustment for bilateral procedures applies, assistant surgeon may not be paid

52327   **Cystoscopy, inject material**   ~ endoscopies or minor procedure - E/M services on the same day generally not paid, special rules for multiple endoscopic procedures apply if billed with another endoscopy in the same family, 150% payment adjustment for bilateral procedures applies, assistant surgeon may not be paid

52330 **Cystoscopy and treatment** ~ endoscopies or minor procedure - E/M services on the same day generally not paid, special rules for multiple endoscopic procedures apply if billed with another endoscopy in the same family, 150% payment adjustment for bilateral procedures applies, assistant surgeon may not be paid

52332 **Cystoscopy and treatment** ~ endoscopies or minor procedure - E/M services on the same day generally not paid, special rules for multiple endoscopic procedures apply if billed with another endoscopy in the same family, 150% payment adjustment for bilateral procedures applies, assistant surgeon may not be paid

52334 **Create passage to kidney** ~ endoscopies or minor procedure - E/M services on the same day generally not paid, special rules for multiple endoscopic procedures apply if billed with another endoscopy in the same family, 150% payment adjustment for bilateral procedures applies, assistant surgeon may not be paid

52341 **Cystoscopy w/ureter stricture tx** ~ endoscopies or minor procedure - E/M services on the same day generally not paid, special rules for multiple endoscopic procedures apply if billed with another endoscopy in the same family, 150% payment adjustment for bilateral procedures applies, assistant surgeon may not be paid

52342 **Cystoscopy w/up stricture tx** ~ endoscopies or minor procedure - E/M services on the same day generally not paid, special rules for multiple endoscopic procedures apply if billed with another endoscopy in the same family, 150% payment adjustment for bilateral procedures applies, assistant surgeon may not be paid

52343 **Cystoscopy w/renal stricture tx** ~ endoscopies or minor procedure - E/M services on the same day generally not paid, special rules for multiple endoscopic procedures apply if billed with another endoscopy in the same family, 150% payment adjustment for bilateral procedures applies, assistant surgeon may not be paid

52344 **Cystoscopy/uretero, stricture tx** ~ endoscopies or minor procedure - E/M services on the same day generally not paid, special rules for multiple endoscopic procedures apply if billed with another endoscopy in the same family, 150% payment adjustment for bilateral procedures applies, assistant surgeon may not be paid

52345 **Cystoscopy/uretero w/up stricture** ~ endoscopies or minor procedure - E/M services on the same day generally not paid, special rules for multiple endoscopic procedures apply if billed with another endoscopy in the same family, 150% payment adjustment for bilateral procedures does not apply, payment for assistant surgeon subject to documentation of medical necessity

52346 **Cystouretero w/renal strict** ~ endoscopies or minor procedure - E/M services on the same day generally not paid, special rules for multiple endoscopic procedures apply if billed with another endoscopy in the same family, 150% payment adjustment for bilateral procedures does not apply, payment for assistant surgeon subject to documentation of medical necessity

52351   **Cystouretero & or pyeloscope**   ~ endoscopies or minor procedure - E/M services on the same day generally not paid, standard payment adjustment rules for multiple procedures apply, 150% payment adjustment for bilateral procedures does not apply, assistant surgeon may not be paid

52352   **Cystouretero w/stone remove**   ~ endoscopies or minor procedure - E/M services on the same day generally not paid, special rules for multiple endoscopic procedures apply if billed with another endoscopy in the same family, 150% payment adjustment for bilateral procedures applies, assistant surgeon may not be paid

52353   **Cystouretero w/lithotripsy**   ~ endoscopies or minor procedure - E/M services on the same day generally not paid, special rules for multiple endoscopic procedures apply if billed with another endoscopy in the same family, 150% payment adjustment for bilateral procedures applies, assistant surgeon may not be paid

52354   **Cystouretero w/biopsy**   ~ endoscopies or minor procedure - E/M services on the same day generally not paid, special rules for multiple endoscopic procedures apply if billed with another endoscopy in the same family, 150% payment adjustment for bilateral procedures applies, assistant surgeon may not be paid

52355   **Cystouretero w/excise tumor**   ~ endoscopies or minor procedure - E/M services on the same day generally not paid, special rules for multiple endoscopic procedures apply if billed with another endoscopy in the same family, 150% payment adjustment for bilateral procedures applies, assistant surgeon may not be paid

Vesical Neck and Prostate

52400   **Cystouretero w/congenital repair**   ~ follow-up period is 90 days, special rules for multiple endoscopic procedures apply if billed with another endoscopy in the same family, 150% payment adjustment for bilateral procedures does not apply, assistant surgeon may not be paid

52402   **Cystouretero cut ejaculatory duct**   ~ endoscopies or minor procedure - E/M services on the same day generally not paid, special rules for multiple endoscopic procedures apply if billed with another endoscopy in the same family, 150% payment adjustment for bilateral procedures does not apply, payment for assistant surgeon subject to documentation of medical necessity

52450   **Incise prostate**   ~ follow-up period is 90 days, standard payment adjustment rules for multiple procedures apply, 150% payment adjustment for bilateral procedures does not apply, assistant surgeon may not be paid

52500   **Revise bladder neck**   ~ follow-up period is 90 days, standard payment adjustment rules for multiple procedures apply, 150% payment adjustment for bilateral procedures does not apply, assistant surgeon may not be paid

    CPT codes and descriptions only copyright American Medical Association

52510 **Dilate prostatic urethra** ~ follow-up period is 90 days, standard payment adjustment rules for multiple procedures apply, 150% payment adjustment for bilateral procedures does not apply, assistant surgeon may not be paid

52601 **Prostatectomy (turp)** ~ follow-up period is 90 days, standard payment adjustment rules for multiple procedures apply, 150% payment adjustment for bilateral procedures does not apply, assistant surgeon may not be paid

52606 **Control postop bleeding** ~ follow-up period is 90 days, standard payment adjustment rules for multiple procedures apply, 150% payment adjustment for bilateral procedures does not apply, assistant surgeon may not be paid

52612 **Prostatectomy, first stage** ~ follow-up period is 90 days, standard payment adjustment rules for multiple procedures apply, 150% payment adjustment for bilateral procedures does not apply, assistant surgeon may not be paid

52614 **Prostatectomy, second stage** ~ follow-up period is 90 days, standard payment adjustment rules for multiple procedures apply, 150% payment adjustment for bilateral procedures does not apply, assistant surgeon may not be paid

52620 **Remove residual prostate** ~ follow-up period is 90 days, standard payment adjustment rules for multiple procedures apply, 150% payment adjustment for bilateral procedures does not apply, assistant surgeon may not be paid

52630 **Remove prostate regrowth** ~ follow-up period is 90 days, standard payment adjustment rules for multiple procedures apply, 150% payment adjustment for bilateral procedures does not apply, assistant surgeon may not be paid

52640 **Relieve bladder contracture** ~ follow-up period is 90 days, standard payment adjustment rules for multiple procedures apply, 150% payment adjustment for bilateral procedures does not apply, assistant surgeon may not be paid

52647 **Laser surgery prostate** ~ follow-up period is 90 days, standard payment adjustment rules for multiple procedures apply, 150% payment adjustment for bilateral procedures does not apply, assistant surgeon may not be paid

52648 **Laser surgery prostate** ~ follow-up period is 90 days, standard payment adjustment rules for multiple procedures apply, 150% payment adjustment for bilateral procedures does not apply, assistant surgeon may not be paid

52700 **Drain prostate abscess** ~ follow-up period is 90 days, standard payment adjustment rules for multiple procedures apply, 150% payment adjustment for bilateral procedures does not apply, payment for assistant surgeon subject to documentation of medical necessity

Urethra

53000   **Incise urethra**   ~ follow-up period is 10 days, standard payment adjustment rules for multiple procedures apply, 150% payment adjustment for bilateral procedures does not apply, assistant surgeon may not be paid

53010   **Incise urethra**   ~ follow-up period is 90 days, standard payment adjustment rules for multiple procedures apply, 150% payment adjustment for bilateral procedures does not apply, assistant surgeon may not be paid

53020   **Incise urethra**   ~ endoscopies or minor procedure - E/M services on the same day generally not paid, standard payment adjustment rules for multiple procedures apply, 150% payment adjustment for bilateral procedures does not apply, assistant surgeon may not be paid

53025   **Incise urethra**   ~ endoscopies or minor procedure - E/M services on the same day generally not paid, standard payment adjustment rules for multiple procedures apply, 150% payment adjustment for bilateral procedures does not apply, payment for assistant surgeon subject to documentation of medical necessity

53040   **Drain urethra abscess**   ~ follow-up period is 90 days, standard payment adjustment rules for multiple procedures apply, 150% payment adjustment for bilateral procedures does not apply, payment for assistant surgeon subject to documentation of medical necessity

53060   **Drain urethra abscess**   ~ follow-up period is 10 days, standard payment adjustment rules for multiple procedures apply, 150% payment adjustment for bilateral procedures does not apply, assistant surgeon may not be paid

53080   **Drain urinary leakage**   ~ follow-up period is 90 days, standard payment adjustment rules for multiple procedures apply, 150% payment adjustment for bilateral procedures does not apply, assistant surgeon may not be paid

53085   **Drain urinary leakage**   ~ follow-up period is 90 days, standard payment adjustment rules for multiple procedures apply, 150% payment adjustment for bilateral procedures does not apply, assistant surgeon may be paid

53200   **Biopsy urethra**   ~ endoscopies or minor procedure - E/M services on the same day generally not paid, standard payment adjustment rules for multiple procedures apply, 150% payment adjustment for bilateral procedures does not apply, assistant surgeon may not be paid

53210   **Remove urethra**   ~ follow-up period is 90 days, standard payment adjustment rules for multiple procedures apply, 150% payment adjustment for bilateral procedures does not apply, assistant surgeon may be paid

53215   **Remove urethra**   ~ follow-up period is 90 days, standard payment adjustment rules for multiple procedures apply, 150% payment adjustment for bilateral procedures does not apply, assistant surgeon may be paid

53220   **Treat urethra lesion**   ~ follow-up period is 90 days, standard payment adjustment rules for multiple procedures apply, 150% payment adjustment for bilateral procedures does not apply, payment for assistant surgeon subject to documentation of medical necessity

53230   **Remove urethra lesion**   ~ follow-up period is 90 days, standard payment adjustment rules for multiple procedures apply, 150% payment adjustment for bilateral procedures does not apply, assistant surgeon may be paid

53235   **Remove urethra lesion**   ~ follow-up period is 90 days, standard payment adjustment rules for multiple procedures apply, 150% payment adjustment for bilateral procedures does not apply, assistant surgeon may be paid

53240   **Surgery for urethra pouch**   ~ follow-up period is 90 days, standard payment adjustment rules for multiple procedures apply, 150% payment adjustment for bilateral procedures does not apply, assistant surgeon may not be paid

53250   **Remove urethra gland**   ~ follow-up period is 90 days, standard payment adjustment rules for multiple procedures apply, 150% payment adjustment for bilateral procedures does not apply, assistant surgeon may not be paid

53260   **Treat urethra lesion**   ~ follow-up period is 10 days, standard payment adjustment rules for multiple procedures apply, 150% payment adjustment for bilateral procedures does not apply, assistant surgeon may not be paid

53265   **Treat urethra lesion**   ~ follow-up period is 10 days, standard payment adjustment rules for multiple procedures apply, 150% payment adjustment for bilateral procedures does not apply, assistant surgeon may not be paid

53270   **Remove urethra gland**   ~ follow-up period is 10 days, standard payment adjustment rules for multiple procedures apply, 150% payment adjustment for bilateral procedures does not apply, assistant surgeon may not be paid

53275   **Repair urethra defect**   ~ follow-up period is 10 days, standard payment adjustment rules for multiple procedures apply, 150% payment adjustment for bilateral procedures does not apply, assistant surgeon may not be paid

53400   **Revise urethra, stage 1**   ~ follow-up period is 90 days, standard payment adjustment rules for multiple procedures apply, 150% payment adjustment for bilateral procedures does not apply, assistant surgeon may be paid

53405　　**Revise urethra, stage 2**　　　　~ follow-up period is 90 days, standard payment adjustment rules for multiple procedures apply, 150% payment adjustment for bilateral procedures does not apply, assistant surgeon may be paid

53410　　**Reconstruct urethra**　　　　~ follow-up period is 90 days, standard payment adjustment rules for multiple procedures apply, 150% payment adjustment for bilateral procedures does not apply, assistant surgeon may be paid

53415　　**Reconstruct urethra**　　　　~ follow-up period is 90 days, standard payment adjustment rules for multiple procedures apply, 150% payment adjustment for bilateral procedures does not apply, assistant surgeon may be paid

53420　　**Reconstruct urethra, stage 1**　　　　~ follow-up period is 90 days, standard payment adjustment rules for multiple procedures apply, 150% payment adjustment for bilateral procedures does not apply, assistant surgeon may not be paid

53425　　**Reconstruct urethra, stage 2**　　　　~ follow-up period is 90 days, standard payment adjustment rules for multiple procedures apply, 150% payment adjustment for bilateral procedures does not apply, assistant surgeon may be paid

53430　　**Reconstruct urethra**　　　　~ follow-up period is 90 days, standard payment adjustment rules for multiple procedures apply, 150% payment adjustment for bilateral procedures does not apply, assistant surgeon may be paid

53431　　**Reconstruct urethra/bladder**　　　　~ follow-up period is 90 days, standard payment adjustment rules for multiple procedures apply, 150% payment adjustment for bilateral procedures does not apply, assistant surgeon may be paid

53440　　**Male sling procedure**　　　　~ follow-up period is 90 days, standard payment adjustment rules for multiple procedures apply, 150% payment adjustment for bilateral procedures does not apply, assistant surgeon may be paid

53442　　**Remove/revise male sling**　　　　~ follow-up period is 90 days, standard payment adjustment rules for multiple procedures apply, 150% payment adjustment for bilateral procedures does not apply, assistant surgeon may be paid

53444　　**Insert tandem cuff**　　　　~ follow-up period is 90 days, standard payment adjustment rules for multiple procedures apply, 150% payment adjustment for bilateral procedures does not apply, assistant surgeon may be paid

53445　　**Insert uro/ves neck sphincter**　　　　~ follow-up period is 90 days, standard payment adjustment rules for multiple procedures apply, 150% payment adjustment for bilateral procedures does not apply, assistant surgeon may be paid

53446　　**Remove uro sphincter**　　　　~ follow-up period is 90 days, standard payment adjustment rules for multiple procedures apply, 150% payment adjustment for bilateral procedures does not apply, assistant surgeon may be paid

53447   **Remove/replace ur sphincter**   ~ follow-up period is 90 days, standard payment adjustment rules for multiple procedures apply, 150% payment adjustment for bilateral procedures does not apply, assistant surgeon may be paid

53448   **Remove/replace ur sphincter comp**   ~ follow-up period is 90 days, standard payment adjustment rules for multiple procedures apply, 150% payment adjustment for bilateral procedures does not apply, assistant surgeon may be paid

53449   **Repair uro sphincter**   ~ follow-up period is 90 days, standard payment adjustment rules for multiple procedures apply, 150% payment adjustment for bilateral procedures does not apply, assistant surgeon may be paid

53450   **Revise urethra**   ~ follow-up period is 90 days, standard payment adjustment rules for multiple procedures apply, 150% payment adjustment for bilateral procedures does not apply, assistant surgeon may not be paid

53460   **Revise urethra**   ~ follow-up period is 90 days, standard payment adjustment rules for multiple procedures apply, 150% payment adjustment for bilateral procedures does not apply, payment for assistant surgeon subject to documentation of medical necessity

53500   **Urethrolysis, transvaginal w/ scope**   ~ follow-up period is 90 days, standard payment adjustment rules for multiple procedures apply, 150% payment adjustment for bilateral procedures does not apply, assistant surgeon may be paid

53502   **Repair urethra injury**   ~ follow-up period is 90 days, standard payment adjustment rules for multiple procedures apply, 150% payment adjustment for bilateral procedures does not apply, assistant surgeon may not be paid

53505   **Repair urethra injury**   ~ follow-up period is 90 days, standard payment adjustment rules for multiple procedures apply, 150% payment adjustment for bilateral procedures does not apply, assistant surgeon may be paid

53510   **Repair urethra injury**   ~ follow-up period is 90 days, standard payment adjustment rules for multiple procedures apply, 150% payment adjustment for bilateral procedures does not apply, assistant surgeon may be paid

53515   **Repair urethra injury**   ~ follow-up period is 90 days, standard payment adjustment rules for multiple procedures apply, 150% payment adjustment for bilateral procedures does not apply, assistant surgeon may be paid

53520   **Repair urethra defect**   ~ follow-up period is 90 days, standard payment adjustment rules for multiple procedures apply, 150% payment adjustment for bilateral procedures does not apply, assistant surgeon may not be paid

53600   **Dilate urethra stricture**   ~ endoscopies or minor procedure - E/M services on the same day generally not paid, standard payment adjustment rules for multiple

procedures apply, 150% payment adjustment for bilateral procedures does not apply, assistant surgeon may not be paid

53601 **Dilate urethra stricture** ~ endoscopies or minor procedure - E/M services on the same day generally not paid, standard payment adjustment rules for multiple procedures apply, 150% payment adjustment for bilateral procedures does not apply, assistant surgeon may not be paid

53605 **Dilate urethra stricture** ~ endoscopies or minor procedure - E/M services on the same day generally not paid, standard payment adjustment rules for multiple procedures apply, 150% payment adjustment for bilateral procedures does not apply, assistant surgeon may not be paid

53620 **Dilate urethra stricture** ~ endoscopies or minor procedure - E/M services on the same day generally not paid, standard payment adjustment rules for multiple procedures apply, 150% payment adjustment for bilateral procedures does not apply, assistant surgeon may not be paid

53621 **Dilate urethra stricture** ~ endoscopies or minor procedure - E/M services on the same day generally not paid, standard payment adjustment rules for multiple procedures apply, 150% payment adjustment for bilateral procedures does not apply, assistant surgeon may not be paid

53660 **Dilate urethra** ~ endoscopies or minor procedure - E/M services on the same day generally not paid, standard payment adjustment rules for multiple procedures apply, 150% payment adjustment for bilateral procedures does not apply, assistant surgeon may not be paid

53661 **Dilate urethra** ~ endoscopies or minor procedure - E/M services on the same day generally not paid, standard payment adjustment rules for multiple procedures apply, 150% payment adjustment for bilateral procedures does not apply, assistant surgeon may not be paid

53665 **Dilate urethra** ~ endoscopies or minor procedure - E/M services on the same day generally not paid, standard payment adjustment rules for multiple procedures apply, 150% payment adjustment for bilateral procedures does not apply, assistant surgeon may not be paid

53850 **Prostatic microwave thermo tx** ~ follow-up period is 90 days, standard payment adjustment rules for multiple procedures apply, 150% payment adjustment for bilateral procedures does not apply, assistant surgeon may not be paid

53852 **Prostatic rf thermo tx** ~ follow-up period is 90 days, standard payment adjustment rules for multiple procedures apply, 150% payment adjustment for bilateral procedures does not apply, assistant surgeon may not be paid

53853   **Prostatic water thermotherapy**   ~ follow-up period is 90 days, standard payment adjustment rules for multiple procedures apply, 150% payment adjustment for bilateral procedures does not apply, assistant surgeon may not be paid

53899   **Urology surgery procedure**   ~ medicare carrier determines global period, standard payment adjustment rules for multiple procedures apply, 150% payment adjustment for bilateral procedures does not apply, payment for assistant surgeon subject to documentation of medical necessity

MALE GENITAL SYSTEM

Penis

54000   **Slitting of prepuce**   ~ follow-up period is 10 days, standard payment adjustment rules for multiple procedures apply, 150% payment adjustment for bilateral procedures does not apply, payment for assistant surgeon subject to documentation of medical necessity

54001   **Slitting of prepuce**   ~ follow-up period is 10 days, standard payment adjustment rules for multiple procedures apply, 150% payment adjustment for bilateral procedures does not apply, assistant surgeon may not be paid

54015   **Drain penis lesion**   ~ follow-up period is 10 days, standard payment adjustment rules for multiple procedures apply, 150% payment adjustment for bilateral procedures does not apply, payment for assistant surgeon subject to documentation of medical necessity

54050   **Destroy penis lesion(s)**   ~ follow-up period is 10 days, standard payment adjustment rules for multiple procedures apply, 150% payment adjustment for bilateral procedures does not apply, assistant surgeon may not be paid

54055   **Destroy penis lesion(s)**   ~ follow-up period is 10 days, standard payment adjustment rules for multiple procedures apply, 150% payment adjustment for bilateral procedures does not apply, assistant surgeon may not be paid

54056   **Cryosurgery, penis lesion(s)**   ~ follow-up period is 10 days, standard payment adjustment rules for multiple procedures apply, 150% payment adjustment for bilateral procedures does not apply, assistant surgeon may not be paid

54057   **Laser surg, penis lesion(s)**   ~ follow-up period is 10 days, standard payment adjustment rules for multiple procedures apply, 150% payment adjustment for bilateral procedures does not apply, assistant surgeon may not be paid

54060   **Excise penis lesion(s)**   ~ follow-up period is 10 days, standard payment adjustment rules for multiple procedures apply, 150% payment adjustment for bilateral procedures does not apply, assistant surgeon may not be paid

54065   **Destroy penis lesion(s)**   ~ follow-up period is 10 days, standard payment adjustment rules for multiple procedures apply, 150% payment adjustment for bilateral procedures does not apply, assistant surgeon may not be paid

54100   **Biopsy penis**   ~ endoscopies or minor procedure - E/M services on the same day generally not paid, standard payment adjustment rules for multiple procedures apply, 150% payment adjustment for bilateral procedures does not apply, assistant surgeon may not be paid

54105   **Biopsy penis**   ~ follow-up period is 10 days, standard payment adjustment rules for multiple procedures apply, 150% payment adjustment for bilateral procedures does not apply, assistant surgeon may not be paid

54110   **Treat penis lesion**   ~ follow-up period is 90 days, standard payment adjustment rules for multiple procedures apply, 150% payment adjustment for bilateral procedures does not apply, assistant surgeon may be paid

54111   **Treat penis lesion, graft**   ~ follow-up period is 90 days, standard payment adjustment rules for multiple procedures apply, 150% payment adjustment for bilateral procedures does not apply, assistant surgeon may be paid

54112   **Treat penis lesion, graft**   ~ follow-up period is 90 days, standard payment adjustment rules for multiple procedures apply, 150% payment adjustment for bilateral procedures does not apply, assistant surgeon may be paid

54115   **Treat penis lesion**   ~ follow-up period is 90 days, standard payment adjustment rules for multiple procedures apply, 150% payment adjustment for bilateral procedures does not apply, assistant surgeon may be paid

54120   **Partial remove penis**   ~ follow-up period is 90 days, standard payment adjustment rules for multiple procedures apply, 150% payment adjustment for bilateral procedures does not apply, assistant surgeon may be paid

54125   **Remove penis**   ~ follow-up period is 90 days, standard payment adjustment rules for multiple procedures apply, 150% payment adjustment for bilateral procedures does not apply, assistant surgeon may be paid

54130   **Remove penis & nodes**   ~ follow-up period is 90 days, standard payment adjustment rules for multiple procedures apply, 150% payment adjustment does not apply - RVUs based on bilateral procedure, assistant surgeon may be paid

54135   **Remove penis & nodes**   ~ follow-up period is 90 days, standard payment adjustment rules for multiple procedures apply, 150% payment adjustment does not apply - RVUs based on bilateral procedure, assistant surgeon may be paid

54150   **Circumcision w/regional block**   ~ endoscopies or minor procedure - E/M services on the same day generally not paid, standard payment adjustment rules for multiple

procedures apply, 150% payment adjustment for bilateral procedures does not apply, payment for assistant surgeon subject to documentation of medical necessity

54160   **Circumcision, neonate**   ~ follow-up period is 10 days, standard payment adjustment rules for multiple procedures apply, 150% payment adjustment for bilateral procedures does not apply, assistant surgeon may not be paid

54161   **Circum 28 days or older**   ~ follow-up period is 10 days, standard payment adjustment rules for multiple procedures apply, 150% payment adjustment for bilateral procedures does not apply, assistant surgeon may not be paid

54162   **Lysis penile circumcise lesion**   ~ follow-up period is 10 days, standard payment adjustment rules for multiple procedures apply, 150% payment adjustment for bilateral procedures does not apply, assistant surgeon may not be paid

54163   **Repair circumcision**   ~ follow-up period is 10 days, standard payment adjustment rules for multiple procedures apply, 150% payment adjustment for bilateral procedures does not apply, assistant surgeon may not be paid

54164   **Frenulotomy of penis**   ~ follow-up period is 10 days, standard payment adjustment rules for multiple procedures apply, 150% payment adjustment for bilateral procedures does not apply, assistant surgeon may not be paid

54200   **Treat penis lesion**   ~ follow-up period is 10 days, standard payment adjustment rules for multiple procedures apply, 150% payment adjustment for bilateral procedures does not apply, assistant surgeon may not be paid

54205   **Treat penis lesion**   ~ follow-up period is 90 days, standard payment adjustment rules for multiple procedures apply, 150% payment adjustment for bilateral procedures does not apply, assistant surgeon may be paid

54220   **Treat penis lesion**   ~ endoscopies or minor procedure - E/M services on the same day generally not paid, standard payment adjustment rules for multiple procedures apply, 150% payment adjustment for bilateral procedures does not apply, assistant surgeon may not be paid

54230   **Prepare penis study**   ~ endoscopies or minor procedure - E/M services on the same day generally not paid, standard payment adjustment rules for multiple procedures apply, 150% payment adjustment for bilateral procedures does not apply, assistant surgeon may not be paid

54231   **Dynamic cavernosometry**   ~ endoscopies or minor procedure - E/M services on the same day generally not paid, standard payment adjustment rules for multiple procedures apply, 150% payment adjustment for bilateral procedures does not apply, assistant surgeon may not be paid

54235 **Penile injection** ~ endoscopies or minor procedure - E/M services on the same day generally not paid, standard payment adjustment rules for multiple procedures apply, 150% payment adjustment for bilateral procedures does not apply, assistant surgeon may not be paid

54240 **Penis study** ~ endoscopies or minor procedure - E/M services on the same day generally not paid, standard payment adjustment rules for multiple procedures apply, 150% payment adjustment for bilateral procedures does not apply, payment for assistant surgeon subject to documentation of medical necessity

54250 **Penis study** ~ endoscopies or minor procedure - E/M services on the same day generally not paid, standard payment adjustment rules for multiple procedures apply, 150% payment adjustment for bilateral procedures does not apply, payment for assistant surgeon subject to documentation of medical necessity

54300 **Revise penis** ~ follow-up period is 90 days, standard payment adjustment rules for multiple procedures apply, 150% payment adjustment for bilateral procedures does not apply, assistant surgeon may be paid

54304 **Revise penis** ~ follow-up period is 90 days, standard payment adjustment rules for multiple procedures apply, 150% payment adjustment for bilateral procedures does not apply, assistant surgeon may be paid

54308 **Reconstruct urethra** ~ follow-up period is 90 days, standard payment adjustment rules for multiple procedures apply, 150% payment adjustment for bilateral procedures does not apply, assistant surgeon may be paid

54312 **Reconstruct urethra** ~ follow-up period is 90 days, standard payment adjustment rules for multiple procedures apply, 150% payment adjustment for bilateral procedures does not apply, assistant surgeon may be paid

54316 **Reconstruct urethra** ~ follow-up period is 90 days, standard payment adjustment rules for multiple procedures apply, 150% payment adjustment for bilateral procedures does not apply, assistant surgeon may be paid

54318 **Reconstruct urethra** ~ follow-up period is 90 days, standard payment adjustment rules for multiple procedures apply, 150% payment adjustment for bilateral procedures does not apply, assistant surgeon may be paid

54322 **Reconstruct urethra** ~ follow-up period is 90 days, standard payment adjustment rules for multiple procedures apply, 150% payment adjustment for bilateral procedures does not apply, assistant surgeon may be paid

54324 **Reconstruct urethra** ~ follow-up period is 90 days, standard payment adjustment rules for multiple procedures apply, 150% payment adjustment for bilateral procedures does not apply, assistant surgeon may be paid

54326   **Reconstruct urethra**   ~ follow-up period is 90 days, standard payment adjustment rules for multiple procedures apply, 150% payment adjustment for bilateral procedures does not apply, assistant surgeon may be paid

54328   **Revise penis/urethra**   ~ follow-up period is 90 days, standard payment adjustment rules for multiple procedures apply, 150% payment adjustment for bilateral procedures does not apply, assistant surgeon may be paid

54332   **Revise penis/urethra**   ~ follow-up period is 90 days, standard payment adjustment rules for multiple procedures apply, 150% payment adjustment for bilateral procedures does not apply, assistant surgeon may be paid

54336   **Revise penis/urethra**   ~ follow-up period is 90 days, standard payment adjustment rules for multiple procedures apply, 150% payment adjustment for bilateral procedures does not apply, assistant surgeon may be paid

54340   **Secondary urethral surgery**   ~ follow-up period is 90 days, standard payment adjustment rules for multiple procedures apply, 150% payment adjustment for bilateral procedures does not apply, assistant surgeon may be paid

54344   **Secondary urethral surgery**   ~ follow-up period is 90 days, standard payment adjustment rules for multiple procedures apply, 150% payment adjustment for bilateral procedures does not apply, assistant surgeon may be paid

54348   **Secondary urethral surgery**   ~ follow-up period is 90 days, standard payment adjustment rules for multiple procedures apply, 150% payment adjustment for bilateral procedures does not apply, assistant surgeon may be paid

54352   **Reconstruct urethra/penis**   ~ follow-up period is 90 days, standard payment adjustment rules for multiple procedures apply, 150% payment adjustment for bilateral procedures does not apply, assistant surgeon may be paid

54360   **Penis plastic surgery**   ~ follow-up period is 90 days, standard payment adjustment rules for multiple procedures apply, 150% payment adjustment for bilateral procedures does not apply, assistant surgeon may be paid

54380   **Repair penis**   ~ follow-up period is 90 days, standard payment adjustment rules for multiple procedures apply, 150% payment adjustment for bilateral procedures does not apply, assistant surgeon may be paid

54385   **Repair penis**   ~ follow-up period is 90 days, standard payment adjustment rules for multiple procedures apply, 150% payment adjustment for bilateral procedures does not apply, assistant surgeon may be paid

54390   **Repair penis and bladder**   ~ follow-up period is 90 days, standard payment adjustment rules for multiple procedures apply, 150% payment adjustment for bilateral procedures does not apply, assistant surgeon may be paid

54400   **Insert semi-rigid prosthesis**   ~ follow-up period is 90 days, standard payment adjustment rules for multiple procedures apply, 150% payment adjustment for bilateral procedures does not apply, assistant surgeon may not be paid

54401   **Insert self-contained prosthesis**   ~ follow-up period is 90 days, standard payment adjustment rules for multiple procedures apply, 150% payment adjustment for bilateral procedures does not apply, assistant surgeon may not be paid

54405   **Insert multi-comp penis pros**   ~ follow-up period is 90 days, standard payment adjustment rules for multiple procedures apply, 150% payment adjustment for bilateral procedures does not apply, assistant surgeon may be paid

54406   **Remove multi-comp penis pros**   ~ follow-up period is 90 days, standard payment adjustment rules for multiple procedures apply, 150% payment adjustment for bilateral procedures does not apply, assistant surgeon may be paid

54408   **Repair multi-comp penis pros**   ~ follow-up period is 90 days, standard payment adjustment rules for multiple procedures apply, 150% payment adjustment for bilateral procedures does not apply, assistant surgeon may be paid

54410   **Remove/replace penis prosth**   ~ follow-up period is 90 days, standard payment adjustment rules for multiple procedures apply, 150% payment adjustment for bilateral procedures does not apply, assistant surgeon may be paid

54411   **Remove/replace penis pros, comp**   ~ follow-up period is 90 days, standard payment adjustment rules for multiple procedures apply, 150% payment adjustment for bilateral procedures does not apply, assistant surgeon may be paid

54415   **Remove self-contained penis pros**   ~ follow-up period is 90 days, standard payment adjustment rules for multiple procedures apply, 150% payment adjustment for bilateral procedures does not apply, assistant surgeon may be paid

54416   **Remove/replace penis contain pros**   ~ follow-up period is 90 days, standard payment adjustment rules for multiple procedures apply, 150% payment adjustment for bilateral procedures does not apply, assistant surgeon may be paid

54417   **Remove/replace penis pros, complete**   ~ follow-up period is 90 days, standard payment adjustment rules for multiple procedures apply, 150% payment adjustment for bilateral procedures does not apply, assistant surgeon may be paid

54420   **Revise penis**   ~ follow-up period is 90 days, standard payment adjustment rules for multiple procedures apply, 150% payment adjustment for bilateral procedures does not apply, assistant surgeon may be paid

54430   **Revise penis**   ~ follow-up period is 90 days, standard payment adjustment rules for multiple procedures apply, 150% payment adjustment does not apply - RVUs based on bilateral procedure, assistant surgeon may be paid

54435 **Revise penis**   ~ follow-up period is 90 days, standard payment adjustment rules for multiple procedures apply, 150% payment adjustment for bilateral procedures does not apply, assistant surgeon may not be paid

54440 **Repair penis**   ~ follow-up period is 90 days, standard payment adjustment rules for multiple procedures apply, 150% payment adjustment for bilateral procedures does not apply, assistant surgeon may be paid

54450 **Preputial stretching**   ~ endoscopies or minor procedure - E/M services on the same day generally not paid, standard payment adjustment rules for multiple procedures apply, 150% payment adjustment for bilateral procedures does not apply, assistant surgeon may not be paid

Testis

54500 **Biopsy testis**   ~ endoscopies or minor procedure - E/M services on the same day generally not paid, standard payment adjustment rules for multiple procedures apply, 150% payment adjustment for bilateral procedures applies, payment for assistant surgeon subject to documentation of medical necessity

54505 **Biopsy testis**   ~ follow-up period is 10 days, standard payment adjustment rules for multiple procedures apply, 150% payment adjustment for bilateral procedures applies, payment for assistant surgeon subject to documentation of medical necessity

54512 **Excise lesion testis**   ~ follow-up period is 90 days, standard payment adjustment rules for multiple procedures apply, 150% payment adjustment for bilateral procedures applies, assistant surgeon may be paid

54520 **Remove testis**   ~ follow-up period is 90 days, standard payment adjustment rules for multiple procedures apply, 150% payment adjustment for bilateral procedures applies, assistant surgeon may not be paid

54522 **Orchiectomy, partial**   ~ follow-up period is 90 days, standard payment adjustment rules for multiple procedures apply, 150% payment adjustment for bilateral procedures applies, assistant surgeon may be paid

54530 **Remove testis**   ~ follow-up period is 90 days, standard payment adjustment rules for multiple procedures apply, 150% payment adjustment for bilateral procedures applies, assistant surgeon may be paid

54535 **Extensive testis surgery**   ~ follow-up period is 90 days, standard payment adjustment rules for multiple procedures apply, 150% payment adjustment for bilateral procedures applies, assistant surgeon may be paid

54550   **Explore for testis**   ~ follow-up period is 90 days, standard payment adjustment rules for multiple procedures apply, 150% payment adjustment for bilateral procedures applies, assistant surgeon may be paid

54560   **Explore for testis**   ~ follow-up period is 90 days, standard payment adjustment rules for multiple procedures apply, 150% payment adjustment for bilateral procedures applies, assistant surgeon may be paid

54600   **Reduce testis torsion**   ~ follow-up period is 90 days, standard payment adjustment rules for multiple procedures apply, 150% payment adjustment for bilateral procedures applies, assistant surgeon may not be paid

54620   **Suspend testis**   ~ follow-up period is 10 days, standard payment adjustment rules for multiple procedures apply, 150% payment adjustment for bilateral procedures applies, assistant surgeon may not be paid

54640   **Suspend testis**   ~ follow-up period is 90 days, standard payment adjustment rules for multiple procedures apply, 150% payment adjustment for bilateral procedures applies, payment for assistant surgeon subject to documentation of medical necessity

54650   **Orchiopexy (fowler-Stephens)**   ~ follow-up period is 90 days, standard payment adjustment rules for multiple procedures apply, 150% payment adjustment for bilateral procedures applies, assistant surgeon may be paid

54660   **Revise testis**   ~ follow-up period is 90 days, standard payment adjustment rules for multiple procedures apply, 150% payment adjustment for bilateral procedures applies, payment for assistant surgeon subject to documentation of medical necessity

54670   **Repair testis injury**   ~ follow-up period is 90 days, standard payment adjustment rules for multiple procedures apply, 150% payment adjustment for bilateral procedures applies, payment for assistant surgeon subject to documentation of medical necessity

54680   **Relocation of testis(es)**   ~ follow-up period is 90 days, standard payment adjustment rules for multiple procedures apply, 150% payment adjustment for bilateral procedures applies, assistant surgeon may be paid

54690   **Laparoscopy, orchiectomy**   ~ follow-up period is 90 days, standard payment adjustment rules for multiple procedures apply, 150% payment adjustment for bilateral procedures applies, assistant surgeon may be paid

54692   **Laparoscopy, orchiopexy**   ~ follow-up period is 90 days, standard payment adjustment rules for multiple procedures apply, 150% payment adjustment for bilateral procedures applies, assistant surgeon may not be paid

54699   **Laparoscope proc, testis**   ~ medicare carrier determines global period, standard payment adjustment rules for multiple procedures apply, 150% payment adjustment for bilateral procedures applies, assistant surgeon may be paid

Epididymis

54700   **Drain scrotum**   ~ follow-up period is 10 days, standard payment adjustment rules for multiple procedures apply, 150% payment adjustment for bilateral procedures does not apply, assistant surgeon may not be paid

54800   **Biopsy epididymis**   ~ endoscopies or minor procedure - E/M services on the same day generally not paid, standard payment adjustment rules for multiple procedures apply, 150% payment adjustment for bilateral procedures does not apply, payment for assistant surgeon subject to documentation of medical necessity

54830   **Remove epididymis lesion**   ~ follow-up period is 90 days, standard payment adjustment rules for multiple procedures apply, 150% payment adjustment for bilateral procedures does not apply, payment for assistant surgeon subject to documentation of medical necessity

54840   **Remove epididymis lesion**   ~ follow-up period is 90 days, standard payment adjustment rules for multiple procedures apply, 150% payment adjustment for bilateral procedures does not apply, assistant surgeon may not be paid

54860   **Remove epididymis**   ~ follow-up period is 90 days, standard payment adjustment rules for multiple procedures apply, 150% payment adjustment for bilateral procedures does not apply, assistant surgeon may not be paid

54861   **Remove epididymis**   ~ follow-up period is 90 days, standard payment adjustment rules for multiple procedures apply, 150% payment adjustment for bilateral procedures does not apply, payment for assistant surgeon subject to documentation of medical necessity

54865   **Explore epididymis**   ~ follow-up period is 90 days, standard payment adjustment rules for multiple procedures apply, 150% payment adjustment for bilateral procedures does not apply, payment for assistant surgeon subject to documentation of medical necessity

54900   **Fuse spermatic ducts**   ~ follow-up period is 90 days, standard payment adjustment rules for multiple procedures apply, 150% payment adjustment for bilateral procedures does not apply, payment for assistant surgeon subject to documentation of medical necessity

54901   **Fuse spermatic ducts**   ~ follow-up period is 90 days, standard payment adjustment rules for multiple procedures apply, 150% payment adjustment does not apply - RVUs based on bilateral procedure, payment for assistant surgeon subject to documentation of medical necessity

---

Tunica Vaginalis

55000   **Drain hydrocele**   ~ endoscopies or minor procedure - E/M services on the same day generally not paid, standard payment adjustment rules for multiple procedures apply, 150% payment adjustment for bilateral procedures does not apply, assistant surgeon may not be paid

55040   **Remove hydrocele**   ~ follow-up period is 90 days, standard payment adjustment rules for multiple procedures apply, 150% payment adjustment for bilateral procedures does not apply, assistant surgeon may not be paid

55041   **Remove hydroceles**   ~ follow-up period is 90 days, standard payment adjustment rules for multiple procedures apply, 150% payment adjustment does not apply - RVUs based on bilateral procedure, assistant surgeon may not be paid

55060   **Repair hydrocele**   ~ follow-up period is 90 days, standard payment adjustment rules for multiple procedures apply, 150% payment adjustment for bilateral procedures applies, payment for assistant surgeon subject to documentation of medical necessity

55100   **Drain scrotum abscess**   ~ follow-up period is 10 days, standard payment adjustment rules for multiple procedures apply, 150% payment adjustment for bilateral procedures does not apply, assistant surgeon may not be paid

55110   **Explore scrotum**   ~ follow-up period is 90 days, standard payment adjustment rules for multiple procedures apply, 150% payment adjustment for bilateral procedures does not apply, assistant surgeon may not be paid

55120   **Remove scrotum lesion**   ~ follow-up period is 90 days, standard payment adjustment rules for multiple procedures apply, 150% payment adjustment for bilateral procedures does not apply, payment for assistant surgeon subject to documentation of medical necessity

55150   **Remove scrotum**   ~ follow-up period is 90 days, standard payment adjustment rules for multiple procedures apply, 150% payment adjustment for bilateral procedures does not apply, assistant surgeon may be paid

55175   **Revise scrotum**   ~ follow-up period is 90 days, standard payment adjustment rules for multiple procedures apply, 150% payment adjustment for bilateral procedures does not apply, payment for assistant surgeon subject to documentation of medical necessity

55180   **Revise scrotum**   ~ follow-up period is 90 days, standard payment adjustment rules for multiple procedures apply, 150% payment adjustment for bilateral procedures does not apply, payment for assistant surgeon subject to documentation of medical necessity

Vas Deferens

55200   **Incise sperm duct**   ~ follow-up period is 90 days, standard payment adjustment rules for multiple procedures apply, 150% payment adjustment does not apply - RVUs based on bilateral procedure, payment for assistant surgeon subject to documentation of medical necessity

55250   **Remove sperm duct(s)**   ~ follow-up period is 90 days, standard payment adjustment rules for multiple procedures apply, 150% payment adjustment does not apply - RVUs based on bilateral procedure, assistant surgeon may not be paid

55300   **Prepare, sperm duct x-ray**   ~ endoscopies or minor procedure - E/M services on the same day generally not paid, standard payment adjustment rules for multiple procedures apply, 150% payment adjustment does not apply - RVUs based on bilateral procedure, payment for assistant surgeon subject to documentation of medical necessity

55400   **Repair sperm duct**   ~ follow-up period is 90 days, standard payment adjustment rules for multiple procedures apply, 150% payment adjustment for bilateral procedures applies, assistant surgeon may be paid

55450   **Ligate sperm duct**   ~ follow-up period is 10 days, standard payment adjustment rules for multiple procedures apply, 150% payment adjustment does not apply - RVUs based on bilateral procedure, payment for assistant surgeon subject to documentation of medical necessity

Spermatic Cord

55500   **Remove hydrocele**   ~ follow-up period is 90 days, standard payment adjustment rules for multiple procedures apply, 150% payment adjustment for bilateral procedures does not apply, payment for assistant surgeon subject to documentation of medical necessity

55520   **Remove sperm cord lesion**   ~ follow-up period is 90 days, standard payment adjustment rules for multiple procedures apply, 150% payment adjustment for bilateral procedures does not apply, assistant surgeon may be paid

55530   **Revise spermatic cord veins**   ~ follow-up period is 90 days, standard payment adjustment rules for multiple procedures apply, 150% payment adjustment for bilateral procedures applies, assistant surgeon may not be paid

55535   **Revise spermatic cord veins**   ~ follow-up period is 90 days, standard payment adjustment rules for multiple procedures apply, 150% payment adjustment for bilateral procedures applies, assistant surgeon may be paid

55540   **Revise hernia & sperm veins**   ~ follow-up period is 90 days, standard payment adjustment rules for multiple procedures apply, 150% payment adjustment for bilateral procedures applies, assistant surgeon may be paid

55550   **Laparo ligate spermatic vein**   ~ follow-up period is 90 days, standard payment adjustment rules for multiple procedures apply, 150% payment adjustment for bilateral procedures applies, assistant surgeon may be paid

55559   **Laparo proc, spermatic cord**   ~ medicare carrier determines global period, standard payment adjustment rules for multiple procedures apply, 150% payment adjustment for bilateral procedures applies, assistant surgeon may be paid

Seminal Vesicles

55600   **Incise sperm duct pouch**   ~ follow-up period is 90 days, standard payment adjustment rules for multiple procedures apply, 150% payment adjustment for bilateral procedures applies, payment for assistant surgeon subject to documentation of medical necessity

55605   **Incise sperm duct pouch**   ~ follow-up period is 90 days, standard payment adjustment rules for multiple procedures apply, 150% payment adjustment for bilateral procedures applies, payment for assistant surgeon subject to documentation of medical necessity

55650   **Remove sperm duct pouch**   ~ follow-up period is 90 days, standard payment adjustment rules for multiple procedures apply, 150% payment adjustment for bilateral procedures applies, assistant surgeon may be paid

55680   **Remove sperm pouch lesion**   ~ follow-up period is 90 days, standard payment adjustment rules for multiple procedures apply, 150% payment adjustment for bilateral procedures does not apply, payment for assistant surgeon subject to documentation of medical necessity

Prostate

55700   **Biopsy prostate**   ~ endoscopies or minor procedure - E/M services on the same day generally not paid, standard payment adjustment rules for multiple procedures apply, 150% payment adjustment for bilateral procedures does not apply, assistant surgeon may not be paid

55705   **Biopsy prostate**   ~ follow-up period is 10 days, standard payment adjustment rules for multiple procedures apply, 150% payment adjustment for bilateral procedures does not apply, assistant surgeon may not be paid

55720   **Drain prostate abscess**   ~ follow-up period is 90 days, standard payment adjustment rules for multiple procedures apply, 150% payment adjustment for bilateral procedures does not apply, assistant surgeon may be paid

55725   **Drain prostate abscess**   ~ follow-up period is 90 days, standard payment adjustment rules for multiple procedures apply, 150% payment adjustment for bilateral procedures does not apply, assistant surgeon may be paid

55801   **Remove prostate**   ~ follow-up period is 90 days, standard payment adjustment rules for multiple procedures apply, 150% payment adjustment for bilateral procedures does not apply, assistant surgeon may be paid

55810   **Extensive prostate surgery**   ~ follow-up period is 90 days, standard payment adjustment rules for multiple procedures apply, 150% payment adjustment for bilateral procedures does not apply, assistant surgeon may be paid

55812   **Extensive prostate surgery**   ~ follow-up period is 90 days, standard payment adjustment rules for multiple procedures apply, 150% payment adjustment for bilateral procedures does not apply, assistant surgeon may be paid

55815   **Extensive prostate surgery**   ~ follow-up period is 90 days, standard payment adjustment rules for multiple procedures apply, 150% payment adjustment does not apply - RVUs based on bilateral procedure, assistant surgeon may be paid

55821   **Remove prostate**   ~ follow-up period is 90 days, standard payment adjustment rules for multiple procedures apply, 150% payment adjustment for bilateral procedures does not apply, assistant surgeon may be paid

55831   **Remove prostate**   ~ follow-up period is 90 days, standard payment adjustment rules for multiple procedures apply, 150% payment adjustment for bilateral procedures does not apply, assistant surgeon may be paid

55840   **Extensive prostate surgery**   ~ follow-up period is 90 days, standard payment adjustment rules for multiple procedures apply, 150% payment adjustment for bilateral procedures does not apply, assistant surgeon may be paid

55842   **Extensive prostate surgery**   ~ follow-up period is 90 days, standard payment adjustment rules for multiple procedures apply, 150% payment adjustment for bilateral procedures does not apply, assistant surgeon may be paid

55845   **Extensive prostate surgery**   ~ follow-up period is 90 days, standard payment adjustment rules for multiple procedures apply, 150% payment adjustment does not apply - RVUs based on bilateral procedure, assistant surgeon may be paid

55860   **Surgical exposure, prostate**   ~ follow-up period is 90 days, standard payment adjustment rules for multiple procedures apply, 150% payment adjustment for bilateral procedures does not apply, assistant surgeon may not be paid

55862   **Extensive prostate surgery**   ~ follow-up period is 90 days, standard payment adjustment rules for multiple procedures apply, 150% payment adjustment for bilateral procedures does not apply, assistant surgeon may be paid

55865   **Extensive prostate surgery**   ~ follow-up period is 90 days, standard payment adjustment rules for multiple procedures apply, 150% payment adjustment does not apply - RVUs based on bilateral procedure, assistant surgeon may be paid

55866   **Laparo radical prostatectomy**   ~ follow-up period is 90 days, standard payment adjustment rules for multiple procedures apply, 150% payment adjustment for bilateral procedures does not apply, assistant surgeon may be paid

55870   **Electroejaculation**   ~ endoscopies or minor procedure - E/M services on the same day generally not paid, standard payment adjustment rules for multiple procedures apply, 150% payment adjustment for bilateral procedures does not apply, assistant surgeon may not be paid

55873   **Cryoablate prostate**   ~ follow-up period is 90 days, standard payment adjustment rules for multiple procedures apply, 150% payment adjustment for bilateral procedures does not apply, assistant surgeon may not be paid

55875   **Transperineal needle place, pros**   ~ follow-up period is 90 days, standard payment adjustment rules for multiple procedures apply, 150% payment adjustment for bilateral procedures does not apply, payment for assistant surgeon subject to documentation of medical necessity

55876   **Place radiation therapy device/marker, pros** ~ endoscopies or minor procedure - E/M services on the same day generally not paid, standard payment adjustment rules for multiple procedures apply, 150% payment adjustment for bilateral procedures does not apply, assistant surgeon may not be paid

55899   **Genital surgery procedure**   ~ medicare carrier determines global period, standard payment adjustment rules for multiple procedures apply, 150% payment adjustment for bilateral procedures does not apply, assistant surgeon may not be paid

Intersex Surgery

55970   **Sex transformation, male to female**   ~ non-covered service, multiple procedure concept does not apply, bilateral surgery concept does not apply, assistant surgery concept does not apply

55980   **Sex transformation, female to male**   ~ non-covered service, multiple procedure concept does not apply, bilateral surgery concept does not apply, assistant surgery concept does not apply

FEMALE GENITAL SYSTEM

Vulva, Perineum, and Introitus

56405   **I & D of vulva/perineum**   ~ follow-up period is 10 days, standard payment adjustment rules for multiple procedures apply, 150% payment adjustment for bilateral procedures does not apply, assistant surgeon may not be paid

56420   **Drain gland abscess**   ~ follow-up period is 10 days, standard payment adjustment rules for multiple procedures apply, 150% payment adjustment for bilateral procedures does not apply, assistant surgeon may not be paid

56440   **Surgery for vulva lesion**   ~ follow-up period is 10 days, standard payment adjustment rules for multiple procedures apply, 150% payment adjustment for bilateral procedures does not apply, assistant surgeon may not be paid

56441   **Lysis of labial lesion(s)**   ~ follow-up period is 10 days, standard payment adjustment rules for multiple procedures apply, 150% payment adjustment for bilateral procedures does not apply, payment for assistant surgeon subject to documentation of medical necessity

56442   **Hymenotomy**   ~ endoscopies or minor procedure - E/M services on the same day generally not paid, standard payment adjustment rules for multiple procedures apply, 150% payment adjustment for bilateral procedures does not apply, payment for assistant surgeon subject to documentation of medical necessity

56501   **Destroy vulva lesions, simple**   ~ follow-up period is 10 days, standard payment adjustment rules for multiple procedures apply, 150% payment adjustment for bilateral procedures does not apply, assistant surgeon may not be paid

56515   **Destroy vulva lesion/s complete**   ~ follow-up period is 10 days, standard payment adjustment rules for multiple procedures apply, 150% payment adjustment for bilateral procedures does not apply, assistant surgeon may not be paid

56605   **Biopsy vulva/perineum**   ~ endoscopies or minor procedure - E/M services on the same day generally not paid, standard payment adjustment rules for multiple procedures apply, 150% payment adjustment for bilateral procedures does not apply, assistant surgeon may not be paid

56606   **Biopsy vulva/perineum**   ~ follow-up period included in another service, no payment adjustment rules for multiple procedures apply, 150% payment adjustment for bilateral procedures does not apply, assistant surgeon may not be paid

56620   **Partial remove vulva**   ~ follow-up period is 90 days, standard payment adjustment rules for multiple procedures apply, 150% payment adjustment for bilateral procedures does not apply, assistant surgeon may be paid

56625   **Complete remove vulva**   ~ follow-up period is 90 days, standard payment adjustment rules for multiple procedures apply, 150% payment adjustment for bilateral procedures does not apply, assistant surgeon may be paid

56630   **Extensive vulva surgery**   ~ follow-up period is 90 days, standard payment adjustment rules for multiple procedures apply, 150% payment adjustment for bilateral procedures does not apply, assistant surgeon may be paid

---

56631   **Extensive vulva surgery**   ~ follow-up period is 90 days, standard payment adjustment rules for multiple procedures apply, 150% payment adjustment for bilateral procedures does not apply, assistant surgeon may be paid

56632   **Extensive vulva surgery**   ~ follow-up period is 90 days, standard payment adjustment rules for multiple procedures apply, 150% payment adjustment does not apply - RVUs based on bilateral procedure, assistant surgeon may be paid

56633   **Extensive vulva surgery**   ~ follow-up period is 90 days, standard payment adjustment rules for multiple procedures apply, 150% payment adjustment for bilateral procedures does not apply, assistant surgeon may be paid

56634   **Extensive vulva surgery**   ~ follow-up period is 90 days, standard payment adjustment rules for multiple procedures apply, 150% payment adjustment for bilateral procedures does not apply, assistant surgeon may be paid

56637   **Extensive vulva surgery**   ~ follow-up period is 90 days, standard payment adjustment rules for multiple procedures apply, 150% payment adjustment for bilateral procedures does not apply, assistant surgeon may be paid

56640   **Extensive vulva surgery**   ~ follow-up period is 90 days, standard payment adjustment rules for multiple procedures apply, 150% payment adjustment for bilateral procedures applies, assistant surgeon may be paid

56700   **Partial remove hymen**   ~ follow-up period is 10 days, standard payment adjustment rules for multiple procedures apply, 150% payment adjustment for bilateral procedures does not apply, assistant surgeon may be paid

56740   **Remove vagina gland lesion**   ~ follow-up period is 10 days, standard payment adjustment rules for multiple procedures apply, 150% payment adjustment for bilateral procedures does not apply, assistant surgeon may not be paid

56800   **Repair vagina**   ~ follow-up period is 10 days, standard payment adjustment rules for multiple procedures apply, 150% payment adjustment for bilateral procedures does not apply, assistant surgeon may be paid

56805   **Repair clitoris**   ~ follow-up period is 90 days, standard payment adjustment rules for multiple procedures apply, 150% payment adjustment for bilateral procedures does not apply, assistant surgeon may be paid

56810   **Repair perineum**   ~ follow-up period is 10 days, standard payment adjustment rules for multiple procedures apply, 150% payment adjustment for bilateral procedures does not apply, assistant surgeon may be paid

56820   **Exam vulva w/scope**   ~ endoscopies or minor procedure - E/M services on the same day generally not paid, standard payment adjustment rules for multiple

procedures apply, 150% payment adjustment for bilateral procedures does not apply, assistant surgeon may not be paid

56821   **Exam/biopsy vulva w/scope**   ~ endoscopies or minor procedure - E/M services on the same day generally not paid, standard payment adjustment rules for multiple procedures apply, 150% payment adjustment for bilateral procedures does not apply, assistant surgeon may not be paid

Vagina

57000   **Explore vagina**   ~ follow-up period is 10 days, standard payment adjustment rules for multiple procedures apply, 150% payment adjustment for bilateral procedures does not apply, payment for assistant surgeon subject to documentation of medical necessity

57010   **Drain pelvic abscess**   ~ follow-up period is 90 days, standard payment adjustment rules for multiple procedures apply, 150% payment adjustment for bilateral procedures does not apply, payment for assistant surgeon subject to documentation of medical necessity

57020   **Drain pelvic fluid**   ~ endoscopies or minor procedure - E/M services on the same day generally not paid, standard payment adjustment rules for multiple procedures apply, 150% payment adjustment for bilateral procedures does not apply, payment for assistant surgeon subject to documentation of medical necessity

57022   **I & D vaginal hematoma, pp**   ~ follow-up period is 10 days, standard payment adjustment rules for multiple procedures apply, 150% payment adjustment for bilateral procedures does not apply, payment for assistant surgeon subject to documentation of medical necessity

57023   **I & D vaginal hematoma, non-ob**   ~ follow-up period is 10 days, standard payment adjustment rules for multiple procedures apply, 150% payment adjustment for bilateral procedures does not apply, payment for assistant surgeon subject to documentation of medical necessity

57061   **Destroy vaginal lesions, simple**   ~ follow-up period is 10 days, standard payment adjustment rules for multiple procedures apply, 150% payment adjustment for bilateral procedures does not apply, assistant surgeon may not be paid

57065   **Destroy vaginal lesions, complex**   ~ follow-up period is 10 days, standard payment adjustment rules for multiple procedures apply, 150% payment adjustment for bilateral procedures does not apply, assistant surgeon may not be paid

57100   **Biopsy vagina**   ~ endoscopies or minor procedure - E/M services on the same day generally not paid, standard payment adjustment rules for multiple procedures apply, 150% payment adjustment for bilateral procedures does not apply, assistant surgeon may not be paid

57105   **Biopsy vagina**   ~ follow-up period is 10 days, standard payment adjustment rules for multiple procedures apply, 150% payment adjustment for bilateral procedures does not apply, assistant surgeon may not be paid

57106   **Remove vagina wall, partial**   ~ follow-up period is 90 days, standard payment adjustment rules for multiple procedures apply, 150% payment adjustment for bilateral procedures does not apply, assistant surgeon may be paid

57107   **Remove vagina tissue, part**   ~ follow-up period is 90 days, standard payment adjustment rules for multiple procedures apply, 150% payment adjustment for bilateral procedures does not apply, assistant surgeon may be paid

57109   **Vaginectomy partial w/nodes**   ~ follow-up period is 90 days, standard payment adjustment rules for multiple procedures apply, 150% payment adjustment does not apply - RVUs based on bilateral procedure, assistant surgeon may be paid

57110   **Remove vagina wall, complete**   ~ follow-up period is 90 days, standard payment adjustment rules for multiple procedures apply, 150% payment adjustment for bilateral procedures does not apply, assistant surgeon may be paid

57111   **Remove vagina tissue, complete**   ~ follow-up period is 90 days, standard payment adjustment rules for multiple procedures apply, 150% payment adjustment does not apply - RVUs based on bilateral procedure, assistant surgeon may be paid

57112   **Vaginectomy w/nodes, complete**   ~ follow-up period is 90 days, standard payment adjustment rules for multiple procedures apply, 150% payment adjustment does not apply - RVUs based on bilateral procedure, assistant surgeon may be paid

57120   **Closure vagina**   ~ follow-up period is 90 days, standard payment adjustment rules for multiple procedures apply, 150% payment adjustment for bilateral procedures does not apply, assistant surgeon may be paid

57130   **Remove vagina lesion**   ~ follow-up period is 10 days, standard payment adjustment rules for multiple procedures apply, 150% payment adjustment for bilateral procedures does not apply, assistant surgeon may be paid

57135   **Remove vagina lesion**   ~ follow-up period is 10 days, standard payment adjustment rules for multiple procedures apply, 150% payment adjustment for bilateral procedures does not apply, assistant surgeon may not be paid

57150   **Treat vagina infection**   ~ endoscopies or minor procedure - E/M services on the same day generally not paid, standard payment adjustment rules for multiple procedures apply, 150% payment adjustment for bilateral procedures does not apply, assistant surgeon may not be paid

57155   **Insert uteri tandems/ovoids**   ~ follow-up period is 90 days, standard payment adjustment rules for multiple procedures apply, 150% payment adjustment for bilateral procedures does not apply, assistant surgeon may not be paid

57160   **Insert pessary/other device**   ~ endoscopies or minor procedure - E/M services on the same day generally not paid, standard payment adjustment rules for multiple procedures apply, 150% payment adjustment for bilateral procedures does not apply, assistant surgeon may not be paid

57170   **Fit diaphragm/cap**   ~ endoscopies or minor procedure - E/M services on the same day generally not paid, standard payment adjustment rules for multiple procedures apply, 150% payment adjustment for bilateral procedures does not apply, payment for assistant surgeon subject to documentation of medical necessity

57180   **Treat vaginal bleeding**   ~ follow-up period is 10 days, standard payment adjustment rules for multiple procedures apply, 150% payment adjustment for bilateral procedures does not apply, assistant surgeon may not be paid

57200   **Repair vagina**   ~ follow-up period is 90 days, standard payment adjustment rules for multiple procedures apply, 150% payment adjustment for bilateral procedures does not apply, assistant surgeon may be paid

57210   **Repair vagina/perineum**   ~ follow-up period is 90 days, standard payment adjustment rules for multiple procedures apply, 150% payment adjustment for bilateral procedures does not apply, assistant surgeon may be paid

57220   **Revise urethra**   ~ follow-up period is 90 days, standard payment adjustment rules for multiple procedures apply, 150% payment adjustment for bilateral procedures does not apply, assistant surgeon may be paid

57230   **Repair urethral lesion**   ~ follow-up period is 90 days, standard payment adjustment rules for multiple procedures apply, 150% payment adjustment for bilateral procedures does not apply, assistant surgeon may be paid

57240   **Repair bladder & vagina**   ~ follow-up period is 90 days, standard payment adjustment rules for multiple procedures apply, 150% payment adjustment for bilateral procedures does not apply, assistant surgeon may be paid

57250   **Repair rectum & vagina**   ~ follow-up period is 90 days, standard payment adjustment rules for multiple procedures apply, 150% payment adjustment for bilateral procedures does not apply, assistant surgeon may be paid

57260   **Repair vagina**   ~ follow-up period is 90 days, standard payment adjustment rules for multiple procedures apply, 150% payment adjustment for bilateral procedures does not apply, assistant surgeon may be paid

57265   **Extensive repair vagina**   ~ follow-up period is 90 days, standard payment adjustment rules for multiple procedures apply, 150% payment adjustment for bilateral procedures does not apply, assistant surgeon may be paid

57267   **Insert mesh/pelvic floor, add-on**   ~ follow-up period included in another service, no payment adjustment rules for multiple procedures apply, 150% payment adjustment for bilateral procedures does not apply, assistant surgeon may be paid, +add-on code (list separately in addition to primary procedure)

57268   **Repair bowel bulge**   ~ follow-up period is 90 days, standard payment adjustment rules for multiple procedures apply, 150% payment adjustment for bilateral procedures does not apply, assistant surgeon may be paid

57270   **Repair bowel pouch**   ~ follow-up period is 90 days, standard payment adjustment rules for multiple procedures apply, 150% payment adjustment for bilateral procedures does not apply, assistant surgeon may be paid

57280   **Suspend vagina**   ~ follow-up period is 90 days, standard payment adjustment rules for multiple procedures apply, 150% payment adjustment for bilateral procedures does not apply, assistant surgeon may be paid

57282   **Colpopexy, extraperitoneal**   ~ follow-up period is 90 days, standard payment adjustment rules for multiple procedures apply, 150% payment adjustment for bilateral procedures does not apply, assistant surgeon may be paid

57283   **Colpopexy, intraperitoneal**   ~ follow-up period is 90 days, standard payment adjustment rules for multiple procedures apply, 150% payment adjustment for bilateral procedures does not apply, assistant surgeon may be paid

57284   **Repair paravaginal defect**   ~ follow-up period is 90 days, standard payment adjustment rules for multiple procedures apply, 150% payment adjustment for bilateral procedures does not apply, assistant surgeon may be paid

57287   **Revise/remove sling repair**   ~ follow-up period is 90 days, standard payment adjustment rules for multiple procedures apply, 150% payment adjustment for bilateral procedures does not apply, assistant surgeon may be paid

57288   **Repair bladder defect**   ~ follow-up period is 90 days, standard payment adjustment rules for multiple procedures apply, 150% payment adjustment for bilateral procedures does not apply, assistant surgeon may be paid

57289   **Repair bladder & vagina**   ~ follow-up period is 90 days, standard payment adjustment rules for multiple procedures apply, 150% payment adjustment for bilateral procedures does not apply, assistant surgeon may be paid

57291   **Construct vagina**   ~ follow-up period is 90 days, standard payment adjustment rules for multiple procedures apply, 150% payment adjustment for bilateral procedures does not apply, assistant surgeon may be paid

57292   **Construct vagina with graft**   ~ follow-up period is 90 days, standard payment adjustment rules for multiple procedures apply, 150% payment adjustment for bilateral procedures does not apply, assistant surgeon may be paid

57295   **Revise vaginal graft via vagina**   ~ follow-up period is 90 days, standard payment adjustment rules for multiple procedures apply, 150% payment adjustment for bilateral procedures does not apply, assistant surgeon may be paid

57296   **Revise vaginal graft, open abdomen**   ~ follow-up period is 90 days, standard payment adjustment rules for multiple procedures apply, 150% payment adjustment for bilateral procedures does not apply, assistant surgeon may be paid

57300   **Repair rectum-vagina fistula**   ~ follow-up period is 90 days, standard payment adjustment rules for multiple procedures apply, 150% payment adjustment for bilateral procedures does not apply, assistant surgeon may be paid

57305   **Repair rectum-vagina fistula**   ~ follow-up period is 90 days, standard payment adjustment rules for multiple procedures apply, 150% payment adjustment for bilateral procedures does not apply, assistant surgeon may be paid

57307   **Fistula repair & colostomy**   ~ follow-up period is 90 days, standard payment adjustment rules for multiple procedures apply, 150% payment adjustment for bilateral procedures does not apply, assistant surgeon may be paid

57308   **Fistula repair, transperine**   ~ follow-up period is 90 days, standard payment adjustment rules for multiple procedures apply, 150% payment adjustment for bilateral procedures does not apply, assistant surgeon may be paid

57310   **Repair urethrovaginal lesion**   ~ follow-up period is 90 days, standard payment adjustment rules for multiple procedures apply, 150% payment adjustment for bilateral procedures does not apply, assistant surgeon may be paid

57311   **Repair urethrovaginal lesion**   ~ follow-up period is 90 days, standard payment adjustment rules for multiple procedures apply, 150% payment adjustment for bilateral procedures does not apply, assistant surgeon may be paid

57320   **Repair bladder-vagina lesion**   ~ follow-up period is 90 days, standard payment adjustment rules for multiple procedures apply, 150% payment adjustment for bilateral procedures does not apply, assistant surgeon may be paid

57330   **Repair bladder-vagina lesion**   ~ follow-up period is 90 days, standard payment adjustment rules for multiple procedures apply, 150% payment adjustment for bilateral procedures does not apply, assistant surgeon may be paid

57335 **Repair vagina** ~ follow-up period is 90 days, standard payment adjustment rules for multiple procedures apply, 150% payment adjustment for bilateral procedures does not apply, assistant surgeon may be paid

57400 **Dilate vagina** ~ endoscopies or minor procedure - E/M services on the same day generally not paid, standard payment adjustment rules for multiple procedures apply, 150% payment adjustment for bilateral procedures does not apply, payment for assistant surgeon subject to documentation of medical necessity

57410 **Pelvic examination** ~ endoscopies or minor procedure - E/M services on the same day generally not paid, standard payment adjustment rules for multiple procedures apply, 150% payment adjustment for bilateral procedures does not apply, assistant surgeon may not be paid

57415 **Remove vaginal foreign body** ~ follow-up period is 10 days, standard payment adjustment rules for multiple procedures apply, 150% payment adjustment for bilateral procedures does not apply, payment for assistant surgeon subject to documentation of medical necessity

57420 **Exam vagina w/scope** ~ endoscopies or minor procedure - E/M services on the same day generally not paid, standard payment adjustment rules for multiple procedures apply, 150% payment adjustment for bilateral procedures does not apply, assistant surgeon may not be paid

57421 **Exam/biopsy vaginal w/scope** ~ endoscopies or minor procedure - E/M services on the same day generally not paid, standard payment adjustment rules for multiple procedures apply, 150% payment adjustment for bilateral procedures does not apply, assistant surgeon may not be paid

57425 **Laparoscopy, surg, colpopexy** ~ follow-up period is 90 days, standard payment adjustment rules for multiple procedures apply, 150% payment adjustment for bilateral procedures does not apply, assistant surgeon may be paid

Cervix Uteri

57452 **Exam cervix w/scope** ~ endoscopies or minor procedure - E/M services on the same day generally not paid, standard payment adjustment rules for multiple procedures apply, 150% payment adjustment for bilateral procedures does not apply, assistant surgeon may not be paid

57454 **Biopsy/curette of cervix w/scope** ~ endoscopies or minor procedure - E/M services on the same day generally not paid, special rules for multiple endoscopic procedures apply if billed with another endoscopy in the same family, 150% payment adjustment for bilateral procedures does not apply, assistant surgeon may not be paid

57455 **Biopsy cervix w/scope** ~ endoscopies or minor procedure - E/M services on the same day generally not paid, special rules for multiple endoscopic

procedures apply if billed with another endoscopy in the same family, 150% payment adjustment for bilateral procedures does not apply, assistant surgeon may not be paid

57456   **Endocervix curettage w/scope**   ~ endoscopies or minor procedure - E/M services on the same day generally not paid, special rules for multiple endoscopic procedures apply if billed with another endoscopy in the same family, 150% payment adjustment for bilateral procedures does not apply, assistant surgeon may not be paid

57460   **Biopsy cervix w/scope, leep**   ~ endoscopies or minor procedure - E/M services on the same day generally not paid, special rules for multiple endoscopic procedures apply if billed with another endoscopy in the same family, 150% payment adjustment for bilateral procedures does not apply, assistant surgeon may not be paid

57461   **Conization of cervix w/scope, leep**   ~ endoscopies or minor procedure - E/M services on the same day generally not paid, special rules for multiple endoscopic procedures apply if billed with another endoscopy in the same family, 150% payment adjustment for bilateral procedures does not apply, assistant surgeon may not be paid

57500   **Biopsy cervix**   ~ endoscopies or minor procedure - E/M services on the same day generally not paid, standard payment adjustment rules for multiple procedures apply, 150% payment adjustment for bilateral procedures does not apply, assistant surgeon may not be paid

57505   **Endocervical curettage**   ~ follow-up period is 10 days, standard payment adjustment rules for multiple procedures apply, 150% payment adjustment for bilateral procedures does not apply, assistant surgeon may not be paid

57510   **Cauterize cervix**   ~ follow-up period is 10 days, standard payment adjustment rules for multiple procedures apply, 150% payment adjustment for bilateral procedures does not apply, assistant surgeon may not be paid

57511   **Cryocautery of cervix**   ~ follow-up period is 10 days, standard payment adjustment rules for multiple procedures apply, 150% payment adjustment for bilateral procedures does not apply, assistant surgeon may not be paid

57513   **Laser surgery cervix**   ~ follow-up period is 10 days, standard payment adjustment rules for multiple procedures apply, 150% payment adjustment for bilateral procedures does not apply, assistant surgeon may not be paid

57520   **Conization of cervix**   ~ follow-up period is 90 days, standard payment adjustment rules for multiple procedures apply, 150% payment adjustment for bilateral procedures does not apply, assistant surgeon may not be paid

57522   **Conization of cervix**   ~ follow-up period is 90 days, standard payment adjustment rules for multiple procedures apply, 150% payment adjustment for bilateral procedures does not apply, assistant surgeon may not be paid

57530   **Remove cervix**   ~ follow-up period is 90 days, standard payment adjustment rules for multiple procedures apply, 150% payment adjustment for bilateral procedures does not apply, assistant surgeon may be paid

57531   **Remove cervix, radical**   ~ follow-up period is 90 days, standard payment adjustment rules for multiple procedures apply, 150% payment adjustment does not apply - RVUs based on bilateral procedure, assistant surgeon may be paid

57540   **Remove residual cervix**   ~ follow-up period is 90 days, standard payment adjustment rules for multiple procedures apply, 150% payment adjustment for bilateral procedures does not apply, assistant surgeon may be paid

57545   **Remove cervix/repair pelvis**   ~ follow-up period is 90 days, standard payment adjustment rules for multiple procedures apply, 150% payment adjustment for bilateral procedures does not apply, assistant surgeon may be paid

57550   **Remove residual cervix**   ~ follow-up period is 90 days, standard payment adjustment rules for multiple procedures apply, 150% payment adjustment for bilateral procedures does not apply, assistant surgeon may be paid

57555   **Remove cervix/repair vagina**   ~ follow-up period is 90 days, standard payment adjustment rules for multiple procedures apply, 150% payment adjustment for bilateral procedures does not apply, assistant surgeon may be paid

57556   **Remove cervix, repair bowel**   ~ follow-up period is 90 days, standard payment adjustment rules for multiple procedures apply, 150% payment adjustment for bilateral procedures does not apply, assistant surgeon may be paid

57558   **D & C cervical stump**   ~ follow-up period is 10 days, standard payment adjustment rules for multiple procedures apply, 150% payment adjustment for bilateral procedures does not apply, assistant surgeon may not be paid

57700   **Revise cervix**   ~ follow-up period is 90 days, standard payment adjustment rules for multiple procedures apply, 150% payment adjustment for bilateral procedures does not apply, payment for assistant surgeon subject to documentation of medical necessity

57720   **Revise cervix**   ~ follow-up period is 90 days, standard payment adjustment rules for multiple procedures apply, 150% payment adjustment for bilateral procedures does not apply, assistant surgeon may be paid

57800   **Dilate cervical canal**   ~ endoscopies or minor procedure - E/M services on the same day generally not paid, standard payment adjustment rules for multiple procedures apply, 150% payment adjustment for bilateral procedures does not apply, assistant surgeon may not be paid

Corpus Uteri

58100   **Biopsy uterus lining**   ~ endoscopies or minor procedure - E/M services on the same day generally not paid, standard payment adjustment rules for multiple procedures apply, 150% payment adjustment for bilateral procedures does not apply, assistant surgeon may not be paid

58110   **Biopsy done w/colposcopy, add-on**   ~ follow-up period included in another service, no payment adjustment rules for multiple procedures apply, 150% payment adjustment for bilateral procedures does not apply, payment for assistant surgeon subject to documentation of medical necessity, +add-on code (list separately in addition to primary procedure)

58120   **Dilate and curettage**   ~ follow-up period is 10 days, standard payment adjustment rules for multiple procedures apply, 150% payment adjustment for bilateral procedures does not apply, assistant surgeon may not be paid

58140   **Myomectomy abdom method**   ~ follow-up period is 90 days, standard payment adjustment rules for multiple procedures apply, 150% payment adjustment for bilateral procedures does not apply, assistant surgeon may be paid

58145   **Myomectomy vaginal method**   ~ follow-up period is 90 days, standard payment adjustment rules for multiple procedures apply, 150% payment adjustment for bilateral procedures does not apply, assistant surgeon may be paid

58146   **Myomectomy abdom complex**   ~ follow-up period is 90 days, standard payment adjustment rules for multiple procedures apply, 150% payment adjustment for bilateral procedures does not apply, assistant surgeon may be paid

58150   **Total hysterectomy**   ~ follow-up period is 90 days, standard payment adjustment rules for multiple procedures apply, 150% payment adjustment for bilateral procedures does not apply, assistant surgeon may be paid

58152   **Total hysterectomy**   ~ follow-up period is 90 days, standard payment adjustment rules for multiple procedures apply, 150% payment adjustment for bilateral procedures does not apply, assistant surgeon may be paid

58180   **Partial hysterectomy**   ~ follow-up period is 90 days, standard payment adjustment rules for multiple procedures apply, 150% payment adjustment for bilateral procedures does not apply, assistant surgeon may be paid

58200   **Extensive hysterectomy**   ~ follow-up period is 90 days, standard payment adjustment rules for multiple procedures apply, 150% payment adjustment for bilateral procedures does not apply, assistant surgeon may be paid

58210   **Extensive hysterectomy**   ~ follow-up period is 90 days, standard payment adjustment rules for multiple procedures apply, 150% payment adjustment does not apply - RVUs based on bilateral procedure, assistant surgeon may be paid

58240   **Remove pelvis contents**   ~ follow-up period is 90 days, standard payment adjustment rules for multiple procedures apply, 150% payment adjustment for bilateral procedures does not apply, assistant surgeon may be paid

58260   **Vaginal hysterectomy**   ~ follow-up period is 90 days, standard payment adjustment rules for multiple procedures apply, 150% payment adjustment for bilateral procedures does not apply, assistant surgeon may be paid

58262   **Vaginal hysterectomy including t/o**   ~ follow-up period is 90 days, standard payment adjustment rules for multiple procedures apply, 150% payment adjustment for bilateral procedures does not apply, assistant surgeon may be paid

58263   **Vaginal hysterectomy w/t/o & vaginal repair** ~ follow-up period is 90 days, standard payment adjustment rules for multiple procedures apply, 150% payment adjustment for bilateral procedures does not apply, assistant surgeon may be paid

58267   **Vaginal hysterectomy w/urinary repair**   ~ follow-up period is 90 days, standard payment adjustment rules for multiple procedures apply, 150% payment adjustment for bilateral procedures does not apply, assistant surgeon may be paid

58270   **Vaginal hysterectomy w/enterocele repair** ~ follow-up period is 90 days, standard payment adjustment rules for multiple procedures apply, 150% payment adjustment for bilateral procedures does not apply, assistant surgeon may be paid

58275   **Hysterectomy/revise vagina**   ~ follow-up period is 90 days, standard payment adjustment rules for multiple procedures apply, 150% payment adjustment for bilateral procedures does not apply, assistant surgeon may be paid

58280   **Hysterectomy/revise vagina**   ~ follow-up period is 90 days, standard payment adjustment rules for multiple procedures apply, 150% payment adjustment for bilateral procedures does not apply, assistant surgeon may be paid

58285   **Extensive hysterectomy**   ~ follow-up period is 90 days, standard payment adjustment rules for multiple procedures apply, 150% payment adjustment for bilateral procedures does not apply, assistant surgeon may be paid

58290   **Vaginal hysterectomy complex**   ~ follow-up period is 90 days, standard payment adjustment rules for multiple procedures apply, 150% payment adjustment for bilateral procedures does not apply, assistant surgeon may be paid

58291   **Vaginal hysterectomy including t/o, complex** ~ follow-up period is 90 days, standard payment adjustment rules for multiple procedures apply, 150% payment adjustment for bilateral procedures does not apply, assistant surgeon may be paid

58292   **Vaginal hysterectomy t/o & repair, complete~** follow-up period is 90 days, standard payment adjustment rules for multiple procedures apply, 150% payment adjustment for bilateral procedures does not apply, assistant surgeon may be paid

58293   **Vaginal hysterectomy w/uro repair, complete~** follow-up period is 90 days, standard payment adjustment rules for multiple procedures apply, 150% payment adjustment for bilateral procedures does not apply, assistant surgeon may be paid

58294   **Vaginal hysterectomy w/enterocele, complete** ~ follow-up period is 90 days, standard payment adjustment rules for multiple procedures apply, 150% payment adjustment for bilateral procedures does not apply, assistant surgeon may be paid

58300   **Insert intrauterine device**   non-covered service, multiple procedure concept does not apply, bilateral surgery concept does not apply, assistant surgery concept does not apply

58301   **Remove intrauterine device**   ~ endoscopies or minor procedure - E/M services on the same day generally not paid, standard payment adjustment rules for multiple procedures apply, 150% payment adjustment for bilateral procedures does not apply, payment for assistant surgeon subject to documentation of medical necessity

58321   **Artificial insemination**   ~ endoscopies or minor procedure - E/M services on the same day generally not paid, standard payment adjustment rules for multiple procedures apply, 150% payment adjustment for bilateral procedures does not apply, payment for assistant surgeon subject to documentation of medical necessity

58322   **Artificial insemination**   ~ endoscopies or minor procedure - E/M services on the same day generally not paid, standard payment adjustment rules for multiple procedures apply, 150% payment adjustment for bilateral procedures does not apply, payment for assistant surgeon subject to documentation of medical necessity

58323   **Sperm washing**   ~ endoscopies or minor procedure - E/M services on the same day generally not paid, standard payment adjustment rules for multiple procedures apply, 150% payment adjustment for bilateral procedures does not apply, payment for assistant surgeon subject to documentation of medical necessity

58340   **Catheter for hysterorrhaphy**   ~ endoscopies or minor procedure - E/M services on the same day generally not paid, standard payment adjustment rules for multiple procedures apply, 150% payment adjustment for bilateral procedures does not apply, assistant surgeon may not be paid

58345   **Reopen fallopian tube**   ~ follow-up period is 10 days, standard payment adjustment rules for multiple procedures apply, 150% payment adjustment for bilateral procedures applies, assistant surgeon may be paid

58346   **Insert heyman uteri capsule**   ~ follow-up period is 90 days, standard payment adjustment rules for multiple procedures apply, 150% payment adjustment for bilateral procedures does not apply, assistant surgeon may not be paid

58350   **Reopen fallopian tube**   ~ follow-up period is 10 days, standard payment adjustment rules for multiple procedures apply, 150% payment adjustment for bilateral procedures does not apply, assistant surgeon may not be paid

58353   **Endometrial ablate, thermal**   ~ follow-up period is 10 days, standard payment adjustment rules for multiple procedures apply, 150% payment adjustment for bilateral procedures applies, assistant surgeon may be paid

58356   **Endometrial cryoablation**   ~ follow-up period is 10 days, standard payment adjustment rules for multiple procedures apply, 150% payment adjustment for bilateral procedures applies, assistant surgeon may be paid

58400   **Suspend uterus**   ~ follow-up period is 90 days, standard payment adjustment rules for multiple procedures apply, 150% payment adjustment for bilateral procedures does not apply, assistant surgeon may be paid

58410   **Suspend uterus**   ~ follow-up period is 90 days, standard payment adjustment rules for multiple procedures apply, 150% payment adjustment for bilateral procedures does not apply, assistant surgeon may be paid

58520   **Repair ruptured uteri**   ~ follow-up period is 90 days, standard payment adjustment rules for multiple procedures apply, 150% payment adjustment for bilateral procedures does not apply, assistant surgeon may be paid

58540   **Revise uterus**   ~ follow-up period is 90 days, standard payment adjustment rules for multiple procedures apply, 150% payment adjustment for bilateral procedures does not apply, assistant surgeon may be paid

58541   **Lsh, uterus 250 g or less**   ~ follow-up period is 90 days, special rules for multiple endoscopic procedures apply if billed with another endoscopy in the same family, 150% payment adjustment for bilateral procedures does not apply, assistant surgeon may be paid

58542   **Lsh w/t/o ut 250 g or less**   ~ follow-up period is 90 days, standard payment adjustment rules for multiple procedures apply, 150% payment adjustment for bilateral procedures does not apply, assistant surgeon may be paid

58543   **Lsh uterus above 250 g**   ~ follow-up period is 90 days, standard payment adjustment rules for multiple procedures apply, 150% payment adjustment for bilateral procedures does not apply, assistant surgeon may be paid

58544   **Lsh w/t/o uterus above 250 g**   ~ follow-up period is 90 days, standard payment adjustment rules for multiple procedures apply, 150% payment adjustment for bilateral procedures does not apply, assistant surgeon may be paid

58545   **Laparoscopic myomectomy**   ~ follow-up period is 90 days, standard payment adjustment rules for multiple procedures apply, 150% payment adjustment for bilateral procedures does not apply, assistant surgeon may be paid

58546   **Laparo-myomectomy, complex**   ~ follow-up period is 90 days, standard payment adjustment rules for multiple procedures apply, 150% payment adjustment for bilateral procedures does not apply, assistant surgeon may be paid

58548   **Laparoscopy radical hysterectomy**   ~ follow-up period is 90 days, standard payment adjustment rules for multiple procedures apply, 150% payment adjustment does not apply - RVUs based on bilateral procedure, assistant surgeon may be paid

58550   **Laparo-asst vaginal hysterectomy**   ~ follow-up period is 90 days, special rules for multiple endoscopic procedures apply if billed with another endoscopy in the same family, 150% payment adjustment for bilateral procedures does not apply, assistant surgeon may be paid

58552   **Laparo-vaginal hysterectomy including t/o** ~ follow-up period is 90 days, standard payment adjustment rules for multiple procedures apply, 150% payment adjustment for bilateral procedures does not apply, assistant surgeon may be paid

58553   **Laparo-vaginal hysterectomy, complex**   ~ follow-up period is 90 days, standard payment adjustment rules for multiple procedures apply, 150% payment adjustment for bilateral procedures does not apply, assistant surgeon may be paid

58554   **Laparo-vaginal hysterectomy w/t/o, complete**~ follow-up period is 90 days, standard payment adjustment rules for multiple procedures apply, 150% payment adjustment for bilateral procedures does not apply, assistant surgeon may be paid

58555   **Hysteroscopy, dx, sep proc**   ~ endoscopies or minor procedure - E/M services on the same day generally not paid, standard payment adjustment rules for multiple procedures apply, 150% payment adjustment for bilateral procedures does not apply, payment for assistant surgeon subject to documentation of medical necessity

58558   **Hysteroscopy, biopsy**   ~ endoscopies or minor procedure - E/M services on the same day generally not paid, special rules for multiple endoscopic procedures apply if billed with another endoscopy in the same family, 150% payment adjustment for bilateral procedures does not apply, assistant surgeon may not be paid

58559   **Hysteroscopy, lysis**   ~ endoscopies or minor procedure - E/M services on the same day generally not paid, special rules for multiple endoscopic procedures apply if billed with another endoscopy in the same family, 150% payment adjustment for bilateral procedures does not apply, assistant surgeon may not be paid

58560   **Hysteroscopy, resect septum**   ~ endoscopies or minor procedure - E/M services on the same day generally not paid, special rules for multiple endoscopic procedures apply if billed with another endoscopy in the same family, 150% payment adjustment for bilateral procedures does not apply, assistant surgeon may be paid

58561   **Hysteroscopy, remove myoma**   ~ endoscopies or minor procedure - E/M services on the same day generally not paid, special rules for multiple endoscopic procedures apply if billed with another endoscopy in the same family, 150% payment adjustment for bilateral procedures does not apply, payment for assistant surgeon subject to documentation of medical necessity

58562   **Hysteroscopy, remove foreign body**   ~ endoscopies or minor procedure - E/M services on the same day generally not paid, special rules for multiple endoscopic procedures apply if billed with another endoscopy in the same family, 150% payment adjustment for bilateral procedures does not apply, assistant surgeon may not be paid

58563   **Hysteroscopy, ablation**   ~ endoscopies or minor procedure - E/M services on the same day generally not paid, special rules for multiple endoscopic procedures apply if billed with another endoscopy in the same family, 150% payment adjustment for bilateral procedures does not apply, payment for assistant surgeon subject to documentation of medical necessity

58565   **Hysteroscopy, sterilization**   ~ follow-up period is 90 days, special rules for multiple endoscopic procedures apply if billed with another endoscopy in the same family, 150% payment adjustment does not apply - RVUs based on bilateral procedure, assistant surgeon may not be paid

58578   **Laparo proc, uterus**   ~ medicare carrier determines global period, standard payment adjustment rules for multiple procedures apply, 150% payment adjustment for bilateral procedures applies, assistant surgeon may be paid

58579   **Hysteroscopic procedure**   ~ medicare carrier determines global period, standard payment adjustment rules for multiple procedures apply, 150% payment adjustment for bilateral procedures applies, assistant surgeon may be paid

58600   **Divide fallopian tube**   ~ follow-up period is 90 days, standard payment adjustment rules for multiple procedures apply, 150% payment adjustment does not apply - RVUs based on bilateral procedure, assistant surgeon may be paid

58605   **Divide fallopian tube**   ~ follow-up period is 90 days, standard payment adjustment rules for multiple procedures apply, 150% payment adjustment does not apply - RVUs based on bilateral procedure, assistant surgeon may be paid

58611   **Ligate oviduct(s), add-on**   ~ follow-up period included in another service, no payment adjustment rules for multiple procedures apply, 150% payment adjustment for bilateral procedures does not apply, assistant surgeon may be paid, +add-on code (list separately in addition to primary procedure)

58615 **Occlude fallopian tube(s)** ~ follow-up period is 10 days, standard payment adjustment rules for multiple procedures apply, 150% payment adjustment for bilateral procedures does not apply, assistant surgeon may be paid

58660 **Laparoscopy, lysis** ~ follow-up period is 90 days, special rules for multiple endoscopic procedures apply if billed with another endoscopy in the same family, 150% payment adjustment for bilateral procedures does not apply, assistant surgeon may be paid

58661 **Laparoscopy, remove adnexa** ~ follow-up period is 10 days, special rules for multiple endoscopic procedures apply if billed with another endoscopy in the same family, 150% payment adjustment for bilateral procedures does not apply, assistant surgeon may be paid

58662 **Laparoscopy, excise lesions** ~ follow-up period is 90 days, special rules for multiple endoscopic procedures apply if billed with another endoscopy in the same family, 150% payment adjustment for bilateral procedures does not apply, assistant surgeon may be paid

58670 **Laparoscopy, tubal cautery** ~ follow-up period is 90 days, special rules for multiple endoscopic procedures apply if billed with another endoscopy in the same family, 150% payment adjustment for bilateral procedures does not apply, assistant surgeon may not be paid

58671 **Laparoscopy, tubal block** ~ follow-up period is 90 days, special rules for multiple endoscopic procedures apply if billed with another endoscopy in the same family, 150% payment adjustment for bilateral procedures does not apply, assistant surgeon may not be paid

58672 **Laparoscopy, fimbrioplasty** ~ follow-up period is 90 days, special rules for multiple endoscopic procedures apply if billed with another endoscopy in the same family, 150% payment adjustment for bilateral procedures applies, assistant surgeon may be paid

58673 **Laparoscopy, salpingostomy** ~ follow-up period is 90 days, special rules for multiple endoscopic procedures apply if billed with another endoscopy in the same family, 150% payment adjustment for bilateral procedures applies, assistant surgeon may be paid

58679 **Laparo proc, oviduct-ovary** ~ medicare carrier determines global period, standard payment adjustment rules for multiple procedures apply, 150% payment adjustment for bilateral procedures applies, assistant surgeon may be paid

58700 **Remove fallopian tube** ~ follow-up period is 90 days, standard payment adjustment rules for multiple procedures apply, 150% payment adjustment does not apply - RVUs based on bilateral procedure, assistant surgeon may be paid

58720 **Remove ovary/tube(s)** ~ follow-up period is 90 days, standard payment adjustment rules for multiple procedures apply, 150% payment adjustment does not apply - RVUs based on bilateral procedure, assistant surgeon may be paid

58740 **Revise fallopian tube(s)** ~ follow-up period is 90 days, standard payment adjustment rules for multiple procedures apply, 150% payment adjustment for bilateral procedures does not apply, assistant surgeon may be paid

58750 **Repair oviduct** ~ follow-up period is 90 days, standard payment adjustment rules for multiple procedures apply, 150% payment adjustment for bilateral procedures does not apply, assistant surgeon may be paid

58752 **Revise ovarian tube(s)** ~ follow-up period is 90 days, standard payment adjustment rules for multiple procedures apply, 150% payment adjustment for bilateral procedures does not apply, assistant surgeon may be paid

58760 **Remove tubal obstruction** ~ follow-up period is 90 days, standard payment adjustment rules for multiple procedures apply, 150% payment adjustment for bilateral procedures applies, assistant surgeon may be paid

58770 **Create new tubal opening** ~ follow-up period is 90 days, standard payment adjustment rules for multiple procedures apply, 150% payment adjustment for bilateral procedures applies, assistant surgeon may be paid

Ovary

58800 **Drain ovarian cyst(s)** ~ follow-up period is 90 days, standard payment adjustment rules for multiple procedures apply, 150% payment adjustment does not apply - RVUs based on bilateral procedure, assistant surgeon may not be paid

58805 **Drain ovarian cyst(s)** ~ follow-up period is 90 days, standard payment adjustment rules for multiple procedures apply, 150% payment adjustment does not apply - RVUs based on bilateral procedure, assistant surgeon may be paid

58820 **Drain ovary abscess, open** ~ follow-up period is 90 days, standard payment adjustment rules for multiple procedures apply, 150% payment adjustment for bilateral procedures does not apply, assistant surgeon may be paid

58822 **Drain ovary abscess, percutaneous** ~ follow-up period is 90 days, standard payment adjustment rules for multiple procedures apply, 150% payment adjustment for bilateral procedures does not apply, assistant surgeon may be paid

58823 **Drain pelvic abscess, percutaneous** ~ endoscopies or minor procedure - E/M services on the same day generally not paid, standard payment adjustment rules for multiple procedures apply, 150% payment adjustment for bilateral procedures does not apply, assistant surgeon may be paid

58825   **Transpose ovary(s)**   ~ follow-up period is 90 days, standard payment adjustment rules for multiple procedures apply, 150% payment adjustment for bilateral procedures does not apply, assistant surgeon may be paid

58900   **Biopsy ovary(s)**   ~ follow-up period is 90 days, standard payment adjustment rules for multiple procedures apply, 150% payment adjustment does not apply - RVUs based on bilateral procedure, assistant surgeon may be paid

58920   **Partial remove ovary(s)**   ~ follow-up period is 90 days, standard payment adjustment rules for multiple procedures apply, 150% payment adjustment does not apply - RVUs based on bilateral procedure, assistant surgeon may be paid

58925   **Remove ovarian cyst(s)**   ~ follow-up period is 90 days, standard payment adjustment rules for multiple procedures apply, 150% payment adjustment does not apply - RVUs based on bilateral procedure, assistant surgeon may be paid

58940   **Remove ovary(s)**   ~ follow-up period is 90 days, standard payment adjustment rules for multiple procedures apply, 150% payment adjustment does not apply - RVUs based on bilateral procedure, assistant surgeon may be paid

58943   **Remove ovary(s)**   ~ follow-up period is 90 days, standard payment adjustment rules for multiple procedures apply, 150% payment adjustment for bilateral procedures does not apply, assistant surgeon may be paid

58950   **Resect ovarian malignancy**   ~ follow-up period is 90 days, standard payment adjustment rules for multiple procedures apply, 150% payment adjustment does not apply - RVUs based on bilateral procedure, assistant surgeon may be paid

58951   **Resect ovarian malignancy**   ~ follow-up period is 90 days, standard payment adjustment rules for multiple procedures apply, 150% payment adjustment does not apply - RVUs based on bilateral procedure, assistant surgeon may be paid

58952   **Resect ovarian malignancy**   ~ follow-up period is 90 days, standard payment adjustment rules for multiple procedures apply, 150% payment adjustment does not apply - RVUs based on bilateral procedure, assistant surgeon may be paid

58953   **Tah, radiation dissect for debulk**   ~ follow-up period is 90 days, standard payment adjustment rules for multiple procedures apply, 150% payment adjustment does not apply - RVUs based on bilateral procedure, assistant surgeon may be paid

58954   **Tah radiation debulk/lymph remove**   ~ follow-up period is 90 days, standard payment adjustment rules for multiple procedures apply, 150% payment adjustment does not apply - RVUs based on bilateral procedure, assistant surgeon may be paid

58956   **Bso, omentectomy w/tah**   ~ follow-up period is 90 days, standard payment adjustment rules for multiple procedures apply, 150% payment adjustment does not apply - RVUs based on bilateral procedure, assistant surgeon may be paid

58957   **Resect recurrent gyn mal**   ~ follow-up period is 90 days, standard payment adjustment rules for multiple procedures apply, 150% payment adjustment does not apply - RVUs based on bilateral procedure, assistant surgeon may be paid

58958   **Resect recur gyn mal w/lymph**   ~ follow-up period is 90 days, standard payment adjustment rules for multiple procedures apply, 150% payment adjustment does not apply - RVUs based on bilateral procedure, assistant surgeon may be paid

58960   **Explore abdomen**   ~ follow-up period is 90 days, standard payment adjustment rules for multiple procedures apply, 150% payment adjustment for bilateral procedures does not apply, assistant surgeon may be paid

In Vitro Fertilization

58970   **Retrieval of oocyte**   ~ endoscopies or minor procedure - E/M services on the same day generally not paid, standard payment adjustment rules for multiple procedures apply, 150% payment adjustment for bilateral procedures does not apply, payment for assistant surgeon subject to documentation of medical necessity

58974   **Transfer of embryo**   ~ endoscopies or minor procedure - E/M services on the same day generally not paid, standard payment adjustment rules for multiple procedures apply, 150% payment adjustment for bilateral procedures does not apply, assistant surgeon may be paid

58976   **Transfer of embryo**   ~ endoscopies or minor procedure - E/M services on the same day generally not paid, standard payment adjustment rules for multiple procedures apply, 150% payment adjustment for bilateral procedures does not apply, assistant surgeon may be paid

58999   **Genital surgery procedure**   ~ medicare carrier determines global period, standard payment adjustment rules for multiple procedures apply, 150% payment adjustment for bilateral procedures does not apply, assistant surgeon may be paid

MATERNITY CARE AND DELIVERY

59000   **Amniocentesis, diagnostic**   ~ endoscopies or minor procedure - E/M services on the same day generally not paid, standard payment adjustment rules for multiple procedures apply, 150% payment adjustment for bilateral procedures does not apply, assistant surgeon may not be paid

59001   **Amniocentesis, therapeutic**   ~ endoscopies or minor procedure - E/M services on the same day generally not paid, standard payment adjustment rules for multiple procedures apply, 150% payment adjustment for bilateral procedures does not apply, assistant surgeon may not be paid

59012   **Fetal cord puncture, prenatal**   ~ endoscopies or minor procedure - E/M services on the same day generally not paid, standard payment adjustment rules for multiple

procedures apply, 150% payment adjustment for bilateral procedures does not apply, payment for assistant surgeon subject to documentation of medical necessity

59015   **Chorionic biopsy**   ~ endoscopies or minor procedure - E/M services on the same day generally not paid, standard payment adjustment rules for multiple procedures apply, 150% payment adjustment for bilateral procedures does not apply, payment for assistant surgeon subject to documentation of medical necessity

59020   **Fetal contract stress test**   ~ endoscopies or minor procedure - E/M services on the same day generally not paid, standard payment adjustment rules for multiple procedures apply, 150% payment adjustment for bilateral procedures does not apply, payment for assistant surgeon subject to documentation of medical necessity

59025   **Fetal non-stress test**   ~ endoscopies or minor procedure - E/M services on the same day generally not paid, standard payment adjustment rules for multiple procedures apply, 150% payment adjustment for bilateral procedures does not apply, payment for assistant surgeon subject to documentation of medical necessity

59030   **Fetal scalp blood sample**   ~ endoscopies or minor procedure - E/M services on the same day generally not paid, standard payment adjustment rules for multiple procedures apply, 150% payment adjustment for bilateral procedures does not apply, payment for assistant surgeon subject to documentation of medical necessity

59050   **Fetal monitor w/report**   ~ no payment adjustment rules for multiple procedures apply, 150% payment adjustment for bilateral procedures does not apply, payment for assistant surgeon subject to documentation of medical necessity

59051   **Fetal monitor/interpret only**   ~ no payment adjustment rules for multiple procedures apply, 150% payment adjustment for bilateral procedures does not apply, payment for assistant surgeon subject to documentation of medical necessity

59070   **Transabdominal amnioinfusion w/us**   ~ endoscopies or minor procedure - E/M services on the same day generally not paid, standard payment adjustment rules for multiple procedures apply, 150% payment adjustment for bilateral procedures does not apply, assistant surgeon may be paid

59072   **Umbilical cord occlusion w/us**   ~ endoscopies or minor procedure - E/M services on the same day generally not paid, standard payment adjustment rules for multiple procedures apply, 150% payment adjustment for bilateral procedures does not apply, assistant surgeon may not be paid

59074   **Fetal fluid drain w/us**   ~ endoscopies or minor procedure - E/M services on the same day generally not paid, standard payment adjustment rules for multiple procedures apply, 150% payment adjustment for bilateral procedures does not apply, assistant surgeon may be paid

59076   **Fetal shunt placement, w/us**   ~ endoscopies or minor procedure - E/M services on the same day generally not paid, standard payment adjustment rules for multiple procedures apply, 150% payment adjustment for bilateral procedures does not apply, assistant surgeon may be paid

59100   **Remove uterus lesion**   ~ follow-up period is 90 days, standard payment adjustment rules for multiple procedures apply, 150% payment adjustment for bilateral procedures does not apply, assistant surgeon may be paid

59120   **Treat ectopic pregnancy**   ~ follow-up period is 90 days, standard payment adjustment rules for multiple procedures apply, 150% payment adjustment for bilateral procedures does not apply, assistant surgeon may be paid

59121   **Treat ectopic pregnancy**   ~ follow-up period is 90 days, standard payment adjustment rules for multiple procedures apply, 150% payment adjustment for bilateral procedures does not apply, assistant surgeon may be paid

59130   **Treat ectopic pregnancy**   ~ follow-up period is 90 days, standard payment adjustment rules for multiple procedures apply, 150% payment adjustment for bilateral procedures does not apply, payment for assistant surgeon subject to documentation of medical necessity

59135   **Treat ectopic pregnancy**   ~ follow-up period is 90 days, standard payment adjustment rules for multiple procedures apply, 150% payment adjustment for bilateral procedures does not apply, payment for assistant surgeon subject to documentation of medical necessity

59136   **Treat ectopic pregnancy**   ~ follow-up period is 90 days, standard payment adjustment rules for multiple procedures apply, 150% payment adjustment for bilateral procedures does not apply, assistant surgeon may be paid

59140   **Treat ectopic pregnancy**   ~ follow-up period is 90 days, standard payment adjustment rules for multiple procedures apply, 150% payment adjustment for bilateral procedures does not apply, assistant surgeon may be paid

59150   **Treat ectopic pregnancy**   ~ follow-up period is 90 days, standard payment adjustment rules for multiple procedures apply, 150% payment adjustment for bilateral procedures does not apply, assistant surgeon may be paid

59151   **Treat ectopic pregnancy**   ~ follow-up period is 90 days, standard payment adjustment rules for multiple procedures apply, 150% payment adjustment for bilateral procedures does not apply, assistant surgeon may be paid

59160   **D & C after delivery**   ~ follow-up period is 10 days, standard payment adjustment rules for multiple procedures apply, 150% payment adjustment for bilateral procedures does not apply, payment for assistant surgeon subject to documentation of medical necessity

59200   **Insert cervical dilator**   ~ endoscopies or minor procedure - E/M services on the same day generally not paid, standard payment adjustment rules for multiple procedures apply, 150% payment adjustment for bilateral procedures does not apply, assistant surgeon may not be paid

59300   **Episiotomy or vaginal repair**   ~ endoscopies or minor procedure - E/M services on the same day generally not paid, standard payment adjustment rules for multiple procedures apply, 150% payment adjustment for bilateral procedures does not apply, payment for assistant surgeon subject to documentation of medical necessity

59320   **Revise cervix**   ~ endoscopies or minor procedure - E/M services on the same day generally not paid, standard payment adjustment rules for multiple procedures apply, 150% payment adjustment for bilateral procedures does not apply, payment for assistant surgeon subject to documentation of medical necessity

59325   **Revise cervix**   ~ endoscopies or minor procedure - E/M services on the same day generally not paid, standard payment adjustment rules for multiple procedures apply, 150% payment adjustment for bilateral procedures does not apply, payment for assistant surgeon subject to documentation of medical necessity

59350   **Repair uterus**   ~ endoscopies or minor procedure - E/M services on the same day generally not paid, standard payment adjustment rules for multiple procedures apply, 150% payment adjustment for bilateral procedures does not apply, assistant surgeon may be paid

59400   **Obstetrical care**   maternity code - global period does not apply, standard payment adjustment rules for multiple procedures apply, 150% payment adjustment for bilateral procedures does not apply, assistant surgeon may not be paid

59409   **Obstetrical care**   maternity code - global period does not apply, standard payment adjustment rules for multiple procedures apply, 150% payment adjustment for bilateral procedures does not apply, payment for assistant surgeon subject to documentation of medical necessity

59410   **Obstetrical care**   maternity code - global period does not apply, standard payment adjustment rules for multiple procedures apply, 150% payment adjustment for bilateral procedures does not apply, assistant surgeon may not be paid

59412   **Antepartum manipulation**   maternity code - global period does not apply, no payment adjustment rules for multiple procedures apply, 150% payment adjustment for bilateral procedures does not apply, payment for assistant surgeon subject to documentation of medical necessity

59414   **Deliver placenta**   maternity code - global period does not apply, standard payment adjustment rules for multiple procedures apply, 150% payment adjustment for bilateral procedures does not apply, payment for assistant surgeon subject to documentation of medical necessity

59425   **Antepartum care only**   maternity code - global period does not apply, no payment adjustment rules for multiple procedures apply, 150% payment adjustment for bilateral procedures does not apply, payment for assistant surgeon subject to documentation of medical necessity

59426   **Antepartum care only**   maternity code - global period does not apply, no payment adjustment rules for multiple procedures apply, 150% payment adjustment for bilateral procedures does not apply, payment for assistant surgeon subject to documentation of medical necessity

59430   **Care after delivery**   maternity code - global period does not apply, standard payment adjustment rules for multiple procedures apply, 150% payment adjustment for bilateral procedures does not apply, assistant surgeon may not be paid

59510   **Cesarean delivery**   maternity code - global period does not apply, standard payment adjustment rules for multiple procedures apply, 150% payment adjustment for bilateral procedures does not apply, assistant surgeon may not be paid

59514   **Cesarean delivery only**   maternity code - global period does not apply, standard payment adjustment rules for multiple procedures apply, 150% payment adjustment for bilateral procedures does not apply, assistant surgeon may be paid

59515   **Cesarean delivery**   maternity code - global period does not apply, standard payment adjustment rules for multiple procedures apply, 150% payment adjustment for bilateral procedures does not apply, assistant surgeon may not be paid

59525   **Remove uterus after cesarean**   ~ follow-up period included in another service, no payment adjustment rules for multiple procedures apply, 150% payment adjustment for bilateral procedures does not apply, assistant surgeon may be paid

59610   **VBAC delivery**   maternity code - global period does not apply, standard payment adjustment rules for multiple procedures apply, 150% payment adjustment for bilateral procedures does not apply, payment for assistant surgeon subject to documentation of medical necessity

59612   **VBAC delivery only**   maternity code - global period does not apply, standard payment adjustment rules for multiple procedures apply, 150% payment adjustment for bilateral procedures does not apply, payment for assistant surgeon subject to documentation of medical necessity

59614   **VBAC care after delivery**   maternity code - global period does not apply, standard payment adjustment rules for multiple procedures apply, 150% payment adjustment for bilateral procedures does not apply, payment for assistant surgeon subject to documentation of medical necessity

59618   **Attempted VBAC delivery**   maternity code - global period does not apply, standard payment adjustment rules for multiple procedures apply, 150% payment adjustment for bilateral procedures does not apply, assistant surgeon may be paid

59620   **Attempted VBAC delivery only**   maternity code - global period does not apply, standard payment adjustment rules for multiple procedures apply, 150% payment adjustment for bilateral procedures does not apply, assistant surgeon may be paid

59622   **Attempted VBAC after care**   maternity code - global period does not apply, standard payment adjustment rules for multiple procedures apply, 150% payment adjustment for bilateral procedures does not apply, assistant surgeon may be paid

59812   **Treat miscarriage**   ~ follow-up period is 90 days, standard payment adjustment rules for multiple procedures apply, 150% payment adjustment for bilateral procedures does not apply, assistant surgeon may not be paid

59820   **Care of miscarriage**   ~ follow-up period is 90 days, standard payment adjustment rules for multiple procedures apply, 150% payment adjustment for bilateral procedures does not apply, assistant surgeon may not be paid

59821   **Treat miscarriage**   ~ follow-up period is 90 days, standard payment adjustment rules for multiple procedures apply, 150% payment adjustment for bilateral procedures does not apply, payment for assistant surgeon subject to documentation of medical necessity

59830   **Treat uterus infection**   ~ follow-up period is 90 days, standard payment adjustment rules for multiple procedures apply, 150% payment adjustment for bilateral procedures does not apply, payment for assistant surgeon subject to documentation of medical necessity

59840   **Abortion**   ~ restricted coverage - special coverage rules apply, follow-up period is 10 days, standard payment adjustment rules for multiple procedures apply, 150% payment adjustment for bilateral procedures does not apply, payment for assistant surgeon subject to documentation of medical necessity

59841   **Abortion**   ~ restricted coverage - special coverage rules apply, follow-up period is 10 days, standard payment adjustment rules for multiple procedures apply, 150% payment adjustment for bilateral procedures does not apply, payment for assistant surgeon subject to documentation of medical necessity

59850   **Abortion**   ~ restricted coverage - special coverage rules apply, follow-up period is 90 days, standard payment adjustment rules for multiple procedures apply, 150% payment adjustment for bilateral procedures does not apply, payment for assistant surgeon subject to documentation of medical necessity

59851   **Abortion**   ~ restricted coverage - special coverage rules apply, follow-up period is 90 days, standard payment adjustment rules for multiple

procedures apply, 150% payment adjustment for bilateral procedures does not apply, payment for assistant surgeon subject to documentation of medical necessity

59852   **Abortion**   ~ restricted coverage - special coverage rules apply, follow-up period is 90 days, standard payment adjustment rules for multiple procedures apply, 150% payment adjustment for bilateral procedures does not apply, payment for assistant surgeon subject to documentation of medical necessity

59855   **Abortion**   ~ restricted coverage - special coverage rules apply, follow-up period is 90 days, standard payment adjustment rules for multiple procedures apply, 150% payment adjustment for bilateral procedures does not apply, payment for assistant surgeon subject to documentation of medical necessity

59856   **Abortion**   ~ restricted coverage - special coverage rules apply, follow-up period is 90 days, standard payment adjustment rules for multiple procedures apply, 150% payment adjustment for bilateral procedures does not apply, payment for assistant surgeon subject to documentation of medical necessity

59857   **Abortion**   ~ restricted coverage - special coverage rules apply, follow-up period is 90 days, standard payment adjustment rules for multiple procedures apply, 150% payment adjustment for bilateral procedures does not apply, payment for assistant surgeon subject to documentation of medical necessity

59866   **Abortion (mpr)**   ~ restricted coverage - special coverage rules apply, endoscopies or minor procedure - E/M services on the same day generally not paid, standard payment adjustment rules for multiple procedures apply, 150% payment adjustment for bilateral procedures does not apply, assistant surgeon may be paid

59870   **Evacuate mole of uterus**   ~ follow-up period is 90 days, standard payment adjustment rules for multiple procedures apply, 150% payment adjustment for bilateral procedures does not apply, assistant surgeon may be paid

59871   **Remove cerclage suture**   ~ endoscopies or minor procedure - E/M services on the same day generally not paid, standard payment adjustment rules for multiple procedures apply, 150% payment adjustment for bilateral procedures does not apply, payment for assistant surgeon subject to documentation of medical necessity

59897   **Fetal invasive procedure w/us**   ~ medicare carrier determines global period, standard payment adjustment rules for multiple procedures apply, 150% payment adjustment for bilateral procedures does not apply, assistant surgeon may not be paid

59898   **Laparo proc, ob care/deliver**   ~ medicare carrier determines global period, standard payment adjustment rules for multiple procedures apply, 150% payment adjustment for bilateral procedures applies, assistant surgeon may be paid

59899   **Maternity care procedure**   ~ medicare carrier determines global period, standard payment adjustment rules for multiple procedures apply, 150% payment adjustment for bilateral procedures does not apply, assistant surgeon may be paid

ENDOCRINE SYSTEM

Thyroid Gland

60000   **Drain thyroid/tongue cyst**   ~ follow-up period is 10 days, standard payment adjustment rules for multiple procedures apply, 150% payment adjustment for bilateral procedures does not apply, payment for assistant surgeon subject to documentation of medical necessity

60001   **Aspirate/inject thyroid cyst**   ~ endoscopies or minor procedure - E/M services on the same day generally not paid, standard payment adjustment rules for multiple procedures apply, 150% payment adjustment for bilateral procedures does not apply, assistant surgeon may not be paid

60100   **Biopsy thyroid**   ~ endoscopies or minor procedure - E/M services on the same day generally not paid, standard payment adjustment rules for multiple procedures apply, 150% payment adjustment for bilateral procedures does not apply, assistant surgeon may not be paid

60200   **Remove thyroid lesion**   ~ follow-up period is 90 days, standard payment adjustment rules for multiple procedures apply, 150% payment adjustment for bilateral procedures does not apply, assistant surgeon may be paid

60210   **Partial thyroid excision**   ~ follow-up period is 90 days, standard payment adjustment rules for multiple procedures apply, 150% payment adjustment for bilateral procedures does not apply, assistant surgeon may be paid

60212   **Partial thyroid excision**   ~ follow-up period is 90 days, standard payment adjustment rules for multiple procedures apply, 150% payment adjustment for bilateral procedures does not apply, assistant surgeon may be paid

60220   **Partial remove thyroid**   ~ follow-up period is 90 days, standard payment adjustment rules for multiple procedures apply, 150% payment adjustment for bilateral procedures does not apply, assistant surgeon may be paid

60225   **Partial remove thyroid**   ~ follow-up period is 90 days, standard payment adjustment rules for multiple procedures apply, 150% payment adjustment for bilateral procedures does not apply, assistant surgeon may be paid

60240   **Remove thyroid**   ~ follow-up period is 90 days, standard payment adjustment rules for multiple procedures apply, 150% payment adjustment for bilateral procedures does not apply, assistant surgeon may be paid

60252   **Remove thyroid**   ~ follow-up period is 90 days, standard payment adjustment rules for multiple procedures apply, 150% payment adjustment for bilateral procedures does not apply, assistant surgeon may be paid

60254   **Extensive thyroid surgery**   ~ follow-up period is 90 days, standard payment adjustment rules for multiple procedures apply, 150% payment adjustment for bilateral procedures does not apply, assistant surgeon may be paid

60260   **Repeat thyroid surgery**   ~ follow-up period is 90 days, standard payment adjustment rules for multiple procedures apply, 150% payment adjustment for bilateral procedures applies, assistant surgeon may be paid

60270   **Remove thyroid**   ~ follow-up period is 90 days, standard payment adjustment rules for multiple procedures apply, 150% payment adjustment for bilateral procedures does not apply, assistant surgeon may be paid

60271   **Remove thyroid**   ~ follow-up period is 90 days, standard payment adjustment rules for multiple procedures apply, 150% payment adjustment for bilateral procedures does not apply, assistant surgeon may be paid

60280   **Remove thyroid duct lesion**   ~ follow-up period is 90 days, standard payment adjustment rules for multiple procedures apply, 150% payment adjustment for bilateral procedures does not apply, assistant surgeon may be paid

60281   **Remove thyroid duct lesion**   ~ follow-up period is 90 days, standard payment adjustment rules for multiple procedures apply, 150% payment adjustment for bilateral procedures does not apply, assistant surgeon may be paid

Parathyroid, Thymus, Adrenal Glands, Pancreas, and Carotid Body

60500   **Explore parathyroid glands**   ~ follow-up period is 90 days, standard payment adjustment rules for multiple procedures apply, 150% payment adjustment for bilateral procedures does not apply, assistant surgeon may be paid

60502   **Re-explore parathyroids**   ~ follow-up period is 90 days, standard payment adjustment rules for multiple procedures apply, 150% payment adjustment for bilateral procedures does not apply, assistant surgeon may be paid

60505   **Explore parathyroid glands**   ~ follow-up period is 90 days, standard payment adjustment rules for multiple procedures apply, 150% payment adjustment for bilateral procedures does not apply, assistant surgeon may be paid

60512   **Autotransplant parathyroid**   ~ follow-up period included in another service, no payment adjustment rules for multiple procedures apply, 150% payment adjustment for bilateral procedures does not apply, assistant surgeon may be paid

60520   **Remove thymus gland**   ~ follow-up period is 90 days, standard payment adjustment rules for multiple procedures apply, 150% payment adjustment for bilateral procedures does not apply, assistant surgeon may be paid

60521   **Remove thymus gland**   ~ follow-up period is 90 days, standard payment adjustment rules for multiple procedures apply, 150% payment adjustment for bilateral procedures does not apply, assistant surgeon may be paid

60522   **Remove thymus gland**   ~ follow-up period is 90 days, standard payment adjustment rules for multiple procedures apply, 150% payment adjustment for bilateral procedures does not apply, assistant surgeon may be paid

60540   **Explore adrenal gland**   ~ follow-up period is 90 days, standard payment adjustment rules for multiple procedures apply, 150% payment adjustment for bilateral procedures applies, assistant surgeon may be paid

60545   **Explore adrenal gland**   ~ follow-up period is 90 days, standard payment adjustment rules for multiple procedures apply, 150% payment adjustment for bilateral procedures does not apply, assistant surgeon may be paid

60600   **Remove carotid body lesion**   ~ follow-up period is 90 days, standard payment adjustment rules for multiple procedures apply, 150% payment adjustment for bilateral procedures does not apply, assistant surgeon may be paid

60605   **Remove carotid body lesion**   ~ follow-up period is 90 days, standard payment adjustment rules for multiple procedures apply, 150% payment adjustment for bilateral procedures does not apply, assistant surgeon may be paid

60650   **Laparoscopy adrenalectomy**   ~ follow-up period is 90 days, standard payment adjustment rules for multiple procedures apply, 150% payment adjustment for bilateral procedures applies, assistant surgeon may be paid

60659   **Laparo proc, endocrine**   ~ medicare carrier determines global period, standard payment adjustment rules for multiple procedures apply, 150% payment adjustment for bilateral procedures applies, assistant surgeon may be paid

60699   **Endocrine surgery procedure**   ~ medicare carrier determines global period, standard payment adjustment rules for multiple procedures apply, 150% payment adjustment for bilateral procedures does not apply, assistant surgeon may be paid

NERVOUS SYSTEM

Skull, Meninges, and Brain

61000   **Remove cranial cavity fluid**   ~ endoscopies or minor procedure - E/M services on the same day generally not paid, standard payment adjustment rules for multiple procedures apply, 150% payment adjustment does not apply - RVUs based on bilateral procedure, assistant surgeon may not be paid

61001   **Remove cranial cavity fluid**   ~ endoscopies or minor procedure - E/M services on the same day generally not paid, standard payment adjustment rules for multiple procedures apply, 150% payment adjustment does not apply - RVUs based on bilateral procedure, assistant surgeon may not be paid

61020   **Remove brain cavity fluid**   ~ endoscopies or minor procedure - E/M services on the same day generally not paid, standard payment adjustment rules for multiple procedures apply, 150% payment adjustment for bilateral procedures does not apply, assistant surgeon may not be paid

61026   **Inject into brain canal**   ~ endoscopies or minor procedure - E/M services on the same day generally not paid, standard payment adjustment rules for multiple procedures apply, 150% payment adjustment for bilateral procedures does not apply, assistant surgeon may not be paid

61050   **Remove brain canal fluid**   ~ endoscopies or minor procedure - E/M services on the same day generally not paid, standard payment adjustment rules for multiple procedures apply, 150% payment adjustment for bilateral procedures does not apply, payment for assistant surgeon subject to documentation of medical necessity

61055   **Inject into brain canal**   ~ endoscopies or minor procedure - E/M services on the same day generally not paid, no payment adjustment rules for multiple procedures apply, 150% payment adjustment for bilateral procedures does not apply, assistant surgeon may not be paid

61070   **Brain canal shunt procedure**   ~ endoscopies or minor procedure - E/M services on the same day generally not paid, standard payment adjustment rules for multiple procedures apply, 150% payment adjustment for bilateral procedures does not apply, assistant surgeon may not be paid

61105   **Twist drill hole**   ~ follow-up period is 90 days, standard payment adjustment rules for multiple procedures apply, 150% payment adjustment for bilateral procedures does not apply, payment for assistant surgeon subject to documentation of medical necessity

61107   **Drill skull for implantation**   ~ endoscopies or minor procedure - E/M services on the same day generally not paid, no payment adjustment rules for multiple procedures apply, 150% payment adjustment for bilateral procedures does not apply, assistant surgeon may not be paid

61108   **Drill skull for drainage**   ~ follow-up period is 90 days, standard payment adjustment rules for multiple procedures apply, 150% payment adjustment for bilateral procedures does not apply, assistant surgeon may not be paid

61120 **Burr hole for puncture** ~ follow-up period is 90 days, standard payment adjustment rules for multiple procedures apply, 150% payment adjustment for bilateral procedures does not apply, payment for assistant surgeon subject to documentation of medical necessity

61140 **Pierce skull for biopsy** ~ follow-up period is 90 days, standard payment adjustment rules for multiple procedures apply, 150% payment adjustment for bilateral procedures does not apply, assistant surgeon may be paid

61150 **Pierce skull for drainage** ~ follow-up period is 90 days, standard payment adjustment rules for multiple procedures apply, 150% payment adjustment for bilateral procedures does not apply, assistant surgeon may not be paid

61151 **Pierce skull for drainage** ~ follow-up period is 90 days, standard payment adjustment rules for multiple procedures apply, 150% payment adjustment for bilateral procedures does not apply, assistant surgeon may not be paid

61154 **Pierce skull & remove clot** ~ follow-up period is 90 days, standard payment adjustment rules for multiple procedures apply, 150% payment adjustment for bilateral procedures applies, assistant surgeon may be paid

61156 **Pierce skull for drainage** ~ follow-up period is 90 days, standard payment adjustment rules for multiple procedures apply, 150% payment adjustment for bilateral procedures does not apply, assistant surgeon may be paid

61210 **Pierce skull, implant device** ~ endoscopies or minor procedure - E/M services on the same day generally not paid, no payment adjustment rules for multiple procedures apply, 150% payment adjustment for bilateral procedures does not apply, assistant surgeon may not be paid

61215 **Insert brain-fluid device** ~ follow-up period is 90 days, standard payment adjustment rules for multiple procedures apply, 150% payment adjustment for bilateral procedures does not apply, assistant surgeon may not be paid

61250 **Pierce skull & explore** ~ follow-up period is 90 days, standard payment adjustment rules for multiple procedures apply, 150% payment adjustment for bilateral procedures applies, assistant surgeon may be paid

61253 **Pierce skull & explore** ~ follow-up period is 90 days, standard payment adjustment rules for multiple procedures apply, 150% payment adjustment does not apply - RVUs based on bilateral procedure, assistant surgeon may be paid

61304 **Open skull for exploration** ~ follow-up period is 90 days, standard payment adjustment rules for multiple procedures apply, 150% payment adjustment for bilateral procedures does not apply, assistant surgeon may be paid

61305   **Open skull for exploration**   ~ follow-up period is 90 days, standard payment adjustment rules for multiple procedures apply, 150% payment adjustment for bilateral procedures does not apply, assistant surgeon may be paid

61312   **Open skull for drainage**   ~ follow-up period is 90 days, standard payment adjustment rules for multiple procedures apply, 150% payment adjustment for bilateral procedures does not apply, assistant surgeon may be paid

61313   **Open skull for drainage**   ~ follow-up period is 90 days, standard payment adjustment rules for multiple procedures apply, 150% payment adjustment for bilateral procedures does not apply, assistant surgeon may be paid

61314   **Open skull for drainage**   ~ follow-up period is 90 days, standard payment adjustment rules for multiple procedures apply, 150% payment adjustment for bilateral procedures does not apply, assistant surgeon may be paid

61315   **Open skull for drainage**   ~ follow-up period is 90 days, standard payment adjustment rules for multiple procedures apply, 150% payment adjustment for bilateral procedures does not apply, assistant surgeon may be paid

61316   **Implant cranial bone flap to abdomen**   ~ follow-up period included in another service, no payment adjustment rules for multiple procedures apply, 150% payment adjustment for bilateral procedures does not apply, assistant surgeon may not be paid

61320   **Open skull for drainage**   ~ follow-up period is 90 days, standard payment adjustment rules for multiple procedures apply, 150% payment adjustment for bilateral procedures does not apply, assistant surgeon may be paid

61321   **Open skull for drainage**   ~ follow-up period is 90 days, standard payment adjustment rules for multiple procedures apply, 150% payment adjustment for bilateral procedures does not apply, assistant surgeon may be paid

61322   **Decompressive craniotomy**   ~ follow-up period is 90 days, standard payment adjustment rules for multiple procedures apply, 150% payment adjustment for bilateral procedures does not apply, assistant surgeon may be paid

61323   **Decompressive lobectomy**   ~ follow-up period is 90 days, standard payment adjustment rules for multiple procedures apply, 150% payment adjustment for bilateral procedures does not apply, assistant surgeon may not be paid

61330   **Decompress eye socket**   ~ follow-up period is 90 days, standard payment adjustment rules for multiple procedures apply, 150% payment adjustment for bilateral procedures applies, assistant surgeon may be paid

61332   **Explore/biopsy eye socket**   ~ follow-up period is 90 days, standard payment adjustment rules for multiple procedures apply, 150% payment adjustment for bilateral procedures does not apply, assistant surgeon may be paid

61333   **Explore orbit/remove lesion**   ~ follow-up period is 90 days, standard payment adjustment rules for multiple procedures apply, 150% payment adjustment for bilateral procedures does not apply, assistant surgeon may be paid

61334   **Explore orbit/remove object**   ~ follow-up period is 90 days, standard payment adjustment rules for multiple procedures apply, 150% payment adjustment for bilateral procedures does not apply, assistant surgeon may be paid

61340   **Subtemporal decompression**   ~ follow-up period is 90 days, standard payment adjustment rules for multiple procedures apply, 150% payment adjustment for bilateral procedures applies, assistant surgeon may be paid

61343   **Incise skull (press relief)**   ~ follow-up period is 90 days, standard payment adjustment rules for multiple procedures apply, 150% payment adjustment for bilateral procedures does not apply, assistant surgeon may be paid

61345   **Relieve cranial pressure**   ~ follow-up period is 90 days, standard payment adjustment rules for multiple procedures apply, 150% payment adjustment for bilateral procedures does not apply, assistant surgeon may be paid

61440   **Incise skull for surgery**   ~ follow-up period is 90 days, standard payment adjustment rules for multiple procedures apply, 150% payment adjustment for bilateral procedures does not apply, assistant surgeon may be paid

61450   **Incise skull for surgery**   ~ follow-up period is 90 days, standard payment adjustment rules for multiple procedures apply, 150% payment adjustment for bilateral procedures does not apply, assistant surgeon may be paid

61458   **Incise skull for brain wound**   ~ follow-up period is 90 days, standard payment adjustment rules for multiple procedures apply, 150% payment adjustment for bilateral procedures does not apply, assistant surgeon may be paid

61460   **Incise skull for surgery**   ~ follow-up period is 90 days, standard payment adjustment rules for multiple procedures apply, 150% payment adjustment for bilateral procedures does not apply, assistant surgeon may be paid

61470   **Incise skull for surgery**   ~ follow-up period is 90 days, standard payment adjustment rules for multiple procedures apply, 150% payment adjustment for bilateral procedures does not apply, assistant surgeon may be paid

61480   **Incise skull for surgery**   ~ follow-up period is 90 days, standard payment adjustment rules for multiple procedures apply, 150% payment adjustment for bilateral procedures does not apply, assistant surgeon may be paid

61490   **Incise skull for surgery**   ~ follow-up period is 90 days, standard payment adjustment rules for multiple procedures apply, 150% payment adjustment for bilateral procedures applies, assistant surgeon may be paid

61500 **Remove skull lesion** ~ follow-up period is 90 days, standard payment adjustment rules for multiple procedures apply, 150% payment adjustment for bilateral procedures does not apply, assistant surgeon may be paid

61501 **Remove infected skull bone** ~ follow-up period is 90 days, standard payment adjustment rules for multiple procedures apply, 150% payment adjustment for bilateral procedures does not apply, assistant surgeon may be paid

61510 **Remove brain lesion** ~ follow-up period is 90 days, standard payment adjustment rules for multiple procedures apply, 150% payment adjustment for bilateral procedures does not apply, assistant surgeon may be paid

61512 **Remove brain lining lesion** ~ follow-up period is 90 days, standard payment adjustment rules for multiple procedures apply, 150% payment adjustment for bilateral procedures does not apply, assistant surgeon may be paid

61514 **Remove brain abscess** ~ follow-up period is 90 days, standard payment adjustment rules for multiple procedures apply, 150% payment adjustment for bilateral procedures does not apply, assistant surgeon may be paid

61516 **Remove brain lesion** ~ follow-up period is 90 days, standard payment adjustment rules for multiple procedures apply, 150% payment adjustment for bilateral procedures does not apply, assistant surgeon may be paid

61517 **Implant brain chemotherapy, add-on** ~ follow-up period included in another service, no payment adjustment rules for multiple procedures apply, 150% payment adjustment for bilateral procedures does not apply, assistant surgeon may not be paid, +add-on code (list separately in addition to primary procedure)

61518 **Remove brain lesion** ~ follow-up period is 90 days, standard payment adjustment rules for multiple procedures apply, 150% payment adjustment for bilateral procedures does not apply, assistant surgeon may be paid

61519 **Remove brain lining lesion** ~ follow-up period is 90 days, standard payment adjustment rules for multiple procedures apply, 150% payment adjustment for bilateral procedures does not apply, assistant surgeon may be paid

61520 **Remove brain lesion** ~ follow-up period is 90 days, standard payment adjustment rules for multiple procedures apply, 150% payment adjustment for bilateral procedures does not apply, assistant surgeon may be paid

61521 **Remove brain lesion** ~ follow-up period is 90 days, standard payment adjustment rules for multiple procedures apply, 150% payment adjustment for bilateral procedures does not apply, assistant surgeon may be paid

61522   **Remove brain abscess**   ~ follow-up period is 90 days, standard payment adjustment rules for multiple procedures apply, 150% payment adjustment for bilateral procedures does not apply, assistant surgeon may be paid

61524   **Remove brain lesion**   ~ follow-up period is 90 days, standard payment adjustment rules for multiple procedures apply, 150% payment adjustment for bilateral procedures does not apply, assistant surgeon may be paid

61526   **Remove brain lesion**   ~ follow-up period is 90 days, standard payment adjustment rules for multiple procedures apply, 150% payment adjustment for bilateral procedures does not apply, assistant surgeon may not be paid

61530   **Remove brain lesion**   ~ follow-up period is 90 days, standard payment adjustment rules for multiple procedures apply, 150% payment adjustment for bilateral procedures does not apply, assistant surgeon may not be paid

61531   **Implant brain electrodes**   ~ follow-up period is 90 days, standard payment adjustment rules for multiple procedures apply, 150% payment adjustment for bilateral procedures does not apply, assistant surgeon may be paid

61533   **Implant brain electrodes**   ~ follow-up period is 90 days, standard payment adjustment rules for multiple procedures apply, 150% payment adjustment for bilateral procedures does not apply, assistant surgeon may be paid

61534   **Remove brain lesion**   ~ follow-up period is 90 days, standard payment adjustment rules for multiple procedures apply, 150% payment adjustment for bilateral procedures does not apply, assistant surgeon may be paid

61535   **Remove brain electrodes**   ~ follow-up period is 90 days, standard payment adjustment rules for multiple procedures apply, 150% payment adjustment for bilateral procedures does not apply, assistant surgeon may be paid

61536   **Remove brain lesion**   ~ follow-up period is 90 days, standard payment adjustment rules for multiple procedures apply, 150% payment adjustment for bilateral procedures does not apply, assistant surgeon may be paid

61537   **Remove brain tissue**   ~ follow-up period is 90 days, standard payment adjustment rules for multiple procedures apply, 150% payment adjustment for bilateral procedures does not apply, assistant surgeon may be paid

61538   **Remove brain tissue**   ~ follow-up period is 90 days, standard payment adjustment rules for multiple procedures apply, 150% payment adjustment for bilateral procedures does not apply, assistant surgeon may be paid

61539   **Remove brain tissue**   ~ follow-up period is 90 days, standard payment adjustment rules for multiple procedures apply, 150% payment adjustment for bilateral procedures does not apply, assistant surgeon may be paid

61540   **Remove brain tissue**   ~ follow-up period is 90 days, standard payment adjustment rules for multiple procedures apply, 150% payment adjustment for bilateral procedures does not apply, assistant surgeon may be paid

61541   **Incise brain tissue**   ~ follow-up period is 90 days, standard payment adjustment rules for multiple procedures apply, 150% payment adjustment for bilateral procedures does not apply, assistant surgeon may be paid

61542   **Remove brain tissue**   ~ follow-up period is 90 days, standard payment adjustment rules for multiple procedures apply, 150% payment adjustment for bilateral procedures does not apply, assistant surgeon may be paid

61543   **Remove brain tissue**   ~ follow-up period is 90 days, standard payment adjustment rules for multiple procedures apply, 150% payment adjustment for bilateral procedures does not apply, assistant surgeon may be paid

61544   **Remove & treat brain lesion**   ~ follow-up period is 90 days, standard payment adjustment rules for multiple procedures apply, 150% payment adjustment for bilateral procedures does not apply, assistant surgeon may be paid

61545   **Excise brain tumor**   ~ follow-up period is 90 days, standard payment adjustment rules for multiple procedures apply, 150% payment adjustment for bilateral procedures does not apply, assistant surgeon may be paid

61546   **Remove pituitary gland**   ~ follow-up period is 90 days, standard payment adjustment rules for multiple procedures apply, 150% payment adjustment for bilateral procedures does not apply, assistant surgeon may be paid

61548   **Remove pituitary gland**   ~ follow-up period is 90 days, standard payment adjustment rules for multiple procedures apply, 150% payment adjustment for bilateral procedures does not apply, assistant surgeon may be paid

61550   **Release skull seams**   ~ follow-up period is 90 days, standard payment adjustment rules for multiple procedures apply, 150% payment adjustment for bilateral procedures does not apply, assistant surgeon may be paid

61552   **Release skull seams**   ~ follow-up period is 90 days, standard payment adjustment rules for multiple procedures apply, 150% payment adjustment for bilateral procedures does not apply, assistant surgeon may be paid

61556   **Incise skull/sutures**   ~ follow-up period is 90 days, standard payment adjustment rules for multiple procedures apply, 150% payment adjustment for bilateral procedures does not apply, assistant surgeon may be paid

61557   **Incise skull/sutures**   ~ follow-up period is 90 days, standard payment adjustment rules for multiple procedures apply, 150% payment adjustment for bilateral procedures does not apply, assistant surgeon may be paid

61558   **Excise skull/sutures**   ~ follow-up period is 90 days, standard payment adjustment rules for multiple procedures apply, 150% payment adjustment for bilateral procedures does not apply, assistant surgeon may be paid

61559   **Excise skull/sutures**   ~ follow-up period is 90 days, standard payment adjustment rules for multiple procedures apply, 150% payment adjustment for bilateral procedures does not apply, assistant surgeon may be paid

61563   **Excise skull tumor**   ~ follow-up period is 90 days, standard payment adjustment rules for multiple procedures apply, 150% payment adjustment for bilateral procedures does not apply, assistant surgeon may be paid

61564   **Excise skull tumor**   ~ follow-up period is 90 days, standard payment adjustment rules for multiple procedures apply, 150% payment adjustment for bilateral procedures does not apply, assistant surgeon may be paid

61566   **Remove brain tissue**   ~ follow-up period is 90 days, standard payment adjustment rules for multiple procedures apply, 150% payment adjustment for bilateral procedures does not apply, assistant surgeon may be paid

61567   **Incise brain tissue**   ~ follow-up period is 90 days, standard payment adjustment rules for multiple procedures apply, 150% payment adjustment for bilateral procedures does not apply, assistant surgeon may be paid

61570   **Remove foreign body brain**   ~ follow-up period is 90 days, standard payment adjustment rules for multiple procedures apply, 150% payment adjustment for bilateral procedures does not apply, assistant surgeon may be paid

61571   **Incise skull for brain wound**   ~ follow-up period is 90 days, standard payment adjustment rules for multiple procedures apply, 150% payment adjustment for bilateral procedures does not apply, assistant surgeon may be paid

61575   **Skull base/brainstem surgery**   ~ follow-up period is 90 days, standard payment adjustment rules for multiple procedures apply, 150% payment adjustment for bilateral procedures does not apply, assistant surgeon may be paid

61576   **Skull base/brainstem surgery**   ~ follow-up period is 90 days, standard payment adjustment rules for multiple procedures apply, 150% payment adjustment for bilateral procedures does not apply, assistant surgeon may be paid

61580   **Craniofacial approach, skull**   ~ follow-up period is 90 days, standard payment adjustment rules for multiple procedures apply, 150% payment adjustment for bilateral procedures applies, assistant surgeon may be paid

61581   **Craniofacial approach, skull**   ~ follow-up period is 90 days, standard payment adjustment rules for multiple procedures apply, 150% payment adjustment for bilateral procedures applies, assistant surgeon may not be paid

61582   **Craniofacial approach, skull**   ~ follow-up period is 90 days, standard payment adjustment rules for multiple procedures apply, 150% payment adjustment for bilateral procedures does not apply, assistant surgeon may be paid

61583   **Craniofacial approach, skull**   ~ follow-up period is 90 days, standard payment adjustment rules for multiple procedures apply, 150% payment adjustment for bilateral procedures does not apply, assistant surgeon may be paid

61584   **Orbitocranial approach/skull**   ~ follow-up period is 90 days, standard payment adjustment rules for multiple procedures apply, 150% payment adjustment for bilateral procedures applies, assistant surgeon may be paid

61585   **Orbitocranial approach/skull**   ~ follow-up period is 90 days, standard payment adjustment rules for multiple procedures apply, 150% payment adjustment for bilateral procedures applies, assistant surgeon may be paid

61586   **Resect nasopharynx, skull**   ~ follow-up period is 90 days, standard payment adjustment rules for multiple procedures apply, 150% payment adjustment for bilateral procedures does not apply, assistant surgeon may be paid

61590   **Infratemporal approach/skull**   ~ follow-up period is 90 days, standard payment adjustment rules for multiple procedures apply, 150% payment adjustment for bilateral procedures applies, assistant surgeon may be paid

61591   **Infratemporal approach/skull**   ~ follow-up period is 90 days, standard payment adjustment rules for multiple procedures apply, 150% payment adjustment for bilateral procedures applies, assistant surgeon may be paid

61592   **Orbitocranial approach/skull**   ~ follow-up period is 90 days, standard payment adjustment rules for multiple procedures apply, 150% payment adjustment for bilateral procedures applies, assistant surgeon may be paid

61595   **Transtemporal approach/skull**   ~ follow-up period is 90 days, standard payment adjustment rules for multiple procedures apply, 150% payment adjustment for bilateral procedures applies, assistant surgeon may be paid

61596   **Transcochlear approach/skull**   ~ follow-up period is 90 days, standard payment adjustment rules for multiple procedures apply, 150% payment adjustment for bilateral procedures applies, assistant surgeon may be paid

61597   **Transcondylar approach/skull**   ~ follow-up period is 90 days, standard payment adjustment rules for multiple procedures apply, 150% payment adjustment for bilateral procedures applies, assistant surgeon may be paid

61598   **Transpetrosal approach/skull**   ~ follow-up period is 90 days, standard payment adjustment rules for multiple procedures apply, 150% payment adjustment for bilateral procedures does not apply, assistant surgeon may be paid

61600   **Resect/excise cranial lesion**   ~ follow-up period is 90 days, standard payment adjustment rules for multiple procedures apply, 150% payment adjustment for bilateral procedures does not apply, assistant surgeon may be paid

61601   **Resect/excise cranial lesion**   ~ follow-up period is 90 days, standard payment adjustment rules for multiple procedures apply, 150% payment adjustment for bilateral procedures does not apply, assistant surgeon may be paid

61605   **Resect/excise cranial lesion**   ~ follow-up period is 90 days, standard payment adjustment rules for multiple procedures apply, 150% payment adjustment for bilateral procedures does not apply, assistant surgeon may be paid

61606   **Resect/excise cranial lesion**   ~ follow-up period is 90 days, standard payment adjustment rules for multiple procedures apply, 150% payment adjustment for bilateral procedures does not apply, assistant surgeon may be paid

61607   **Resect/excise cranial lesion**   ~ follow-up period is 90 days, standard payment adjustment rules for multiple procedures apply, 150% payment adjustment for bilateral procedures does not apply, assistant surgeon may be paid

61608   **Resect/excise cranial lesion**   ~ follow-up period is 90 days, standard payment adjustment rules for multiple procedures apply, 150% payment adjustment for bilateral procedures does not apply, assistant surgeon may be paid

61609   **Transect artery, sinus**   ~ follow-up period included in another service, no payment adjustment rules for multiple procedures apply, 150% payment adjustment for bilateral procedures does not apply, assistant surgeon may be paid

61610   **Transect artery, sinus**   ~ follow-up period included in another service, no payment adjustment rules for multiple procedures apply, 150% payment adjustment for bilateral procedures does not apply, assistant surgeon may be paid

61611   **Transect artery, sinus**   ~ follow-up period included in another service, no payment adjustment rules for multiple procedures apply, 150% payment adjustment for bilateral procedures does not apply, assistant surgeon may be paid

61612   **Transect artery, sinus**   ~ follow-up period included in another service, no payment adjustment rules for multiple procedures apply, 150% payment adjustment for bilateral procedures does not apply, assistant surgeon may be paid

61613   **Remove aneurysm, sinus**   ~ follow-up period is 90 days, standard payment adjustment rules for multiple procedures apply, 150% payment adjustment for bilateral procedures applies, assistant surgeon may be paid

61615   **Resect/excise lesion, skull**   ~ follow-up period is 90 days, standard payment adjustment rules for multiple procedures apply, 150% payment adjustment for bilateral procedures does not apply, assistant surgeon may be paid

61616   **Resect/excise lesion, skull**   ~ follow-up period is 90 days, standard payment adjustment rules for multiple procedures apply, 150% payment adjustment for bilateral procedures does not apply, assistant surgeon may be paid

61618   **Repair dura**   ~ follow-up period is 90 days, standard payment adjustment rules for multiple procedures apply, 150% payment adjustment for bilateral procedures does not apply, assistant surgeon may be paid

61619   **Repair dura**   ~ follow-up period is 90 days, standard payment adjustment rules for multiple procedures apply, 150% payment adjustment for bilateral procedures does not apply, assistant surgeon may be paid

61623   **Endovascular temporary vessel occlusion** ~ endoscopies or minor procedure - E/M services on the same day generally not paid, standard payment adjustment rules for multiple procedures apply, 150% payment adjustment for bilateral procedures does not apply, assistant surgeon may not be paid

61624   **Transcatheter occlusion, cns**   ~ endoscopies or minor procedure - E/M services on the same day generally not paid, standard payment adjustment rules for multiple procedures apply, 150% payment adjustment for bilateral procedures does not apply, assistant surgeon may not be paid

61626   **Transcatheter occlusion, non-cns**   ~ endoscopies or minor procedure - E/M services on the same day generally not paid, standard payment adjustment rules for multiple procedures apply, 150% payment adjustment for bilateral procedures does not apply, assistant surgeon may not be paid

61630   **Intracranial angioplasty**   non-covered service, follow-up period is 90 days, multiple procedure concept does not apply, bilateral surgery concept does not apply, assistant surgery concept does not apply

61635   **Intracranial angioplasty w/stent**   non-covered service, follow-up period is 90 days, multiple procedure concept does not apply, bilateral surgery concept does not apply, assistant surgery concept does not apply

61640   **Dilate ic vasospasm, init**   non-covered service, endoscopies or minor procedure - E/M services on the same day generally not paid, multiple procedure concept does not apply, bilateral surgery concept does not apply, assistant surgery concept does not apply

61641   **Dilate ic vasospasm, add-on**   non-covered service, follow-up period included in another service, multiple procedure concept does not apply, bilateral surgery concept does not apply, assistant surgery concept does not apply, +add-on code (list separately in addition to primary procedure)

61642   **Dilate ic vasospasm, add-on**   non-covered service, follow-up period included in another service, multiple procedure concept does not apply, bilateral surgery concept does not apply, assistant surgery concept does not apply, +add-on code (list separately in addition to primary procedure)

61680 **Intracranial vessel surgery** ~ follow-up period is 90 days, standard payment adjustment rules for multiple procedures apply, 150% payment adjustment for bilateral procedures does not apply, assistant surgeon may be paid

61682 **Intracranial vessel surgery** ~ follow-up period is 90 days, standard payment adjustment rules for multiple procedures apply, 150% payment adjustment for bilateral procedures does not apply, assistant surgeon may be paid

61684 **Intracranial vessel surgery** ~ follow-up period is 90 days, standard payment adjustment rules for multiple procedures apply, 150% payment adjustment for bilateral procedures does not apply, assistant surgeon may be paid

61686 **Intracranial vessel surgery** ~ follow-up period is 90 days, standard payment adjustment rules for multiple procedures apply, 150% payment adjustment for bilateral procedures does not apply, assistant surgeon may be paid

61690 **Intracranial vessel surgery** ~ follow-up period is 90 days, standard payment adjustment rules for multiple procedures apply, 150% payment adjustment for bilateral procedures does not apply, assistant surgeon may be paid

61692 **Intracranial vessel surgery** ~ follow-up period is 90 days, standard payment adjustment rules for multiple procedures apply, 150% payment adjustment for bilateral procedures does not apply, assistant surgeon may be paid

61697 **Brain aneurysm repair, complex** ~ follow-up period is 90 days, standard payment adjustment rules for multiple procedures apply, 150% payment adjustment for bilateral procedures does not apply, assistant surgeon may be paid

61698 **Brain aneurysm repair, complex** ~ follow-up period is 90 days, standard payment adjustment rules for multiple procedures apply, 150% payment adjustment for bilateral procedures does not apply, assistant surgeon may be paid

61700 **Brain aneurysm repair, simple** ~ follow-up period is 90 days, standard payment adjustment rules for multiple procedures apply, 150% payment adjustment for bilateral procedures does not apply, assistant surgeon may be paid

61702 **Inner skull vessel surgery** ~ follow-up period is 90 days, standard payment adjustment rules for multiple procedures apply, 150% payment adjustment for bilateral procedures does not apply, assistant surgeon may be paid

61703 **Clamp neck artery** ~ follow-up period is 90 days, standard payment adjustment rules for multiple procedures apply, 150% payment adjustment for bilateral procedures does not apply, assistant surgeon may be paid

61705 **Revise circulation to head** ~ follow-up period is 90 days, standard payment adjustment rules for multiple procedures apply, 150% payment adjustment for bilateral procedures does not apply, assistant surgeon may be paid

61708 **Revise circulation to head** ~ follow-up period is 90 days, standard payment adjustment rules for multiple procedures apply, 150% payment adjustment for bilateral procedures does not apply, assistant surgeon may be paid

61710 **Revise circulation to head** ~ follow-up period is 90 days, standard payment adjustment rules for multiple procedures apply, 150% payment adjustment for bilateral procedures does not apply, payment for assistant surgeon subject to documentation of medical necessity

61711 **Fuse skull arteries** ~ follow-up period is 90 days, standard payment adjustment rules for multiple procedures apply, 150% payment adjustment for bilateral procedures does not apply, assistant surgeon may be paid

61720 **Incise skull/brain surgery** ~ follow-up period is 90 days, standard payment adjustment rules for multiple procedures apply, 150% payment adjustment for bilateral procedures does not apply, assistant surgeon may not be paid

61735 **Incise skull/brain surgery** ~ follow-up period is 90 days, standard payment adjustment rules for multiple procedures apply, 150% payment adjustment for bilateral procedures does not apply, assistant surgeon may not be paid

61750 **Incise skull/brain biopsy** ~ follow-up period is 90 days, standard payment adjustment rules for multiple procedures apply, 150% payment adjustment for bilateral procedures does not apply, assistant surgeon may not be paid

61751 **Brain biopsy w/ct/mr guide** ~ follow-up period is 90 days, standard payment adjustment rules for multiple procedures apply, 150% payment adjustment for bilateral procedures does not apply, assistant surgeon may not be paid

61760 **Implant brain electrodes** ~ follow-up period is 90 days, standard payment adjustment rules for multiple procedures apply, 150% payment adjustment for bilateral procedures does not apply, assistant surgeon may not be paid

61770 **Incise skull for treatment** ~ follow-up period is 90 days, standard payment adjustment rules for multiple procedures apply, 150% payment adjustment for bilateral procedures does not apply, assistant surgeon may not be paid

61790 **Treat trigeminal nerve** ~ follow-up period is 90 days, standard payment adjustment rules for multiple procedures apply, 150% payment adjustment for bilateral procedures does not apply, assistant surgeon may not be paid

61791 **Treat trigeminal tract** ~ follow-up period is 90 days, standard payment adjustment rules for multiple procedures apply, 150% payment adjustment for

bilateral procedures does not apply, payment for assistant surgeon subject to documentation of medical necessity

61793   **Focus radiation beam**   ~ follow-up period is 90 days, standard payment adjustment rules for multiple procedures apply, 150% payment adjustment for bilateral procedures does not apply, assistant surgeon may not be paid

61795   **Brain surgery using computer**   ~ follow-up period included in another service, no payment adjustment rules for multiple procedures apply, 150% payment adjustment for bilateral procedures does not apply, assistant surgeon may not be paid

61850   **Implant neuroelectrodes**   ~ follow-up period is 90 days, standard payment adjustment rules for multiple procedures apply, 150% payment adjustment for bilateral procedures does not apply, assistant surgeon may be paid

61860   **Implant neuroelectrodes**   ~ follow-up period is 90 days, standard payment adjustment rules for multiple procedures apply, 150% payment adjustment for bilateral procedures does not apply, assistant surgeon may be paid

61863   **Implant neuroelectrode**   ~ follow-up period is 90 days, standard payment adjustment rules for multiple procedures apply, 150% payment adjustment for bilateral procedures applies, assistant surgeon may be paid

61864   **Implant neuroelectrode, added**   ~ follow-up period included in another service, no payment adjustment rules for multiple procedures apply, 150% payment adjustment for bilateral procedures does not apply, assistant surgeon may be paid, +add-on code (list separately in addition to primary procedure)

61867   **Implant neuroelectrode**   ~ follow-up period is 90 days, standard payment adjustment rules for multiple procedures apply, 150% payment adjustment for bilateral procedures applies, assistant surgeon may be paid

61868   **Implant neuroelectrode, added**   ~ follow-up period included in another service, no payment adjustment rules for multiple procedures apply, 150% payment adjustment for bilateral procedures does not apply, assistant surgeon may be paid, +add-on code (list separately in addition to primary procedure)

61870   **Implant neuroelectrodes**   ~ follow-up period is 90 days, standard payment adjustment rules for multiple procedures apply, 150% payment adjustment for bilateral procedures does not apply, assistant surgeon may be paid

61875   **Implant neuroelectrodes**   ~ follow-up period is 90 days, standard payment adjustment rules for multiple procedures apply, 150% payment adjustment for bilateral procedures does not apply, assistant surgeon may be paid

61880   **Revise/remove neuroelectrode**   ~ follow-up period is 90 days, standard payment adjustment rules for multiple procedures apply, 150% payment adjustment for bilateral procedures applies, assistant surgeon may be paid

61885   **Insert/redo neurostim 1 array**   ~ follow-up period is 90 days, standard payment adjustment rules for multiple procedures apply, 150% payment adjustment for bilateral procedures applies, payment for assistant surgeon subject to documentation of medical necessity

61886   **Implant neurostim arrays**   ~ follow-up period is 90 days, standard payment adjustment rules for multiple procedures apply, 150% payment adjustment for bilateral procedures does not apply, payment for assistant surgeon subject to documentation of medical necessity

61888   **Revise/remove neuroreceiver**   ~ follow-up period is 10 days, standard payment adjustment rules for multiple procedures apply, 150% payment adjustment for bilateral procedures applies, assistant surgeon may not be paid

62000   **Treat skull fracture**   ~ follow-up period is 90 days, standard payment adjustment rules for multiple procedures apply, 150% payment adjustment for bilateral procedures does not apply, assistant surgeon may not be paid

62005   **Treat skull fracture**   ~ follow-up period is 90 days, standard payment adjustment rules for multiple procedures apply, 150% payment adjustment for bilateral procedures does not apply, assistant surgeon may be paid

62010   **Treat head injury**   ~ follow-up period is 90 days, standard payment adjustment rules for multiple procedures apply, 150% payment adjustment for bilateral procedures does not apply, assistant surgeon may be paid

62100   **Repair brain fluid leakage**   ~ follow-up period is 90 days, standard payment adjustment rules for multiple procedures apply, 150% payment adjustment for bilateral procedures does not apply, assistant surgeon may be paid

62115   **Reduce skull defect**   ~ follow-up period is 90 days, standard payment adjustment rules for multiple procedures apply, 150% payment adjustment for bilateral procedures does not apply, assistant surgeon may be paid

62116   **Reduce skull defect**   ~ follow-up period is 90 days, standard payment adjustment rules for multiple procedures apply, 150% payment adjustment for bilateral procedures does not apply, assistant surgeon may be paid

62117   **Reduce skull defect**   ~ follow-up period is 90 days, standard payment adjustment rules for multiple procedures apply, 150% payment adjustment for bilateral procedures does not apply, assistant surgeon may be paid

62120   **Repair skull cavity lesion**   ~ follow-up period is 90 days, standard payment adjustment rules for multiple procedures apply, 150% payment adjustment for bilateral procedures does not apply, assistant surgeon may be paid

62121   **Incise skull repair**   ~ follow-up period is 90 days, standard payment adjustment rules for multiple procedures apply, 150% payment adjustment for bilateral procedures does not apply, assistant surgeon may be paid

62140   **Repair skull defect**   ~ follow-up period is 90 days, standard payment adjustment rules for multiple procedures apply, 150% payment adjustment for bilateral procedures does not apply, assistant surgeon may be paid

62141   **Repair skull defect**   ~ follow-up period is 90 days, standard payment adjustment rules for multiple procedures apply, 150% payment adjustment for bilateral procedures does not apply, assistant surgeon may be paid

62142   **Remove skull plate/flap**   ~ follow-up period is 90 days, standard payment adjustment rules for multiple procedures apply, 150% payment adjustment for bilateral procedures does not apply, assistant surgeon may be paid

62143   **Replace skull plate/flap**   ~ follow-up period is 90 days, standard payment adjustment rules for multiple procedures apply, 150% payment adjustment for bilateral procedures does not apply, assistant surgeon may be paid

62145   **Repair skull & brain**   ~ follow-up period is 90 days, standard payment adjustment rules for multiple procedures apply, 150% payment adjustment for bilateral procedures does not apply, assistant surgeon may be paid

62146   **Repair skull with graft**   ~ follow-up period is 90 days, standard payment adjustment rules for multiple procedures apply, 150% payment adjustment for bilateral procedures does not apply, assistant surgeon may be paid

62147   **Repair skull with graft**   ~ follow-up period is 90 days, standard payment adjustment rules for multiple procedures apply, 150% payment adjustment for bilateral procedures does not apply, assistant surgeon may be paid

62148   **Retrieve bone flap to fix skull**   ~ follow-up period included in another service, no payment adjustment rules for multiple procedures apply, 150% payment adjustment for bilateral procedures does not apply, assistant surgeon may not be paid

62160   **Neuroendoscopy, add-on**   ~ follow-up period included in another service, no payment adjustment rules for multiple procedures apply, 150% payment adjustment for bilateral procedures does not apply, assistant surgeon may not be paid, +add-on code (list separately in addition to primary procedure)

62161 **Dissect brain w/scope** ~ follow-up period is 90 days, standard payment adjustment rules for multiple procedures apply, 150% payment adjustment for bilateral procedures does not apply, assistant surgeon may be paid

62162 **Remove colloid cyst w/scope** ~ follow-up period is 90 days, standard payment adjustment rules for multiple procedures apply, 150% payment adjustment for bilateral procedures does not apply, assistant surgeon may be paid

62163 **Neuroendoscopy w/foreign body remove** ~ follow-up period is 90 days, standard payment adjustment rules for multiple procedures apply, 150% payment adjustment for bilateral procedures does not apply, assistant surgeon may be paid

62164 **Remove brain tumor w/scope** ~ follow-up period is 90 days, standard payment adjustment rules for multiple procedures apply, 150% payment adjustment for bilateral procedures does not apply, assistant surgeon may be paid

62165 **Remove pituitary tumor w/scope** ~ follow-up period is 90 days, standard payment adjustment rules for multiple procedures apply, 150% payment adjustment for bilateral procedures does not apply, payment for assistant surgeon subject to documentation of medical necessity

62180 **Establish brain cavity shunt** ~ follow-up period is 90 days, standard payment adjustment rules for multiple procedures apply, 150% payment adjustment for bilateral procedures does not apply, assistant surgeon may be paid

62190 **Establish brain cavity shunt** ~ follow-up period is 90 days, standard payment adjustment rules for multiple procedures apply, 150% payment adjustment for bilateral procedures does not apply, assistant surgeon may not be paid

62192 **Establish brain cavity shunt** ~ follow-up period is 90 days, standard payment adjustment rules for multiple procedures apply, 150% payment adjustment for bilateral procedures does not apply, assistant surgeon may be paid

62194 **Replace/irrigate catheter** ~ follow-up period is 10 days, standard payment adjustment rules for multiple procedures apply, 150% payment adjustment for bilateral procedures does not apply, payment for assistant surgeon subject to documentation of medical necessity

62200 **Establish brain cavity shunt** ~ follow-up period is 90 days, standard payment adjustment rules for multiple procedures apply, 150% payment adjustment for bilateral procedures does not apply, assistant surgeon may be paid

62201 **Brain cavity shunt w/scope** ~ follow-up period is 90 days, standard payment adjustment rules for multiple procedures apply, 150% payment adjustment for bilateral procedures does not apply, assistant surgeon may not be paid

62220   **Establish brain cavity shunt**   ~ follow-up period is 90 days, standard payment adjustment rules for multiple procedures apply, 150% payment adjustment for bilateral procedures does not apply, assistant surgeon may be paid

62223   **Establish brain cavity shunt**   ~ follow-up period is 90 days, standard payment adjustment rules for multiple procedures apply, 150% payment adjustment for bilateral procedures does not apply, assistant surgeon may be paid

62225   **Replace/irrigate catheter**   ~ follow-up period is 90 days, standard payment adjustment rules for multiple procedures apply, 150% payment adjustment for bilateral procedures does not apply, assistant surgeon may not be paid

62230   **Replace/revise brain shunt**   ~ follow-up period is 90 days, standard payment adjustment rules for multiple procedures apply, 150% payment adjustment for bilateral procedures does not apply, assistant surgeon may be paid

62252   **Csf shunt reprogram**   ~ no payment adjustment rules for multiple procedures apply, 150% payment adjustment for bilateral procedures does not apply, payment for assistant surgeon subject to documentation of medical necessity

62256   **Remove brain cavity shunt**   ~ follow-up period is 90 days, standard payment adjustment rules for multiple procedures apply, 150% payment adjustment for bilateral procedures does not apply, assistant surgeon may be paid

62258   **Replace brain cavity shunt**   ~ follow-up period is 90 days, standard payment adjustment rules for multiple procedures apply, 150% payment adjustment for bilateral procedures does not apply, assistant surgeon may be paid

Spine and Spinal Cord

62263   **Epidural lysis multiple sessions**   ~ follow-up period is 10 days, standard payment adjustment rules for multiple procedures apply, 150% payment adjustment for bilateral procedures does not apply, assistant surgeon may not be paid

62264   **Epidural lysis on single day**   ~ follow-up period is 10 days, standard payment adjustment rules for multiple procedures apply, 150% payment adjustment for bilateral procedures does not apply, assistant surgeon may not be paid

62268   **Drain spinal cord cyst**   ~ endoscopies or minor procedure - E/M services on the same day generally not paid, standard payment adjustment rules for multiple procedures apply, 150% payment adjustment for bilateral procedures does not apply, assistant surgeon may not be paid

62269   **Needle biopsy spinal cord**   ~ endoscopies or minor procedure - E/M services on the same day generally not paid, standard payment adjustment rules for multiple procedures apply, 150% payment adjustment for bilateral procedures does not apply, payment for assistant surgeon subject to documentation of medical necessity

---

62270   **Spinal fluid tap, diagnostic**   ~ endoscopies or minor procedure - E/M services on the same day generally not paid, standard payment adjustment rules for multiple procedures apply, 150% payment adjustment for bilateral procedures does not apply, assistant surgeon may not be paid

62272   **Drain cerebrospinal fluid**   ~ endoscopies or minor procedure - E/M services on the same day generally not paid, standard payment adjustment rules for multiple procedures apply, 150% payment adjustment for bilateral procedures does not apply, assistant surgeon may not be paid

62273   **Inject epidural patch**   ~ endoscopies or minor procedure - E/M services on the same day generally not paid, standard payment adjustment rules for multiple procedures apply, 150% payment adjustment for bilateral procedures does not apply, assistant surgeon may not be paid

62280   **Treat spinal cord lesion**   ~ follow-up period is 10 days, standard payment adjustment rules for multiple procedures apply, 150% payment adjustment for bilateral procedures does not apply, assistant surgeon may not be paid

62281   **Treat spinal cord lesion**   ~ follow-up period is 10 days, standard payment adjustment rules for multiple procedures apply, 150% payment adjustment for bilateral procedures does not apply, assistant surgeon may not be paid

62282   **Treat spinal canal lesion**   ~ follow-up period is 10 days, standard payment adjustment rules for multiple procedures apply, 150% payment adjustment for bilateral procedures does not apply, assistant surgeon may not be paid

62284   **Inject for myelogram**   ~ endoscopies or minor procedure - E/M services on the same day generally not paid, no payment adjustment rules for multiple procedures apply, 150% payment adjustment for bilateral procedures does not apply, assistant surgeon may not be paid

62287   **Percutaneous diskectomy**   ~ follow-up period is 90 days, standard payment adjustment rules for multiple procedures apply, 150% payment adjustment for bilateral procedures does not apply, assistant surgeon may not be paid

62290   **Inject for spine disk x-ray**   ~ endoscopies or minor procedure - E/M services on the same day generally not paid, standard payment adjustment rules for multiple procedures apply, 150% payment adjustment for bilateral procedures does not apply, assistant surgeon may not be paid

62291   **Inject for spine disk x-ray**   ~ endoscopies or minor procedure - E/M services on the same day generally not paid, standard payment adjustment rules for multiple procedures apply, 150% payment adjustment for bilateral procedures does not apply, assistant surgeon may not be paid

62292 Inject into disk lesion ~ follow-up period is 90 days, standard payment adjustment rules for multiple procedures apply, 150% payment adjustment for bilateral procedures does not apply, payment for assistant surgeon subject to documentation of medical necessity

62294 Inject into spinal artery ~ follow-up period is 90 days, standard payment adjustment rules for multiple procedures apply, 150% payment adjustment for bilateral procedures does not apply, assistant surgeon may not be paid

62310 Inject spine c/t ~ endoscopies or minor procedure - E/M services on the same day generally not paid, standard payment adjustment rules for multiple procedures apply, 150% payment adjustment for bilateral procedures does not apply, assistant surgeon may not be paid

62311 Inject spine l/s (cd) ~ endoscopies or minor procedure - E/M services on the same day generally not paid, standard payment adjustment rules for multiple procedures apply, 150% payment adjustment for bilateral procedures does not apply, assistant surgeon may not be paid

62318 Inject spine w/cath, c/t ~ endoscopies or minor procedure - E/M services on the same day generally not paid, standard payment adjustment rules for multiple procedures apply, 150% payment adjustment for bilateral procedures does not apply, assistant surgeon may not be paid

62319 Inject spine w/cath l/s (cd) ~ endoscopies or minor procedure - E/M services on the same day generally not paid, standard payment adjustment rules for multiple procedures apply, 150% payment adjustment for bilateral procedures does not apply, assistant surgeon may not be paid

62350 Implant spinal canal cath ~ follow-up period is 90 days, standard payment adjustment rules for multiple procedures apply, 150% payment adjustment for bilateral procedures does not apply, assistant surgeon may not be paid

62351 Implant spinal canal cath ~ follow-up period is 90 days, standard payment adjustment rules for multiple procedures apply, 150% payment adjustment for bilateral procedures does not apply, assistant surgeon may be paid

62355 Remove spinal canal catheter ~ follow-up period is 90 days, standard payment adjustment rules for multiple procedures apply, 150% payment adjustment for bilateral procedures does not apply, payment for assistant surgeon subject to documentation of medical necessity

62360 Insert spine infuse device ~ follow-up period is 90 days, standard payment adjustment rules for multiple procedures apply, 150% payment adjustment for bilateral procedures does not apply, payment for assistant surgeon subject to documentation of medical necessity

62361 **Implant spine infuse pump** ~ follow-up period is 90 days, standard payment adjustment rules for multiple procedures apply, 150% payment adjustment for bilateral procedures does not apply, payment for assistant surgeon subject to documentation of medical necessity

62362 **Implant spine infuse pump** ~ follow-up period is 90 days, standard payment adjustment rules for multiple procedures apply, 150% payment adjustment for bilateral procedures does not apply, payment for assistant surgeon subject to documentation of medical necessity

62365 **Remove spine infuse device** ~ follow-up period is 90 days, standard payment adjustment rules for multiple procedures apply, 150% payment adjustment for bilateral procedures does not apply, payment for assistant surgeon subject to documentation of medical necessity

62367 **Analyze spine infuse pump** ~ no payment adjustment rules for multiple procedures apply, 150% payment adjustment for bilateral procedures does not apply, payment for assistant surgeon subject to documentation of medical necessity

62368 **Analyze spine infuse pump** ~ no payment adjustment rules for multiple procedures apply, 150% payment adjustment for bilateral procedures does not apply, payment for assistant surgeon subject to documentation of medical necessity

63001 **Remove spinal lamina** ~ follow-up period is 90 days, standard payment adjustment rules for multiple procedures apply, 150% payment adjustment for bilateral procedures does not apply, assistant surgeon may be paid

63003 **Remove spinal lamina** ~ follow-up period is 90 days, standard payment adjustment rules for multiple procedures apply, 150% payment adjustment for bilateral procedures does not apply, assistant surgeon may be paid

63005 **Remove spinal lamina** ~ follow-up period is 90 days, standard payment adjustment rules for multiple procedures apply, 150% payment adjustment for bilateral procedures does not apply, assistant surgeon may be paid

63011 **Remove spinal lamina** ~ follow-up period is 90 days, standard payment adjustment rules for multiple procedures apply, 150% payment adjustment for bilateral procedures does not apply, assistant surgeon may be paid

63012 **Remove spinal lamina** ~ follow-up period is 90 days, standard payment adjustment rules for multiple procedures apply, 150% payment adjustment for bilateral procedures does not apply, assistant surgeon may be paid

63015 **Remove spinal lamina** ~ follow-up period is 90 days, standard payment adjustment rules for multiple procedures apply, 150% payment adjustment for bilateral procedures does not apply, assistant surgeon may be paid

63016   **Remove spinal lamina**   ~ follow-up period is 90 days, standard payment adjustment rules for multiple procedures apply, 150% payment adjustment for bilateral procedures does not apply, assistant surgeon may be paid

63017   **Remove spinal lamina**   ~ follow-up period is 90 days, standard payment adjustment rules for multiple procedures apply, 150% payment adjustment for bilateral procedures does not apply, assistant surgeon may be paid

63020   **Neck spine disk surgery**   ~ follow-up period is 90 days, standard payment adjustment rules for multiple procedures apply, 150% payment adjustment for bilateral procedures applies, assistant surgeon may be paid

63030   **Low back disk surgery**   ~ follow-up period is 90 days, standard payment adjustment rules for multiple procedures apply, 150% payment adjustment for bilateral procedures applies, assistant surgeon may be paid

63035   **Spinal disk surgery, add-on**   ~ follow-up period included in another service, no payment adjustment rules for multiple procedures apply, 150% payment adjustment for bilateral procedures applies, assistant surgeon may be paid, +add-on code (list separately in addition to primary procedure)

63040   **Laminotomy, single cervical**   ~ follow-up period is 90 days, standard payment adjustment rules for multiple procedures apply, 150% payment adjustment for bilateral procedures applies, assistant surgeon may be paid

63042   **Laminotomy, single lumbar**   ~ follow-up period is 90 days, standard payment adjustment rules for multiple procedures apply, 150% payment adjustment for bilateral procedures applies, assistant surgeon may be paid

63043   **Laminotomy, added cervical**   ~ follow-up period included in another service, no payment adjustment rules for multiple procedures apply, 150% payment adjustment for bilateral procedures applies, assistant surgeon may be paid, +add-on code (list separately in addition to primary procedure)

63044   **Laminotomy, added lumbar**   ~ follow-up period included in another service, no payment adjustment rules for multiple procedures apply, 150% payment adjustment for bilateral procedures applies, assistant surgeon may be paid, +add-on code (list separately in addition to primary procedure)

63045   **Remove spinal lamina**   ~ follow-up period is 90 days, standard payment adjustment rules for multiple procedures apply, 150% payment adjustment does not apply - RVUs based on bilateral procedure, assistant surgeon may be paid

63046   **Remove spinal lamina**   ~ follow-up period is 90 days, standard payment adjustment rules for multiple procedures apply, 150% payment adjustment does not apply - RVUs based on bilateral procedure, assistant surgeon may be paid

---

63047 **Remove spinal lamina** ~ follow-up period is 90 days, standard payment adjustment rules for multiple procedures apply, 150% payment adjustment does not apply - RVUs based on bilateral procedure, assistant surgeon may be paid

63048 **Remove spinal lamina, add-on** ~ follow-up period included in another service, no payment adjustment rules for multiple procedures apply, 150% payment adjustment for bilateral procedures does not apply, assistant surgeon may be paid, +add-on code (list separately in addition to primary procedure)

63050 **Cervical laminoplasty** ~ follow-up period is 90 days, standard payment adjustment rules for multiple procedures apply, 150% payment adjustment for bilateral procedures does not apply, assistant surgeon may be paid

63051 **Cervical laminoplasty w/graft/plate** ~ follow-up period is 90 days, standard payment adjustment rules for multiple procedures apply, 150% payment adjustment for bilateral procedures does not apply, assistant surgeon may be paid

63055 **Decompress spinal cord** ~ follow-up period is 90 days, standard payment adjustment rules for multiple procedures apply, 150% payment adjustment for bilateral procedures does not apply, assistant surgeon may be paid

63056 **Decompress spinal cord** ~ follow-up period is 90 days, standard payment adjustment rules for multiple procedures apply, 150% payment adjustment for bilateral procedures does not apply, assistant surgeon may be paid

63057 **Decompress spine cord, add-on** ~ follow-up period included in another service, no payment adjustment rules for multiple procedures apply, 150% payment adjustment for bilateral procedures does not apply, assistant surgeon may be paid, +add-on code (list separately in addition to primary procedure)

63064 **Decompress spinal cord** ~ follow-up period is 90 days, standard payment adjustment rules for multiple procedures apply, 150% payment adjustment for bilateral procedures does not apply, assistant surgeon may be paid

63066 **Decompress spine cord, add-on** ~ follow-up period included in another service, no payment adjustment rules for multiple procedures apply, 150% payment adjustment for bilateral procedures does not apply, assistant surgeon may be paid, +add-on code (list separately in addition to primary procedure)

63075 **Neck spine disk surgery** ~ follow-up period is 90 days, standard payment adjustment rules for multiple procedures apply, 150% payment adjustment for bilateral procedures does not apply, assistant surgeon may be paid

63076 **Neck spine disk surgery** ~ follow-up period included in another service, no payment adjustment rules for multiple procedures apply, 150% payment adjustment for bilateral procedures does not apply, assistant surgeon may be paid

63077 **Spine disk surgery, thorax**   ~ follow-up period is 90 days, standard payment adjustment rules for multiple procedures apply, 150% payment adjustment for bilateral procedures does not apply, assistant surgeon may be paid

63078 **Spine disk surgery, thorax**   ~ follow-up period included in another service, no payment adjustment rules for multiple procedures apply, 150% payment adjustment for bilateral procedures does not apply, assistant surgeon may be paid

63081 **Remove vertebral body**   ~ follow-up period is 90 days, standard payment adjustment rules for multiple procedures apply, 150% payment adjustment for bilateral procedures does not apply, assistant surgeon may be paid

63082 **Remove vertebral body, add-on**   ~ follow-up period included in another service, no payment adjustment rules for multiple procedures apply, 150% payment adjustment for bilateral procedures does not apply, assistant surgeon may be paid, +add-on code (list separately in addition to primary procedure)

63085 **Remove vertebral body**   ~ follow-up period is 90 days, standard payment adjustment rules for multiple procedures apply, 150% payment adjustment for bilateral procedures does not apply, assistant surgeon may be paid

63086 **Remove vertebral body, add-on**   ~ follow-up period included in another service, no payment adjustment rules for multiple procedures apply, 150% payment adjustment for bilateral procedures does not apply, assistant surgeon may be paid, +add-on code (list separately in addition to primary procedure)

63087 **Remove vertebral body**   ~ follow-up period is 90 days, standard payment adjustment rules for multiple procedures apply, 150% payment adjustment for bilateral procedures does not apply, assistant surgeon may be paid

63088 **Remove vertebral body, add-on**   ~ follow-up period included in another service, no payment adjustment rules for multiple procedures apply, 150% payment adjustment for bilateral procedures does not apply, assistant surgeon may be paid, +add-on code (list separately in addition to primary procedure)

63090 **Remove vertebral body**   ~ follow-up period is 90 days, standard payment adjustment rules for multiple procedures apply, 150% payment adjustment for bilateral procedures does not apply, assistant surgeon may be paid

63091 **Remove vertebral body, add-on**   ~ follow-up period included in another service, no payment adjustment rules for multiple procedures apply, 150% payment adjustment for bilateral procedures does not apply, assistant surgeon may be paid, +add-on code (list separately in addition to primary procedure)

63101 **Remove vertebral body**   ~ follow-up period is 90 days, standard payment adjustment rules for multiple procedures apply, 150% payment adjustment for bilateral procedures does not apply, assistant surgeon may be paid

---

CPT codes and descriptions only copyright American Medical Association

63102   **Remove vertebral body**   ~ follow-up period is 90 days, standard payment adjustment rules for multiple procedures apply, 150% payment adjustment for bilateral procedures does not apply, assistant surgeon may be paid

63103   **Remove vertebral body, add-on**   ~ follow-up period included in another service, no payment adjustment rules for multiple procedures apply, 150% payment adjustment for bilateral procedures does not apply, assistant surgeon may be paid, +add-on code (list separately in addition to primary procedure)

63170   **Incise spinal cord tract(s)**   ~ follow-up period is 90 days, standard payment adjustment rules for multiple procedures apply, 150% payment adjustment for bilateral procedures does not apply, assistant surgeon may be paid

63172   **Drain spinal cyst**   ~ follow-up period is 90 days, standard payment adjustment rules for multiple procedures apply, 150% payment adjustment for bilateral procedures does not apply, assistant surgeon may be paid

63173   **Drain spinal cyst**   ~ follow-up period is 90 days, standard payment adjustment rules for multiple procedures apply, 150% payment adjustment for bilateral procedures does not apply, assistant surgeon may be paid

63180   **Revise spinal cord ligaments**   ~ follow-up period is 90 days, standard payment adjustment rules for multiple procedures apply, 150% payment adjustment for bilateral procedures does not apply, assistant surgeon may be paid

63182   **Revise spinal cord ligaments**   ~ follow-up period is 90 days, standard payment adjustment rules for multiple procedures apply, 150% payment adjustment for bilateral procedures does not apply, assistant surgeon may be paid

63185   **Incise spinal column/nerves**   ~ follow-up period is 90 days, standard payment adjustment rules for multiple procedures apply, 150% payment adjustment for bilateral procedures does not apply, assistant surgeon may be paid

63190   **Incise spinal column/nerves**   ~ follow-up period is 90 days, standard payment adjustment rules for multiple procedures apply, 150% payment adjustment for bilateral procedures does not apply, assistant surgeon may be paid

63191   **Incise spinal column/nerves**   ~ follow-up period is 90 days, standard payment adjustment rules for multiple procedures apply, 150% payment adjustment for bilateral procedures applies, assistant surgeon may be paid

63194   **Incise spinal column & cord**   ~ follow-up period is 90 days, standard payment adjustment rules for multiple procedures apply, 150% payment adjustment for bilateral procedures does not apply, assistant surgeon may be paid

63195   **Incise spinal column & cord**   ~ follow-up period is 90 days, standard payment adjustment rules for multiple procedures apply, 150% payment adjustment for bilateral procedures does not apply, assistant surgeon may be paid

63196   **Incise spinal column & cord**   ~ follow-up period is 90 days, standard payment adjustment rules for multiple procedures apply, 150% payment adjustment for bilateral procedures does not apply, assistant surgeon may be paid

63197   **Incise spinal column & cord**   ~ follow-up period is 90 days, standard payment adjustment rules for multiple procedures apply, 150% payment adjustment for bilateral procedures does not apply, assistant surgeon may be paid

63198   **Incise spinal column & cord**   ~ follow-up period is 90 days, standard payment adjustment rules for multiple procedures apply, 150% payment adjustment for bilateral procedures does not apply, assistant surgeon may be paid

63199   **Incise spinal column & cord**   ~ follow-up period is 90 days, standard payment adjustment rules for multiple procedures apply, 150% payment adjustment for bilateral procedures does not apply, assistant surgeon may be paid

63200   **Release spinal cord**   ~ follow-up period is 90 days, standard payment adjustment rules for multiple procedures apply, 150% payment adjustment for bilateral procedures does not apply, assistant surgeon may be paid

63250   **Revise spinal cord vessels**   ~ follow-up period is 90 days, standard payment adjustment rules for multiple procedures apply, 150% payment adjustment for bilateral procedures does not apply, assistant surgeon may be paid

63251   **Revise spinal cord vessels**   ~ follow-up period is 90 days, standard payment adjustment rules for multiple procedures apply, 150% payment adjustment for bilateral procedures does not apply, assistant surgeon may be paid

63252   **Revise spinal cord vessels**   ~ follow-up period is 90 days, standard payment adjustment rules for multiple procedures apply, 150% payment adjustment for bilateral procedures does not apply, assistant surgeon may be paid

63265   **Excise intraspinal lesion**   ~ follow-up period is 90 days, standard payment adjustment rules for multiple procedures apply, 150% payment adjustment for bilateral procedures does not apply, assistant surgeon may be paid

63266   **Excise intraspinal lesion**   ~ follow-up period is 90 days, standard payment adjustment rules for multiple procedures apply, 150% payment adjustment for bilateral procedures does not apply, assistant surgeon may be paid

63267   **Excise intraspinal lesion**   ~ follow-up period is 90 days, standard payment adjustment rules for multiple procedures apply, 150% payment adjustment for bilateral procedures does not apply, assistant surgeon may be paid

63268 **Excise intraspinal lesion** ~ follow-up period is 90 days, standard payment adjustment rules for multiple procedures apply, 150% payment adjustment for bilateral procedures does not apply, assistant surgeon may be paid

63270 **Excise intraspinal lesion** ~ follow-up period is 90 days, standard payment adjustment rules for multiple procedures apply, 150% payment adjustment for bilateral procedures does not apply, assistant surgeon may be paid

63271 **Excise intraspinal lesion** ~ follow-up period is 90 days, standard payment adjustment rules for multiple procedures apply, 150% payment adjustment for bilateral procedures does not apply, assistant surgeon may be paid

63272 **Excise intraspinal lesion** ~ follow-up period is 90 days, standard payment adjustment rules for multiple procedures apply, 150% payment adjustment for bilateral procedures does not apply, assistant surgeon may be paid

63273 **Excise intraspinal lesion** ~ follow-up period is 90 days, standard payment adjustment rules for multiple procedures apply, 150% payment adjustment for bilateral procedures does not apply, assistant surgeon may be paid

63275 **Biopsy/excise spinal tumor** ~ follow-up period is 90 days, standard payment adjustment rules for multiple procedures apply, 150% payment adjustment for bilateral procedures does not apply, assistant surgeon may be paid

63276 **Biopsy/excise spinal tumor** ~ follow-up period is 90 days, standard payment adjustment rules for multiple procedures apply, 150% payment adjustment for bilateral procedures does not apply, assistant surgeon may be paid

63277 **Biopsy/excise spinal tumor** ~ follow-up period is 90 days, standard payment adjustment rules for multiple procedures apply, 150% payment adjustment for bilateral procedures does not apply, assistant surgeon may be paid

63278 **Biopsy/excise spinal tumor** ~ follow-up period is 90 days, standard payment adjustment rules for multiple procedures apply, 150% payment adjustment for bilateral procedures does not apply, assistant surgeon may be paid

63280 **Biopsy/excise spinal tumor** ~ follow-up period is 90 days, standard payment adjustment rules for multiple procedures apply, 150% payment adjustment for bilateral procedures does not apply, assistant surgeon may be paid

63281 **Biopsy/excise spinal tumor** ~ follow-up period is 90 days, standard payment adjustment rules for multiple procedures apply, 150% payment adjustment for bilateral procedures does not apply, assistant surgeon may be paid

63282 **Biopsy/excise spinal tumor** ~ follow-up period is 90 days, standard payment adjustment rules for multiple procedures apply, 150% payment adjustment for bilateral procedures does not apply, assistant surgeon may be paid

63283   **Biopsy/excise spinal tumor**   ~ follow-up period is 90 days, standard payment adjustment rules for multiple procedures apply, 150% payment adjustment for bilateral procedures does not apply, assistant surgeon may be paid

63285   **Biopsy/excise spinal tumor**   ~ follow-up period is 90 days, standard payment adjustment rules for multiple procedures apply, 150% payment adjustment for bilateral procedures does not apply, assistant surgeon may be paid

63286   **Biopsy/excise spinal tumor**   ~ follow-up period is 90 days, standard payment adjustment rules for multiple procedures apply, 150% payment adjustment for bilateral procedures does not apply, assistant surgeon may be paid

63287   **Biopsy/excise spinal tumor**   ~ follow-up period is 90 days, standard payment adjustment rules for multiple procedures apply, 150% payment adjustment for bilateral procedures does not apply, assistant surgeon may be paid

63290   **Biopsy/excise spinal tumor**   ~ follow-up period is 90 days, standard payment adjustment rules for multiple procedures apply, 150% payment adjustment for bilateral procedures does not apply, assistant surgeon may be paid

63295   **Repair laminectomy defect**   ~ follow-up period included in another service, no payment adjustment rules for multiple procedures apply, 150% payment adjustment does not apply - RVUs based on bilateral procedure, assistant surgeon may be paid

63300   **Remove vertebral body**   ~ follow-up period is 90 days, standard payment adjustment rules for multiple procedures apply, 150% payment adjustment for bilateral procedures does not apply, assistant surgeon may be paid

63301   **Remove vertebral body**   ~ follow-up period is 90 days, standard payment adjustment rules for multiple procedures apply, 150% payment adjustment for bilateral procedures does not apply, assistant surgeon may be paid

63302   **Remove vertebral body**   ~ follow-up period is 90 days, standard payment adjustment rules for multiple procedures apply, 150% payment adjustment for bilateral procedures does not apply, assistant surgeon may be paid

63303   **Remove vertebral body**   ~ follow-up period is 90 days, standard payment adjustment rules for multiple procedures apply, 150% payment adjustment for bilateral procedures does not apply, assistant surgeon may be paid

63304   **Remove vertebral body**   ~ follow-up period is 90 days, standard payment adjustment rules for multiple procedures apply, 150% payment adjustment for bilateral procedures does not apply, assistant surgeon may be paid

63305   **Remove vertebral body**   ~ follow-up period is 90 days, standard payment adjustment rules for multiple procedures apply, 150% payment adjustment for bilateral procedures does not apply, assistant surgeon may be paid

63306   **Remove vertebral body**   ~ follow-up period is 90 days, standard payment adjustment rules for multiple procedures apply, 150% payment adjustment for bilateral procedures does not apply, assistant surgeon may be paid

63307   **Remove vertebral body**   ~ follow-up period is 90 days, standard payment adjustment rules for multiple procedures apply, 150% payment adjustment for bilateral procedures does not apply, assistant surgeon may be paid

63308   **Remove vertebral body, add-on**   ~ follow-up period included in another service, no payment adjustment rules for multiple procedures apply, 150% payment adjustment for bilateral procedures does not apply, assistant surgeon may be paid, +add-on code (list separately in addition to primary procedure)

63600   **Remove spinal cord lesion**   ~ follow-up period is 90 days, standard payment adjustment rules for multiple procedures apply, 150% payment adjustment for bilateral procedures does not apply, payment for assistant surgeon subject to documentation of medical necessity

63610   **Stimulation of spinal cord**   ~ endoscopies or minor procedure - E/M services on the same day generally not paid, standard payment adjustment rules for multiple procedures apply, 150% payment adjustment for bilateral procedures does not apply, payment for assistant surgeon subject to documentation of medical necessity

63615   **Remove lesion of spinal cord**   ~ follow-up period is 90 days, standard payment adjustment rules for multiple procedures apply, 150% payment adjustment for bilateral procedures does not apply, assistant surgeon may not be paid

63650   **Implant neuroelectrodes**   ~ follow-up period is 90 days, standard payment adjustment rules for multiple procedures apply, 150% payment adjustment for bilateral procedures does not apply, assistant surgeon may not be paid

63655   **Implant neuroelectrodes**   ~ follow-up period is 90 days, standard payment adjustment rules for multiple procedures apply, 150% payment adjustment for bilateral procedures does not apply, assistant surgeon may be paid

63660   **Revise/remove neuroelectrode**   ~ follow-up period is 90 days, standard payment adjustment rules for multiple procedures apply, 150% payment adjustment for bilateral procedures does not apply, assistant surgeon may not be paid

63685   **Insert/redo spine n generator**   ~ follow-up period is 90 days, standard payment adjustment rules for multiple procedures apply, 150% payment adjustment for bilateral procedures does not apply, assistant surgeon may be paid

63688   **Revise/remove neuroreceiver**   ~ follow-up period is 90 days, standard payment adjustment rules for multiple procedures apply, 150% payment adjustment for bilateral procedures does not apply, assistant surgeon may not be paid

63700 **Repair spinal herniation** ~ follow-up period is 90 days, standard payment adjustment rules for multiple procedures apply, 150% payment adjustment for bilateral procedures does not apply, assistant surgeon may be paid

63702 **Repair spinal herniation** ~ follow-up period is 90 days, standard payment adjustment rules for multiple procedures apply, 150% payment adjustment for bilateral procedures does not apply, assistant surgeon may be paid

63704 **Repair spinal herniation** ~ follow-up period is 90 days, standard payment adjustment rules for multiple procedures apply, 150% payment adjustment for bilateral procedures does not apply, assistant surgeon may be paid

63706 **Repair spinal herniation** ~ follow-up period is 90 days, standard payment adjustment rules for multiple procedures apply, 150% payment adjustment for bilateral procedures does not apply, assistant surgeon may be paid

63707 **Repair spinal fluid leakage** ~ follow-up period is 90 days, standard payment adjustment rules for multiple procedures apply, 150% payment adjustment for bilateral procedures does not apply, assistant surgeon may be paid

63709 **Repair spinal fluid leakage** ~ follow-up period is 90 days, standard payment adjustment rules for multiple procedures apply, 150% payment adjustment for bilateral procedures does not apply, assistant surgeon may be paid

63710 **Graft repair spine defect** ~ follow-up period is 90 days, standard payment adjustment rules for multiple procedures apply, 150% payment adjustment for bilateral procedures does not apply, assistant surgeon may be paid

63740 **Install spinal shunt** ~ follow-up period is 90 days, standard payment adjustment rules for multiple procedures apply, 150% payment adjustment for bilateral procedures does not apply, assistant surgeon may be paid

63741 **Install spinal shunt** ~ follow-up period is 90 days, standard payment adjustment rules for multiple procedures apply, 150% payment adjustment for bilateral procedures does not apply, assistant surgeon may be paid

63744 **Revise spinal shunt** ~ follow-up period is 90 days, standard payment adjustment rules for multiple procedures apply, 150% payment adjustment for bilateral procedures does not apply, assistant surgeon may be paid

63746 **Remove spinal shunt** ~ follow-up period is 90 days, standard payment adjustment rules for multiple procedures apply, 150% payment adjustment for bilateral procedures does not apply, payment for assistant surgeon subject to documentation of medical necessity

Extracranial Nerves, Peripheral Nerves, and Autonomic Nervous System

64400   **Nerve block inject, trigeminal**   ~ endoscopies or minor procedure - E/M services on the same day generally not paid, standard payment adjustment rules for multiple procedures apply, 150% payment adjustment for bilateral procedures does not apply, assistant surgeon may not be paid

64402   **Nerve block inject, facial**   ~ endoscopies or minor procedure - E/M services on the same day generally not paid, standard payment adjustment rules for multiple procedures apply, 150% payment adjustment for bilateral procedures does not apply, assistant surgeon may not be paid

64405   **Nerve block inject, occipital**   ~ endoscopies or minor procedure - E/M services on the same day generally not paid, standard payment adjustment rules for multiple procedures apply, 150% payment adjustment for bilateral procedures does not apply, assistant surgeon may not be paid

64408   **Nerve block inject, vagus**   ~ endoscopies or minor procedure - E/M services on the same day generally not paid, standard payment adjustment rules for multiple procedures apply, 150% payment adjustment for bilateral procedures does not apply, payment for assistant surgeon subject to documentation of medical necessity

64410   **Nerve block inject, phrenic**   ~ endoscopies or minor procedure - E/M services on the same day generally not paid, standard payment adjustment rules for multiple procedures apply, 150% payment adjustment for bilateral procedures does not apply, payment for assistant surgeon subject to documentation of medical necessity

64412   **Nerve block inject, spinal accessory**   ~ endoscopies or minor procedure - E/M services on the same day generally not paid, standard payment adjustment rules for multiple procedures apply, 150% payment adjustment for bilateral procedures does not apply, assistant surgeon may not be paid

64413   **Nerve block inject, cervical plexus**   ~ endoscopies or minor procedure - E/M services on the same day generally not paid, standard payment adjustment rules for multiple procedures apply, 150% payment adjustment for bilateral procedures does not apply, assistant surgeon may not be paid

64415   **Nerve block inject, brachial plexus**   ~ endoscopies or minor procedure - E/M services on the same day generally not paid, standard payment adjustment rules for multiple procedures apply, 150% payment adjustment for bilateral procedures does not apply, assistant surgeon may not be paid

64416   **Nerve block cont infuse, b plex**   ~ follow-up period is 10 days, standard payment adjustment rules for multiple procedures apply, 150% payment adjustment for bilateral procedures does not apply, assistant surgeon may not be paid

64417   **Nerve block inject, axillary**   ~ endoscopies or minor procedure - E/M services on the same day generally not paid, standard payment adjustment rules for multiple procedures apply, 150% payment adjustment for bilateral procedures does not apply, assistant surgeon may not be paid

64418   **Nerve block inject, suprascapular**   ~ endoscopies or minor procedure - E/M services on the same day generally not paid, standard payment adjustment rules for multiple procedures apply, 150% payment adjustment for bilateral procedures does not apply, assistant surgeon may not be paid

64420   **Nerve block inject, intercostal, single**   ~ endoscopies or minor procedure - E/M services on the same day generally not paid, standard payment adjustment rules for multiple procedures apply, 150% payment adjustment for bilateral procedures does not apply, assistant surgeon may not be paid

64421   **Nerve block inject, intercostal, multiple**   ~ endoscopies or minor procedure - E/M services on the same day generally not paid, standard payment adjustment rules for multiple procedures apply, 150% payment adjustment for bilateral procedures does not apply, assistant surgeon may not be paid

64425   **Nerve block inject, ilio-ing/hypogi**   ~ endoscopies or minor procedure - E/M services on the same day generally not paid, standard payment adjustment rules for multiple procedures apply, 150% payment adjustment for bilateral procedures does not apply, assistant surgeon may not be paid

64430   **Nerve block inject, pudendal**   ~ endoscopies or minor procedure - E/M services on the same day generally not paid, standard payment adjustment rules for multiple procedures apply, 150% payment adjustment for bilateral procedures does not apply, assistant surgeon may not be paid

64435   **Nerve block inject, paracervical**   ~ endoscopies or minor procedure - E/M services on the same day generally not paid, standard payment adjustment rules for multiple procedures apply, 150% payment adjustment for bilateral procedures does not apply, assistant surgeon may not be paid

64445   **Nerve block inject, sciatic, single**   ~ endoscopies or minor procedure - E/M services on the same day generally not paid, standard payment adjustment rules for multiple procedures apply, 150% payment adjustment for bilateral procedures does not apply, assistant surgeon may not be paid

64446   **N block inject, sciatic, cont inf**   ~ follow-up period is 10 days, standard payment adjustment rules for multiple procedures apply, 150% payment adjustment for bilateral procedures does not apply, assistant surgeon may not be paid

64447   **Nerve block inject fem, single**   ~ endoscopies or minor procedure - E/M services on the same day generally not paid, standard payment adjustment rules for multiple

procedures apply, 150% payment adjustment for bilateral procedures does not apply, assistant surgeon may not be paid

64448 **Nerve block inject fem, cont inf** ~ follow-up period is 10 days, standard payment adjustment rules for multiple procedures apply, 150% payment adjustment for bilateral procedures does not apply, assistant surgeon may not be paid

64449 **Nerve block inject, lumbar plexus** ~ follow-up period is 10 days, standard payment adjustment rules for multiple procedures apply, 150% payment adjustment for bilateral procedures does not apply, assistant surgeon may not be paid

64450 **Nerve block, other peripheral** ~ endoscopies or minor procedure - E/M services on the same day generally not paid, standard payment adjustment rules for multiple procedures apply, 150% payment adjustment for bilateral procedures applies, assistant surgeon may not be paid

64470 **Inject paravertebral c/t** ~ endoscopies or minor procedure - E/M services on the same day generally not paid, standard payment adjustment rules for multiple procedures apply, 150% payment adjustment for bilateral procedures applies, assistant surgeon may not be paid

64472 **Inject paravertebral c/t, add-on** ~ follow-up period included in another service, no payment adjustment rules for multiple procedures apply, 150% payment adjustment for bilateral procedures applies, assistant surgeon may not be paid, +add-on code (list separately in addition to primary procedure)

64475 **Inject paravertebral l/s** ~ endoscopies or minor procedure - E/M services on the same day generally not paid, standard payment adjustment rules for multiple procedures apply, 150% payment adjustment for bilateral procedures applies, assistant surgeon may not be paid

64476 **Inject paravertebral l/s, add-on** ~ follow-up period included in another service, no payment adjustment rules for multiple procedures apply, 150% payment adjustment for bilateral procedures applies, assistant surgeon may not be paid, +add-on code (list separately in addition to primary procedure)

64479 **Inject foramen epidural c/t** ~ endoscopies or minor procedure - E/M services on the same day generally not paid, standard payment adjustment rules for multiple procedures apply, 150% payment adjustment for bilateral procedures applies, assistant surgeon may not be paid

64480 **Inject foramen epidural, add-on** ~ follow-up period included in another service, no payment adjustment rules for multiple procedures apply, 150% payment adjustment for bilateral procedures applies, assistant surgeon may not be paid, +add-on code (list separately in addition to primary procedure)

64483   **Inject foramen epidural l/s**   ~ endoscopies or minor procedure - E/M services on the same day generally not paid, standard payment adjustment rules for multiple procedures apply, 150% payment adjustment for bilateral procedures applies, assistant surgeon may not be paid

64484   **Inject foramen epidural, add-on**   ~ follow-up period included in another service, no payment adjustment rules for multiple procedures apply, 150% payment adjustment for bilateral procedures applies, assistant surgeon may not be paid, +add-on code (list separately in addition to primary procedure)

64505   **Nerve block, sphenopalatine ganglia**   ~ endoscopies or minor procedure - E/M services on the same day generally not paid, standard payment adjustment rules for multiple procedures apply, 150% payment adjustment for bilateral procedures does not apply, assistant surgeon may not be paid

64508   **Nerve block, carotid sinus s/p**   ~ endoscopies or minor procedure - E/M services on the same day generally not paid, standard payment adjustment rules for multiple procedures apply, 150% payment adjustment for bilateral procedures does not apply, payment for assistant surgeon subject to documentation of medical necessity

64510   **Nerve block, stellate ganglion**   ~ endoscopies or minor procedure - E/M services on the same day generally not paid, standard payment adjustment rules for multiple procedures apply, 150% payment adjustment for bilateral procedures does not apply, assistant surgeon may not be paid

64517   **Nerve block inject, hypogas plexus**   ~ endoscopies or minor procedure - E/M services on the same day generally not paid, standard payment adjustment rules for multiple procedures apply, 150% payment adjustment for bilateral procedures does not apply, assistant surgeon may not be paid

64520   **Nerve block, lumbar/thoracic**   ~ endoscopies or minor procedure - E/M services on the same day generally not paid, standard payment adjustment rules for multiple procedures apply, 150% payment adjustment for bilateral procedures does not apply, assistant surgeon may not be paid

64530   **Nerve block inject, celiac plexus**   ~ endoscopies or minor procedure - E/M services on the same day generally not paid, standard payment adjustment rules for multiple procedures apply, 150% payment adjustment for bilateral procedures does not apply, assistant surgeon may not be paid

64550   **Apply neurostimulator**   ~ endoscopies or minor procedure - E/M services on the same day generally not paid, no payment adjustment rules for multiple procedures apply, 150% payment adjustment for bilateral procedures does not apply, assistant surgeon may not be paid

64553   **Implant neuroelectrodes**   ~ follow-up period is 10 days, standard payment adjustment rules for multiple procedures apply, 150% payment adjustment for

bilateral procedures does not apply, payment for assistant surgeon subject to documentation of medical necessity

64555   **Implant neuroelectrodes**   ~ follow-up period is 10 days, standard payment adjustment rules for multiple procedures apply, 150% payment adjustment for bilateral procedures does not apply, assistant surgeon may not be paid

64560   **Implant neuroelectrodes**   ~ follow-up period is 10 days, standard payment adjustment rules for multiple procedures apply, 150% payment adjustment for bilateral procedures does not apply, payment for assistant surgeon subject to documentation of medical necessity

64561   **Implant neuroelectrodes**   ~ follow-up period is 10 days, standard payment adjustment rules for multiple procedures apply, 150% payment adjustment for bilateral procedures does not apply, assistant surgeon may not be paid

64565   **Implant neuroelectrodes**   ~ follow-up period is 10 days, standard payment adjustment rules for multiple procedures apply, 150% payment adjustment for bilateral procedures does not apply, assistant surgeon may not be paid

64573   **Implant neuroelectrodes**   ~ follow-up period is 90 days, standard payment adjustment rules for multiple procedures apply, 150% payment adjustment for bilateral procedures does not apply, payment for assistant surgeon subject to documentation of medical necessity

64575   **Implant neuroelectrodes**   ~ follow-up period is 90 days, standard payment adjustment rules for multiple procedures apply, 150% payment adjustment for bilateral procedures does not apply, assistant surgeon may not be paid

64577   **Implant neuroelectrodes**   ~ follow-up period is 90 days, standard payment adjustment rules for multiple procedures apply, 150% payment adjustment for bilateral procedures does not apply, assistant surgeon may not be paid

64580   **Implant neuroelectrodes**   ~ follow-up period is 90 days, standard payment adjustment rules for multiple procedures apply, 150% payment adjustment for bilateral procedures does not apply, assistant surgeon may be paid

64581   **Implant neuroelectrodes**   ~ follow-up period is 90 days, standard payment adjustment rules for multiple procedures apply, 150% payment adjustment for bilateral procedures does not apply, assistant surgeon may not be paid

64585   **Revise/remove neuroelectrode**   ~ follow-up period is 10 days, standard payment adjustment rules for multiple procedures apply, 150% payment adjustment for bilateral procedures does not apply, assistant surgeon may be paid

64590   **Insert/redo pn/gastric stimuli**   ~ follow-up period is 10 days, standard payment adjustment rules for multiple procedures apply, 150% payment adjustment for bilateral procedures does not apply, assistant surgeon may be paid

64595 **Revise/remove pn/gastric stimuli** ~ follow-up period is 10 days, standard payment adjustment rules for multiple procedures apply, 150% payment adjustment for bilateral procedures does not apply, assistant surgeon may not be paid

64600 **Injection treat nerve** ~ follow-up period is 10 days, standard payment adjustment rules for multiple procedures apply, 150% payment adjustment does not apply - RVUs based on bilateral procedure, assistant surgeon may not be paid

64605 **Injection treat nerve** ~ follow-up period is 10 days, standard payment adjustment rules for multiple procedures apply, 150% payment adjustment for bilateral procedures does not apply, payment for assistant surgeon subject to documentation of medical necessity

64610 **Injection treat nerve** ~ follow-up period is 10 days, standard payment adjustment rules for multiple procedures apply, 150% payment adjustment for bilateral procedures does not apply, assistant surgeon may not be paid

64612 **Destroy nerve, face muscle** ~ follow-up period is 10 days, standard payment adjustment rules for multiple procedures apply, 150% payment adjustment for bilateral procedures applies, assistant surgeon may not be paid

64613 **Destroy nerve, neck muscle** ~ follow-up period is 10 days, standard payment adjustment rules for multiple procedures apply, 150% payment adjustment for bilateral procedures does not apply, assistant surgeon may not be paid

64614 **Destroy nerve, extremity muscle** ~ follow-up period is 10 days, standard payment adjustment rules for multiple procedures apply, 150% payment adjustment for bilateral procedures applies, assistant surgeon may not be paid

64620 **Injection treat nerve** ~ follow-up period is 10 days, standard payment adjustment rules for multiple procedures apply, 150% payment adjustment for bilateral procedures does not apply, assistant surgeon may not be paid

64622 **Destroy paravertebral nerve l/s** ~ follow-up period is 10 days, standard payment adjustment rules for multiple procedures apply, 150% payment adjustment for bilateral procedures applies, assistant surgeon may not be paid

64623 **Destroy paravertebral n, add-on** ~ follow-up period included in another service, no payment adjustment rules for multiple procedures apply, 150% payment adjustment for bilateral procedures applies, assistant surgeon may not be paid, +add-on code (list separately in addition to primary procedure)

64626 **Destroy paravertebral nerve c/t** ~ follow-up period is 10 days, standard payment adjustment rules for multiple procedures apply, 150% payment adjustment for bilateral procedures applies, assistant surgeon may not be paid

---

64627   **Destroy paravertebral n, add-on**   ~ follow-up period included in another service, no payment adjustment rules for multiple procedures apply, 150% payment adjustment for bilateral procedures applies, assistant surgeon may not be paid, +add-on code (list separately in addition to primary procedure)

64630   **Injection treat nerve**   ~ follow-up period is 10 days, standard payment adjustment rules for multiple procedures apply, 150% payment adjustment for bilateral procedures does not apply, payment for assistant surgeon subject to documentation of medical necessity

64640   **Injection treat nerve**   ~ follow-up period is 10 days, standard payment adjustment rules for multiple procedures apply, 150% payment adjustment for bilateral procedures applies, assistant surgeon may not be paid

64650   **Chemodenervation eccrine glands**   ~ endoscopies or minor procedure - E/M services on the same day generally not paid, standard payment adjustment rules for multiple procedures apply, 150% payment adjustment for bilateral procedures does not apply, payment for assistant surgeon subject to documentation of medical necessity

64653   **Chemodenervation eccrine glands**   ~ endoscopies or minor procedure - E/M services on the same day generally not paid, standard payment adjustment rules for multiple procedures apply, 150% payment adjustment for bilateral procedures does not apply, payment for assistant surgeon subject to documentation of medical necessity

64680   **Injection treat nerve**   ~ follow-up period is 10 days, standard payment adjustment rules for multiple procedures apply, 150% payment adjustment for bilateral procedures does not apply, assistant surgeon may not be paid

64681   **Injection treat nerve**   ~ follow-up period is 10 days, standard payment adjustment rules for multiple procedures apply, 150% payment adjustment for bilateral procedures does not apply, assistant surgeon may not be paid

64702   **Revise finger/toe nerve**   ~ follow-up period is 90 days, standard payment adjustment rules for multiple procedures apply, 150% payment adjustment for bilateral procedures does not apply, assistant surgeon may not be paid

64704   **Revise hand/foot nerve**   ~ follow-up period is 90 days, standard payment adjustment rules for multiple procedures apply, 150% payment adjustment for bilateral procedures does not apply, assistant surgeon may be paid

64708   **Revise arm/leg nerve**   ~ follow-up period is 90 days, standard payment adjustment rules for multiple procedures apply, 150% payment adjustment for bilateral procedures does not apply, assistant surgeon may be paid

64712   **Revise sciatic nerve**   ~ follow-up period is 90 days, standard payment adjustment rules for multiple procedures apply, 150% payment adjustment for bilateral procedures does not apply, assistant surgeon may be paid

64713 **Revise arm nerve(s)** ~ follow-up period is 90 days, standard payment adjustment rules for multiple procedures apply, 150% payment adjustment for bilateral procedures does not apply, assistant surgeon may be paid

64714 **Revise low back nerve(s)** ~ follow-up period is 90 days, standard payment adjustment rules for multiple procedures apply, 150% payment adjustment for bilateral procedures does not apply, assistant surgeon may be paid

64716 **Revise cranial nerve** ~ follow-up period is 90 days, standard payment adjustment rules for multiple procedures apply, 150% payment adjustment for bilateral procedures does not apply, assistant surgeon may be paid

64718 **Revise ulnar nerve at elbow** ~ follow-up period is 90 days, standard payment adjustment rules for multiple procedures apply, 150% payment adjustment for bilateral procedures does not apply, payment for assistant surgeon subject to documentation of medical necessity

64719 **Revise ulnar nerve at wrist** ~ follow-up period is 90 days, standard payment adjustment rules for multiple procedures apply, 150% payment adjustment for bilateral procedures does not apply, assistant surgeon may not be paid

64721 **Carpal tunnel surgery** ~ follow-up period is 90 days, standard payment adjustment rules for multiple procedures apply, 150% payment adjustment for bilateral procedures applies, assistant surgeon may not be paid

64722 **Relieve pressure on nerve(s)** ~ follow-up period is 90 days, standard payment adjustment rules for multiple procedures apply, 150% payment adjustment for bilateral procedures does not apply, assistant surgeon may be paid

64726 **Release foot/toe nerve** ~ follow-up period is 90 days, standard payment adjustment rules for multiple procedures apply, 150% payment adjustment for bilateral procedures does not apply, assistant surgeon may not be paid

64727 **Internal nerve revision** ~ follow-up period included in another service, no payment adjustment rules for multiple procedures apply, 150% payment adjustment for bilateral procedures does not apply, assistant surgeon may not be paid

64732 **Incise brow nerve** ~ follow-up period is 90 days, standard payment adjustment rules for multiple procedures apply, 150% payment adjustment for bilateral procedures does not apply, assistant surgeon may be paid

64734 **Incise cheek nerve** ~ follow-up period is 90 days, standard payment adjustment rules for multiple procedures apply, 150% payment adjustment for bilateral procedures does not apply, payment for assistant surgeon subject to documentation of medical necessity

64736   **Incise chin nerve**   ~ follow-up period is 90 days, standard payment adjustment rules for multiple procedures apply, 150% payment adjustment for bilateral procedures does not apply, assistant surgeon may be paid

64738   **Incise jaw nerve**   ~ follow-up period is 90 days, standard payment adjustment rules for multiple procedures apply, 150% payment adjustment for bilateral procedures does not apply, assistant surgeon may be paid

64740   **Incise tongue nerve**   ~ follow-up period is 90 days, standard payment adjustment rules for multiple procedures apply, 150% payment adjustment for bilateral procedures does not apply, assistant surgeon may be paid

64742   **Incise facial nerve**   ~ follow-up period is 90 days, standard payment adjustment rules for multiple procedures apply, 150% payment adjustment for bilateral procedures does not apply, assistant surgeon may be paid

64744   **Incise nerve, back of head**   ~ follow-up period is 90 days, standard payment adjustment rules for multiple procedures apply, 150% payment adjustment for bilateral procedures applies, payment for assistant surgeon subject to documentation of medical necessity

64746   **Incise diaphragm nerve**   ~ follow-up period is 90 days, standard payment adjustment rules for multiple procedures apply, 150% payment adjustment for bilateral procedures does not apply, assistant surgeon may be paid

64752   **Incise vagus nerve**   ~ follow-up period is 90 days, standard payment adjustment rules for multiple procedures apply, 150% payment adjustment for bilateral procedures does not apply, assistant surgeon may be paid

64755   **Incise stomach nerves**   ~ follow-up period is 90 days, standard payment adjustment rules for multiple procedures apply, 150% payment adjustment for bilateral procedures does not apply, assistant surgeon may be paid

64760   **Incise vagus nerve**   ~ follow-up period is 90 days, standard payment adjustment rules for multiple procedures apply, 150% payment adjustment for bilateral procedures does not apply, assistant surgeon may be paid

64761   **Incise pelvis nerve**   ~ follow-up period is 90 days, standard payment adjustment rules for multiple procedures apply, 150% payment adjustment for bilateral procedures applies, assistant surgeon may be paid

64763   **Incise hip/thigh nerve**   ~ follow-up period is 90 days, standard payment adjustment rules for multiple procedures apply, 150% payment adjustment for bilateral procedures applies, assistant surgeon may be paid

64766   **Incise hip/thigh nerve**   ~ follow-up period is 90 days, standard payment adjustment rules for multiple procedures apply, 150% payment adjustment for bilateral procedures applies, assistant surgeon may be paid

64771   **Sever cranial nerve**   ~ follow-up period is 90 days, standard payment adjustment rules for multiple procedures apply, 150% payment adjustment for bilateral procedures does not apply, assistant surgeon may be paid

64772   **Incise spinal nerve**   ~ follow-up period is 90 days, standard payment adjustment rules for multiple procedures apply, 150% payment adjustment for bilateral procedures does not apply, assistant surgeon may be paid

64774   **Remove skin nerve lesion**   ~ follow-up period is 90 days, standard payment adjustment rules for multiple procedures apply, 150% payment adjustment for bilateral procedures does not apply, assistant surgeon may not be paid

64776   **Remove digit nerve lesion**   ~ follow-up period is 90 days, standard payment adjustment rules for multiple procedures apply, 150% payment adjustment for bilateral procedures does not apply, payment for assistant surgeon subject to documentation of medical necessity

64778   **Digit nerve surgery, add-on**   ~ follow-up period included in another service, no payment adjustment rules for multiple procedures apply, 150% payment adjustment for bilateral procedures does not apply, assistant surgeon may not be paid, +add-on code (list separately in addition to primary procedure)

64782   **Remove limb nerve lesion**   ~ follow-up period is 90 days, standard payment adjustment rules for multiple procedures apply, 150% payment adjustment for bilateral procedures does not apply, assistant surgeon may not be paid

64783   **Limb nerve surgery, add-on**   ~ follow-up period included in another service, no payment adjustment rules for multiple procedures apply, 150% payment adjustment for bilateral procedures does not apply, assistant surgeon may not be paid, +add-on code (list separately in addition to primary procedure)

64784   **Remove nerve lesion**   ~ follow-up period is 90 days, standard payment adjustment rules for multiple procedures apply, 150% payment adjustment for bilateral procedures does not apply, payment for assistant surgeon subject to documentation of medical necessity

64786   **Remove sciatic nerve lesion**   ~ follow-up period is 90 days, standard payment adjustment rules for multiple procedures apply, 150% payment adjustment for bilateral procedures does not apply, assistant surgeon may be paid

64787   **Implant nerve end**   ~ follow-up period included in another service, no payment adjustment rules for multiple procedures apply, 150% payment adjustment for

---

bilateral procedures does not apply, payment for assistant surgeon subject to documentation of medical necessity

64788   **Remove skin nerve lesion**   ~ follow-up period is 90 days, standard payment adjustment rules for multiple procedures apply, 150% payment adjustment for bilateral procedures does not apply, assistant surgeon may not be paid

64790   **Remove nerve lesion**   ~ follow-up period is 90 days, standard payment adjustment rules for multiple procedures apply, 150% payment adjustment for bilateral procedures does not apply, payment for assistant surgeon subject to documentation of medical necessity

64792   **Remove nerve lesion**   ~ follow-up period is 90 days, standard payment adjustment rules for multiple procedures apply, 150% payment adjustment for bilateral procedures does not apply, assistant surgeon may be paid

64795   **Biopsy nerve**   ~ endoscopies or minor procedure - E/M services on the same day generally not paid, standard payment adjustment rules for multiple procedures apply, 150% payment adjustment for bilateral procedures does not apply, assistant surgeon may not be paid

64802   **Remove sympathetic nerves**   ~ follow-up period is 90 days, standard payment adjustment rules for multiple procedures apply, 150% payment adjustment for bilateral procedures applies, assistant surgeon may be paid

64804   **Remove sympathetic nerves**   ~ follow-up period is 90 days, standard payment adjustment rules for multiple procedures apply, 150% payment adjustment for bilateral procedures applies, assistant surgeon may be paid

64809   **Remove sympathetic nerves**   ~ follow-up period is 90 days, standard payment adjustment rules for multiple procedures apply, 150% payment adjustment for bilateral procedures applies, assistant surgeon may be paid

64818   **Remove sympathetic nerves**   ~ follow-up period is 90 days, standard payment adjustment rules for multiple procedures apply, 150% payment adjustment for bilateral procedures applies, assistant surgeon may be paid

64820   **Remove sympathetic nerves**   ~ follow-up period is 90 days, standard payment adjustment rules for multiple procedures apply, 150% payment adjustment for bilateral procedures does not apply, assistant surgeon may not be paid

64821   **Remove sympathetic nerves**   ~ follow-up period is 90 days, standard payment adjustment rules for multiple procedures apply, 150% payment adjustment for bilateral procedures applies, assistant surgeon may not be paid

64822   **Remove sympathetic nerves**   ~ follow-up period is 90 days, standard payment adjustment rules for multiple procedures apply, 150% payment adjustment for bilateral procedures applies, assistant surgeon may not be paid

64823   **Remove sympathetic nerves**   ~ follow-up period is 90 days, standard payment adjustment rules for multiple procedures apply, 150% payment adjustment for bilateral procedures applies, assistant surgeon may not be paid

64831   **Repair digit nerve**   ~ follow-up period is 90 days, standard payment adjustment rules for multiple procedures apply, 150% payment adjustment for bilateral procedures does not apply, assistant surgeon may not be paid

64832   **Repair nerve, add-on**   ~ follow-up period included in another service, no payment adjustment rules for multiple procedures apply, 150% payment adjustment for bilateral procedures does not apply, payment for assistant surgeon subject to documentation of medical necessity, +add-on code (list separately in addition to primary procedure)

64834   **Repair hand or foot nerve**   ~ follow-up period is 90 days, standard payment adjustment rules for multiple procedures apply, 150% payment adjustment for bilateral procedures does not apply, payment for assistant surgeon subject to documentation of medical necessity

64835   **Repair hand or foot nerve**   ~ follow-up period is 90 days, standard payment adjustment rules for multiple procedures apply, 150% payment adjustment for bilateral procedures does not apply, assistant surgeon may be paid

64836   **Repair hand or foot nerve**   ~ follow-up period is 90 days, standard payment adjustment rules for multiple procedures apply, 150% payment adjustment for bilateral procedures does not apply, assistant surgeon may be paid

64837   **Repair nerve, add-on**   ~ follow-up period included in another service, no payment adjustment rules for multiple procedures apply, 150% payment adjustment for bilateral procedures does not apply, assistant surgeon may be paid, +add-on code (list separately in addition to primary procedure)

64840   **Repair leg nerve**   ~ follow-up period is 90 days, standard payment adjustment rules for multiple procedures apply, 150% payment adjustment for bilateral procedures does not apply, assistant surgeon may be paid

64856   **Repair/transpose nerve**   ~ follow-up period is 90 days, standard payment adjustment rules for multiple procedures apply, 150% payment adjustment for bilateral procedures does not apply, assistant surgeon may not be paid

64857   **Repair arm/leg nerve**   ~ follow-up period is 90 days, standard payment adjustment rules for multiple procedures apply, 150% payment adjustment for bilateral procedures does not apply, assistant surgeon may be paid

64858   **Repair sciatic nerve**   ~ follow-up period is 90 days, standard payment adjustment rules for multiple procedures apply, 150% payment adjustment for bilateral procedures does not apply, assistant surgeon may be paid

64859   **Nerve surgery**   ~ follow-up period included in another service, no payment adjustment rules for multiple procedures apply, 150% payment adjustment for bilateral procedures does not apply, assistant surgeon may be paid

64861   **Repair arm nerves**   ~ follow-up period is 90 days, standard payment adjustment rules for multiple procedures apply, 150% payment adjustment for bilateral procedures does not apply, assistant surgeon may be paid

64862   **Repair low back nerves**   ~ follow-up period is 90 days, standard payment adjustment rules for multiple procedures apply, 150% payment adjustment for bilateral procedures does not apply, assistant surgeon may be paid

64864   **Repair facial nerve**   ~ follow-up period is 90 days, standard payment adjustment rules for multiple procedures apply, 150% payment adjustment for bilateral procedures does not apply, assistant surgeon may be paid

64865   **Repair facial nerve**   ~ follow-up period is 90 days, standard payment adjustment rules for multiple procedures apply, 150% payment adjustment for bilateral procedures does not apply, assistant surgeon may be paid

64866   **Fuse facial/other nerve**   ~ follow-up period is 90 days, standard payment adjustment rules for multiple procedures apply, 150% payment adjustment for bilateral procedures does not apply, assistant surgeon may be paid

64868   **Fuse facial/other nerve**   ~ follow-up period is 90 days, standard payment adjustment rules for multiple procedures apply, 150% payment adjustment for bilateral procedures does not apply, assistant surgeon may be paid

64870   **Fuse facial/other nerve**   ~ follow-up period is 90 days, standard payment adjustment rules for multiple procedures apply, 150% payment adjustment for bilateral procedures does not apply, assistant surgeon may be paid

64872   **Subsequent repair nerve**   ~ follow-up period included in another service, no payment adjustment rules for multiple procedures apply, 150% payment adjustment for bilateral procedures does not apply, assistant surgeon may be paid

64874   **Repair & revise nerve, add-on**   ~ follow-up period included in another service, no payment adjustment rules for multiple procedures apply, 150% payment adjustment for bilateral procedures does not apply, assistant surgeon may be paid, +add-on code (list separately in addition to primary procedure)

64876   **Repair nerve/shorten bone**   ~ follow-up period included in another service, no payment adjustment rules for multiple procedures apply, 150% payment adjustment for bilateral procedures does not apply, assistant surgeon may be paid

64885   **Nerve graft, head or neck**   ~ follow-up period is 90 days, standard payment adjustment rules for multiple procedures apply, 150% payment adjustment for bilateral procedures does not apply, assistant surgeon may be paid

64886   **Nerve graft, head or neck**   ~ follow-up period is 90 days, standard payment adjustment rules for multiple procedures apply, 150% payment adjustment for bilateral procedures does not apply, assistant surgeon may be paid

64890   **Nerve graft, hand or foot**   ~ follow-up period is 90 days, standard payment adjustment rules for multiple procedures apply, 150% payment adjustment for bilateral procedures does not apply, assistant surgeon may be paid

64891   **Nerve graft, hand or foot**   ~ follow-up period is 90 days, standard payment adjustment rules for multiple procedures apply, 150% payment adjustment for bilateral procedures does not apply, assistant surgeon may be paid

64892   **Nerve graft, arm or leg**   ~ follow-up period is 90 days, standard payment adjustment rules for multiple procedures apply, 150% payment adjustment for bilateral procedures does not apply, assistant surgeon may be paid

64893   **Nerve graft, arm or leg**   ~ follow-up period is 90 days, standard payment adjustment rules for multiple procedures apply, 150% payment adjustment for bilateral procedures does not apply, assistant surgeon may be paid

64895   **Nerve graft, hand or foot**   ~ follow-up period is 90 days, standard payment adjustment rules for multiple procedures apply, 150% payment adjustment for bilateral procedures does not apply, assistant surgeon may be paid

64896   **Nerve graft, hand or foot**   ~ follow-up period is 90 days, standard payment adjustment rules for multiple procedures apply, 150% payment adjustment for bilateral procedures does not apply, assistant surgeon may be paid

64897   **Nerve graft, arm or leg**   ~ follow-up period is 90 days, standard payment adjustment rules for multiple procedures apply, 150% payment adjustment for bilateral procedures does not apply, assistant surgeon may be paid

64898   **Nerve graft, arm or leg**   ~ follow-up period is 90 days, standard payment adjustment rules for multiple procedures apply, 150% payment adjustment for bilateral procedures does not apply, assistant surgeon may be paid

64901   **Nerve graft, add-on**   ~ follow-up period included in another service, no payment adjustment rules for multiple procedures apply, 150% payment adjustment for

bilateral procedures does not apply, assistant surgeon may be paid, +add-on code (list separately in addition to primary procedure)

64902   **Nerve graft, add-on**   ~ follow-up period included in another service, no payment adjustment rules for multiple procedures apply, 150% payment adjustment for bilateral procedures does not apply, assistant surgeon may be paid, +add-on code (list separately in addition to primary procedure)

64905   **Nerve pedicle transfer**   ~ follow-up period is 90 days, standard payment adjustment rules for multiple procedures apply, 150% payment adjustment for bilateral procedures does not apply, assistant surgeon may be paid

64907   **Nerve pedicle transfer**   ~ follow-up period is 90 days, standard payment adjustment rules for multiple procedures apply, 150% payment adjustment for bilateral procedures does not apply, assistant surgeon may be paid

64910   **Nerve repair w/allograft**   ~ follow-up period is 90 days, standard payment adjustment rules for multiple procedures apply, 150% payment adjustment for bilateral procedures does not apply, assistant surgeon may be paid

64911   **Neurorrhaphy w/vein autograft**   ~ follow-up period is 90 days, standard payment adjustment rules for multiple procedures apply, 150% payment adjustment for bilateral procedures does not apply, assistant surgeon may be paid

64999   **Nervous system surgery**   ~ medicare carrier determines global period, standard payment adjustment rules for multiple procedures apply, 150% payment adjustment for bilateral procedures does not apply, payment for assistant surgeon subject to documentation of medical necessity

65091   **Revise eye**   ~ follow-up period is 90 days, standard payment adjustment rules for multiple procedures apply, 150% payment adjustment for bilateral procedures applies, payment for assistant surgeon subject to documentation of medical necessity

65093   **Revise eye with implant**   ~ follow-up period is 90 days, standard payment adjustment rules for multiple procedures apply, 150% payment adjustment for bilateral procedures applies, assistant surgeon may not be paid

EYE AND OCULAR ADNEXA

Eyeball

65101   **Remove eye**   ~ follow-up period is 90 days, standard payment adjustment rules for multiple procedures apply, 150% payment adjustment for bilateral procedures applies, assistant surgeon may not be paid

65103   **Remove eye/insert implant**   ~ follow-up period is 90 days, standard payment adjustment rules for multiple procedures apply, 150% payment adjustment for bilateral procedures applies, assistant surgeon may not be paid

65105   **Remove eye/attach implant**   ~ follow-up period is 90 days, standard payment adjustment rules for multiple procedures apply, 150% payment adjustment for bilateral procedures applies, assistant surgeon may be paid

65110   **Remove eye**   ~ follow-up period is 90 days, standard payment adjustment rules for multiple procedures apply, 150% payment adjustment for bilateral procedures applies, assistant surgeon may be paid

65112   **Remove eye/revise socket**   ~ follow-up period is 90 days, standard payment adjustment rules for multiple procedures apply, 150% payment adjustment for bilateral procedures applies, assistant surgeon may be paid

65114   **Remove eye/revise socket**   ~ follow-up period is 90 days, standard payment adjustment rules for multiple procedures apply, 150% payment adjustment for bilateral procedures applies, assistant surgeon may be paid

65125   **Revise ocular implant**   ~ follow-up period is 90 days, standard payment adjustment rules for multiple procedures apply, 150% payment adjustment for bilateral procedures applies, assistant surgeon may not be paid

65130   **Insert ocular implant**   ~ follow-up period is 90 days, standard payment adjustment rules for multiple procedures apply, 150% payment adjustment for bilateral procedures applies, assistant surgeon may not be paid

65135   **Insert ocular implant**   ~ follow-up period is 90 days, standard payment adjustment rules for multiple procedures apply, 150% payment adjustment for bilateral procedures applies, assistant surgeon may not be paid

65140   **Attach ocular implant**   ~ follow-up period is 90 days, standard payment adjustment rules for multiple procedures apply, 150% payment adjustment for bilateral procedures applies, assistant surgeon may not be paid

65150   **Revise ocular implant**   ~ follow-up period is 90 days, standard payment adjustment rules for multiple procedures apply, 150% payment adjustment for bilateral procedures applies, payment for assistant surgeon subject to documentation of medical necessity

65155   **Reinsert ocular implant**   ~ follow-up period is 90 days, standard payment adjustment rules for multiple procedures apply, 150% payment adjustment for bilateral procedures applies, assistant surgeon may not be paid

65175   **Remove ocular implant**   ~ follow-up period is 90 days, standard payment adjustment rules for multiple procedures apply, 150% payment adjustment for bilateral procedures applies, assistant surgeon may not be paid

65205   **Remove foreign body eye**   ~ endoscopies or minor procedure - E/M services on the same day generally not paid, standard payment adjustment rules for multiple procedures apply, 150% payment adjustment for bilateral procedures applies, assistant surgeon may not be paid

65210   **Remove foreign body eye**   ~ endoscopies or minor procedure - E/M services on the same day generally not paid, standard payment adjustment rules for multiple procedures apply, 150% payment adjustment for bilateral procedures applies, assistant surgeon may not be paid

65220   **Remove foreign body eye**   ~ endoscopies or minor procedure - E/M services on the same day generally not paid, standard payment adjustment rules for multiple procedures apply, 150% payment adjustment for bilateral procedures applies, assistant surgeon may not be paid

65222   **Remove foreign body eye**   ~ endoscopies or minor procedure - E/M services on the same day generally not paid, standard payment adjustment rules for multiple procedures apply, 150% payment adjustment for bilateral procedures applies, assistant surgeon may not be paid

65235   **Remove foreign body eye**   ~ follow-up period is 90 days, standard payment adjustment rules for multiple procedures apply, 150% payment adjustment for bilateral procedures applies, payment for assistant surgeon subject to documentation of medical necessity

65260   **Remove foreign body eye**   ~ follow-up period is 90 days, standard payment adjustment rules for multiple procedures apply, 150% payment adjustment for bilateral procedures applies, assistant surgeon may be paid

65265   **Remove foreign body eye**   ~ follow-up period is 90 days, standard payment adjustment rules for multiple procedures apply, 150% payment adjustment for bilateral procedures applies, assistant surgeon may be paid

65270   **Repair eye wound**   ~ follow-up period is 10 days, standard payment adjustment rules for multiple procedures apply, 150% payment adjustment for bilateral procedures applies, payment for assistant surgeon subject to documentation of medical necessity

65272   **Repair eye wound**   ~ follow-up period is 90 days, standard payment adjustment rules for multiple procedures apply, 150% payment adjustment for bilateral procedures applies, assistant surgeon may not be paid

65273   **Repair eye wound**   ~ follow-up period is 90 days, standard payment adjustment rules for multiple procedures apply, 150% payment adjustment for bilateral procedures applies, assistant surgeon may not be paid

65275   **Repair eye wound**   ~ follow-up period is 90 days, standard payment adjustment rules for multiple procedures apply, 150% payment adjustment for bilateral procedures applies, payment for assistant surgeon subject to documentation of medical necessity

65280   **Repair eye wound**   ~ follow-up period is 90 days, standard payment adjustment rules for multiple procedures apply, 150% payment adjustment for bilateral procedures applies, payment for assistant surgeon subject to documentation of medical necessity

65285   **Repair eye wound**   ~ follow-up period is 90 days, standard payment adjustment rules for multiple procedures apply, 150% payment adjustment for bilateral procedures applies, assistant surgeon may be paid

65286   **Repair eye wound**   ~ follow-up period is 90 days, standard payment adjustment rules for multiple procedures apply, 150% payment adjustment for bilateral procedures applies, assistant surgeon may not be paid

65290   **Repair eye socket wound**   ~ follow-up period is 90 days, standard payment adjustment rules for multiple procedures apply, 150% payment adjustment for bilateral procedures applies, assistant surgeon may not be paid

65400   **Remove eye lesion**   ~ follow-up period is 90 days, standard payment adjustment rules for multiple procedures apply, 150% payment adjustment for bilateral procedures applies, assistant surgeon may not be paid

65410   **Biopsy cornea**   ~ endoscopies or minor procedure - E/M services on the same day generally not paid, standard payment adjustment rules for multiple procedures apply, 150% payment adjustment for bilateral procedures applies, payment for assistant surgeon subject to documentation of medical necessity

65420   **Remove eye lesion**   ~ follow-up period is 90 days, standard payment adjustment rules for multiple procedures apply, 150% payment adjustment for bilateral procedures applies, assistant surgeon may not be paid

65426   **Remove eye lesion**   ~ follow-up period is 90 days, standard payment adjustment rules for multiple procedures apply, 150% payment adjustment for bilateral procedures applies, assistant surgeon may not be paid

65430   **Corneal smear**   ~ endoscopies or minor procedure - E/M services on the same day generally not paid, standard payment adjustment rules for multiple procedures apply, 150% payment adjustment for bilateral procedures applies, assistant surgeon may not be paid

---

65435   **Curette/treat cornea**   ~ endoscopies or minor procedure - E/M services on the same day generally not paid, standard payment adjustment rules for multiple procedures apply, 150% payment adjustment for bilateral procedures applies, assistant surgeon may not be paid

65436   **Curette/treat cornea**   ~ follow-up period is 90 days, standard payment adjustment rules for multiple procedures apply, 150% payment adjustment for bilateral procedures applies, assistant surgeon may not be paid

65450   **Treat corneal lesion**   ~ follow-up period is 90 days, standard payment adjustment rules for multiple procedures apply, 150% payment adjustment for bilateral procedures applies, assistant surgeon may not be paid

65600   **Revise cornea**   ~ follow-up period is 90 days, standard payment adjustment rules for multiple procedures apply, 150% payment adjustment for bilateral procedures applies, assistant surgeon may not be paid

65710   **Corneal transplant**   ~ follow-up period is 90 days, standard payment adjustment rules for multiple procedures apply, 150% payment adjustment for bilateral procedures applies, assistant surgeon may be paid

65730   **Corneal transplant**   ~ follow-up period is 90 days, standard payment adjustment rules for multiple procedures apply, 150% payment adjustment for bilateral procedures applies, assistant surgeon may be paid

65750   **Corneal transplant**   ~ follow-up period is 90 days, standard payment adjustment rules for multiple procedures apply, 150% payment adjustment for bilateral procedures applies, assistant surgeon may be paid

65755   **Corneal transplant**   ~ follow-up period is 90 days, standard payment adjustment rules for multiple procedures apply, 150% payment adjustment for bilateral procedures applies, assistant surgeon may be paid

65760   **Revise cornea**   non-covered service, multiple procedure concept does not apply, bilateral surgery concept does not apply, assistant surgery concept does not apply

65765   **Revise cornea**   non-covered service, multiple procedure concept does not apply, bilateral surgery concept does not apply, assistant surgery concept does not apply

65767   **Corneal tissue transplant**   non-covered service, multiple procedure concept does not apply, bilateral surgery concept does not apply, assistant surgery concept does not apply

65770   **Revise cornea with implant**   ~ follow-up period is 90 days, standard payment adjustment rules for multiple procedures apply, 150% payment adjustment for bilateral procedures applies, assistant surgeon may be paid

65771   **Radial keratotomy**   non-covered service, multiple procedure concept does not apply, bilateral surgery concept does not apply, assistant surgery concept does not apply

65772   **Correct astigmatism**   ~ follow-up period is 90 days, standard payment adjustment rules for multiple procedures apply, 150% payment adjustment for bilateral procedures applies, assistant surgeon may not be paid

65775   **Correct astigmatism**   ~ follow-up period is 90 days, standard payment adjustment rules for multiple procedures apply, 150% payment adjustment for bilateral procedures applies, assistant surgeon may not be paid

65780   **Ocular reconstruct transplant**   ~ follow-up period is 90 days, standard payment adjustment rules for multiple procedures apply, 150% payment adjustment for bilateral procedures applies, assistant surgeon may be paid

65781   **Ocular reconstruct transplant**   ~ follow-up period is 90 days, standard payment adjustment rules for multiple procedures apply, 150% payment adjustment for bilateral procedures applies, assistant surgeon may be paid

65782   **Ocular reconstruct transplant**   ~ follow-up period is 90 days, standard payment adjustment rules for multiple procedures apply, 150% payment adjustment for bilateral procedures applies, assistant surgeon may be paid

65800   **Drain eye**   ~ endoscopies or minor procedure - E/M services on the same day generally not paid, standard payment adjustment rules for multiple procedures apply, 150% payment adjustment for bilateral procedures applies, assistant surgeon may not be paid

65805   **Drain eye**   ~ endoscopies or minor procedure - E/M services on the same day generally not paid, standard payment adjustment rules for multiple procedures apply, 150% payment adjustment for bilateral procedures applies, assistant surgeon may not be paid

65810   **Drain eye**   ~ follow-up period is 90 days, standard payment adjustment rules for multiple procedures apply, 150% payment adjustment for bilateral procedures applies, assistant surgeon may not be paid

65815   **Drain eye**   ~ follow-up period is 90 days, standard payment adjustment rules for multiple procedures apply, 150% payment adjustment for bilateral procedures applies, assistant surgeon may not be paid

65820   **Relieve inner eye pressure**   ~ follow-up period is 90 days, standard payment adjustment rules for multiple procedures apply, 150% payment adjustment for bilateral procedures applies, payment for assistant surgeon subject to documentation of medical necessity

65850   **Incise eye**   ~ follow-up period is 90 days, standard payment adjustment rules for multiple procedures apply, 150% payment adjustment for bilateral procedures applies, assistant surgeon may not be paid

65855   **Laser surgery eye**   ~ follow-up period is 10 days, standard payment adjustment rules for multiple procedures apply, 150% payment adjustment for bilateral procedures applies, assistant surgeon may not be paid

65860   **Incise inner eye adhesions**   ~ follow-up period is 90 days, standard payment adjustment rules for multiple procedures apply, 150% payment adjustment for bilateral procedures applies, payment for assistant surgeon subject to documentation of medical necessity

65865   **Incise inner eye adhesions**   ~ follow-up period is 90 days, standard payment adjustment rules for multiple procedures apply, 150% payment adjustment for bilateral procedures applies, assistant surgeon may not be paid

65870   **Incise inner eye adhesions**   ~ follow-up period is 90 days, standard payment adjustment rules for multiple procedures apply, 150% payment adjustment for bilateral procedures applies, assistant surgeon may not be paid

65875   **Incise inner eye adhesions**   ~ follow-up period is 90 days, standard payment adjustment rules for multiple procedures apply, 150% payment adjustment for bilateral procedures applies, assistant surgeon may not be paid

65880   **Incise inner eye adhesions**   ~ follow-up period is 90 days, standard payment adjustment rules for multiple procedures apply, 150% payment adjustment for bilateral procedures applies, assistant surgeon may not be paid

65900   **Remove eye lesion**   ~ follow-up period is 90 days, standard payment adjustment rules for multiple procedures apply, 150% payment adjustment for bilateral procedures applies, assistant surgeon may be paid

65920   **Remove implant of eye**   ~ follow-up period is 90 days, standard payment adjustment rules for multiple procedures apply, 150% payment adjustment for bilateral procedures applies, assistant surgeon may not be paid

65930   **Remove blood clot from eye**   ~ follow-up period is 90 days, standard payment adjustment rules for multiple procedures apply, 150% payment adjustment for bilateral procedures applies, assistant surgeon may not be paid

66020 **Injection treat eye** ~ follow-up period is 10 days, standard payment adjustment rules for multiple procedures apply, 150% payment adjustment for bilateral procedures applies, assistant surgeon may not be paid

66030 **Injection treat eye** ~ follow-up period is 10 days, standard payment adjustment rules for multiple procedures apply, 150% payment adjustment for bilateral procedures applies, assistant surgeon may not be paid

66130 **Remove eye lesion** ~ follow-up period is 90 days, standard payment adjustment rules for multiple procedures apply, 150% payment adjustment for bilateral procedures applies, payment for assistant surgeon subject to documentation of medical necessity

66150 **Glaucoma surgery** ~ follow-up period is 90 days, standard payment adjustment rules for multiple procedures apply, 150% payment adjustment for bilateral procedures applies, assistant surgeon may not be paid

66155 **Glaucoma surgery** ~ follow-up period is 90 days, standard payment adjustment rules for multiple procedures apply, 150% payment adjustment for bilateral procedures applies, assistant surgeon may not be paid

66160 **Glaucoma surgery** ~ follow-up period is 90 days, standard payment adjustment rules for multiple procedures apply, 150% payment adjustment for bilateral procedures applies, assistant surgeon may not be paid

66165 **Glaucoma surgery** ~ follow-up period is 90 days, standard payment adjustment rules for multiple procedures apply, 150% payment adjustment for bilateral procedures applies, assistant surgeon may be paid

66170 **Glaucoma surgery** ~ follow-up period is 90 days, standard payment adjustment rules for multiple procedures apply, 150% payment adjustment for bilateral procedures applies, assistant surgeon may be paid

66172 **Incise eye** ~ follow-up period is 90 days, standard payment adjustment rules for multiple procedures apply, 150% payment adjustment for bilateral procedures applies, assistant surgeon may be paid

66180 **Implant eye shunt** ~ follow-up period is 90 days, standard payment adjustment rules for multiple procedures apply, 150% payment adjustment for bilateral procedures applies, assistant surgeon may be paid

66185 **Revise eye shunt** ~ follow-up period is 90 days, standard payment adjustment rules for multiple procedures apply, 150% payment adjustment for bilateral procedures applies, assistant surgeon may be paid

66220 **Repair eye lesion** ~ follow-up period is 90 days, standard payment adjustment rules for multiple procedures apply, 150% payment adjustment for bilateral procedures applies, assistant surgeon may be paid

66225 **Repair/graft eye lesion** ~ follow-up period is 90 days, standard payment adjustment rules for multiple procedures apply, 150% payment adjustment for bilateral procedures applies, assistant surgeon may be paid

66250 **Follow-up surgery eye** ~ follow-up period is 90 days, standard payment adjustment rules for multiple procedures apply, 150% payment adjustment for bilateral procedures applies, assistant surgeon may not be paid

Iris, Ciliary Body

66500 **Incise iris** ~ follow-up period is 90 days, standard payment adjustment rules for multiple procedures apply, 150% payment adjustment for bilateral procedures applies, assistant surgeon may not be paid

66505 **Incise iris** ~ follow-up period is 90 days, standard payment adjustment rules for multiple procedures apply, 150% payment adjustment for bilateral procedures applies, assistant surgeon may not be paid

66600 **Remove iris and lesion** ~ follow-up period is 90 days, standard payment adjustment rules for multiple procedures apply, 150% payment adjustment for bilateral procedures applies, assistant surgeon may not be paid

66605 **Remove iris** ~ follow-up period is 90 days, standard payment adjustment rules for multiple procedures apply, 150% payment adjustment for bilateral procedures applies, assistant surgeon may not be paid

66625 **Remove iris** ~ follow-up period is 90 days, standard payment adjustment rules for multiple procedures apply, 150% payment adjustment for bilateral procedures applies, assistant surgeon may not be paid

66630 **Remove iris** ~ follow-up period is 90 days, standard payment adjustment rules for multiple procedures apply, 150% payment adjustment for bilateral procedures applies, assistant surgeon may not be paid

66635 **Remove iris** ~ follow-up period is 90 days, standard payment adjustment rules for multiple procedures apply, 150% payment adjustment for bilateral procedures applies, assistant surgeon may not be paid

66680 **Repair iris & ciliary body** ~ follow-up period is 90 days, standard payment adjustment rules for multiple procedures apply, 150% payment adjustment for bilateral procedures applies, assistant surgeon may not be paid

66682 **Repair iris & ciliary body** ~ follow-up period is 90 days, standard payment adjustment rules for multiple procedures apply, 150% payment adjustment for bilateral procedures applies, assistant surgeon may not be paid

66700 **Destroy ciliary body** ~ follow-up period is 90 days, standard payment adjustment rules for multiple procedures apply, 150% payment adjustment for bilateral procedures applies, payment for assistant surgeon subject to documentation of medical necessity

66710 **Ciliary transscleral therapy** ~ follow-up period is 90 days, standard payment adjustment rules for multiple procedures apply, 150% payment adjustment for bilateral procedures applies, assistant surgeon may not be paid

66711 **Ciliary endoscopic ablation** ~ follow-up period is 90 days, special rules for multiple endoscopic procedures apply if billed with another endoscopy in the same family, 150% payment adjustment for bilateral procedures applies, assistant surgeon may not be paid

66720 **Destroy ciliary body** ~ follow-up period is 90 days, standard payment adjustment rules for multiple procedures apply, 150% payment adjustment for bilateral procedures applies, assistant surgeon may not be paid

66740 **Destroy ciliary body** ~ follow-up period is 90 days, standard payment adjustment rules for multiple procedures apply, 150% payment adjustment for bilateral procedures applies, assistant surgeon may not be paid

66761 **Revise iris** ~ follow-up period is 90 days, standard payment adjustment rules for multiple procedures apply, 150% payment adjustment for bilateral procedures applies, assistant surgeon may not be paid

66762 **Revise iris** ~ follow-up period is 90 days, standard payment adjustment rules for multiple procedures apply, 150% payment adjustment for bilateral procedures applies, assistant surgeon may not be paid

66770 **Remove inner eye lesion** ~ follow-up period is 90 days, standard payment adjustment rules for multiple procedures apply, 150% payment adjustment for bilateral procedures applies, assistant surgeon may not be paid

66820 **Incise secondary cataract** ~ follow-up period is 90 days, standard payment adjustment rules for multiple procedures apply, 150% payment adjustment for bilateral procedures applies, assistant surgeon may not be paid

66821 **After cataract laser surgery** ~ follow-up period is 90 days, standard payment adjustment rules for multiple procedures apply, 150% payment adjustment for bilateral procedures applies, assistant surgeon may not be paid

66825   **Reposition intraocular lens**   ~ follow-up period is 90 days, standard payment adjustment rules for multiple procedures apply, 150% payment adjustment for bilateral procedures applies, payment for assistant surgeon subject to documentation of medical necessity

66830   **Remove lens lesion**   ~ follow-up period is 90 days, standard payment adjustment rules for multiple procedures apply, 150% payment adjustment for bilateral procedures applies, assistant surgeon may not be paid

66840   **Remove lens material**   ~ follow-up period is 90 days, standard payment adjustment rules for multiple procedures apply, 150% payment adjustment for bilateral procedures applies, assistant surgeon may not be paid

66850   **Remove lens material**   ~ follow-up period is 90 days, standard payment adjustment rules for multiple procedures apply, 150% payment adjustment for bilateral procedures applies, assistant surgeon may not be paid

66852   **Remove lens material**   ~ follow-up period is 90 days, standard payment adjustment rules for multiple procedures apply, 150% payment adjustment for bilateral procedures applies, payment for assistant surgeon subject to documentation of medical necessity

66920   **Extraction of lens**   ~ follow-up period is 90 days, standard payment adjustment rules for multiple procedures apply, 150% payment adjustment for bilateral procedures applies, payment for assistant surgeon subject to documentation of medical necessity

66930   **Extraction of lens**   ~ follow-up period is 90 days, standard payment adjustment rules for multiple procedures apply, 150% payment adjustment for bilateral procedures applies, payment for assistant surgeon subject to documentation of medical necessity

66940   **Extraction of lens**   ~ follow-up period is 90 days, standard payment adjustment rules for multiple procedures apply, 150% payment adjustment for bilateral procedures applies, payment for assistant surgeon subject to documentation of medical necessity

66982   **Cataract surgery, complex**   ~ follow-up period is 90 days, standard payment adjustment rules for multiple procedures apply, 150% payment adjustment for bilateral procedures applies, assistant surgeon may not be paid

66983   **Cataract surg w/iol, 1 stage**   ~ follow-up period is 90 days, standard payment adjustment rules for multiple procedures apply, 150% payment adjustment for bilateral procedures applies, assistant surgeon may not be paid

66984 **Cataract surg w/iol, 1 stage** ~ follow-up period is 90 days, standard payment adjustment rules for multiple procedures apply, 150% payment adjustment for bilateral procedures applies, assistant surgeon may not be paid

66985 **Insert lens prosthesis** ~ follow-up period is 90 days, standard payment adjustment rules for multiple procedures apply, 150% payment adjustment for bilateral procedures applies, assistant surgeon may not be paid

66986 **Exchange lens prosthesis** ~ follow-up period is 90 days, standard payment adjustment rules for multiple procedures apply, 150% payment adjustment for bilateral procedures applies, assistant surgeon may not be paid

66990 **Ophthalmic endoscope, add-on** ~ follow-up period included in another service, no payment adjustment rules for multiple procedures apply, 150% payment adjustment for bilateral procedures does not apply, assistant surgeon may not be paid, +add-on code (list separately in addition to primary procedure)

66999 **Eye surgery procedure** ~ medicare carrier determines global period, standard payment adjustment rules for multiple procedures apply, 150% payment adjustment for bilateral procedures applies, payment for assistant surgeon subject to documentation of medical necessity

Posterior Segment

67005 **Partial remove eye fluid** ~ follow-up period is 90 days, standard payment adjustment rules for multiple procedures apply, 150% payment adjustment for bilateral procedures applies, assistant surgeon may not be paid

67010 **Partial remove eye fluid** ~ follow-up period is 90 days, standard payment adjustment rules for multiple procedures apply, 150% payment adjustment for bilateral procedures applies, assistant surgeon may be paid

67015 **Release eye fluid** ~ follow-up period is 90 days, standard payment adjustment rules for multiple procedures apply, 150% payment adjustment for bilateral procedures applies, assistant surgeon may not be paid

67025 **Replace eye fluid** ~ follow-up period is 90 days, standard payment adjustment rules for multiple procedures apply, 150% payment adjustment for bilateral procedures applies, assistant surgeon may not be paid

67027 **Implant eye drug system** ~ follow-up period is 90 days, standard payment adjustment rules for multiple procedures apply, 150% payment adjustment for bilateral procedures applies, assistant surgeon may be paid

67028 **Inject eye drug** ~ endoscopies or minor procedure - E/M services on the same day generally not paid, standard payment adjustment rules for multiple

procedures apply, 150% payment adjustment for bilateral procedures applies, assistant surgeon may not be paid

67030   **Incise inner eye strands**   ~ follow-up period is 90 days, standard payment adjustment rules for multiple procedures apply, 150% payment adjustment for bilateral procedures applies, assistant surgeon may be paid

67031   **Laser surgery, eye strands**   ~ follow-up period is 90 days, standard payment adjustment rules for multiple procedures apply, 150% payment adjustment for bilateral procedures applies, assistant surgeon may not be paid

67036   **Remove inner eye fluid**   ~ follow-up period is 90 days, standard payment adjustment rules for multiple procedures apply, 150% payment adjustment for bilateral procedures applies, assistant surgeon may be paid

67038   **Strip retinal membrane**   ~ follow-up period is 90 days, standard payment adjustment rules for multiple procedures apply, 150% payment adjustment for bilateral procedures applies, assistant surgeon may be paid

67039   **Laser treat retina**   ~ follow-up period is 90 days, standard payment adjustment rules for multiple procedures apply, 150% payment adjustment for bilateral procedures applies, assistant surgeon may be paid

67040   **Laser treat retina**   ~ follow-up period is 90 days, standard payment adjustment rules for multiple procedures apply, 150% payment adjustment for bilateral procedures applies, assistant surgeon may be paid

67101   **Repair detached retina**   ~ follow-up period is 90 days, standard payment adjustment rules for multiple procedures apply, 150% payment adjustment for bilateral procedures applies, assistant surgeon may not be paid

67105   **Repair detached retina**   ~ follow-up period is 90 days, standard payment adjustment rules for multiple procedures apply, 150% payment adjustment for bilateral procedures applies, assistant surgeon may not be paid

67107   **Repair detached retina**   ~ follow-up period is 90 days, standard payment adjustment rules for multiple procedures apply, 150% payment adjustment for bilateral procedures applies, assistant surgeon may be paid

67108   **Repair detached retina**   ~ follow-up period is 90 days, standard payment adjustment rules for multiple procedures apply, 150% payment adjustment for bilateral procedures applies, assistant surgeon may be paid

67110   **Repair detached retina**   ~ follow-up period is 90 days, standard payment adjustment rules for multiple procedures apply, 150% payment adjustment for bilateral procedures applies, assistant surgeon may not be paid

67112 **Rerepair detached retina** ~ follow-up period is 90 days, standard payment adjustment rules for multiple procedures apply, 150% payment adjustment for bilateral procedures applies, assistant surgeon may be paid

67115 **Release encircling material** ~ follow-up period is 90 days, standard payment adjustment rules for multiple procedures apply, 150% payment adjustment for bilateral procedures applies, assistant surgeon may not be paid

67120 **Remove eye implant material** ~ follow-up period is 90 days, standard payment adjustment rules for multiple procedures apply, 150% payment adjustment for bilateral procedures applies, assistant surgeon may not be paid

67121 **Remove eye implant material** ~ follow-up period is 90 days, standard payment adjustment rules for multiple procedures apply, 150% payment adjustment for bilateral procedures applies, assistant surgeon may be paid

67141 **Treat retina** ~ follow-up period is 90 days, standard payment adjustment rules for multiple procedures apply, 150% payment adjustment for bilateral procedures applies, assistant surgeon may not be paid

67145 **Treat retina** ~ follow-up period is 90 days, standard payment adjustment rules for multiple procedures apply, 150% payment adjustment for bilateral procedures applies, assistant surgeon may not be paid

67208 **Treat retinal lesion** ~ follow-up period is 90 days, standard payment adjustment rules for multiple procedures apply, 150% payment adjustment for bilateral procedures applies, assistant surgeon may not be paid

67210 **Treat retinal lesion** ~ follow-up period is 90 days, standard payment adjustment rules for multiple procedures apply, 150% payment adjustment for bilateral procedures applies, assistant surgeon may not be paid

67218 **Treat retinal lesion** ~ follow-up period is 90 days, standard payment adjustment rules for multiple procedures apply, 150% payment adjustment for bilateral procedures applies, assistant surgeon may not be paid

67220 **Treat choroid lesion** ~ follow-up period is 90 days, standard payment adjustment rules for multiple procedures apply, 150% payment adjustment for bilateral procedures applies, assistant surgeon may not be paid

67221 **Ocular photodynamic therapeutic** ~ restricted coverage - special coverage rules apply, endoscopies or minor procedure - E/M services on the same day generally not paid, standard payment adjustment rules for multiple procedures apply, 150% payment adjustment for bilateral procedures does not apply, assistant surgeon may not be paid

67225 **Eye photodynamic therapeutic, add-on** ~ follow-up period included in another service, no payment adjustment rules for multiple procedures apply, 150% payment adjustment for

---

bilateral procedures does not apply, assistant surgeon may not be paid, +add-on code (list separately in addition to primary procedure)

67227 **Treat retinal lesion** ~ follow-up period is 90 days, standard payment adjustment rules for multiple procedures apply, 150% payment adjustment for bilateral procedures applies, assistant surgeon may not be paid

67228 **Treat retinal lesion** ~ follow-up period is 90 days, standard payment adjustment rules for multiple procedures apply, 150% payment adjustment for bilateral procedures applies, assistant surgeon may not be paid

67250 **Reinforce eye wall** ~ follow-up period is 90 days, standard payment adjustment rules for multiple procedures apply, 150% payment adjustment for bilateral procedures applies, assistant surgeon may not be paid

67255 **Reinforce/graft eye wall** ~ follow-up period is 90 days, standard payment adjustment rules for multiple procedures apply, 150% payment adjustment for bilateral procedures applies, assistant surgeon may be paid

67299 **Eye surgery procedure** ~ medicare carrier determines global period, standard payment adjustment rules for multiple procedures apply, 150% payment adjustment for bilateral procedures applies, payment for assistant surgeon subject to documentation of medical necessity

Ocular Adnexa

67311 **Revise eye muscle** ~ follow-up period is 90 days, standard payment adjustment rules for multiple procedures apply, 150% payment adjustment for bilateral procedures applies, assistant surgeon may not be paid

67312 **Revise two eye muscles** ~ follow-up period is 90 days, standard payment adjustment rules for multiple procedures apply, 150% payment adjustment for bilateral procedures applies, assistant surgeon may not be paid

67314 **Revise eye muscle** ~ follow-up period is 90 days, standard payment adjustment rules for multiple procedures apply, 150% payment adjustment for bilateral procedures applies, assistant surgeon may not be paid

67316 **Revise two eye muscles** ~ follow-up period is 90 days, standard payment adjustment rules for multiple procedures apply, 150% payment adjustment for bilateral procedures applies, payment for assistant surgeon subject to documentation of medical necessity

67318 **Revise eye muscle(s)** ~ follow-up period is 90 days, standard payment adjustment rules for multiple procedures apply, 150% payment adjustment for bilateral procedures applies, assistant surgeon may not be paid

67320   **Revise eye muscle(s), add-on**   ~ follow-up period included in another service, no payment adjustment rules for multiple procedures apply, 150% payment adjustment for bilateral procedures does not apply, assistant surgeon may not be paid, +add-on code (list separately in addition to primary procedure)

67331   **Eye surgery follow-up, add-on**   ~ follow-up period included in another service, no payment adjustment rules for multiple procedures apply, 150% payment adjustment for bilateral procedures does not apply, assistant surgeon may not be paid, +add-on code (list separately in addition to primary procedure)

67332   **Rerevise eye muscles, add-on**   ~ follow-up period included in another service, no payment adjustment rules for multiple procedures apply, 150% payment adjustment for bilateral procedures does not apply, assistant surgeon may be paid, +add-on code (list separately in addition to primary procedure)

67334   **Revise eye muscle w/suture**   ~ follow-up period included in another service, no payment adjustment rules for multiple procedures apply, 150% payment adjustment for bilateral procedures does not apply, assistant surgeon may not be paid

67335   **Eye suture during surgery**   ~ follow-up period included in another service, no payment adjustment rules for multiple procedures apply, 150% payment adjustment for bilateral procedures does not apply, assistant surgeon may not be paid

67340   **Revise eye muscle, add-on**   ~ follow-up period included in another service, no payment adjustment rules for multiple procedures apply, 150% payment adjustment for bilateral procedures does not apply, assistant surgeon may be paid, +add-on code (list separately in addition to primary procedure)

67343   **Release eye tissue**   ~ follow-up period is 90 days, standard payment adjustment rules for multiple procedures apply, 150% payment adjustment for bilateral procedures applies, assistant surgeon may be paid

67345   **Destroy nerve of eye muscle**   ~ follow-up period is 10 days, standard payment adjustment rules for multiple procedures apply, 150% payment adjustment for bilateral procedures applies, assistant surgeon may not be paid

67346   **Biopsy eye muscle**   ~ endoscopies or minor procedure - E/M services on the same day generally not paid, standard payment adjustment rules for multiple procedures apply, 150% payment adjustment for bilateral procedures applies, payment for assistant surgeon subject to documentation of medical necessity

67399   **Eye muscle surgery procedure**   ~ medicare carrier determines global period, standard payment adjustment rules for multiple procedures apply, 150% payment adjustment for bilateral procedures applies, assistant surgeon may be paid

67400   **Explore/biopsy eye socket**   ~ follow-up period is 90 days, standard payment adjustment rules for multiple procedures apply, 150% payment adjustment for bilateral procedures applies, assistant surgeon may be paid

67405   **Explore/drain eye socket**   ~ follow-up period is 90 days, standard payment adjustment rules for multiple procedures apply, 150% payment adjustment for bilateral procedures applies, assistant surgeon may be paid

67412   **Explore/treat eye socket**   ~ follow-up period is 90 days, standard payment adjustment rules for multiple procedures apply, 150% payment adjustment for bilateral procedures applies, assistant surgeon may be paid

67413   **Explore/treat eye socket**   ~ follow-up period is 90 days, standard payment adjustment rules for multiple procedures apply, 150% payment adjustment for bilateral procedures applies, assistant surgeon may be paid

67414   **Explore/decompress eye socket**   ~ follow-up period is 90 days, standard payment adjustment rules for multiple procedures apply, 150% payment adjustment for bilateral procedures applies, assistant surgeon may be paid

67415   **Aspiration, orbital contents**   ~ endoscopies or minor procedure - E/M services on the same day generally not paid, standard payment adjustment rules for multiple procedures apply, 150% payment adjustment for bilateral procedures applies, payment for assistant surgeon subject to documentation of medical necessity

67420   **Explore/treat eye socket**   ~ follow-up period is 90 days, standard payment adjustment rules for multiple procedures apply, 150% payment adjustment for bilateral procedures applies, assistant surgeon may be paid

67430   **Explore/treat eye socket**   ~ follow-up period is 90 days, standard payment adjustment rules for multiple procedures apply, 150% payment adjustment for bilateral procedures applies, assistant surgeon may be paid

67440   **Explore/drain eye socket**   ~ follow-up period is 90 days, standard payment adjustment rules for multiple procedures apply, 150% payment adjustment for bilateral procedures applies, assistant surgeon may be paid

67445   **Explore/decompress eye socket**   ~ follow-up period is 90 days, standard payment adjustment rules for multiple procedures apply, 150% payment adjustment for bilateral procedures applies, assistant surgeon may be paid

67450   **Explore/biopsy eye socket**   ~ follow-up period is 90 days, standard payment adjustment rules for multiple procedures apply, 150% payment adjustment for bilateral procedures applies, assistant surgeon may be paid

67500   **Inject/treat eye socket**   ~ endoscopies or minor procedure - E/M services on the same day generally not paid, standard payment adjustment rules for multiple

procedures apply, 150% payment adjustment for bilateral procedures applies, assistant surgeon may not be paid

67505   **Inject/treat eye socket**   ~ endoscopies or minor procedure - E/M services on the same day generally not paid, standard payment adjustment rules for multiple procedures apply, 150% payment adjustment for bilateral procedures applies, assistant surgeon may not be paid

67515   **Inject/treat eye socket**   ~ endoscopies or minor procedure - E/M services on the same day generally not paid, standard payment adjustment rules for multiple procedures apply, 150% payment adjustment for bilateral procedures applies, assistant surgeon may not be paid

67550   **Insert eye socket implant**   ~ follow-up period is 90 days, standard payment adjustment rules for multiple procedures apply, 150% payment adjustment for bilateral procedures applies, assistant surgeon may not be paid

67560   **Revise eye socket implant**   ~ follow-up period is 90 days, standard payment adjustment rules for multiple procedures apply, 150% payment adjustment for bilateral procedures applies, payment for assistant surgeon subject to documentation of medical necessity

67570   **Decompress optic nerve**   ~ follow-up period is 90 days, standard payment adjustment rules for multiple procedures apply, 150% payment adjustment for bilateral procedures applies, assistant surgeon may be paid

67599   **Orbit surgery procedure**   ~ medicare carrier determines global period, standard payment adjustment rules for multiple procedures apply, 150% payment adjustment for bilateral procedures applies, assistant surgeon may be paid

67700   **Drain eyelid abscess**   ~ follow-up period is 10 days, standard payment adjustment rules for multiple procedures apply, 150% payment adjustment for bilateral procedures applies, assistant surgeon may not be paid

67710   **Incise eyelid**   ~ follow-up period is 10 days, standard payment adjustment rules for multiple procedures apply, 150% payment adjustment for bilateral procedures applies, assistant surgeon may not be paid

67715   **Incise eyelid fold**   ~ follow-up period is 10 days, standard payment adjustment rules for multiple procedures apply, 150% payment adjustment for bilateral procedures applies, assistant surgeon may not be paid

67800   **Remove eyelid lesion**   ~ follow-up period is 10 days, standard payment adjustment rules for multiple procedures apply, 150% payment adjustment for bilateral procedures does not apply, assistant surgeon may not be paid

---

67801   **Remove eyelid lesions**   ~ follow-up period is 10 days, standard payment adjustment rules for multiple procedures apply, 150% payment adjustment for bilateral procedures does not apply, assistant surgeon may not be paid

67805   **Remove eyelid lesions**   ~ follow-up period is 10 days, standard payment adjustment rules for multiple procedures apply, 150% payment adjustment for bilateral procedures does not apply, assistant surgeon may not be paid

67808   **Remove eyelid lesion(s)**   ~ follow-up period is 90 days, standard payment adjustment rules for multiple procedures apply, 150% payment adjustment for bilateral procedures does not apply, assistant surgeon may not be paid

67810   **Biopsy eyelid**   ~ endoscopies or minor procedure - E/M services on the same day generally not paid, standard payment adjustment rules for multiple procedures apply, 150% payment adjustment for bilateral procedures applies, assistant surgeon may not be paid

67820   **Revise eyelashes**   ~ endoscopies or minor procedure - E/M services on the same day generally not paid, standard payment adjustment rules for multiple procedures apply, 150% payment adjustment for bilateral procedures applies, assistant surgeon may not be paid

67825   **Revise eyelashes**   ~ follow-up period is 10 days, standard payment adjustment rules for multiple procedures apply, 150% payment adjustment for bilateral procedures applies, assistant surgeon may not be paid

67830   **Revise eyelashes**   ~ follow-up period is 10 days, standard payment adjustment rules for multiple procedures apply, 150% payment adjustment for bilateral procedures applies, assistant surgeon may not be paid

67835   **Revise eyelashes**   ~ follow-up period is 90 days, standard payment adjustment rules for multiple procedures apply, 150% payment adjustment for bilateral procedures applies, payment for assistant surgeon subject to documentation of medical necessity

67840   **Remove eyelid lesion**   ~ follow-up period is 10 days, standard payment adjustment rules for multiple procedures apply, 150% payment adjustment for bilateral procedures applies, assistant surgeon may not be paid

67850   **Treat eyelid lesion**   ~ follow-up period is 10 days, standard payment adjustment rules for multiple procedures apply, 150% payment adjustment for bilateral procedures applies, assistant surgeon may not be paid

67875   **Closure eyelid by suture**   ~ endoscopies or minor procedure - E/M services on the same day generally not paid, standard payment adjustment rules for multiple procedures apply, 150% payment adjustment for bilateral procedures applies, assistant surgeon may not be paid

67880 **Revise eyelid** ~ follow-up period is 90 days, standard payment adjustment rules for multiple procedures apply, 150% payment adjustment for bilateral procedures applies, assistant surgeon may not be paid

67882 **Revise eyelid** ~ follow-up period is 90 days, standard payment adjustment rules for multiple procedures apply, 150% payment adjustment for bilateral procedures applies, assistant surgeon may not be paid

67900 **Repair brow defect** ~ follow-up period is 90 days, standard payment adjustment rules for multiple procedures apply, 150% payment adjustment for bilateral procedures applies, assistant surgeon may not be paid

67901 **Repair eyelid defect** ~ follow-up period is 90 days, standard payment adjustment rules for multiple procedures apply, 150% payment adjustment for bilateral procedures applies, assistant surgeon may not be paid

67902 **Repair eyelid defect** ~ follow-up period is 90 days, standard payment adjustment rules for multiple procedures apply, 150% payment adjustment for bilateral procedures applies, assistant surgeon may not be paid

67903 **Repair eyelid defect** ~ follow-up period is 90 days, standard payment adjustment rules for multiple procedures apply, 150% payment adjustment for bilateral procedures applies, assistant surgeon may not be paid

67904 **Repair eyelid defect** ~ follow-up period is 90 days, standard payment adjustment rules for multiple procedures apply, 150% payment adjustment for bilateral procedures applies, assistant surgeon may not be paid

67906 **Repair eyelid defect** ~ follow-up period is 90 days, standard payment adjustment rules for multiple procedures apply, 150% payment adjustment for bilateral procedures applies, assistant surgeon may not be paid

67908 **Repair eyelid defect** ~ follow-up period is 90 days, standard payment adjustment rules for multiple procedures apply, 150% payment adjustment for bilateral procedures applies, assistant surgeon may not be paid

67909 **Revise eyelid defect** ~ follow-up period is 90 days, standard payment adjustment rules for multiple procedures apply, 150% payment adjustment for bilateral procedures applies, assistant surgeon may not be paid

67911 **Revise eyelid defect** ~ follow-up period is 90 days, standard payment adjustment rules for multiple procedures apply, 150% payment adjustment for bilateral procedures applies, assistant surgeon may not be paid

67912 **Correct eyelid w/implant** ~ follow-up period is 90 days, standard payment adjustment rules for multiple procedures apply, 150% payment adjustment for bilateral procedures applies, assistant surgeon may not be paid

67914   **Repair eyelid defect**   ~ follow-up period is 90 days, standard payment adjustment rules for multiple procedures apply, 150% payment adjustment for bilateral procedures applies, assistant surgeon may not be paid

67915   **Repair eyelid defect**   ~ follow-up period is 90 days, standard payment adjustment rules for multiple procedures apply, 150% payment adjustment for bilateral procedures applies, assistant surgeon may not be paid

67916   **Repair eyelid defect**   ~ follow-up period is 90 days, standard payment adjustment rules for multiple procedures apply, 150% payment adjustment for bilateral procedures applies, assistant surgeon may not be paid

67917   **Repair eyelid defect**   ~ follow-up period is 90 days, standard payment adjustment rules for multiple procedures apply, 150% payment adjustment for bilateral procedures applies, assistant surgeon may not be paid

67921   **Repair eyelid defect**   ~ follow-up period is 90 days, standard payment adjustment rules for multiple procedures apply, 150% payment adjustment for bilateral procedures applies, assistant surgeon may not be paid

67922   **Repair eyelid defect**   ~ follow-up period is 90 days, standard payment adjustment rules for multiple procedures apply, 150% payment adjustment for bilateral procedures applies, assistant surgeon may not be paid

67923   **Repair eyelid defect**   ~ follow-up period is 90 days, standard payment adjustment rules for multiple procedures apply, 150% payment adjustment for bilateral procedures applies, assistant surgeon may not be paid

67924   **Repair eyelid defect**   ~ follow-up period is 90 days, standard payment adjustment rules for multiple procedures apply, 150% payment adjustment for bilateral procedures applies, assistant surgeon may not be paid

67930   **Repair eyelid wound**   ~ follow-up period is 10 days, standard payment adjustment rules for multiple procedures apply, 150% payment adjustment for bilateral procedures applies, assistant surgeon may not be paid

67935   **Repair eyelid wound**   ~ follow-up period is 90 days, standard payment adjustment rules for multiple procedures apply, 150% payment adjustment for bilateral procedures applies, assistant surgeon may not be paid

67938   **Remove eyelid foreign body**   ~ follow-up period is 10 days, standard payment adjustment rules for multiple procedures apply, 150% payment adjustment for bilateral procedures applies, assistant surgeon may not be paid

67950   **Revise eyelid**   ~ follow-up period is 90 days, standard payment adjustment rules for multiple procedures apply, 150% payment adjustment for bilateral procedures applies, assistant surgeon may not be paid

    CPT codes and descriptions only copyright American Medical Association

67961 **Revise eyelid**   ~ follow-up period is 90 days, standard payment adjustment rules for multiple procedures apply, 150% payment adjustment for bilateral procedures applies, payment for assistant surgeon subject to documentation of medical necessity

67966 **Revise eyelid**   ~ follow-up period is 90 days, standard payment adjustment rules for multiple procedures apply, 150% payment adjustment for bilateral procedures applies, assistant surgeon may not be paid

67971 **Reconstruct eyelid**   ~ follow-up period is 90 days, standard payment adjustment rules for multiple procedures apply, 150% payment adjustment for bilateral procedures applies, assistant surgeon may be paid

67973 **Reconstruct eyelid**   ~ follow-up period is 90 days, standard payment adjustment rules for multiple procedures apply, 150% payment adjustment for bilateral procedures applies, assistant surgeon may be paid

67974 **Reconstruct eyelid**   ~ follow-up period is 90 days, standard payment adjustment rules for multiple procedures apply, 150% payment adjustment for bilateral procedures applies, assistant surgeon may be paid

67975 **Reconstruct eyelid**   ~ follow-up period is 90 days, standard payment adjustment rules for multiple procedures apply, 150% payment adjustment for bilateral procedures applies, assistant surgeon may not be paid

67999 **Revise eyelid**   ~ medicare carrier determines global period, standard payment adjustment rules for multiple procedures apply, 150% payment adjustment for bilateral procedures applies, payment for assistant surgeon subject to documentation of medical necessity

Conjunctiva

68020 **Incise/drain eyelid lining**   ~ follow-up period is 10 days, standard payment adjustment rules for multiple procedures apply, 150% payment adjustment for bilateral procedures applies, assistant surgeon may not be paid

68040 **Treat eyelid lesions**   ~ endoscopies or minor procedure - E/M services on the same day generally not paid, standard payment adjustment rules for multiple procedures apply, 150% payment adjustment for bilateral procedures applies, assistant surgeon may not be paid

68100 **Biopsy eyelid lining**   ~ endoscopies or minor procedure - E/M services on the same day generally not paid, standard payment adjustment rules for multiple procedures apply, 150% payment adjustment for bilateral procedures applies, assistant surgeon may not be paid

---

68110   **Remove eyelid lining lesion**   ~ follow-up period is 10 days, standard payment adjustment rules for multiple procedures apply, 150% payment adjustment for bilateral procedures applies, assistant surgeon may not be paid

68115   **Remove eyelid lining lesion**   ~ follow-up period is 10 days, standard payment adjustment rules for multiple procedures apply, 150% payment adjustment for bilateral procedures applies, assistant surgeon may not be paid

68130   **Remove eyelid lining lesion**   ~ follow-up period is 90 days, standard payment adjustment rules for multiple procedures apply, 150% payment adjustment for bilateral procedures applies, assistant surgeon may not be paid

68135   **Remove eyelid lining lesion**   ~ follow-up period is 10 days, standard payment adjustment rules for multiple procedures apply, 150% payment adjustment for bilateral procedures applies, assistant surgeon may not be paid

68200   **Treat eyelid by injection**   ~ endoscopies or minor procedure - E/M services on the same day generally not paid, standard payment adjustment rules for multiple procedures apply, 150% payment adjustment for bilateral procedures applies, assistant surgeon may not be paid

68320   **Revise/graft eyelid lining**   ~ follow-up period is 90 days, standard payment adjustment rules for multiple procedures apply, 150% payment adjustment for bilateral procedures applies, assistant surgeon may not be paid

68325   **Revise/graft eyelid lining**   ~ follow-up period is 90 days, standard payment adjustment rules for multiple procedures apply, 150% payment adjustment for bilateral procedures applies, assistant surgeon may not be paid

68326   **Revise/graft eyelid lining**   ~ follow-up period is 90 days, standard payment adjustment rules for multiple procedures apply, 150% payment adjustment for bilateral procedures applies, assistant surgeon may not be paid

68328   **Revise/graft eyelid lining**   ~ follow-up period is 90 days, standard payment adjustment rules for multiple procedures apply, 150% payment adjustment for bilateral procedures applies, payment for assistant surgeon subject to documentation of medical necessity

68330   **Revise eyelid lining**   ~ follow-up period is 90 days, standard payment adjustment rules for multiple procedures apply, 150% payment adjustment for bilateral procedures applies, payment for assistant surgeon subject to documentation of medical necessity

68335   **Revise/graft eyelid lining**   ~ follow-up period is 90 days, standard payment adjustment rules for multiple procedures apply, 150% payment adjustment for bilateral procedures applies, assistant surgeon may not be paid

68340   **Separate eyelid adhesions**   ~ follow-up period is 90 days, standard payment adjustment rules for multiple procedures apply, 150% payment adjustment for bilateral procedures applies, payment for assistant surgeon subject to documentation of medical necessity

68360   **Revise eyelid lining**   ~ follow-up period is 90 days, standard payment adjustment rules for multiple procedures apply, 150% payment adjustment for bilateral procedures applies, assistant surgeon may not be paid

68362   **Revise eyelid lining**   ~ follow-up period is 90 days, standard payment adjustment rules for multiple procedures apply, 150% payment adjustment for bilateral procedures applies, assistant surgeon may not be paid

68371   **Harvest eye tissue, allograft**   ~ follow-up period is 10 days, standard payment adjustment rules for multiple procedures apply, 150% payment adjustment for bilateral procedures applies, assistant surgeon may not be paid

68399   **Eyelid lining surgery**   ~ medicare carrier determines global period, standard payment adjustment rules for multiple procedures apply, 150% payment adjustment for bilateral procedures applies, payment for assistant surgeon subject to documentation of medical necessity

68400   **Incise/drain tear gland**   ~ follow-up period is 10 days, standard payment adjustment rules for multiple procedures apply, 150% payment adjustment for bilateral procedures applies, assistant surgeon may not be paid

68420   **Incise/drain tear sac**   ~ follow-up period is 10 days, standard payment adjustment rules for multiple procedures apply, 150% payment adjustment for bilateral procedures applies, assistant surgeon may not be paid

68440   **Incise tear duct opening**   ~ follow-up period is 10 days, standard payment adjustment rules for multiple procedures apply, 150% payment adjustment for bilateral procedures applies, assistant surgeon may not be paid

68500   **Remove tear gland**   ~ follow-up period is 90 days, standard payment adjustment rules for multiple procedures apply, 150% payment adjustment for bilateral procedures applies, assistant surgeon may not be paid

68505   **Partial remove tear gland**   ~ follow-up period is 90 days, standard payment adjustment rules for multiple procedures apply, 150% payment adjustment for bilateral procedures applies, assistant surgeon may not be paid

68510   **Biopsy tear gland**   ~ endoscopies or minor procedure - E/M services on the same day generally not paid, standard payment adjustment rules for multiple procedures apply, 150% payment adjustment for bilateral procedures applies, payment for assistant surgeon subject to documentation of medical necessity

68520   **Remove tear sac**   ~ follow-up period is 90 days, standard payment adjustment rules for multiple procedures apply, 150% payment adjustment for bilateral procedures applies, payment for assistant surgeon subject to documentation of medical necessity

68525   **Biopsy tear sac**   ~ endoscopies or minor procedure - E/M services on the same day generally not paid, standard payment adjustment rules for multiple procedures apply, 150% payment adjustment for bilateral procedures applies, assistant surgeon may not be paid

68530   **Clear tear duct**   ~ follow-up period is 10 days, standard payment adjustment rules for multiple procedures apply, 150% payment adjustment for bilateral procedures applies, assistant surgeon may not be paid

68540   **Remove tear gland lesion**   ~ follow-up period is 90 days, standard payment adjustment rules for multiple procedures apply, 150% payment adjustment for bilateral procedures applies, assistant surgeon may not be paid

68550   **Remove tear gland lesion**   ~ follow-up period is 90 days, standard payment adjustment rules for multiple procedures apply, 150% payment adjustment for bilateral procedures applies, assistant surgeon may not be paid

68700   **Repair tear ducts**   ~ follow-up period is 90 days, standard payment adjustment rules for multiple procedures apply, 150% payment adjustment for bilateral procedures applies, assistant surgeon may not be paid

68705   **Revise tear duct opening**   ~ follow-up period is 10 days, standard payment adjustment rules for multiple procedures apply, 150% payment adjustment for bilateral procedures applies, assistant surgeon may not be paid

68720   **Create tear sac drain**   ~ follow-up period is 90 days, standard payment adjustment rules for multiple procedures apply, 150% payment adjustment for bilateral procedures applies, assistant surgeon may be paid

68745   **Create tear duct drain**   ~ follow-up period is 90 days, standard payment adjustment rules for multiple procedures apply, 150% payment adjustment for bilateral procedures applies, assistant surgeon may be paid

68750   **Create tear duct drain**   ~ follow-up period is 90 days, standard payment adjustment rules for multiple procedures apply, 150% payment adjustment for bilateral procedures applies, assistant surgeon may be paid

68760   **Close tear duct opening**   ~ follow-up period is 10 days, standard payment adjustment rules for multiple procedures apply, 150% payment adjustment for bilateral procedures applies, assistant surgeon may not be paid

68761   **Close tear duct opening**   ~ follow-up period is 10 days, standard payment adjustment rules for multiple procedures apply, 150% payment adjustment for bilateral procedures applies, payment for assistant surgeon subject to documentation of medical necessity

68770   **Close tear system fistula**   ~ follow-up period is 90 days, standard payment adjustment rules for multiple procedures apply, 150% payment adjustment for bilateral procedures applies, payment for assistant surgeon subject to documentation of medical necessity

68801   **Dilate tear duct opening**   ~ follow-up period is 10 days, standard payment adjustment rules for multiple procedures apply, 150% payment adjustment for bilateral procedures applies, assistant surgeon may not be paid

68810   **Probe nasolacrimal duct**   ~ follow-up period is 10 days, standard payment adjustment rules for multiple procedures apply, 150% payment adjustment for bilateral procedures applies, assistant surgeon may not be paid

68811   **Probe nasolacrimal duct**   ~ follow-up period is 10 days, standard payment adjustment rules for multiple procedures apply, 150% payment adjustment for bilateral procedures applies, assistant surgeon may not be paid

68815   **Probe nasolacrimal duct**   ~ follow-up period is 10 days, standard payment adjustment rules for multiple procedures apply, 150% payment adjustment for bilateral procedures applies, assistant surgeon may not be paid

68840   **Explore/irrigate tear ducts**   ~ follow-up period is 10 days, standard payment adjustment rules for multiple procedures apply, 150% payment adjustment for bilateral procedures applies, assistant surgeon may not be paid

68850   **Inject for tear sac x-ray**   ~ endoscopies or minor procedure - E/M services on the same day generally not paid, standard payment adjustment rules for multiple procedures apply, 150% payment adjustment for bilateral procedures applies, assistant surgeon may not be paid

68899   **Tear duct system surgery**   ~ medicare carrier determines global period, standard payment adjustment rules for multiple procedures apply, 150% payment adjustment for bilateral procedures applies, payment for assistant surgeon subject to documentation of medical necessity

AUDITORY SYSTEM

External Ear

69000 **Drain external ear lesion** ~ follow-up period is 10 days, standard payment adjustment rules for multiple procedures apply, 150% payment adjustment for bilateral procedures does not apply, assistant surgeon may not be paid

69005 **Drain external ear lesion** ~ follow-up period is 10 days, standard payment adjustment rules for multiple procedures apply, 150% payment adjustment for bilateral procedures does not apply, assistant surgeon may not be paid

69020 **Drain outer ear canal lesion** ~ follow-up period is 10 days, standard payment adjustment rules for multiple procedures apply, 150% payment adjustment for bilateral procedures does not apply, assistant surgeon may not be paid

69090 **Pierce earlobes** non-covered service, multiple procedure concept does not apply, bilateral surgery concept does not apply, assistant surgery concept does not apply

69100 **Biopsy external ear** ~ endoscopies or minor procedure - E/M services on the same day generally not paid, standard payment adjustment rules for multiple procedures apply, 150% payment adjustment for bilateral procedures does not apply, assistant surgeon may not be paid

69105 **Biopsy external ear canal** ~ endoscopies or minor procedure - E/M services on the same day generally not paid, standard payment adjustment rules for multiple procedures apply, 150% payment adjustment for bilateral procedures does not apply, assistant surgeon may not be paid

69110 **Remove external ear, partial** ~ follow-up period is 90 days, standard payment adjustment rules for multiple procedures apply, 150% payment adjustment for bilateral procedures does not apply, assistant surgeon may not be paid

69120 **Remove external ear** ~ follow-up period is 90 days, standard payment adjustment rules for multiple procedures apply, 150% payment adjustment for bilateral procedures does not apply, assistant surgeon may not be paid

69140 **Remove ear canal lesion(s)** ~ follow-up period is 90 days, standard payment adjustment rules for multiple procedures apply, 150% payment adjustment for bilateral procedures does not apply, payment for assistant surgeon subject to documentation of medical necessity

69145 **Remove ear canal lesion(s)** ~ follow-up period is 90 days, standard payment adjustment rules for multiple procedures apply, 150% payment adjustment for bilateral procedures does not apply, assistant surgeon may not be paid

69150   **Extensive ear canal surgery**   ~ follow-up period is 90 days, standard payment adjustment rules for multiple procedures apply, 150% payment adjustment for bilateral procedures does not apply, assistant surgeon may not be paid

69155   **Extensive ear/neck surgery**   ~ follow-up period is 90 days, standard payment adjustment rules for multiple procedures apply, 150% payment adjustment for bilateral procedures does not apply, assistant surgeon may be paid

69200   **Clear outer ear canal**   ~ endoscopies or minor procedure - E/M services on the same day generally not paid, standard payment adjustment rules for multiple procedures apply, 150% payment adjustment for bilateral procedures does not apply, assistant surgeon may not be paid

69205   **Clear outer ear canal**   ~ follow-up period is 10 days, standard payment adjustment rules for multiple procedures apply, 150% payment adjustment for bilateral procedures does not apply, assistant surgeon may not be paid

69210   **Remove impacted ear wax**   ~ endoscopies or minor procedure - E/M services on the same day generally not paid, standard payment adjustment rules for multiple procedures apply, 150% payment adjustment does not apply - RVUs based on bilateral procedure, assistant surgeon may not be paid

69220   **Clean out mastoid cavity**   ~ endoscopies or minor procedure - E/M services on the same day generally not paid, standard payment adjustment rules for multiple procedures apply, 150% payment adjustment for bilateral procedures applies, assistant surgeon may not be paid

69222   **Clean out mastoid cavity**   ~ follow-up period is 10 days, standard payment adjustment rules for multiple procedures apply, 150% payment adjustment for bilateral procedures applies, assistant surgeon may not be paid

69300   **Revise external ear**   ~ restricted coverage @~ medicare carrier determines global period, standard payment adjustment rules for multiple procedures apply, 150% payment adjustment for bilateral procedures applies, payment for assistant surgeon subject to documentation of medical necessity

69310   **Rebuild outer ear canal**   ~ follow-up period is 90 days, standard payment adjustment rules for multiple procedures apply, 150% payment adjustment for bilateral procedures does not apply, assistant surgeon may not be paid

69320   **Rebuild outer ear canal**   ~ follow-up period is 90 days, standard payment adjustment rules for multiple procedures apply, 150% payment adjustment for bilateral procedures does not apply, assistant surgeon may be paid

69399   **Outer ear surgery procedure**   ~ medicare carrier determines global period, standard payment adjustment rules for multiple procedures apply, 150% payment

adjustment for bilateral procedures does not apply, payment for assistant surgeon subject to documentation of medical necessity

Middle Ear

69400   **Inflate middle ear canal**   ~ endoscopies or minor procedure - E/M services on the same day generally not paid, standard payment adjustment rules for multiple procedures apply, 150% payment adjustment for bilateral procedures does not apply, assistant surgeon may not be paid

69401   **Inflate middle ear canal**   ~ endoscopies or minor procedure - E/M services on the same day generally not paid, standard payment adjustment rules for multiple procedures apply, 150% payment adjustment for bilateral procedures does not apply, assistant surgeon may not be paid

69405   **Catheterize middle ear canal**   ~ follow-up period is 10 days, standard payment adjustment rules for multiple procedures apply, 150% payment adjustment for bilateral procedures does not apply, payment for assistant surgeon subject to documentation of medical necessity

69420   **Incise eardrum**   ~ follow-up period is 10 days, standard payment adjustment rules for multiple procedures apply, 150% payment adjustment for bilateral procedures applies, assistant surgeon may not be paid

69421   **Incise eardrum**   ~ follow-up period is 10 days, standard payment adjustment rules for multiple procedures apply, 150% payment adjustment for bilateral procedures applies, assistant surgeon may not be paid

69424   **Remove ventilating tube**   ~ endoscopies or minor procedure - E/M services on the same day generally not paid, standard payment adjustment rules for multiple procedures apply, 150% payment adjustment for bilateral procedures applies, assistant surgeon may not be paid

69433   **Create eardrum opening**   ~ follow-up period is 10 days, standard payment adjustment rules for multiple procedures apply, 150% payment adjustment for bilateral procedures applies, assistant surgeon may not be paid

69436   **Create eardrum opening**   ~ follow-up period is 10 days, standard payment adjustment rules for multiple procedures apply, 150% payment adjustment for bilateral procedures applies, assistant surgeon may not be paid

69440   **Explore middle ear**   ~ follow-up period is 90 days, standard payment adjustment rules for multiple procedures apply, 150% payment adjustment for bilateral procedures applies, assistant surgeon may not be paid

69450   **Eardrum revision**   ~ follow-up period is 90 days, standard payment adjustment rules for multiple procedures apply, 150% payment adjustment for

bilateral procedures applies, payment for assistant surgeon subject to documentation of medical necessity

69501   **Mastoidectomy**   ~ follow-up period is 90 days, standard payment adjustment rules for multiple procedures apply, 150% payment adjustment for bilateral procedures applies, assistant surgeon may not be paid

69502   **Mastoidectomy**   ~ follow-up period is 90 days, standard payment adjustment rules for multiple procedures apply, 150% payment adjustment for bilateral procedures applies, payment for assistant surgeon subject to documentation of medical necessity

69505   **Remove mastoid structures**   ~ follow-up period is 90 days, standard payment adjustment rules for multiple procedures apply, 150% payment adjustment for bilateral procedures applies, payment for assistant surgeon subject to documentation of medical necessity

69511   **Extensive mastoid surgery**   ~ follow-up period is 90 days, standard payment adjustment rules for multiple procedures apply, 150% payment adjustment for bilateral procedures applies, payment for assistant surgeon subject to documentation of medical necessity

69530   **Extensive mastoid surgery**   ~ follow-up period is 90 days, standard payment adjustment rules for multiple procedures apply, 150% payment adjustment for bilateral procedures applies, assistant surgeon may be paid

69535   **Remove part of temporal bone**   ~ follow-up period is 90 days, standard payment adjustment rules for multiple procedures apply, 150% payment adjustment for bilateral procedures applies, assistant surgeon may not be paid

69540   **Remove ear lesion**   ~ follow-up period is 10 days, standard payment adjustment rules for multiple procedures apply, 150% payment adjustment for bilateral procedures applies, assistant surgeon may not be paid

69550   **Remove ear lesion**   ~ follow-up period is 90 days, standard payment adjustment rules for multiple procedures apply, 150% payment adjustment for bilateral procedures applies, assistant surgeon may be paid

69552   **Remove ear lesion**   ~ follow-up period is 90 days, standard payment adjustment rules for multiple procedures apply, 150% payment adjustment for bilateral procedures applies, assistant surgeon may be paid

69554   **Remove ear lesion**   ~ follow-up period is 90 days, standard payment adjustment rules for multiple procedures apply, 150% payment adjustment for bilateral procedures applies, assistant surgeon may be paid

69601   **Mastoid surgery revision**   ~ follow-up period is 90 days, standard payment adjustment rules for multiple procedures apply, 150% payment adjustment for bilateral procedures applies, payment for assistant surgeon subject to documentation of medical necessity

69602   **Mastoid surgery revision**   ~ follow-up period is 90 days, standard payment adjustment rules for multiple procedures apply, 150% payment adjustment for bilateral procedures applies, payment for assistant surgeon subject to documentation of medical necessity

69603   **Mastoid surgery revision**   ~ follow-up period is 90 days, standard payment adjustment rules for multiple procedures apply, 150% payment adjustment for bilateral procedures applies, payment for assistant surgeon subject to documentation of medical necessity

69604   **Mastoid surgery revision**   ~ follow-up period is 90 days, standard payment adjustment rules for multiple procedures apply, 150% payment adjustment for bilateral procedures applies, assistant surgeon may not be paid

69605   **Mastoid surgery revision**   ~ follow-up period is 90 days, standard payment adjustment rules for multiple procedures apply, 150% payment adjustment for bilateral procedures applies, assistant surgeon may be paid

69610   **Repair eardrum**   ~ follow-up period is 10 days, standard payment adjustment rules for multiple procedures apply, 150% payment adjustment for bilateral procedures applies, assistant surgeon may not be paid

69620   **Repair eardrum**   ~ follow-up period is 90 days, standard payment adjustment rules for multiple procedures apply, 150% payment adjustment for bilateral procedures applies, assistant surgeon may not be paid

69631   **Repair eardrum structures**   ~ follow-up period is 90 days, standard payment adjustment rules for multiple procedures apply, 150% payment adjustment for bilateral procedures applies, assistant surgeon may not be paid

69632   **Rebuild eardrum structures**   ~ follow-up period is 90 days, standard payment adjustment rules for multiple procedures apply, 150% payment adjustment for bilateral procedures applies, assistant surgeon may not be paid

69633   **Rebuild eardrum structures**   ~ follow-up period is 90 days, standard payment adjustment rules for multiple procedures apply, 150% payment adjustment for bilateral procedures applies, assistant surgeon may not be paid

69635   **Repair eardrum structures**   ~ follow-up period is 90 days, standard payment adjustment rules for multiple procedures apply, 150% payment adjustment for bilateral procedures applies, assistant surgeon may not be paid

69636   **Rebuild eardrum structures**   ~ follow-up period is 90 days, standard payment adjustment rules for multiple procedures apply, 150% payment adjustment for bilateral procedures applies, payment for assistant surgeon subject to documentation of medical necessity

69637   **Rebuild eardrum structures**   ~ follow-up period is 90 days, standard payment adjustment rules for multiple procedures apply, 150% payment adjustment for bilateral procedures applies, payment for assistant surgeon subject to documentation of medical necessity

69641   **Revise middle ear & mastoid**   ~ follow-up period is 90 days, standard payment adjustment rules for multiple procedures apply, 150% payment adjustment for bilateral procedures applies, assistant surgeon may not be paid

69642   **Revise middle ear & mastoid**   ~ follow-up period is 90 days, standard payment adjustment rules for multiple procedures apply, 150% payment adjustment for bilateral procedures applies, assistant surgeon may not be paid

69643   **Revise middle ear & mastoid**   ~ follow-up period is 90 days, standard payment adjustment rules for multiple procedures apply, 150% payment adjustment for bilateral procedures applies, assistant surgeon may not be paid

69644   **Revise middle ear & mastoid**   ~ follow-up period is 90 days, standard payment adjustment rules for multiple procedures apply, 150% payment adjustment for bilateral procedures applies, assistant surgeon may not be paid

69645   **Revise middle ear & mastoid**   ~ follow-up period is 90 days, standard payment adjustment rules for multiple procedures apply, 150% payment adjustment for bilateral procedures applies, assistant surgeon may not be paid

69646   **Revise middle ear & mastoid**   ~ follow-up period is 90 days, standard payment adjustment rules for multiple procedures apply, 150% payment adjustment for bilateral procedures applies, payment for assistant surgeon subject to documentation of medical necessity

69650   **Release middle ear bone**   ~ follow-up period is 90 days, standard payment adjustment rules for multiple procedures apply, 150% payment adjustment for bilateral procedures applies, assistant surgeon may not be paid

69660   **Revise middle ear bone**   ~ follow-up period is 90 days, standard payment adjustment rules for multiple procedures apply, 150% payment adjustment for bilateral procedures applies, assistant surgeon may not be paid

69661   **Revise middle ear bone**   ~ follow-up period is 90 days, standard payment adjustment rules for multiple procedures apply, 150% payment adjustment for bilateral procedures applies, payment for assistant surgeon subject to documentation of medical necessity

69662   **Revise middle ear bone**   ~ follow-up period is 90 days, standard payment adjustment rules for multiple procedures apply, 150% payment adjustment for bilateral procedures applies, assistant surgeon may not be paid

69666   **Repair middle ear structures**   ~ follow-up period is 90 days, standard payment adjustment rules for multiple procedures apply, 150% payment adjustment for bilateral procedures applies, payment for assistant surgeon subject to documentation of medical necessity

69667   **Repair middle ear structures**   ~ follow-up period is 90 days, standard payment adjustment rules for multiple procedures apply, 150% payment adjustment for bilateral procedures applies, payment for assistant surgeon subject to documentation of medical necessity

69670   **Remove mastoid air cells**   ~ follow-up period is 90 days, standard payment adjustment rules for multiple procedures apply, 150% payment adjustment for bilateral procedures applies, assistant surgeon may be paid

69676   **Remove middle ear nerve**   ~ follow-up period is 90 days, standard payment adjustment rules for multiple procedures apply, 150% payment adjustment for bilateral procedures applies, assistant surgeon may not be paid

69700   **Close mastoid fistula**   ~ follow-up period is 90 days, standard payment adjustment rules for multiple procedures apply, 150% payment adjustment for bilateral procedures applies, assistant surgeon may not be paid

69710   **Implant/replace hearing aid**   non-covered service, multiple procedure concept does not apply, bilateral surgery concept does not apply, assistant surgery concept does not apply

69711   **Remove/repair hearing aid**   ~ follow-up period is 90 days, standard payment adjustment rules for multiple procedures apply, 150% payment adjustment for bilateral procedures applies, assistant surgeon may be paid

69714   **Implant temple bone w/stimuli**   ~ follow-up period is 90 days, standard payment adjustment rules for multiple procedures apply, 150% payment adjustment for bilateral procedures applies, assistant surgeon may not be paid

69715   **Temple bone implant w/stimulate**   ~ follow-up period is 90 days, standard payment adjustment rules for multiple procedures apply, 150% payment adjustment for bilateral procedures applies, assistant surgeon may not be paid

69717   **Temple bone implant revision**   ~ follow-up period is 90 days, standard payment adjustment rules for multiple procedures apply, 150% payment adjustment for bilateral procedures applies, assistant surgeon may not be paid

69718   **Revise temple bone implant**   ~ follow-up period is 90 days, standard payment adjustment rules for multiple procedures apply, 150% payment adjustment for bilateral procedures applies, assistant surgeon may not be paid

69720   **Release facial nerve**   ~ follow-up period is 90 days, standard payment adjustment rules for multiple procedures apply, 150% payment adjustment for bilateral procedures applies, payment for assistant surgeon subject to documentation of medical necessity

69725   **Release facial nerve**   ~ follow-up period is 90 days, standard payment adjustment rules for multiple procedures apply, 150% payment adjustment for bilateral procedures applies, assistant surgeon may be paid

69740   **Repair facial nerve**   ~ follow-up period is 90 days, standard payment adjustment rules for multiple procedures apply, 150% payment adjustment for bilateral procedures applies, assistant surgeon may be paid

69745   **Repair facial nerve**   ~ follow-up period is 90 days, standard payment adjustment rules for multiple procedures apply, 150% payment adjustment for bilateral procedures applies, assistant surgeon may be paid

69799   **Middle ear surgery procedure**   ~ medicare carrier determines global period, standard payment adjustment rules for multiple procedures apply, 150% payment adjustment for bilateral procedures applies, payment for assistant surgeon subject to documentation of medical necessity

Inner Ear

69801   **Incise inner ear**   ~ follow-up period is 90 days, standard payment adjustment rules for multiple procedures apply, 150% payment adjustment for bilateral procedures applies, payment for assistant surgeon subject to documentation of medical necessity

69802   **Incise inner ear**   ~ follow-up period is 90 days, standard payment adjustment rules for multiple procedures apply, 150% payment adjustment for bilateral procedures applies, assistant surgeon may be paid

69805   **Explore inner ear**   ~ follow-up period is 90 days, standard payment adjustment rules for multiple procedures apply, 150% payment adjustment for bilateral procedures applies, assistant surgeon may be paid

69806   **Explore inner ear**   ~ follow-up period is 90 days, standard payment adjustment rules for multiple procedures apply, 150% payment adjustment for bilateral procedures applies, assistant surgeon may not be paid

69820   **Establish inner ear window**   ~ follow-up period is 90 days, standard payment adjustment rules for multiple procedures apply, 150% payment adjustment for bilateral procedures applies, assistant surgeon may be paid

69840   **Revise inner ear window**   ~ follow-up period is 90 days, standard payment adjustment rules for multiple procedures apply, 150% payment adjustment for bilateral procedures applies, assistant surgeon may be paid

69905   **Remove inner ear**   ~ follow-up period is 90 days, standard payment adjustment rules for multiple procedures apply, 150% payment adjustment for bilateral procedures applies, assistant surgeon may not be paid

69910   **Remove inner ear & mastoid**   ~ follow-up period is 90 days, standard payment adjustment rules for multiple procedures apply, 150% payment adjustment for bilateral procedures applies, payment for assistant surgeon subject to documentation of medical necessity

69915   **Incise inner ear nerve**   ~ follow-up period is 90 days, standard payment adjustment rules for multiple procedures apply, 150% payment adjustment for bilateral procedures applies, assistant surgeon may be paid

69930   **Implant cochlear device**   ~ follow-up period is 90 days, standard payment adjustment rules for multiple procedures apply, 150% payment adjustment for bilateral procedures applies, payment for assistant surgeon subject to documentation of medical necessity

69949   **Inner ear surgery procedure**   ~ medicare carrier determines global period, standard payment adjustment rules for multiple procedures apply, 150% payment adjustment for bilateral procedures applies, payment for assistant surgeon subject to documentation of medical necessity

Temporal Bone, Middle Fossa Approach

69950   **Incise inner ear nerve**   ~ follow-up period is 90 days, standard payment adjustment rules for multiple procedures apply, 150% payment adjustment for bilateral procedures applies, assistant surgeon may be paid

69955   **Release facial nerve**   ~ follow-up period is 90 days, standard payment adjustment rules for multiple procedures apply, 150% payment adjustment for bilateral procedures applies, assistant surgeon may be paid

69960   **Release inner ear canal**   ~ follow-up period is 90 days, standard payment adjustment rules for multiple procedures apply, 150% payment adjustment for bilateral procedures applies, assistant surgeon may be paid

69970   **Remove inner ear lesion** ~ follow-up period is 90 days, standard payment adjustment rules for multiple procedures apply, 150% payment adjustment for bilateral procedures applies, assistant surgeon may be paid

69979   **Temporal bone surgery** ~ medicare carrier determines global period, standard payment adjustment rules for multiple procedures apply, 150% payment adjustment for bilateral procedures applies, payment for assistant surgeon subject to documentation of medical necessity

Operating Microscope

69990   **Microsurgery, add-on** ~ restricted coverage - special coverage rules apply, follow-up period included in another service, no payment adjustment rules for multiple procedures apply, 150% payment adjustment for bilateral procedures does not apply, assistant surgeon may be paid, +add-on code (list separately in addition to primary procedure)

MEDICINE

Immunization Administration For Vaccines/Toxoids

90465   **Immune admin 1 inject, < 8 years** ~ no payment adjustment rules for multiple procedures apply

90466   **Immune admin added inject, < 8 years** ~ follow-up period included in another service, no payment adjustment rules for multiple procedures apply, +add-on code (list separately in addition to primary procedure)

90467   **Immune admin oral or intranasal, < 8 years** ~ no payment adjustment rules for multiple procedures apply

90468   **Immune admin oral or intranasal, added < 8 years** ~ no payment adjustment rules for multiple procedures apply, +add-on code (list separately in addition to primary procedure)

90471   **Immunization admin** ~ no payment adjustment rules for multiple procedures apply

90472   **Immunization admin, each added** ~ no payment adjustment rules for multiple procedures apply, +add-on code (list separately in addition to primary procedure)

90473   **Immune admin oral/nasal** ~ no payment adjustment rules for multiple procedures apply

90474   **Immune admin oral/nasal added** ~ no payment adjustment rules for multiple procedures apply, +add-on code (list separately in addition to primary procedure)

Hydration, Therapeutic, Prophylactic, And Diagnostic Injections And Infusions (Excludes Chemotherapy)

90760   **Hydration iv infuse initial**   ~ no payment adjustment rules for multiple
         procedures apply

90761   **Hydration iv infuse, add-on**   ~ no payment adjustment rules for multiple
         procedures apply, +add-on code (list separately in addition to primary procedure)

Therapeutic, Prophylactic, And Diagnostic Injections And Infusions

90765   **Intravenous infusion; initial, to 1 hour**
         ~ no payment adjustment rules for multiple procedures apply

90766   **Intravenous infusion; each added hour**
         ~ no payment adjustment rules for multiple procedures apply, +add-on code (list separately
         in addition to primary procedure)

90767   **Intravenous infusion; added seq, to 1 hr**
         ~ no payment adjustment rules for multiple procedures apply, +add-on code (list separately
         in addition to primary procedure)

90768   **Intravenous infusion; concurrent**   ~ no payment adjustment rules for multiple
         procedures apply, +add-on code (list separately in addition to primary procedure)

90772   **Therapeutic, prophy, diag inject, sc/im**
         ~ no payment adjustment rules for multiple procedures apply

90773   **Therapeutic, prophy, diag inject, intraart**
         ~ no payment adjustment rules for multiple procedures apply

90774   **Therapeutic, prophy, diag inject, iv push**
         ~ no payment adjustment rules for multiple procedures apply

90775   **Therapeutic, prophy, diag inject, add-on**
         ~ no payment adjustment rules for multiple procedures apply, +add-on code (list separately
         in addition to primary procedure)

Psychiatry

90801   **Psychiatric diagnostic interview**   ~ no payment adjustment rules for multiple
         procedures apply

90802   **Interact psychiatric diagnostic interview**   ~

no payment adjustment rules for multiple procedures apply

90804 **Psychotherapy, office, 20-30 min**
procedures apply

~ no payment adjustment rules for multiple

90805 **Psychotherapy, office, 20-30 min**
procedures apply

~ no payment adjustment rules for multiple

90806 **Psychotherapy, office, 45-50 min**
procedures apply

~ no payment adjustment rules for multiple

90807 **Psychotherapy, office, 45-50 min**
procedures apply,

~ no payment adjustment rules for multiple

90808 **Psychotherapy, office, 75-80 min**
procedures apply

~ no payment adjustment rules for multiple

90809 **Psychotherapy, office, 75-80**
procedures apply

~ no payment adjustment rules for multiple

90810 **Interact psych, office, 20-30 min**
procedures apply

~ no payment adjustment rules for multiple

90811 **Interact psychotherapy, 20-30**
procedures apply

~ no payment adjustment rules for multiple

90812 **Interact psych, office, 45-50 min**
procedures apply

~ no payment adjustment rules for multiple

90813 **Interact psych, 45-50 min**
procedures apply

~ no payment adjustment rules for multiple

90814 **Interact psych, office, 75-80 min**
procedures apply

~ no payment adjustment rules for multiple

90815 **Interact psych, 75-80 w/e & m**
procedures apply

~ no payment adjustment rules for multiple

90816 **Psychotherapy, hosp, 20-30 min**
procedures apply

~ no payment adjustment rules for multiple

90817 **Psych, hosp, 20-30 min w/e & m**
procedures apply

~ no payment adjustment rules for multiple

90818 **Psychotherapy, hosp, 45-50 min**
procedures apply

~ no payment adjustment rules for multiple

90819	**Psych, hosp, 45-50 min w/e & m** procedures apply	~ no payment adjustment rules for multiple
90821	**Psychotherapy, hosp, 75-80 min** procedures apply	~ no payment adjustment rules for multiple
90822	**Psych, hosp, 75-80 min w/e & m** procedures apply	~ no payment adjustment rules for multiple
90823	**Interact psych, hosp, 20-30 min** procedures apply	~ no payment adjustment rules for multiple
90824	**Interact psych, hosp 20-30 w/e & m** procedures apply	~ no payment adjustment rules for multiple
90826	**Interact psych, hosp, 45-50 min** procedures apply	~ no payment adjustment rules for multiple
90827	**Interact psych, hosp 45-50 w/e & m** procedures apply	~ no payment adjustment rules for multiple
90828	**Interact psych, hosp, 75-80 min** procedures apply	~ no payment adjustment rules for multiple
90829	**Interact psych, hosp 75-80 w/e & m** procedures apply	~ no payment adjustment rules for multiple
90845	**Psychoanalysis** procedures apply	~ no payment adjustment rules for multiple
90846	**Family psych w/o patient** apply, no payment adjustment rules for multiple procedures apply	~ restricted coverage - special coverage rules
90847	**Family psychotherapy w/patient** apply, no payment adjustment rules for multiple procedures apply	~ restricted coverage - special coverage rules
90849	**Mult family group psychotherapy** apply, no payment adjustment rules for multiple procedures apply	~ restricted coverage - special coverage rules
90853	**Group psychotherapy** procedures apply	~ no payment adjustment rules for multiple
90857	**Interact group psychotherapy** procedures apply	~ no payment adjustment rules for multiple
90862	**Medication management** procedures apply	~ no payment adjustment rules for multiple

| 90865 | **Narcosynthesis** | ~ no payment adjustment rules for multiple |
| | procedures apply | |

90870 **Electroconvulsive therapy** ~ endoscopies or minor procedure - E/M services on the same day generally not paid, no payment adjustment rules for multiple procedures apply

90875 **Psychophysiological therapy** ~ non-covered service, multiple procedure concept does not apply

90876 **Psychophysiological therapy** ~ non-covered service, multiple procedure concept does not apply

90880 **Hypnotherapy** ~ no payment adjustment rules for multiple procedures apply

90882 **Environmental manipulation** ~ non-covered service, multiple procedure concept does not apply

90885 **Psychiatric evaluation of records** ~ bundled code - no separate payment made, multiple procedure concept does not apply

90887 **Consultation with family** ~ bundled code - no separate payment made, multiple procedure concept does not apply

90889 **Prepare report** ~ bundled code - no separate payment made, multiple procedure concept does not apply

90899 **Unlisted psychiatric service/therapy** ~ no payment adjustment rules for multiple procedures apply

Biofeedback

90901 **Biofeedback training, any method** ~ endoscopies or minor procedure - E/M services on the same day generally not paid, no payment adjustment rules for multiple procedures apply

90911 **Biofeedback peri/uro/rectal** ~ endoscopies or minor procedure - E/M services on the same day generally not paid, no payment adjustment rules for multiple procedures apply

Dialysis

90918 **ESRD related services, month** ~ not valid for Medicare, multiple procedure concept does not apply

90919 **ESRD related services, month** ~ not valid for Medicare, multiple procedure
concept does not apply

90920 **ESRD related services, month** ~ not valid for Medicare, multiple procedure
concept does not apply

90921 **ESRD related services, month** ~ not valid for Medicare, multiple procedure
concept does not apply

90922 **ESRD related services, day** ~ not valid for Medicare, multiple procedure
concept does not apply

90923 **ESRD related services, day** ~ not valid for Medicare, multiple procedure
concept does not apply

90924 **ESRD related services, day** ~ not valid for Medicare, multiple procedure
concept does not apply

90925 **ESRD related services, day** ~ not valid for Medicare, multiple procedure
concept does not apply

90935 **Hemodialysis, one evaluation** ~ endoscopies or minor procedure - E/M
services on the same day generally not paid, no payment adjustment rules for multiple
procedures apply

90937 **Hemodialysis, repeated evaluate** ~ endoscopies or minor procedure - E/M
services on the same day generally not paid, no payment adjustment rules for multiple
procedures apply

90940 **Hemodialysis access study** ~ multiple procedure concept does not apply

90945 **Dialysis, one evaluation** ~ endoscopies or minor procedure - E/M
services on the same day generally not paid, no payment adjustment rules for multiple
procedures apply

90947 **Dialysis, repeated evaluate** ~ endoscopies or minor procedure - E/M
services on the same day generally not paid, no payment adjustment rules for multiple
procedures apply

90989 **Dialysis training, complete** ~ multiple procedure concept does not apply

90993 **Dialysis training, incomplete** ~ multiple procedure concept does not apply

90997 **Hemoperfusion** ~ endoscopies or minor procedure - E/M
services on the same day generally not paid, no payment adjustment rules for multiple
procedures apply, 150% payment adjustment for bilateral procedures does not apply,
payment for assistant surgeon subject to documentation of medical necessity

90999   **Dialysis procedure**   ~ no payment adjustment rules for multiple procedures apply, 150% payment adjustment for bilateral procedures does not apply, payment for assistant surgeon subject to documentation of medical necessity

Gastroenterology

91000   **Esophageal intubation**   ~ endoscopies or minor procedure - E/M services on the same day generally not paid, no payment adjustment rules for multiple procedures applypayment for assistant surgeon subject to documentation of medical necessity

91010   **Esophagus motility study**   ~ endoscopies or minor procedure - E/M services on the same day generally not paid, no payment adjustment rules for multiple procedures apply

91011   **Esophagus motility study**   ~ endoscopies or minor procedure - E/M services on the same day generally not paid, no payment adjustment rules for multiple procedures apply

91012   **Esophagus motility study**   ~ endoscopies or minor procedure - E/M services on the same day generally not paid, no payment adjustment rules for multiple procedures apply

91020   **Gastric motility studies**   ~ endoscopies or minor procedure - E/M services on the same day generally not paid, no payment adjustment rules for multiple procedures apply

91022   **Duodenal motility study**   ~ endoscopies or minor procedure - E/M services on the same day generally not paid, no payment adjustment rules for multiple procedures apply

91030   **Acid perfuse esophagus**   ~ endoscopies or minor procedure - E/M services on the same day generally not paid, no payment adjustment rules for multiple procedures apply

91034   **Gastroesophageal reflux test**   ~ endoscopies or minor procedure - E/M services on the same day generally not paid, no payment adjustment rules for multiple procedures apply

91035   **G-esophagus reflux test w/electrode**   ~ endoscopies or minor procedure - E/M services on the same day generally not paid, no payment adjustment rules for multiple procedures apply

91037   **Esophagus impedance funct test**   ~ endoscopies or minor procedure - E/M services on the same day generally not paid, no payment adjustment rules for multiple procedures apply

---

91038 **Esophagus imped funct test > 1h**   ~ endoscopies or minor procedure - E/M services on the same day generally not paid, no payment adjustment rules for multiple procedures apply

91040 **Esophagus balloon distension test**   ~ endoscopies or minor procedure - E/M services on the same day generally not paid, no payment adjustment rules for multiple procedures apply

91052 **Gastric analysis test**   ~ endoscopies or minor procedure - E/M services on the same day generally not paid, no payment adjustment rules for multiple procedures apply

91055 **Gastric intubation for smear**   ~ endoscopies or minor procedure - E/M services on the same day generally not paid, no payment adjustment rules for multiple procedures apply

91065 **Breath hydrogen test**   ~ endoscopies or minor procedure - E/M services on the same day generally not paid, no payment adjustment rules for multiple procedures apply

91100 **Pass intestine bleeding tube**   ~ endoscopies or minor procedure - E/M services on the same day generally not paid, no payment adjustment rules for multiple procedures apply

91105 **Gastric intubation treatment**   ~ endoscopies or minor procedure - E/M services on the same day generally not paid, no payment adjustment rules for multiple procedures apply

91110 **GI tract capsule endoscopy**   ~ no payment adjustment rules for multiple procedures apply

91111 **Esophageal capsule endoscopy**   ~ no payment adjustment rules for multiple procedures apply

91120 **Rectal sensation test**   ~ no payment adjustment rules for multiple procedures apply

91122 **Anal pressure record**   ~ endoscopies or minor procedure - E/M services on the same day generally not paid, no payment adjustment rules for multiple procedures apply

91123 **Irrigate fecal impaction**   ~ bundled code - no separate payment made, multiple procedure concept does not apply, bilateral surgery concept does not apply, assistant surgery concept does not apply

91132 **Electrogastrography**   ~ no payment adjustment rules for multiple procedures apply

---

91133 **Electrogastrography w/test** ~ no payment adjustment rules for multiple
procedures apply

91299 **Gastroenterology procedure** ~ no payment adjustment rules for multiple
procedures apply

Ophthalmology

92002 **Eye exam new patient** ~ no payment adjustment rules for multiple
procedures apply, 150% payment adjustment does not apply - RVUs based on bilateral
procedure

92004 **Eye exam new patient** ~ no payment adjustment rules for multiple
procedures apply, 150% payment adjustment does not apply - RVUs based on bilateral
procedure

92012 **Eye exam established pat** ~ no payment adjustment rules for multiple
procedures apply, 150% payment adjustment does not apply - RVUs based on bilateral
procedure

92014 **Eye exam & treatment** ~ no payment adjustment rules for multiple
procedures apply, 150% payment adjustment does not apply - RVUs based on bilateral
procedure

92015 **Refraction** ~ non-covered service, multiple procedure
concept does not apply, bilateral surgery concept does not apply, assistant surgery concept
does not apply

92018 **New eye exam & treatment** ~ no payment adjustment rules for multiple
procedures apply

92019 **Eye exam & treatment** ~ no payment adjustment rules for multiple
procedures apply

92020 **Special eye evaluation** ~ no payment adjustment rules for multiple
procedures apply, 150% payment adjustment does not apply - RVUs based on bilateral
procedure

92025 **Corneal topography** ~ no payment adjustment rules for multiple
procedures apply

92060 **Special eye evaluation** ~ no payment adjustment rules for multiple
procedures apply, 150% payment adjustment does not apply - RVUs based on bilateral
procedure

92065   **Orthoptic/pleoptic training**   ~ no payment adjustment rules for multiple procedures apply, 150% payment adjustment does not apply - RVUs based on bilateral procedure

92070   **Fit contact lens**   ~ no payment adjustment rules for multiple procedures apply, the usual payment adjustment for bilateral procedures does not apply

92081   **Visual field examination(s)**   ~ no payment adjustment rules for multiple procedures apply, 150% payment adjustment does not apply - RVUs based on bilateral procedure

92082   **Visual field examination(s)**   ~ no payment adjustment rules for multiple procedures apply, 150% payment adjustment does not apply - RVUs based on bilateral procedure

92083   **Visual field examination(s)**   ~ no payment adjustment rules for multiple procedures apply, 150% payment adjustment does not apply - RVUs based on bilateral procedure

92100   **Serial tonometry exam(s)**   ~ no payment adjustment rules for multiple procedures apply, 150% payment adjustment does not apply - RVUs based on bilateral procedure

92120   **Tonography & eye evaluation**   ~ no payment adjustment rules for multiple procedures apply, 150% payment adjustment does not apply - RVUs based on bilateral procedure

92130   **Water provocation tonography**   ~ no payment adjustment rules for multiple procedures apply, 150% payment adjustment does not apply - RVUs based on bilateral procedure

92135   **Ophthalmic dx imaging**   ~ no payment adjustment rules for multiple procedures apply, the usual payment adjustment for bilateral procedures does not apply, assistant surgeon may not be paid

92136   **Ophthalmic biometry**   ~ no payment adjustment rules for multiple procedures apply, 150% payment adjustment does not apply - RVUs based on bilateral procedure

92140   **Glaucoma provocative tests**   ~ no payment adjustment rules for multiple procedures apply, 150% payment adjustment does not apply - RVUs based on bilateral procedure

92225   **Special eye exam initial**   ~ no payment adjustment rules for multiple procedures apply, the usual payment adjustment for bilateral procedures does not apply

92226   **Special eye exam subsequent**   ~ no payment adjustment rules for multiple procedures apply, the usual payment adjustment for bilateral procedures does not apply

92230   **Eye exam with photos**   ~ no payment adjustment rules for multiple procedures apply, the usual payment adjustment for bilateral procedures does not apply

92235   **Eye exam with photos**   ~ no payment adjustment rules for multiple procedures apply, the usual payment adjustment for bilateral procedures does not apply

92240   **Icg angiography**   ~ no payment adjustment rules for multiple procedures apply, the usual payment adjustment for bilateral procedures does not apply

92250   **Eye exam with photos**   ~ no payment adjustment rules for multiple procedures apply, 150% payment adjustment does not apply - RVUs based on bilateral procedure

92260   **Ophthalmoscopy/dynamometry**   ~ no payment adjustment rules for multiple procedures apply, 150% payment adjustment does not apply - RVUs based on bilateral procedure

92265   **Eye muscle evaluation**   ~ no payment adjustment rules for multiple procedures apply, 150% payment adjustment does not apply - RVUs based on bilateral procedure

92270   **Electro-oculography**   ~ no payment adjustment rules for multiple procedures apply, 150% payment adjustment does not apply - RVUs based on bilateral procedure

92275   **Electroretinography**   ~ no payment adjustment rules for multiple procedures apply, 150% payment adjustment does not apply - RVUs based on bilateral procedure

92283   **Color vision examination**   ~ no payment adjustment rules for multiple procedures apply, 150% payment adjustment does not apply - RVUs based on bilateral procedure

92284   **Dark adaptation eye exam**   ~ no payment adjustment rules for multiple procedures apply, 150% payment adjustment does not apply - RVUs based on bilateral procedure

92285   **Eye photography**   ~ no payment adjustment rules for multiple procedures apply, 150% payment adjustment does not apply - RVUs based on bilateral procedure

92286   **Internal eye photography**   ~ no payment adjustment rules for multiple procedures apply, 150% payment adjustment does not apply - RVUs based on bilateral procedure

---

92287   **Internal eye photography**   ~ no payment adjustment rules for multiple procedures apply, 150% payment adjustment does not apply - RVUs based on bilateral procedure

92310   **Contact lens fitting**   ~ non-covered service, multiple procedure concept does not apply, bilateral surgery concept does not apply, assistant surgery concept does not apply

92311   **Contact lens fitting**   ~ no payment adjustment rules for multiple procedures apply

92312   **Contact lens fitting**   ~ no payment adjustment rules for multiple procedures apply, 150% payment adjustment does not apply - RVUs based on bilateral procedure

92313   **Contact lens fitting**   ~ no payment adjustment rules for multiple procedures apply

92314   **Prescribe contact lens**   ~ non-covered service, multiple procedure concept does not apply, bilateral surgery concept does not apply, assistant surgery concept does not apply

92315   **Prescribe contact lens**   ~ no payment adjustment rules for multiple procedures apply

92316   **Prescribe contact lens**   ~ no payment adjustment rules for multiple procedures apply, 150% payment adjustment does not apply - RVUs based on bilateral procedure

92317   **Prescribe contact lens**   ~ no payment adjustment rules for multiple procedures apply

92325   **Modification of contact lens**   ~ no payment adjustment rules for multiple procedures apply

92326   **Replace contact lens**   ~ no payment adjustment rules for multiple procedures apply

92340   **Fit spectacles**   ~ non-covered service, multiple procedure concept does not apply, bilateral surgery concept does not apply, assistant surgery concept does not apply

92341   **Fit spectacles**   ~ non-covered service, multiple procedure concept does not apply, bilateral surgery concept does not apply, assistant surgery concept does not apply

92342   **Fit spectacles**   ~ non-covered service, multiple procedure concept does not apply, bilateral surgery concept does not apply, assistant surgery concept does not apply

92352   **Special spectacles fitting**   ~ bundled code - no separate payment made, multiple procedure concept does not apply, bilateral surgery concept does not apply, assistant surgery concept does not apply

92353   **Special spectacles fitting**   ~ bundled code - no separate payment made, multiple procedure concept does not apply, bilateral surgery concept does not apply, assistant surgery concept does not apply

92354   **Special spectacles fitting**   ~ bundled code - no separate payment made, multiple procedure concept does not apply, bilateral surgery concept does not apply, assistant surgery concept does not apply

92355   **Special spectacles fitting**   ~ bundled code - no separate payment made, multiple procedure concept does not apply, bilateral surgery concept does not apply, assistant surgery concept does not apply

92358   **Eye prosthesis service**   ~ bundled code - no separate payment made, multiple procedure concept does not apply, bilateral surgery concept does not apply, assistant surgery concept does not apply

92370   **Repair & adjust spectacles**   ~ non-covered service, multiple procedure concept does not apply, bilateral surgery concept does not apply, assistant surgery concept does not apply

92371   **Repair & adjust spectacles**   ~ bundled code - no separate payment made, multiple procedure concept does not apply, bilateral surgery concept does not apply, assistant surgery concept does not apply

92499   **Eye service or procedure**   ~ no payment adjustment rules for multiple procedures apply

Special Otorhinolaryngologic Services

92502   **Ear and throat examination**   ~ endoscopies or minor procedure - E/M services on the same day generally not paid, no payment adjustment rules for multiple procedures apply

92504   **Ear microscopy examination**   ~ no payment adjustment rules for multiple procedures apply

92506   **Speech/hearing evaluation**   ~ no payment adjustment rules for multiple procedures apply

---

| 92507 | **Speech/hearing therapy** | ~ no payment adjustment rules for multiple |
| | procedures apply | |

| 92508 | **Speech/hearing therapy** | ~ no payment adjustment rules for multiple |
| | procedures apply | |

| 92511 | **Nasopharyngoscopy** | ~ endoscopies or minor procedure - E/M |

services on the same day generally not paid, no payment adjustment rules for multiple procedures apply

| 92512 | **Nasal function studies** | ~ no payment adjustment rules for multiple |
| | procedures apply | |

| 92516 | **Facial nerve function test** | ~ no payment adjustment rules for multiple |
| | procedures apply | |

| 92520 | **Laryngeal function studies** | ~ no payment adjustment rules for multiple |
| | procedures apply | |

| 92526 | **Oral function therapy** | ~ no payment adjustment rules for multiple |
| | procedures apply | |

| 92531 | **Spontaneous nystagmus study** | ~ bundled code - no separate payment made, |
| | multiple procedure concept does not apply | |

| 92532 | **Positional nystagmus test** | ~ bundled code - no separate payment made, |
| | multiple procedure concept does not apply | |

| 92533 | **Caloric vestibular test** | ~ bundled code - no separate payment made, |
| | multiple procedure concept does not apply | |

| 92534 | **Optokinetic nystagmus test** | ~ bundled code - no separate payment made, |

multiple procedure concept does not apply, bilateral surgery concept does not apply, assistant surgery concept does not apply

| 92541 | **Spontaneous nystagmus test** | ~ no payment adjustment rules for multiple |
| | procedures apply | |

| 92542 | **Positional nystagmus test** | ~ no payment adjustment rules for multiple |
| | procedures apply | |

| 92543 | **Caloric vestibular test** | ~ no payment adjustment rules for multiple |
| | procedures apply | |

| 92544 | **Optokinetic nystagmus test** | ~ no payment adjustment rules for multiple |
| | procedures apply | |

92545 **Oscillating tracking test** ~ no payment adjustment rules for multiple procedures apply

92546 **Sinusoidal rotational test** ~ no payment adjustment rules for multiple procedures apply

92547 **Supplemental electrical test** ~ follow-up period included in another service, no payment adjustment rules for multiple procedures apply

92548 **Posturography** ~ no payment adjustment rules for multiple procedures apply

92551 **Pure tone hearing test, air** ~ non-covered service, multiple procedure concept does not apply, bilateral surgery concept does not apply, assistant surgery concept does not apply

92552 **Pure tone audiometry, air** ~ no payment adjustment rules for multiple procedures apply, 150% payment adjustment does not apply - RVUs based on bilateral procedure

92553 **Audiometry, air & bone** ~ no payment adjustment rules for multiple procedures apply, 150% payment adjustment does not apply - RVUs based on bilateral procedure

92555 **Speech threshold audiometry** ~ no payment adjustment rules for multiple procedures apply, 150% payment adjustment does not apply - RVUs based on bilateral procedure

92556 **Speech audiometry, complete** ~ no payment adjustment rules for multiple procedures apply, 150% payment adjustment does not apply - RVUs based on bilateral procedure

92557 **Comprehensive hearing test** ~ no payment adjustment rules for multiple procedures apply, 150% payment adjustment does not apply - RVUs based on bilateral procedure

92559 **Group audiometric testing** ~ non-covered service, multiple procedure concept does not apply, bilateral surgery concept does not apply, assistant surgery concept does not apply

92560 **Bekesy audiometry, screen** ~ non-covered service, multiple procedure concept does not apply, bilateral surgery concept does not apply, assistant surgery concept does not apply

92561 **Bekesy audiometry, diagnosis** ~ no payment adjustment rules for multiple procedures apply, 150% payment adjustment does not apply - RVUs based on bilateral procedure

92562 **Loudness balance test**   ~ no payment adjustment rules for multiple procedures apply, 150% payment adjustment does not apply - RVUs based on bilateral procedure

92563 **Tone decay hearing test**   ~ no payment adjustment rules for multiple procedures apply, 150% payment adjustment does not apply - RVUs based on bilateral procedure

92564 **Sisi hearing test**   ~ no payment adjustment rules for multiple procedures apply, 150% payment adjustment does not apply - RVUs based on bilateral procedure

92565 **Stenger test, pure tone**   ~ no payment adjustment rules for multiple procedures apply, 150% payment adjustment does not apply - RVUs based on bilateral procedure

92567 **Tympanometry**   ~ no payment adjustment rules for multiple procedures apply, 150% payment adjustment does not apply - RVUs based on bilateral procedure

92568 **Acoustic reflex threshold test**   ~ no payment adjustment rules for multiple procedures apply, 150% payment adjustment does not apply - RVUs based on bilateral procedure

92569 **Acoustic reflex decay test**   ~ no payment adjustment rules for multiple procedures apply, 150% payment adjustment does not apply - RVUs based on bilateral procedure

92571 **Filtered speech hearing test**   ~ no payment adjustment rules for multiple procedures apply, 150% payment adjustment does not apply - RVUs based on bilateral procedure

92572 **Staggered spondaic word test**   ~ no payment adjustment rules for multiple procedures apply, 150% payment adjustment does not apply - RVUs based on bilateral procedure

92575 **Sensorineural acuity test**   ~ no payment adjustment rules for multiple procedures apply, 150% payment adjustment does not apply - RVUs based on bilateral procedure

92576 **Synthetic sentence test**   ~ no payment adjustment rules for multiple procedures apply, 150% payment adjustment does not apply - RVUs based on bilateral procedure

92577 **Stenger test, speech**   ~ no payment adjustment rules for multiple procedures apply, 150% payment adjustment does not apply - RVUs based on bilateral procedure

92579 **Visual audiometry (vra)** ~ no payment adjustment rules for multiple procedures apply, 150% payment adjustment does not apply - RVUs based on bilateral procedure

92582 **Conditioning play audiometry** ~ no payment adjustment rules for multiple procedures apply, 150% payment adjustment does not apply - RVUs based on bilateral procedure

92583 **Select picture audiometry** ~ no payment adjustment rules for multiple procedures apply, 150% payment adjustment does not apply - RVUs based on bilateral procedure

92584 **Electrocochleography** ~ no payment adjustment rules for multiple procedures apply, 150% payment adjustment does not apply - RVUs based on bilateral procedure

92585 **Auditor evoke potent, comprehensive** ~ no payment adjustment rules for multiple procedures apply, 150% payment adjustment does not apply - RVUs based on bilateral procedure

92586 **Auditor evoke potent, limit** ~ no payment adjustment rules for multiple procedures apply, 150% payment adjustment does not apply - RVUs based on bilateral procedure

92587 **Evoked auditory test** ~ no payment adjustment rules for multiple procedures apply, 150% payment adjustment does not apply - RVUs based on bilateral procedure

92588 **Evoked auditory test** ~ no payment adjustment rules for multiple procedures apply, 150% payment adjustment does not apply - RVUs based on bilateral procedure

92590 **Hearing aid exam one ear** ~ non-covered service, multiple procedure concept does not apply, bilateral surgery concept does not apply, assistant surgery concept does not apply

92591 **Hearing aid exam both ears** ~ non-covered service, multiple procedure concept does not apply, bilateral surgery concept does not apply, assistant surgery concept does not apply

92592 **Hearing aid check, one ear** ~ non-covered service, multiple procedure concept does not apply, bilateral surgery concept does not apply, assistant surgery concept does not apply

92593 **Hearing aid check, both ears** ~ non-covered service, multiple procedure concept does not apply, bilateral surgery concept does not apply, assistant surgery concept does not apply

92594   **Electro hearing aid test, one**   ~ non-covered service, multiple procedure concept does not apply, bilateral surgery concept does not apply, assistant surgery concept does not apply

92595   **Electro hearing aid test, both**   ~ non-covered service, multiple procedure concept does not apply, bilateral surgery concept does not apply, assistant surgery concept does not apply

92596   **Ear protector evaluation**   ~ no payment adjustment rules for multiple procedures apply, 150% payment adjustment does not apply - RVUs based on bilateral procedure

92597   **Oral speech device evaluate**   ~ no payment adjustment rules for multiple procedures apply

92601   **Cochlear implant f/up exam < 7 years**   ~ no payment adjustment rules for multiple procedures apply

92602   **Reprogram cochlear implant < 7 years**   ~ no payment adjustment rules for multiple procedures apply

92603   **Cochlear implant f/up exam 7 years or >**   ~ no payment adjustment rules for multiple procedures apply

92604   **Reprogram cochlear implant 7 years or >** ~ no payment adjustment rules for multiple procedures apply

92605   **Evaluate for nonspeech device rx**   ~ bundled code - no separate payment made, multiple procedure concept does not apply

92606   **Non-speech device service**   ~ bundled code - no separate payment made, multiple procedure concept does not apply, bilateral surgery concept does not apply, assistant surgery concept does not apply

92607   **Ex for speech device rx, 1hr**   ~ no payment adjustment rules for multiple procedures apply

92608   **Ex for speech device rx added**   ~ no payment adjustment rules for multiple procedures apply, +add-on code (list separately in addition to primary procedure)

92609   **Use of speech device service**   ~ no payment adjustment rules for multiple procedures apply

92610   **Evaluate swallowing function**   ~ no payment adjustment rules for multiple procedures apply

92611	**Motion fluoroscopy/swallow** procedures apply	~ no payment adjustment rules for multiple
92612	**Endoscopy swallow test (fees)** procedures apply	~ no payment adjustment rules for multiple
92613	**Endoscopy swallow test (fees)** procedures apply	~ no payment adjustment rules for multiple
92614	**Laryngoscopic sensory test** procedures apply	~ no payment adjustment rules for multiple
92615	**Evaluate laryngoscopy sense test** procedures apply	~ no payment adjustment rules for multiple
92616	**Fees w/laryngeal sense test** procedures apply	~ no payment adjustment rules for multiple
92617	**Interpretation fees/laryngeal test** procedures apply	~ no payment adjustment rules for multiple

92620 **Auditory function, initial 60 min** ~ no payment adjustment rules for multiple procedures apply, 150% payment adjustment does not apply - RVUs based on bilateral procedure

92621 **Auditory function, added 15 min** ~ follow-up period included in another service, no payment adjustment rules for multiple procedures apply, 150% payment adjustment does not apply - RVUs based on bilateral procedure

92625 **Tinnitus assessment** ~ no payment adjustment rules for multiple procedures apply, 150% payment adjustment does not apply - RVUs based on bilateral procedure

92626 **Evaluate auditory rehab status** ~ no payment adjustment rules for multiple procedures apply, 150% payment adjustment does not apply - RVUs based on bilateral procedure

92627 **Eval auditory status rehab, add-on** ~ follow-up period included in another service, no payment adjustment rules for multiple procedures apply, 150% payment adjustment does not apply - RVUs based on bilateral procedure , +add-on code (list separately in addition to primary procedure)

92630 **Auditory rehab pre-ling hear loss** ~ not valid for Medicare, multiple procedure concept does not apply, bilateral surgery concept does not apply, assistant surgery concept does not apply

92633   **Auditory rehab postlingual hear loss**   ~ not valid for Medicare, multiple procedure concept does not apply, bilateral surgery concept does not apply, assistant surgery concept does not apply

92640   **Auditory brainstem implant program**   ~ no payment adjustment rules for multiple procedures apply, 150% payment adjustment does not apply - RVUs based on bilateral procedure

92700   **Unlisted ENT procedure/service**   ~ no payment adjustment rules for multiple procedures apply

Cardiovascular

92950   **Heart/lung resuscitation cpr**   ~ endoscopies or minor procedure - E/M services on the same day generally not paid, no payment adjustment rules for multiple procedures applypayment for assistant surgeon subject to documentation of medical necessity

92953   **Temporary external pacing**   ~ endoscopies or minor procedure - E/M services on the same day generally not paid, no payment adjustment rules for multiple procedures applypayment for assistant surgeon subject to documentation of medical necessity

92960   **Cardioversion electric, external**   ~ endoscopies or minor procedure - E/M services on the same day generally not paid, no payment adjustment rules for multiple procedures applypayment for assistant surgeon subject to documentation of medical necessity

92961   **Cardioversion, electric, internal**   ~ endoscopies or minor procedure - E/M services on the same day generally not paid, multiple procedure concept does not apply, bilateral surgery concept does not apply, assistant surgery concept does not apply

92970   **Cardioassist, internal**   ~ endoscopies or minor procedure - E/M services on the same day generally not paid, no payment adjustment rules for multiple procedures applypayment for assistant surgeon subject to documentation of medical necessity

92971   **Cardioassist, external**   ~ endoscopies or minor procedure - E/M services on the same day generally not paid, no payment adjustment rules for multiple procedures applypayment for assistant surgeon subject to documentation of medical necessity

92973   **Percutaneous coronary thrombectomy**   ~ follow-up period included in another service, no payment adjustment rules for multiple procedures applypayment for assistant surgeon subject to documentation of medical necessity

92974   **Cath place, cardio brachytherapy**   ~ follow-up period included in another service, no payment adjustment rules for multiple procedures applypayment for assistant surgeon subject to documentation of medical necessity

92975   **Dissolve clot, heart vessel**   ~ endoscopies or minor procedure - E/M services on the same day generally not paid, standard payment adjustment rules for multiple procedures applypayment for assistant surgeon subject to documentation of medical necessity

92977   **Dissolve clot, heart vessel**   ~ no payment adjustment rules for multiple procedures applypayment for assistant surgeon subject to documentation of medical necessity

92978   **Intravascular us, heart, add-on**   ~ follow-up period included in another service, no payment adjustment rules for multiple procedures applypayment for assistant surgeon subject to documentation of medical necessity, +add-on code (list separately in addition to primary procedure)

92979   **Intravascular us, heart, add-on**   ~ follow-up period included in another service, no payment adjustment rules for multiple procedures applypayment for assistant surgeon subject to documentation of medical necessity, +add-on code (list separately in addition to primary procedure)

92980   **Insert intracoronary stent**   ~ endoscopies or minor procedure - E/M services on the same day generally not paid, standard payment adjustment rules for multiple procedures applypayment for assistant surgeon subject to documentation of medical necessity

92981   **Insert intracoronary stent**   ~ follow-up period included in another service, no payment adjustment rules for multiple procedures applypayment for assistant surgeon subject to documentation of medical necessity

92982   **Coronary artery dilate**   ~ endoscopies or minor procedure - E/M services on the same day generally not paid, standard payment adjustment rules for multiple procedures applypayment for assistant surgeon subject to documentation of medical necessity

92984   **Coronary artery dilate**   ~ follow-up period included in another service, no payment adjustment rules for multiple procedures applypayment for assistant surgeon subject to documentation of medical necessity

92986   **Revise aortic valve**   ~ follow-up period is 90 days, standard payment adjustment rules for multiple procedures applypayment for assistant surgeon subject to documentation of medical necessity

---

92987   **Revise mitral valve**   ~ follow-up period is 90 days, standard payment adjustment rules for multiple procedures applypayment for assistant surgeon subject to documentation of medical necessity

92990   **Revise pulmonary valve**   ~ follow-up period is 90 days, standard payment adjustment rules for multiple procedures applypayment for assistant surgeon subject to documentation of medical necessity

92992   **Revise heart chamber**   ~ follow-up period is 90 days, standard payment adjustment rules for multiple procedures applyassistant surgeon may be paid

92993   **Revise heart chamber**   ~ follow-up period is 90 days, standard payment adjustment rules for multiple procedures applyassistant surgeon may be paid

92995   **Coronary atherectomy**   ~ endoscopies or minor procedure - E/M services on the same day generally not paid, standard payment adjustment rules for multiple procedures applypayment for assistant surgeon subject to documentation of medical necessity

92996   **Coronary atherectomy, add-on**   ~ follow-up period included in another service, no payment adjustment rules for multiple procedures applypayment for assistant surgeon subject to documentation of medical necessity, +add-on code (list separately in addition to primary procedure)

92997   **Pulmonary art balloon repair, percutaneous** ~ endoscopies or minor procedure - E/M services on the same day generally not paid, standard payment adjustment rules for multiple procedures applypayment for assistant surgeon subject to documentation of medical necessity

92998   **Pulmonary art balloon repair, percutaneous** ~ follow-up period included in another service, no payment adjustment rules for multiple procedures applypayment for assistant surgeon subject to documentation of medical necessity

93000   **Electrocardiogram, complete**   ~ no payment adjustment rules for multiple procedures applypayment for assistant surgeon subject to documentation of medical necessity

93005   **Electrocardiogram, tracing**   ~ no payment adjustment rules for multiple procedures apply

93010   **Electrocardiogram report**   ~ no payment adjustment rules for multiple procedures apply

93012   **Transmission of ECG**   ~ no payment adjustment rules for multiple procedures apply

93014	**Report on transmitted ECG** procedures apply	~ no payment adjustment rules for multiple
93015	**Cardiovascular stress test** procedures apply	~ no payment adjustment rules for multiple
93016	**Cardiovascular stress test** procedures apply	~ no payment adjustment rules for multiple
93017	**Cardiovascular stress test** procedures apply	~ no payment adjustment rules for multiple
93018	**Cardiovascular stress test** procedures apply	~ no payment adjustment rules for multiple
93024	**Cardiac drug stress test** procedures apply	~ no payment adjustment rules for multiple
93025	**Microvolt t-wave assess** procedures apply	~ no payment adjustment rules for multiple
93040	**Rhythm ECG with report** procedures apply	~ no payment adjustment rules for multiple
93041	**Rhythm ECG, tracing** procedures apply	~ no payment adjustment rules for multiple
93042	**Rhythm ECG, report** procedures apply	~ no payment adjustment rules for multiple
93224	**ECG monitor/report, 24 hrs** procedures apply	~ no payment adjustment rules for multiple
93225	**ECG monitor/record, 24 hrs** procedures apply	~ no payment adjustment rules for multiple
93226	**ECG monitor/report, 24 hrs** procedures apply	~ no payment adjustment rules for multiple
93227	**ECG monitor/review, 24 hrs** procedures apply	~ no payment adjustment rules for multiple
93230	**ECG monitor/report, 24 hrs** procedures apply	~ no payment adjustment rules for multiple
93231	**ECG monitor/record, 24 hrs** procedures apply	~ no payment adjustment rules for multiple

93232	ECG monitor/report, 24 hrs procedures apply	~ no payment adjustment rules for multiple
93233	ECG monitor/review, 24 hrs procedures apply	~ no payment adjustment rules for multiple
93235	ECG monitor/report, 24 hrs procedures apply	~ no payment adjustment rules for multiple
93236	ECG monitor/report, 24 hrs procedures apply	~ no payment adjustment rules for multiple
93237	ECG monitor/review, 24 hrs procedures apply	~ no payment adjustment rules for multiple
93268	ECG record/review procedures apply	~ no payment adjustment rules for multiple
93270	ECG recording procedures apply	~ no payment adjustment rules for multiple
93271	ECG/monitoring and analysis procedures apply	~ no payment adjustment rules for multiple
93272	ECG/review, interpret only procedures apply	~ no payment adjustment rules for multiple
93278	ECG/signal-averaged procedures apply	~ no payment adjustment rules for multiple
93303	Echo transthoracic procedures apply	~ no payment adjustment rules for multiple
93304	Echo transthoracic procedures apply	~ no payment adjustment rules for multiple
93307	Echo exam heart procedures apply	~ no payment adjustment rules for multiple
93308	Echo exam heart procedures apply	~ no payment adjustment rules for multiple
93312	Echo transesophageal procedures apply	~ no payment adjustment rules for multiple
93313	Echo transesophageal procedures apply	~ no payment adjustment rules for multiple

93314 **Echo transesophageal**   ~ no payment adjustment rules for multiple
procedures apply

93315 **Echo transesophageal**   ~ no payment adjustment rules for multiple
procedures apply

93316 **Echo transesophageal**   ~ no payment adjustment rules for multiple
procedures apply

93317 **Echo transesophageal**   ~ no payment adjustment rules for multiple
procedures apply

93318 **Echo transesophageal intraop**   ~ no payment adjustment rules for multiple
procedures apply

93320 **Doppler echo exam heart**   ~ follow-up period included in another service,
no payment adjustment rules for multiple procedures apply

93321 **Doppler echo exam heart**   ~ follow-up period included in another service,
no payment adjustment rules for multiple procedures apply

93325 **Doppler color flow, add-on**   ~ follow-up period included in another service,
no payment adjustment rules for multiple procedures apply, +add-on code (list separately in
addition to primary procedure)

93350 **Echo transthoracic**   ~ no payment adjustment rules for multiple
procedures apply

93501 **Right heart catheterization**   ~ endoscopies or minor procedure - E/M
services on the same day generally not paid, standard payment adjustment rules for multiple
procedures applypayment for assistant surgeon subject to documentation of medical
necessity

93503 **Insert/place heart catheter**   ~ endoscopies or minor procedure - E/M
services on the same day generally not paid, no payment adjustment rules for multiple
procedures applypayment for assistant surgeon subject to documentation of medical
necessity

93505 **Biopsy heart lining**   ~ endoscopies or minor procedure - E/M
services on the same day generally not paid, standard payment adjustment rules for multiple
procedures applypayment for assistant surgeon subject to documentation of medical
necessity

93508 **Cath placement, angiography**   ~ endoscopies or minor procedure - E/M
services on the same day generally not paid, standard payment adjustment rules for multiple
procedures applypayment for assistant surgeon subject to documentation of medical
necessity

93510   **Left heart catheterization**   ~ endoscopies or minor procedure - E/M services on the same day generally not paid, standard payment adjustment rules for multiple procedures applypayment for assistant surgeon subject to documentation of medical necessity

93511   **Left heart catheterization**   ~ endoscopies or minor procedure - E/M services on the same day generally not paid, standard payment adjustment rules for multiple procedures applypayment for assistant surgeon subject to documentation of medical necessity

93514   **Left heart catheterization**   ~ endoscopies or minor procedure - E/M services on the same day generally not paid, standard payment adjustment rules for multiple procedures applypayment for assistant surgeon subject to documentation of medical necessity

93524   **Left heart catheterization**   ~ endoscopies or minor procedure - E/M services on the same day generally not paid, standard payment adjustment rules for multiple procedures applypayment for assistant surgeon subject to documentation of medical necessity

93526   **Right & left heart catheters**   ~ endoscopies or minor procedure - E/M services on the same day generally not paid, standard payment adjustment rules for multiple procedures applypayment for assistant surgeon subject to documentation of medical necessity

93527   **Right & left heart catheters**   ~ endoscopies or minor procedure - E/M services on the same day generally not paid, standard payment adjustment rules for multiple procedures applypayment for assistant surgeon subject to documentation of medical necessity

93528   **Right & left heart catheters**   ~ endoscopies or minor procedure - E/M services on the same day generally not paid, standard payment adjustment rules for multiple procedures applypayment for assistant surgeon subject to documentation of medical necessity

93529   **Right, left heart catheterization**   ~ endoscopies or minor procedure - E/M services on the same day generally not paid, standard payment adjustment rules for multiple procedures applypayment for assistant surgeon subject to documentation of medical necessity

93530   **Right heart cath, congenital**   ~ endoscopies or minor procedure - E/M services on the same day generally not paid, standard payment adjustment rules for multiple procedures applypayment for assistant surgeon subject to documentation of medical necessity

93531   **Right & left heart cath, congenital**   ~ endoscopies or minor procedure - E/M services on the same day generally not paid, standard payment adjustment rules for multiple

procedures applypayment for assistant surgeon subject to documentation of medical necessity

93532   **Right & left heart cath, congenital**   ~ endoscopies or minor procedure - E/M services on the same day generally not paid, standard payment adjustment rules for multiple procedures applypayment for assistant surgeon subject to documentation of medical necessity

93533   **Right & left heart cath, congenital**   ~ endoscopies or minor procedure - E/M services on the same day generally not paid, standard payment adjustment rules for multiple procedures applypayment for assistant surgeon subject to documentation of medical necessity

93539   **Injection, cardiac cath**   ~ endoscopies or minor procedure - E/M services on the same day generally not paid, no payment adjustment rules for multiple procedures applypayment for assistant surgeon subject to documentation of medical necessity

93540   **Injection, cardiac cath**   ~ endoscopies or minor procedure - E/M services on the same day generally not paid, no payment adjustment rules for multiple procedures applypayment for assistant surgeon subject to documentation of medical necessity

93541   **Inject for lung angiogram**   ~ endoscopies or minor procedure - E/M services on the same day generally not paid, no payment adjustment rules for multiple procedures applypayment for assistant surgeon subject to documentation of medical necessity

93542   **Inject for heart x-rays**   ~ endoscopies or minor procedure - E/M services on the same day generally not paid, no payment adjustment rules for multiple procedures applypayment for assistant surgeon subject to documentation of medical necessity

93543   **Inject for heart x-rays**   ~ endoscopies or minor procedure - E/M services on the same day generally not paid, no payment adjustment rules for multiple procedures applypayment for assistant surgeon subject to documentation of medical necessity

93544   **Inject for aortography**   ~ endoscopies or minor procedure - E/M services on the same day generally not paid, no payment adjustment rules for multiple procedures applypayment for assistant surgeon subject to documentation of medical necessity

93545   **Inject for coronary x-rays**   ~ endoscopies or minor procedure - E/M services on the same day generally not paid, no payment adjustment rules for multiple procedures applypayment for assistant surgeon subject to documentation of medical necessity

93555 **Imaging, cardiac cath** ~ no payment adjustment rules for multiple procedures applypayment for assistant surgeon subject to documentation of medical necessity

93556 **Imaging, cardiac cath** ~ no payment adjustment rules for multiple procedures applypayment for assistant surgeon subject to documentation of medical necessity

93561 **Cardiac output measurement** ~ endoscopies or minor procedure - E/M services on the same day generally not paid, no payment adjustment rules for multiple procedures applypayment for assistant surgeon subject to documentation of medical necessity

93562 **Cardiac output measurement** ~ endoscopies or minor procedure - E/M services on the same day generally not paid, no payment adjustment rules for multiple procedures applypayment for assistant surgeon subject to documentation of medical necessity

93571 **Heart flow reserve measure** ~ follow-up period included in another service, no payment adjustment rules for multiple procedures applypayment for assistant surgeon subject to documentation of medical necessity

93572 **Heart flow reserve measure** ~ follow-up period included in another service, no payment adjustment rules for multiple procedures applypayment for assistant surgeon subject to documentation of medical necessity

93580 **Transcatheter closure asd** ~ endoscopies or minor procedure - E/M services on the same day generally not paid, standard payment adjustment rules for multiple procedures applypayment for assistant surgeon subject to documentation of medical necessity

93581 **Transcatheter closure vsd** ~ endoscopies or minor procedure - E/M services on the same day generally not paid, standard payment adjustment rules for multiple procedures applypayment for assistant surgeon subject to documentation of medical necessity

93600 **Bundle of his recording** ~ endoscopies or minor procedure - E/M services on the same day generally not paid, no payment adjustment rules for multiple procedures applypayment for assistant surgeon subject to documentation of medical necessity

93602 **Intra-atrial recording** ~ endoscopies or minor procedure - E/M services on the same day generally not paid, no payment adjustment rules for multiple procedures applypayment for assistant surgeon subject to documentation of medical necessity

93603   **Right ventricular recording**   ~ endoscopies or minor procedure - E/M services on the same day generally not paid, no payment adjustment rules for multiple procedures applypayment for assistant surgeon subject to documentation of medical necessity

93609   **Map tachycardia, add-on**   ~ follow-up period included in another service, no payment adjustment rules for multiple procedures applypayment for assistant surgeon subject to documentation of medical necessity, +add-on code (list separately in addition to primary procedure)

93610   **Intra-atrial pacing**   ~ endoscopies or minor procedure - E/M services on the same day generally not paid, no payment adjustment rules for multiple procedures applypayment for assistant surgeon subject to documentation of medical necessity

93612   **Intraventricular pacing**   ~ endoscopies or minor procedure - E/M services on the same day generally not paid, no payment adjustment rules for multiple procedures applypayment for assistant surgeon subject to documentation of medical necessity

93613   **Electrophys map 3d, add-on**   ~ follow-up period included in another service, no payment adjustment rules for multiple procedures applypayment for assistant surgeon subject to documentation of medical necessity, +add-on code (list separately in addition to primary procedure)

93615   **Esophageal recording**   ~ endoscopies or minor procedure - E/M services on the same day generally not paid, no payment adjustment rules for multiple procedures applypayment for assistant surgeon subject to documentation of medical necessity

93616   **Esophageal recording**   ~ endoscopies or minor procedure - E/M services on the same day generally not paid, no payment adjustment rules for multiple procedures applypayment for assistant surgeon subject to documentation of medical necessity

93618   **Heart rhythm pacing**   ~ endoscopies or minor procedure - E/M services on the same day generally not paid, no payment adjustment rules for multiple procedures applypayment for assistant surgeon subject to documentation of medical necessity

93619   **Electrophysiology evaluation**   ~ endoscopies or minor procedure - E/M services on the same day generally not paid, no payment adjustment rules for multiple procedures applypayment for assistant surgeon subject to documentation of medical necessity

93620   **Electrophysiology evaluation**   ~ endoscopies or minor procedure - E/M services on the same day generally not paid, no payment adjustment rules for multiple

procedures applypayment for assistant surgeon subject to documentation of medical necessity

93621   **Electrophysiology evaluation**   ~ follow-up period included in another service, no payment adjustment rules for multiple procedures applypayment for assistant surgeon subject to documentation of medical necessity

93622   **Electrophysiology evaluation**   ~ follow-up period included in another service, no payment adjustment rules for multiple procedures applypayment for assistant surgeon subject to documentation of medical necessity

93623   **Stimulation, pacing heart**   ~ follow-up period included in another service, no payment adjustment rules for multiple procedures applypayment for assistant surgeon subject to documentation of medical necessity

93624   **Electrophysiologic study**   ~ endoscopies or minor procedure - E/M services on the same day generally not paid, no payment adjustment rules for multiple procedures applypayment for assistant surgeon subject to documentation of medical necessity

93631   **Heart pacing, mapping**   ~ endoscopies or minor procedure - E/M services on the same day generally not paid, no payment adjustment rules for multiple procedures applypayment for assistant surgeon subject to documentation of medical necessity

93640   **Evaluation heart device**   ~ endoscopies or minor procedure - E/M services on the same day generally not paid, no payment adjustment rules for multiple procedures applypayment for assistant surgeon subject to documentation of medical necessity

93641   **Electrophysiology evaluation**   ~ endoscopies or minor procedure - E/M services on the same day generally not paid, no payment adjustment rules for multiple procedures applypayment for assistant surgeon subject to documentation of medical necessity

93642   **Electrophysiology evaluation**   ~ endoscopies or minor procedure - E/M services on the same day generally not paid, no payment adjustment rules for multiple procedures applypayment for assistant surgeon subject to documentation of medical necessity

93650   **Ablate heart dysrhythm focus**   ~ endoscopies or minor procedure - E/M services on the same day generally not paid, no payment adjustment rules for multiple procedures applypayment for assistant surgeon subject to documentation of medical necessity

93651   **Ablate heart dysrhythm focus**   ~ endoscopies or minor procedure - E/M services on the same day generally not paid, no payment adjustment rules for multiple

procedures applypayment for assistant surgeon subject to documentation of medical necessity

93652   **Ablate heart dysrhythm focus**   ~ endoscopies or minor procedure - E/M services on the same day generally not paid, no payment adjustment rules for multiple procedures applypayment for assistant surgeon subject to documentation of medical necessity

93660   **Tilt table evaluation**   ~ endoscopies or minor procedure - E/M services on the same day generally not paid, no payment adjustment rules for multiple procedures applypayment for assistant surgeon subject to documentation of medical necessity

93662   **Intracardiac ECG (ice)**   ~ follow-up period included in another service, no payment adjustment rules for multiple procedures applypayment for assistant surgeon subject to documentation of medical necessity

93668   **Peripheral vascular rehab**   ~ non-covered service, multiple procedure concept does not apply, bilateral surgery concept does not apply, assistant surgery concept does not apply

93701   **Bioimpedance, thoracic**   ~ no payment adjustment rules for multiple procedures applypayment for assistant surgeon subject to documentation of medical necessity

93720   **Total body plethysmography**   ~ no payment adjustment rules for multiple procedures applypayment for assistant surgeon subject to documentation of medical necessity

93721   **Plethysmography tracing**   ~ no payment adjustment rules for multiple procedures applypayment for assistant surgeon subject to documentation of medical necessity

93722   **Plethysmography report**   ~ no payment adjustment rules for multiple procedures applypayment for assistant surgeon subject to documentation of medical necessity

93724   **Analyze pacemaker system**   ~ endoscopies or minor procedure - E/M services on the same day generally not paid, no payment adjustment rules for multiple procedures applypayment for assistant surgeon subject to documentation of medical necessity

93727   **Analyze ilr system**   ~ multiple procedure concept does not apply, assistant surgery concept does not apply

93731   **Analyze pacemaker system**   ~ no payment adjustment rules for multiple procedures apply

93732   **Analyze pacemaker system**   ~ no payment adjustment rules for multiple
procedures apply

93733   **Telephone analysis, pacemaker**   ~ no payment adjustment rules for multiple
procedures apply

93734   **Analyze pacemaker system**   ~ no payment adjustment rules for multiple
procedures apply

93735   **Analyze pacemaker system**   ~ no payment adjustment rules for multiple
procedures apply

93736   **Telephonic analysis, pacemaker**   ~ no payment adjustment rules for multiple
procedures apply

93740   **Temperature gradient studies**   ~ bundled code - no separate payment made,
multiple procedure concept does not apply, bilateral surgery concept does not apply,
assistant surgery concept does not apply

93741   **Analyze heart pace device single**   ~ multiple procedure concept does not apply,
bilateral surgery concept does not apply, assistant surgery concept does not apply

93742   **Analyze heart pace device single**   ~ multiple procedure concept does not apply,
bilateral surgery concept does not apply, assistant surgery concept does not apply

93743   **Analyze heart pace device dual**   ~ multiple procedure concept does not apply,
bilateral surgery concept does not apply, assistant surgery concept does not apply

93744   **Analyze heart pace device dual**   ~ multiple procedure concept does not apply,
bilateral surgery concept does not apply, assistant surgery concept does not apply

93745   **Set-up cardiovert-defibrill**   ~ no payment adjustment rules for multiple
procedures apply

93760   **Cephalic thermogram**   ~ non-covered service, multiple procedure
concept does not apply, bilateral surgery concept does not apply, assistant surgery concept
does not apply

93762   **Peripheral thermogram**   ~ non-covered service, multiple procedure
concept does not apply, bilateral surgery concept does not apply, assistant surgery concept
does not apply

93770   **Measure venous pressure**   ~ bundled code - no separate payment made,
multiple procedure concept does not apply, bilateral surgery concept does not apply,
assistant surgery concept does not apply

93784	**Ambulatory bp monitoring** procedures apply	~ no payment adjustment rules for multiple
93786	**Ambulatory bp recording** procedures apply	~ no payment adjustment rules for multiple
93788	**Ambulatory bp analysis** procedures apply	~ no payment adjustment rules for multiple
93790	**Review/report bp recording** procedures apply	~ no payment adjustment rules for multiple
93797	**Cardiac rehab** services on the same day generally not paid, no payment adjustment rules for multiple procedures apply	~ endoscopies or minor procedure - E/M
93798	**Cardiac rehab/monitor** services on the same day generally not paid, no payment adjustment rules for multiple procedures apply	~ endoscopies or minor procedure - E/M
93799	**Unlisted cardiovascular procedure** procedures applypayment for assistant surgeon subject to documentation of medical necessity	~ no payment adjustment rules for multiple

Noninvasive Vascular Diagnostic Studies

93875	**Extracranial study** procedures apply, 150% payment adjustment does not apply - RVUs based on bilateral procedure	~ no payment adjustment rules for multiple
93880	**Extracranial study** procedures apply, 150% payment adjustment does not apply - RVUs based on bilateral procedure	~ no payment adjustment rules for multiple
93882	**Extracranial study** procedures apply	~ no payment adjustment rules for multiple
93886	**Intracranial study** procedures apply	~ no payment adjustment rules for multiple
93888	**Intracranial study** procedures apply	~ no payment adjustment rules for multiple
93890	**TCD, vasoreactivity study** procedures apply	~ no payment adjustment rules for multiple

93892 **TCD, emboli detect w/o inject** ~ no payment adjustment rules for multiple
procedures apply

93893 **TCD, emboli detect w/inject** ~ no payment adjustment rules for multiple
procedures apply

93922 **Extremity study** ~ no payment adjustment rules for multiple
procedures apply, 150% payment adjustment does not apply - RVUs based on bilateral
procedure

93923 **Extremity study** ~ no payment adjustment rules for multiple
procedures apply, 150% payment adjustment does not apply - RVUs based on bilateral
procedure

93924 **Extremity study** ~ no payment adjustment rules for multiple
procedures apply, 150% payment adjustment does not apply - RVUs based on bilateral
procedure

93925 **Lower extremity study** ~ no payment adjustment rules for multiple
procedures apply, 150% payment adjustment does not apply - RVUs based on bilateral
procedure

93926 **Lower extremity study** ~ no payment adjustment rules for multiple
procedures apply

93930 **Upper extremity study** ~ no payment adjustment rules for multiple
procedures apply, 150% payment adjustment does not apply - RVUs based on bilateral
procedure

93931 **Upper extremity study** ~ no payment adjustment rules for multiple
procedures apply

93965 **Extremity study** ~ no payment adjustment rules for multiple
procedures apply, 150% payment adjustment does not apply - RVUs based on bilateral
procedure

93970 **Extremity study** ~ no payment adjustment rules for multiple
procedures apply, 150% payment adjustment does not apply - RVUs based on bilateral
procedure

93971 **Extremity study** ~ no payment adjustment rules for multiple
procedures apply

93975 **Vascular study** ~ no payment adjustment rules for multiple
procedures apply

| 93976 | **Vascular study** procedures apply | ~ no payment adjustment rules for multiple |

| 93978 | **Vascular study** procedures apply | ~ no payment adjustment rules for multiple |

| 93979 | **Vascular study** procedures apply | ~ no payment adjustment rules for multiple |

| 93980 | **Penile vascular study** procedures apply | ~ no payment adjustment rules for multiple |

| 93981 | **Penile vascular study** procedures apply | ~ no payment adjustment rules for multiple |

| 93990 | **Doppler flow testing** procedures apply | ~ no payment adjustment rules for multiple |

Pulmonary

| 94002 | **Ventilation management inpat, initial day** procedures apply | ~ no payment adjustment rules for multiple |

| 94003 | **Ventilation management inpat, added day** procedures apply | ~ no payment adjustment rules for multiple |

| 94004 | **Ventilation management nurse fac, per day** procedures apply | ~ no payment adjustment rules for multiple |

| 94005 | **Home ventilation management supervision** ~ bundled code - no separate payment made, multiple procedure concept does not apply, bilateral surgery concept does not apply, assistant surgery concept does not apply |

| 94010 | **Breathing capacity test** procedures apply | ~ no payment adjustment rules for multiple |

| 94014 | **Patient recorded spirometry** procedures apply | ~ no payment adjustment rules for multiple |

| 94015 | **Patient recorded spirometry** procedures apply | ~ no payment adjustment rules for multiple |

| 94016 | **Review patient spirometry** procedures apply | ~ no payment adjustment rules for multiple |

| 94060 | **Evaluation of wheezing** procedures apply | ~ no payment adjustment rules for multiple |

94070   **Evaluation of wheezing**   ~ no payment adjustment rules for multiple
procedures apply

94150   **Vital capacity test**   ~ bundled code - no separate payment made,
multiple procedure concept does not apply, bilateral surgery concept does not apply,
assistant surgery concept does not apply

94200   **Lung function test (mbc/mvv)**   ~ no payment adjustment rules for multiple
procedures apply

94240   **Residual lung capacity**   ~ no payment adjustment rules for multiple
procedures apply

94250   **Expired gas collection**   ~ no payment adjustment rules for multiple
procedures apply

94260   **Thoracic gas volume**   ~ no payment adjustment rules for multiple
procedures apply

94350   **Lung nitrogen washout curve**   ~ no payment adjustment rules for multiple
procedures apply

94360   **Measure airflow resistance**   ~ no payment adjustment rules for multiple
procedures apply

94370   **Breath airway closing volume**   ~ no payment adjustment rules for multiple
procedures apply

94375   **Respiratory flow volume loop**   ~ no payment adjustment rules for multiple
procedures apply

94400   **C02 breathing response curve**   ~ no payment adjustment rules for multiple
procedures apply

94450   **Hypoxia response curve**   ~ no payment adjustment rules for multiple
procedures apply

94452   **Hast w/report**   ~ no payment adjustment rules for multiple
procedures apply

94453   **Hast w/oxygen titrate**   ~ no payment adjustment rules for multiple
procedures apply

94610   **Surfactant admin thru tube**   ~ no payment adjustment rules for multiple
procedures apply

94620   **Pulmonary stress test/simple**   ~ no payment adjustment rules for multiple
              procedures apply

94621   **Pulmonary stress test/complex**   ~ no payment adjustment rules for multiple
              procedures apply

94640   **Airway inhalation treatment**   ~ no payment adjustment rules for multiple
              procedures apply

94642   **Aerosol inhalation treatment**   ~ no payment adjustment rules for multiple
              procedures apply

94644   **Cbt, 1st hour**   ~ no payment adjustment rules for multiple
              procedures apply

94645   **Cbt, each added hour**   ~ no payment adjustment rules for multiple
              procedures apply, +add-on code (list separately in addition to primary procedure)

94660   **Pos airway pressure, cpap**   ~ no payment adjustment rules for multiple
              procedures apply

94662   **Neg press ventilation, cnp**   ~ no payment adjustment rules for multiple
              procedures apply

94664   **Evaluate pt use of inhaler**   ~ no payment adjustment rules for multiple
              procedures apply

94667   **Chest wall manipulation**   ~ no payment adjustment rules for multiple
              procedures apply

94668   **Chest wall manipulation**   ~ no payment adjustment rules for multiple
              procedures apply

94680   **Exhaled air analysis, O2**   ~ no payment adjustment rules for multiple
              procedures apply

94681   **Exhaled air analysis, O2/CO2**   ~ no payment adjustment rules for multiple
              procedures apply

94690   **Exhaled air analysis**   ~ no payment adjustment rules for multiple
              procedures apply

94720   **Monoxide diffusing capacity**   ~ no payment adjustment rules for multiple
              procedures apply

94725   **Membrane diffuse capacity**   ~ no payment adjustment rules for multiple
              procedures apply

94750	**Pulmonary compliance study** procedures apply	~ no payment adjustment rules for multiple
94760	**Measure blood oxygen level** procedures apply	~ no payment adjustment rules for multiple
94761	**Measure blood oxygen level** procedures apply	~ no payment adjustment rules for multiple
94762	**Measure blood oxygen level** procedures apply	~ no payment adjustment rules for multiple
94770	**Exhaled carbon dioxide test** procedures apply	~ no payment adjustment rules for multiple
94772	**Breath recording, infant** procedures apply	~ no payment adjustment rules for multiple
94774	**Ped home apnea rec, complete** no payment adjustment rules for multiple procedures apply	~ medicare carrier determines global period,
94775	**Ped home apnea rec, hook-up** no payment adjustment rules for multiple procedures apply	~ medicare carrier determines global period,
94776	**Ped home apnea rec, download** no payment adjustment rules for multiple procedures apply	~ medicare carrier determines global period,
94777	**Ped home apnea rec, report** no payment adjustment rules for multiple procedures apply	~ medicare carrier determines global period,
94799	**Pulmonary service/procedure** procedures apply	~ no payment adjustment rules for multiple

Allergy And Clinical Immunology

95004	**Percutaneous allergy skin tests** procedures apply	~ no payment adjustment rules for multiple
95010	**Percutaneous allergy titrate test** procedures apply	~ no payment adjustment rules for multiple
95012	**Exhaled nitric oxide measure** procedures apply	~ no payment adjustment rules for multiple
95015	**Intradermal allergy titrate-drug/bug** procedures apply	~ no payment adjustment rules for multiple

95024   **Intradermal allergy test, drug/bug**   ~ no payment adjustment rules for multiple
procedures apply

95027   **Intradermal allergy titrate-airborne**   ~ no payment adjustment rules for multiple
procedures apply

95028   **Intradermal allergy test-delayed type**   ~ no payment adjustment rules for multiple
procedures apply

95044   **Allergy patch tests**   ~ no payment adjustment rules for multiple
procedures apply

95052   **Photo patch test**   ~ no payment adjustment rules for multiple
procedures apply

95056   **Photosensitivity tests**   ~ no payment adjustment rules for multiple
procedures apply

95060   **Eye allergy tests**   ~ no payment adjustment rules for multiple
procedures apply

95065   **Nose allergy test**   ~ no payment adjustment rules for multiple
procedures apply

95070   **Bronchial allergy tests**   ~ no payment adjustment rules for multiple
procedures apply

95071   **Bronchial allergy tests**   ~ no payment adjustment rules for multiple
procedures apply

95075   **Ingestion challenge test**   ~ no payment adjustment rules for multiple
procedures apply

95115   **Immunotherapy, one injection**   ~ no payment adjustment rules for multiple
procedures apply

95117   **Immunotherapy injections**   ~ no payment adjustment rules for multiple
procedures apply

95120   **Immunotherapy, one injection**   ~ not valid for Medicare, multiple procedure
concept does not apply, bilateral surgery concept does not apply, assistant surgery concept
does not apply

95125   **Immunotherapy, many antigens**   ~ not valid for Medicare, multiple procedure
concept does not apply, bilateral surgery concept does not apply, assistant surgery concept
does not apply

95130 **Immunotherapy, insect venom** ~ not valid for Medicare, multiple procedure concept does not apply, bilateral surgery concept does not apply, assistant surgery concept does not apply

95131 **Immunotherapy, insect venoms** ~ not valid for Medicare, multiple procedure concept does not apply, bilateral surgery concept does not apply, assistant surgery concept does not apply

95132 **Immunotherapy, insect venoms** ~ not valid for Medicare, multiple procedure concept does not apply, bilateral surgery concept does not apply, assistant surgery concept does not apply

95133 **Immunotherapy, insect venoms** ~ not valid for Medicare, multiple procedure concept does not apply, bilateral surgery concept does not apply, assistant surgery concept does not apply

95134 **Immunotherapy, insect venoms** ~ not valid for Medicare, multiple procedure concept does not apply, bilateral surgery concept does not apply, assistant surgery concept does not apply

95144 **Antigen therapy services** ~ no payment adjustment rules for multiple procedures apply

95145 **Antigen therapy services** ~ no payment adjustment rules for multiple procedures apply

95146 **Antigen therapy services** ~ no payment adjustment rules for multiple procedures apply

95147 **Antigen therapy services** ~ no payment adjustment rules for multiple procedures apply

95148 **Antigen therapy services** ~ no payment adjustment rules for multiple procedures apply

95149 **Antigen therapy services** ~ no payment adjustment rules for multiple procedures apply

95165 **Antigen therapy services** ~ no payment adjustment rules for multiple procedures apply

95170 **Antigen therapy services** ~ no payment adjustment rules for multiple procedures apply

95180 **Rapid desensitization** ~ no payment adjustment rules for multiple procedures apply

| 95199 | Allergy immunology services procedures apply | ~ no payment adjustment rules for multiple |

Endocrinology

| 95250 | Glucose monitoring, cont procedures apply | ~ no payment adjustment rules for multiple |
| 95251 | Glucose monitor, cont, phys i & r procedures apply | ~ no payment adjustment rules for multiple |

Neurology And Neuromuscular Procedures

95805	Multiple sleep latency test procedures apply	~ no payment adjustment rules for multiple
95806	Sleep study, unattended procedures apply	~ no payment adjustment rules for multiple
95807	Sleep study, attended procedures apply	~ no payment adjustment rules for multiple
95808	Polysomnography, 1-3 procedures apply	~ no payment adjustment rules for multiple
95810	Polysomnography, 4 or more procedures apply	~ no payment adjustment rules for multiple
95811	Polysomnography w/cpap procedures apply	~ no payment adjustment rules for multiple
95812	EEG, 41-60 minutes procedures apply	~ no payment adjustment rules for multiple
95813	EEG, over 1 hour procedures apply	~ no payment adjustment rules for multiple
95816	EEG, awake and drowsy procedures apply	~ no payment adjustment rules for multiple
95819	EEG, awake and asleep procedures apply	~ no payment adjustment rules for multiple
95822	EEG, coma or sleep only procedures apply	~ no payment adjustment rules for multiple

95824	EEG, cerebral death only procedures apply	~ no payment adjustment rules for multiple
95827	EEG, all night recording procedures apply	~ no payment adjustment rules for multiple
95829	Surgery electrocorticogram procedures apply	~ no payment adjustment rules for multiple
95830	Insert electrodes for EEG procedures apply	~ no payment adjustment rules for multiple
95831	Limb muscle testing, manual procedures apply	~ no payment adjustment rules for multiple
95832	Hand muscle testing, manual procedures apply	~ no payment adjustment rules for multiple
95833	Body muscle testing, manual procedures apply	~ no payment adjustment rules for multiple
95834	Body muscle testing, manual procedures apply	~ no payment adjustment rules for multiple
95851	Range of motion measurements procedures apply	~ no payment adjustment rules for multiple
95852	Range of motion measurements procedures apply	~ no payment adjustment rules for multiple
95857	Tensilon test procedures apply	~ no payment adjustment rules for multiple
95860	Muscle test, one limb procedures apply	~ no payment adjustment rules for multiple
95861	Muscle test, 2 limbs procedures apply	~ no payment adjustment rules for multiple
95863	Muscle test, 3 limbs procedures apply	~ no payment adjustment rules for multiple
95864	Muscle test, 4 limbs procedures apply	~ no payment adjustment rules for multiple

95865   **Muscle test, larynx**   ~ no payment adjustment rules for multiple procedures apply, 150% payment adjustment does not apply - RVUs based on bilateral procedure

95866   **Muscle test, hemidiaphragm**   ~ no payment adjustment rules for multiple procedures apply, 150% payment adjustment for bilateral procedures applies

95867   **Muscle test cranial nerve unilat**   ~ no payment adjustment rules for multiple procedures apply

95868   **Muscle test cranial nerve bilat**   ~ no payment adjustment rules for multiple procedures apply, 150% payment adjustment does not apply - RVUs based on bilateral procedure

95869   **Muscle test, thor paraspinal**   ~ no payment adjustment rules for multiple procedures apply

95870   **Muscle test, nonparaspinal**   ~ no payment adjustment rules for multiple procedures apply

95872   **Muscle test, one fiber**   ~ no payment adjustment rules for multiple procedures apply

95873   **Guide nerve destroy, elect stim**   ~ follow-up period included in another service, no payment adjustment rules for multiple procedures apply

95874   **Guide nerve destroy, needle emg**   ~ follow-up period included in another service, no payment adjustment rules for multiple procedures apply

95875   **Limb exercise test**   ~ no payment adjustment rules for multiple procedures apply

95900   **Motor nerve conduction test**   ~ no payment adjustment rules for multiple procedures apply

95903   **Motor nerve conduction test**   ~ no payment adjustment rules for multiple procedures apply

95904   **Sense nerve conduction test**   ~ no payment adjustment rules for multiple procedures apply

95920   **Intraop nerve test, add-on**   ~ follow-up period included in another service, no payment adjustment rules for multiple procedures apply, +add-on code (list separately in addition to primary procedure)

95921   **Autonomic nerve function test**   ~ no payment adjustment rules for multiple procedures apply

95922 **Autonomic nerve function test**   ~ no payment adjustment rules for multiple
procedures apply

95923 **Autonomic nerve function test**   ~ no payment adjustment rules for multiple
procedures apply

95925 **Somatosensory testing**   ~ no payment adjustment rules for multiple
procedures apply, 150% payment adjustment does not apply - RVUs based on bilateral
procedure

95926 **Somatosensory testing**   ~ no payment adjustment rules for multiple
procedures apply, 150% payment adjustment does not apply - RVUs based on bilateral
procedure

95927 **Somatosensory testing**   ~ no payment adjustment rules for multiple
procedures apply

95928 **C motor evoked, upper limbs**   ~ no payment adjustment rules for multiple
procedures apply

95929 **C motor evoked, lower limbs**   ~ no payment adjustment rules for multiple
procedures apply

95930 **Visual evoked potential test**   ~ no payment adjustment rules for multiple
procedures apply, 150% payment adjustment does not apply - RVUs based on bilateral
procedure

95933 **Blink reflex test**   ~ no payment adjustment rules for multiple
procedures apply

95934 **H-reflex test**   ~ no payment adjustment rules for multiple
procedures apply, 150% payment adjustment for bilateral procedures applies

95936 **H-reflex test**   ~ no payment adjustment rules for multiple
procedures apply, 150% payment adjustment for bilateral procedures applies

95937 **Neuromuscular junction test**   ~ no payment adjustment rules for multiple
procedures apply

95950 **Ambulatory EEG monitoring**   ~ no payment adjustment rules for multiple
procedures apply

95951 **EEG monitoring/video record**   ~ no payment adjustment rules for multiple
procedures apply

95953 **EEG monitoring/computer**   ~ no payment adjustment rules for multiple
procedures apply

95954	**EEG monitoring/giving drugs** procedures apply	~ no payment adjustment rules for multiple

95955	**EEG during surgery** procedures apply	~ no payment adjustment rules for multiple

95956	**EEG monitoring, cable/radio** procedures apply	~ no payment adjustment rules for multiple

95957	**EEG digital analysis** procedures apply	~ no payment adjustment rules for multiple

95958	**EEG monitoring/function test** procedures apply	~ no payment adjustment rules for multiple

95961	**Electrode stimulation, brain** procedures apply	~ no payment adjustment rules for multiple

95962   **Electrode stim, brain, add-on**   ~ follow-up period included in another service, no payment adjustment rules for multiple procedures apply, +add-on code (list separately in addition to primary procedure)

95965	**Meg, spontaneous** procedures apply	~ no payment adjustment rules for multiple

95966	**Meg, evoked, single** procedures apply	~ no payment adjustment rules for multiple

95967   **Meg, evoked, each added**   ~ follow-up period included in another service, no payment adjustment rules for multiple procedures apply, +add-on code (list separately in addition to primary procedure)

95970	**Analyze neurostim, no prog** procedures apply	~ no payment adjustment rules for multiple

95971	**Analyze neurostim, simple** procedures apply	~ no payment adjustment rules for multiple

95972	**Analyze neurostim, complex** procedures apply	~ no payment adjustment rules for multiple

95973   **Analyze neurostim, complex**   ~ follow-up period included in another service, no payment adjustment rules for multiple procedures apply

95974	**Cranial neurostim, complex** procedures apply	~ no payment adjustment rules for multiple

95975   **Cranial neurostim, complex**   ~ follow-up period included in another service, no payment adjustment rules for multiple procedures apply

95978   **Analyze neurostim brain/1h**   ~ no payment adjustment rules for multiple procedures apply

95979   **Analyze neurostim brain, add-on**   ~ follow-up period included in another service, no payment adjustment rules for multiple procedures apply, +add-on code (list separately in addition to primary procedure)

95990   **Spin/brain pump refill & main**   ~ no payment adjustment rules for multiple procedures apply

95991   **Spin/brain pump refill & main**   ~ no payment adjustment rules for multiple procedures apply

95999   **Neurological procedure**   ~ no payment adjustment rules for multiple procedures apply

96000   **Motion analysis, video/3d**   ~ no payment adjustment rules for multiple procedures apply, 150% payment adjustment does not apply - RVUs based on bilateral procedure

96001   **Motion test w/ft press measure**   ~ no payment adjustment rules for multiple procedures apply, 150% payment adjustment does not apply - RVUs based on bilateral procedure

96002   **Dynamic surface emg**   ~ no payment adjustment rules for multiple procedures apply, 150% payment adjustment does not apply - RVUs based on bilateral procedure

96003   **Dynamic fine wire emg**   ~ no payment adjustment rules for multiple procedures apply, 150% payment adjustment does not apply - RVUs based on bilateral procedure

96004   **Phys review of motion tests**   ~ no payment adjustment rules for multiple procedures apply, 150% payment adjustment does not apply - RVUs based on bilateral procedure

96020   **Functional brain mapping**   ~ no payment adjustment rules for multiple procedures apply

Medical Genetics And Genetic Counseling Services

96040   **Genetic counseling, 30 min**   ~ bundled code - no separate payment made, multiple procedure concept does not apply

Central Nervous System Assessments/Tests

96101	Psychological testing by psych/phys procedures apply	~ no payment adjustment rules for multiple
96102	Psychological testing by technician procedures apply	~ no payment adjustment rules for multiple
96103	Psychological testing admin by comp procedures apply	~ no payment adjustment rules for multiple
96105	Assess aphasia procedures apply	~ no payment adjustment rules for multiple
96110	Developmental test, limited procedures apply	~ no payment adjustment rules for multiple
96111	Developmental test, extended procedures apply	~ no payment adjustment rules for multiple
96116	Neurobehavioral status exam procedures apply	~ no payment adjustment rules for multiple
96118	Neuropsych test by psych/phys procedures apply	~ no payment adjustment rules for multiple
96119	Neuropsych testing by tech procedures apply	~ no payment adjustment rules for multiple
96120	Neuropsych test admin w/comp procedures apply	~ no payment adjustment rules for multiple

Health And Behavior Assessment/Intervention

96150	Assess health/behave, initial procedures apply	~ no payment adjustment rules for multiple
96151	Assess health/behave, subseq procedures apply	~ no payment adjustment rules for multiple
96152	Intervene health/behave, individual procedures apply	~ no payment adjustment rules for multiple
96153	Intervene health/behave, group procedures apply	~ no payment adjustment rules for multiple
96154	Intervene health/behavior, family w/pat procedures apply	~ no payment adjustment rules for multiple

96155   **Intervene health/behavior family no pat** ~ non-covered service, multiple procedure concept does not apply, bilateral surgery concept does not apply, assistant surgery concept does not apply

Chemotherapy Administration

96401   **Chemotherapy anti-neoplasm, sq/im** ~ no payment adjustment rules for multiple procedures apply

96402   **Chemotherapy hormone antineoplastic sq/im** ~ no payment adjustment rules for multiple procedures apply

96405   **Chemotherapy intrales, up to 7 yrs** ~ endoscopies or minor procedure - E/M services on the same day generally not paid, standard payment adjustment rules for multiple procedures applyassistant surgeon may not be paid

96406   **Chemotherapy intrales over 7 yrs** ~ endoscopies or minor procedure - E/M services on the same day generally not paid, standard payment adjustment rules for multiple procedures applyassistant surgeon may not be paid

96409   **Chemotherapy iv push, single drug** ~ no payment adjustment rules for multiple procedures apply

96411   **Chemotherapy iv push, added drug** ~ follow-up period included in another service, no payment adjustment rules for multiple procedures apply, +add-on code (list separately in addition to primary procedure)

96413   **Chemotherapy iv infuse 1 hour** ~ no payment adjustment rules for multiple procedures apply

96415   **Chemotherapy iv infuse added hour** ~ follow-up period included in another service, no payment adjustment rules for multiple procedures apply, +add-on code (list separately in addition to primary procedure)

96416   **Chemotherapy prolong infuse w/pump** ~ no payment adjustment rules for multiple procedures apply

96417   **Chemotherapy iv infusion added seq** ~ follow-up period included in another service, no payment adjustment rules for multiple procedures apply, +add-on code (list separately in addition to primary procedure)

96420   **Chemotherapy ia, push technique** ~ no payment adjustment rules for multiple procedures apply

96422   **Chemotherapy ia infuse up to 1 hr** ~ no payment adjustment rules for multiple procedures apply

| 96423 | **Chemotherapy ia infuse added hr** | ~ follow-up period included in another service, no payment adjustment rules for multiple procedures apply, +add-on code (list separately in addition to primary procedure) |

| 96425 | **Chemotherapy, infuse method** | ~ no payment adjustment rules for multiple procedures apply |

| 96440 | **Chemotherapy, intracavitary** | ~ endoscopies or minor procedure - E/M services on the same day generally not paid, no payment adjustment rules for multiple procedures apply |

| 96445 | **Chemotherapy, intracavitary** | ~ endoscopies or minor procedure - E/M services on the same day generally not paid, no payment adjustment rules for multiple procedures apply |

| 96450 | **Chemotherapy, into cns** | ~ endoscopies or minor procedure - E/M services on the same day generally not paid, no payment adjustment rules for multiple procedures apply |

| 96521 | **Refill/maintain, portable pump** | ~ no payment adjustment rules for multiple procedures apply |

| 96522 | **Refill/maintain pump/reservoir system** | ~ no payment adjustment rules for multiple procedures apply |

| 96523 | **Irrigation drug delivery device** | T ~ no payment adjustment rules for multiple procedures apply |

| 96542 | **Chemotherapy injection** | ~ no payment adjustment rules for multiple procedures apply |

| 96549 | **Chemotherapy, unspecified** | ~ no payment adjustment rules for multiple procedures apply |

Photodynamic Therapy

| 96567 | **Photodynamic therapy, skin** | ~ no payment adjustment rules for multiple procedures apply |

| 96570 | **Photodynamic therapy, 30 min** | ~ no payment adjustment rules for multiple procedures apply |

| 96571 | **Photodynamic therapy, added 15 min** | ~ no payment adjustment rules for multiple procedures apply, +add-on code (list separately in addition to primary procedure) |

| 96900 | **Ultraviolet light therapy** | ~ no payment adjustment rules for multiple procedures apply |

96902   **Trichogram**   ~ bundled code - no separate payment made,
              multiple procedure concept does not apply

96904   **Whole body photography**   ~ restricted coverage - special coverage rules
              apply, no payment adjustment rules for multiple procedures apply

96910   **Photochemotherapy with uv-b**   ~ no payment adjustment rules for multiple
              procedures apply

96912   **Photochemotherapy with uv-a**   ~ no payment adjustment rules for multiple
              procedures apply

96913   **Photochemotherapy, uv-a or b**   ~ no payment adjustment rules for multiple
              procedures apply

96920   **Laser treatment, skin < 250 sq cm**   ~ endoscopies or minor procedure - E/M
              services on the same day generally not paid, standard payment adjustment rules for multiple
              procedures applyassistant surgeon may not be paid

96921   **Laser treatment, skin 250-500 sq cm**   ~ endoscopies or minor procedure - E/M
              services on the same day generally not paid, standard payment adjustment rules for multiple
              procedures applyassistant surgeon may not be paid

96922   **Laser treatment, skin > 500 sq cm**   ~ endoscopies or minor procedure - E/M
              services on the same day generally not paid, standard payment adjustment rules for multiple
              procedures applyassistant surgeon may not be paid

96999   **Dermatological procedure**   ~ no payment adjustment rules for multiple
              procedures apply

Physical Medicine And Rehabilitation

97001   **Physical therapy evaluation**   ~ no payment adjustment rules for multiple
              procedures apply

97002   **Physical therapy re-evaluation**   ~ no payment adjustment rules for multiple
              procedures apply

97003   **Occupational therapy evaluation**   ~ no payment adjustment rules for multiple
              procedures apply

97004   **Occupational therapy re-evaluation**   ~ no payment adjustment rules for multiple
              procedures apply

97005 **Athletic training evaluation** ~ not valid for Medicare, multiple procedure concept does not apply, bilateral surgery concept does not apply, assistant surgery concept does not apply

97006 **Athletic training reevaluation** ~ not valid for Medicare, multiple procedure concept does not apply, bilateral surgery concept does not apply, assistant surgery concept does not apply

97010 **Hot or cold packs therapy** ~ bundled code - no separate payment made, multiple procedure concept does not apply, bilateral surgery concept does not apply, assistant surgery concept does not apply

97012 **Mechanical traction therapy** ~ no payment adjustment rules for multiple procedures apply

97014 **Electric stimulation therapy** ~ not valid for Medicare, multiple procedure concept does not apply, bilateral surgery concept does not apply, assistant surgery concept does not apply

97016 **Vasopneumatic device therapy** ~ no payment adjustment rules for multiple procedures apply

97018 **Paraffin bath therapy** ~ no payment adjustment rules for multiple procedures apply

97022 **Whirlpool therapy** ~ no payment adjustment rules for multiple procedures apply

97024 **Diathermy eg, microwave** ~ no payment adjustment rules for multiple procedures apply

97026 **Infrared therapy** ~ no payment adjustment rules for multiple procedures apply

97028 **Ultraviolet therapy** ~ no payment adjustment rules for multiple procedures apply

97032 **Electrical stimulation** ~ no payment adjustment rules for multiple procedures apply

97033 **Electric current therapy** ~ no payment adjustment rules for multiple procedures apply

97034 **Contrast bath therapy** ~ no payment adjustment rules for multiple procedures apply

97035	**Ultrasound therapy** procedures apply	~ no payment adjustment rules for multiple
97036	**Hydrotherapy** procedures apply	~ no payment adjustment rules for multiple
97039	**Physical therapy treatment** procedures apply	~ no payment adjustment rules for multiple
97110	**Therapeutic exercises** procedures apply	~ no payment adjustment rules for multiple
97112	**Neuromuscular reeducation** procedures apply	~ no payment adjustment rules for multiple
97113	**Aquatic therapy/exercises** procedures apply	~ no payment adjustment rules for multiple
97116	**Gait training therapy** procedures apply	~ no payment adjustment rules for multiple
97124	**Massage therapy** procedures apply	~ no payment adjustment rules for multiple
97139	**Physical medicine procedure** procedures apply	~ no payment adjustment rules for multiple
97140	**Manual therapy** procedures apply	~ no payment adjustment rules for multiple
97150	**Group therapeutic procedures** procedures apply	~ no payment adjustment rules for multiple
97530	**Therapeutic activities** procedures apply	~ no payment adjustment rules for multiple
97532	**Cognitive skills development** procedures apply	~ no payment adjustment rules for multiple
97533	**Sensory integration** procedures apply	~ no payment adjustment rules for multiple
97535	**Self care management training** procedures apply	~ no payment adjustment rules for multiple
97537	**Community/work reintegration** procedures apply	~ no payment adjustment rules for multiple

| 97542 | **Wheelchair management training** procedures apply | ~ no payment adjustment rules for multiple |

97542 **Wheelchair management training** ~ no payment adjustment rules for multiple
procedures apply

97545 **Work hardening** ~ restricted coverage - special coverage rules
apply, no payment adjustment rules for multiple procedures apply

97546 **Work hardening, add-on** ~ restricted coverage - special coverage rules
apply, no payment adjustment rules for multiple procedures apply, +add-on code (list
separately in addition to primary procedure)

97597 **Active wound care/20 cm or <** ~ no payment adjustment rules for multiple
procedures apply

97598 **Active wound care > 20 cm** ~ no payment adjustment rules for multiple
procedures apply

97602 **Wound(s) care non-selective** ~ bundled code - no separate payment made,
multiple procedure concept does not apply, bilateral surgery concept does not apply,
assistant surgery concept does not apply

97605 **Neg press wound tx, < 50 cm** ~ no payment adjustment rules for multiple
procedures apply

97606 **Neg press wound tx, > 50 cm** ~ no payment adjustment rules for multiple
procedures apply

97750 **Physical performance test** ~ no payment adjustment rules for multiple
procedures apply

97755 **Assistive technology assess** ~ no payment adjustment rules for multiple
procedures apply

97760 **Orthotic mgmt and training** ~ no payment adjustment rules for multiple
procedures apply

97761 **Prosthetic training** ~ no payment adjustment rules for multiple
procedures apply

97762 **C/o for orthotic/prosth use** ~ no payment adjustment rules for multiple
procedures apply

97799 **Unlisted physical medicine procedure** ~ no payment adjustment rules for multiple
procedures apply

Medical Nutrition Therapy

97802   **Medical nutrition, individual, in**   ~ no payment adjustment rules for multiple
procedures apply

97803   **Medical nutrition, individual, subseq**   ~ no payment adjustment rules for multiple
procedures apply

97804   **Medical nutrition, group**   ~ no payment adjustment rules for multiple
procedures apply

Acupuncture

97810   **Acupuncture w/o stimuli 15 min**   ~ non-covered service, multiple procedure
concept does not apply

97811   **Acupuncture w/o stimuli added 15m**   ~ non-covered service, +add-on code (list
separately in addition to primary procedure)

97813   **Acupuncture w/stimuli 15 min**   ~ non-covered service, multiple procedure
concept does not apply

97814   **Acupuncture w/stimuli added 15 min**   ~ non-covered service, +add-on code (list
separately in addition to primary procedure)

Osteopathic Manipulation

98925   **Osteopathic manipulation; 1-2 regions**   ~ endoscopies or minor procedure - E/M
services on the same day generally not paid, no payment adjustment rules for multiple
procedures apply

98926   **Osteopathic manipulation; 3-4 regions**   ~ endoscopies or minor procedure - E/M
services on the same day generally not paid, no payment adjustment rules for multiple
procedures apply

98927   **Osteopathic manipulation; 5-6 regions**   ~ endoscopies or minor procedure - E/M
services on the same day generally not paid, no payment adjustment rules for multiple
procedures apply

98928   **Osteopathic manipulation; 7-8 regions**   ~ endoscopies or minor procedure - E/M
services on the same day generally not paid, no payment adjustment rules for multiple
procedures apply

98929   **Osteopathic manipulation; 9-10 regions**   ~ endoscopies or minor procedure - E/M
services on the same day generally not paid, no payment adjustment rules for multiple
procedures apply

Chiropractic Manipulation

98940 **Chiropractic manipulation; 1-2 regions** ~ endoscopies or minor procedure - E/M services on the same day generally not paid, no payment adjustment rules for multiple procedures apply

98941 **Chiropractic manipulation; 3-4 regions** ~ endoscopies or minor procedure - E/M services on the same day generally not paid, no payment adjustment rules for multiple procedures apply

98942 **Chiropractic manipulation; 5 regions** ~ endoscopies or minor procedure - E/M services on the same day generally not paid, no payment adjustment rules for multiple procedures apply

98943 **Chiropractic manipulation; 1+ regions** ~ non-covered service, multiple procedure concept does not apply

Education And Training For Patient Self Management

98960 **Self-managed educ & train, 1 pat** ~ bundled code - no separate payment made, multiple procedure concept does not apply, bilateral surgery concept does not apply, assistant surgery concept does not apply

98961 **Self-managed educ & train, 2-4 pat** ~ bundled code - no separate payment made, multiple procedure concept does not apply, bilateral surgery concept does not apply, assistant surgery concept does not apply

98962 **Self-managed educ & train, 5-8 pat** ~ bundled code - no separate payment made, multiple procedure concept does not apply, bilateral surgery concept does not apply, assistant surgery concept does not apply

Special Services, Procedures And Report

99000 **Specimen handling** ~ bundled code - no separate payment made, multiple procedure concept does not apply

99001 **Specimen handling** ~ bundled code - no separate payment made, multiple procedure concept does not apply

99002 **Device handling** ~ bundled code - no separate payment made, multiple procedure concept does not apply

99024 **Postop follow-up visit** ~ bundled code - no separate payment made, multiple procedure concept does not apply

99026 **In-hospital on call service** ~ non-covered service, multiple procedure concept does not apply

99027	**Out-of-hosp on call service** concept does not apply	~ non-covered service, multiple procedure
99050	**Medical services after hours** multiple procedure concept does not apply	~ bundled code - no separate payment made,
99051	**Medical service, eve/weekend/holiday** multiple procedure concept does not apply	~ bundled code - no separate payment made,
99053	**Medical service 10pm-8am, 24 hr fac** multiple procedure concept does not apply	~ bundled code - no separate payment made,
99056	**Medical service out of office** multiple procedure concept does not apply	~ bundled code - no separate payment made,
99058	**Office emergency care** multiple procedure concept does not apply	~ bundled code - no separate payment made,
99060	**Out of office emergency med service** multiple procedure concept does not apply	~ bundled code - no separate payment made,
99070	**Special supplies** multiple procedure concept does not apply	~ bundled code - no separate payment made,
99071	**Patient education materials** multiple procedure concept does not apply	~ bundled code - no separate payment made,
99075	**Medical testimony** concept does not apply	~ non-covered service, multiple procedure
99078	**Group health education** multiple procedure concept does not apply	~ bundled code - no separate payment made,
99080	**Special reports or forms** multiple procedure concept does not apply	~ bundled code - no separate payment made,
99082	**Unusual physician travel** procedures apply	~ no payment adjustment rules for multiple
99090	**Computer data analysis** multiple procedure concept does not apply	~ bundled code - no separate payment made,
99091	**Collect/review data from patient** multiple procedure concept does not apply	~ bundled code - no separate payment made,

Qualifying Circumstances For Anesthesia

99100   **Special anesthesia service**   ~ bundled code - no separate payment made,
follow-up period included in another service

99116   **Anesthesia with hypothermia**   ~ bundled code - no separate payment made,
follow-up period included in another service

99135   **Special anesthesia procedure**   ~ bundled code - no separate payment made,
follow-up period included in another service

99140   **Emergency anesthesia**   ~ bundled code - no separate payment made,
follow-up period included in another service

Moderate (Conscious) Sedation

99143   **Mod conscious sedation by same phys, < 5 yrs**
~ no payment adjustment rules for multiple procedures apply

99144   **Mod conscious sedation by same phys, 5 yrs +**
~ no payment adjustment rules for multiple procedures apply

99145   **Mod conscious sedation by same phys, add-on**
~ follow-up period included in another service, no payment adjustment rules for multiple
procedures apply, +add-on code (list separately in addition to primary procedure)

99148   **Mod conscious sedation diff phys < 5 yrs**
~ no payment adjustment rules for multiple procedures apply

99149   **Mod conscious sedation diff phys 5 yrs +**
~ no payment adjustment rules for multiple procedures apply

99150   **Mod conscious sedation diff phys, add-on**
~ follow-up period included in another service, no payment adjustment rules for multiple
procedures apply, +add-on code (list separately in addition to primary procedure)

Other Services And Procedures

99170   **Anogenital exam child**   ~ endoscopies or minor procedure - E/M
services on the same day generally not paid, standard payment adjustment rules for multiple
procedures apply

99172   **Ocular function screen**   ~ non-covered service, multiple procedure
concept does not apply

99173   **Visual acuity screen**   ~ non-covered service, multiple procedure
concept does not apply

99175	Induction of vomiting procedures apply	~ no payment adjustment rules for multiple
99183	Hyperbaric oxygen therapy procedures apply	~ no payment adjustment rules for multiple
99185	Regional hypothermia procedures apply	~ no payment adjustment rules for multiple
99186	Total body hypothermia procedures apply	~ no payment adjustment rules for multiple
99190	Special pump services; each hour	~ multiple procedure concept does not apply
99191	Special pump services; 45 minutes	~ multiple procedure concept does not apply
99192	Special pump services; 30 minutes	~ multiple procedure concept does not apply
99195	Phlebotomy procedures apply	~ no payment adjustment rules for multiple
99199	Unlisted special service/proc/report procedures apply	~ no payment adjustment rules for multiple

Home Health Procedures/Services

99500	Home visit, prenatal	~ not valid for Medicare
99501	Home visit, postnatal	~ not valid for Medicare
99502	Home visit, nb care	~ not valid for Medicare
99503	Home visit, respiratory therapy	~ not valid for Medicare
99504	Home visit mechanical ventilator	~ not valid for Medicare
99505	Home visit, stoma care	~ not valid for Medicare
99506	Home visit, im injection	~ not valid for Medicare
99507	Home visit, cath maintain	~ not valid for Medicare
99509	Home visit day life activity	~ not valid for Medicare
99510	Home visit, sing/m/family counsel	~ not valid for Medicare
99511	Home visit, fecal/enema mgmt	~ not valid for Medicare

99512	Home visit for hemodialysis	~ not valid for Medicare
99600	Home visit nos	~ not valid for Medicare
99601	Home infuse/visit, 2 hrs	~ not valid for Medicare
99602	Home infuse each added hr separately in addition to primary procedure)	~ not valid for Medicare, +add-on code (list

EVALUATION & MANAGEMENT

Office Or Other Outpatient Services

99201	Office/outpatient visit, new patient procedures apply	~ no payment adjustment rules for multiple
99202	Office/outpatient visit, new patient procedures apply	~ no payment adjustment rules for multiple
99203	Office/outpatient visit, new patient procedures apply	~ no payment adjustment rules for multiple
99204	Office/outpatient visit, new patient procedures apply	~ no payment adjustment rules for multiple
99205	Office/outpatient visit, new patient procedures apply	~ no payment adjustment rules for multiple
99211	Office/outpatient visit, est patient procedures apply	~ no payment adjustment rules for multiple
99212	Office/outpatient visit, est patient procedures apply	~ no payment adjustment rules for multiple
99213	Office/outpatient visit, est patient procedures apply	~ no payment adjustment rules for multiple
99214	Office/outpatient visit, est patient procedures apply	~ no payment adjustment rules for multiple
99215	Office/outpatient visit, est patient procedures apply	~ no payment adjustment rules for multiple

Hospital Observation Services

99217	**Observation care discharge** procedures apply	~ no payment adjustment rules for multiple
99218	**Observation care** procedures apply	~ no payment adjustment rules for multiple
99219	**Observation care** procedures apply	~ no payment adjustment rules for multiple
99220	**Observation care** procedures apply	~ no payment adjustment rules for multiple

Hospital Inpatient Services

99221	**Initial hospital care** procedures apply	~ no payment adjustment rules for multiple
99222	**Initial hospital care** procedures apply	~ no payment adjustment rules for multiple
99223	**Initial hospital care** procedures apply	~ no payment adjustment rules for multiple
99231	**Subsequent hospital care** procedures apply	~ no payment adjustment rules for multiple
99232	**Subsequent hospital care** procedures apply	~ no payment adjustment rules for multiple
99233	**Subsequent hospital care** procedures apply	~ no payment adjustment rules for multiple
99234	**Observe/hosp same date** procedures apply	~ no payment adjustment rules for multiple
99235	**Observe/hosp same date** procedures apply	~ no payment adjustment rules for multiple
99236	**Observe/hosp same date** procedures apply	~ no payment adjustment rules for multiple
99238	**Hospital discharge day** procedures apply	~ no payment adjustment rules for multiple

99239   **Hospital discharge day**
         procedures apply

~ no payment adjustment rules for multiple

Consultations

99241   **Office consultation**
         procedures apply

~ no payment adjustment rules for multiple

99242   **Office consultation**
         procedures apply

~ no payment adjustment rules for multiple

99243   **Office consultation**
         procedures apply

~ no payment adjustment rules for multiple

99244   **Office consultation**
         procedures apply

~ no payment adjustment rules for multiple

99245   **Office consultation**
         procedures apply

~ no payment adjustment rules for multiple

99251   **Inpatient consultation**
         procedures apply

~ no payment adjustment rules for multiple

99252   **Inpatient consultation**
         procedures apply

~ no payment adjustment rules for multiple

99253   **Inpatient consultation**
         procedures apply

~ no payment adjustment rules for multiple

99254   **Inpatient consultation**
         procedures apply

~ no payment adjustment rules for multiple

99255   **Inpatient consultation**
         procedures apply

~ no payment adjustment rules for multiple

Emergency Department Services

99281   **Emergency dept visit**
         procedures apply

~ no payment adjustment rules for multiple

99282   **Emergency dept visit**
         procedures apply

~ no payment adjustment rules for multiple

99283   **Emergency dept visit**
         procedures apply

~ no payment adjustment rules for multiple

99284   **Emergency dept visit**   ~ no payment adjustment rules for multiple
         procedures apply

99285   **Emergency dept visit**   ~ no payment adjustment rules for multiple
         procedures apply

99288   **Direct advanced life support**   ~ bundled code - no separate payment made,
         multiple procedure concept does not apply

Pediatric Critical Care Patient Transport

99289   **Ped critical care transport**   ~ no payment adjustment rules for multiple
         procedures apply

99290   **Ped critical care transport added**   ~ follow-up period included in another service,
         no payment adjustment rules for multiple procedures apply, +add-on code (list separately in
         addition to primary procedure)

Critical Care Services

99291   **Critical care, first hour**   ~ no payment adjustment rules for multiple
         procedures apply

99292   **Critical care, added 30 min**   ~ follow-up period included in another service,
         no payment adjustment rules for multiple procedures apply, +add-on code (list separately in
         addition to primary procedure)

Inpatient Neonatal And Pediatric Critical Care Services

99293   **Pediatric critical care, initial**   ~ no payment adjustment rules for multiple
         procedures apply

99294   **Pediatric critical care, subseq**   ~ no payment adjustment rules for multiple
         procedures apply

99295   **Neonate critical care, initial**   ~ no payment adjustment rules for multiple
         procedures apply

99296   **Neonate critical care subseq**   ~ no payment adjustment rules for multiple
         procedures apply

99298   **Intensive care low birth wgt infant < 1500 gm**
         ~ no payment adjustment rules for multiple procedures apply

99299   **Intensive care low birth wgt infant 1500-2500 gm**
         ~ no payment adjustment rules for multiple procedures apply

99300   **Intensive care infant pbw 2501-5000 gm**
~ no payment adjustment rules for multiple procedures apply

Nursing Facility Services

99304	**Nursing facility care, init** procedures apply	~ no payment adjustment rules for multiple
99305	**Nursing facility care, init** procedures apply	~ no payment adjustment rules for multiple
99306	**Nursing facility care, init** procedures apply	~ no payment adjustment rules for multiple
99307	**Nursing facility care, subseq** procedures apply	~ no payment adjustment rules for multiple
99308	**Nursing facility care, subseq** procedures apply	~ no payment adjustment rules for multiple
99309	**Nursing facility care, subseq** procedures apply	~ no payment adjustment rules for multiple
99310	**Nursing facility care, subseq** procedures apply	~ no payment adjustment rules for multiple
99315	**Nursing facility discharge day** procedures apply	~ no payment adjustment rules for multiple
99316	**Nursing facility discharge day** procedures apply	~ no payment adjustment rules for multiple
99318	**Annual nursing facility assessment** procedures apply	~ no payment adjustment rules for multiple

Domiciliary, Rest Home Or Custodial Care Services

99324	**Domiciliary/rest home visit new patient** procedures apply	~ no payment adjustment rules for multiple
99325	**Domiciliary/rest home visit new patient** procedures apply	~ no payment adjustment rules for multiple
99326	**Domiciliary/rest home visit new patient** procedures apply	~ no payment adjustment rules for multiple

99327	**Domiciliary/rest home visit new patient** procedures apply	~ no payment adjustment rules for multiple
99328	**Domiciliary/rest home visit new patient** procedures apply	~ no payment adjustment rules for multiple
99334	**Domiciliary/rest home visit est patient** procedures apply	~ no payment adjustment rules for multiple
99335	**Domiciliary/rest home visit est patient** procedures apply	~ no payment adjustment rules for multiple
99336	**Domiciliary/rest home visit est patient** procedures apply	~ no payment adjustment rules for multiple
99337	**Domiciliary/rest home visit est patient** procedures apply	~ no payment adjustment rules for multiple

Domiciliary, Rest Home, Or Home Care Plan Oversight Services

99339	**Domiciliary/rest home care supervise** multiple procedure concept does not apply	~ bundled code - no separate payment made,
99340	**Domiciliary/rest home care supervise** multiple procedure concept does not apply	~ bundled code - no separate payment made,

Home Visit

99341	**Home visit, new patient** procedures apply	~ no payment adjustment rules for multiple
99342	**Home visit, new patient** procedures apply	~ no payment adjustment rules for multiple
99343	**Home visit, new patient** procedures apply	~ no payment adjustment rules for multiple
99344	**Home visit, new patient** procedures apply	~ no payment adjustment rules for multiple
99345	**Home visit, new patient** procedures apply	~ no payment adjustment rules for multiple
99347	**Home visit, est patient** procedures apply	~ no payment adjustment rules for multiple

99348	**Home visit, est patient** procedures apply	~ no payment adjustment rules for multiple

99349	**Home visit, est patient** procedures apply	~ no payment adjustment rules for multiple

99350	**Home visit, est patient** procedures apply	~ no payment adjustment rules for multiple

Prolonged Services

99354	**Prolonged service, office** no payment adjustment rules for multiple procedures apply	~ follow-up period included in another service,

99355	**Prolonged service, office** no payment adjustment rules for multiple procedures apply	~ follow-up period included in another service,

99356	**Prolonged service, inpatient** no payment adjustment rules for multiple procedures apply	~ follow-up period included in another service,

99357	**Prolonged service, inpatient** no payment adjustment rules for multiple procedures apply	~ follow-up period included in another service,

99358	**Prolonged service, w/o contact** follow-up period included in another service, multiple procedure concept does not apply	~ bundled code - no separate payment made,

99359	**Prolonged service, w/o contact** follow-up period included in another service, multiple procedure concept does not apply	~ bundled code - no separate payment made,

99360	**Physician standby services**	~ multiple procedure concept does not apply,

Case Management Services

99361	**Physician/team conference** multiple procedure concept does not apply	~ bundled code - no separate payment made,

99362	**Physician/team conference** multiple procedure concept does not apply	~ bundled code - no separate payment made,

99363	**Anticoagulant management, init** multiple procedure concept does not apply	~ bundled code - no separate payment made,

99364	**Anticoagulant management, subseq** multiple procedure concept does not apply	~ bundled code - no separate payment made,

99371	**Physician phone consultation** multiple procedure concept does not apply	~ bundled code - no separate payment made,

| 99372 | **Physician phone consultation** multiple procedure concept does not apply | ~ bundled code - no separate payment made, |
| 99373 | **Physician phone consultation** multiple procedure concept does not apply | ~ bundled code - no separate payment made, |

Care Plan Oversight Services

99374	**Home health care supervision** multiple procedure concept does not apply	~ bundled code - no separate payment made,
99375	**Home health care supervision** concept does not apply	~ not valid for Medicare, multiple procedure
99377	**Hospice care supervision** multiple procedure concept does not apply	~ bundled code - no separate payment made,
99378	**Hospice care supervision** concept does not apply	~ not valid for Medicare, multiple procedure
99379	**Nursing facility care supervision** multiple procedure concept does not apply	~ bundled code - no separate payment made,
99380	**Nursing facility care supervision** multiple procedure concept does not apply	~ bundled code - no separate payment made,

Preventive Medicine Services

99381	**Preventive visit new patient, < 1 yr** concept does not apply	~ non-covered service, multiple procedure
99382	**Preventive visit new patient 1-4 yrs** concept does not apply	~ non-covered service, multiple procedure
99383	**Preventive visit new patient 5-11 yrs** concept does not apply	~ non-covered service, multiple procedure
99384	**Preventive visit new patient,12-17 yrs** concept does not apply	~ non-covered service, multiple procedure
99385	**Preventive visit new patient 18-39 yrs** concept does not apply	~ non-covered service, multiple procedure
99386	**Preventive visit new patient 40-64 yrs** concept does not apply	~ non-covered service, multiple procedure

CPT codes and descriptions only copyright American Medical Association